S0-CVK-643

Primary Health Care of the Young

Primary Health Care of the Young

Jane A. Fox R.N., M.S., P.N.P.

Instructor, Pediatric and Primary Health Care Nursing
Graduate Division, Lienhard School of Nursing
Pace University, Briarcliff Manor, New York

Instructor, Continuing Education for Health Providers
Teachers College, Columbia University
New York, New York

McGRAW-HILL BOOK COMPANY
New York St. Louis San Francisco Auckland Bogotá Hamburg
Johannesburg London Madrid Mexico Montreal New Delhi Panama
Paris São Paulo Singapore Sydney Tokyo Toronto

NOTICE

Medicine is an ever-changing science. As new research and clinical experience broaden our knowledge, changes in treatment and drug therapy are required. The editors and the publisher of this work have made every effort to ensure that the drug dosage schedules herein are accurate and in accord with the standards accepted at the time of publication. Readers are advised, however, to check the product information sheet included in the package of each drug they plan to administer to be certain that changes have not been made in the recommended dose or in the contraindications for administration. This recommendation is of particular importance in regard to new or infrequently used drugs.

PRIMARY HEALTH CARE OF THE YOUNG

1 2 3 4 5 6 7 8 9 0 R M R M 8 9 8 7 6 5 4 3 2 1

This book was set in Caledonia by the Clarinda Company. The editors were David P. Carroll and Irene Curran; the production supervisor was Jeanne Skahan. The design was done by Caliber Design Planning.
Rand McNally & Company was printer and binder.

Library of Congress Cataloging in Publication Data

Main entry under title:

Primary health care of the young.

Includes bibliographies and index.

1. Pediatric nursing. 2. Ambulatory medical care for children. I. Fox, Jane A.
RJ245.P74   610.73′62   80-367
ISBN 0-07-021741-6

To my husband, Jack, and my parents, Ann and Arthur

Contents

Part 3

Common Symptoms and Problems

List of Contributors

R. Evelyn Aabel, R.N., M.P.H., P.N.P.
Clinical Nurse Specialist
in Pediatrics
Duchess County Department
of Health
Poughkeepsie, New York

Joan Hagan Arnold, R.N., M.A.
Assistant Professor
Adelphi University School of Nursing
Garden City, New York;
Consultant, New York City
Information and Counseling Program
for Sudden Infant Death

Eldon H. "Bud" Baker, Jr., M.A., C.C.C.
Speech, Hearing, and Language
Specialist
Chula Vista School District
Chula Vista, California

Karen A. Ballard, R.N., M.A.
Clinical Nurse Specialist, Pediatric
Mental Health
The New York Hospital–Cornell
University Medical Center
New York, New York;
Instructor, Department of Continuing
Nursing Education
Division of Nursing
New York Hospital
New York, New York

Carol Ann Brown, R.N., B.S.N., P.N.P.
Pediatric Nurse Practitioner
Columbia Presbyterian Hospital
Pediatric Clinic
New York, New York

Marie Scott Brown, R.N., Ph.D.,
P.N.P.
Associate Professor, Parent-Child
Nursing
University of Colorado Health
Sciences Center
School of Nursing
Denver, Colorado

Kathleen M. Buckley, R.N., M.S.
Instructor
Division of Adolescent Medicine,
Department of Pediatrics, and
Division of Maternal Child Nursing,
School of Nursing
University of Maryland
Baltimore, Maryland

Rita M. Carty, R.N., D.N.Sc.
Coordinator, Graduate Nursing
Program
George Mason University
Fairfax, Virginia

Colleen Caulfield, R.N., M.N., P.N.P.
Pediatric Pulmonary Clinical Nurse
Specialist
Department of Pediatrics
School of Medicine;
Clinical Assistant Professor
Department of Maternal Child
Nursing
School of Nursing
University of Washington
Seattle, Washington

Harriett S. Chaney, R.N., Ph.D.
Assistant Professor
University of Texas School of
Nursing at Galveston

Dian Norton Chiamulera, R.N., M.A.
Instructor, Parent Child Nursing
Herbert H. Lehman College
Bronx, New York

Barbara J. Choplin, R. N., M.Ed.
Assistant Professor, Maternal Health
Nursing
School of Nursing
University of Kansas College of
Health Sciences
Kansas City, Kansas

Maureen Collar, R.N., M.S., P.N.P.
Professional Research Assistant
University of Colorado Health
Sciences Center
School of Nursing
Denver, Colorado

Carolyn B. Colwell, R.N., M.A.
Instructor, Child Health Nursing
San Diego State University
San Diego, California

Lois Kopp Daniels, R.N., M.S.N.,
C.N.M.
Certified Nurse-Midwife
Department of Obstetrics and
Gynecology
Grove Hill Clinic, P.C.
New Britain, Connecticut

Nancy E. DeVore, R.N., M.S., M.S.N.,
C.N.M.
Certified Nurse-Midwife
Hospital of the Albert Einstein
College of Medicine
Bronx, New York;
Clinical Instructor, Graduate Program
in Nurse-Midwifery
Columbia University
New York, New York

Linda Myer Dite, R.N., M.S.N.
Maternal-Child Clinical Specialist
Mercer Medical Center
Trenton, New Jersey

Jacalyn Peck Dougherty, R.N., M.S.,
P.N.P.
Assistant Professor
University of Colorado Health
Sciences Center
School of Nursing
Denver, Colorado

Theresa M. Eldridge, R.N., M.S., P.N.P.
Assistant Professor
University of Colorado Health Sciences Center
School of Nuring
Denver, Colorado

Charlotte Cram Elsberry, R.N., M.S.N., C.N.M.
Certified Nurse-Midwife
Coordinator of Education, Nurse Midwifery Service
Montefiore Hospital Medical Center–North Central Bronx Hospital
Bronx, New York;
Assistant Clinical Professor
Yale University School of Nursing
New Haven, Connecticut

Jane Cooper Evans, R.N., M.S.N.
Associate Professor
College of Nursing
University of Texas at El Paso

Jane A. Fox, R.N., M.S., P.N.P.
Instructor, Pediatric and Primary Health Care Nursing
Graduate Division, Lienhard School of Nursing
Pace University
Briarcliff Manor, New York;
Instructor, Continuing Education for Health Providers
Teachers College
Columbia University
New York, New York

Rachael Feldman Frank, R.N., B.S.
Staff Nurse
Pediatric Endocrinology and Nephrology
Long Island Jewish-Hillside Medical Center
New Hyde Park, New York

Martha Frisby, R.N., M.S., P.N.P.
Pediatric Nurse Practitioner
Fresno County Department of Education
Migrant Education Division
Fresno, California

Mary J. Giuffra, R.N., Ph.D.
Professor and Director, Nursing Program
College of Mount St. Vincent
Riverdale, New York

Ilene Burson Gottesfeld, R.N., M.N.
Instructor
Adelphi University School of Nursing
Garden City, New York

Christina M. Graf, R.N., M.S.
Director, Maternal Child Nursing
Methodist Hospitals of Dallas
Dallas, Texas

Nancy Graham, R.N., Dr. P.H.
Assistant Professor of Public Health
Assistant Professor of Nursing
Columbia University School of Public Health and School of Nursing
New York, New York

Marilyn Grebin, R.N., P.N.P.
Nurse Practitioner Director
Roosevelt Hospital–Staten Island Developmental Center
Staten Island, New York;
Instructor, Continuing Education for Health Providers
Teachers College
Columbia University
New York, New York

Sheryl Groninga, R.N., B.S., S.N.P.
School Nurse Practitioner
Child Resource Team, Jefferson County Schools
Denver, Colorado;
Instructor
School Nurse Practitioner Program
University of Colorado
Denver, Colorado

Carol Ann Grunfeld, R.N., M.S., P.N.P.
Instructor
University of Colorado Health Sciences Center
School of Nursing
Denver, Colorado

Diana W. Guthrie, R.N., M.S.P.H., F.A.A.N., C.
Assistant Professor
University of Kansas School of Medicine
Wichita, Kansas;
Department of Nursing
Wichita State University
Wichita, Kansas

Nancy Ann Calland Hart, R.N., M.A.
Inservice Instructor
Suburban Hospital
Bethesda, Maryland

Elizabeth Hawkins-Walsh, R.N., M.S., P.N.P.
Family Liaison, Neonatology
Georgetown University Hospital
Washington, D.C.

Judith Ballaire Igoe, R.N., M.S., P.N.P.
Associate Professor and Project Director
School Nurse Practitioner Program
University of Colorado Health Sciences Center
Denver, Colorado

Paulene S. Johnson, R.N., M.S., M.Ed.
Instructor
Pace University
Graduate Division, Lienhard School of Nursing
Briarcliff Manor, New York

Mary Ann Kasper, R.N., M.Ed.
Assistant Professor, Maternal Health Nursing
School of Nursing
University of Kansas College of Health Sciences
Kansas City, Kansas

Michaeline Kelley, R.N., M.S., F.N.P.
Family Nurse Practitioner
Staten Island Developmental Center
Staten Island, New York

Helen M. Lerner, R.N., M.Ed.
Instructor, Parent-Child Nursing
Herbert H. Lehman College
Bronx, New York

Leslie Lieth, R.N., M.A., P.N.P.
Pediatric Nurse Practitioner
New York Medical College
New York, New York

Carla North Littlefield, R.N., M.A., P.N.P.
Assistant Professor
University of Colorado Health Sciences Center
School of Nursing
Denver, Colorado

Anthony S. Manoguerra, Jr., Pharm.D.
Director for Professional Services
San Diego Regional Poison Center
San Diego, California;
Assistant Clinical Professor
Division of Clinical Pharmacy
School of Pharmacy
University of California at San Francisco;
Assistant Professor
Department of Pediatrics
School of Medicine
University of California at San Diego

Jane Ellen Mead, R.N., M.S.N.
Assistant Professor, Pediatric Nursing
Catholic University of America
School of Nursing
Washington, D.C.

Mary Alexander Murphy, R.N., M.S.N., P.N.P.
Instructor, Department of Pediatrics
University of Colorado Health Sciences Center
School of Nursing
Denver, Colorado

Ann M. Newman, R.N., M.S., F.N.P.
Family Nurse Practitioner
Hurtado Health Center
Rutgers University
New Brunswick, New Jersey

Carol R. Notaro, R.N., M.A.
Nursing Supervisor
Perth Amboy General Hospital
Perth Amboy, New Jersey

Julie Cowan Novak, R.N., M.A., P.N.P.
Pediatric Nurse Practitioner Coordinator
University of California at San Diego
Adult-Child Health Nurse Practitioner Program;
Pediatric Nurse Practitioner
Chicano Community Health Clinic
San Diego, California;
Assistant Professor
San Diego State University
School of Nursing
San Diego, California

Elizabeth Ormond, R.N., M.N.
Staff Nurse, Neonatal Intensive Care Unit
Group Health Cooperative of Puget Sound
Seattle, Washington

Marjorie Peck, R.N., M.S.
Head Nurse, Neonatal Intensive Care Unit
Children's Hospital and Health Center
San Diego, California

Penelope S. Peckos, M.S., R.D.
Associate Member of Staff
Forsyth Dental Center
Boston, Massachusetts;
Consultant in Nutrition
Camp Seascape
Brewster, Massachusetts

Claire F. Pettrone, R.N., M.S., P.N.P.
Pediatric Nurse Practitioner
Georgetown Community Health Program
Reston, Virginia

Jennifer L. Piersma, R.N., M.S., P.N.P.
Assistant Professor
University of Colorado Health Sciences Center
School of Nursing
Denver, Colorado

Sister Penny Prophit, R.N., D.N.Sc.
Assistant Professor of Psychiatric-Mental Health Nursing
Catholic University of America
School of Nursing
Washington, D.C.;
Consultant, National Institute of Mental Health;
Consultant, The National Institutes of Health;
Consultant on International Nursing
George Mason University

Teri Richards, R.N., M.S.N.
Genetic Nurse Consultant
Department of Medicine
School of Medicine
University of California at San Diego
La Jolla, California

Eleanor Rudick, R.N., Ed.D.
Associate Professor
Mercy College
Dobbs Ferry, New York

M. Constance Salerno, R.N., M.S., S.N.P.
Professor of Child Health Nursing
San Diego State University School of Nursing
San Diego, California

Carole Stone, R.N., M.S.N., P.N.P.
Pediatric Nurse Practitioner
Georgetown University Hospital
Washington, D.C.

Barbara Tai, R.N., M.A., C.N.M.
Certified Nurse-Midwife
Private Nurse Midwifery Practice
Stamford, Connecticut

Isobel H. Thorp, R.N., M.A.
Associate Professor
Community Health Nursing
School of Nursing
University of Alabama at Birmingham

Ericka K. Leibold Waidley, R.N., M.S.N.
Instructor, Staff Development
Nursing Service
University of California at San Francisco
San Francisco, California;
Assistant Clinical Professor
Department of Biological Dysfunction
School of Nursing
University of California at San Francisco

John Wallach, R.N., M.S., F.N.P.
Resident Nurse Supervisor
Westchester Developmental Services
Tarrytown, New York

Asher H. Weinstein, R.P.A.-C.
Physicians Assistant, Surgery
Community Health Program of Queens-Nassau
New Hyde Park, New York;
Manhasset Medical Center Hospital
Manhasset, New York;
Long Island Jewish–Hillside Medical Center
New Hyde Park, New York

Preface

Every individual in this country has a right to quality health care. The need to make health care more accessible has caused dramatic changes within the health care delivery system and within the nursing profession.

The nurse as a primary health care practitioner is often the initial contact for the client and family within the health care delivery system. She or he has a responsibility to educate and counsel both client and family in making knowledgeable decisions about health care and to assist the client and the family in assuming greater responsibility for their own health.

The nurse practitioner's expertise is health maintenance and health promotion. It is in this area that she or he functions most independently. Common health problems and illnesses are also assessed and managed by nurse practitioners; collaboration with physicians and other health team members is encouraged and necessary in providing optimum health care.

Few books today meet the needs of nurse practitioners. This text was written for two reasons. First, to provide a comprehensive, clinically oriented reference text for primary health care practitioners, educators, and students who care for infants, children, adolescents, young adults, and their families. Second, to introduce into the literature a family-centered, health-oriented text which discusses, in detail, those areas of health care for which the nurse practitioner can and does assume responsibility. The book is the collaborative effort of nurse practitioners, educators, and clinicians from all parts of the country.

The text has many unique features. It progresses from health to illness and stresses health promotion, counselling, and prevention. Areas of particular interest to practitioners, such as well-child care, psychological assessment, parenting, behavioral concerns, assessing school readiness, and family assessment, are covered in depth. Common symptoms frequently encountered in clinical practice, chronic long-term problems managed in collaboration with a physician, emergencies, and preparation for hospitalization are discussed. Tables are provided at the end of many chapters for those diagnoses which require referral to and/or consultation with a physician. Other unique features include chapters on the dying child, adoption, foster care, the gifted child, a developmental approach to administering medications, and radiologic procedures.

The text is divided into seven parts. Part 1, Health Maintenance and Health Promotion, provides a data base for the reader in using the other parts of the text. It includes chapters on family assessment, newborn assessment, developmental assessment, genetic evaluation, health history and physical examination, and well-child care. Part 2, Families with Special Needs, discusses health concerns for which the practitioner may be called upon for guidance, such as birth control, foster care, and infant death. This part should be referred to as the need arises within the practitioner's clinical practice. Part 3 discusses common symptoms and problems within a body system. Sections in Parts 3 and 4 contain broad *Subjective Data,* information the practitioner needs from the client and/or parent(s), and *Objective Data,* the physical examination and laboratory data required. At the beginning of each chapter in Parts 3, 4, 5 is an *Alert,* which informs the practitioner of certain signs and symptoms that require careful evaluation and possible physician consultation/referral. Chapters in Parts 3 and 4 are divided into three areas:

(1) Etiology: causes of the symptom/problem.

(2) Assessment: including problems/illnesses diagnosed and managed by the practitioner. There are two areas for each assessment: *subjective data,* pertinent information gathered from the history, and *objective data,* significant physical findings and laboratory data.

(3) Management: treatments/medications, counselling/prevention, follow-up, and consultations/referrals. At the end of each chapter, when needed, is a medical referral/consultation table. This table contains those diagnoses which require physician input. Information important to the practitioner is included in the table.

Part 4, Communicable Diseases, includes chapters on chickenpox, rubella, etc. Part 5 is Conditions Requiring Long-Term Management (diseases, developmental disabilities, and social disorders). Chapters on cystic fibrosis, learning disabilities, Down's syndrome, drug abuse, and rape are included. Although the practitioner will not manage these conditions independently, she or he will play a significant role in prevention, early detection, and long-term compliance with treatment. Part 6, Emergencies, such as burns, drowning, poisoning, and choking, should be especially helpful to school and camp nurses. Each chapter is divided into two areas:

(1) Assessment and management: specific guidelines to follow, areas to assess to determine extent of injury, and treatment.

(2) Counselling/prevention: areas to discuss with client/family and suggestions for prevention.

Part 7, Preparation for Hospitalization, provides a developmental approach to preparing a client for hospitalization, whether a planned or an emergency admission. Since hospitalization can be traumatic for both client and family, the practitioner should be actively involved and available to both client, family, and hospital staff throughout the hospital stay.

Treatments for various problems often vary, and different approaches have been included by the different authors.

This book will help the practitioner in providing optimal health care. It is a text which contains useful information presented in a unique and usable way.

ACKNOWLEDGMENTS

This text required the help and support of many people in the five years from conception to publication. I would like to acknowledge some of them. A sincere thank you to all the contributors for their support and hard work; Judi Reginna for typing the manuscript; and the editorial staff at McGraw-Hill: David Carroll, Irene Curran, and Joseph Brehm for their guidance, support, and enthusiasm.

A special mention and thank you to my parents, family, and friends for their patience, love, and most of all for encouraging me when I needed it most.

My deepest love and appreciation to my husband, Jack Riordan, for his support, encouragement, and confidence in my ability to successfully complete this project.

I would also like to express appreciation to the following people for reviewing and critiquing various chapters of the manuscript: Lottie Flater-Benz, M.S.W.; Alice Liebman Bromberg, R.N., B.S.; Doris Brotman, R.P.T., M.P.S.; Deborah Bublitz, M.D.; Mary Elizabeth Carey, R.N., M.N.; Jack Frankel, M.D.; J. Gorvoy, M.D.; Burton Grebin, M.D.; Kathleen Polowy Kavanaugh, R.N., M.A.; Richard D. Krugman, M.D.; J. Ann LeMoine, R.N., M.S., P.N.P.; John Nicoletti, Ph.D.; Susan Panny, M.D.; and Edward J. Ruley, M.D.

Jane A. Fox

Introduction

NANCY GRAHAM

The need to improve the delivery of health care to the youth of the United States has been documented repeatedly. Some of the causes of this health care crisis have been identified as the shortage, maldistribution, and inefficient utilization of the health work force. Principal proposals for solving the work force problems include increasing the supply, improving the distribution, and encouraging better utilization of health workers. Some of the strategies employed in attaining these goals have been the formation of health maintenance organizations (HMOs); the funding of training for physician's assistants and nurse practitioners, the initiation of the National Health Services Corps, the approval of special grants to support residency training programs for family practitioners, and the forgiveness of certain loans for the education of health personnel according to the type and location of practice.

Other recommended strategies for improving the utilization of the health work force include (1) integrating technology effectively in the health care system, (2) utilizing new categories of nursing and allied health personnel, (3) redefining professional roles in the delivery of personal health services, and (4) incorporating the concept of health care teams.

Until the present century, the health care of children was primarily in the hands of mothers or midwives. Physicians essentially were not trained in this area and families did not expect to consult a doctor except under unusual circumstances. Currently, American professional nurses and other types of health workers have not been as widely utilized to give counsel and advice regarding child care and common health problems as have been women in countries where pediatrics is less firmly entrenched as a specialty. The Western European pediatrician functions as a consultant and is usually hospital-based. In contrast, the American pediatrician is often a generalist delivering primary care—the vast majority of the pediatrician's time is spent in office practice giving care to ambulatory patients.

The Department of Health, Education, and Welfare (HEW) report *Extending the Scope of Nursing Practice (1971)* states that as health care becomes increasingly valued in our society, nurses will be expected to take more responsibility for the delivery of primary health and nursing care. Nurses constitute the largest group of licensed practitioners prepared in health care. Nurses' education already covers a broad base of knowledge and consists of information which is basic to understanding health care, yet the nurse remains the most obviously underutilized resource for improving this care to children. During the present century, the focus of pediatrics has shifted from the treatment of serious acute illnesses to the maintenance and promotion of health. This also has implications for the use of nurses in primary care.

The introduction of new and expanding roles for health workers represents an important innovation in health personnel policy in the United States. The philosophy behind the concept of the *primary health care practitioner*—a term which encompasses the two generic terms *nurse practitioner* and *physician's assistant*—is that nonphysician personnel can manage a large portion of preventative, acute, and restorative client care. This term (primary health care practitioner) is used to denote both new and expanded roles of health professionals, with an awareness that the programs preparing such personnel differ in scope and philosophy. The concept of physicians delegating tasks is not new; what is new is the growth of formal education and training programs for the primary health care practitioner.

The following definition of a physician's assistant was adapted by the American Medical Association House of Delegates in 1970. A *physician's assistant* is "a skilled person qualified by academic and practical on the job training to provide patient services under the supervision and direction of a licensed physician, who is responsible for the performance of that assistant."

The extent of the training programs ranges from the 4-month health assistant program to the 15-month Medex program to the 24-month physician's associate program. In addition, there is a 3-year program for the child health associate which trains the health worker to assume primary responsibility for the ambulatory pediatric patient.

The nurses graduating from nurse practitioner programs are identified by a variety of titles, including nurse practitioner, primary care nurse, primary health practitioner, community nurse clinician, advanced and specialized registered nurse. Among the programs that award certificates to nurse practitioners in pediatrics alone there are a variety of occupational titles: child nurse associate, pediatric nurse clinician, pediatric nurse practitioner, and pediatric nurse associate.

The element common to the training of each of these groups of nurse practitioners appears to be the incorporation of theoretical and experimental learning in the following areas: the development of a health history, physical and development assessment skills, interpretations of the findings of laboratory procedures, counselling, selected aspects of clinical medicine including diagnosis and treatment, and assessments of community resources and health care needs. The development of the nurse practitioner role is described as follows:

> Today's nurse, operating in an expanding role as a professional nurse practitioner provides direct patient care to individuals, families and other groups in a variety of settings. . . . The nurse practitioner engages in independent decision making about nursing care needs of clients and collaborates with other health professionals in making decisions about health care needs. The nurse working in an expanded role practices in primary, acute and chronic health care settings. As a member of the health care team the nurse practitioner plans and institutes health care programs. (USDHEW, 1973–1974)

The origin of the nurse practitioner concept probably lies in the roles assumed out of necessity by public health nurses. In the late nineteenth century, Lillian Wald, a pioneer in public health nursing, made house calls, prescribed and dispensed medications and treatments, and counselled her client families as needed. In 1915 Mary Breckenridge founded the Frontier Nursing Service in Kentucky. It was noted for its "nursing on horseback" midwifery services, which gradually expanded to include overall family services.

The first formal pediatric nurse practitioner (PNP) program in the United States was started in Denver in 1965 by Dr. Henry Silver and Loretta Ford, R.N. Dr. Silver felt that the lack of adequate care for children was in part due to the decrease in family practitioners, which put more burdens on the overworked pediatrician. Yet in analyzing the tasks of pediatricians, it was found that over half of their time was devoted to well-child supervision, while another one-fifth was required for management of minor respiratory infections. Dr. Silver felt that the care of these children could be carried out with skill and competence by nurses with additional preparation. Thus, he and Loretta Ford developed the short-term PNP program under the joint auspices of the Schools of Medicine and Nursing of the University of Colorado.

There are many changing and challenging issues related to primary care and the role of nurse practitioners.

A major factor that would appear to influence the scope and function of nurse practitioners is the type and level of preparation. The programs as presently constituted are offered within the framework of continuing education, undergraduate and master's level preparation. They vary in length from short-term in-service education to 2-

year programs, some programs awarding the graduates a certificate and others a master's degree.

Increased use of nurse practitioners has been impeded by uncertainty about the legal implications and liabilities inherent in positions with delegated medical responsibilities. The diversity in program development has contributed to the complexities of legal issues surrounding the use of nurse practitioners. One major difference between a nurse practitioner and a physician's assistant is that the nurse practitioner, unlike most physicians' assistants, is a licensed professional who practices under the nurse practice act (licensure law).

In response to the expansion of nursing roles, the laws and regulations are changing rapidly, but inconsistently. Generally these changes fall into two categories: definitions of nursing practice that are being rewritten or provisions that are being made in the rules and regulations to permit nurses to perform additional acts. The most obvious generalization which can be made is that there exists a wide range of diversity in the approach of giving legal recognition to nurses who are practicing in expanded roles. Because of the variety of approaches to this problem, the laws are confusing both to practitioners who may choose to move from state to state and to consumers. Professional certification may serve as the only logical or consistent way to recognize those nurses who have the qualifications to practice expanding roles.

In 1973 the American Nurses' Association (ANA) certification of excellence for PNPs was established. A licensed PNP in ambulatory care, regardless of the basic nursing program from which the nurse was graduated, was eligible for certification. Only clinical practitioners of nursing qualified. In July of 1976, a new certification approach was initiated by the National Association of Pediatric Nurse Associates and Practitioners (NAPNAP) and the American Academy of Pediatrics (AAP), which recognizes beginning competence in nursing practice.

Currently, professional certification is sponsored by the Divisions of Practice of the ANA, the American College of Nurse Midwives (ACNM), American Association of Nurse Anesthetists (AANA), and NAPNAP. The question is raised as to who is the appropriate certifying body and what criteria are to be used.

The federal government has subsidized training programs for nurse practitioners but initially left unresolved the questions of reimbursement for services. The paradox of federal support for the training programs and lack of support for payment of services can be attributed partly to differences in jurisdiction of congressional committees over health personnel resource development and subsequent financing of health services. The issue of reimbursement has been complicated by the diversity of training programs, the informal nature of many in-service programs, and the general lack of knowledge regarding differences in competence among personnel performing the same task.

The Rural Health Clinics Services Act was signed into law on December 13, 1977. This act represents a significant milestone in the recognition of the expanded role that nurse practitioners and physician's assistants may have as health care providers, since it offers them an opportunity to take a prominent and leading role in the development and operation of rural health clinics. A major innovation accomplished by the act is to make available Medicare and Medicaid funds for reimbursement of clinics in rural areas for "medical services provided by qualified nurse practitioners and physician's assistants." This act permits the nurse practitioner or physician's assistant to furnish a wide variety of diagnostic and therapeutic services under the medical direction of a physician who need only be present as infrequently as once every 2 weeks. This act also allows a nurse practitioner to be the owner of the clinic and it also states that a clinic can operate only if it has a nurse practitioner or physician's assistant on its staff.

Attitudes of physicians, other health personnel, and consumers, as well as the satisfaction and role perception of nurse practitioners, have a definite impact on the success or failure of the introduction of new occupations. The ease and rapidity with which new health professionals are introduced into medical and health care delivery depends heavily upon physicians' attitudes, because physicians frequently make the decisions about whether or not and how the nurse practitioners are to be used.

The effectiveness of nurse practitioners in providing care depends not only on physician acceptance but also on client acceptance of their role. The results of numerous research efforts suggest that client reaction is generally positive. Cohen et al. (1974) found that research has identified a number of factors that potentially determine the degree of client acceptance. These factors have been suggested, but not empirically studied as determinants of client attitudes: the physician's acceptance and endorsement of the primary health care practitioner, the personal qualities and characteristics of such personnel, and the manner in which their qualifications and the benefits of their services have been explained to the client. Other factors affecting the acceptance of new health practitioners, e.g., availability of physicians' services, severity of the health problem, changes in fee structure, and a decrease in waiting time, can be tested relatively easily, yet few studies have attempted to determine empirically how these factors influence acceptance of the new worker.

The organizational aspects of the health care system on the macro level is a critical factor in the employment and utilization of nurse practitioners. Our present system, which is hospital-based, specialist-intensive, and resource-rich, acts as a deterrent to the best utilization of nurse practitioners. The specific structural and organizational characteristics of the individual delivery sites on the macro level have been recognized as critical factors in determining the successful integration of the nurse practitioner role in a particular practice setting. If the nurse practitioner is to practice efficiently and competently, she or he must have available examining rooms, clerical assistance, diagnostic and treatment equipment, and physician backup.

The passage of PL 93-641, the National Health Planning and Resources Development Act of 1974, acknowledges that the health care providers should actively participate in developing health policies. Since at least one-half of the 10 national health priorities specified in the act are related to primary health care and since nurse practitioners are actively involved in this, participation in the local health systems agency would seem to be one of many logical political involvements.

Psychological, legal, reimbursement, organizational, and attitudinal barriers to the development of a full role for the nurse practitioner do exist. In spite of these barriers substantial progress has been made. There has been an increasing amount of facilitating state and federal legislation and the capabilities of the nurse practitioners have been demonstrated. Physician resistance may be expected to subside as the issues of legal liability, reimbursement policies, and interprofessional practice relationships are worked out.

A substantial need for nurse practitioners exists, and society wants high-quality personalized health care. The potential exists for providing this kind of care by the utilization of nurse practitioners and other primary health care practitioners functioning as colleagues in the health care team.

references

Cohen, Eva, et al. *An evaluation of policy related research on new and expanded roles of health workers.* New Haven: Yale, October 1974.

De Angelis, Catherine. *Pediatric primary care* (2d ed). Boston: Little, Brown, 1979.

George, Virginia. P.L. 93-641 Title XV and Title XVI Public Health Service Act. *Nurse Practitioner,* September–October: 7–19 (1976).

Jelinek, Darlene. The longitudinal study of nurse practitioners: Report of phase II. *Nurse Practitioner,* January–February: 17–19 (1977).

Kelly, Lucie Young. Nursing practice acts. *American Journal of Nursing,* **74**(7):1310–1319 (1974).

Leitch, Cynthia, and Mitchell, Ellen. A state-by-state report: The legal accommodation of nurses practicing expanded roles. *Nurse Practitioner,* November–December: 19–30 (1977).

Mauksch, Ingeborg. The nurse practitioner movement—Where does it go from here? *American Journal of Public Health,* **68**(11):1074–1075 (1978).

Ross, Shirley. The clinical nurse practitioners in ambulatory care service. *Bulletin of the New York*

Academy of Medicine, **49**(5):393–402 (1973).

Silver, Henry, and McAtee, Patricia. The rural health clinic services act of 1977. *Nurse Practitioner*, September–October: 30–32 (1978).

Simpson, James. Reimbursement to physician's assistants and nurse practitioners under medicaid. *National Health Law Program Newsletter*, November 25, 1974.

Sullivan, J., Dachelet, C., Saltz, H., Henry, M., and Carrol, H. Overcoming barriers to the employment and utilization of the nurse practitioner. *American Journal of Public Health*, **68**(11):1097–1103 (1978).

Yankauer, A., Connelly, J. P., and Feldman, J. J. Pediatric practice in the U.S. *Pediatrics* (suppl.) **45**:521–554 (1970.)

PART 1

health maintenance and health promotion

1 Family Assessment

MARY J. GIUFFRA

I. Ancestral History

- **A.** Genogram of family (see Fig. 3-2)
- **B.** Symbols used to complete genogram (see Fig. 3-1)

II. Information Recorded on Genogram

- **A.** Family titles; siblings placed in order with oldest on left
  1. First names, nicknames, labels (little mother, troublemaker, family nurse or lawyer, peacemaker, actress, etc.)
  2. Privileges and/or difficulties passed on from generation to generation with the name or title
- **B.** Ages of all members
- **C.** Dates of births
  1. Family changes required by births
  2. Difficulty of births
  3. Planned or unplanned
  4. Nodal events taking place in family at the time of the birth, i.e., deaths, promotions, etc.
- **D.** Dates of marriages, separations, or divorces
  1. Family reaction
  2. Changes required
  3. Changes in contact with family or mate's family following marriages, separations, or divorces
- **E.** Physical location of family members
  1. Closest family member
  2. Most distant family member
  3. Frequency of contact among family and extended family
  4. How contact is made, i.e., by visit, mail, phone
- **F.** Connections to roots
  1. Knowledge of ethnic background
  2. Interest in connectedness with roots
  3. Influence of both extended family cultures on family
     - a. Complimentary
     - b. Openly conflictual
     - c. Reactive distance
  4. Values influenced by extended families in following areas:
     - a. Parenting and childbearing
     - b. Spouse relationships
     - c. Sexual relationships
     - d. Religious orientations and practices
     - e. Educational goals and attitudes
     - f. Money and its function
  5. Careers
     - a. Job satisfaction
     - b. Job stresses
  6. Socioeconomic status
     - a. Similarity to status of extended family
     - b. Family reaction to mobility
- **G.** Important family themes
  1. Education
  2. Money
  3. Religion
  4. Alcoholism
  5. Power
  6. Occupation
  7. Social acceptability
  8. Health/illness
  9. Success/failure
  10. Death
  11. Sex
  12. Drugs
  13. Gambling
  14. Other
- **H.** Family health history
  1. Dates of serious physical and emotional illness or surgery
  2. Diagnoses

3. Impact of illness on family system and individual members
4. Changes required by illness
5. If child was hospitalized, how it later affected child's functioning in the family and the family functioning in general
6. If parent hospitalized, who fulfilled parental role; family reaction
7. Socially deviant behavior related to school, police, community, i.e., delinquency, truancy, etc.; dates
8. Impact of socially deviant behavior on family and community

III. Evaluative Family Outline

A. Family roles

1. Satisfaction of members with roles
2. How are members assigned to roles
   a. Mutual discussion
   b. Power plays
   c. Inaction
3. Sexual approach to role assignment, i.e., males: instrumental roles, females: expressive roles
4. Blurring of generational boundaries in role assignment
5. Clarity of roles and their assignments
6. Manner in which roles are changed
7. Complementarity of roles
8. Rules for changing roles
9. Consequences of role change
10. Relationship of roles to current crisis
    a. Functional
    b. Dysfunctional

B. Family myths

1. Do all members accept the myth?
2. Reactions to demythologizing by family members

C. Communication patterns

1. Content
   a. What topics are child-centered?
   b. What topics are health- or illness-centered?
   c. Do members talk about themselves or do they always talk about other people?
   d. Do members make "I" statements or only "we" statements?
   e. What are the major topics discussed?
   f. What are taboo topics?
2. Process
   a. Is there clarity of communication?
   b. Do family members listen to one another?
   c. Do family members speak for one another?
   d. Are members supportive of one another?
   e. Do members separate thoughts from feelings?
   f. Do they express thoughts as thoughts and not as feelings?
   g. Are there family rules?
   h. Do they fit the current family situation?
   i. Is communication direct, clear, specific, congruent, and growth-producing?
   j. Do family members validate one another's communication?
   k. Is communication used to share separateness or to control other members?
   l. Do family members listen to one another when they speak?
   m. Is there a family spokesperson?
   n. Who speaks for whom?
   o. Are family members free to say what they really think?
   p. Is body language congruent with spoken language?
   q. Are members free to express fear, helplessness, anger, need for comfort, loneliness, tenderness, or aggression?
   r. To whom can they say it?
   s. How does family cope with disagreement?
   t. Do family members talk about themselves or about other people?
   u. Do members scapegoat one another?

IV. Presenting Concern

A. Clarity of presenting issue

1. Coherent statement of chief concern
2. Focus of chief complaint
   a. Identified patient
   b. Outside the family
   c. Entire family

B. History of presenting concern

1. Factor(s) that precipitated it
2. Shifts in individual or family life recently, i.e., loss of family member due to death, desertion, divorce, chronic illness
3. Changes in family composition through
   a. Births
   b. Adoptions
   c. Marriages
4. New members who might exceed operative resources of family

V. Assessment

A. Family problem-solving style

1. Direct confrontation
2. Considers alternate solutions
3. Seeks advice

a. From extended family
b. From friends
c. From professionals
d. Within nuclear family
4. Denial and avoidance of problem
5. Scapegoating
a. Within family—focus on one person, or shifting focus
b. Outside family—focus on one person or group; focus shifts depending on problem

B. Excessive environmental pressures or handicaps
1. Severe poverty
2. Community disorganization
3. Social discrimination

C. Family members who might have severely limited coping or adaptive capacity
1. Insufficient income
2. Insufficient schooling
3. Social handicaps
4. Physical handicaps
5. Personality handicaps

D. Normal developmental crises that surpass the family's coping abilities
1. Birth of child
2. Toddler period
3. School entrance
4. Adolescence
5. Marriage
6. Pregnancy
7. Climacteric
8. Member in nursing home
9. Situational crises that tax the family's coping ability
a. Death of close friend
b. Personal injuries
c. Marital reconciliation
d. Jail term
e. Acquisition of debts
f. Outstanding personal achievement
g. Change in living conditions
h. Holidays
i. Trouble with in-laws
j. Change in residence
k. Change in schools
l. Change in recreation
m. Change in church activities
n. Change in social activities
o. Change in eating habits
p. Change in sleeping habits
10. Work-related changes
a. Fired at work
b. New job
c. First job
d. Wife begins or stops work
e. Retirement
f. Business readjustment
g. Change in financial state
h. Change to different line of work
i. Change in work responsibilities
j. Trouble with boss
k. Change in work hours or conditions

E. Family coping
1. Family reaction to increasing internal or external pressures
2. Extent of family support system
a. Extended family
b. Friends
c. Community support system
d. Professional support system
3. Family reaction to increased pressure and stress
a. Boundaries around family system made rigid
b. Family becomes disorganized
c. Family becomes more organized
d. Stress expressed as physical illness in member(s)
e. Stress expressed as emotional illness in member(s)

F. Family emotional climate
1. Is there sense of tension in atmosphere?
2. Family anxiety level. Is there disparity in family anxiety level, i.e., some members extremely calm, other members extremely anxious?
3. Is overall atmosphere serious, playful, or mixed?
4. Do members seem to enjoy one another?
5. Is there an atmosphere of disparagement and faultfinding?
6. Are members supportive of one another?

G. Family level of differentiation
1. Is there a family "we" position on most issues?
2. Is individuality or deviance from family belief or value system tolerated?
3. Do parents maintain a "we" position in child rearing?
4. Is any deviation permitted either of the parents?
5. Are there alliances between or among members?
Parent—parent
Parent—child
Child—child
6. Is grieving permitted in reorganizing following loss of a member?

7. Does reorganization take place after loss of a family member?
8. Does family system attempt to fill in the empty space created by the loss in lieu of reorganizing?
9. Is there fluidity in changing roles to accommodate loss?
10. What is the family's capacity for change?

H. Family boundaries
1. Rigid and relatively impervious to outside influence
2. Loose and undifferentiated; tending to merge with the environment
3. Flexible; can accommodate change

I. Family attitudes towards
1. Sex
2. Money
3. Power

J. Current family functioning
1. Marital relationships
   a. Description of interaction as marital partners; roles played
   b. Overfunctioning and underfunctioning of partners
   c. Mutually supportive
   d. Competing identities
   e. Patterns of communication
   f. Satisfaction with partner on social and emotional level
   g. Image of future relationship with and without children
   h. Recreation spent alone as husband and wife
   i. Sexual relationship satisfactory to
      (1) Both
      (2) Husband
      (3) Wife
      (4) Neither
2. Parent-child relationship
   a. What are the relations of parental pair and each parent with child?
   b. What is influence of parental pair and each parent on child and vice versa?
   c. Who plays what role with children?
      (1) Disciplinarian
      (2) Emotional supporter
      (3) Teacher
   d. Is the family child centered in its focus?
   e. Do the parents overfunction for the child?
3. Sibling relationships
   a. Description of relationship between each sibling and other siblings
   b. Influence of siblings on each other

K. Major triangles in family
1. Do members talk about absent family member?
2. Do members talk through other members?
3. Is a child pulled into parental focus in lieu of dealing with parental conflicts?
4. Is illness, alcoholism, drug addiction, affairs, gambling, excessive work used as an avoidance phenomenon between two members of the family?
5. Who are the family pursuers?
6. Who are the family distancers?

L. Major stresses in the family (include dates)

M. Relationship of physical or emotional illness to family dynamics

N. Analysis of family strengths
1. Coping mechanisms that have worked
2. Those which have not worked
3. Family functions that engender growth
4. Those which hamper it
5. Strengths that can be mobilized in intervention

O. Analysis of major family weaknesses

P. Analysis of family's probable response to intervention

Q. Prospects for change—direction

VI. Intervention Plan

A. Assessment data

B. Analysis of data

C. Intervention in terms of family system and how it operates

D. Evaluation of intervention in terms of family system; intervention functional or dysfunctional to family system

bibliography

Bowen, Murray. The use of family theory in clinical practice. *Comprehensive Psychiatry,* **7** (5) (1966).

Fogarty, Thomas. Evolution of a systems thinker. *The Family,* **1** (2) (1974).

———. The emotional climate in the family and therapy. *The Family,* **2** (1) (1974).

———. Triangles. *The Family,* **2** (2) (1975).

Giuffra, Mary J. Demystifying adolescent behavior. *American Journal of Nursing,* **75** (10) (1975).

———. Family therapy: A therapeutic vehicle for all families. In *Building for the future* (No. NP-47,

2N). Kansas City: American Nurses' Association, April 1975.

Guerin, Philip J. *Family therapy: theory and practice.* New York: Gardner Press, 1977.

———. System, system who's got the system. *The Family,* (**3**) (1) (1976).

Handel, Gerald. *Psychosocial interior of the family.* Chicago: Aldine, 1967.

Holmes, Thomas, and Masuda, Bivorn. Life change and illness susceptibility. In *separation and depression* (AAAS, 1973).

Pendagast, Eileen, and Sherman, Charles. A guide to the genogram, family systems training. *The Family,* **5** (1):101–102 (1977).

Rahe, R. H., Mahan, J. L., and Arthur, R. J. Prediction of near-future health changes from subjects preceeding life changes. *Journal of Psychosomatic Research,* **14**:401–406 (1970).

2 Psychological Assessment

SISTER PENNY PROPHIT

The main purpose of this chapter is to provide a systematic method for the primary nurse to assess the psychological dimensions of the developing person.

To *assess* means to analyze critically, to appraise, to judge the nature, significance, or status of a phenomenon. Assessment is the first step of a systematic ordering of cognitive actions that provide the bases for nursing practice.

Psychological assessment is the critical analysis of human behavior; it involves several components, or partial processes, which must be learned. Each component is inherent to the process and vital to the accomplishment of the goals of assessment.

The essential goal of psychological assessment is to accurately perceive the other person's world, to understand the other through an organized and precise method for collecting, validating, analyzing, and interpreting information.

The belief system which guides the primary health care practitioner's approach to psychological assessment must include a respect for the unique identity of the individual. Every human person is a mystery that must be learned slowly, reverently, and with care.

Table 2-1 Components of Psychological Assessment, Related Goals, and Challenges

Components (partial processes)	Related Goals	Challenges (related tasks for primary practitioners)
Communication for relationship building	To accurately perceive To understand	To learn the other from the other's frame of reference To recognize the possible discrepancy between the subjective and objective frames of reference To include perceptions of others regarding the persons' strengths, needs, and goals for care
Norming/standard setting for the identification of the need for intervention	To identify existing norms and to establish norms where lacking To formulate decisions regarding how much deviation from health and what kinds constitute a pattern requiring intervention To make decisions concerning appropriateness of behavior with regard to health/illness dimensions	To develop awareness and appreciation of the interrelated dynamic: which norms set by whom in what setting To develop knowledge concerning an awareness of the shifting and overlapping ranges of "normal" within the dynamics of the developing person To avoid psychological "shoulds" which are unrelated to the qualities and capacities of the human person

Table 2-1 Components of Psychological Assessment, Related Goals, and Challenges *(continued)*

Components (partial processes)	Related Goals	Challenges (related tasks for primary practitioners)
Framework for focused observations and/or focal questions	To increase precision in observation and interaction	To develop a repertoire of questions or situational challenges which reflect developmental status through related tasks
	To focus cognitive actions for specific, sequential areas of assessment	To identify mechanisms to support and enhance the wellness/strengths dimension of human behavior
	To give perspective of nursing focus on health and strength building	To develop skills in the use of questions to elicit responses which reflect developmental task behaviors
	To raise levels of consciousness and intentional operations, such as experiencing, understanding, judging, and deciding	

FORMAT AND CONTENT OF PSYCHOLOGICAL ASSESSMENT FRAMEWORK

The general framework forming the bases for anchoring psychological assessment was adapted from Jahoda's (1958) classic concepts of positive mental health:

Attitudes toward the self
Accessibility to the self
Correctness
Feelings about the self
Sense of identity and autonomy

Growth and development
Motivational processes (Maslow, 1954)
Psychosocial developmental tasks, challenges and virtue (Erikson, 1963)
Moral development (Kohlberg, 1971; Duska and Whelan, 1975)

Cognition
Language, time, and space (Piaget, 1954)

Environmental mastery
Ability and adequacy in love, work, play
Adequacy in interpersonal relationships
Meeting situational requirements
Adaptation and adjustment
Problem solving

These essential elements for assessment are presented within the generally accepted categories for the chronological periods:

1. Infancy (from birth to 12 months)
2. Toddler (from 12 months to 3 years)
3. Preschool (from 3 to 6 years)
4. School (from 6 to 12 years)
5. Adolescent (from 12 to 20 years)

Each period is considered separately. The general framework is consistently utilized across the developmental periods, though emphasis varies because of the specific normed tasks of the particular stage of development. Focused questions and observations (when the developing person is in the preverbal phase, or for family perceptions) are suggested for the assessment of various components of the framework. (See Table 2-2, pages 16 through 27.)

Table 2-2 Psychological Assessment Framework

Component	Norms	Observations/Questions
	Infancy (birth to 12 mo)	
THE SELF		
Accessibility Correctness Feelings about Sense of identity/autonomy	At birth and up to the approach of the first birthday, there is little normal awareness of the self or the "me," rather, only diffuse feelings of hunger, pain, and comfort	
GROWTH AND DEVELOPMENT		
Motivational processes	Oral-respiratory-sensory-kinesthetic stage Incorporative mode Task of trust vs. mistrust Virtue of hope	Ease of feeding, depth of sleep, relaxation of bowels, and overall appearance of contentment
PERCEPTION OF REALITY		
ENVIRONMENTAL MASTERY		
Love		
Work		
Play		Self-playing with hands, feet, rolling, getting into various positions
COGNITION	Primary circular reactions	
Language development	Vocalization First 4 mo: Undifferentiated, cooing, babbling 6 mo: Babbling intensifies, lalling, m-m-m sounds when crying 9–12 mo: Language comprehension, responds to "no," and beginning attempts to articulate words; syllable "la" used	
Time Space	Radius of significant relations: Parental figures	
Moral development	Infant acts to experience good, that which is pleasant, and to avoid bad, that which is painful	

DEVELOPMENTAL TASKS OF INFANCY

1. Becoming aware of the self as animate vs. inanimate and of the familiar vs. the unfamiliar, and developing rudimentary social interaction
2. Developing feeling of and desire for affection and response from others

Table 2-2 Psychological Assessment Framework *(continued)*

Component	Norms	Observations/Questions
	Infancy (birth to 12 mo) (continued)	
	3. Developing beginning symbol system, preverbal communication 4. Directing emotional expression to indicate needs/wishes 5. Developing eye-hand coordination, rest-activity rhythm 6. Beginning establishment of self as dependent person, but separate from others	
	Toddler (12 mo to 3 yr)	
THE SELF		
Accessibility	Dim perception but developing sense of self; forming opinion about self, and aware of gradients of anxiety	Self-loving, uninhibited, dominating, energetic little person absorbed in own importance, always seeking attention, approval, and own goals
Correctness	Appraisals of others cause formation of "good-me" or "bad-me" concept	
Feelings about	Likes self because others do	
Sense of identity/autonomy	Primary identification; imitates parents and responds to their encouragement and discouragement	
GROWTH AND DEVELOPMENT		
	Urethral-muscular-anal stage	
	Retentive-eliminative mode	
	Task of autonomy vs. shame and doubt	
	Virtue of willpower	Sometimes cuddly and loving; other times bites, pinches, and is almost sadistic
		Lacks control of exploratory impulses
		Learning sense of self-control
		Shame and doubt evidenced by feelings of being fooled, embarrassed, exposed, small, uncertain, fearful, and no good
PERCEPTION OF REALITY		
	Need for security, safety, love, and belonging	Experiences world in parataxic mode: wholeness of experience and cause-effect relationships do not exist
ENVIRONMENTAL MASTERY		
Love	Attachment behavior most evident during this period; close bond to those who care for toddler	Eye contact with, smiling to, babbling at, and reaching toward care giver

Table 2-2 Psychological Assessment Framework *(continued)*

Component	Norms	Observations/Questions
	Toddler (12 mo to 3 yr) (continued)	
Work Play	Self-loving uninhibited, dominating, energetic little person absorbed in own importance, always seeking attention, approval	
COGNITION		
Language development	Preconceptual phase: thinking concrete and literal Uses syncretic speech where one word stands for certain object; single words represent entire sentences; uses telegraphic speech at 2 yr, at 3 yr will introduce additional words; vocabulary of hundreds of words	
Time	Experiences most things in present Attention span about 1–2 min	
Space	Limited: radius still parental persons	
Moral development	Preconventional stage of moral reasoning, stage 1: the punishment and obedience orientation (results from consequences of actions and from physical power of those in authority)	
	DEVELOPMENTAL TASKS OF TODDLER 1. Settling into healthy daily routines 2. Mastering basic toilet training 3. Becoming an active family member 4. Learning to communicate efficiently, with increasing numbers of others	
	Preschooler (3 to 6 yr)	
THE SELF		
Accessibility Correctness Feelings about Sense of identity/autonomy	At 3 yr knows self as separate person; knows sex and sex differences; body boundaries now definite At 4 yr senses self as one among many; self-critical; appraises self as good and bad; desires to please At 5 yr aware of cultural and other differences in people	
GROWTH AND DEVELOPMENT		
	Infantile-genital-locomotor stage Intrusive-inclusive mode Tasks of initiative vs. guilt Virtue of purpose	Curious, moves independently and vigorously; makes comparisons and develops untiring curiosity, particularly about sexual differences

Table 2-2 Psychological Assessment Framework *(continued)*

Component	Norms	Observations/Questions
	Preschooler (3 to 6 yr) (continued)	
	Sense of planning or undertaking; begins moving out	Enjoyment of energy displayed in action; assertive; increasing dependability and ability to plan Guilt evidenced by being easily frightened, feeling bad about self, shameful, deserving punishment, defeated, feeling responsible for things not responsible for
PERCEPTION OF REALITY	Concepts of relationships: time, causation, space, and number becoming more meaningful Adults seem changeless Cause-effect thinking magical Some fluctuation between reality and fantasy; materialistic and animistic view of the world	"What do you do during the day?" "Tell me a story."
ENVIRONMENTAL MASTERY		
Love	Time for making friends; going out to others	
Work		
Play	At 3 yr is active/sedentary; solitary/gregarious; dramatic play involved and enjoyed; frequently changes activity; listens to nursery rhymes; rides tricycle At 4 yr is imaginative and dramatic; play in groups of two to three enjoyed, often with companions of own sex, but imaginary playmates sometimes Likes to help with household tasks; likes to dress up; likes to play simple puzzles with trial-and-error method At 5 yr more varied activity; graceful in play; realistic; plays in groups of five to six; chooses friends of like interest; generous with toys; wants rules and to do things right; rhythmic motion to music; likes excursions; likes to run, jump, play with bicycle, wagon, sled, etc.	Observations based on norms indicated Questions based on norms might be asked of family, significant others
COGNITION	Intuitive thought (can be reasoned with logically)	
Language development	At 3 yr 900 words, repeats three	

Table 2-2 Psychological Assessment Framework *(continued)*

Component	Norms	Observations/Questions
	Preschooler (3 to 6 yr) (continued)	
	numbers; uses language to communicate	
	At 4 yr 1500 words; counts to 5	
	At 5 yr 2100 words and counts to 10	
Time	At 3 yr attention span 1–15 min	
	At 4 yr attention span 20 min; conception of time, days of week, birthday	
	At 5 yr attention span 30 min; understands week as unit of time; knows days of the week; memory very accurate	
Space	Radius of significant relations: basic family	
Moral development	Preconventional stage 1 (continued): Beginning to ask questions like "Why am I here?" "Where did I come from?" "Why did the bird die?" "Why is it wrong to . . .?"	
	Development of conscience through contact with significant others	
	DEVELOPMENTAL TASKS OF THE PRESCHOOLER 1. Settling into healthful daily routine of eating, exercising, and resting 2. Becoming a participant member of the family 3. Conforming to others' expectations 4. Expressing emotional feelings healthfully and for wide variety of experiences 5. Communicating effectively with increasing number of others 6. Using initiative tempered by conscience	
	Schoolchild (juvenile, latency, preadolescent period, 6–12 yr)	
THE SELF Accessibility Correctness Feelings about Sense of identity/autonomy	At school, child compares self with and is compared by peers in cognitive, language, and social skills	"Tell me about yourself. How would you describe yourself? Who are some of the people you like? What sorts of things do you think about?"
	At 6 yr self-centered; likes to be in control of self, situations, and possessions	
	At 7 yr more modest and aware of self	
	At 8 yr redefines sense of status with others	
	At 9–10 yr relatively content with and confident of self	

Table 2-2 Psychological Assessment Framework *(continued)*

Component	Norms	Observations/Questions
Schoolchild (juvenile, latency, preadolescent period, 6–12 yr) (continued)		
	At 11–12 yr states self is in heart, head, face, or body part most actively expressing; feels more self-conscious with physical changes occurring	
GROWTH AND DEVELOPMENT	Latency stage Tasks of industry vs. inferiority Virtue of competence Foundation of responsible work habits, work attitudes	Interest in doing work, feeling can learn and solve problems; sense of being useful, being busy with something
PERCEPTION OF REALITY	Needs for esteem highlighted At 6 yr learns through automatic imitations and incidental suggestions At 7 yr more reflective, deeper understanding of meanings and feelings At 8 yr less animistic, more aware of impersonal forces of nature; intellectually expansive; learns from own experience At 9 yr realistic, reasonable, self-motivated, intellectually energetic and curious; likes to plan in advance, to classify, identify, and to make inventories At 10 yr thinking is concrete and matter-of-fact; likes to memorize, to identify facts, to think in terms of cause-effect At 11 yr has boundless curiosity, but thinking is concrete and specific; understands relationship terms such as weight and size At 12 yr likes to learn and to consider all sides of a situation; more independent in homework; likes group work; likes to discuss and debate	Inferiority manifested by expressions of inadequacy, defeat, inability to learn or to do, laziness, inability to compete, to compromise, or to cooperate Again, key questions based on content of norms
ENVIRONMENTAL MASTERY		
Love	"Chumship" period; time of the special, same-sex friend through which learns self-acceptance; foundation of intimacy with opposite sex	
Work	Enjoys peer group work; the "work" phase	

Table 2-2 Psychological Assessment Framework *(continued)*

Component	Norms	Observations/Questions
Schoolchild (juvenile, latency, preadolescent period, 6–12 yr) (continued)		
Play	Peer group play, including gang, with peer teaching of new roles, with much giggling during the play of healthy schoolchildren At 6–8 yr enjoys playing with peers and occasionally enjoys having parent as "child"; enjoys painting, cutting, pasting, reading, simple table games, TV, swimming, bicycling, running games, etc. At 9–12 yr more interested in active sports, but continues reading, TV, table games, and enjoys adult-organized games; Creative talents appear; may be interested in music, dance, and art At 10 yr sex-differentiated play may become pronounced Gang becomes important for teaching competition, morality of constraint, compromise, cooperation	
COGNITION		
Language development	Period of concrete operations Beginning of conceptual thinking and abstract defining; verbal, formal reasoning possible now Systematic reasoning about actual or imagined situations: Classification: placing objects in groups according to attributes Seriation: arranging objects in increasing series according to relative characteristics Multiplication: simultaneously placing into classifications and series Reversibility: performing opposite operations or actions with same problem Conservation: ability to see constancy during transformations	Observations made and questions asked based on norms
Time	Time of transition to logical thinking occurring slowly At 8 yr interested in present; likes own watch; punctuality very important At 9 yr can tell time without	

Table 2-2 Psychological Assessment Framework *(continued)*

Component	Norms	Observations/Questions
Schoolchild (juvenile, latency, preadolescent period, 6–12 yr) (continued)		
	difficulty; interested in ancient times At 10 yr is able to get places on time; own initiative; feels relentless passing of time At 11–12 yr plans ahead so time can be under control; radius of significant relations: neighborhood or school	
Space	At 7 yr space sense becoming more realistic At 8 yr expanding, goes more places by self At 9 yr includes whole earth, geography, history At 10 yr specific as to where things are At 11–12 yr considers space as nothingness that goes on forever; space is abstract, difficult to define	
Moral development	Preconventional stage 2 and conventional stages 3 and 4: Stage 2: Moral reasoning; necessity to satisfy one's own needs forms the basis for moral decisions; interest in needs of others is viewed pragmatically Sees moral of story; capacity for reverence, awe; asks questions about religious teaching and God; can be taught through stories which employ moral qualities Stage 3: The interpersonal concordance of "Good-boy–nice-girl" orientation Moral reasoning in terms of that which pleases or helps others and is approved by them; becomes the basis for moral decisions, and behavior is frequently judged by the intention "the person means well," which becomes important for first time Stage 4: The law-and-order orientation: Moral reasoning based on obeying rules and authority	Questions are based on norms indicated. Conventional stage is one in which the individual through moral reasoning considers the expectations of the social group as vital. What is the moral of this story? (Tell a story.)

Table 2-2 Psychological Assessment Framework *(continued)*

Component	Norms	Observations/Questions
Schoolchild (juvenile, latency, preadolescent period, 6–12 yr) (continued)		
	and maintaining social order, and is basis for moral decisions with law and order as important ends in themselves	
	DEVELOPMENTAL TASKS OF THE SCHOOLCHILD 1. Decreasing dependence upon the family; gaining satisfaction from peers and other adults 2. Learning basic adult concepts and knowledge and being able to reason and engage in tasks of everyday living 3. Learning ways to communicate with others realistically 4. Giving and receiving affection from family and friends 5. Learning socially acceptable ways of handling strong feelings and impulses 6. Adjusting to a changing body image and self-concept in order to come to terms with masculine and feminine roles 7. Discovering healthy ways of becoming acceptable as a person; developing positive attitudes toward self and toward one's own and other social, racial, ethnic, economic, and religious groups	
Adolescent (12 to 20 yr)		
THE SELF Accessibility Correctness Feelings about Sense of identity/autonomy	Three types of identity or self-forming: Real: what adolescent believes self to be Ideal: what adolescent would like to be Claimed: what adolescent wants others to think about self Questions of "Who am I?" "How do I feel?" "Where am I going?" "What meaning is there in life?" Development of self-concept and body image closely related to identity formation Emotional characteristics: Mood swings Extremes of behaviors which are contrasting or polar and exemplify the independent vs. dependent strain	"What kind of person would you say you are?" "How do you feel about yourself?" "What is life like for you now?" "Do you see yourself as mostly positive, mostly negative, or maybe mixed between the two?" "What do you think of your body? Do you like it?" (Focused questions by practitioner may be similar to perceive the adolescent's world.) "If you could change your body, how would you change it?"
GROWTH AND DEVELOPMENT	Puberty stage	Changing physical body image with initial awkwardness, clumsiness

Table 2-2 Psychological Assessment Framework *(continued)*

Component	Norms	Observations/Questions
	Adolescent (12 to 20 yr) (continued)	
	Task of identity formation vs. identity diffusion or confusion Virtue of fidelity Period of life which begins with puberty and extends for 8–10 years until the person is physically and psychologically mature; ready to assume adult responsibility and be self-sufficient because of changes in the intellect, attitudes, and interests Early period: begins with puberty, when reproductive organs functionally operative (12–14 for females and 14–18 for males) Late period: when physical growth completed (usually extends from age 15 to 18 for females and from 16 to 20 for males	Achievement of identity, internal stability, sameness, continuity which resists extreme change and preserves itself in the face of stress and contradiction Diffusion reflected by feelings of self-consciousness, doubts, and confusions about the self as a human being and about roles in life; impotent, insecure, disillusioned, alienated; appears brazen, arrogant, and defensive to protect insecurity; avoids adult behavior; gives up, feels defeated, pursues antisocial behavior: "It's better to be bad than to be nobody at all."
PERCEPTION OF REALITY	Great need for privacy and isolation as well as belonging; values independence but conforms readily to group norms	"Tell me about your friends. Do you have one really good friend?" "They say that a friend is someone with whom you can think out loud; do you have someone like this?"
ENVIRONMENTAL MASTERY Love	Achievement of heterosexual relationships Importance of peer group; progression of peer group mix: Unisexual preadolescent Unisexual but mixing with opposite sex Heterosexual Heterosexual with paired couples Paired couples, going steady, engaged, disintegration of total group Characterized also by clique formation in which member commitment is based on social status, the sharing of intimate thoughts and plans Characterized by crowd formation: together not because of mutual liking but because of mutual interests, social ideals	"Have you ever been told stories about yourself when you were a baby or before you went to school? Tell me about them." "Have you tended to doubt yourself lately or feel ashamed?" "Who was and is your favorite older person?" "Tell me about school. Do you like it?"
Work	Beginning tasks for eventual	

Table 2-2 Psychological Assessment Framework *(continued)*

Component	Norms	Observations/Questions
	Adolescent (12 to 20 yr) (continued)	
	selection of occupation or profession	
Play	More time away from home as successfully achieves greater identity	
	Leisure activities: sports, dating, hobbies, reading, listening to radio, TV, talking, daydreaming, loafing	"How do you spend your days?"
COGNITION		
	Formal operations	Observations and questions focused upon operation norms
	Tests of mental ability indicate adolescence time when mind has the greatest ability to acquire and utilize knowledge	
	Capable of highly imaginative thinking, problem solving; projects thinking into future and tries to categorize thoughts	
	Theories may be oversimplified and lack originality, but time of setting up structure for adult thinking patterns	
Language development	Although no overall differences, females—greater verbal skills, males—more facility with quantitative and spatial problems	
	Peer group dialect and highly informal language, coined terminology, and new or extended interpretations attached to traditional terms	
	Slang used to provide a sense of belonging and to exclude "authority" persons	
Space	Radius of significant relations: peer groups and out-groups	
	Changing physical body image and initial awkwardness and clumsiness in process of readjusting spatial relationships ("my feet just seem so far away from my head these days")	
Moral development	Postconventional or principled level: Social control and legalistic orientation Moral reasoning includes realization of universal moral principles which supercede authority of groups. Reasoning is based on	

Table 2-2 Psychological Assessment Framework *(continued)*

Component	Norms	Observations/Questions
	Adolescent (12 to 20 yr) (continued)	
	personal views and opinions in moral decision making; however, individual is seen as member of a group which democratically makes rules based on the opinions of the individual members and allows these rules to be altered by the individuals involved. Adolescent examines parental morality and religion and the verbal standards against practice to decide if real and worth it; By 16 yr the adolescent will make a decision and may accept or reject family religion; individual may have own religious awakening experience which is called by some the crisis of "conversion," suggesting that the adolescent who can find strength in God can rely on power greater than self, can find much consolation in this turbulent period	

DEVELOPMENTAL TASKS OF THE ADOLESCENT

1. Accepting changing body size, shape, function; understanding the meaning of maturity
2. Achieving satisfying social acceptance of female or male role, recognizing how roles have similarities and differences
3. Finding self as member of one or more peer groups and developing skills in relating to variety of persons, including those of opposite sex
4. Achieving independence from parents and other adults while maintaining mature affection for and interdependence with them
5. Selecting satisfying beginning interest in occupational lines
6. Developing intellectual and work skills and social sensitivities for competent citizenship
7. Developing workable philosophy of life, mature set of values, and worthy ideals

summary

As indicated in the initial discussion, an assessment form is an instrument for ordering or systematizing data for the analysis of a phenomenon, in this case the analysis of the psychological health of the developing person. A framework based on the concepts of mental health was presented. Focused observations and questions were suggested; however, the clinician is encouraged to develop a repertoire of questions which may further reflect the status of the person assessed. Suggested norms for growth and development were also presented.

Utilization of a systematic means of observation must be combined with a systematized method of recording data. The written report of data is essential for the evaluation of interrelated variables both in the development of improved assessment methods and in the research of the effectiveness of related modalities for intervention.

Every human person
Is a mystery
That must be learned
slowly, reverently,
With care, tenderness and pain
and never learned
Completely.

references

Duska, R. and Whelan, M. *Moral development: A guide to Piaget and Kohlberg.* New York: Paulist Press, 1975.

Erikson, E. *Childhood and society.* New York: Norton, 1963.

Francis, G. M., and Munjas, B. *Manual of socialpsychologic assessment.* New York: Appleton-Century-Crofts, 1976.

Jahoda, M. *Current concepts of positive mental health.* New York: Basic Books, 1958.

Kohlberg, L. Moral development. *International encyclopedia of social science.* New York: Macmillan, 1968.

Maslow, A. H. *Motivation and personality.* New York: Harper, 1954.

Murray, R., and Zentner, J. *Nursing assessment and health promotion through the life span.* Englewood Cliffs, N.J.: Prentice-Hall, 1975.

Piaget, J. *The construction of reality in the child.* New York: Basic Books, 1954.

3 Genetic Evaluation

TERI RICHARDS

Genetics may be defined as the study of inheritance; *genetic counselling* might be described as a communication process concerned with the occurrence or risk of occurrence of a hereditary disorder within a family. The primary goal of such counselling is to provide the client with an understanding of the disorder and its implications. The counsellor provides information regarding the risk of recurrence of the disorder in future offspring or other family members. The family is helped to make the best possible adjustment in terms of decision making, management, and referrals to appropriate community resources.

GENETIC COUNSELLING PROCESS

Fraser describes four steps in the genetic counselling process: (1) establishing the risk of recurrence of the disorder in question, (2) interpreting the risk in meaningful terms to the client, (3) assisting the client in evaluating the risks in personal yet practical terms, and (4) follow-up counselling to reinforce or provide additional information to evaluate the client's response. In order to establish the risk of recurrence, an accurate diagnosis must be established or inaccurate counselling will be given. The diagnosis is established by utilizing several methodologies. Initially, a thorough history and medical examination, laboratory tests, x-rays, etc., are obtained. A second tool utilized in establishing the risk of recurrence is the *pedigree*, which is a detailed family history. The pedigree may be very helpful in confirming a diagnosis and in establishing the pattern of inheritance. The subject of pedigrees will be expanded upon later in this chapter. Finally the pertinent literature regarding the diagnosis or tentative diagnosis must be reviewed so that counselling will be based upon up-to-date and thoroughly documented studies. After the diagnosis is determined, its implications and the risk of recurrence must be explained to the client in a meaningful manner so that planning and decision making may begin. The client may require assistance in evaluating all options; he or she will have many feelings which must be considered. Holmes and Hecht (1972) have stated that the lessening of guilt and denial and the venting of anger and other emotional responses must first take place prior to rational planning for the future. Then the family will need to evaluate various options with regard to future offspring. Options may include prenatal diagnosis for specified disorders, adoption, artificial insemination, having children even though a risk is present, having no further children, or aborting a fetus. The decision made by each client is highly individualized; many studies have shown that the risk factor may be less important than the burden which would be imposed should a child be affected. Thus a 1 percent risk may be very high for one couple while a 50 percent risk is acceptable to another couple faced with a different disorder. Finally, the initial counselling should be followed by one or more counselling sessions. As stated by Sly, follow-up is essential for several reasons: (1) The client's attitudes may change, and the family situation changes with time; thus genetic risks may need to be reevaluated. (2) With rapid advances in the field of genetics, new developments may be available to the family and be of importance to family planning. (3) Because families may misinterpret the counselling given them, follow-up is necessary to clarify any misconceptions. (4) New information regarding the family and the given disorder may become available in future sessions. (5) Follow-up allows the counsellor to evaluate the counselling given and allows for improvement in the counselling technique. Throughout the counselling process a nondirective approach is utilized which allows the families to make their own decisions.

PEDIGREES

A basic requirement for any type of genetic counselling is a carefully derived and recorded family history. It is essential to have detailed background information about the client's relatives, especially when the client is affected with a genetic disorder for which the mode of inheritance is not established.

Pedigree Construction

In order to observe the distribution pattern of a specific trait in a family, the construction of a family tree, or pedigree, is indicated. The methods utilized in gathering this information are unique for this purpose and there are certain principles to be employed. Initially, the counsellor should plan for adequate time in which to obtain the data, as it is important that a comprehensive data base be accumulated. Both parents or pertinent family members should be included in the systematic data collection; also, it is usually necessary to consult other family members and family records for additional information. Medical records are an essential source of data regarding the family's health history; however, the consent to release the records of a particular family member must be obtained and time allotted for the receipt of such medical information. Pertinent data to be obtained from various family members should include the following: name, maiden name, place of birth, present address, physician's name and address, pertinent medical data, relevant information regarding the specific genetic disorder, and in cases where the client has died, time of death and cause of death. It is important that any family member who has congenital anomalies, is mentally retarded, or exhibits other noted differences in appearance or behavior be investigated. The records of family members who died at an early age should also be investigated. Autopsy reports are the most helpful sources of information in such cases.

The family pedigree can be summarized by the utilization of a chart that has symbols to designate family members, relationships between family members, and other pertinent information. These symbols are depicted in Fig. 3-1. The construction of the pedigree begins with the affected person, who is referred to as the *proband* or *propositus* (*proposita* if female) and designated by an arrow. All persons who possess the trait which is being investigated are designated by a black

Figure 3-1 Common symbols used in construction of a pedigree chart.

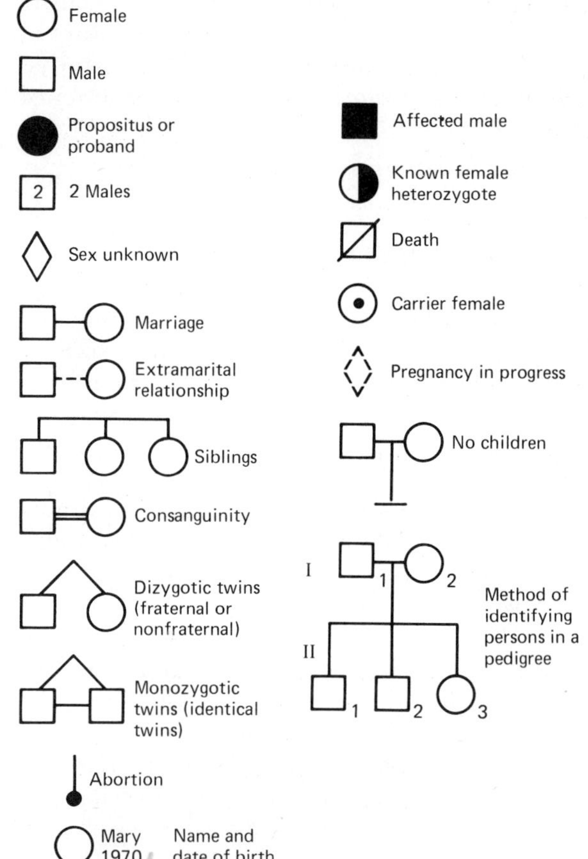

symbol; a blank symbol represents a person who is not affected. Death is signified by a line drawn through the symbolized male or female. In most cases, the cause of death is included in the pedigree as are various other conditions which are significant or inherited, such as diabetes or hypertension, even though such disorders may not be present in the proband. Other important symbols which are commonly utilized include circles for females and squares for males. A marriage is represented by a bar, with males positioned on the left; a marriage between blood relatives, or a *consanguineous* marriage, is indicated by a double bar. Generations are represented by roman numerals and persons within a generation by arabic numbers. The children of a parental couple form a *sibship* and are called *siblings* regardless of sex. In a pedigree the siblings are placed from left to right in order of birth. A sample pedigree which includes these and other symbols may be found in Fig. 3-2.

The guidelines to be utilized in recording a pedigree might be summarized as follows:

1. The pedigree must include all the members of a sibship, normal and abnormal. If the number of siblings, their sex, or knowledge of them is lacking, this also must be noted. Stillbirths, miscarriages, or elective abortions must be included.

2. For clarity, it is best to arrange the paternal siblings on the left and the maternal siblings on the right. The husband and wife may be placed outside the birth order of their respective siblings to simplify the recording of the pedigree.

3. Names and dates of births are usually recorded next to the appropriate symbol.

4. It is often necessary to obtain an extensive family history going back several generations in order to clarify the mode of inheritance. The extent of the pedigree will depend upon the disorder in question, the knowledge of the mode of transmission, and the certainty of the diagnosis. It is generally indicated to obtain a detailed history of the probands' siblings and their offspring, the parents, the parents' siblings, their offspring, and the grandparents.

5. It is essential that a history of consanguinity be investigated and defined. Designating the birthplace of the parents may be of assistance in determining whether the couple might be unknowingly related.

6. It is assumed that the person seeking genetic counselling will provide as much information as possible in an accurate manner. However, other family members should be consulted to supply additional information and to verify information already given. Members of the older generation may provide valuable information that would otherwise be unobtainable because of unavailable medical records. However, some relatives may be less open and even refuse to participate in a discussion with a genetic counsellor.

7. When evaluating genetic conditions, the basic procedure of eliciting a medical history and establishing a medical diagnosis is followed although certain areas will be emphasized. In the history-gathering process, it is essential that the history be comprehensively and systematically derived, as serious genetic disorders may not be disclosed with a brief history. Since the pregnancy history is so important, the outcome of the client's pregnancies must be reviewed for the following information: normal or abnormal outcomes; miscarriages, abortions, stillbirths, infant deaths; exposure to medications, radiation, or illnesses during the pregnancy; adverse occur-

Figure 3-2 Construction of a pedigree chart utilizing common symbols. The pattern of inheritance shown is an autosomal dominant trait.

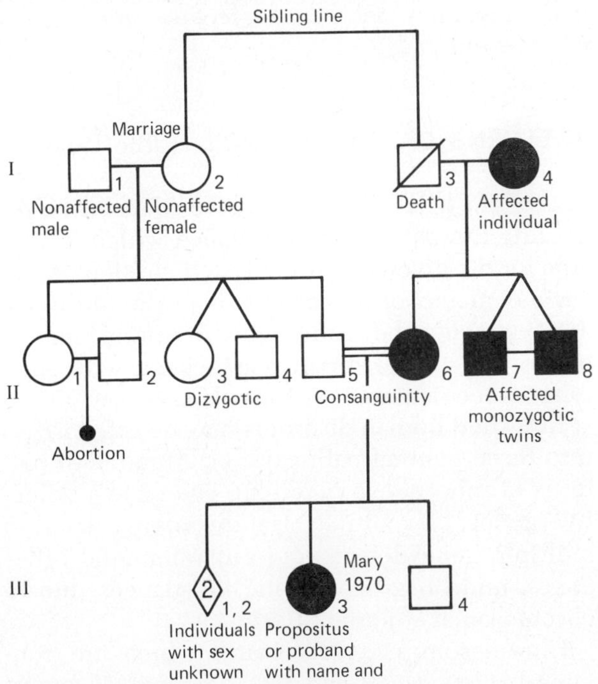

rences during the pregnancy, and the labor and delivery history. With regard to the client's offspring, it is important to discuss any congenital anomalies or neonatal problems in detail, to explore the growth and developmental process, and to assess pertinent childhood illnesses or other health problems. This type of information should also be obtained from other family members, if indicated.

Genetic Analysis

After reviewing the pedigree, it is always important that the individual(s) designated as having the genetic defect be medically examined. If there are medical records available, these need to be reviewed for pertinent data. A thorough physical examination is performed, and additional follow-up by medical specialists, laboratory testing, x-rays, or other measures are obtained, as necessary, in order to comprehensively evaluate the client. It is possible for a person to have a defective gene which is not fully expressed; this is called *incomplete genetic penetrance* and occurs primarily in dominant gene disorders. A medical examination may reveal minor expressions of the gene, and so the person is identified as carrying the gene. This person's children are at risk for inheriting the dominant gene, which may be fully expressed in them.

The genetic counsellor now must integrate all data derived from the family history, medical records, the medical evaluation, and current literature in order to arrive at a diagnosis. It then is his or her responsibility to inform the client and other family members about their potential genetic risks. As it may be impossible to obtain and verify all pertinent data, the genetic counselling will then be based upon limited information. Also, the diagnosis may remain tentative or unknown rather than definite. The client must be so informed and told that the counselling could change if further data becomes available.

GENETIC PRENATAL DIAGNOSIS

Mid-second trimester amniocentesis is considered to be a relatively safe procedure as a part of prenatal care for specific high-risk pregnancies. Many couples are fearful of pregnancy because previous pregnancies resulted in children with chromosome abnormalities, neural tube defects, or certain metabolic disorders; others are fearful because there is risk of having offspring with chromosome abnormalities as a result of advanced maternal age. Amniocentesis can offer reassurance to those couples: if a fetal disorder is detected during the second trimester, the option of terminating the pregnancy is available.

The process of amniocentesis involves inserting a needle through the abdomen into the uterus and withdrawing a small sample of amniotic fluid which contains fetal cells. These fetal cells are capable of growing in culture and providing a source of material for biochemical and/or chromosomal analysis. Chromosome abnormalities, open neural tube defects, and approximately 60 to 70 biochemical disorders can be detected through this means.

The majority of referrals for amniocentesis are for pregnancies at risk for a chromosomal abnormality, more than half for maternal age alone. Amniocentesis may also be considered for sex-linked disorders by determining the fetal sex.

Although minimal, there are risks associated with the amniocentesis procedure. The major complication is miscarriage (1:300). This and all other risks are discussed with the parents prior to the amniocentesis.

For the majority, the amniocentesis provides a means of reassuring parents facing a high-risk pregnancy that the defect in question is not present.

PATTERNS OF INHERITANCE (Table 3-1)

The client will require extensive counselling regarding the pattern of inheritance which is specific for the given disorder. This dicussion on the various modes of inheritance is presented in order to provide the reader with an understanding of the basic characteristics associated with each inheritance pattern.

Inherited human disorders may be categorized into three general pathways: (1) Mendelian patterns of inheritance involving one or two defective genes, (2) multifactorial disorders related to multiple gene defects and environmental influences, and (3) gross genetic imbalances due to chromosomal abnormalities.

Chromosomes are structures which are contained in each cell and are composed of genes.

All cells except gametes, sperm and ova, contain a total of 46 chromosomes. These include 22 pairs which are alike in males and females and are called *autosomes* plus two sex chromosomes. Each autosome appears identical to its partner but each pair is different from all other chromosomes in its genetic content and appearance. A defective gene(s) on one of the paired chromosomes would have an entirely different effect on the individual than a defective gene(s) on another chromosome. The sex chromosomes differ from the autosomes: they are *not* alike in both sexes. A male has one X chromosome and one Y chromosome. A female has two X chromosomes. A female may be homozygous for genes located on the two X chromosomes. A male can be only heterozygous as he has only one X chromosome.

The Mendelian disorders may be subdivided into four distinct patterns of inheritance involving one or two defective genes. These four patterns of inheritance are autosomal dominant, autosomal recessive, X-linked recessive, and X-linked dominant.

summary

The field of genetics and genetic counselling is now a vital part of health care and must be incorporated into preventative health care and health maintenance activities. The genetic counselling process, which includes the systematic collection of data to assess the family's genetic history, will assist the family in evaluating the potential risk of having an offspring with a given disorder, in understanding the natural history of the disorder, and in considering the various alternatives available to the family. The material presented in this chapter will contribute toward achieving a basic understanding of genetic inheritance patterns and the genetic counselling process. This knowledge may then be utilized in eliciting a comprehensive family history, recording the data, and interpreting the data to the family.

Table 3-1 Characteristics of Common Genetic Disorders

Patterns of Inheritance	Characteristics	Common Disorders
MENDELIAN INHERITANCE PATTERNS		
Autosomal dominant inheritance 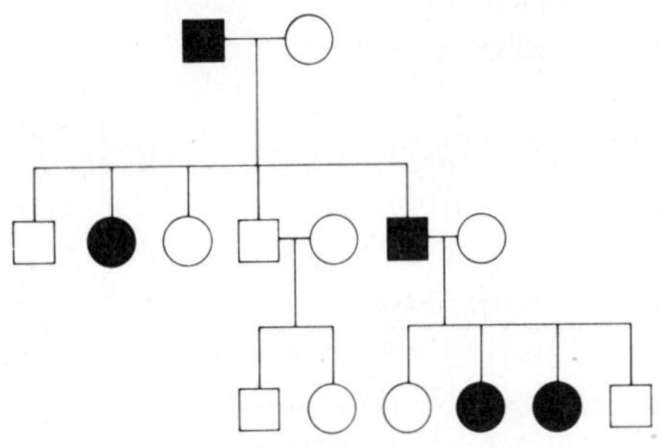	The first case in a family appears as a new mutation, and depending on reproductivity of the individual will either be transmitted to next generation or end with this person. Males and females are equally affected. Each offspring of the affected person has a 50% chance of being affected. Unaffected persons do not transmit the disorder to the next generation. (However, it is possible that the individual will carry the gene even though the condition is not recognized; this is called nonpenetrance.) Transmission of the disorder occurs from one generation to the next. Affected children usually have one affected parent. The physical manifestations which are associated with a specific condition vary in their expressivity. New mutations have been associated with advanced paternal age.	Achondroplastic dwarfism Huntington's chorea Marfan's syndrome Neurofibromatosis Retinoblastoma Tuberous sclerosis

●■ = Affected female, male. ○□ = Unaffected female, male. ◐◨ = Carriers of recessive gene.
◐=◨ = Consanguineous first-cousin marriage. ⊙ = Female carrier of X-linked recessive trait.

Table 3-1 Characteristics of Common Genetic Disorders *(continued)*

Patterns of Inheritance	Characteristics	Common Disorders
Automosal recessive inheritance 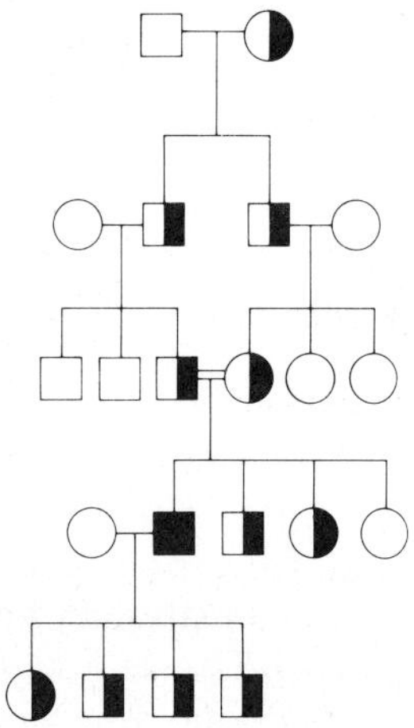	Males and females are equally affected. Each child has a 25% chance of being affected 50% chance of being a carrier 25% chance of not inheriting the gene from either parent Affected persons usually have unaffected parents who are carriers of the gene for that disorder. Affected children whose mates do not carry this gene will have children who will all be carriers of the gene. Transmission occurs in a horizontal manner, as it appears primarily in one generation and may skip one or more generations and appear later. Consanguinity (parents share common ancestor and gene pool) predisposes to this type of inheritance.	Tay-Sachs disease Cystic fibrosis Sickle cell anemia Phenylketonuria Adrenogenital syndrome Albinism Diastrophic dwarfism
X-linked recessive 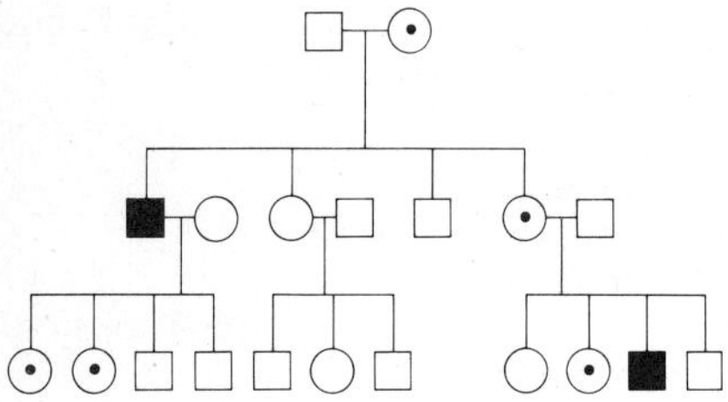	Affected males inherit X-linked genes from their mothers when the mother is a carrier of the disorder, or the gene defect may occur as a fresh gene mutation. Each male child of a female carrier has a 50% chance of being affected. Each female child has a 50% chance of being a carrier. There is no male-to-male transmission as the father gives only male offspring a Y chromosome. Female offspring of affected males are all carriers; they inherit their father's only X chromosome with the defective recessive gene. Transmission occurs from one generation to the next; only males are affected in a majority of families. The disorder may skip a generation if only females inherit the recessive gene and the males are unaffected.	Hemophilia Duchenne's muscular dystrophy Lesh-Nyhan syndrome Hurler's syndrome Agammaglobulinemia
X-linked dominant 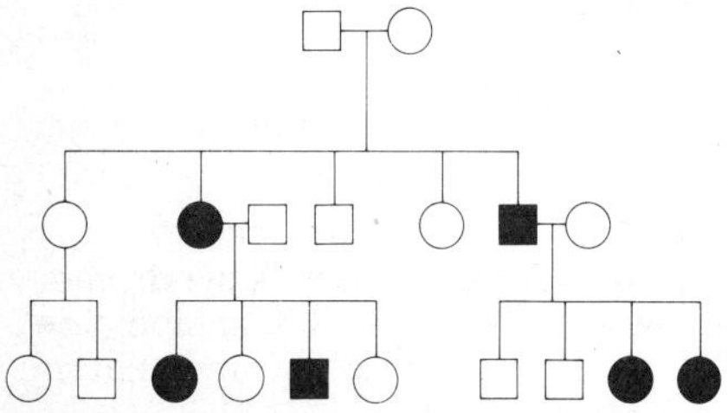	The affected male will have no affected sons; all daughters will be affected. The affected female's offspring will have a 50% chance of being affected whether male or female. There is positive family history where the gene is transmitted from one generation to the next unless it represents a new mutation. Twice as many females are affected as males.	Vitamin D–resistant rickets

● ■ = Affected female, male. ○ □ = Unaffected female, male. ◑ ◨ = Carriers of recessive gene.
◑–◨ = Consanguineous first-cousin marriage. ⊙ = Female carrier of X-linked recessive trait.

Table 3-1 Characteristics of Common Genetic Disorders *(continued)*

Patterns of Inheritance	Characteristics	Common Disorders
MULTIFACTORIAL INHERITANCE	These disorders are a result of interaction between multiple defective genes and the environment. A thorough analysis of family pedigree will not reveal a distinctive mode of inheritance. There is an increased incidence rate in relatives of affected persons. The recurrence risk depends upon The number of affected persons within a family How closely related the affected persons are to the person seeking genetic counselling The sex of affected individuals Certain multifactorial disorders occur more often in one sex than another. In general, the recurrence risk for parents with an affected child is 3–5%. If one parent is affected, the risk for the offspring is also 3–5%.	Cleft lip Cleft palate Spina bifida and anencephaly Congenital dislocated hip Clubfoot Congenital heart malformations
CHROMOSOMAL ABNORMALITIES	The most common type of chromosome abnormality is simply a change in total chromosome number. These abnormalities result from a sporadic defect in chromosome separation, usually during meiosis, called *nondisjunction.* In general, reduction of the total number of autosomes is incompatible with life.	
	An increase in total number of autosomes results in multiple physical abnormalities, mental retardation, and often a limited life span.	Trisomy 13 Trisomy 18
	Advanced maternal age is a definite factor in the increased frequency of trisomy 21 syndrome.	Trisomy 21 (Downs syndrome)
	Another type of chromosome abnormality is structural rearrangement of the chromosomes. In general, this includes deletions, duplications, inversions, and, most often, translocations. In *translocation* chromosome breakage occurs and there is an exchange of material between two chromosomes. In *Balanced translocation* all chromosomal material is present but not located in the normal position.	
	In *Unbalanced translocation* a portion of chromosomal material is lost or additional material is gained and is associated with severe defects.	Translocation Down's syndrome (D/G Translocation) (G/G Translocation)

● ■ = Affected female, male. ○ □ = Unaffected female, male. ◑ ◨ = Carriers of recessive gene.
◑═◨ = Consanguineous first-cousin marriage. ⊙ = Female carrier of X-linked recessive trait.

Table 3-1 Characteristics of Common Genetic Disorders *(continued)*

Patterns of Inheritance	Characteristics	Common Disorders
	A parent carrying a balanced translocation, although normal, is at risk for producing offspring with unbalanced translocations.	
	Sex chromosome abnormalities may result from nondisjunction or structural rearrangements.	XO Turners syndrome
	Depending on the type of sex chromosome anomaly, various forms of gonadal dysgenesis are noted. Physical alterations may include impaired development of secondary sexual characteristics, short or tall stature, and infertility.	XXY Klinefelter's syndrome XXX XYY
	As the total number of sex chromosomes increases, there is an increased prevalence of associated birth defects and mental retardation.	XXXY XXXX XXXXX
	Chromosome abnormalities can be detected in the developing fetus by the sixteenth to eighteenth week of gestation through amniocentesis.	
	Approximately 50% of all recognized spontaneous abortions are chromosomally abnormal.	

● ■ = Affected female, male. ○ □ = Unaffected female, male. ◑ ◨ = Carriers of recessive gene.
◑═◨ = Consanguineous first-cousin marriage. ⊙ = Female carrier of X-linked recessive trait.

references

Fraser, F. C. Counseling in genetics: Its content and scope. Baltimore: Williams and Wilkins. National Foundation March of Dimes, **VI**(1):7 (1970).

Hecht, F., and Holmes, L. What we don't know about genetic counseling, *New England Journal of Medicine*, **287**:464 (1972).

Sly, William S. What is genetic counseling. In D. Bergsma(ed.), *Birth Defects Original Article Series.* New York: National Foundation March of Dimes, 1973, pp. 5–18.

bibliography

deGrouchy, J., and Turleu, C., *Clinical atlas of human chromosomes.* New York: Wiley, 1977.

Fahrmann, Walter, and Vogel, Friedrich. *Genetic counseling.* New York: Springer-Verlag, 1976.

Horan, Mary. Genetic counselling: Helping the family. *JOGN,* pp. 25–29 (1977).

Lub, Herbert, and de la Cruz, Felix. *Genetic counseling.* New York: Raven Press, 1977.

McKusick, Victor A. *Mendelian inheritance in man.* Baltimore: Johns Hopkins, 1978.

Milunsky, Aubrey. *The prevention of genetic disease and mental retardation.* Philadelphia: W. B. Saunders, Co., 1975, pp. 64–89.

Nitowsky, Harold M. Genetic counseling: objectives, principles and procedures. *Clinical Obstetrics and Gynecology,* **19**:919–939 (1976).

Sahin, Selcuk T. The multifaceted role of the nurse as genetic counselor, *Maternal Child Nursing* **1**:211–216 (1976).

Smith, David. *Recognizable patterns of human malformation.* Philadelphia: Saunders, 1976.

Whaley, Lucille. *Understanding inherited disorders.* St. Louis: St. Louis, 1974.

4 Counselling/Guidance/ Education: An Overview

SHERYL GRONINGA

Counselling is a very broad term defined in *Webster's New Collegiate Dictionary,* second edition, as "advising, recommending or deliberating together." Deciding how to use counselling for emotional and physical problems can be very confusing. The following chapter will give you some hints, but keep in mind that you need to develop your own technique for integrating counselling into your practice. Use whatever is comfortable for you and helps the client achieve positive results.

Use the following outline as a guide for counselling a child, adolescent, adult, or family.

I. Evaluate the client's life system
  A. Developmental changes
  B. Family system adaptation
  C. Situational factors
II. Help the client define the problem
III. Set and implement goals
IV. Evaluate the effectiveness of your counselling or teaching

EVALUATION OF THE CLIENT'S LIFE SYSTEM

Life system essentially means how the client's time is spent, with whom, and the feelings about that time. Three areas which affect the client's life system are developmental changes, family adaptation, and situational factors.

Developmental Changes

Development includes not only social and physical growth but cognitive ability, motor skills, and language skills. This chapter will deal mainly with social development, but all the above areas need to be considered when counselling and teaching children and adults. Every person is different and may be going through a suggested stage earlier or later, but the cycle or rotation generally stays in the same order. A good equilibrium cycle will be followed by a breaking up or disruptive period and then will start again. The following table gives you a general outline of the cycles.

Ages	
2,5,10	United, smooth
2½, 5½, 11	Disruptive
3, 6½, 12	Poised, rounded
3½, 7, 13	Indwelling, inward-looking
4, 8, 14	Vigorous, extending
4½, 9, 15	Ambivalent, troubled, "neurotic"
5, 10, 16–17	Consolidated, smooth
18–22	Independence/dependence
22–30	"I should," making choices
The thirties	"I want," disruptive
The forties	"I must," restless
The fifties	New warmth and mellowing
The sixties and over	Integrity, satisfaction, or extreme bitterness

Since most counselling to children below 5 years of age is given to parents, the detailed description of each age will start at 5 years.

5-year-old: Delightfully even-tempered. Secure within, calm and friendly without. Likes to be near mother and likes to be instructed.

6-year-old: Violently emotional, tumultuous, egocentric, demanding of others, rigid, unable to adapt, and negative. Is ready for anything new, wants all of everything, has to be right, has to be praised. Works well with outsiders and less well with mom.

7-year-old: Withdrawn, complaining, mopey, moody. Likes to be alone, likes to watch and listen. Is busy touching and exploring. Demands too much of self. Is somewhat paranoid, and feels "nobody loves me"

8-year-old: Nothing too difficult. Will not always follow through. Is expansive, speedy, and excessively self-critical. Wants two-way relationships.

9-year-old: Lives more within self, is extremely independent. Feels opinions of friends are more important than those of parents. Wants the need for separateness from adults respected. Tends to worry, complains (sometimes physical), and rebels against authority. Develops solid skills.

10-year-old: Parent(s)' word is law. Pleased with life, matter-of-fact, straightforward, and flexible. Is in comfortable equilibrium.

11-year-old: Increase in energy level and activity, self-doubts and insecurity. Finds much to criticize in parents, is impatient with school, feels discriminated against, and likes materials that can be memorized. Loud in actions.

12-year-old: Outgoing, enthusiastic, and generous. Beginning to assert feelings of no longer being a child. Is critical of appearance and has difficulty accepting praise. Romantically interested, eager friend-maker. Restless and daydreaming in school, likes sports and adventure stories.

13-year-old: Period of introspection. Worries, is touchy, more shy. Diminution of friendships. Reading increases, telephoning and outdoor activities increase. Reclusion is a constructive and necessary period that requires some freedom to proceed.

14-year-old: Outgoing, happy, more mature, and self-confident. Likes to express feelings. Friendships blossom, talking and socializing are most important. Works well in groups, gets along better with parents. Plans out long-term activities.

15-year-old: Somber, quiet demeanor. Mental withdrawal seen by adults as sign of being lazy and uncooperative. Independence and liberty are most important goals. Absent from home, functions in groups, has heterosexual relationships, and is greatly concerned with definitions and details.

16–17-year-old: Remarkably even disposition. Receptive to constructive criticism, less sensitive, more sociable and outgoing, accepts self. More responsible and feels more equal to parents. Likes magazines and socializing with friends.

18–22-year-old: Motto: "I have to get away from my parents." Independence/dependence struggle. An identity crisis is normal; if not, it will erupt later and be more severe. Tasks: search for self-identity in peer group situations, establish sex role, anticipate occupation, and form a world view.

22–30-year-old: Motto: "I should." Focus shifts from internal to external turmoils. Tasks: prepare for a life work, find a mentor, develop capacity for intimacy. Fear of getting "locked into" a life pattern. The twenties set a life pattern into motion, but it is not irrevocable.

The thirties: Motto: "I want." Aware of restrictions of career and personal choices of the twenties. Period of great change, turmoil, and often crisis with the urge to bust out. Dreams of "being president," for instance, are turned into more realistic goals. Competency proven, now more self-concern. Example: single, find a partner: married, child care giver, with kids off to school now ventures into the world. Childless couples reconsider children. Many discontents and recommitments lead to divorce or review of marriage and career. In late thirties diminishing physical powers, vulnerability to criticism, and realization that we are basically alone.

The forties: Motto: "I must." Often feels stale, restless, burdened, and unappreciated. Worries about health. "Is this all there is?" Many shift away from a sense of being driven to a more feeling attitude toward life. Mid-forties equilibrium regained. New stability achieved that is more or less satisfying. Most persons in forties take one of two paths:

1. Mate will go away or stay away; career is viewed as just a job; children become strangers; feelings of abandonment are experienced.

2. There is a renewal of purpose. Children can be let go and a new life begun. Accept fact: "I can't expect anyone to fully understand me."

The fifties: Motto: "No more searching." New warmth and mellowing. Friends are more important than ever, but so is privacy. Feels "younger persons may have the power but I have influence." Secondary interests developed as "drivenness" of primary career fades somewhat.

The sixties and over: The age of integrity. Either feelings of a life basically well spent, or feelings of emptiness and bitterness. Increased ability to laugh at life and see it in perspective.

If more detail is needed about any age please refer to the bibliography at the end of this chapter.

Family System Adaptation

The primary group for most individuals is the family. Classically this means the father, mother, and children. When interviewing your client clarify who the client's family is. The client may never see or talk to natural parents, but may instead consider the little old lady down the street or a roommate "family."

The principle of *hemeostasis* applies to social systems such as families. The steady state of the family is not motionless. There is a continuous inflow and outflow of energy from the external environment, but the character of the system stays the same. As the family responds to these constant changes, it does not simply return to its prior equilibrium. A new, more complex and comprehensive equilibrium is established.

It is important to help the client and his or her family consider and deal with the effect on each person of a family that is growing and changing. As children pass through their developmental stages, there is a stress on the family system. Likewise, adults continue to move through their own developmental stages, often husband and wife at different times. Each additional child effects a new change and stress on each family member, with each responding differently. Husbands, wives, and children often assume new roles in the family or bring in outside values, which affects homeostasis. Outside forces intrude on the family system, as in the case of a wife who goes back to work or a teenager who is influenced by group pressure. Thus family stresses are present.

How family system changes are processed is extremely important. Sometimes having the client and his or her family identify the following principles and discussing how to accept or to influence change can be comforting and have positive results. Use the following guide for stimulating discussion:

1. Developmental changes—Have each person identify or have other members help identify the developmental changes he or she is going through.
2. Family norms—Identify past norms, present norms, and future goals.
3. Decision making—How are decisions made? As children grow older and/or as women's liberation becomes more prevalent in our culture, changes in family decision-making models may be necessary.
4. Communications—Is there always a win-lose situation? Do people state clearly what they want? What "games" do they play?

Encourage the client and family to continue discussions at home. Setting a definite day or time of the week for the family to meet helps everyone make a firm commitment. Review the situation with the client and family on return visits.

Situational Factors Affecting Life-System Changes

Everyday Situational Factors The stresses of daily life affect all of us differently. One way of decreasing that stress is to use deep muscle relaxation techniques. This will not be discussed in this chapter, but a long and short form of deep muscle relaxation on audio tape may be obtained from Nicoletti-Benz Associates, P.O. Box 318 Conifer, Colorado 80433.

Life-Changing Events One way to help your client identify changes is to use the Life Event Chart (see Table 4-1).

Table 4-1 Life Event Chart

Rank	Life Event	Mean Value
1	Death of a spouse	100
2	Divorce	73
3	Marital separation	65
4	Jail term	63
5	Death of a close family member	63
6	Personal injury or illness	53
7	Marriage	50
8	Fired at work	47
9	Marital reconciliation	45
10	Retirement	45
11	Change in health of a family member	44
12	Pregnancy	40
13	Sex difficulties	39
14	Gain of new family member	39
15	Business readjustment	39
16	Change in financial state	38
17	Death of close friend	37
18	Change to different line of work	36
19	Change in number of arguments with spouse	35
20	Mortgage over $10,000	31
21	Foreclosure of mortgage or loan	30
22	Change in responsibilities at work	29
23	Son or daughter leaving home	29
24	Trouble with in-laws	29
25	Outstanding personal achievement	28
26	Spouse begins or stops work	26
27	Begin or end school	26
28	Change in living conditions	25
29	Revision of personal habits	24
30	Trouble with boss	23
31	Change in work hours or conditions	20
32	Change in residence	20
33	Change in schools	20
34	Change in recreation	19
35	Change in church activities	19
36	Change in social activities	18
37	Mortgage or loan less than $10,000	17
38	Change in sleeping habits	16
39	Change in number of family get-togethers	15
40	Change in eating habits	15
41	Vacation	13
42	Christmas	12
43	Minor violations of the law	11

Source: Gunderson, E. K., and Rahe, Richard. *Life, stress, and illness.* Springfield, Ill.: Charles C Thomas, 1974, pp. 150-151.

Have the client circle the numbers to the left of the Life Events column in Table 4-1 that correspond to the events which have happened to him or her in the past 2 years. Some numbers may be circled more than once if the events associated with them have occurred frequently in this period of time. Then add up all the numbers in the Mean Value column which correspond to those in the Rank column.

Above 500:	High risk; too many life-changing events for most people to handle comfortably
300–500:	Large amount of change
150–300:	Moderate amount of change
Below 150:	Little change

Let's say that your client circles numbers 3, 13, 16, 18, 24, 27, 32, 36, 38, 39, 42 twice, and 43 three times. Add up the numbers in the right-hand column opposite those in the Rank column.

65
39
38
36
29
26
20
18
16
15
24 (12 × 2)
33 (11 × 3)
———
359

You then discover that 359 is in the large amount of change area. This does not necessarily

mean that the client is uncomfortable with this high rate of change. Some persons function at a high rate of change all their lives and enjoy it. Others function regularly below the 150 level and are suddenly thrust above 500. Then the client will have difficulty dealing with such a large amount of change. The same may happen in reverse, such as a top executive functioning at a 600 level and retiring to a 100 level. The importance is not in the number itself but what it means to the client. The Life Event table will give you a common starting point for discussion with the client. It may be revised for use with children and adolescents.

Another technique that may be used to look at life system changes is to divide the client's life into typical sections and have the client assign percentages to each section. One column should have the percentage of a "normal" present week that is spent in each area and the next column should have the percentage goal for the future. The following table and definitions may be used as a guide.

Definition	*% Now*	*% Future*
Work		
Education		
Spouse		
Parent		
Recreation		
Maintenance		
Social		
Child		

Work: This means not only a paid job but housework, extra jobs, etc.

Education: Time spent in educating self.

Spouse: Time spent with spouse or "significant other" person.

Parent: Time spent in parenting own child or being a parental figure.

Recreation: Exercise and other types of recreation. Performing an activity for a recreational purpose, not a social purpose.

Maintenance: Sleeping, keeping self clean and neat, doing housework, etc.

Social: Dinners, parties, church. For adolescents it would be time spent "hanging around" with friends.

Child: Time spent in the child role such as visiting parents if it is viewed as an obligation.

By reviewing the client's percentages in each column you may find a significant difference between the amounts of time spent in each area. Table 4-3 can give the client a "bird's-eye view" of the areas that he or she wishes to concentrate on changing. For example, if the percentage in the now column after the word *spouse* is 5 and in the future column it is 15, this could stimulate a discussion not only about change but about problem areas with a mate. You now have the opportunity to help the client define the problem more clearly and set goals.

HELPING THE CLIENT DEFINE THE PROBLEM

In defining a problem the following model may be used:

1. The problem should be defined or stated in specific, concrete, and behavioral terms.
2. All problems should be dealt with individually.
3. The problem should be analyzed according to who is doing (or not doing) what to whom, why, where, when, and how often.

For instance, after the evaluation of a client's system and following the discussion, the client may decide that her problem is in the area of not spending enough time with her husband and that the time spent is usually in silence or arguing. The problem or problems may be defined as follows:

1. I do not spend enough time with my husband.
   a. I avoid him by doing housework.
   b. He works late and spends time with friends on weekends.
2. When we are together we can't communicate appropriately or positively. There is too much silence or arguing.

The problems have been stated individually, behaviorally, and objectively. Now you are ready for goal setting.

SETTING AND IMPLEMENTING GOALS

When setting and implementing goals the following model may be used:

I. Goal Setting
Set a *goal,* or a general statement of what you want to accomplish.

II. Establishing Objectives
- **A.** Set *Objectives,* or specific and behavioral intentions of what needs to be accomplished or changed.
- **B.** Whenever possible, objectives should be stated in the positive.
- **C.** If there is more than one objective, you should establish priorities.

III. Generating Alternatives
- **A.** Discussion approach
- **B.** Brainstorming approach

IV. Critiquing and Establishing Priorities
- **A.** Evaluation of alternatives
- **B.** Elimination of inappropriate choices
- **C.** Ranking of appropriate solutions

V. Selecting and Implementing
- **A.** Choose first alternative or combination of top choices.
- **B.** Identify who will be doing what, where, when, and how often.
- **C.** Establish evaluation time line.

VI. Evaluating and Readjusting
- **A.** Evaluate results.
- **B.** If results are negative, assess breakdown of steps in problem-solving and goal-setting models.
- **C.** Readjust models.

In dealing with the client's problems mentioned before in this chapter, goal setting and implementation would proceed as follows. In this case the client does not spend enough time with her husband. The solution to her problem might take the following form.

I. Goal Setting
Increase time spent with husband.

II. Establishing Objectives
- **A.** Increase time spent with husband from 5 to 15 percent of the week.
- **B.** Decrease time spent in doing housework from 25 to 15 percent of week.
- **C.** Increase time spent together on weekends.
- **D.** Decrease time husband spends at work.

III. Generating Alternatives
Client chooses brainstorming rather than discussion; lists brainstorming ideas.
1. Get housekeeper.
2. Have husband quit job.
3. Get a divorce.
4. Wash and wax floors less often.
5. Ask husband to spend 1 hour per night talking to me.
6. Decrease value attached to a clean house.
7. Have kids help with housework.
8. Go with husband and friends on weekends.
9. Take a vacation together.
10. Ask husband to play tennis once a week.
11. Get marriage counselling.

IV. Critiquing and Establishing Priorities
- **A.** Client eliminated the following brainstorming ideas in III.A: no. 2, 3, and 9.
- **B.** Client gave priority to the following; no. 1, 4 to 8, 10, and 11.

V. Selecting and Implementing
Client selected the following brainstorming ideas in III.A: no. 5, 6, 7, 10, and 11. A plan was drawn up.
1. Accept that the house will be less clean.
2. Ask husband to talk with me from 9 to 10 P.M. Monday through Friday in the study with the door closed for privacy.
3. Ask children to do dishes and clean own rooms.
4. Ask husband to play tennis each Thursday from 6 to 7 P.M., and have a late dinner.

VI. Evaluating and Readjusting
Will call and/or see practitioner in 1 week to evaluate results and to readjust. If there

are no improvements in 6 weeks, ask practitioner to refer me to a marriage counsellor.

EVALUATING THE EFFECTIVENESS OF YOUR COUNSELLING OR TEACHING

There are numerous ways to evaluate your effectiveness. If you formulate and record the goals of your counselling, you can check back with the client immediately to see if the material you presented can be recalled. Also on subsequent visits you can refer to previous goals. The chart or folder may take this form:

GOALS:

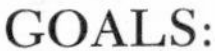

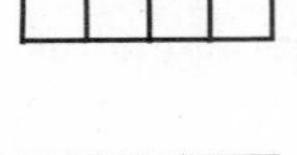

1. Teach client steps in the problem-solving method. (Increase time with husband.)
2. Teach client four food groups and how to balance diet.

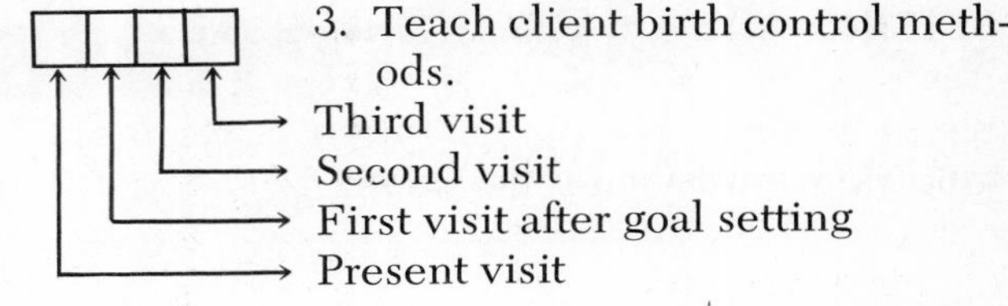

3. Teach client birth control methods.

A check in the square means the client has understood and recalled your teaching. If, for instance, you have no checks in the boxes on the second visit, you will know that you will have to do some repeat teaching or change your methods of teaching. You may want to use a separate sheet for counselling and teaching goals in the front of the client's chart so that new goals can be added at each visit.

When deciding on a method of evaluating the effectiveness of your teaching or counselling, be sure to include your co-workers in your planning and review. They may be able to give you some good hints, and you may be able to share your new ideas with them.

bibliography

Brown, Marie Scott, and Murphy, Mary Alexander. *Ambulatory pediatrics for nurses.* New York: McGraw-Hill, 1975.

Carkhuff, Robert R. *The art of helping.* Amherst, Mass.: Human Resource Development Press, 1972.

Elkind, David. *A sympathetic understanding of the child six to sixteen.* Boston: Allyn and Bacon, 1971.

Ilg, Frances L., and Ames, Louise Bates. *Child behavior.* New York: Harper & Row, 1955.

Josselyn, Irene M. *The adolescent and his world.* New York: Family Service Association of America, 1972.

McQuade, Walter, and Aikman. *Stress.* New York: Dutton, 1974.

Richmond, Julius B., et al. *The health and growth program.* Glenview, Ill.: Scott, Foresman, 1974.

Sheehy, Gail. *Passages.* New York: Bantam, 1977.

5 PNP Prenatal Interview

CAROL ANN BROWN

I. Purpose of Prenatal Assessment Interview

A. Obtain base-line information.

B. Acquaint yourself with expectant parent(s).

C. Begin identifying potential problems.

D. Assess expectant parent(s)' readiness to parent.

E. Initiate counselling.

II. Areas To Cover While Obtaining Base-line Information

A. Family history (interview with both expectant parents preferable)

1. Family health history: maternal and paternal
2. General health of parent(s)
3. Expectant parental age(s)
4. Other children
   a. Ages
   b. Pregnancy, birth, and neonatal—details of each
   c. Developmental progress
   d. Health problems
   e. Problems in infancy
   f. Difficulties parent(s) had adjusting to the child
   g. Parental anticipation of response of sibling(s) to new baby

B. Social history

1. Living conditions—apartment or house
   a. Walk-up or elevators
   b. Number of rooms
   c. Condition of apartment, e.g., peeling paint, window guards
   d. Heat
   e. Hot water
   f. Neighborhood
   g. Crib, cradle
2. Person(s) living in home with mother—baby's father, siblings, her mother, other relatives, supportive others
3. Educational level achieved by parent(s)
4. Source(s) and amount of income
5. Medical insurance—Medicaid
6. Type of job and hours working

III. Assessing Readiness to Parent

A. See Parenting, Chap. 11.

B. Plans made for arrival of new infant

1. Selection of feeding method; see Nutritional Assessment, Chap. 9.
2. Materials read about pregnancy, labor, delivery, and children
3. Supportive person to help mother after baby is born
4. Sleeping arrangements for infant
5. Equipment at home for infant
6. Parent(s) taken or enrolled in classes for childbirth and infant care

C. Parental feelings and fears about this pregnancy; pregnancy planned or unplanned

D. Parental expectations of this pregnancy, of this child

E. Description of childhood of parent(s)

1. How discipline was handled
2. Possible change in the way children will be raised from the way parent(s) was raised

F. Identifying potential risk factors; see Parenting, Chap. 11.

IV. Counselling

A. Make parent(s) aware of delivery room and nursery procedures for all types of deliveries and of rationale for procedures.

B. Stress the need for help at home.

1. Husband (father) should take time off.
2. Ask grandparent(s), friends for assistance.

3. Hire nurse—visiting nurse service or public health nurse.
4. Hire housekeeper—someone to do housework, shopping, cleaning, etc., giving parent(s) time to care for infant.

C. Review methods of feeding—advantages and disadvantages.
1. Discuss bottle feeding and breast feeding.
2. If parent(s) adamant about a particular method, do not coerce.
3. Advise about schedule versus demand feeding.
4. Caution against addition of solid food before 3 months, not necessary before 6 months.

D. Review sleeping arrangements, problems with same, and offer suggestions for better arrangements.

E. Advise parent(s) on what to expect of sibling rivalry and how to handle problems (see Sibling Rivalry, Chap. 116).

F. Advise on what to expect of new infant.
1. Discuss behavior: crying, sleeping, noises, grimaces, feeding, and individuality of all babies.
2. Talk about physical appearance of infant and changes throughout first 2 weeks.

G. Counsel mother about postpartum blues.

H. Introduce parent(s) to the pediatrician if possible, and give information about ways and means to contact the pediatric nurse practitioner (PNP) and pediatrician.

V. Follow-up

A. Get referral from nursery or call from parent(s) after child is born. Determine if any problems exist.

B. Schedule first well-child care visit at 2 weeks of age.

VI. Referrals

A. Social problems—social service department, social workers, visiting nurse service, or public health nurse

B. Childbirth classes
1. Hospital classes
2. Private classes—American Society for Psychoprophylaxis in Obstetrics (ASPO)

C. Breast feeding—LaLeche League

D. Bottle feeding—infant care programs for women, if available, for free formula where need exists

6 Developmental Assessment

ISOBEL H. THORP

Developmental assessment is an integral part of all child health care. The development of a child is affected by and affects the health of each child. Table 6-1 is designed to be used with other health assessment tools, since development is affected by the nutritional status, the psychosocial adaptation, and the physical status of each child.

Developmental assessment forms the data base from which behavior management can be planned and implemented. By working with developmental assessment the primary health care practitioner can provide the counselling necessary for the child's maximum development and adaptation. Although behavior management may be the best reason for using developmental assessment, the assessment can also be used in the early detection of developmental problems, in forming a basis for counselling and anticipatory guidance, in encouraging developmental tasks, and in assisting the parent(s) to understand how to promote development.

The tests identified in this chart are not designed to provide predictive value for later development by providing a numerical standard, but are designed to alert the practitioner to deviations of behavior which are not consistent with average behavior for age. The practitioner is required to examine the variables which contribute to abnormal behavior and provide referral or counselling as indicated.

It is recommended that a longitudinal record of development be maintained in order to assist the practitioner in identifying deviations and exploring causal factors. When consistent negative deviations are encountered, a complete psychological test should be administered by a qualified professional.

The Denver Developmental Screening Test (DDST) (see Appendix 5), easily administered and probably best known, can be utilized as identified in the charts. Overutilization often causes excessive anxiety in parent(s) when it is not fully explained. The test can be used reliably through the child's fourth year, but it has no screening validity after age 5.

The developmental profile is an easily administered, self-report type of assessment. It provides descriptions of behavior for each chronological age and can also provide a numerical profile. In use with children with mild deviations, it gives directions to the parent(s) for guiding the child's development and provides behavior norms through 15 years of age.

Any assessment of development should be as extensive and complete as possible. A thorough examination of many variables and/or combinations of these variables often leads to more comprehensive decision making in behavior management.

It is recommended that the health care provider keep in mind when specific lags might occur within the normal developmental process, prompted by either physical malfunction or the child's inability to deal with what appears to be an increasingly enlarging world.

Table 6-1 Developmental Assessment

Normal				Lags	
Subjective	Objective	Tests	Areas of counselling	Assessment	Recommendations
			Neonate		
Gestational history Labor history Mother's perception	Tonus Symmetry Alertness	Dubowitz gestational age Neurological and physical	Mother-infant bonding Feeding Behavior awareness Stimulation	Abnormal reflexes Abnormal tonus Nonadaptation to extrauterine life	Refer client. Make daily/weekly observations and assessments.
			2–3 mo		
Has normal rooting-sucking-eating cycle—MA Responds to voice—L Makes "oh-ah" sounds—L Has normal sleep-wake cycle	Does not raise head when lying on stomach—M Makes symmetrical movements—MA Head turns toward sound—L Eyes follow object past midline—MA Is alert	Neurological and physical	Stimulation Feeding Sleep-wake cycle Family adaptation	Muscular control inadequate to lift head when on stomach Abnormal tonus Lack of response to stimuli Multiple lags in all areas	Give neurological exam and check related systems (neurological endocrine, or other). Check hearing, using stimulus-response. Stay alert for serious problems.
			4–5 mo		
Holds and looks at objects—MA Squeals, babbles—L Is active when picked up—MA Responds to mother's presence—PS Laughs—PS	Keeps head erect when sitting—M Makes symmetrical movements—M Eyes follow 180°—MA Grasps bottle—MA Transfers objects from hand to hand—MA Laughs—L	Sight/hearing	Stimulation Disease prevention Safety Sleep-activity cycle	Poor muscle tone; asymmetry—MA Poor response to stimuli—L Rejecting behavior—PS Multiple lags	Give neurological-orthopedic-endocrine exam—MA. Check hearing, using stimulus-response—L. Observe mothering. Observe interaction with objects—PS. Give Denver Developmental Screening Test (DDST). Refer client.

M—Motor
PS—Personal Social
L—Language
MA—Adaptive
A—Academic

Table 6-1 Developmental Assessment (*continued*)

Normal				Lags	
Subjective	Objective	Tests	Areas of counselling	Assessment	Recommendations
			6–7 mo		
Rolls from back to stomach and vice versa—MA Puts hand to mouth—MA Vocalizes to objects—L Responds to care giver—PS	Bounces feet when held standing—M Pulls to sit; no head lag—M Grasps cube with palm—MA Localizes source of sound—L Responds to examiner, slowly—PS	DDST	Verbal stimulation Simple games, e.g., peek-a-boo Strange-person contact Limited self-feeding	M (as in DDST) MA L PS Multiple lags	Give neurological exam. Increase opportunity to practice the specific task. Check hearing, sight. Observe interaction with objects and people. Refer for complete testing.
			9–10 mo		
Sits without support—M Says "dada-mama"—L Imitates sounds—L Tries to crawl—M Drinks from cup—MA Is initially shy with strangers—PS	Holds two cubes—MA Stands, holding onto support—M Sits without support—M Is interested in instruments—PS Is receptive to behavior after warm-up—PS Responds to sounds and imitates—L	DDST if not tested previously or if lags in development occur	Motor practice with safety parameters Few, familiar toys Simple games, e.g., pat-a-cake Behavior to imitate Speech to imitate Exploration/safety	M (as in DDST) MA L PS	Give neurological exam. Practice specific or related task. Give hearing tests; verbal stimulation. Gradually introduce to new objects and people one at a time.

M—Motor
PS—Personal Social
L—Language
MA—Adaptive
A—Academic

Table 6-1 Developmental Assessment (*continued*)

Normal				Lags	
Subjective	Objective	Tests	Areas of counselling	Assessment	Recommendations
			1 yr		
Walks, cruises with support—M Holds cup to drink—MA Uses apposition grasp—MA Responds to specific nouns—L Experiments with sound—L	Responds when called—PS Waves bye-bye—MA Shakes and nods head: no, yes—MA Cooperates with dressing—MA Explores instrument—PS	DDST Hearing Sight	Setting limits in behavior Books, pictures, nouns Self-feeding Exploration with safety parameters Safety, ingestion and injury Dental care (Chap. 9)	M MA L PS; rejection or ignoring behavior	Practice/experience of tasks not accomplished/introduction to new experiences Encourage games, e.g., simple "goneness"/return, picking up/letting go. Practice hearing tests, sight test. Expose to new words and behaviors. Assess mothering; if consistent with everything, refer client.
			18 mo		
Walks without support—M Imitates behavior—PS Feeds self—MA Follows simple instructions—L Has temper tantrums—PS	Unwraps candy—MA Scribbles—MA Takes off shoes and socks—MA Responds to directions—L Interest overcomes shyness—PS	DDST Hearing Sight	Handling negativism—see Chap. 120 Handling temper tantrum—see Chap. 121 Stimulation with books, sights, sounds Parameters for activity Cues for readiness of toilet training Dental care	M MA L PS Multiple lags	Practice tasks not accomplished. Check for wide variations in fine motor coordination, thought, and action—important. Check stimulus-response, hearing, previous exposure to tasks, testing. Encourage familiarity. Encourage increased interest, a few toys. Refer client.

M—Motor
PS—Personal Social
L—Language
MA—Adaptive
A—Academic

Table 6-1 Developmental Assessment (*continued*)

Normal				Lags	
Subjective	Objective	Tests	Areas of counselling	Assessment	Recommendations
			2 yr		
Walks up stairs—M	Builds tower with three to four blocks—MA	DDST	Manipulative behavior	M	Practice tasks not accomplished; make orthopedic assessment.
Uses nouns and verbs—L	Follows and gives directions (3 yr on)—L	Hearing	Safety	MA	Encourage demonstration and practice of tasks.
Dresses self: pulls up pants, puts on hat—PS	Imitates circle—MA	Sight	Stimulation; rhymes	L	Require language; encourage mother to require child to ask, not point, use language and imitation; check hearing.
			Discipline	PS	Encourage increased exposure beyond family.
				Multiple lags	Refer client.
			30 mo		
Jumps on both feet—M	Imitates vertical and horizontal stroke—MA	DDST	Picture identification	M	Make orthopedic assessment.
Holds crayon between thumb and finger—MA	Says first and last name—L	Vision	Contact with other children	MA	Use repetition to increase ability to pass DDST items; refer client if no results.
Uses "I, me"—PS	Uses "small, big" correctly—L	Hearing	Self-help skills	L	Require use of language, stimulation, imitation.
Identifies need to go to toilet—PS			Safety	PS	Encourage simple tasks to completion, additional encounters.
Aware of meaning of hot, cold, burn, heights					

M—Motor
PS—Personal Social
L—Language
MA—Adaptive
A—Academic

Table 6-1 Developmental Assessment (*continued*)

Normal				Lags	
Subjective	Objective	Tests	Areas of counselling	Assessment	Recommendations
3 yr					
Hops on one foot—M	Imitates cross—MA	DDST	Time and attention for verbal expression	M	Opportunity to practice task.
Understands "taking turns"—PS	Identifies by pointing; knows two colors—MA	Denver Screening Inventory (DSI)	Group activity	MA	Practice; provide stimulating activity for task; check for minimal brain dysfunction.
Follows rules for group—PS	Undoes buttons, zippers—MA	Good-Enough Harris "Draw a person" test	Self-help skills	L	Encourage correct use of language and articulation.
Washes and dries hands—MA	Knows a few rhymes	Hearing	Supervised use of scissors, pencils, crayons, etc.	PS	Encourage responsibility, simple tasks to be completed.
		Vision			
		Denver Articulation Screening Exam (DASE)			
4 yr					
Sings songs—MA	Names nickels, dimes, pennies—A	"Draw a person" test	Increasing independence	PS	Encourage group play, sharing, responsibility.
Responds to discipline, limits—PS	Copies square—M	Vision	Assuming simple family responsibility	L	Check hearing and articulation.
Engages in dramatic play—PS, M, A, L		Hearing	Self-expression with some limits	A	Check stimulation to do tasks.
Engages in group play; needs less supervision—PS		DDST		MA	Check for possible dyslexia.
		Dental			Refer when no response to repetitive exposure to tasks.

M—Motor
PS—Personal Social
L—Language
MA—Adaptive
A—Academic

Table 6-1 Developmental Assessment (*continued*)

Normal				Lags	
Subjective	Objective	Tests	Areas of counselling	Assessment	Recommendations
		5 yr			
Tells nursery stories—A Argues, using simple cause and effect—A Hops and jumps with skill—M Has longer periods of prolonged activity—MA	Copies triangle—MA Relates daily activity—L Responds to conversation—L	"Draw a person" test Vision Hearing Dental	Independence Responsibility Listening/interacting Safety	M MA L A PS	Check orthopedic and neurological factors. Counsel, practice tasks required. Practice; encourage responsibility. Encourage stimulation. Suggest discipline with parameters. Encourage decision making with parameters. Refer when repetition and opportunity do not result in improvement.
		6–9 yr			
Develops reading, writing, and math ability—A Interacts with friends—PS Participates in group games—PS Assists with household responsibilities—PS	Verbally expresses self—L Responds to environment, examiner, and parent(s)—MA	Depends on reported problems Vision Hearing Dental	Family responsibility Decision making with parameters Handling money with responsibility Enrichment of interests	M L PS	Check orthopedic and neurological factors. Explore cause and effect. Encourage use of language, reading; "Tell a story." Explore problems.
		10–15 yr			
Makes progress in school—A Is attached to peer group—PS Is involved with opposite sex—PS Has self-identity—PS	Discusses career goals and plans for attainment—L, A, PS Interacts with others—PS	Vision Hearing Dental	Sexual orientation Family decision making Encouraging responsibility and self-concept	A PS Identity	Counsel with school. Ascertain problem as seen by client. Examine family-client negotiations. Decide if counsellor is needed.

M—Motor
PS—Personal Social
L—Language
MA—Adaptive
A—Academic

references

Alpern, Gerald D., and Boll, Thomas. *Developmental profile.* Aspen, Colo.: Psychological Development Publications, 1972.

Barnard, Kathryn E., and Erickson, Marcene. *Teaching children with developmental problems.* St. Louis: Mosby, 1976.

Brazelton, T. Berry. *The neonatal behavioral assessment scale.* Philadelphia: Lippincott, 1973.

Council on Pediatric Practice—American Academy of Pediatrics. *Suggested Schedule for Preventive Child Health Care.* Evanston, Ill., 1972.

Dubowitz, L., Dubowitz, V., and Goldberg, C. Clinical assessment of gestational age. *Journal of Pediatrics,* 77:1–10 (1970).

Erickson, Marcene L. *Assessment and management of developmental changes in children.* St. Louis: Mosby, 1976.

Frankenburg, William K., and Dodds, Joseah. *Denver developmental screening test.* Denver: University of Colorado Medical Center, 1969.

Johnson, Orval. *Tests and measurements* (Vol. 1 and 2) San Francisco: Jossey-Bass, 1976.

Knoblock, Hilda and Pasamanick, Benjamin. (Eds.) *Gessell and Arma Trude's developmental diagnosis.* New York: Harper & Row, 1975.

Tudor, Mary. Developmental screening. *Issues in Comprehensive Pediatric Nursing.* New York: McGraw-Hill, 1977.

7 Health History and Physical Examination

MARIE SCOTT BROWN/JUDITH BELLAIRE IGOE

An accurate determination of the health status of an individual depends upon a data collection process involving the investigative procedures of history taking and physical examination. Only when both these two techniques are used does the health information accumulated become sufficiently explicit, detailed, and extensive to reveal the actual state of the child's health. Therefore, it is most important that anyone who must make judgments about the health of children have the knowledge and skills to competently and confidently take a health history and conduct a physical examination.

This chapter presents the component parts and information ordinarily included in a comprehensive health history and systematic physical examination. For the individual interested in learning these data collection procedures, prior knowledge of interviewing methods and of the principles of anatomy and physiology is essential. In addition, supervised clinical practice in taking health histories and performing physical examinations must accompany classroom study if performance proficiency is to be gained. Finally, one will discover that the skills of history taking and physical examination develop gradually. Initially the content described in this chapter must be committed to memory.

Next this information has to be well integrated to the point that the examiner no longer has to think consciously about what step is next in the evaluation. Having achieved this ability, the examiner is then free to fully consider the findings obtained from the history and physical examination for the purpose of recognizing normal and abnormal results.

Eventually, with continuous supervised practice, the skill of efficiently and effectively arriving at correct decisions about the child's health will be acquired. Physicians and nurses alike perform physical examinations and obtain health histories to collect whatever information is necessary to determine the individual's state of health. Nurses, however, have another important responsibility to fulfill as they carry out these procedures. As a health consumer advocate, each nurse has an obligation to increase the understanding and knowledge of parent and child about health and to assist these consumers with the development of active and participatory roles in their own health care. At the time of a visit for health services, there is frequently a readiness on the part of consumers to learn new information about their health and to adopt new attitudes about their personal responsibilities in this regard. Children as well as adults should be encouraged to take an active part in their own health care and their relationships with health professionals.

There has been increasing concern and support for consumer participation in health care and the need to develop more active rather than passive roles for health consumers. Critics of the present health care system believe, for example, the poorly informed and passive health consumers have significantly contributed to the skyrocketing health costs in this country. Specifically, the inappropriate patterns of consumer utilization of community health services are cited as a problem with serious economic ramifications. On the one hand, individuals are seeking expensive professional help for minor health problems which they could easily handle themselves if proper health education were provided. On the other hand, consumers delay seeking health care frequently out of ignorance, with the result that the health condition becomes more severe over time, thereby requiring expensive medical treatment including hospitalization. And, of course, additional costs are always involved when the health consumer with an illness fails to follow a prescribed medical regime and the progress of the disease continues. Noncompliance or the failure to follow the physician's instructions is a common occurrence. Several studies report that 50 percent of professional health service visits result in noncompliance (Gillum and Barsky, 1974). While many factors contribute to this phenomenon, the traditional passive role of the health consumer cannot be overlooked as a contributing force in maintaining this problem. People just don't ask questions of the professional from whom they are receiving health services. Timidity also prevents them from explaining that a particular medical treatment will be necessary. Without the assertiveness necessary to bring their personal concerns to the attention of the health professional, the consumer's response is noncompliance—an expensive retort to the situation.

In addition to the concern for containment of health costs, the other argument strongly in support of increased health consumer participation is that the control of the present major health problems in the United States depends directly on modification of the consumer's behavior and habits of living. No health professional can or should have control over such matters. Therefore, successful preventive health measures depend heavily upon the ability of the consumer to maintain health on a day-to-day basis.

All consumers should become fully familiar with the activities involved in histories and physical examinations for two major reasons. First, it is important that parents and children be able to assess the quality of the health services provided to them. Only through knowledge of the activities which constitute an adequate health history and physical examination is it possible for consumers to make such judgments.

The second reason for acquainting the parents and child with the procedures involved in a health evaluation is to encourage their use of such techniques as history taking as an objective basis for reaching decisions about the need for professional health services and when these services should be sought.

Contained in this chapter are a number of suggestions for increasing the educational value of health evaluations for the consumer. As these ideas are implemented, it is highly recommended that this teaching extend beyond providing new health information to include also efforts directed at the development of more assertive and participatory health consumer roles. Igoe and her associates at the University of Colorado have identified the following behaviors as major constituents of an active health consumer role, and it is suggested that primary care examiners try to elicit and reward this type of consumer participation at the time health services are provided (Igoe, 1977). The consumer should be taught to:

1. Ask questions for the purposes of clarification and improved understanding.
2. Personally communicate information about one's own health.
3. Expect to acquire pertinent health information simultaneously with the delivery of service.
4. Participate in the decision-making activity with regard to one's own health at the time health services are rendered.
5. Assume responsibility for certain tasks related to the maintenance of one's own health.

The role of the nurse in conducting physical examinations and obtaining health histories has been delineated so far as serving two useful functions: (1) data collection so that an accurate determination of the child's health status can be made, and (2) health education for the consumer (parent and child) so that additional personal responsibility for health will emerge. Another significant function of the nurses performing these evaluations is the development of a client profile. Essentially this profile consists of a descriptive account of the health practices and beliefs of the parent(s) and child, including interest in preventive health measures, prior experience in dealing with health problems, previous health education, personal understanding of the roles of health professionals and the preferred ways to utilize these individuals, sources of support when health problems arise, and problem-solving techniques employed for resolving health difficulties. Every nurse will wish to gather this type of information during the course of the evaluation because of its relevance to effective health planning

A special set of guidelines for history taking and physical examination follows. Basically, this information is designed to assist the examiner with health evaluation by providing direction in four areas:

1. Outlining the component parts of the history and physical ("what to ask")
2. Relating the specific instances, by age and type of chief complaint, when certain health history questions and particular examinations should be included in the health evaluation ("when to ask")
3. Presenting practical advice with respect to the actual conduct of the evaluation in order to enhance the quality of the nurse's clinical performance ("practical hints")
4. Offering various ideas for health education and counselling to accompany the evaluation of different body parts

TABLE 7-1 Guidelines to History Taking

What to Ask	When to Ask: Age*	Chief Complaint†: Learning Disability	Nausea and Vomiting	Constipation	Headache	Practical Hints	Education/Counselling
INTRODUCTION							
CHIEF COMPLAINT							
PAST HISTORY							
Birth							
Prenatal: Chronological order of this pregnancy; any other births, stillbirths, abortions, or miscarriages; length of gestation; known family history of genetic defects; prenatal care: when and where; health of mother during pregnancy: bleeding, blood pressure, illness, x-ray, infection, vomiting, fever, rashes, medications,	Should be recorded once in health history	X					Explanation of the relation between such prenatal events as nutrition, drug ingestion, exposure to infectious diseases, x-rays, etc., can be important to the parent(s) in terms of preventive care for future pregnancies and often alleviation of guilt for things the parent(s) did or didn't do during this child's gestation which may be unrelated to current problem. Of prime importance is discussion of rubella, with rubella

*Age should be recorded at every well-child visit and when client presents with illness.

†Any chief complaint necessitates obtaining the following information in addition to that noted in this table: onset and progress of symptoms (chronology, positive and negative signs and symptoms), aggravating and alleviating factors, health immediately prior to onset, health status in general, medical attention or self-medication; behavior connected with present complaint; health of contacts; immunization status.

TABLE 7-1 Guidelines to History Taking *(continued)*

What to Ask	When to Ask: Age*	When to Ask: Chief Complaint†				Practical Hints	Education/Counselling
accidents, hospitalizations, diet, weight gain; blood type (father also)							immunization *between* pregnancies for unprotected women. When dealing with the child, this is a particularly important category for adolescents who are interested in their babyhood and its relation to their present health and who themselves may soon be making decisions regarding their own pregnancies.
Natal: Length of labor and difficulty, breech or cephalic, Apgar, analgesia, anesthesia, hospital, birth weight, birth injuries, condition of baby (cry, color, incubator, oxygen, etc.)	Recorded once	X				Except in the case of the very young infant, this information may be difficult for the parent to remember. A form mailed out beforehand may help the parent sort through memories before coming to the office. For the adolescent, this will afford an opportunity to obtain the information from the parent(s)—often an ideal situation for sex education.	Explanation of the relation of length and type of labor, drugs, anesthesia may be helpful preventive counselling for the next pregnancy; again, it is particularly important when dealing directly with the adolescent.
Postnatal: Any problems in the nursery, went home with mother, twitching, cry, jaundice, cyanosis, feeding problems, rashes, weight gain, excessive mucus, paralysis, convulsions, hemorrhage, fever, congenital anomalies, difficulty in sucking	Recorded once	X				In some situations, a request for medical records from the hospital may be necessary. Be sure to phrase your questions in terms of signs and symptoms that parents will remember rather than a medical diagnosis that a physician or nurse would remember, for example, "Was your child's skin yellow?"	May provide an opportunity to clear up misconceptions about early infancy care for future children or to allay guilt feelings about early care. Also highly relevant to adolescents.

*Age should be recorded at every well-child visit and when client presents with illness.

†Any chief complaint necessitates obtaining the following information in addition to that noted in this table: onset and progress of symptoms (chronology, positive and negative signs and symptoms), aggravating and alleviating factors, health immediately prior to onset, health status in general, medical attention or self-medication; behavior connected with present complaint; health of contacts; immunization status.

TABLE 7-1 Guidelines to History Taking *(continued)*

What to Ask	When to Ask: Age*	Chief Complaint†: Learning Disability	Chief Complaint†: Nausea and Vomiting	Chief Complaint†: Constipation	Chief Complaint†: Headache	Practical Hints	Education/Counselling
Allergies List of specific allergies, reactions, and timing (food, medications, insects, animals, seasons); history of rashes	Recorded annually	X	X	X	X		Education regarding avoidance of specific allergens as well as care for allergic reactions ("home remedies" such as cornstarch baths for itching versus recognizing serious reactions which require immediate or eventual medical treatment or emergency intervention) may be indicated. In highly allergic children, counselling regarding how to keep the child's life as "normal" as possible may be necessary. Teaching the child directly about developing an awareness of the body and its reactions to certain allergies and related self-care measures is important for the older child. Counselling regarding the need for specialized care may be indicated.
Accidents When, where, what happened; treatment: immediate and long-term; follow-up; child's reaction	Recorded annually	X	X		X	Particularly with very traumatic accidents, there is usually a period of amnesia for the accident itself and often for subsequent events. This amnesia could be	Preventive safety education (about car seats, locked medicine cabinets, ipecac, burn prevention, swimming classes) may be indicated. Discussion of

*Age should be recorded at every well-child visit and when client presents with illness.

†Any chief complaint necessitates obtaining the following information in addition to that noted in this table: onset and progress of symptoms (chronology, positive and negative signs and symptoms), aggravating and alleviating factors, health immediately prior to onset, health status in general, medical attention or self-medication; behavior connected with present complaing; health of contacts; immunization status.

TABLE 7-1 Guidelines to History Taking *(continued)*

What to Ask	When to Ask: Age*	Chief Complaint†				Practical Hints	Education/Counselling
						permanent or temporary. It is more common for the child, but may involve the parent(s) also. Be alert to "accident prone" children; this may be a symptom of psychological problems within the child or family. Be alert to the possibility of child abuse when there are inadequate explanations for many accidents.	behavior problems to be expected after major traumas and developmentally appropriate ways of "working through" these residual effects (e.g., "talking it out" for the adolescent; "playing it out" through puppet, dramatic, or artistic play for the preschooler) are important.
Illnesses Childhood diseases (measles, rubella, roseola, mumps, chickenpox, whooping cough, undiagnosed rashes, or fever); any other illnesses or infections; when, where, severity, treatment, follow-up, reactions to follow-up	Recorded annually	X	X	X	X	For a child under 10 years, memory of both parent and child may be vague. Again, results may be better if the parent or child has been alerted beforehand that these questions will be asked. Ask in terms of signs and symptons as well as diagnosis. Explaining why it is important to remember if there were any reactions usually improves recall.	Recognition of the importance of home care for various "childhood diseases" may be appropriate; as may be counselling on fever control, pruritis control, control of infection in the home by isolation, handwashing, etc. Counselling concerning immunization may be appropriate. Suggestions of particularly good self-care books, such as *Mommy, I Don't Feel Good* by Gerald Vaughan, Sir Josephy Causton & Sons, 1970; and *The Sick Book* by Marie Winn, Four Winds Press, 1976, are also worthwhile, though it is important to evaluate style and content of the book to be sure it's compatible with the child's level of understanding.

*Age should be recorded at every well-child visit and when client presents with illness.

†Any chief complaint necessitates obtaining the following information in addition to that noted in this table: onset and progress of symptoms (chronology, positive and negative signs and symptoms), aggravating and alleviating factors, health immediately prior to onset, health status in general, medical attention or self-medication; behavior connected with present complaint; health of contacts; immunization status.

TABLE 7-1 Guidelines to History Taking *(continued)*

What to Ask	When to Ask: Age*	Chief Complaint†: Learning Disability	Chief Complaint†: Nausea and Vomiting	Chief Complaint†: Constipation	Chief Complaint†: Headache	Practical Hints	Education/Counselling
Operations What, when, where, why, outcome, child's reactions, temporary or permanent residual	Recorded annually	X	X			May need to get a consent for release of information to be sent to the operating hospital. Fears or phobias, particularly fear of the dark and castration anxieties, are common in preschoolers. Their problems and fears usually relate to body image and health care.	Discussion of any residual effects of a specific type of surgery is important. For the young child, parental education concerning the normal childhood response to parental separation and surgery as well as appropriate methods of helping the child work through these reactions is essential. (Reliving it through "playacting" allows a chance for catharsis as well as a chance for parent(s) to clear up childhood misinterpretations.) Children very often feel operations or hospitalizations are punishments because they are "bad."
Hospitalizations What, when, why, where, follow-up, child's reaction, temporary or permanent physical or psychological residual	Recorded annually	X	X			May need to get a consent for release to be sent to the hospital to receive details of the problem. Fears or phobias, particularly fear of the dark and castration anxieties, are common in preschoolers. Younger children's problems and fears may relate more	Education may be indicated related to the cause for hospitalization. With a young child, the normal reaction to hospitalization and ways to handle this are important (e.g., reliving it through playacting). Numerous programs for familiarizing children with

*Age should be recorded at every well-child visit and when client presents with illness.

†Any chief complaint necessitates obtaining the following information in addition to that noted in this table: onset and progress of symptoms (chronology, positive and negative signs and symptoms), aggravating and alleviating factors, health immediately prior to onset, health status in general, medical attention or self-medication; behavior connected with present complaint; health of contacts; immunization status.

TABLE 7-1 Guidelines to History Taking *(continued)*

What to Ask	When to Ask					Practical Hints	Education/Counselling
	Age*	Chief Complaint†					
						specifically to body image and health care.	the hospital environment prior to hospitalization now are available and should be utilized.
Immunizations and tests Age of child; type and timing of tests; location of injection and reactions; TB test, x-rays, laboratory tests. Other screening tests for vision, speech, and development	Recorded annually	X				Most clinics and offices now provide the parent(s) with a copy of the immunization record, which simplifies changes from one health facility to another. Other screening tests, however, are usually not included.	Parent(s) should be taught to hold the child during or immediately following an immunization as it has been shown to significantly reduce the stress of the situation. Need for immunizations, watching for and handling untoward effects (i.e., recognition and control of fever, etc.) are important. School-age children and adolescents are in many instances mature enough to carry their own immunization record and should be encouraged to do so as well as to be aware when boosters are needed.
FAMILY HISTORY		X		X	X	May be recorded in graphic form on a "family tree" (see Figs. 3-1 and 3-2).	
Family members Mother's age and state of health, father's age and health, siblings, other members ("Who is at home with you?")						In many cultural groups, the extended family or even good friends can be as important as or even more important than the nuclear family. Be sure to inquire about nonnuclear relatives living in or coming often to the house. Remember the possibility of communes or other living arrangements.	

*Age should be recorded at every well-child visit and when client presents with illness.

†Any chief complaint necessitates obtaining the following information in addition to that noted in this table: onset and progress of symptoms (chronology, positive and negative signs and symptoms), aggravating and alleviating factors, health immediately prior to onset, health status in general, medical attention or self-medication; behavior connected with present complaint; health of contacts; immunization status.

TABLE 7-1 Guidelines to History Taking *(continued)*

What to Ask	When to Ask: Age*	Chief Complaint†: Learning Disability	Nausea and Vomiting	Constipation	Headache	Practical Hints	Education/Counselling
Family health history: any of the following conditions *Eyes, ears, nose, and throat (EENT):* Nosebleeds, sinus problems, glaucoma, cataracts, myopia, strabismus, other problems related to EENT *Cardiorespiratory:* TB, asthma, hay fever, hypertension, heart murmurs, heart attacks, strokes, anemia, rheumatic fever, leukemia, pneumonia, emphysema, high cholesterol levels, other problems *Gastrointestinal:* Ulcers, colitis, vomiting, diarrhea, other problems *Genitourinary:* Kidney infections, bladder problems, congenital abnormalities *Skeletomuscular:* Congenital hip or foot problems, muscular dystrophy, arthritis, other problems *Neurological:* Convulsions, seizures, epilepsy, nervous disorder, mental retardation, mental problems, comas, other problems *Chronic disease:* Diabetes, jaundice,	Recorded in detail once; updated annually					It may be useful to take this in *review of systems* format so that all diseases are covered systematically. The primary purpose is to discover genetic diseases which may have an effect on the child at a particular time (i.e., juvenile onset of diabetes in the case of an adolescent). To elicit complete information it is often helpful to begin with a general question (i.e., "Are there any neurological problems in the family?") followed by specific ones ("like epilepsy, or headaches?"). Common synonyms as well as medical terms should be included (i.e., "Does anyone have convulsions? Fits? Seizures?" "Does anyone have hypertension? High blood pressure?"). In addition to revealing potential diseases related to family genetics, these questions may also elicit factors of psychosocial concern, e.g., if a family member is very ill or handicapped, the child is likely to be affected in some way; the child may worry or be frightened or feel guilty; normal childhood experiences may be more limited than usual.	The genetic potential for all the diseases found in the family history need to be discussed. In those (such as myopia) where early detection can provide remediation, appropriate screening or diagnostic studies should be encouraged. Genetic counselling may be appropriate if future pregnancies are being considered. Discussion of how serious illness or handicaps in important family members can affect children and how to handle these (direct discussions with the older child, perhaps with the help of the primary care giver; dollplay, playacting, or drawing to elicit the younger child's feelings and interpretations) is important; it can be particularly important when there is serious mental illness in the family. Certain children's books, such as *About Handicaps* by Sara Bonnettsten, Walker & Co., 1974, may be suggested for the older child. Mental health prevention measures for the child may be appropriate. Counselling regarding how to ensure adequate childhood experiences is

*Age should be recorded at every well-child visit and when client presents with illness.

†Any chief complaint necessitates obtaining the following information in addition to that noted in this table: onset and progress of symptoms (chronology, positive and negative signs and symptoms), aggravating and alleviating factors, health immediately prior to onset, health status in general, medical attention or self-medication; behavior connected with present complaint; health of contacts; immunization status.

TABLE 7-1 Guidelines to History Taking *(continued)*

What to Ask	When to Ask: Age*	Chief Complaint†				Practical Hints	Education/Counselling
cancer, tumors, thyroid problems, congenital disorders *Special senses:* "Is anyone deaf or blind?" *Miscellaneous:* "Any other medical problems not mentioned?"						If a form or checklist is filled out beforehand by the child or caregiver, it must be discussed in detail during the visit since written forms related to family history are frequently misunderstood. Always explain to the informant that these questions (like all other questions in the history) are standard and not unique to this informant's particular circumstances. All too often parents and children worry that a certain condition is suspected because the examiner says, "Does anyone have diabetes?" Frequently children with learning disabilities have a relative with a similar problem. Nocturnal enuresis commonly occurs in a number of family members rather than just in the designated client.	appropriate if major health problems of the child's care givers exist. Children of 10 or older should know their own family history as one means of assuming personal responsibility for their own health. Efforts should be made to facilitate this type of learning.
Family social history *Residence:* Apartment or house, size, yard, stairs, proximity to transportation and shopping, safe neighborhood, city water *Financial situation:* Who works, where, occupation, income, welfare, food stamps, spending habits, debts, major expenditures, health insurance						Some of this information may be considered personal; it may not be appropriate to elicit it until the rapport of several visits has been established. When eliciting, it is often helpful to justify the need for it (i.e., "In taking care of your child, it is helpful to me to know a little about the persons outside the family with whom he has contact. Do	Counselling concerning safety hazards of particular residences may be indicated, e.g., traffic, drinking water, structural problems, high lead content. Referrals to appropriate community resources may be indicated if a precarious financial situation is endangering the child's health. Guidelines for choosing

*Age should be recorded at every well-child visit and when client presents with illness.

†Any chief complaint necessitates obtaining the following information in addition to that noted in this table: onset and progress of symptoms (chronology, positive and negative signs and symptoms), aggravating and alleviating factors, health immediately prior to onset, health status in general, medical attention or self-medication; behavior connected with present complaint; health of contacts; immunization status.

TABLE 7-1 Guidelines to History Taking *(continued)*

What to Ask	When to Ask: Age*	Chief Complaint†: Learning Disability	Nausea and Vomiting	Constipation	Headache	Practical Hints	Education/Counselling
Outside help: Baby-sitters, day-care center, preschool, teen center *Family interrelationships:* Happy, cooperative, antagonistic, chaotic, multiproblem, violent, etc. *School:* Preschool, number of schools attended, long periods of time expended for transportation to and from school						you use a baby-sitter? A day-care home?" "It is also helpful if I understand the kinds of places your child can play and grow up in. Do you have a backyard? Is it fenced?" "It is also helpful to me to understand how things are going in your family. Do you feel that Jimmy and his dad get along pretty well?"). Some of this information may be filled out by the parent(s) or child before the visit on a form mailed beforehand or given out in the waiting room (e.g., occupation, address). It should be read before the visit and clarifying or elaborating information then sought. This is an excellent opportunity to point out interrelatedness of health and social events.	caretakers, day-care homes, or preschools are often important. A significant amount of counselling regarding how family interrelationships (parent-parent, parent-child, child-child) affect the child's mental health and how good relationships can be fostered is often important.
REVIEW OF SYSTEMS (for child) Ear, eye, nose, throat Eyes ever cross? Unilateral tearing? Foreign object in eye? Redness? Burning? Earaches, ear infections, colds, strep throats, nosebleeds, congestion, postnasal drip, sneezing, sore throat, stuffy nose, otitis, snoring, adenitis, mouth breathing?		X	X	X	X	A useful technique is beginning with a general question, i.e., "Has Jimmy had any trouble with his bones or joints?" and then proceeding to specifics, i.e., "Has he had painful joints, sprains?" Questions using both the names of diseases and a description of the symptoms are helpful.	Discussion of particular diseases found is indicated. Knowledge, is important concerning how to recognize various diseases, when home remedies may be appropriate, and what signs, symptoms, or circumstances indicate a need for eventual or immediate medical intervention.

*Age should be recorded at every well-child visit and when client presents with illness.

†Any chief complaint necessitates obtaining the following information in addition to that noted in this table: onset and progress of symptoms (chronology, positive and negative signs and symptoms), aggravating and alleviating factors, health immediately prior to onset, health status in general, medical attention or self-medication; behavior connected with present complaint; health of contacts; immunization status.

TABLE 7-1 Guidelines to History Taking *(continued)*

What to Ask	When to Ask: Age*	When to Ask: Chief Complaint†	Practical Hints	Education/Counselling
Teeth Age of eruption of deciduous and permanent; number at 1 yr; comparison with siblings Cardiorespiratory Heart murmurs, blue baby, asthma, pneumonia, frequent URI's, cystic fibrosis, congenital heart defect, rheumatic fever, trouble breathing, turning blue, tires easily, cough (when, where, what position, wet or dry) Gastrointestinal Diarrhea, constipation, vomiting, abdominal pain, bloody stools, bleeding from rectum, fissures, ulcer, pyloric stenosis, jaundice Genitourinary Urinary system: period of dryness (as of urine); color, odor, and frequency; pain, bleeding; menstruation: how often, problems (pain, increased flow, etc.); urinary tract infection (UTI), enuresis, dysuria, frequency, polyuria, pyuria, hematuria, character of stream, vaginal discharge, menstrual history, bladder control, abnormalities of penis or testes	Recorded annually or at the time of complaint		"Has Jimmy ever had a urinary tract infection? Have you ever noticed that there have been times when it seems to hurt him or make him cry when he passes water? Or times when he has a fever that you can't explain or that he wets his bed or pants when you don't expect it?" Children over 10 can usually be asked these questions directly with some assurance that their memories are accurate enough that they can be considered reliable informants. At even earlier ages, the examiner should encourage the child's participation in his or her own health care by including the child in the questioning process ("Mrs. Jones and Jane—do either of you recall if Jane has had frequent nosebleeds?") Initiating this practice as young as in the preschool years is most important in promoting the development of active (as opposed to passive) health consumer roles.	Counselling regarding disease prevention may be appropriate (e.g., not propping a milk bottle for children with frequent otitis media, diet modifications for children with frequent diarrhea or constipation, safety precautions for children with seizure disorders). Explanations of disease etiologies may be of interest to some parents. Children are interested in different parts of their bodies at different ages. Hence, the examiner should choose to discuss and explain those sections of the review of systems segment of the history about which the child is most curious. See *Teach Us What We Want To Know,* by Gertrude Lewis and Ruth Totman, Mental Health Materials Center, New York, 1969.

*Age should be recorded at every well-child visit and when client presents with illness.

†Any chief complaint necessitates obtaining the following information in addition to that noted in this table: onset and progress of symptoms (chronology, positive and negative signs and symptoms), aggravating and alleviating factors, health immediately prior to onset, health status in general, medical attention or self-medication; behavior connected with present complaint; health of contacts; immunization status.

TABLE 7-1 Guidelines to History Taking *(continued)*

What to Ask	When to Ask: Age*	Chief Complaint†: Learning Disability	Nausea and Vomiting	Constipation	Headache	Practical Hints	Education/Counselling
Neurological Convulsions, fainting, tremors, twitches, blackouts, dizziness, headaches, and their frequency Skeletal History of fractures, sprains, painful joints, swelling or redness around joints, posture/ exercise tolerance, gait Endocrine Any diagnosed thyroid or adrenal problems or diabetes Senses Do parent(s) and child think child can see and hear well? Is child clumsy? Uncoordinated? Does muscle strength seem adequate for age? Any numbness? Any difficulty in seeing blackboards? Does child sit too close to the television or radio? Does child "ignore" voices, not react to loud sounds?							
HABITS Diet If formula, what kind, how much, how mixed, frequency of feedings, how much in 24-h period; if taking solids, look for sources of vitamin C, calcium, protein, and iron in diet; what size	Recorded at each visit	X	X	X	X	There are two general categories of information important in diet history—one pertains to nutrient intake and one to diet habits and attitudes. Nutrients most likely to be lacking are iron, calcium, vitamins A and C, and	Education regarding nutrition is one of the foundations of well-child care. Discussion is needed about the appropriate intake of required nutrients, the avoidance of empty calories, and the

*Age should be recorded at every well-child visit and when client presents with illness.

†Any chief complaint necessitates obtaining the following information in addition to that noted in this table: onset and progress of symptoms (chronology, positive and negative signs and symptoms), aggravating and alleviating factors, health immediately prior to onset, health status in general, medical attention or self-medication; behavior connected with present complaint; health of contacts; immunization status.

TABLE 7-1 Guidelines to History Taking *(continued)*

What to Ask	When to Ask: Age*	Chief Complaint†				Practical Hints	Education/Counselling
portions, frequency of snacks; self-help skills; use of a cup, spoon, knife, fork; how messy; what kind of vitamins, how often, how much; likes and dislikes; meal pattern/constant snacking; food attitude: use as a symbol for love or as a reward; food deprivation as a punishment						protein. It is helpful to ascertain vitamin C intake in a typical day and the rest in a typical week. If a child is getting sufficient milk, then calcium and protein intake are usually adequate. Iron and vitamins C and A may be taken separately; a system according to the "daily 4" is also sometimes useful. Discussion of appetite and education about it must be developmentally appropriate. (These questions should be asked separately and viewed in a context of the family meal, food habits, and attitudes.)	formation of good food habits. Discussion of methods of recognizing and dealing with normal developmental problems and changes in eating habits is important (e.g., the nursing infant's 2-wk and 2-mo appetite spurt that may temporarily outstrip the mother's milk supply, or the 1-yr-old's decrease in appetite, or the toddler's need for finger food, or the adolescent's need to learn to blend solid nutrition with peer socialization). Instruction about nutritional sources of iron is frequently important. Discussion about avoiding high-carbohydrate foods, which predispose to caries and obesity, is appropriate.
Elimination Bowel patterns: frequency, consistency, color, discomfort; when toilet trained, any accidents, by day or night or both	Recorded at each visit	X	X	X	X	For some cultural groups or certain individuals, questioning in this area may cause embarrassment. Tact and an explanation of why this information is needed may be important. Many synonyms are used when talking to the child directly. Words like "wee wee," "pop," "tinkle" may be needed. This is also true for some adults.	Discussion of regulation of bowel movements by dietary measures rather than by enemas, laxatives, etc., is important. Anticipatory guidance may be needed regarding toilet training. Knowledge of "normal" daytime or nighttime accidents is indicated for the toddler, preschooler, and early school-age child. Wiping front to back should be mentioned.

*Age should be recorded at every well-child visit and when client presents with illness.

†Any chief complaint necessitates obtaining the following information in addition to that noted in this table: onset and progress of symptoms (chronology, positive and negative signs and symptoms), aggravating and alleviating factors, health immediately prior to onset, health status in general, medical attention or self-medication; behavior connected with present complaint; health of contacts; immunization status.

TABLE 7-1 Guidelines to History Taking *(continued)*

What to Ask	When to Ask: Age*	Chief Complaint†: Learning Disability	Nausea and Vomiting	Constipation	Headache	Practical Hints	Education/Counselling
							Counselling related to toilet training may be done at this time. It is important to help parents avoid conveying to their children the idea that this part of them is "dirty." Need to help new mothers understand meaning of words "constipation" and "diarrhea."
Exercise Sports, hobbies, tolerance for exercise; amount of exercise; school-related activities	Recorded annually or at the time of complaint	X	X	X	X	Parental expectations for the child in sports is important to determine. Leg cramps are a common complaint among children with the habit of constant exercise, more so than for children who take intermittent rest periods. Exercise is an important area to explore when a child is labeled "hyperactive." How purposeful is exercise and activity? Explore social relationships connected with exercise.	Physical fitness plans should begin in infancy through parental instruction. Adaptive physical education plans should be encouraged for children with motor problems. These programs allow the child to experience success at the child's own individual rate of development, thereby promoting a positive response to physical exercise. These programs will, one hopes, reduce situations in which children are ridiculed for poor motor performance by peers, and grow up to become very sedentary adults at risk for numerous health problems.
Sleep When to bed, sleep through night, frequency of awakening during night, what does mother do, nightmares, night terrors	Recorded at each visit	X	X		X	Research has not validated the idea that early feeding of solids helps the average baby sleep through the night, although this may work for individual children.	Discussion is important regarding normal developmental patterns of sleep, e.g., the toddler's refusal to go to bed. Determine if there are sleep problems

*Age should be recorded at every well-child visit and when client presents with illness.

†Any chief complaint necessitates obtaining the following information in addition to that noted in this table: onset and progress of symptoms (chronology, positive and negative signs and symptoms), aggravating and alleviating factors, health immediately prior to onset, health status in general, medical attention or self-medication; behavior connected with present complaint; health of contacts; immunization status.

TABLE 7-1 Guidelines to History Taking *(continued)*

What to Ask	When to Ask: Age*	Chief Complaint†				Practical Hints	Education/Counselling
Naps: when, how long; where does child sleep, own bed, number of hours, slept in 24 h, tired during the day						It may be helpful to get a baby over 6 mo out of parent(s) room if child has slept there since birth.	(nightmares, night terrors, bruxism). Discuss the need for adequate sleep and sleeping arrangements
Development							
Ordinal position compared with siblings, age when developmental tasks achieved (rolled over, sat alone, stood, walked, talked); if in school, what grade, does child like it, have playmates, what activities does child enjoy in school, after school; what special services at school utilized by child (e.g., speech, counselling)	Recorded at each visit	X	X		X		
Personality							
Self-image; relationships with peers, parents, siblings; hallucinations, obsessions, delusions; fears, anxieties, sensitivities; depression, acting out, or withdrawal; temper tantrums; recent changes in behavior	Recorded at each visit	X		X		Data is best obtained from both parent and child. Child under 10 best expresses self through play, drawings, or telling stories about pictures presented. For a young adolescent who is uncomfortable with his or her body, it may be easiest to express self through writing of poems, stories, or interpretation of best-liked movies. Any child having personality changes, or whose personality is consistently incompatible with others, may have fears of being "crazy."	It is important for the parent(s) to have an awareness of the child's personality. The examiner is in a position to stimulate awareness through discussion. Schools have on staff psychologists and counsellors who are capable of providing psychosocial evaluations. Many parents are unaware this service is available to their child. The child needs self-awareness of his or her personality strengths. These can be identified during the evaluation and positively reinforced.

*Age should be recorded at every well-child visit and when client presents with illness.

†Any chief complaint necessitates obtaining the following information in addition to that noted in this table: onset and progress of symptoms (chronology, positive and negative signs and symptoms), aggravating and alleviating factors, health immediately prior to onset, health status in general, medical attention or self-medication; behavior connected with present complaint; health of contacts; immunization status.

TABLE 7-1 Guidelines to History Taking *(continued)*

What to Ask	When to Ask: Age*	Chief Complaint†				Practical Hints	Education/Counselling
						Presenting reality for children is most important so they may have help in realizing their impressions of a situation are accurate or inaccurate. Depression is increasing in children/adolescents. Do not heed lightly threats by a child to harm self.	Parents need help in identifying and consistently reinforcing positively those strengths within the child's personality.

*Age should be recorded at every well-child visit and when client presents with illness.

†Any chief complaint necessitates obtaining the following information in addition to that noted in this table: onset and progress of symptoms (chronology, positive and negative signs and symptoms), aggravating and alleviating factors, health immediately prior to onset, health status in general, medical attention or self-medication; behavior connected with present complaint; health of contacts; immunization status.

TABLE 7-2 Guidelines to Physical Examination

What to Examine	When: Age	Chief Complaint: Learning Disability	Nausea and Vomiting	Constipation	Headache	Practical Hints	Education/Counselling
VITAL SIGNS Temperature, pulse rate, and respiratory rate (TPR); blood pressure, weight, and height	Any age; all exams	X	X	X	X	The height, weight, and head circumference of the child should be compared with standard charts and the approximate percentiles recorded. Multiple measurements at intervals are of much greater value than single ones since they give information regarding the pattern of growth that cannot be determined by single measurements.	It is very important that all parents be taught how to take and read an infant's temperature during the postpartum stay in the hospital. As the child gets older, parents should be taught to take the temperature orally. Parents should be taught how high a temperature should be allowed to go before calling for medical help.

TABLE 7-2 Guidelines to Physical Examination *(continued)*

What to Examine	When: Age	When: Chief Complaint				Practical Hints	Education/Counselling
						Rectal temperatures: During the first years of life the temperature should be taken rectally (except for routine temperatures of the premature infant, where axillary temperatures are sufficiently accurate). The child should be laid face down across the parent's lap and held firmly with the left forearm placed flat across the child's back; with the thumb and index finger he or she can separate the buttocks and insert the lubricated thermometer with the right hand. Rectal temperature may be 1°F higher than oral temperature; a rectal temperature up to 100°F (37.8°C) may be considered normal in a child. Apprehension and activity may elevate the temperature.	Fever control measures (antipyretics, sponge baths, etc.) should be taught. If baby aspirins are used, poison prevention measures should be included.
GENERAL APPEARANCE Child appearing well or ill; degree of prostration, cooperation, comfort, nutrition, and consciousness; abnormalities; gait, posture, and coordination; estimate of intelligence; reaction to parent(s), examiner, and examination; nature of cry and degree of facial activity and facial expression	Each exam	X	X	X	X		

TABLE 7-2 Guidelines to Physical Examination *(continued)*

What to Examine	When: Age	Chief Complaint: Learning Disability	Chief Complaint: Nausea and Vomiting	Chief Complaint: Constipation	Chief Complaint: Headache	Practical Hints	Education/Counselling
SKIN Color: cyanosis, jaundice, pallor, erythema; texture: eruptions, hydration, edema, hemorrhagic manifestations, scars, dilated vessels and direction of blood flow, hemangiomas, cafe-au-lait areas and nevi, Mongolian (blue-black) spots, pigmentation, turgor, elasticity, and subcutaneous nodules; striae and wrinkling perhaps indicating rapid weight gain or loss; sensitivity, hair distribution and character, and desquamation	Each exam	X	X	X	X	Loss of turgor, especially of the calf muscles and skin over the abdomen, is evidence of dehydration. The soles and palms are often bluish and cold in early infancy; this is of no significance. The degree of anemia cannot be determined reliably by inspection since pallor (even in the newborn) may be normal and not due to anemia. To demonstrate pitting edema in a child, it may be necessary to exert prolonged pressure. A few small pigmented nevi are commonly found, particularly in older children. Spider nevi occur in about one-sixth of children under 5 yr and almost half of older children. "Mongolian spots" (large flat black or blue-black areas) are frequently present over the lower back and buttocks; in non-Caucasian children they have no pathologic significance; be sure to distinguish them from the ecchymosis of child abuse.	Parents of infants are particularly likely to be interested in skin care—should they use baby powder? Baby ointment? How often should they bathe their babies? Discussion of these subjects is often useful to parents. Parents are also very interested in any unusual or different markings on their infants—are they serious? Will they disappear? Do they mean disease? Very common markings such as milia, miliaria, or stork bites will cause these concerns, as will slightly less common markings like cavernous hemangioma and port-wine stains and cafe-au-lait marks. Adolescents are attentive audiences concerning skin care.

TABLE 7-2 Guidelines to Physical Examination *(continued)*

What to Examine	When: Age	Chief Complaint				Practical Hints	Education/Counselling
						Cyanosis will not be evident unless at least 5 g of reduced hemoglobin are present; therefore, it develops less easily in an anemic child. Carotenemic pigmentation is usually most prominent over the palms and soles and around the nose, and spares the conjunctivas; it is absent in the sclera; conversely, jaundice is present in the sclera. Note birthmarks.	
HAIR Texture, distribution, parasites	Annually	X	X			Normal infants may lose their hair around 3 mo of age; this is of no significance. Familial balding may begin in adolescence.	How and with what to shampoo infants' hair is a frequent concern of parents. Most adolescents are very interested in hair care measures. Appearance of axillary, facial, and pubic hair in adolescents warrants anticipatory guidance and reassurance about the normality of the body changes which will occur.
LYMPH NODES Location, size, mobility, consistency; routine attempts to palpate suboccipital, preauricular, anterior cervical, posterior cervical, submaxillary, sublingual, axillary, epitrochlear, and inguinal lymph nodes	Annually	X	X		X	Enlargement of the lymph nodes occurs much more readily in children than in adults. Small inguinal lymph nodes are palpable in almost all healthy young children. Small, mobile, nontender shotty nodes are commonly found as residua of previous infections.	Older children—school age and adolescent—will frequently be surprised to feel a lymph node someplace in their bodies. A discussion of its normality and the purpose of the lymphatic system may be very helpful.

TABLE 7-2 Guidelines to Physical Examination *(continued)*

What to Examine	When: Age	Chief Complaint: Learning Disability	Chief Complaint: Nausea and Vomiting	Chief Complaint: Constipation	Chief Complaint: Headache	Practical Hints	Education/Counselling
HEAD Size, shape, circumference, asymmetry, **cephalhe**matoma, **bosses**, craniotabes, **control**, molding, bruit, **fontanel** (size, tension, **number**, abnormally late or early closure), sutures, dilated veins, scalp, face, transillumination	Each visit during infancy, then annually	X	X		X	The head is measured at its greatest circumference, which is usually at the midforehead. It is done anteriorly and around to the most prominent portion of the occiput posteriorly. The ratio of head circumference to circumference of the chest or abdomen is usually of little value. Fontanel tension is best determined with the child quiet and in the sitting position. Slight pulsations over the anterior fontanel may occur in normal infants. Although bruits may be heard over the temporal areas in normal children, the possibility of an existing abnormality should not be overlooked. Craniotabes may be found in the normal newborn infant (especially the premature) and for the first 2–4 mo, but they may also indicate rickets. A positive Macewen's sign ("cracked pot" sound when skull is percussed with one finger) may be	Parents of infants are often interested to learn more about the baby's "soft spot." Many parents are unduly concerned about the vulnerability of this spot and will even avoid washing the hair over it. Counselling about this can be very helpful.

TABLE 7-2 Guidelines to Physical Examination *(continued)*

	When						
What to Examine	Age	Chief Complaint				Practical Hints	Education/Counselling
						present normally as long as the fontanel is open. Transillumination of the skull can be performed by means of a flashlight with a sponge rubber collar so that it forms a tight fit when held against the head; this should be done in a completely dark room; several minutes should be allowed for the examiner's eyes to accommodate to the dark.	
FACE Symmetry, paralysis, distance between nose and mouth, depth of nasolabial folds, bridge of nose, distribution of hair, size of mandible, swellings, hypertelorism, Chvostek's sign, tenderness of sinuses	Annually	X	X		X	Normal infants have a very large forehead relative to the adult standard. Frontal sinuses do not develop until 7 or 8 yr, so there is no need to percuss these in the younger child.	
EYES Photophobia, visual acuity, muscular control, nystagmus, Mongolian slant, Brushfield spots, epicanthus folds, lacrimation, discharge, lids, exophthalmos or enophthalmos, conjunctivas; pupillary size, shape, and reaction to light and accommodation; media (corneal opacities, cataracts), fundi, visual fields (in older children)	Annually					The newborn infant usually will open the eyes if placed prone, supported with one hand on the abdomen, and lifted over the examiner's head. Not infrequently, one pupil is normally larger than the other. This sometimes occurs only in bright or in subdued light. "Hippus" (a phenomenon in which the pupils alternately constrict and dilate when a light is shined on them) is not uncommon in the adolescent.	Parents of newborns are always interested to find out when and how much their babies can see. They will often be interested in receiving counselling in regard to how they can stimulate their baby's vision through the use of brightly colored moving mobiles at about 14 in away. They will probably also be interested a few weeks later in helping baby learn to follow by tracking objects (or their own faces) slowly from one side to the other.

TABLE 7-2 Guidelines to Physical Examination *(continued)*

What to Examine	When: Age	Chief Complaint: Learning Disability	Nausea and Vomiting	Constipation	Headache	Practical Hints	Education/Counselling
						Vision evaluation is essential in all children. Dark blotches are commonly present in the sclera of black children. The retinas of black children are darker than those of white children. Oriental children usually have some degree of epiblepharon; as long as it does not irritate the cornea, it should be considered normal.	There are many myths in this country about how too much reading or reading in a car can damage the eye. Parents are often interested in discussing these myths. Parents of infants often ask when their babies will achieve their final eye color (about 50% do so by 6 mo; over 90% by 1 yr). Questions of the inheritability of eye disease and vision problems can provide very important opportunities for counselling. As children who wear glasses become adolescents, a variety of questions arise about the possibility of contact lenses.
NOSE Exterior, shape, mucosa, patency, discharge, bleeding, pressure over sinuses, flaring of nostrils, septum, turbinates	Annually	X	X		X	A head mirror and nasal speculum or the largest otoscope speculum may aid visualization. Pushing the nose tip with your thumb so that it flattens against the face also aids visualization.	Education concerning how to stop nosebleed (by pinching at the base of the nose without releasing or holding ice at this point—the point of Kiesselbach's Triangle) is important for some children and their parents.
MOUTH Lips (thinness, down-turning, fissures, color, cleft), teeth (number, position, caries, mottling, discoloration, notching, malocclusion or malalignment),	Annually	X	X	X	X	If the tongue can be extended as far as the alveolar ridge, there will be no interference with nursing or speaking.	Dental hygiene is important, since caries are the leading childhood disease. Tooth cleansing should begin with the eruption of the first tooth with the parent(s) using a

TABLE 7-2 Guidelines to Physical Examination *(continued)*

What to Examine	When: Age	When: Chief Complaint				Practical Hints	Education/Counselling
mucosa (color, redness of Stensen's duct, enanthems, Bohn's nodules, Epstein's pearls), gums, palate, tongue, uvula, mouth breathing, geographic tongue (usually normal)							washcloth to cleanse the tooth. Brushing becomes possible later, but for the job to be done well, the parent(s) must at least finish it after the child has begun until about age 7—children below this age are not manually dexterous enough to do a complete job. Flossing must also be done by the parent(s) until about age 10–11, when the child can be taught. Topical, systemic, and water supply fluoride are also topics of educational importance. A healthy preparation of the child for dentist visits is important. An excellent book is *My Friend the Dentist* by Jane Watson and Robert Switzer, Golden Press, NY, 1972. Teething control is an important area for health education until all primary teeth have erupted (by about 2 to 2½ yr). The contribution of high-carbohydrate foods to caries must be stressed. Emergency care for tooth evulsion may be appropriate in certain cases.
THROAT Tonsils (size, inflammation, exudate, crypts, inflammation of the anterior pillars), mucosa, hypertrophic	Annually	X	X		X	Before examining a child's throat it is advisable to examine the mouth first and permit the child to handle the tongue blade,	Education concerning tonsils is frequently appropriate. Many parents want children's tonsils pulled out

TABLE 7-2 Guidelines to Physical Examination *(continued)*

What to Examine	When: Age	Chief Complaint: Learning Disability	Nausea and Vomiting	Constipation	Headache	Practical Hints	Education/Counselling
lymphoid tissue, postnasal drip, epiglottis, voice (hoarseness, stridor, grunting, type of cry, speech)						nasal speculum, and flashlight to help overcome fear of the instruments. Then ask the child to stick out the tongue and say "ah", louder and louder. In some cases this may allow an adequate examination. In others, if the child is cooperative enough, you may ask the child to "pant like a puppy"; while doing this, the tongue blade is applied firmly to the rear of the tongue. Gagging need not usually be elicited in order to obtain a satisfactory examination. In still other cases, it may be expedient to examine one side of the tongue at a time, pushing the base of the tongue to one side and then to the other. This may be less unpleasant and is less apt to cause gagging. Young children may have to be restrained to obtain an adequate examination of the throat. Eliciting a gag reflex may be necessary if the oral pharynx is to be adequately seen. The small child's head may be restrained satisfactorily if the parent's hands are placed at the level of the child's elbows while the child's arms are held firmly against the sides of the head.	thinking this will stop frequent colds. The way a child is handled for this type of procedure can provide the care giver an opportunity to give the parent(s) an example of the appropriate way to handle things which are unpleasant (but necessary) for the child. An age-appropriate brief explanation followed by a firm but quick examination ending with a chance for the child to express feelings in an age-appropriate manner is important. Respect for the child and the child's feelings must be maintained, and cuddling or other age-appropriate reassurance should be given after the examination.

TABLE 7-2 Guidelines to Physical Examination *(continued)*

What to Examine	When					Practical Hints	Education/Counselling
	Age	Chief Complaint					
						If the child can sit up, the parent is asked to hold the child erect in her or his lap with the back against the parent's chest. The child's left hand is then held in the parent's left hand and the right hand in the parent's right hand. The parent places them against the child's groin or lower thigh to prevent the child's slipping down from the lap. If the throat is to be examined in natural light, the parent faces the light. If the artificial light and a head mirror are used, the parent sits with her or his back to the light. In either case, the physician or nurse uses one hand to hold the child's head in position and the other to manipulate the tongue blade. Young children seldom complain of sore throats even in the presence of significant infection of the pharynx and tonsils. The present of a clean tongue blade to bring home and use on a doll is usually appreciated by the preschooler.	
EARS Pinnas (position, size), canals, tympanic membranes (landmarks, mobility, perforation, inflammation, discharge), mastoid tenderness and swelling, hearing	Annually	X	X		X	An evaluation of hearing is an important part of the physical examination of every child. The ears of all sick children should be examined.	Cleaning of ears is a subject which often comes up, particularly if a child's ears must be curetted. It is important to help the parents realize the wax you are

TABLE 7-2 Guidelines to Physical Examination *(continued)*

What to Examine	When: Age	Chief Complaint: Learning Disability	Nausea and Vomiting	Constipation	Headache	Practical Hints	Education/Counselling
						Before actually examining the ears, it is often helpful to place the speculum just within the canal, remove it and place it lightly in the other ear, remove it again, and proceed in this way from one ear to the other, gradually going farther and farther, until a satisfactory examination is completed. In examining the ears, as large a speculum as possible should be used and should be inserted no farther than necessary, to avoid both discomfort and pushing wax in front of the speculum so that it obscures the field. The otoscope should be held balanced in the hand by holding the handle at the end nearest the speculum. One finger should rest against the head to prevent injury resulting from sudden movement by the child. Pneumoscopy should always be performed. The most common difficulty in getting the tympanic membrane (TM) to move is failing to get an airtight seal because the speculum used is too small. The sound of air whistling back out the canal indicates this is the case. A child may be restrained most easily when he or	removing is not dirt and the fact that it is there does not indicate they are doing a poor job cleaning their child's ears. Careful instructions to avoid pointed and small objects such as cotton swabs and bobby pins are important since damage of the tympanic membrane is possible. Hydrogen peroxide is occasionally suggested if the child has bothersome wax; otherwise removal of the wax is not really necessary. Again, a good example of how to handle a child during a potentially uncomfortable experience can be very helpful to the parents. Older children will be interested to see pictures or models of what you are looking at in their ears. School-age children often have many misconceptions about this part of their anatomy. Discussion of how to protect hearing may be appropriate to adolescents interested in rock music.

TABLE 7-2 Guidelines to Physical Examination *(continued)*

What to Examine	When					Practical Hints	Education/Counselling
	Age	Chief Complaint					
						she is lying on the abdomen. Low-set ears are present in a number of congenital syndromes, including several that are associated with mental retardation. The ears may be considered low set if they are below a line drawn from the lateral angle of the eye and the external occipital protuberance. Congenital anomalies of the urinary tract are frequently associated with abnormalities of the pinnas. To examine the ears of an infant it is usually necessary to pull the auricle backward and downward; in the older child the external ear is pulled backward and upward. "Examining" the parent's ears first is often very helpful in allaying the child's fears; so is allowing handling of the instruments and "blowing out" the light.	
NECK Position (torticollis, opisthotonos, inability to support head, mobility), swelling, thyroid (size, contour, bruit, isthmus, nodules, tenderness), lymph nodes, veins, position of trachea, sternocleidomastoid	Annually	X	X		X	In the older child, the size and shape of the thyroid gland may be more clearly defined if the gland is palpated from behind. Full range of motion (ROM) is elicited in the infant most easily by getting the child to follow	Older schoolchildren are often interested in the anatomy of the thyroid and larynx.

TABLE 7-2 Guidelines to Physical Examination *(continued)*

What to Examine	When: Age	Chief Complaint: Learning Disability	Nausea and Vomiting	Constipation	Headache	Practical Hints	Education/Counselling
(swelling, shortening), webbing, edema, auscultation, movement, tonic neck reflex						an object with the eyes. Pushing the head from side to side often elicits the rooting reflex or resistance.	
THORAX Shape and symmetry, veins, retractions and pulsations, beading; Harrison's groove, flaring of ribs, pigeon breast, funnel shape, size and position of nipples and breasts, length of sternum, intercostal and substernal retraction, asymmetry, scapulas, clavicles		X	X		X	At puberty, in normal children, one breast usually begins to develop before the other. In both sexes tenderness of the breasts is relatively common. Gynecomastia is not uncommon in the male. Some male or female newborns will have engorged and occasionally secreting breasts. This occurs because of passage of maternal hormones and generally lasts only a day or two.	Breast development in girls and gynecomastia in boys are an extremely important topic of health education for adolescents. They are frequently too embarrassed to ask questions, and the examiner should take the initiative in this discussion. Reassurance of the normality of this development is vital. Parents of newborns with breast engorgement also need to be reassured that this is normal, and "milking" the breasts will not stop the secretion.
LUNGS Type of breathing, dyspnea, prolongation of expiration, cough, expansion, fremitus, flatness or dullness to percussion, resonance, breath and voice sounds, rales, wheezing	X	X		X		Breath sounds in infants and children are normally more intense and more bronchial than in adults, and expiration is more prolonged. Most of the young child's respiratory movement is produced by abdominal movement; there is very little intercostal motion. If one places the stethoscope over the mouth and subtracts the sounds heard by this route from the sounds heard through the chest	Parents of young infants are likely to be interested in learning the early signs of respiratory infections, what measures they can take at home, and when they should call for professional help concerning such problems. They are also likely to be interested in learning what measures to take to prevent the spread of such infections. Because of the current publicity, parents of young children may also

TABLE 7-2 Guidelines to Physical Examination *(continued)*

What to Examine	When: Age	When: Chief Complaint				Practical Hints	Education/Counselling
						wall, the difference usually represents the amount produced intrathoracically. Allowing the child to listen to his or her own lungs often helps rapport tremendously. The preschooler will often understand the analogy between the stethoscope and listening on a telephone. Patting the bell of the stethoscope first on the child's hand and "listening" may help allay fears. The fearful child should always be allowed to touch and handle the stethoscope first.	be interested in discussing what effect their own smoking or living in polluted areas has on the health of their children's respiratory systems. Adolescents are highly conscious of their bodies. Particularly those interested in sports will be motivated to learn how to keep their lungs in good condition. Avoidance of smoking is often a topic of interest at this time. By school age, children are becoming more interested in the inner workings of their bodies and are able to understand simple cause-and-effect relationships. This is an ideal time to discuss the basic workings of the lungs and how to prevent their injury by avoiding habits such as smoking. In certain situations, parents will be interested in discussing the inheritability of diseases of the respiratory tract which may exist in their family tree, such as asthma, hay fever, or cystic fibrosis.
HEART Location and intensity of apex beat, precordial bulging, pulsation of vessels, thrills, size, shape, auscultation (rate, rhythm, force, quality of sounds—	Annually	X	X		X	Many children normally have sinus arrhythmia. The child should be asked to hold his or her breath to determine its effect on the rhythm.	Parents of newborns are very interested in their infants' bodies and will often be delighted to have the opportunity to listen to their children's hearts.

TABLE 7-2 Guidelines to Physical Examination *(continued)*

What to Examine	When: Age	Chief Complaint: Learning Disability	Chief Complaint: Nausea and Vomiting	Chief Complaint: Constipation	Chief Complaint: Headache	Practical Hints	Education/Counselling
compare with pulse as to rate and rhythm; friction rub-variation with pressure), murmurs (location, position in cycle, intensity, pitch, effect of change of position, transmission, effect of exercise)						Extrasystoles are not uncommon in childhood. The heart should be examined with the child erect, recumbent, and turned to the left.	Preschoolers will be interested in listening to their own hearts. At this age they can learn some very basic concepts about their hearts, like the fact that the heart pumps blood around the body. By the school years, the child becomes much more interested in the parts of the body which cannot be seen (toddlers and preschoolers are more interested in the surface characteristics of their bodies), and can learn a great deal about the heart's functions. Plastic models kept in the examining room for explanations may help in this teaching. Children of this age will also enjoy listening to their hearts. School-age children are good candidates for learning about the effect of diet and exercise on the well-being of their hearts; they are old enough to begin to understand this kind of cause-and-effect reasoning, and they are usually highly motivated in learning to care for their bodies. Adolescents are highly concerned about all parts of their bodies. Constant reassurance is necessary. This is particularly true if any concerns are elicited from the client—

TABLE 7-2 Guidelines to Physical Examination *(continued)*

What to Examine	When: Age	Chief Complaint				Practical Hints	Education/Counselling
							adolescents are often frightened, for instance, by the pounding of their hearts or other sensations they feel are associated with their hearts. If an innocent murmur is found and mentioned, it must be made very clear that this does *not* mean anything is wrong. Teaching about the effect of such things as smoking, diet, and exercise on the health of the heart can be very effective with adolescents.
ABDOMEN Size and contour, visible peristalsis, respiratory movements, veins (distention, direction of flow), umbilicus, hernia, musculature, tenderness and rigidity, tympany, shifting dullness, tenderness, rebound tenderness, pulsation, palpable organs, or masses (size, shape, position, mobility), fluid wave, reflexes, femoral pulsations, bowel sounds	Annually	X	X	X	X	The abdomen may be examined while the child is lying prone in the mother's lap, or held over her shoulder, or seated on the examining table with the back to the doctor or nurse. These positions may be particularly helpful where tenderness, rigidity, or a mass must be palpated. In the infant the examination may be aided by having the child suck at a "sugar tip" or at a bottle. Light palpation, especially for the spleen, often will give more information than deep. Umbilical hernias are common during the first 2 yr of life. They usually disappear spontaneously.	

TABLE 7-2 Guidelines to Physical Examination *(continued)*

What to Examine	When: Age	Chief Complaint: Learning Disability	Nausea and Vomiting	Constipation	Headache	Practical Hints	Education/Counselling
						"Let me feel what you had for breakfast" often helps allay the child's fears. Distraction and the use of the child's own hand to palpate may avoid the ticklish reaction many children have.	
RECTUM AND ANUS Irritation, fissures, prolapse, imperforate anus; the rectal examination should be performed with the little finger (inserted slowly); note muscle tone, character of stool, masses, tenderness, sensation; examine stool on glove finger (gross, microscopic, culture, guaiac) as indicated.	Annually	X	X	X	X		Education concerning hygiene may be indicated for parents of diaper-age children. Questions about diaper rash, wiping from front to back, and care of the diapers may come up. For older children, teaching about washing hands after bowel movements and wiping from front to back may be appropriate. Helping parents avoid conveying the idea of "dirtiness" to their young children concerning any part of the body is important. This is particularly troublesome if it is directed toward bowel movements since the child may generalize this to their genitals because of the proximity. Everything "down there" may become associated with dirt. Discussion related to potty training may be very important in that age group and may come up naturally during this part of the physical exam.

TABLE 7-2 Guidelines to Physical Examination *(continued)*

What to Examine	When: Age	When: Chief Complaint				Practical Hints	Education/Counselling
EXTREMITIES General Deformity, hemiatrophy, bowlegs, knock-knees, paralysis, gait, stance, asymmetry Joints Swelling, redness, pain, limitation, tenderness, motion, rheumatic nodules, carrying angle of elbows, tibial torsion Hands and feet Extra digits, clubbing, simian lines, curvature of little finger, deformity of nails, splinter hemorrhages, flat feet, abnormalities of feet, dermatoglyphics, width of thumbs and big toes, syndactyly, length of various segments, dimpling of dorsa, temperature Peripheral vessels Presence, absence, or diminution of arterial pulses	Annually	X				Children can seldom understand directions about how to move their bodies; it is generally easiest to demonstrate and play the "just like me" game. When observing the gait of a toddler, remember that the toddler won't walk *away* from the parents, but will walk *toward* them; pick the child up and put him or her down several yards from the parent. Feet commonly appear flat during the first 2 yr. Intrauterine position results in many contortions of the limbs, particularly of the feet; generally, if you can passively overcorrect an abnormal position the child will outgrow it.	Parents of young toddlers are often not aware of the normal stages of bowleggedness occurring at this age. It is often helpful to point this out to them. Parents of preschoolers are often not aware that in this stage children are often naturally knock-kneed, and most will outgrow it. Reassurance is often helpful. Parents of newborns are sometimes concerned about the normal hyperflexibility of joints (a newborn's wrist can be flexed flat against the forearm, for instance). Reassurance that this is normal may be useful. Children are often interested in their own growth patterns, e.g., how much more they will grow. Children of later school age are often very interested in first aid for such things as fractures. Advice on posture may be appropriate for the school-age child and adolescent. Discussion of the normal "flat feet of infancy" or defects from intrauterine position is often important for parents of infants.
SPINE AND BACK Posture, curvatures, rigidity, webbed neck, spina bifida, pilonidal	Annually	X				Black children normally have an exaggerated lumbar curve.	

TABLE 7-2 Guidelines to Physical Examination *(continued)*

What to Examine	When: Age	Chief Complaint: Learning Disability	Chief Complaint: Nausea and Vomiting	Chief Complaint: Constipation	Chief Complaint: Headache	Practical Hints	Education/Counselling
dimple or cyst, tufts of hair, mobility, Mongolian spot; tenderness over spine, pelvis, or kidneys						If an apparent scoliosis corrects itself when the child bends over, it is functional; if it does not, it is organic.	
MALE GENITALIA Circumcision, meatal opening, hypospadias, phimosis, adherent foreskin, size of testes, cryptorchidism, scrotum, hydrocele, hernia, pubertal changes	Annually	X				In examining a suspected case of cryptorchidism, palpation for the testicles should be done before the child has fully undressed or become chilled or had the cremasteric reflex stimulated. In some cases, examination while the child is in a hot bath may be helpful. The boy should also be examined while sitting in a chair holding his knees with his heels on the seat; the increased intraabdominal pressure may push the testes into the scrotum. To examine for cryptorchidism, start above the inguinal canal and work downward to prevent pushing the testes up into the canal or abdomen. In the obese boy, the penis may be so obscured by fat as to appear abnormally small. If this fat is pushed back, a penis of normal size is usually found.	The following applies to both male and female genitalia in the physical exam. *Infancy and toddlerhood:* Parents may need education regarding hygiene of the genital areas—wiping from front to back in little girls to prevent urinary tract infections, and gradual retraction of the foreskin of little boys (authorities differ on the best time to retract the foreskin of infant boys, but once it is retracted, it is important to continue to retract it to prevent it from becoming adherent to the shaft due to the formation of adhesions). Parents of infants need to understand that infants often play with their genitals in much the same way that they play with their ears or hands. This is not true masturbation. *Preschoolers and school-age children:* Parents may need help realizing that their own reactions to their children's genitals will form the foundation for

TABLE 7-2 Guidelines to Physical Examination *(continued)*

What to Examine	When					Practical Hints	Education/Counselling
	Age	Chief Complaint					
							the children's reactions to them now and to their sexuality now and later. Parents need to know that masturbation, "playing doctor," concerns of the boy that his penis will be cut off and of the girl that she has already had a penis cut off are all normal, as long as the child is not totally preoccupied with these activities. Parents may need help in handling these matters. *Adolescents* This age group needs a great deal of education and counselling concerning changing genitals and changing sexuality. The sequence of changes in the bodies of adolescents is often of interest to them and provides an opportune time for anticipatory guidance.
FEMALE GENITALIA Vagina (imperforate, discharge, adhesions), hypertrophy of clitoris, pubertal changes		X				Digital or speculum examination is rarely done until after puberty.	
NEUROLOGIC EXAMINATION Cerebral function General behavior, level of consciousness, intelligence, emotional status, memory, orientation, illusions, hallucinations,	Annually	X			X	Because this part of the exam can so easily be made into a game, doing it at the beginning before undressing can help establish a rapport for the rest of the exam. A 4-yr-old can be expected	The nervous system is one of the last systems of the body with which children become familiar. Usually their interest in this system peaks around 9 yr; at this time, explanations of what you

TABLE 7-2 Guidelines to Physical Examination *(continued)*

What to Examine	When: Age	Chief Complaint: Learning Disability	Chief Complaint: Nausea and Vomiting	Chief Complaint: Constipation	Chief Complaint: Headache	Practical Hints	Education/Counselling
cortical sensory interpretation, cortical motor integration, language, ability to understand and communicate, auditory/verbal and visual/verbal comprehension, recognition of visual object, speech, ability to write, performance of skilled motor acts Cranial nerves *I (olfactory):* identify odors, disorders of smell *II (optic):* visual acuity, visual fields, opthalmoscopic examinations, retina *III (oculomotor), IV (trochlear),* and *VI (abducens):* ocular movements,ptosis, dilatation of pupil, nystagmus, pupillary accommodation, and pupillary light reflexes *V (trigeminal):* sensation of face, corneal reflex, masseter and temporal muscles, maxillary reflex (jaw jerk) *VII (facial);* wrinkle forehead, frown smile, raise eyebrows, asymmetry of face, strength of eyelid muscles, taste on anterior portion of tongue *VIII (acoustic):* Cochlear portion: hearing						to repeat three digits or words after the examiner; the 5-yr-old can do four and the 6-yr-old five. Familiar words, such as cat, dog, or pig, often hold the younger child's interest better than numbers. Bottlecaps, coins, and buttons often work well when testing the young child for stereognosis. Schoolchildren can usually identify the numbers 0, 7, 3, 8, and 1 when testing graphesthesia; preschoolers do better with squares and circles or parallel and crossing lines. When testing the kinesthetic sense using the up/down position of the toes, the examiner must be sure to hold the sides of the toes, not the top and bottom; otherwise the pressure sensation may give the answer away. Handclaps and bells work well with young children when testing auditory recognition. Folding a piece of paper is a good test for the young child when testing for control motor integration. Orange peel and peanut butter are more likely than coffee smell to be recognized by the young child when testing the Ist cranial nerve.	are doing and why you are doing it during the neuromuscular examination are usually well received. Children's interest in mental health also peaks around age 9 or fourth grade, and they will often associate this with the brain, so questions about mental health and mental illness as well as mental retardation may occur during this examination. It is a very useful time to help children begin to understand these very complex ideas and some preventive mental health concepts in relation to handling emotions, etc. Questions about sensations are likely to occur during the sensory part of the examination, and children can be encouraged to use their senses fully and appreciate the information brought to them by their senses. Certain of the infantile reflexes may cause concern. One example is the Moro. Infants with a very strong Moro reflex often alarm their parents. Education as to the normality and healthfulness of this response (i.e., primarily loss of support and loud noises) can also be useful. Learning about the expected times of the

TABLE 7-2 Guidelines to Physical Examination *(continued)*

What to Examine	When: Age	When: Chief Complaint				Practical Hints	Education/Counselling
lateralization, air, and bone, conduction, tinnitus vestibular: caloric tests *IX (glossopharyngeal), X (vagus):* pharyngeal gag reflex, ability to swallow and speak clearly; sensation of mucosa of pharynx, larynx, and soft palate; autonomic functions *XI (accessory):* strength of trapezius and sternocleidomastoid muscles *XII (hypoglossal):* protrusion of tongue, tremor, strength of tongue Cerebellar function Finger to nose; finger to examiner's finger; rapidly altering pronation and supination of hands; ability to run heel down other shin and to make a requested motion with foot; ability to stand with eyes closed; walk; heel-to-toe walk; tremor; ataxia; posture; arm swing when walking; nystagmus abnormalities of muscle tone or speech Motor system Muscle size, consistency, and						The "Let's-Make-a-Face" game for the VIIth cranial nerve and the "Tell-Me-Where-the-Goblin-Touches-You" game for testing sensations are examples of how this part of the exam can be made interesting to the young child. Young children do not have enough sense of direction to be able to perform Weber's test accurately. Remember that the infant's cry may be a danger sign related to neurological problems—high-pitched shrieking may indicate intracranial damage, a "cat's cry" is associated with the cri-du-chat syndrome, a hoarse cry may indicate cretinism, and a weak cry may indicate neurological problems. If two adults are present, visual fields may be more accurately assessed from behind. When testing for cerebellar functions, it is useful to know that a 4-yr-old can stand on one foot for about 5 s; a 6-yr-old can stand on one foot with arms crossed for 5 s, and a 7-yr-old can do it with eyes closed for 5 s.	appearance and disappearance of certain reflexes can add to the parents' understanding of and interest in their growing baby. A developmental examination is often considered the best neurological examination at this age. Parents are usually highly interested in their baby's development and counselling about what kinds of developments are expected and what kinds of developmental stimulation are appropriate can be very important.

TABLE 7-2 Guidelines to Physical Examination *(continued)*

What to Examine	When: Age	When: Chief Complaint — Learning Disability	Nausea and Vomiting	Constipation	Headache	Practical Hints	Education/Counselling
tone; muscle contours and outlines, muscle strength; myotonic contraction; slow relaxation; symmetry of posture; fasciculations; tremor; resistance to passive movement; involuntary movement							
Reflexes							
Deep reflexes: biceps, brachioradialis, triceps, patellar, Achilles; rapidity and strength of contraction and relaxation							
Superficial reflexes: abdominals, cremasteric, plantar, gluteal							
Pathologic reflexes: Babinski, Chaddock, Oppenheim, Gordon							
Infantile reflexes (See Table 3 in the introduction to Part 3, Section 8, The Neuropsychiatric System.)							

summary

This chapter delineates the information to be obtained during the course of a health history and a physical examination. The nurse, in performing these functions, has been identified as (1) a decision maker with regard to the child's health status; (2) a health educator, and (3) an inquirer into the consumer's health practices and beliefs. The health evaluation as conducted by the nurse can be a meaningful experience for every health consumer. The overall health of the child is clarified, the participation of consumers in their own health care is encouraged, and the plans for future health care are derived from the preferred health practices and beliefs of parent and child.

references

Gillum, Richard, and Barsky, Arthur. Diagnosis and management of patient non-compliance. *Journal of the American Medical Association,* June:1563 (1974).

Igoe, Judith. A program to expand the role of the adolescent health consumer. Narrative portion of grant awarded by the Office of Consumer Education, HEW, December 1977. Copies available upon request from School Nurse Practitioner Program, University of Colorado Medical Center, 4200 E. 9th Ave., Container #C287, Denver, CO. 80262.

8 Newborn Assessment

Jane Cooper Evans

Management of the newborn will, of course, depend upon the age at which the client is first seen. The practitioner may see the newborn in the nursery or delivery room, or the initial visit may be days or weeks after birth; many practitioners have contact with the family during the prenatal period, especially when there are other children in the family. The earliest possible contact with the infant and family is desirable.

Since each practitioner has already been educated in the care of the newborn, this chapter will illuminate only the latest developments in prenatal assessment and promotion of parent-infant bonding; protocol changes; physical, psychosocial, and environmental assessment; and counselling for the parent(s) of an atypical newborn.

For quick reference purposes, this chapter has been divided into six sections:

Section 1 covers changes in prenatal management and postnatal management protocols.

Section 2 covers new, evolving assessment criteria and techniques.

Section 3 is a reference table for newborn physical norms and for abnormalities and their possible causes in the newborn.

Section 4 covers psychosocial assessment and parent-child adjustment.

Section 5 is an overview of two environmental assessment tools.

Section 6 includes counselling for the parents of atypical newborns.

Management of common newborn problems such as diarrhea, vomiting, sleeping, etc., and new information on feeding are each covered in separate chapters and, therefore, will not be mentioned here.

SECTION 1: PRENATAL MANAGEMENT AND POSTNATAL PROTOCOL

PRENATAL MANAGEMENT

Management of the normal newborn begins prior to birth with the assessment of parental acceptance of the pregnancy and of the individuality of the fetus after quickening. Prenatal acceptance and preparedness lays the foundation for a successful relationship with the baby and the development of a healthy child.

Prenatal Maternal Rejection Behaviors (after first trimester)

1. Negative self-perception and body image—anger over "fat," facial changes, etc.
2. Preoccupation with physical appearance—makeup, clothes, etc.
3. Excessive mood swings or emotional withdrawal
4. Excessive physical complaints—excessive fatigue, aches, pains, etc.
5. Lack of response or negative response to quickening—does not touch abdomen or respond to kicking, or may bruise abdomen hitting baby when it kicks
6. Absence of any preparatory behavior during the last trimester—no purchase of equipment

or clothes for baby, etc. (Some religious groups discourage buying articles for the baby prior to the birth.)

7. Violent accidents or physical abuse of her body—falling down stairs or ramming soda bottles up vagina
8. Lack of desire for knowledge of labor and delivery; perhaps excessive anxiety and fear of labor and delivery

Prenatal Paternal Rejection Behaviors (after first trimester)

1. Negative self-perception—feels unqualified and unable to meet societal and his own expectations of a father
2. Negative preoccupation with wife's physical appearance—"She's too fat, ugly, etc."
3. Emotional withdrawal from wife—anger at lack of attention from wife, failure to meet wife's dependency needs
4. *Excessive* physical complaints—low back pain, fatigue, abdominal cramps, etc.
5. Unwillingness to touch abdomen, no desire to feel fetal movements
6. Refusal to attend prenatal classes and to allow wife to make preparatory purchases
7. Unwillingness to accept responsibility—excessive drinking with male cronies, excessive purchase of personal or household items not infant-related, quits job, etc.
8. Physical abuse of wife directed toward abdomen
9. Insistance on repeated savage intercourse near delivery date

Normal Causes of Rejection Behaviors

1. Stress which causes parent to feel
   a. Unloved or unsupported
   b. Concern for health and survival of self and infant
2. Source(s) of stress may be
   a. Marital problems
   b. Geographic change of residence
   c. Death of a close friend or relative
   d. Previous abortions
   e. Loss of previous children or multiple pregnancies
   f. Age of mother
   g. Lack of successful coping mechanisms
   h. Financial problems
   i. Lack of support system (friend or supportive family member, same sex is preferable)
   j. Poor state of health (weak from malnutrition, having babies too close together, excessive fatigue)
   k. Unwanted pregnancy

Prenatal Intervention

1. Identify source(s) of stress.
2. Counsel and support mother and father psychologically toward acceptance of pregnancy and of fetus as an individual.
   a. Discuss feelings and explore stress.
   b. Reassure parent(s) that feelings are normal in view of stresses (if they are).
   c. Grant parent(s)' desire in fantasy ("Pretend. . . . How would you feel if. . . .")
   d. Discuss problems and explore possible solutions and alternatives.
   e. Promote discussion with other parents if desirable and appropriate.
3. Emphasize positive parenting skills.
4. Mobilize additional support for parent(s) with family, friends, or community groups.

Abnormal Causes of Rejection Behaviors

1. Poor relationship with own parent(s)
2. Emotionally deprived childhood
3. Unresolved grief over death or illness of prior child
4. Long-term emotional disorder or medical illness

Prenatal Intervention

Psychiatric consultation is recommended for the management of these abnormal causes of rejection behaviors.

A sample prenatal and delivery history form is shown in Fig. 8-1.

POSTNATAL PROTOCOL

The general protocol for management of the normal newborn will not be included here because each practitioner and each hospital has an established protocol. Included are two important protocol changes and their rationale and the seven

Figure 8–1: PRENATAL AND DELIVERY HISTORY FORM

Name ______________________ Mother's name ______________________

Address ______________________

Date of delivery ________ Hour ________ Sex _____ Race _____

Paternal History

Father's name ______________________

Age ________ Health status ______________________

Blood type ________ Rh: ☐ Positive ☐ Negative

Congenital anomalies/Familial disorders ______________________

____

Chronic illness/Surgical events ______________________

____

Maternal History

Mother's age ________ Health status ______________________

Parity ____________ Gestation ____________ Weeks ____________

EDC ____________

Blood type ________ Rh: ☐ Positive ☐ Negative

Antibodies: ☐ Negative ☐ Positive

Date of last titer ____________

S.T.S.: ☐ Negative ☐ Positive

If positive: ☐ No Rx ☐ Rx Date ______________________

Type of prenatal care ______________________
(midwife, friend, physician, etc.)

Drugs ingested during pregnancy ______________________
(e.g., aspirin, steroids, alcohol, marijuana, etc.)

____

Congenital anomalies/Familial disorders ______________________

____

Chronic illness/Surgical events ______________________

____

Figure 8–1: PRENATAL AND DELIVERY HISTORY FORM (continued)

History of Previous Pregnancies

No.	Length of labor	Anesthesia/ Sedation	Route of delivery	Complications	Birth weights	Problems during first week of life (jaundice, infection, RDS, etc.)
1.						
2.						
3.						
4.						
5.						

Prenatal care ______________________________
(midwife, friend, physician)

Place of birth ______________________________
(home, hospital)

Labor History

Membranes ruptured ____________________ ☐ spontaneous ☐ artificial
(date and time)

Duration of labor ______________________________ 1st stage __________

2d stage __________

3d stage __________

Complications: ______________________________

____

Delivery History

Position ____________________ Analgesia ______________________________
(type, time, dose, and route)

Anesthesia ______________________________
(type and duration)

Abnormality of placenta ______________________________
(too large, too small, infarcts, previa, etc.)

____

Color of amniotic fluid ______________________________

Type of delivery ______________________________
(spontaneous, C-section, vacuum)

Forceps used ☐ yes ☐ no

Figure 8–1: PRENATAL AND DELIVERY HISTORY FORM (continued)

Vitamin K administered ☐ no ☐ yes ______________________________
(time and date)

Eyes treated ☐ no ☐ yes ______________________________
(name of medication)

Apgar score: ______________ 1 minute ______________ 5 minutes

Complications: ______________________________

____

Resuscitative measures: ______________________________

____

crucial principles of mother-infant attachment which affect protocol.

Protocol Changes

1. DO NOT treat infants' eyes with $AgNO_3$ or anything else until *after* first prolonged interaction with mother.
2. Facilitate *prolonged* mother-infant interaction within first 30 min after birth, including
   a. Skin-to-skin contact
   b. Good eye contact
   c. Nutritive suck (preferably breast-feed)

Rationale for Protocol Changes

1. Eye contact is vital and essential to the bonding process, and the critical period for optimal bonding is shortly after birth.
2. Multiple research studies indicate that mothers who receive skin-to-skin contact with their infants and/or breast-feed within the first 30 min after birth tend to breast-feed longer and show more attachment behaviors.
3. Research at the University of Utah indicates that infants who receive a *nutritive* suck within the first hour after birth are more responsive to their environment and do not necessarily lose weight. If weight loss occurs, it does not usually exceed 3 oz.

Crucial Principles of Parent-Infant Attachment

The following principles are developed from Klaus and Kennell (1976).

1. The first minutes and hours of life are a sensitive period during which it is necessary that the mother and father have close contact with their neonate for later development to be optimal.
2. Species-specific responses to the infant are exhibited in the human mother and father when they are first given their infant (unwrapping baby, exploring infant's body with a finger, etc.).
3. The attachment process is structured so that the father and mother will become optimally attached to only one infant at a time (this creates problems when twins are born).
4. During the process of the parental attachment to the infant, it is essential for the infant to respond to the parent(s) by some signal such as body or eye movements. This is sometimes described as "You can't love a dishrag."
5. People who see the actual birth process become strongly attached to the infant.
6. It is difficult to become attached to an infant while simultaneously going through the process of detachment (grief), that is, to develop an attachment to one person while mourning the loss or threatened loss of the same or another person. (Example: The death of a parent or close friend or a premature birth may interfere with the ability to attach. Also, maternal grief over the loss of a "fantasy" child and the loss of a body part, fetus or placenta, may interfere initially with attachment.) A parent may experience guilt because he or she is *expected* to love the infant but is not yet ready

to feel love. The parent may question whether in fact this is really his or her child.

7. Early events may have long-lasting effects. Anxieties about the well-being of a baby with a temporary disorder (premature birth) in the first day may result in long-lasting concerns which may cast long shadows and adversely shape the development of the child (Kennell and Rolnick, 1960). Parent(s) may stereotype a premature as "sickly and delicate" and treat the child that way for life.

SECTION 2: PHYSICAL ASSESSMENT TECHNIQUES

A great deal of emphasis has been placed on the physical assessment of newborns as a valuable means of detecting abnormalities and ill health and providing preventive intervention (see the newborn assessment guide, Fig. 8-2, and Table 8-2). Skills in assessing newborns have improved radically in the last decade or two, and care has improved accordingly. This section covers some

Figure 8-2: NEWBORN ASSESSMENT GUIDE

Child's name ______________________ Date ______________________

	Normal	Abnormal	Comments
I. General			
A. Birth weight _____			
Today's weight _____			
B. Birth length _____			
Today's length _____			
C. T. _____ P. _____			
R. _____ BP _____			
D. Age _____			
Date of Birth _____			
Gestational age _____			
E. Position/Posture			
F. Activity level/Seizures, tremors			
G. Appearance/Body proportion/Symmetry			
H. Cry			
II. Skin			
A. Color			
B. Texture			
C. Opacity			
D. Lanugo			
E. Vernix			
F. Pigmentation			
G. Wrinkling/Peeling			

	Normal	Abnormal	Comments
III. Head			
A. Circumference			
B. Shape/Symmetry			
C. Size: Anterior fontanel			
D. Size: Posterior fontanel			
E. Head lag			
F. Hair distribution			
1. Whorls			
2. Fine and/or electric			
G. Cm of transillumination			
Anterior _____			
Parietal _____			
Posterior _____			
IV. Ears			
A. Shape/Symmetry			
B. Alignment with eyes			
C. Rotation			
D. Cartilage development			
E. Tympanic membrane			
F. Adherent lobes			
V. Face			
A. Symmetry/Feature placement			
B. Shape			
C. Expression/Movement			
D. Depth nasolabial fold			
VI. Eyes			
A. Size/Slant			
B. Placement/Symmetry			
C. Color: Sclera/Conjunctiva			

Figure 8-2: NEWBORN ASSESSMENT GUIDE (continued)

	Normal	Abnormal	Comments
D. Cornea clarity/ Luster			
E. Pupil reaction			
F. Blink reflex			
G. Eyelids/Lashes			
H. Discharge/Tearing			
I. Muscular control			
VII. Nose			
A. Patent nares			
B. Milia			
C. Discharge			
D. Septum			
E. Breadth of bridge			
VIII. Mouth			
A. Size/Symmetry			
B. Shape of hard and soft palate			
C. Rooting reflex			
D. Strong suck			
E. Saliva			
F. Lip margins			
G. Mucous membranes			
H. Tonsils			
IX. Tongue			
A. Size/Grooves			
B. Color/Coating			
C. Mobility			
D. Tongue retrusion			
X. Neck/Chin			
A. Shape/Size			
B. Masses			
C. Movement			
D. Flexion			
E. Chin size and distance from lips			
XI. Chest			
A. Circumference			
B. Shape/Symmetry			
C. Pulsations or retractions			
D. Nipple size/Position/ Distance between			
E. Length of sternum			
F. Breath sounds/ Diaphragmatic			
G. PMI			
H. Cardiac rhythm/ Heart sounds			
XII. Abdomen			
A. Shape/Size			

	Normal	Abnormal	Comments
B. Peristalsis			
C. Tension/Pulsations			
D. Umbilicus/Hernia			
E. Organs			
XIII. Genitalia			
A. Female			
1. Labia size/Symmetry			
2. Discharge			
B. Male			
1. Meatus			
2. Foreskin/Circumcision			
3. Size/Color scrotum			
4. Testes descended			
XIV. Anus Patent			
XV. Extremities			
A. Range of motion, hip click			
B. Length/Symmetry			
C. Dermatoglyphics			
D. Number of digits			
E. Nail quality			
F. Movement/Tremors			
G. Gluteal folds even			
XVI. Back			
A. Symmetry/Curvature			
B. Alignment of scapulae			
C. Mobility			
XVII. Reflexes/Symmetrical responses			
A. Grasp			
B. Scarf sign			
C. Tonic neck			
D. Plantar			
E. Babinski			
F. Moro			
G. Stepping			
H. Ankle dorsiflexion			
I. Rooting			
J. Sucking			
XVIII. Other			
A. Stools			
1. Number/day			
2. Color/Consistency			
3. Odor			
B. Urine/Voidings			
1. Number/day			
2. Color/Odor			
C. Feedings			
1. Number/day			

Figure 8-2: NEWBORN ASSESSMENT GUIDE (continued)

	Normal	Abnormal	Comments
2. Formula			
a. Kind			
b. Preparation			
3. Breast—length of feeding at each breast			
4. Calories/day			
5. Fluid/day			
6. Beikost (solid food)			
D. Sleep Pattern/Facilities			
E. Disposition			
1. Happy			
2. Fussy			

	Normal	Abnormal	Comments
3. Sleepy			
F. Drugs			
1. Vitamins			
2. ________ (sleep)			
3. ________ (diarrhea/colic)			
4. ________			
G. Lab data			
1. CBC ________			
2. Hgb ________			
3. Hct ________			

of the new, evolving assessment criteria and techniques which are now receiving more emphasis in assessment. Primary health care practitioners are already proficient in performing a physical examination and taking a health history. Therefore, *only* newer assessment techniques and criteria will be included in this section. Some of them may be familiar, but because of regional differences in education and practice they have been included.

Apgar Score

While the Apgar score developed by Virginia Apgar has been in universal use for some time, Chamberlain and Banks (1974) have developed what they feel is a quick, accurate, and more simplified method of predicting neonates at risk. Their tool is based on heart rate and the time from birth to the neonates' first cry or first breath. The heart rate is scored exactly as it is for an Apgar rating, and time of first cry or first breath is scored as follows: 0 = 1 min, 1 = 30 to 60 s, and 2 = 30 s. Therefore, maximum score is 4. Roberts (1975) uses only the Apgar heart and respiratory scores for a maximum score of 4. Other than the routine brief suctioning of the oropharynx and nostrils, infants with a score of 4 (using either the Roberts or the Banks system) receive no treatment. Oxygen and stimulation are given for a score of 3, ventilation with bag and mask for a score of 2, and immediate intubation and ventilation is recommended for those with a score of 1 or 0. If there is no improvement after 1 to 1½ min, 1 is substracted from the score and the new indicated treatment is begun and continued until a score of 4 is reached.

Gestational Age

The Dubowitz scale (see Appendix 5) and the Lubchenco scale for determination of gestational

Table 8-1 Mean Gestational Ages Derived from the Total Scores of Skin Color, Skin Texture, Ear Firmness, Breast Size

Score	Gestational Age	
	Days	Weeks
1	190	27
2	210	30
3	230	33
4	240	34½
5	250	36
6	260	37
7	270	38½
8	276	39½
9	281	40
10	285	41
11	290	41½
12	295	42

Source: Parkin, J. M., Hey, E. N., and Clowes, J. S. Rapid assessment of gestational age at birth. *Archives of Diseases in Childhood,* **5**:262 (1976).

age have been in use for some years now but are lengthy and involve handling the neonate, which produces some undesirable stress in an ill neonate. Recent research by Parkin, Hey, and Clowes (1976) has validated a quick means of estimating gestational age with 95 percent confidence limits of ±15 days. Parkin et al. found that by using the standard Dubowitz scoring (Dubowitz et al.) for skin color, skin texture, breast size, and ear firmness they could accurately estimate gestational age. The beauty of this system lies in the fact that it can be performed on a very ill neonate in less than 1 min without producing stress. Table 8-1 shows the mean gestational ages associated with the *total scores* of skin texture, skin color, breast size, and ear firmness.

Measurements

Weight/Height/Head Circumference Measuring postnatal growth of preterm infants by standard charts is not satisfactory because of the differences in size and greater velocity of growth in the preterm infant. This is particularly true with the preterm infant who is small for gestational age after nutritional requirements are met. Babson and Benda (1976) have published growth graphs revised for infants of varying gestational ages, which provide for more accurate evaluation of disproportionate growth in infants. Sitting height or crown-rump length should comprise 70 percent of total height at birth and should be roughly equivalent to head circumference.

Temperature Axillary temperatures are now recommended for the newborn rather than rectal temperatures because there is no danger of perforation and they provide an earlier indication of cold stress. The neonate attempts (and is often able) to maintain a near normal core temperature in response to cold stress, therefore a normal rectal temperature can be misleading. The normal axillary temperature range for neonates is 97.6 to 98.6°F, or 36.5 to 37.0°C.

Blood Pressure Since the discovery of hypertension in infants and young children, the measurement of blood pressure has become routine in infant assessment. The "flush method" may be used in early infancy or systolic measurement may be obtained by palpating the radial pulse. When using the palpation technique, the first pulsation is roughly 10 mm below the true systolic pressure.

The Doppler ultrasound technique is the most accurate means of measuring neonatal systolic blood pressure. It is accurate within a range of +20 to −10 mmHg for diastolic blood pressure.

Skin Simply stroking the skin gently over the abdomen, back, or chest with a fingernail can provide diagnostic information. Tache cérébrale is a red streak flanked by pale, thin margins. It develops within 30 s of the stroking and lasts several minutes. Particularly during the neonatal period it serves as an early sign of meningitis. Dermatographia is a white or pale line with red margins that is produced by stroking. This wheal is common in clients with fair skin, vasomotor instability, or urticaria pigmentosa (Barness, 1972).

It is important to use blanching technique to get true assessment of skin color.

Head Increasing significance is being attached to transillumination of the skull. A special flexible black "collar" is attached to a flashlight so that there is no light leak around the cone. A Chun transillumination gun is better but is also more expensive.

Start with the frontal area of the head. Usually there is only one finger breadth (1 to 2 cm) visible in the frontal area. Slide the light toward the occipital area; normally there is only 1 cm or less of transillumination in the parietal and temporal areas, and the occipital area should be 0.5 cm to none. Each hemisphere should be visualized in this fashion. The transillumination area is increased in prematures and in congenital anomalies of the brain. A sharply delineated area of increased light transmission may indicate a subdural hygroma, subdural hematoma, or effusion.

Anterior/posterior and lateral measurements of both fontanels are now recommended. The two most common methods of recording these measurements are mean and actual fontanel size.

Mean fontanel size may be defined as length and width divided by 2 [(L + W)/2], whereas the actual fontanel size is measured from apex to apex for both lateral and anterior-posterior measurements. The range for mean anterior fontanel size in the newborn is 1 to 3.5 cm. Mean fontanel diameters greater than 3.5 cm indicate skeletal disorders, chromosomal disorders, or conditions such as malnutrition, rubella, progeria, hypothyroidism, Russell-Silver or Hallermann-Streiff-François syndrome. Disorders associated with small-for-age fontanel include craniosynostosis, hyperthyroidism, microcephaly, and a high calcium–vitamin D ratio in pregnancy (McMillan, Neiburg, and Oski, 1977).

With severe or unusual molding, the head diameter should be measured with calipers so that the resolution of the molding can be monitored. Measurements should be taken both anterior-posterior and side to side at the same level.

Ears The tragus of the ear should be level with the eye as measured by an imaginary line drawn from inner to outer canthus of the eye. If the ears are lower than this imaginary line and/or are rotated more than 20° from perpendicular, eponym or chromosomal anomalies and/or renal anomalies should be suspected. Peaking of the upper helix or other malformations of the ear may indicate possible congenital renal anomalies; however, these malformations occur as "variants of normal" in many otherwise healthy infants.

One innovation in the removal of wax from the ear canal is the use of a Water Pik dental hygiene pump with warm water to flush excess wax.

Eyes Interpupillary and inner canthal distances should be measured to confirm the presence of hypo- and hypertelorism which is useful in syndrome identification. The normal distance between the center of each pupil ranges from 1.4 to 1.75 cm, while the normal distance between the inner canthi is 1.5 to 2.5 cm.

Note: Epicanthal folds are common in chromosomal anomalies and occasionally lead to a misdiagnosis of strabismus.

Face Average width of the face in the newborn is 8 cm. The length of the face is approximately 9 cm (5 cm from top of skull to upper margin or orbit and 4 cm from upper orbit margin to lower edge of the mandible). Prominent or narrow or flat foreheads and flat, round, or depressed faces are associated with chromosomal anomalies. The distance between the nose and lips and the depth of the nasolabial fold should be noted. Short or long distances between the nose and lips and/or deep nasolabial folds may signal chromosomal anomalies.

Mouth Note particularly high narrow arches of the palate, which are associated with several eponym syndromes.

Neck Clavicles should be carefully palpated, especially in a neonate weighing more than 4 kg. An effective palpation method is to place the fingers over the lateral and medial ends of the clavicle and "wiggle" them. Crepitus usually occurs with this maneuver in the presence of a fractured clavicle. Note short or long necks; check for bruits over the thyroid and for unilateral carotid bruits.

Chest Increased anteroposterior diameter suggests an aspiration syndrome. Note that a wide sternum may occur before the anteroposterior chest diameter increases in infants with a left-to-right cardiac shunt and pulmonary hypertension. An intermamillary index [distance between nipples, cm × 100/circumference of chest, cm] above 28 indicates a chromosomal anomaly.

Extremities The average distance from hip joint to extended heel is 16.5 cm in the neonate. The average ankle-to-knee measurement is 7.5 cm. The average length of the upper extremities is roughly the same as that of the lower extremities, 16.5 cm. Short extremities, small hands and/or feet, incurving or hypoplasia of the fifth finger, broad thumb or hypoplasia, broad toes, polydactyly, or syndactyly indicate chromosomal anomalies.

Hands/Feet/Fingers/Toes Average foot length is 6.5 cm. The hand measures roughly the same from heel of the palm to tip of the middle finger. The length of the middle finger averages about 2.2 cm. Note long, short, large, broad, clawlike, overlapping, tapering, unusual placement, etc., or wide spaces between fingers and toes.

To test feet that seem out of alignment, rest feet in palms of your hands and note their position. If the malposition is corrected by spontaneous movement, it is probably due to the fetal position and will correct itself spontaneously. However, if spontaneous movement increases the defect, further evaluation is required. If there is little improvement after 3 months, treatment is required.

Nails Nail color, length, convexity, concavity, pitting, etc., should be noted, as increasing correlations have been determined between nail abnormalities and chromosomal and systemic disorders.

Dermatoglyphics and Creases Examination of dermatoglyphics in the neonate is difficult. The easiest method of study is to take hand and foot prints while the neonate is in deep sleep and study them with a magnifying glass. A magnifying glass can be used with a strong light to study the fingers themselves. This is an especially important feature of the examination when other signs of chromosomal anomalies have been detected (see Table 8-2, Skin, for dematoglyphic normals).

SECTION 3: REFERENCE TABLE FOR PHYSICAL NORMS AND ABNORMALITIES

Table 8-2

Physical Exam	Normal	Abnormal
General		
Gestational age	See Dubowitz scale, Appendix 5	
Weight	Average = 3400 g	Less than 2500 g (premature)
	Range = 2500–4300 g	Over 4300 g (diabetes, postmature)
	Percent of weight loss more important than actual weight loss	Small or large for gestational age
	Stabilized by age 4 days	Loss of 3% birth weight during first 24 h or loss > 6% of birth weight during first 13 days (small cleft palate, congenital heart disease, infection, stress, etc.)
Length	Average = 49.6 cm	Less than 45 cm (premature)
	Range = 48–54 cm	Long (Marfan's syndrome)
		Short (dwarfism, osteogenesis imperfecta)
Vital signs		
Axillary temperature	97.7–98.6°F (36.5–37.2°C)	Too high or low (cold, severe infection, CNS injury)
Pulse	Apical/femoral pulse = 120–140 per min	Above 160 per min (cardiac or respiratory distress; metabolic, hematologic, or infectious disease)
		Below 100 per min (hypoxia, heart block, intracranial disorders)
		Pulsus alternans (cardiac failure)
		Corrigan's "water hammer" pulse (aortic regurgitation, patent ductus arteriosus)
		Pulsus paradoxus (pericardial fluid)
		Dicrotic pulse (aortic stenosis or hyperthyroidism)

Table 8-2 *(continued)*

Physical Exam	Normal	Abnormal
		Gallop rhythm (congestive heart failure, valve disease) Wide bounding pulse (aortic regurgitation) Narrow thready pulse (severe aortic stenosis or congestive failure)
Respiration	Abdominal, irregular in depth and rate, transient tachypnea normal Rate = 30–50 per min Ratio of respiration to pulse = 1:4 Respiratory increase with fever = 4 respirations per 1° above normal	Below 30 per min (alkalosis, drug intoxication, brain tumor, anoxia, impending failure) Weak, slow, or very rapid (brain damage) Above 60 per min *without* retractions (congenital heart disease) Above 60 per min sustained (pneumonia, fever, heart failure, aspirin poisoning, shock, meningitis) Deep sighing respirations (acidosis) Weak, groaning respirations (hypoxia or brain damage) Grunting, rapid respirations (anemia, distended abdomen, severe lung, heart, or brain disease) Decreased abdominal respirations (distended abdomen, pulmonary disease) Thoracic breathing/asymmetrical chest motion (diaphragmatic hernia, massive atelectasis, phrenic nerve paralysis) Head rocking, nasal flaring, retractions, sudden increase in heart rate (impending failure)
Blood pressure	Average blood pressure according to birth weight (Kitterman et al., 1969) (12 h to 5 days old): Birth Weight / Syst. / Dias. / Mean 1000–2000 / 50 / 30 / 38 2001–3000 / 59 / 35 / 42 Over 3000 / 66 / 41 / 50 Range 60/20 to 90/60 ± 16 Thigh and arm systolic pressure equal Normal pulse pressure = ½ systolic pressure; range = 20–50 mmHg	Premature: 70/ (hypertension/hypernatremia, hypoxia) Full term: 89/ (coarctation of aorta, renovascular problems or intracranial hemorrhage, hypoxia) 45/20 or ↓ (shock, hemorrhage, hypoxia) Wide pulse pressure (aortic regurgitation, patent ductus arteriosus, complete heart block) Persistent high systolic with a wide pulse pressure (hyperthyroidism or cardiovascular problems) Narrow pulse pressure (aortic stenosis, pericardial tamponade) Thigh systolic pressure ↓ arm pressure (coarctation)

Table 8-2 *(continued)*

Physical Exam	Normal	Abnormal
Position/posture	Tense with flexion or partial flexion of extremities (pithed "frog" position); muscle tone consistent and firm; assumes fetal position for comfort	Opisthotonus (CNS infection, tetanus) Spasticity, flaccidity, extension of extremities (CNS injury, illness) Head held to one side (torticollis, dislocation, spasm nutans)
Activity level/ disposition	Spontaneous movement Happy, quiet, content	Lethargic or absent movement (infection, CNS lesions) Jittery (hypocalcemia, hypoglycemia, CNS damage, drug withdrawal, hypoxic encephalopathy) Irritable (meningitis, increased intracranial pressure, drug withdrawal, CNS damage) Increased muscle tone (significant CNS damage, cerebral palsy) Hypotonic, perhaps "floppy" (hypermagnesemia, hypoxia, hypothyroidism, hypoglycemia, myasthenia gravis neonatorum, Down's syndrome, myotonic dystrophy, Werdig-Hoffman disease, CNS anomalies, or cerebral hepatorenal syndrome) Convulsions (kernicterus, CNS injury, hyperthermia, allergy) Fussy or crying and cannot soothe (pain somewhere) Quiet, sad expression, no eye contact (autism, bonding problem) Fatigue with slight exertion (congenital heart disease, respiratory disease)
Appearance and body proportion, symmetry of body parts	Trunk longer than extremities, arms longer than legs, head ¼ of total length Short neck, or no neck appearance	Asymmetry (birth trauma, congenital defects) Flattened face (Down's syndrome) Continuous eyebrows, thin upper lip (Cornelia de Lange's syndrome) Paralysis (birth trauma, abuse) Cretinism
Cry	Vigorous, especially after stimulation; tone and pitch moderate Quiets when left alone, no tearing, crying periods average 3.7 min before consoling measures are necessary	Absent or continuous at birth (brain injury) Weak (seriously ill infant) Hoarse (laryngitis, foreign body, epiglottitis, hypothyroidism, hypocalcemic tetany, heart disease, tracheomalacia, stenosis, tumor, laryngeal paralysis) Low raucous cry (hypothyroidism) Growling cry (Cornelia de Lange's syndrome)

Table 8-2 *(continued)*

Physical Exam	Normal	Abnormal
		Hoarse cry at 2–5 days of age (hypocalcemic laryngospasm) Too strong (pain) Sharp, whining cry (intussusception, peritonitis, or severe GI disturbance) High pitched, piercing (CNS pathology) Excessive (parental anxiety, colic, maladjustment) Infrequent (hypothyroidism, Down's syndrome) Unusual (cri-du-chat syndrome) Moaning (meningitis) Grunting (respiratory distress) Two-tone cry (congestive heart failure, congenital anomaly of larynx)
SKIN *Color*	Pink, acrocyanosis (normal first week only) Transient harlequin pattern or transient mottling Occasional petechiae	Dusky color, circumoral cyanosis (hypoxia, respiratory or cardiac in origin) Circumoral pallor with red chin and cheeks, (hypoglycemia, scarlet or rheumatic fever) Generalized cyanosis (severe cardiopulmonary distress) Overly red (hypoglycemia, immature vasomotor reflexes, cardiac anomaly, or cord was "milked") Multiple petechiae, ecchymosis (birth trauma, infection, congenital capillary fragility, drugs, hemorrhagic disease, thrombocytopenia, etc.) Pale yellow–orange tint to palms, nasolabial folds (carotenemia) Jaundice: Prior to 48 h (blood incompatibility, hepatitis) After 48 h (physiological, hepatic lesion or obstruction) Pallor (circulatory failure, edema, shock) With tachycardia (anemia) With bradycardia (anoxia) > 7 café au lait patches (fibromas, neurofibromatosis) Spider nevi on chest and shoulders (liver disease)
	Telangiectasia	Multiple hemangiomas (congenital vascular anomalies, Sturge-Weber disease, etc.) Tache cérébrale (meningitis, febrile illnesses, hydrocephalus)

Table 8-2 *(continued)*

Physical Exam	Normal	Abnormal
Texture	Thin, delicate, soft, and smooth, with evidence of fat pads	Firm (cold stress, shock, infection)
		Hard (sclerema)
		Lacks "baby fat" (premature, malnutrition, retarded intrauterine growth—susceptible to cold stress)
		Perspiring (neonatal narcotic abstinence, CNS injury)
	Resilient, elastic—good turgor	Hyperelastic (Ehlers-Danlos syndrome)
		Nonresilient (dehydration, inadequate nutrition)
		Edema (anemia, RDS, heart failure)
		Nonpitting edema (cretinism)
		Excessively dry (dehydration)
		Shagreen patches (Adenoma sebaceum)
	Dry and peeling, third day	Massive peeling (generalized edema, postmaturity, prematurity, congenital ichthyosis, diabetic mother, kidney dysfunction, blood incompatibility)
		Profuse scaling on palms, soles (scarlet fever)
Opacity	Opaque	Very thin, translucent (prematurity)
Lanugo/hair distribution	Back, face, shoulders covered in fine downy hair	Pronounced in premature
		Hirsutism(adrenocortical problems)
Dermatoglyphics	Whorls common to thumbs and ring finger	Radial loops on fourth or fifth finger (trisomy 21)
	Radial loops and arches on index finger	Simian crease, arches and whorls or ulnar loops on all 10 fingers (trisomy 21)
	Ulnar loop on little finger	Simian crease and distorted patterns, large thenar patterns (trisomy 13)
		Arches on all 10 fingers (trisomy 18)
		Large fingertip loops and whorls (Turner's syndrome)
		Small fingertip patterns with lower ridge count (Klinefelter's syndrome)
Vernix caseosa	White, cheesy protective coating on skin, especially in creases	Absence (postmature)
		Excessive (premature)
		Yellow vernix (hyperbilirubinemia)
		Meconium stained (intrauterine distress)
Pigmentation	Mongolian spots (common to dark-skinned neonates)	Normal only over sacrum, buttocks, shoulders, and/or back; other distribution (hemorrhagic disease)
		Port-wine stain
Lesions	Birth marks—milia	Hemangioma
	Telangiectasia ("stork bites")	Pustules, rash (impetigo, infection)
	Erythema toxicum rash	Bruises (underlying fracture, abuse)

Table 8-2 *(continued)*

Physical Exam	Normal	Abnormal
	Red-mauve blotches Xanthomas	
HEAD		
Circumference	Range: 32–38 cm (40 wk gestational age) Average male: 34.5–35.5 in Average female: 33.5–34.5 in Average: In occipitofrontal circumference (OFC)/week during first 8 wk of life Gestational age = Head growth 38–40 wk = 0.5 cm/wk 34–37 wk = 0.8 cm/wk 30–33 wk = 1.1 cm/wk "Sick" premature = 0.25 cm/wk Head 1–2 cm larger than chest	>35.5 cm (hydrocephaly, tumor, increased intracranial pressure) <31 cm (microcephaly, anencephaly, congenital infections, polymicogyria,trisomies 13–15, 18) Head circumference below 3d percentile for age = mental retardation > or < = intracranial pathology
Shape/symmetry	Molded up to 4 wk, caput succedaneum Intermittent, movable nodes	Cephalohematoma (possible fracture) Conical shape (oxycephaly) Nonmovable nodes (tumors, hematoma, cysts) Small, shallow, conical pits (rickets) Broad, short cephalic index 81.0–85.4 (brachycephalia) Long, narrow cephalic index 75.9 or less (dolichocephaly) Flat occiput (Down's syndrome) Craniotabes (premature, syphilis, hydrocephalus, osteogenesis imperfecta, etc.)
Fontanels	Open, soft, flat; may see slight pulsation Average size Anterior fontanel = 4–6 cm anterior/posterior and lateral measurement Posterior fontanel = 0.5–1 cm	Anterior fontanel closed or small, less than 1 cm (cranial synostosis, microcephaly, high Ca^{2+}–vitamin D ratio in pregnancy, hyperthyroidism) Large anterior: greater than 5 cm fontanel (hydrocephaly, anchodrophasia, hypothyroidism, malnourishment) Bulging, tense (meningitis, encephalitis) Depressed (dehydration, inanition) Marked pulsation (↑ intracranial pressure, venous sinus thrombosis, patent ductus arteriosus, obstructed venous return) Third fontanel (possible Down's syndrome) Large posterior fontanel (hypothyroidism)

Table 8-2 *(continued)*

Physical Exam	Normal	Abnormal
Transillumination	Frontal transillumination of 1 cm or less decreasing to minimal or none in occipital area (premature has periosteal thinning and will look anencephalic)	No transillumination (craniosynostosis) Increased transillumination > 1 cm (anencephaly, microcephaly, gross CNS disorders) Asymmetrical transillumination (brain anomalies)
Bruit	Normal in 50% infants	Bruit (meningitis, subdural effusion, thyrotoxicosis, cerebral aneurysm, intracranial pressure, fever, anemia) Percussion dullness near saggital sinus (subdural hematoma)
Hair	Coarse, evenly distributed, growing toward face and neck	Fine, electric (premature 27–38 weeks) Hair won't comb down (chromosomal anomalies) Silky hair (premature 37–41 wk) Uneven distribution (CNS disorder, chromosomal anomalies) Hair growing toward crown (chromosomal anomalies) Diffuse hair loss (induced by drugs, malnutrition, anemia, high fever) Scalp hair on cheeks (Treacher Collins syndrome) Very brittle, dry coarse (hypothyroidism)
	Long lashes and eyebrows, perhaps familial	Long eyebrows and lashes (chronic or wasting diseases) Alopecia with scaling (fungus) Alopecia with scarring (trauma, Darier's disease, icthyosis, sarcoid, lupus, etc.) Alopecia (Hutchinson-Gilford syndrome, ringworm, monilethrix, pili torti, ectodermal dysplasia, progeria) White forelock (Waardenburg's syndrome, deafness) Low-set hairline (Turner's syndrome) Two-color hair: red and regular color (Kwashiorkor)
Scalp	Smooth, intact, free from lesions and crusting	Scalp defects (trisomy 13) Cradle cap Dandruff, lice Scaliness, especially over anterior fontanel with rash elsewhere (seborrhea) Dimples (hemangiomas, dermal sinus) Dilated scalp veins (hydrocephalus, tumors, subdural hematoma, congenital vascular anomalies)

Table 8-2 *(continued)*

Physical Exam	Normal	Abnormal
		Scalp pain (cerebral hemorrhage, trauma, hypertension) Occipital tenderness, pain (brain tumor, abscess)
EARS		
Alignment/shape	Symmetrical, aligned with eyes, well-developed cartilage, ruddy earlobes	Large and/or low-set ears (trisomies and/or renal anomalies) Malformed, asymmetrical, large or small ears (renal anomalies, chromosomal anomalies) Soft, pliable ears (chromosomal anomalies) Failure to respond to loud environmental sounds or awaken or move in response to speech in quiet room (hearing loss) Defects of pinnae, nose, lips, or palate (hearing loss) Dimples or periauricular skin tags (sinus, chromsomal anomalies 4,5,22) Sagging of posterior canal wall (mastoiditis) Discharge (external otitis, otitis media or perforation) Pale lobes (anemia) Adherent lobes (chromosomal anomalies)
Tympanic membrane	Pearly gray, translucent, light reflex present, mobile	Redness, induration or bulging, short light reflex, perforation, discharge (otitis media) Opaque, yellow, or blue light reflex, malpositioned landmarks, perforation, occasionally cholesteatoma (serous otitis media) Immobile or jerky movement (fluid in middle ear)
Hearing	Blinking or Moro reflex reaction to loud noise or to stimulus using neometer 70-80-90-100 dB at a distance of 12 in	No response (deafness, syphilis, kernicterus, full ear canals)
FACE		
Symmetry, shape; facial expression	Symmetrical, regular features; average size = 8 cm wide; alert, interested	Prominent forehead (chromosomal anomalies 7q+, 8+, 9p−, 11p+, 13)* Narrow forehead (chromosomal anomalies 13+, 13q+, and 15q+)* Flat forehead (chromosomal anomalies 9, 13, 15, and 21)*

*Lewandowski and Yunis, 1975.

Table 8-2 *(continued)*

Physical Exam	Normal	Abnormal
		Facial asymmetry (low birth weight, molding, Silver's syndrome, cranial nerve V injury); infants with facial nerve injuries usually *not* asymmetrical at birth Scalp hair on cheeks (Treacher-Collins syndrome) "Funny-looking-kid" syndrome (rule out chromosomal anomalies) Flat round or depressed face (chromosomal anomalies) Anxious (respiratory, emotional problems)
EYES		
	Corneal reflex, ability to follow to midline or 60 degrees Blink reflex to light, pupils reacting to light	Delayed pupil reaction (CNS injury, possibly emergency) No blink reflex (impaired vision) Microphthalmia (chromosomal anomalies 4,10, 13, and 14)
Sclera, iris color	Sclera Bluish tint Iris Caucasian—grayish blue Other races—grayish brown	Jaundice *Blue* sclera (osteogenesis imperfecta, Ehlers-Danlos syndrome) Brushfield spots (trisomy 21) Hyphema (blunt trauma, leukemia, hemophilia, retrolental fibroplasia, *retinoblastoma,* iritis, retinoschisis, hyperplastic vitreous) Coloboma (chromosomal anomalies 4, 13, and 22) Palpebral hematoma "black eye" (trauma, nasal or skull fracture) Scleral protrusion (trauma, increased intraocular pressure)
Distance between	Normal interpupillary distance: 1.4–1.75 cm Normal inner canthal distance: 1.5–2.5 cm	↑ interpupillary or inner canthal distance = hypertelorism (Apert's syndrome, Pyle's disease, hypertelorism-hypospadias syndrome, otopalatodigital syndrome, chromosomal anomalies 4, 5, 9, 13, 18, 21, 22)* Hypotelorism (chromosomal anomalies 13, 15, 21)* Mongoloid slant (chromosomal anomalies 9, 15, 21)* Antimongoloid slant (chromosomal anomalies 4, 5, 10, 11, 15, 21, and 22)*

*Lewandowski and Yunis, 1975.

Table 8-2 *(continued)*

Physical Exam	Normal	Abnormal
		Narrow palpebral fissures (trisomy 18)*
Movements	Nonparalytic strabismus, incoordinate eye movement, Dolls eye movements Strabismus up to 6 mo	Nystagmus (chromosomal anomalies 11, 18, 21, or may represent seizures)* Paralytic strabismus (brainstem lesion and ↑ intracranial pressure) Setting sun (hydrocephalus)
Optic disc	Red reflex	White disc (optic atrophy, neurofibroma of optic nerve, optic neuritis, methyl alcohol poisoning) Gray stippling around disc (lead poisoning) Unilateral papilledema with contralateral atrophy (Foster Kennedy syndrome, frontal lobe tumor)
Cornea, lens	Clear, bright, shiny	Cataract, dull, hazy (rubella, Hurler's syndrome, Lowe's syndrome, congenital hypoparathyroidism, chromosomal anomalies 15 and 21)
Eyelashes	Medium length, upward curved; very long eyelashes perhaps familial	Long incurved lashes (chromosomal anomaly 13) Very long eyelashes (chronic illness, degenerative disease) Absence of lower lashes (Treacher-Collins syndrome)
Eyebrows		Arched and widespread (trisomy 10) Bushy, confluent eyebrows (Cornelia de Lange's syndrome)
Eyelids	No ptosis, symmetrical blink Lid edema with facial presentation Chemical irritation from eye drop instillation at birth	Ptosis, asymmetrical blink (cranial nerve III damage) Edema beyond 1 wk (contact dermatitis, early indication roseola infantum) Pustule (sty) Unilateral enophthalmos (trauma, inflammation) Bilateral enophthalmos (chromosomal anomalies 9, 11, 15, 18; inanition; dehydration; cervical spine; brachial plexus; brain damage) Unilateral exophthalmos (cellulitis, abscess, hemangioma, gumma, neoplasm, fracture, mucocele, hyperthyroidism) Bilateral exophthalmos (glaucoma, congenital acromegaly, lymphomas, hyperthyroidism, leukemia, oxycephaly)

*Lewandowski and Yunis, 1975.

Table 8-2 *(continued)*

Physical Exam	Normal	Abnormal
Conjunctiva	Dark pink and moist	Pale (anemia) Red (conjunctivitis) Purulent discharge (gonorrhea) Scleral hemorrhage (trauma) Tearing (narcotic withdrawal syndrome) Yellow sclera (hyperbilirubinemia, liver disease)
NOSE	Patent, low, broad, and relatively long; average length = 18–19 mm; greatest width = 1.1 cm; height 1.4 cm	Edema (rhinitis, allergy) Obstructed nares (choanal atresia, tumor, foreign body, trauma, encephalocele, deviated septum, inflammation) Flaring nares (respiratory distress) Nosebleed (syphilis, trauma, hypertension, kidney disease, tuberculosis)
Shape/placement	Located centrally in middle to upper section of face; septum is straight	Peak shape (chromosomal anomalies 1 or 4)* Broad nose (chromosomal anomalies 5, 9, 11, 22)* Small nose (trisomies 7, 10, 18, 21)*
Bridge		Broad nasal bridge (chromosomal anomalies 4, 5, 9, 13, 21)* Flat nasal bridge (chromosomal anomalies 9, 14, 18, 22)* Depressed nasal bridge (chromosomal anomalies 10, 18, 21; syphilis, fracture)*
MOUTH		
Symmetry, size	Symmetrical grimace	Asymmetry, paralysis of mouth alone (peripheral trigeminal nerve lesion)
Reflexes	Strong suck, rooting reflex	Weak suck (prematurity, cardiopulmonary problems, CNS depression—drugs, anorexia, or CNS defects)
Palate	Arched palate, short, wide Average size = 2.3 cm long × 2.2 cm wide	Cleft palate Exceptionally high narrow arch (Treacher-Collins syndrome, Ehlers-Danlos syndrome, Turner's syndrome, Marfan's syndrome, arachnodactyly)
Tonsils	No tonsils, scant saliva, teeth may be present, tumors, epulis, retention cysts, ulcers, Epstein's pearls, pink mucous membranes	Profuse saliva (tracheoesophageal fistula, cystic fibrosis, tracheal aspiration) Drooling (esophageal atresia)

*Lewandowski and Yunis, 1975.

Table 8-2 *(continued)*

Physical Exam	Normal	Abnormal
		Flat, thick white plaques (thrush)
		Pale mucous membranes (anemia)
		Enlarged stensen's duct (mumps)
		Brown/black/blue spots (Addison's disease, intestinal polyposis)
		Black line around gums (metal poisoning)
		Purple, bleeding gums (scurvy, leukemia, poor hygiene)
	Uvula midline	Uvula deviates to one side with gag reflex (cranial nerve IX, X injury)
Lips	Moist, pink, smooth	Cleft lip
		Scaly patches at corner (vitamin nutritional deficiencies)
		Gray-blue lips (cardiopulmonary problems, methemoglobinemia, poisons, or anoxia)
		Bright red lips (acidosis, ingestion of aspirin, diabetes, carbon monoxide poisoning)
Odor	Not remarkable	Halitosis (any illness, foreign body, sinusitis, poor hygiene)
		Sweet, acetone (dehydration, diabetic acidosis, malnourishment)
		Ammonia odor (kidney failure)
Mandible	In proportion with face	Small mandible, or micrognathia (birdface syndrome, juvenile rheumatoid arthritis, chromosomal anomalies)
		Large mandible (Crouzon's disease, chondrodystrophy)
TONGUE		
Size/grooves	Congenital transverse furrows	Large and protruding (cretinism, Down's syndrome, Beckwith's syndrome, tumor)
	Average size = 4 cm long × 2.5 cm wide + 1 cm thick	Glossoptosis with micrognathia (Pierre Robin syndrome)
		Protruding, snake tongue (brain damage)
		Atrophy (Möbius syndrome, injury to cranial nerves VI and VII)
Color/coating	Pink, no coating, geographic tongue	Dry without furrows (Sjögren's syndrome, mouth breathing)
		Dry with furrows (dehydration)
		Desquamation with longitudinal furrows (syphilitic glossitis)
		Coated tongue (infection, poor hygiene)

Table 8-2 *(continued)*

Physical Exam	Normal	Abnormal
		Hairy, black tongue *(Candida albicans* or *Aspergillus niger)* Magenta cobblestone tongue (riboflavin deficiency) Canker sores (food allergy, herpes simplex)
Mobility	Symmetrical fasciculations with cry	Asymmetrical (damage to XIIth cranial nerve) Unequal fasciculation (degenerative disease) Fasciculations at rest (Wernid Hoffman disease, Pompe's disease)
Reflexes	Gag and swallow reflex present	Absent (jaundice, prematurity, damage to cranial nerves IX and X)
Throat	Pink, no swelling	Dull red throat, some edema (viral inflammation) Bright red, swollen, swollen uvula studded with white or yellow follicles (strep or staph infection) Dull red with white, grey, or yellow patch membrane (diptheria)
NECK/CHIN		
Shape/size/movement	Not visible in supine position; short, straight, has complete range of motion, flexes easily	Mastoid skinfolds (gonadal dysgenesis) Webbing of neck and/or excess skin on posterior neck (Turner's syndrome) Stiff neck (meningitis, torticollis, pharyngitis, trauma, arthritis) Wry neck (congenital torticollis, trauma) Very short, poor range of motion (Klippel-Feil syndrome)
Masses		Distended neck veins (mass in pneumomediastinum or chest, or congestive heart disease, pulmonary disease, liver problems) Mass in the lower third of the sternocleidomastoid muscle (congenital torticollis) Midline mass (thyroglossal duct, cyst, or congenital goiter) Clavicular mass Soft (cystic hygroma) Hard (fracture) Crepitus over clavicle (fracture) Branchial cyst Generalized adenopathy (leukemia, Hodgkin's disease, serum sickness) Absence of lymph nodes (agammaglobulinemia)

Table 8-2 *(continued)*

Physical Exam	Normal	Abnormal
		Occipital or postauricular node enlargement (scalp infection, external otitis, varicella, pediculosis, rubella) Periauricular node enlargement (sties, conjunctivitis) Cervical adenopathy (infection of throat, mouth, teeth, ears, sinuses)
Reflex	Tonic neck present	Absence (CNS damage)
Bruit	None	To and fro bruit over thyroid (enlarged thyroid) Unilateral bruit over carotid (vascular insufficiency)
CHEST		
Size/shape/symmetry	Circular, 1–2 cm smaller than head circumference, symmetrical Sternum = 5 cm long	Increased A-P diameter (aspiration syndrome) Depressed sternum (respiratory distress syndrome, funnel chest, atelectasis)
Inspection		Retractions (respiratory distress, usually upper airway obstruction) Asymmetry (pneumothorax, emphysema, tension cysts, pleural effusion, pneumonia, pulmonary agenesis, diaphragmatic paralysis or hernia) Abnormal ribs (chromosome anomalies 4, 7, 8, 10, 13, 14, and 18) Wide sternum (pulmonary hypertension, L → R shunt, cystic fibrosis, emphysema) Funnel breast (rickets, Marfan's syndrome) Short sternum (trisomy 18) Pigeon chest (rickets, Marfan's syndrome, upper airway obstruction, or Morquio's disease) Barrel chest (asthma, cystic fibrosis, emphysema, pulmonary hypertension with L → R shunt) Left parasternal bulge (ventricular hypertrophy) Precordial bulge (biventricular hypertrophy) Visible pulse in suprasternal notch (aortic insufficiency, patent ductus arteriosus, or coarctation of the aorta) Harrison's groove (rickets, congenital syphilis)
Palpation	Fremitus	Rachitic rosary (vitamin C deficiency, hypophosphatasia, chondrodystrophy)

Table 8-2 *(continued)*

Physical Exam	Normal	Abnormal
		Increased fremitus (atelectasis, pneumonia)
		Decreased or absent fremitus (pneumothorax, asthma, emphysema, bronchial obstruction, pleural effusion)
		Pleural friction rub/crepitation (fractured rib, lung puncture)
	No thrills	Suprasternal thrill (aortic stenosis, patent ductus, pulmonary stenosis, coarctation)
		Other thrills (ventricular septal defect, aortic or pulmonary stenosis)
		Epigastric pulsations (ventricular hypertrophy)
		Tap sensation (right ventricular hypertrophy)
		Heaving sensation (left ventricular hypertrophy)
	Apex heart (PMI) at fourth intercostal space, left of midclavicular line	PMI fifth or sixth intercostal space and further left of midclavicular line (left ventricular hypertrophy, diabetic mother, erythroblastosis fetalis, von Gierke's disease)
		PMI in back (dextrocardia)
		PMI further "R" or "L" (dextrocardia, atelectasis, pneumothorax)
Percussion	Resonant	Hyperresonance (pneumothorax, diaphragmatic hernia, emphysema, pneumomediastinum, asthma, pneumonia)
		Decreased resonance (pneumonia, atelectasis, empyema or respiratory distress syndrome, hernia, neoplasm, pleural effusion)
Breath sounds	Easy air entry	Delayed or barely audible air entry (pneumonia, atelectasis, etc.)
	Bilateral bronchial breath sounds, rub sounds are common, rales may be present with normal newborn atelectasis	Peristaltic sounds in chest (diaphragmatic hernia)
		Expiratory grunt (pneumonitis, (L) heart failure and/or respiratory distress syndrome)
		Amphoric (pneumothorax, pleural effusion, bronchopleural fistula)
		Absent/decreased (bronchial obstruction, diaphragmatic hernia, fluid or air in pleura, thickened pleura)
		Wet rales (pneumonia, bronchitis, bronchiectasis, atelectasis, pulmonary edema, heart failure)
		Dry rales (edema, bronchospasm, foreign body, asthma, bronchitis)

Table 8-2 *(continued)*

Physical Exam	Normal	Abnormal
Heart sounds	S_1 louder than S_2 S_2 shorter and pitched higher than S_1 S_3 normal Sinus arrhythmia normal, otherwise rhythm is normal Low systolic murmurs may be normal, venous hum may be normal	Decreased heart sounds (cardiac failure, pneumothorax, CNS injury, pneumomediastinum) Varying rhythm (cerebral defects, anoxia, increased intracranial pressure) Cracking sounds with heart beat (mediastinal emphysema)
Breasts	Full areola, 5–10 mm bud Symmetrical placement (distance between) Some breast engorgement is normal Milk after 3 days normal Extra nipples	Asymmetrical placement (fractured clavicle) Wide-set nipples (Turner's syndrome, chromosomal anomalies 4, 18) Low-set nipples (chromosome anomaly 22) Dark nipples (adrenogenital syndrome) Red, firmness around nipples (abscess, mastitis)
ABDOMEN		
Shape/size/symmetry	Same as chest circumference Cylindrical with slight protrusion, symmetrical Bowel sounds within 2–3 h of birth Femoral pulses present	Absent femoral pulses (coarctation of the aorta) Distention (lower bowel obstruction, paralytic ileus, peritonitis, tracheoesophageal fistula, omphalocele, Hirschsprung's disease, atresia, imperforate anus, prune belly) Localized flank bulging (enlarged kidneys, hydronephrosis) Engorged abdominal vessels (pylephlebitis, peritonitis) Reverse filling of abdominal veins (vena cava obstruction) Visible peristalsis (intestinal obstruction) Peristaltic waves from "L → R" (pyloric stenosis, malrotation of bowel, urinary tract infection, gastrointestinal allergy, duodenal ulcer or stenosis) Flat abdomen (tracheoesophageal fistula) Scaphoid abdomen (if bowel sounds in chest—diaphragmatic hernia, malnutrition) Ascites (liver or kidney disease, ruptured viscus, necrotizing enterocolitis, obstruction portal vein, urethral obstruction, peritonitis) Tympanitic, distended, tender, silent (peritonitis) Pulsating (aortic aneurysm)

Table 8-2 *(continued)*

Physical Exam	Normal	Abnormal
		Venous hum (umbilical or portal vein anomalies, liver hemangioma) Umbilical area murmur (renal artery anomaly) Mass with plastic feel (megacolon) Sausage shape mass (intussusception) Rubbery or hard masses (meconium ileus) Purple scars (adrenal problems) Grey Turner's sign (abdominal hemorrhage) Friction rub (peritoneal obstruction, inflamed spleen, or liver with a tumor) Bruit (aneurysm; dilated, distorted, or constricted vessel)
Umbilicus	Translucent or dry, no bleeding Two arteries and one vein Ventral hernias and diastasis recti may be present Normal umbilical hernia = 2–5 cm	One artery (kidney or cardiovascular problems; CNS, GU, or GI anomalies) Large, flabby umbilicus (patent urachus) "Blue" umbilicus—Cullen's sign (intra-abdominal hemorrhage) Green, yellow, or meconium stained (fetal distress) Wet, red, odiferous stump (omphalitis) Serous or serosanquineous discharge (granuloma) Cord present after 2 wk and/or drainage after 3 wk (sinus or urachal cyst) Umbilical fecal discharge (Meckel's diverticulum, omphalomesenteric duct, ileal prolapse) Dark red with mucoid discharge (umbilical polyp) Pus (urachal cyst or abscess)
Liver/spleen	Liver palpable 2–3 cm below right costal margin Spleen tip is palpable after 1 wk of age	Enlarged liver/spleen (sepsis, erythroblastosis fetalis, trauma, syphilis, hemolytic icterus, biliary atresia, infants of diabetic mothers, Riedel's lobe, glycogen storage disease, rubella, cytomegalic inclusion disease) Left side liver (situs inversus) Systolic liver pulsations (cardiac anomalies) Tenderness (abscess, hepatitis, mononucleosis)
Kidney/bladder	Kidneys may or may not be palpable. Bladder is palpable 1–4 cm above symphysis pubis	Enlarged kidneys (Wilm's tumor, neuroblastoma, hydronephrosis, polycystic kidneys; unilateral = renal vein thrombosis)

Table 8-2 *(continued)*

Physical Exam	Normal	Abnormal
		Distended bladder (bladder neck obstruction, urethral obstruction, spina bifida)
Masses	None	Tumors, localized hemmorhage, meconium ileus, cysts, fecal masses Pyloric tumor (pyloric stenosis)
GENITALIA *Female*	Hymenal tag, large clitoris in premature, mucoid or sanguineous vaginal discharge, large labia minora (2.5 mm thick) Vaginal orifice = 0.5 cm	Dark pigmentation (adrenal hyperplasia) Epispadias (hermaphroditism) Very large clitoris (pseudohermaphroditism, adrenal hyperplasia, small penis) Imperforate hymen (hydrocolpos) Vaginal atresia Ulcerations (venereal disease, chancres, granuloma, herpes, etc.) Red swollen labia (vulvitis, vulvovaginitis, cellulitis) Foul discharge (gonorrhea, trichomonas, foreign body) Fecal urethral discharge (fistulas) Masses (condyloma latum or acuminatum, neoplasms, inguinal hernia) Lymphedema (lymphatic obstruction) Hematoma Varicosities (tumors, enlarged organs) Bartholin or Skene enlargement (gonorrhea, infection) Adhesions Grape-like growth (sarcoma botryoides)
Male	Slender penis 2.5 cm long and 1 cm wide; scrotum length 3 cm by 2 cm wide; testes should be descended and average 10 mm in length and 5 cm in width at birth; the glans should be tapered at the tip, with the meatal opening in the center; foreskin may not retract easily; erection and priapism may occur	Penis $<$ 2 cm in length (hermaphroditism, chromosomal anomalies 9, 15, 18, 21) Enlarged scrotum (hydrocele, orchitis, hernia, hematocele, chylocele) Fecal-urethral discharge (fistula) Ventral meatus (hypospadius) Dorsal meatus (epispadias) Phimosis/stenosis/meatal atresia Preputial adhesions Ulceration of meatus (circumcision, balanitis) Unilateral dark swollen testis (infarction) Absent testis (cryptorchidism, intersex chromosomal anomalies 4, 9, 13, 14, 15, 18, 21)

Table 8-2 *(continued)*

Physical Exam	Normal	Abnormal
		Red, edematous glans (infection, balanoposthitis)
		Urethritis, conjunctivitis, arthritis (Reiter's syndrome)
		Warts (condyloma acuminatum or latum)
		Swollen penis with soft midline mass (diverticulum)
		Mass in Littré's follicle (periurethral abscess)
		Inflamed glans with palpable cord in shaft (dorsal vein thrombosis)
		Varicosities/cavernositis (thrombosis, septicemia, leukemia, infection, or trauma)
		Priapism (lesions of spinal cord or cerebrum, neoplasms, hemorrhage, inflammation, thrombosis)
		Red, shiny scrotum (orchitis)
		Very dark scrotum (adrenal hyperplasia)
		Epididymal mass (retention cyst, spermatocele, neoplasm)
		Epididymal nodules (syphilis)
		Scrotal nodules (tuberculosis)
		Epididymitis
		Thick vas deferens (inflammation, syphilis, tuberculosis)
		Boggy mass (hematoma)
		Sausage bulge over testes (hydrocele of cord)
		"Bag of worms" mass (varicocele)
		Inquinal hernias
Anus	Patent	Imperforate anus/fistula
		Urine/fecal drainage (fistula)
		Anal atresia (chromosomal anomalies 13, 22)
EXTREMITIES		
Arms	Full ROM	Limited ROM (fracture, dislocation, paralysis, osteogenesis imperfecta)
Hands/fingers		Polydactyly (trisomy 13)*
		Extended, pronated (brachial plexus, injury)
		Inability to flex or abduct (Erbs palsy, Klumpke's palsy, C5–7, T1 injury)
		Syndactyly (chromosomal anomalies 5, 22)*
		Camptodactyly (trisomy 4, 8, 10, 13, 18)*

*Lewandowski and Yunis, 1975.

Table 8-2 *(continued)*

Physical Exam	Normal	Abnormal
		Thumbs absent (chromosomal anomaly 13)*
		Thumbs located distally (trisomy 18)*
		Thumbs located proximally (trisomy 10, 18)*
		Short fingers (myositis ossificans, pseudohypoparathyroidism)*
		Short, broad, clawlike hand (Hurler's syndrome, gangliosidoses, Scheie's syndrome, Hunter's syndrome Type II)*
		Short, broad, equal length of three middle fingers and space between first three fingers (chondrodystrophy)*
		Large fingers (neurofibromatosis)*
		Incurved fifth finger (chromosomal anomalies 13, 21, 22)*
		Short fifth finger (trisomy 8, 15, 21)*
		Fingers overlapping (trisomy 10, 13, 18)*
		Long tapering fingers (trisomy 1, 18)*
		Cortical thumb with extension of index and middle finger (decreased nonprotein bound calcium)*
		Hypoplastic phalanges (trisomy 8, 9, 13, 21)*
		Wide wrists (rickets)*
Fingernails/toenails	Pink, convex, length to edge of fingers	Long nails, yellow beds (postmaturity)
	Possible cyanosis during first hours of life	Absence/defect of nails (ichthyosis, ectodermal dysplasia)
		Hyperconvex nails (trisomy 4, 13)
		Square, round nails (cretinism, acromegaly)
		Nail hypoplasia (trisomies 8, 9, 13, 21)
		Long narrow nails (Marfan's syndrome, hypopituitarism)
		Pitted nails (fungal infections)
		Paronychia
		Dark nail beds (porphyria)
		Clubbing (pulmonary disease, cardiac disease, chronic obstruction, jaundice, hyperthyroidism)
		Concave nails (hypochromic anemia, iron deficiency, syphilis, rheumatic fever)
		Nailbed splinter hemorrhages (trichinosis, subacute bacterial endocarditis)

*Lewandowski and Yunis, 1975.

Table 8-2 *(continued)*

Physical Exam	Normal	Abnormal
		White proximal nail beds 80% bed white (hepatic cirrhosis) 50% bed white (renal disease) Red lunulae (cardiac failure) Light-blue lunulae (Wilson's disease) Blue-green (pseudomonas infection) Brown-black (fungal infection) Brown-yellow (phenindione ingestion) Blue-gray (argyria)
Legs	Full ROM, slightly bowed legs, positional deformities corrected with ROM Average length is 16.5 cm	Limited ROM (fracture, dislocation, paralysis, osteogenesis imperfecta) Patella absent (trisomy 8)* Hyperextensible joints (trisomy 15, 21, 22)* Dislocated hips (trisomy 7, 9, 13, 18)* Pes cavus (chromosomal anomalies 5, 7)* Tibial torsion Scissoring (cerebral palsy) Metatarsus valgus/varus
Feet/toes	Foot length averages 6.5 cm from heel to tip of big toe Width averages 1 cm	Pes valgus/varus Edema hands and feet (Milroy's disease, Turner's syndrome) Pretibial edema (hypothyroidism) Syndactyly (trisomy 10, 22)* Polydactyly (trisomy 13)* Rocker bottom feet (trisomy 13, 18)* Wide spaces between toes (trisomy 10, 21)* Big Toe syndrome* Short feet (trisomy 15)* Third toe equal to or longer than second toe (chromosomal anomaly)*
BACK	No curve or slight lumbar lordosis Sacral dimple without hair tufts or nevus flammeus are usually benign	Nevus flammeus on spine (underlying defect) Cysts, dimple, tufts of hair, discoloration over coccygeal area (spina bifida, spina bifida occulta) Scoliosis Pilonidal sinus
REFLEXES (see Table 3 in the introduction to The Neuropsychiatric System, Sec.8)	Moro, rooting, sucking, tonic neck, stepping, palmer and plantar grasp The tonic neck reflex is frequently absent or incomplete in normal infants.	Moro present at birth but disappears shortly (cerebral hemorrhage) Moro slow or absent (severe CNS injury, debilitation)

*Lewandowski and Yunis, 1975.

Table 8-2 *(continued)*

Physical Exam	Normal	Abnormal
		Tonic plantar grasp (hypoxia, hypertonia) Slow or absent grasp reflex (cervical or spinal cord lesions, malformations, hypertonia, lower brachial plexus injury, or lumbosacral plexus injury) Absent cremasteric reflex (spinal cord lesion) Weak, absent rooting (infant just fed, bulbar lesion, sleepy infant) Continuous tonic neck position (CNS injury)

*(Lewandowski and Yunis 1975)

SECTION 4: PSYCHOSOCIAL ASSESSMENT OF THE NEWBORN

Psychosocial assessment is as important as physical assessment in detecting the infant at risk. Multiple clues have been identified to assist us in early intervention with rejection, potential for child abuse, and emotional disturbances. They are summarized below.

Clues to Early Rejection of Infant by Postpartum Mother/Father

1. Attempts to avoid or is indifferent to arrival of infant for feeding
2. Holds infant away from body
3. Is repulsed by infant's excretory processes
4. Talks very little to or about infant
5. Discusses infant *excessively* ("supermother")
6. Exhibits depression; exhibits little or no sensitivity in handling infant or in meeting infant's needs
7. Is disturbed unduly by infant's crying
8. Is upset by idea of being alone with infant
9. Does not think baby is better than others; may perceive baby as ugly or unattractive
10. Holds infant so eye contact with infant is not possible
11. Suspects (*without* evidence) that infant has an illness or defect, and cannot be reassured when none is found
12. Exhibits conflicting attitudes and inconsistent behaviors toward infant

Cropley et al. (1976) have developed a tool for assessing a maternal attachment which is promising but has not yet been standardized. This tool measures the mother's identification of the infant's place in the social system, modalities of interaction, and care-giving behaviors. Observation of early mother-infant interaction at feeding times is essential.

I. Categories of Maladaptive Mothering Behaviors (Harrison, 1976)

A. Feeding behaviors

1. Provides inadequate types or amounts of food for infant
2. Does not hold infant, or holds in uncomfortable position during feeding
3. Does not burp infant
4. Prepares food inappropriately
5. Offers food at pace too rapid or slow for infant's comfort

B. Infant stimulation

1. Provides no or only aggressive verbal stimulation for infant during visit
2. Does not provide tactile stimulation or only that of aggressive handling of infant
3. No evidence of age-appropriate toys
4. Frustrates infant during interactions (excessive tickling, bouncing, etc.)

C. Infant rest

1. Does not provide quiet environment or schedule rest periods according to child's need

2. Does not attend to infant's needs for food, warmth, and/or dryness before sleep

D. Perception
1. Shows unrealistic perception of infant's condition
2. Demonstrates unrealistic expectations of infant
3. Has no awareness of infant's development
4. Shows unrealistic perception of own mothering

E. Initiative

Shows no initiative in attempts to meet infant's needs or to manage problems; does not follow through with plans

F. Recreation

Does not provide positive outlets for own recreation or relaxation

G. Interaction with other children

Demonstrates hostile/aggressive (sibling) interaction with other children in home (sarcasm or passive/aggressive behavior)

H. Mothering role

Expresses dissatisfaction with mothering

II. Parent Behaviors that Signal High Risk (Dubois, 1975)

The parent(s) who exhibits the following behaviors is at high risk for future problems. The parent(s) should receive counselling from the practitioner or be referred for professional counselling.

1. Unable to express feelings of guilt and responsibility for baby's early arrival
2. Has no visible anxiety about the infant's survival, denies the reality of danger, or displaces anxiety onto less threatening matters
3. Consistently misinterprets or exaggerates either positive or negative information about the baby's condition; unable to respond with hope as improvement occurs
4. Appears unable or unwilling to share fears about the baby with spouse
5. Emotional and practical support and help from spouse, family, friends, and community services is lacking
6. Unable to accept and use offered help

III. Behavioral Patterns/Structures Known to Breed Maltreatment of Children

A. Documented drug or alcohol addiction of one or both parents

B. Documented neurosis, psychosis, or mental deficiency in one or both parents

C. Authoritarian, highly structured, inflexibly disciplined family

D. Emotionally immature parents with loose, ill-defined structure

E. Poor maternal-infant bonding

IV. Indices of Emotional Maladjustment during First Year of Life

A. *Excessive*
1. Vomiting
2. Insomnia (less than 16 h of sleep per day)
3. Crying
4. Head rolling/banging
5. Sadness/apathy
6. Hyperactivity/inactivity
7. Apprehension
8. Irritability

B. Resists cuddling—stiffens when held, or fails to respond to being held

C. Exhibits lack of clinging behavior (arms in air like puppet)

D. No or few vocalizations

E. Indifferent to environment

F. No or few smiles

G. Feeding problems, including
1. Poor suck
2. Resisting food
3. No pleasure from feeding—remains fussy after adequate feeding
4. Rumination

In addition to the above cues, a number of tools are available to assist the practitioner in a systematic evaluation of an infant's psychosocial uniqueness, the parental perception of the infant, and the interactions between the two, thereby determining potential or actual risk to the infant and to the relationship.

Some of the tools, such as the Neonatal Perception Inventories (see Appendix 5) and the Infant Temperament Questionnaire[1] are concerned with the mother's perceptions of her infant or his or her temperament. These are important because research indicates that the mother's perception of her infant at 1 month of age is a *critical* variable associated with the need for later intervention for a child. The mother should perceive

[1]Sample copies of the questionnaire, scoring sheet, and profile sheet can be purchased from:
William B. Carey, M.D.
319 West Front Street
Media, PA 19063

her infant as generally better than other infants by 1 month of age.

Other tools, such as Brazelton's Neonatal Behavioral Assessment Scale and Erickson's Parent-Infant Care Record (Appendix 5) are more objective and based on the infant's behavior. These are particularly helpful to the practitioner and the mother in helping the mother identify and cope with the unique personality of her infant. These tools also assist the practitioner in identifying the mother's need for support and reassurance regarding her mothering skills.

A comparison of tools is presented in Table 8-3.

Table 8-3 Comparison of Psychosocial Assessment Tools

Assessment Tools	Neonatal Perception Inventories (NPI)	Infant Temperament Questionnaire	Parent-Infant Care Record	Neonatal Behavioral Assessment Scale
Developer/author	Elsie Broussard	William B. Carey and Sean C. McDevitt (revised 1977)	Marcene L. Erickson (1976, pp. 110–114)	T. Berry Brazelton
Advantages	Identifies maternal base-line perceptions Detects developmental disturbances early Determines priorities for intervention in maternal-infant interactions Is quick and easy to administer	Is an objective identification of individual infant's temperament Is basis for discussing the individual infant's needs Identifies parental concerns without creating feelings of guilt, incompetence, or responsibility for infant's temperament Minimizes parental biases Can be assessed on a continuing basis	Data more accurate than perceptions Is a systematic approach that is sensitive to needs of infant and parent Identifies learning needs of parent Acquaints parent with infant's actual behaviors Assists parent in developing objective ways of describing infant's behavior and communicating problems	Is most extensive assessment tool available Provides specific objective data regarding infant's unique interactive behaviors Is invaluable in early detection, prevention, and management of concerns or problems between infant and parent(s) Is valuable in predicting developmental outcomes in the neonatal period Is a useful resource and guideline for teaching parent(s) about infant's state changes, temperament, and individual behavior patterns *prior* to the infant's discharge home
Disadvantages	Entirely subjective Not balanced with infant observation	Standardized only for use between 4 and 8 mo of age Time-consuming if given in person, and parent may not return it if it is sent home	Parents may find it tedious, confusing, or time-consuming. Results are totally based on parental word and perceptions.	Takes up to an hour to administer and score Repeated assessments more valuable than a single assessment

Table 8-3 Comparison of Psychosocial Assessment Tools *(continued)*

Assessment Tools	Neonatal Perception Inventories (NPI)	Infant Temperament Questionnaire	Parent-Infant Care Record	Neonatal Behavioral Assessment Scale
		Scoring sometimes complicated		Requires special training to administer and score accurately
Administration time	5 min per test	25 min	5–7 days	30–60 min including scoring time
Scoring time	2 min per test	8–10 min	10–20 min	
Interpretation	A zero or negative score at 3 days and again at 1 mo is desirable. Assess infants for physical, developmental, or psychological delays. Negative maternal perceptions of an infant require immediate attention. Suggest that mother keep records of undesirable behavior. Discuss her views and perceptions in depth. Attempt to free parent(s) of stereotypes of "good/bad." Reassure mother regarding her ability to keep records, the importance of her observations, and the fact that change is possible.	Determine the mother's interpretation of language in the tool by asking her to describe a normal infant, how hers differs, what she would like to change, etc. (Erickson 1976, has an extensive list of questions which may be used in conjunction with the tool.) A difficult baby is more "at risk" depending on parental perception and acceptance. Stress the baby's positive points, and discuss ways of working with the difficult areas. Parents of irritable and difficult babies need support for the energy they invest in attempting to console them. Difficult infants with a low sensory threshold are more likely to have colic. Explore the implications for the parent(s) of an infant who is inactive or has a "slow to warm up"	Determine from the record whether the parent(s) is making too much or too little effort with the infant. Validate parental concerns with data. Determine learning needs of parent(s).	Special preparation is required to interpret the Brazelton tool, so interpretation is not included here.

Table 8-3 Comparison of Psychosocial Assessment Tools *(continued)*

Assessment Tools	Neonatal Perception Inventories (NPI)	Infant Temperament Questionnaire	Parent-Infant Care Record	Neonatal Behavioral Assessment Scale
		approach, or who is very active, persistent, and extremely distractible. Discuss parental perceptions and expectations regarding the infant's development, and introduce the fact that infants with different temperaments differ in their rates of development. According to Carey, very active infants walk sooner than inactive ones.		

Neonatal Behavioral Assessment Scale

A copy of Brazelton's Neonatal Behavioral Assessment scale is not included in this text because Dr. Brazelton feels that anyone using the tool should first receive specialized training in its application and in the interpretation of the results. Two-day training workshops are available.

The Brazelton tool covers 27 infant behavioral responses and is divided into the following six categories:

1. *Habitation*—the length of time it takes for infants to diminish response to light, sound, and heel pinch
2. *Orientation*—how much and when infant attends to, focuses on, and gives feedback in response to auditory and visual animate or inanimate stimuli
3. *Motor maturity*—degree and organization of coordination and control of motor activity
4. *Variation*—amount and rate of change during alert periods, and states, activity, color, and peaks of excitement throughout the examination
5. *Self-quieting activities*—how soon, how much, and how effectively the infant quiets and consoles self when distressed
6. *Social behaviors*—smiling and cuddling behaviors of the infant

The most profound result of Brazelton's research is that we now know that infants are already individuals at birth, with unique patterns of response, and that they attempt to control their environment.

MANAGEMENT

Major Concerns of New Parent(s)

Feeding How much, how often, what kind, what amount and type of vitamins are desirable? (For details, see Well-Child Care, Nutritional Assessment, Chap. 9.)

Sleep An interruption of parental patterns and loss of sleep is to be expected. The parent(s) needs reassurance that infants do learn to sleep through the night, usually by 3 months of age.

Normal Sleep Pattern for the Newborn				
		Longest Period during Day of		
Age, wk	Average Sleep, h/day	Wakefulness	Sleep	Abnormal Sleep Pattern
1–3	16–17	2.5	4–4½	Lack of diurnal pattern by 16 wk (CNS disorders)
4–12	15–16	3	6–7	Insomnia (emotional, tension)
12–16	15	4	7–8	Not sleeping through night by 5 mo (complete physical, CNS evaluation)
Diurnal cycle of sleep by 16 wk with more sleep at night				Short sleep cycles, long cycles, or lack of cyclic organization sleep (CNS disorders)

Adapted from Erickson, 1976, pp. 85–86.

Crying The parent(s) may need advice about how to interpret and handle crying, and how to cope with it. Observe the infant and teach the parent(s) about the infant's unique personality, consoling pattern, etc.

Counselling

Parents need counselling and/or support to reinforce parenting skills and promote better parent-child relations. The sooner consonance is developed between parental perceptions and expectations and their infants' unique abilities, the sooner more positive infant development occurs. The more confident a parent is with parenting skills, the more secure the infant is, and the faster the infant will develop. Using the information gathered from the psychosocial assessment tools, discuss the following with the parent(s) *prior to discharge* and as needed thereafter:

I. Teach the parent(s) about the infant's temperament and behavior patterns, and discuss an individualized approach.

A. what the infant's crying means
B. when to hold and console a crying infant
C. when to reduce or present stimuli to infant
D. position infant likes best, etc.
E. feeding techniques
F. how infant responds to care-giving activities such as bathing

II. Discuss the infant's attachment behaviors.

III. Give the opportunity for the parent(s) to discuss perceptions and concerns.

IV. Orient the parent(s) to the infant's positive attributes.

V. Reinforce parenting skills.

VI. Reinforce and encourage parent(s) to maintain a consistent approach.

VII. If the parental perception of the infant is negative, or if the infant is difficult,

A. Discuss with the parent(s).
   1. When did the parent begin to view the baby this way?
   2. What are the reasons why the parent views the baby as not better than average?
   3. What does the parent think would make it easier to stand the crying or feeding or whatever the major problem is?
   4. What does the parent think would help the infant with the problem?
   5. What does the parent expect of the infant at this time?
   6. What particular things about the infant has the parent noticed since the concern first arose?

B. Explore the parent(s)' feelings and reassure appropriately.

C. Suggest that the parent keep records of the infant's undesirable behavior for 4 to 5 days, noting the difficulties experienced, how long they last, how often they occur, and what the parent does to alleviate the situation.

D. Reassure the parent regarding the ability to keep records, the importance of these observations, the fact that change is possible, and that the parent can discuss any further concerns that may arise.

E. Use records to validate the parental concerns, support the parent(s), and give assistance in trying various techniques to alter the infant's behavior.

F. Use records to reinforce parenting skills (e.g., if the mother feels she's not a good mother, point out how quickly the infant is consoled, how well the infant sleeps, etc.).

G. Mobilize resources to support the mothers of difficult infants—an exhausted parent cannot cope well.

VIII. Use questionnaire as a base for *mutual* problem solving with parent(s) to develop intervention techniques and illuminate the parental role in changing and/or responding to that infant's unique behavior.

IX. If the mother is exhibiting rejection behaviors or the infant is abused or displaying maladjustment behaviors,

A. Assess the infant for physical, developmental, or psychological delays.

B. Assess the parent-infant attachment.

C. Explore the parent(s)' feelings and reinforce appropriately.

D. Counsel the parent(s), depending on what you perceive to be the causative factors.

1. Draw parent(s) out about expectations for this child, reasons for expectations, perceptions, etc.
2. Where appropriate, point out the infant's assets and positive attributes.
3. Suggest alternative methods of achieving changes in undesirable behavior.
4. Reassure parent(s) that change is possible.

E. As necessary, refer parent(s) to

1. Parents Anonymous
2. Psychotherapy
3. A child welfare organization
4. An adoption agency

F. Mobilize community resources to support the parent(s).

X. A thorough examination and evaluation should be performed on any infant not sleeping through the night after 5 months of age.

SECTION 5: ENVIRONMENTAL ASSESSMENT

Enriching an infant's environment promotes the child's development and is particularly beneficial to the infant at risk in reaching full developmental potential. However, it is important that the stimuli provided for each infant be neither excessive nor deficient for that baby's individual needs. Tools which may be of assistance in assessing an infant's environment and identifying problem areas are Erickson's Assessment of the Infant's Animate and Inanimate Environment (see Appendix 5) and Caldwell's Home Observation for Measurement of the Environment (HOME) (see Appendix 5). Research using HOME has shown that an optimal environment during a child's first year of life has a dramatic influence on that child's cognitive performance at 3 years of age. The two environmental assessment tools are compared in Table 8-4.

Management

I. Use observations as guidelines to provide verbal support for parents regarding their provision of appropriate and inappropriate stimuli. They want to know if they are doing the right things for their child.

II. Encourage and reinforce parental sensitivity to the developmental needs of the infant.

III. Educate parents regarding the developmental needs of infant *based on the parental value system* (e.g., if the parents value intelligence, stress how appropriate stimuli improve development).

Table 8-4 Comparison of Environmental Assessment Tools

Assessment Tools	Assessment of Animate and Inanimate Environment*	Home Observation for Measurement of the Environment*
Advantages	Provides objective baseline data on an infant's environment, both animate and inanimate Covers infant's development, stimuli, mother-infant interaction, physical environment, and mother's assessment of infant's stimulation Direct observation validating or invalidating mother's reports Serves as valuable adjunct to Parent-Infant Care Record Serves as useful guideline for assessment and counselling regarding parenting skills	*Predicts* developmental risk with accuracy Can be used to assess any environment in which the infant spends time Covers subtle aspects of an infant's environment Is standardized Evaluates environment from child's point of view Measures animate and inanimate aspects with direct observation Determines frequency of contact between care givers and infant, positive or negative emotional climate, adequacy of stimuli provided, and strengths and weaknesses in the family
Disadvantages	Not standardized Primarily concerned with excessive or inadequate stimuli for infant Time-consuming	Time-consuming—must be conducted while child is awake, which may mean several appointments must be made/broken Formal training or an "apprenticeship" desirable to achieve a 90% level of agreement between raters Health and nutritional status not included "Yes or no" scoring, without formal provision for finer gradations
Administration time	1–2 h in the home	1 h in the home
Scoring time	10–15 min	5 min

*Adapted from Erickson, 1976, pp. 110–115.

IV. Stress the positive aspects of their infant's development.

V. Assist parents to relax if they are trying "too hard" to provide the right stimuli at the right time. Praise positive efforts.

VI. Provide anticipatory guidance in relation to safety hazards.

VII. If a good environment is lacking,

A. Discuss positive findings *first.*

B. Reinforce parenting skills.

C. Ask parent(s)

1. If they have thought about the kinds of toys they select, the variety, etc.
2. If they have noticed how they respond to their infant
3. If their observations are congruent with the assessment guide
4. If there is anything they would like to change about the environment, and their first priority for change
5. If they have thought of ways to change the environment to benefit child or themselves

D. Use discussion for mutual problem solving with parents.

E. Discuss setting limits, and reassure parents that this is a common problem.

F. Discuss parental concerns, and assist parents to differentiate concerns and set priorities.

G. Repeat HOME on routine basis to monitor changes when change is recommended.

H. Encourage parents to identify alternative ways of dealing with problems.

SECTION 6: COUNSELLING FOR PARENTS WITH ATYPICAL NEWBORNS

The birth of an atypical child (a premature or a child with an anomaly) represents an object loss to the parent(s), loss of a desired goal (that is, delivery of a perfect infant), loss of the fantasized "perfect" infant, loss of self-esteem, and loss of satisfaction in the birth process. This precipitates a grief response, an overwhelming sense of failure in both parents, and a subsequent crisis reaction. Since attachment cannot take place in the presence of grieving, atypical infants are at high risk for rejection by parents and siblings.

The initial reactions of parents to a premature birth or to the birth of a child with a congenital anomaly are essentially the same; however, the degree of the reaction is greater in parents of infants with visible congenital defects. Mothers tend to see their preterm children as weaker than their term children and experience two periods of pronounced anxiety: the first is immediately after birth and the second is upon the infant's return home (Bidder, 1974).

Initial Reactions of Parent(s) to Premature Birth

1. Disbelief, shock, disorganization
2. Grief over loss of "perfect" baby
3. Inability to absorb explanations
4. Fear of being alone when seeing child for first time
5. Impaired perceptions due to high anxiety level—focus on detail rather than on whole (e.g., can only see baby's leg with IV, or heaving chest)
6. Need contact with other parents of prematures in intensive care nursery (it is well documented in the literature that contact with other parents in same situation is great source of strength)
7. Fear that touching infant might cause child to stop breathing or die
8. Fear of leaving hospital because if anything happens they "wouldn't be there"

Concerns of Parents of Prematures after Infant Outlook Improves

1. What kind of long-term complications will there be?
2. Will infant be mentally retarded?
3. Could infant be blind?
4. Will infant ever catch up in growth and development?
5. Will the baby ever be "normal"?
6. Is there anything else wrong with the baby? Are you sure?

Anxieties/Guilt over Premature Birth

Anxiety and guilt are the two most prominent emotions in the parents of prematures.

Maternal Anxieties/Guilt

1. Feels heightened concern over whether baby is alive and will live
2. Feels lonely and lost, "unable to *do* anything"
3. Expects to hear any moment that baby has died
4. Feels she's an inadequate mother, a failure, because she didn't carry infant to term (or because infant has defect); feels loss of self-esteem
5. Feels anxious and guilty that nurses care for infant better than she; worries whether or not child will love her
6. Feels angry that the infant "belongs" to nurses and doctors, and guilty because she feels this way

Paternal Anxieties/Guilt

1. Guilt over his involvement in child's prematurity/defect; worry about what he could have done differently
2. Guilt because he is father but cannot help his child
3. May feel premature delivery/defect reflects on his masculinity
4. Jealousy toward infant because of diminished attentions from his wife
5. Fear of the social stigma of "defect," which influences the responses of others

6. Concern over inability to meet financial responsibility for infant
7. Guilt over revulsion he feels when he sees defect
8. Afraid mother will be unable to care for baby at home
9. Guilt over feeling of revulsion mother experiences when she sees the defect

Counselling

Counselling parents of prematures is similar to counselling parents of infants with defects.

Parents of premature infants and parents of newborns with congenital defects experience similar shock and grief. There is the anxiety that the infant will die and the grief over the loss of the "perfect" baby they had desired and envisioned. However, the parents of children with congenital defects are unable to resolve their acute grief and progress into chronic sorrow.

Marital discord is much more pronounced in families following the birth of a defective child than it is with a premature birth. Depending on the parent(s)' level of emotional maturity and self-esteem, there is a great tendency to blame the other parent for the anomaly. In fact, more than 50 percent of the families of children with a defect end in divorce within 2 years of the birth. Supportive counselling from a practitioner, or in severe cases from psychiatrists or marriage counsellors, can do much to assist parents in coping with defective children.

Parental Responses to Infant with Defect

The first responses are the same as those for a premature infant, and then the following responses are more descriptive.

1. Shock, disbelief; dazed look; verbal and nonverbal denial; withdrawal
2. Anger (rarely directed toward infant): "*Why* did this happen to me?" Anger turned toward others
3. Grief, depression, anger turned inward, decreased self-esteem, shame
4. Constant anxiety over cause: "What did I do to cause this?" "Maybe if I hadn't taken aspirin. . ."
5. Initial revulsion, shame, an unwillingness to "claim" the infant (no claiming behaviors such as "He looks just like. . . He definitely has your eyes and nose. . ." etc.)
6. Twice as much expression of interest in infant's functional ability as in appearance
7. Each new development—such as hospitalization or surgery—perhaps precipitating another crisis and grief response
8. Fear that child will be mentally retarded
9. If parent(s) knew genetic risk, feeling of tremendous remorse: "What have we done to you?"
10. Hopelessness about future children
11. Fear of establishing bond with infant because afraid baby will die
12. Escalation of maternal fear responses during first 3 months of life
13. Acutely sensitive to attitudes of others
14. May also feel resentment, isolation, and/or alienation

Counselling

1. Be aware of your own feelings—practitioners normally experience the same shock, disbelief, and anger as do parents.
2. Talk to the parents *together*, assisting each to appreciate, understand, and deal with the other's feelings.
3. Create an environment in which parents feel free to express their feelings, both positive and negative.
   a. Express your warmth, concern, and caring—perhaps through touch, by just "being there," or by your tears—in whatever way you feel is best.
   b. Help parents to realize you accept their feelings *and* that their feelings are normal; this relieves some guilt and hastens resolution.
   c. Parents need to feel they are not alone.
   d. Reply to hostility with understanding: "You must feel dreadfully hurt and disappointed that this has happened to you."
   e. Provide hope with factual information rather than reassure with platitudes and cliches. However, if there is no hope, don't instill false hope.
   f. Many parents tend to blame each other for the defect.
4. Allow parents to proceed at their own pace—

they may need to withdraw (not see or handle baby) for awhile. However, consultation is indicated if parents show little progress toward acceptance and adaptation after a reasonable period of time.

5. Encourage parents to participate in the care of the infant as soon as possible. Facilitate this, and give constant feedback to the parents about the infant when care cannot be given by them. The feedback can consist of information about
   a. Weight gain
   b. What baby looks like
   c. Quality of suck, feeding
   d. What tests have been done
   e. Who is caring for infant
   f. What care has been given
   g. Baby's unique characteristics

   This information assures the parents that care is being given and progress is being made.
6. Compliment parents on positive care provided by them, and reinforce parenting skills. This is particularly important after discharge.
7. Assess family strengths and weaknesses, and mobilize outside support when necessary.
   a. Friends or relations
   b. Church groups
   c. Community organizations
8. After the parents begin to ask questions about the defect, arrange for them to talk with other parents who have had similar experiences.
9. If parents seem overly concerned about mental retardation, discuss it with them. Explore ramifications. Give pointers about what to look for in infant development.
10. Discuss child-rearing practices, since there is little or no transference of child-rearing practices suitable for the normal child to the atypical child without special guidance or instruction from outside the family unit.
11. Inform parents about available community resources and the services they provide.
12. Assist parents in finding capable baby-sitters (perhaps a senior citizen may want to make a contribution). The parents need time together alone.
13. Genetic counselling may be appropriate.

references

Babson, S. G., and Benda, G. I. Growth graphs for the clinical assessment of infants of varying gestational age. *Journal of Pediatrics* **89**(5):814–820 (1976).

Bidder, R. T., et al. Mothers' attitudes to preterm infants. *Archives of Diseases in Childhood,* **49:**766–769 (1974).

Carey, William B. Clinical application of infant temperament measurements. *Journal of Pediatrics,* **81:**824 (1972).

Chamberlain, G., and Banks, J. Assessment of the Apgar score. *The Lancet 2,* (7891):1225–1228 (1974).

Cropley, C., et al. Assessment tool for measuring maternal assessment behaviors. In L. K. McNall and J. T. Galeener (eds.), *Current practice in obstetric and gynecologic nursing.* St. Louis: Mosby, 1976.

Dubois, Don R. Indications of an unhealthy relationship between parents and premature infant. *Journal of GN Nursing,* May-June: 21–23 (1975).

Dubowitz, Lilly M. S., et al. Clinical assessment of gestational age in the newborn infant. *Journal of Pediatrics,* **77**:1–10 (1970).

Erickson, Marcene L. *Assessment and management of developmental changes in children.* St. Louis: Mosby, 1976, pp. 16–136.

Harrison, L. H. Nursing intervention with the failure to thrive family. *American Journal of Maternal Child Nursing* **1**(2):111–116 (1976).

Kitterman, J. A., Phibbs, R. H., and Tooley, W. H. Diastolic and mean blood pressures during the first 12 hours of life in normal newborns grouped according to birthweight. *Pediatrics* **44**:959 (1969).

Klaus, Marshall H., and Kennell, John H. *Maternal-infant bonding.* St. Louis: Mosby, 1976, p. 14.

Lewandowski, R. C., and Yunis, L. J. New chromosomal syndromes. *American Journal of Diseases in Children,* **129:**515–527 (1975).

McMillan, J. A., Neiburg, P. I., and Oski, F. A. *The whole pediatrician catalog.* Philadelphia: Saunders, 1977, pp. 3–6, 9–10.

Parkin, J. M., Hey, E. N., and Clowes, J. S. Rapid assessment of gestational age at birth. *Archives of Diseases in Childhood* **51:**259 (1976).

Roberts, R. B. Assessment of the Apgar score. *The Lancet 1,* (7899):164–165 (1975).

bibliography

Alexander, Mary M., and Brown, Marie Scott. *Pediatric history taking and physical diagnosis for nurses.* New York: McGraw-Hill, 1979.

Allen, J. E., Guruaj, V. J., and Russo, R. M. *Practical points in pediatrics.* Flushing, N. Y.: Medical Examination Publishing Company, 1977.

Barnard, Martha Underwood. Supportive nursing care for the mother and newborn who are separated from each other. *The American Journal of Maternal Child Nursing,* March-April:107–110 (1976).

Barness, Lewis A. *Manual of pediatric physical diagnosis* (4th ed.). Chicago: Year Book, 1972.

Crelin, Edmund S. *Functional anatomy of the newborn.* New Haven: Yale, 1973.

Harper, Rita G., and Yoon, Jing Ja. *Handbook of neonatology.* Chicago: Year Book, 1974.

Holt, Sarah B. Dermatoglyphics. *Nursing Mirror,* July:16–19 (1973).

Levison, H., et al. Blood pressure in normal, full term and premature infants. *American Journal of Diseases in Children,* **111**:374 (1966).

Lewandowski, R. C., and Yunis, J. J.: New chromosomal syndromes. *American Journal of Diseases in Children* **129**:516–528 (1975).

Mercer, Ramona T. Mothers' responses to their infants with defects. *Nursing Research* **23**(2):133–137 (1974).

———. Nursing care for parents at risk. Thorofare: Charles B. Slack, 1977.

Schwartz, Jane L., and Schwartz, Lawrence H. *Vulnerable infants—A psychosocial dilemma.* New York: McGraw-Hill, 1977.

Uchida, Irene A., and Soltan, Hubert C. Dermatoglyphics in medical genetics. *Endocrine and Genetic Diseases of Childhood,* Philadelphia: Saunders, 1969.

Waechter, Eugenia H. Bonding problems of infants with congenital anomalies. *Nursing Forum,* **16**(3-4):298–317 (1977).

9 Well-Child Care

Introduction LESLIE LIETH

Well-child care involves both health maintenance or health promotion and prevention of disease. For the primary health care practitioner working in a pediatric ambulatory setting, an understanding of and interest in disease prevention and health promotion is an essential part of daily work.

This section is outlined by the age of the child (newborn to 17 years) to help the practitioner systematically assess the total child and provide appropriate management and planning. The needed subjective and objective information for each visit is covered, as well as treatments, immunizations, anticipatory guidance, counselling, referrals, and follow-up. Table 9-1 is based on the assumption that a complete data base has been collected.

Table 9-1 Well-Child Care

	Age					
	Newborn to 1½ mo	2 mo	4 mo	6 mo	9 mo	12 mo
			Subjective Data			
Interval History	Since hospital discharge	X*	X	X	X	X
Nutritional History (see "Nutritional Assessment," (Chap. 9)	X	X	X	X	X	X
Elimination History	X	X	X	X	X	X
Habits	Sleeping, crying, pacifier, thumb	Same as newborn to 1½ mo col.	Sleeping, crying, thumb vs. pacifier, teething	Same as 4 mo col.	Sleeping, thumb vs. pacifier, teething, temper	Same as 9 mo col.
Psycho/Social History (see Family Assessment, Chap. 1; Psychological Assessment, Chap. 2)	Mother's emotional condition	X	X	X	X	X
Developmental Milestones (see Developmental Assessment, Chap. 6)	X	X	X	X	X	X
Present Complaints	X	X	X	X	X	X
Review of Systems	X	X	X	X	X	X
Other	Skin, bath care Note birth history					
			Objective Data			
Physical Examination	Complete physical exam	Complete physical exam	Skin, lymph, head, eyes, ears, nose, throat, cardiovascular, pulmonary, abdomen	Complete physical exam	See 4 mo col.	Complete physical exam
Measurement (plot on graph)	Weight, height, head and chest circumference, temperature	Same as 2 mo col.	Same as 2 mo col.	Same as 2 mo col.	Same as 2 mo col.	Same as 2 mo col.
Developmental Assessment (see	X	X	X	X	X	X

*Indicates to be done at this time.

Table 9-1 Well-Child Care *(continued)*

Age					
15–18 mo	2–3 yr	4–5 yr	6–8 yr	9–12 yr	13–17 yr
		Subjective Data			
X	X	X	X	X	X
X	X	X	X	X	X
X	X	X	X	X	X
Sleeping, thumb-sucking, temper tantrums, pica	See 15–18 mo col. Head-banging, nightmares	Sleeping, discipline, temper, fears, masturbation	Same as 4–5 yr col.	Sleeping, temper, nail-biting	See 9–12 yr col. Smoking, drug/alcohol use or abuse
Presence of sources of lead (see Lead Poisoning, Chap. 155)	X	Socialization with peers Family relationships	Same as 4–5 yr col.	See 4–5 yr col. Clubs, interests	See 9–12 yr col. Interview of child with parents, then alone Level of sexual activity, if any
X	X	School adjustment	Same as 4–5 yr col.	School grades: best and worst subjects	See 9–12 yr col.
X	X	X	X	X	X
X	X	X	X	X	X
Toilet trained?		Dental checkup last 12 mo?	Same as 4–5 yr col.	Dental history Menstrual history	See 9–12 yr col. Use of birth control Vocational plans
		Objective Data			
Same as 4 mo col.	Complete physical exam Blood pressure at 3 yr and older	Same as 2–3 yr col.	Same as 2–3 yr col.	Same as 2–3 yr col.	Same as 2–3 yr col.
Same as 2 mo col.	Weight, height, temperature	Same as 2–3 yr col.	Same as 2–3 yr col.	Same as 2–3 yr col.	Same as 2–3 yr col.
X	X	X	X	X	X

Table 9-1 Well-Child Care *(continued)*

	Age					
	Newborn to 1½ mo	2 mo	4 mo	6 mo	9 mo	12 mo
			Objective Data (continued)			
Developmental Assessment, Chap. 6)						
Parent-Child Interaction	X	X	X	X	X	X
Laboratory Data	Since hospital discharge, check for phenylketonuria (PKU)	Record results since last visit	Records results since last visit	Record results since last visit	Record results since last visit	Record results since last visit
Vision Screening	X	X	X	X	X	X
Hearing Screening	X	X	X	X	X	X
			Management: Treatments/Medications			
Vitamins	Vitamins A, D, C, and E, with iron and fluoride if indicated by diet and water supply	Same as Newborn to 1½ mo col.	Same as Newborn to 1½ mo col.	Multivitamins, iron, fluoride if indicated	Same as 6 mo col.	Same as 6 mo col.
Antipyretic		Acetaminophen: ½ grain po, q4h, if needed	Same as 2 mo col.	Same as 2 mo col.	Same as 2 mo col.	Acetaminophen: 1 grain, po, q4h, if needed
Immunizations (see immunization schedules, Tables 9-2 and 9-3)		X	X	X		X
Hemoglobin	Done in nursery			To be done once during first year	Same as 6 mo col.	Same as 6 mo col.
Urinalysis				To be done once during first year	Same as 6 mo col.	Same as 6 mo col.
Other				Sickle cell screening		
			Management: Counselling/Prevention			
Nutrition (see Nutritional Assessment in Chap. 9)	X	X	X	X	X	X
Side Effects of Immunization		X	X	X	X	X

Table 9-1 Well-Child Care (*continued*)

Age					
15–18 mo	2–3 yr	4–5 yr	6–8 yr	9–12 yr	13–17 yr
			Objective Data (continued)		
X	X	X	X	X	X
Record results since last visit	Record results since last visit	Record results since last visit	Record results since last visit	Record results since last visit	Record results since last visit
X	At 3 yr visit use eye chart	Every 2–3 yr	Every 2–3 yr	Every 2–3 yr	Every 2–3 yr
X	At 3 yr visit—audiometry	Every 2–3 yr	Every 2–3 yr	Every 2–3 yr	Every 2–3 yr
			Management: Treatments/Medications		
Same as 6 mo col.	Same as 6 mo col.	As indicated by diet history	Same as 4–5 yr col.	Same as 4–5 yr col.	Same as 4–5 yr col.
Same as 12 mo col.	Aspirin or Acetaminophen (see Oral Medication Appendix 2)	Same as 2–3 yr col.	Same as 2–3 yr col.	Same as 2–3 yr col.	Same as 2–3 yr col.
	Tine test annually if city dweller Others, as indicated	Same as 2–3 yr col.	Same as 2–3 yr col.	Same as 2–3 yr col.	Same as 2–3 yr col.
	Check every 1–2 yr	Check every 1–2 yr	Check every 1–2 yr	Check every 1–2 yr	Check every 1–2 yr
	Check every 1–2 yr	Same as 1–2 yr col.	Same as 1–2 yr col.	Same as 1–2 yr col.	Same as 1–2 yr col.
F.E.P. or lead screening if indicated					Syphilis screening if indicated
			Management: Counselling/Prevention		
X	X	X	X	X	X
X	X	X	X	X	X

Table 9-1 Well-Child Care *(continued)*

	Age					
	Newborn to 1½ mo	2 mo	4 mo	6 mo	9 mo	12 mo
			Management: Counselling/Prevention (continued)			
(see "Immunization," Chap. 9)						
Accident Prevention (see "Accident Prevention," Chap. 9)	X	X	X	X	X	X
Address Special Concerns	X	X	X	X	X	X
Dental Care (see "Dental Health" in Chap. 9)				Clean teeth with gauze daily.	Same as 6 mo col.	See 6 mo col. Decrease use of bottle- and sugar-containing foods.
Anticipatory Guidance	Sleep and activity Sibling rivalry Sleeping arrangements Immunizations Common illnesses	Same as Newborn to 1½ mo col.	Teething	Teething Baby's increased activity, mobility Temper tantrums Initial discussion of discipline	Shy stage Messiness during meals (can put plastic tablecloth under high chair for easy cleanup) Discussion of buying footware	Negativism Increase in child's activity Exploring toilet training Normal decrease in appetite coming year Discipline
Growth and Development	X	X	X	X	X	X
Stimulation	Pictures on wall near crib Playing radio Talking and singing to baby Exercising arms and legs while bathing Placing baby in room with family	See Newborn to 1½ mo col.	See Newborn to 1½ mo col. Rattles Well-anchored squeak toy Peekaboo Infant seat	Starting on cup Toys that make noise Finger and toe games Mirror play Pat-a-cake Supervised play with paper Tying balloons on feet and wrists Soft toys Vocal games	See 6 mo col. Water play Pots and pans to bang Crawling on different surfaces Continuing talking and singing to baby Tying toys to high chair or walker	Fill and dump toys Large, soft ball Pots and pans, rolling pin Pointing to objects and body parts and naming them Feeling different kinds of food Encouraging to walk on variety of surfaces

Table 9-1 Well-Child Care (*continued*)

Age					
15–18 mo	2–3 yr	4–5 yr	6–8 yr	9–12 yr	13–17 yr
Management: Counselling/Prevention (continued)					
X	X	X	X	X	X
X	X	X	X	X	X
No bottle should be given baby at sleep except water.	Parent(s) should brush child's teeth twice daily. Avoidance of sugar-containing foods Visit dentist	Child and parent(s) should brush child's teeth twice daily. Avoidance of sugar-containing foods. Visit to dentist twice a yr	Child should brush at least twice daily. Use floss daily. Visit to dentist twice a year	Same as 6–8 yr col.	Same as 6–8 yr col.
See 9 and 12 mo col.	Temper tantrums Biting Negativism Development of rituals Not dry at night Normal changes in appetite	Explain questions about sex; help to establish gender identity Tastes for food change Discourage child's wish to sleep with parent(s) Explain death	Increased peer involvement School adjustment School failures Personality development	Need for sex education Increased interest in opposite sex Increased involvement in groups	Exploring relationships with friends of both sexes Discussing vocational plans Adolescent's need for privacy Discussing feelings of independence Discussing feelings and knowledge about parenthood, marriage
X	X	X	X	X	X
Toy phone Reading picture books with child Pull or push toys Paper and crayon for scribbling Pounding toys, drum Letting child help around house Simple jigsaw puzzles Having child say word for objects	Puppet play Dress-up games Finger painting Records that tell stories Rocking horse Stacking toys Simple puzzles Sand play Riding tricycle Dressing self Playing with clay	Group play Big boxes Pasting pictures in scrapbook Painting Ball games More books Care for a plant Board games More puzzles Counting games Jumping rope	Board games More ball games Trips to zoo, museums, etc. Dancing Books Crossword, jigsaw puzzles Bicycle Encouraging homework Learning use of money	After school and summer programs Woodworking, crafts Sports, dancing Books More board games Balancing TV habits Encouraging homework Realistic chores around house	After school, weekend, and summer programs, clubs Responsibilities and chores around house Part-time job

Table 9-1 Well-Child Care *(continued)*

	Age					
	Newborn to 1½ mo	2 mo	4 mo	6 mo	9 mo	12 mo
	Management: Counselling/Prevention (continued)					
Other Topics	Skin, bath Bottle sterilization Family planning	Baby-sitting Family planning Reading thermometer				
	Management: Follow-up					
	Revisit 2 mo of age Stress importance of visit Give information regarding emergency or episodic care	Revisit 6–8 wk	Revisit 6–8 wk	Revisit 2–3 mo	Revisit 3 mo	Revisit 3 mo
	Management: Consultations/Referrals					
	Visiting nurse if parents overwhelmed Social worker if necessary Mental health clinician for postpartum depression MD as indicated	MD as indicated Available community resources, (e.g., mothers' groups)	Same as 2 mo col.	Same as 2 mo col.	Same as 2 mo col.	Same as 2 mo col.

Table 9-1 Well-Child Care (*continued*)

Age					
15–18 mo	2–3 yr	4–5 yr	6–8 yr	9–12 yr	13–17 yr
		Management: Counselling/Prevention (continued)			
	Following the leader Coloring books Teaching colors Musical instruments More books	Dressing self Singing games Bicycle Small tasks around house Using scissors	Balancing T.V. habits Simple chores around the house Arts/crafts		
	Discussing nursery school, day care			Discussing need for proper amount of sleep	Discussing birth control, venereal disease Acne and skin care Need for sleep Teaching breast self-exam
		Management: Follow-up			
Revisit 3–6 mo	Revisit 1 yr	Revisit 1 yr	Revisit 1 yr	Revisit 1 yr	Revisit 1 yr
		Management: Consultations/Referrals			
Same as 2 mo col.	MD as indicated Available community resources Dental checkup every 6–12 mo (3 yr and older)	Same as 2–3 yr col.	See 2–3 yr col. Community centers for children, pertinent to child's interests (e.g. boys' and girls' club, scouts, YMCA, YWCA)	Same as 6–8 yr col.	MD as indicated Dentist every 6–12 mo School guidance counsellor for vocational guidance After-school community centers Youth centers for jobs Gynecology if necessary

bibliography

American Academy of Pediatrics. *Standards of child health care* (3rd ed.). Evanston, Ill. Author, 1977.

Barnwell, Elizabeth, et al. *Infant and preschool assessment and counselling guide for nurses.* Lansing, Mich., Michigan Dept. of Health, 1972.

Chinn, Peggy L., and Leitch, Cynthia J. *Child health maintenance.* St. Louis: Mosby, 1974.

Hoole, Azalla J., et al. *Patient care guidelines for family nurse practitioners.* Boston: Little, Brown, 1976.

Immunizations M. CONSTANCE SALERNO

ACTIVE IMMUNIZATION

The brilliant success achieved in conquering the classic contagious diseases of childhood is attributed to immunization. Active immunization (artificial) is achieved when antigens are injected into the body to stimulate the production of antibodies. Antibodies that are present will injure or destroy the disease-producing agent or neutralize its toxins. By means of immunoprophylaxis, many formerly dreaded diseases such as poliomyelitis, diphtheria, and measles have been prevented. Immunization is the most routine procedure in preventive pediatrics and is the most effective, yet least expensive, method of preventing illness.

Although many vaccines are available for use, only seven are recommended for routine use. Before recommending any vaccine, the practitioner should know the composition of the agent and how it should be administered. The package insert is the best guide and should be read before administering immunizing agents. Because the concentration of antigen varies in different products, the insert should be consulted regarding the volume of individual doses of vaccines needed. The manufacturer's recommendations for optimal storage conditions (e.g., temperature, light) should be carefully followed since the stability of various products differs. Failure to observe these precautions may significantly reduce the potency and effectiveness of the vaccines.

Clients and parent(s) should be informed of any possible side effects or adverse reactions. They should be counselled regarding the benefits of the vaccine versus the risks of the disease. All healthy infants and children should be routinely immunized as part of well-child care. Im-

Table 9-2 Recommended Schedule for Active Immunization of Normal Infants and Children

2 mo	DTP[a]	TOPV[b]
4 mo	DTP	TOPV
6 mo	DTP	[c]
1 yr		Tuberculin test[d]
15 mo	Measles,[e] Rubella[e]	Mumps[e]
1½ yr	DTP	TOPV
4–6 yr	DTP	TOPV
14–16 yr	Td[f]—repeat every 10 yr	

[a]DTP—diphtheria and tetanus toxoids combined with pertussis vaccine.

[b]TOPV—trivalent oral poliovirus vaccine. This recommendation is suitable for breast-fed as well as bottle-fed infants.

[c]A third dose of TOPV is optional but may be given in areas of high endemicity of poliomyelitis.

[d]Frequency of repeated tuberculin tests depends on risk of exposure of the child and on the prevalence of tuberculosis in the population group. For the pediatrician's office or outpatient clinic, an annual or biennial tuberculin test, unless local circumstances clearly indicate otherwise, is appropriate. The initial test should be done at the time of, or preceding, the measles immunization.

[e]May be given at 15 mo as measles-rubella or measles-mumps-rubella vaccines.

[f]Td—combined tetanus and diphtheria toxoids (adult type) for those more than 6 yr of age, in contrast to diphtheria and tetanus (DT) toxoids which contain a larger amount of diphtheria antigen. *Tetanus toxoid at time of injury:* For clean, minor wounds, no booster dose is needed by a fully immunized child unless more than 10 yr have elapsed since the last dose. For contaminated wounds, a booster dose should be given if more than 5 yr have elapsed since the last dose.

Source: Report of the Committee on the Control of Infectious Diseases. *Red book.* Evanston, Ill.: American Academy of Pediatrics, 1977, p. 3.

munization should be initiated as early as possible, since there is great variability in passive protection in the young infant and no passive immunity against pertussis. Current practice begins immunization when the infant is between 8 and 12 weeks of age. A "triple" toxoid of diphtheria, pertussis, and tetanus antigens in one injection and a concurrent feeding of oral polio vaccine are given. This procedure is repeated 3 times at intervals of not less than 1 month. Combined antigens reduce the number of injections, enhance the action of each, and establish a desired immunity within the first 6 months of life. After the initial series of immunizations, "recall," or "booster," doses are given to stimulate high antibody levels and maintain maximum immunity. The schedules for active immunization proposed by the American Academy of Pediatrics Committee on Infectious Diseases are listed in Tables 9-2 and 9-3. The schedule in Table 9-2 is recommended for normal infants during the first year of life. The schedule in Table 9-3 is recommended for children who receive their first immunization after 1 year of age.

Table 9-3 Primary Immunization for Children Not Immunized in Early Infancy*

Under 6 Yr	
First visit	DTP, TOPV, tuberculin test
Interval after first visit	
1 mo	Measles,† mumps, rubella
2 mo	DTP, TOPV
4 mo	DTP, TOPV‡
10–16 mo or preschool	DTP, TOPV
Age 14—16 yr	Td—repeat every 10 yr
6 Yr and Over	
First visit	Td, TOPV, tuberculin test
Interval after first visit	
1 mo	Measles, mumps, rubella
2 mo	Td, TOPV
8–14 mo	Td, TOPV
Age 14–16 yr	Td—repeat every 10 yr

*Physicians may choose to alter the sequence of these schedules if specific infections are prevalent at the time. For example, measles vaccine might be given on the first visit if an epidemic is underway in the community.

†Measles vaccine is not routinely given before 15 mo of age.

‡Optional.

Source: Report of the Committee on the Control of Infectious Diseases. *Red book.* Evanston, Ill.: American Academy of Pediatrics, 1977, p. 11.

CONTRAINDICATIONS

1. Acute febrile illness. (A delay between doses does not interfere with the final immunity.)
2. If the child has an *evolving* neurologic disorder, it may be necessary to avoid all immunizations.
3. Immunizations are deferred during the administration of steroids, irradiation, and anticancer drug therapy. They should also be deferred if the child has received within 8 weeks immune serum globulin, plasma, or blood.
4. Immunizations are *not* given to persons with generalized malignancy.
5. Measles, mumps, and rubella vaccine are *not* given during pregnancy.
6. If allergic reactions were experienced, the same or related vaccines should be avoided.

DIPHTHERIA, TETANUS TOXOIDS, AND PERTUSSIS VACCINE

Diphtheria and tetanus toxoids and pertussis vaccine are available in various combinations and concentrations for specific purposes.

1. Diphtheria and tetanus toxoids and pertussis vaccine (DTP)
2. Diphtheria and tetanus toxoids (DT)
3. Tetanus and diphtheria toxoids (Td)—adult type (small "d" indicates 10–25% of that in standard DTP)
4. Tetanus toxoid (T)

Diphtheria

Several hundred cases of diphtheria are reported annually in the United States. Most cases occur in partially or unimmunized children. Diphtheria is a very serious disease, and 10 percent of respiratory diphtheria cases are fatal. Immunization against diphtheria is combined with pertussis and tetanus and given at 2, 4, and 6 months. The toxoid has few side effects, although severe local reactions have been reported with increasing age.

Tetanus

Immunization with tetanus toxoid should begin in infancy, continue through childhood, and extend into adult life. The initial dose of the primary series is given at 2 months, together with the diphtheria and pertussis vaccine. Tetanus toxoid is an excellent immunizing agent and provides long-lasting protection. It is unnecessary to give booster doses less than once every 10 years. Although side effects are uncommon with primary immunization, persons who have received an excessive number of booster injections occasionally manifest hypersensitivity reactions. (See Table 9-4 for tetanus immunization in wound management.)

Pertussis

The severe complications and high mortality from pertussis in infancy are the major reasons for immunizing early in life. Common side effects from the vaccine include low-grade fever, malaise, local tenderness, and induration. These may occur 4 to 6 hours after immunization and subside within 24 to 48 hours. Pertussis immunization should not be repeated if a history of fever 105°F (40.5°C) or over, severe screaming episodes, symptoms of CNS involvement (e.g., stupor, coma, or convulsions), or platelet destruction (e.g., petechiae or bruising) has been noted after DTP injection. DT should be used instead. Because the incidence, severity, and fatality of pertussis decreases with age, routine pertussis vaccination is not generally needed or recommended for persons 7 years of age or older.

Table 9-4 Recommended Use of Tetanus Toxoid and Tetanus Immune Globulin (Human)—TIG—in Wound Management

Type of Wound*	Immunization Status
Unimmunized, Uncertain, or Incomplete (one or two doses of toxoid)	
Low-risk wound	One dose of TD† or DT‡ followed by completion of immunization; booster every 10 yr thereafter
Tetanus-prone wounds and wounds neglected for > 24 h	One dose of Td† or DT‡ plus 250–500 U TIG followed by completion of immunization.§
Full Primary Immunization with Booster Dose within 10 Yr of Wound	
Low-risk wounds	No toxoid necessary
Tetanus-prone wounds	If > 5 yr since last dose, one dose of Td;† > 5 yr, no toxoid necessary
Wound neglected > 24 h	One dose of Td plus 250–500 U TIG
Full Primary Immunization with No Booster Doses or Last Booster Dose > 10 Yr	
Low-risk wounds	One dose of Td
Tetanus-prone wounds	One dose of Td
Wounds neglected > 24 h	One dose of Td plus 250–500 U TIG

*Wound definition—It is impossible to categorize all clinical situations by a terminology. In this scheme "tetanus-prone" refers to wounds which yield anaerobic conditions or were incurred in circumstances yielding the probability of exposure to tetanus spores. Examples include severe necrotizing machinery injuries, puncture wounds, wounds heavily contaminated with animal excreta, and so forth. All others are to be considered low-risk from the standpoint of tetanus. Neglected wounds are at greater risk.

†Td—(adult) should be used in individuals more than 6 yr old.

‡DT—(pediatric) should be used in individuals less than 6 yr old.

§Use separate syringe and sites for TIG and toxoid.

Source: Report of the Committee on the Control of Infectious Diseases. *Red book.* Evanston, Ill.: American Academy of Pediatrics, 1977, p. 283.

TRIVALENT ORAL POLIO VACCINE (TOPV-SABIN)

Poliovirus vaccines have dramatically reduced the incidence of paralytic poliomyelitis in the United States. Live attenuated oral poliovirus vaccine (TOPV) is preferable to inactive poliomyelitis vaccine (IPV), because it produces an immune response equivalent to that induced by natural poliovirus infection. It is simple to administer, well accepted by the client, and it does not require booster doses. The first dose of TOPV is commonly given to infants at the same time as the first dose of DTP. The vaccine usually has no side effects; however, in rare instances oral polio vaccine has been associated temporarily with paralytic disease in healthy recipients or their close contacts. Although the risk of vaccine-associated paralysis is extremely small (1 in 9 million), the benefits and risk of the vaccine should be stated so that vaccination is carried out among persons who are fully informed.

MEASLES VACCINE

Measles is often a severe disease with frequent complications. One successful inoculation with live attenuated measles virus vaccine confers lifelong protection against the disease. Measles vaccine produces a mild, noncommunicable infection. About 15 percent of vaccinated children have fever beginning about 6 days after vaccination and lasting up to 5 days. Transient atypical rashes have been reported, and subacute sclerosing encephalopathy has occurred, though rarely, following vaccination. Live measles virus vaccine should be given to all children over 15 months of age unless documented evidence of the disease exists, to children who have been immunized against measles with either gamma globulin or inactivated measles vaccines, and to children who were immunized before 15 months of age with live measles virus vaccine. Live measles vaccine may be given as early as 6 to 9 months of age if exposure of the infant is probable. A second dose is given after 15 months of age.

MUMPS VACCINE

Live attenuated mumps virus vaccine is recommended for all susceptible children and especially for preadolescent males and men who have not had the disease. The vaccine produces a subclinical, noncommunicable infection without any adverse side effects. One inoculation is protective and long-lasting. Mumps virus vaccine is available alone or in combination with measles and rubella vaccines and should be given at 15 months.

RUBELLA VACCINE

The principal objective of rubella (German measles) control is preventing infection of the fetus and the congenital rubella syndrome. This can best be achieved by eliminating the transmission of the virus among children, who are the major source of infection for pregnant women. All children between 15 months of age and puberty should receive the live rubella virus vaccine. It is not recommended for younger infants because of possible interference in active antibody formation by persisting maternal rubella antibody. Side effects from the vaccine include rash and lymphadenopathy. Transient pain in the small peripheral joints has been noted in up to 5 percent of vaccinated children. Children of pregnant women may be given rubella vaccine, since the vaccine virus is noncommunicable. However, immunization with live virus vaccine during pregnancy should be *avoided* because of the possible risk to the fetus.

RECORD KEEPING

A continuous written record of the type of protection the child has received and the dates of administration should be given to the parent(s). The date and time of the next appointment should be clearly understood. It is also important to record all immunizations received on the client's hospital record or clinic folder. Immunization status should be reviewed at the time of each health assessment, illness, or injury.

PASSIVE IMMUNIZATION

Immune serum globulin (ISG), commonly known as gamma globulin, is an antibody-rich fraction of pooled plasma from donors who have desired plasma levels of antibodies. It confers temporary immunity that is attained in approximately 2 days and lasts from 2 to 6 weeks. ISG should be administered immediately upon exposure. It is a viscous solution which must be given intramuscularly with an 18- or 20-gauge needle. A large dose should be divided and given at two different sites.

ISG is limited in supply and has been clearly documented to be of value in (1) prevention or modification of measles, (2) prevention or modification of viral hepatitis type A (HAV), (3) viral hepatitis type B (HBV) prevention when hepatitis B virus immune globulin is indicated but not available, and (4) treatment of certain antibody deficiency diseases.

Special human immune globulins are available (in limited supply) and are useful in several disorders in which ISG is of no value. Specific human immune globulins are derived from the sera of hyperimmunized persons or from individuals convalescing from specific infections. The following preparations have documented proven value.

Several other preparations of human immune globulin are available, but these are of unproven value or are under investigation.

Human Immune Serum Globulin	*Purpose*
Tetanus Immune Globulin (TIG)	Prophylaxis and treatment of tetanus
Rabies Immune Globulin (RIG)	Prophylaxis of rabies after exposure
Zoster Immune Globulin (ZIG)	Prophylaxis or modification of varicella-zoster infection of high-risk susceptible children
Hepatitis B Immune Globulin (HBIG)	Prophylaxis for accidental parenteral exposure to hepatitis B or intimate contact with infected person

references

Benenson, A. (ed.). *Control of communicable diseases in man* (12th ed.). Washington, D.C.: American Public Health Association, 1975.

Fannin, S. L. Immunization Practice. In S. S. Gellis and B. M. Kagan (eds.), *Current pediatric therapy* (8th ed.). Philadelphia: Saunders, 1978, pp. 668–674.

Krugman, S., Ward, R., and Katz, S. L. *Infectious diseases of children* (6th ed.). St. Louis: Mosby, 1977, pp. 481–514.

Steigman, A. J. (ed.). *Report of the committee on infectious diseases* (18th ed.). The American Academy of Pediatrics, 1977, pp. 1–34; 282–285.

Accident Prevention

THERESA M. ELDRIDGE

Table 9-5 Safety Tips to Remember for Prevention of Accidental Poisoning

Young children will eat and drink almost anything—keep all liquid and solids that may be poisonous out of their reach.

Of all cases of accidental poisoning 90% involve children under 5 yr of age.

The following are the most commonly ingested items
- Aspirin (most common cause of accidental poisoning)
- Soaps, detergents, cleaners
- Plants
- Vitamins
- Antihistamines and cold medicines
- Disinfectants and deodorizers
- Miscellaneous medicines
- Perfume and toilet water

Most accidents (up to 90%) are preventable.

Keep all medicines and hazardous products locked away when not in use.

Never call medicine "candy."

Table 9-5 Safety Tips to Remember for Prevention of Accidental Poisoning (*continued*)

Keep all products in original containers.

Read labels on all household products and medicines and follow directions carefully.

Destroy old products.

Keep foods and household products separated.

Always turn on the lights when giving or taking medicine.

Since children imitate adults, avoid taking medicines in their presence.

Use safety closures on as many products as possible, but realize that children may still be able to open them.

Keep a bottle of syrup of ipecac for each child and Epsom salts at home. Do not use unless instructed by a physician or poison center.

Accidental poisonings often occur when the usual household routine is upset (e.g., holidays, relatives or friends visiting, a new baby at home, a family move).

Holidays often present special poisoning problems. Christmas ornaments, such as lights, bulbs, tinsel, "snow," angel hair, etc., may cause injury or contain poisonous materials. Christmas plants such as poinsettia, holly, mistletoe, and Christmas greens may be harmful if swallowed.

Remember that many poisonings occur in the homes of babysitters, relatives, and friends, so help them "poison-proof" their homes.

Utilize safety stickers on poisonous items and teach children to recognize and avoid items with safety stickers. (Stickers can be obtained from local poison centers.)

Keep the telephone numbers of the family doctor, poison center, hospital, police, and fire department near the telephone.

Table 9-6 Checklist for Poison-Proofing at Home

Area of House	Recommendations	Check Here
Kitchen	No medicines on counters, open areas, refrigerator top, or windowsills	☐
	All cleaners, household products, and medications locked away or out of reach	☐
	No household products under the sink	☐
	All medicines, cleaners, and household products in original, safety-top containers	☐
Bathroom	All medicines in original safety-top containers	☐
	Medicine chest cleaned out routinely	☐
	All old medications flushed down toilet	☐
	All medicines, powders, sprays, cosmetics, hair-care products, mouthwash locked in medicine chest or out of reach	☐
Bedroom	No medicines in or on dresser or bedside table	☐
	All perfumes, cosmetics, etc., out of reach	☐
Laundry Area	All products in original containers	☐
	All bleaches, soaps, detergents, fabric softeners, etc., out of reach or locked away	☐
Garage/ Basement	Insect sprays and weed killers locked up	☐
	Gasoline and car products locked up	☐
	Paints, turpentine, paint products locked up	☐
	All products in original containers	☐
	All gardening and workshop tools out of reach or locked up	☐

Table 9-6 Checklist for Poison-Proofing at Home (*continued*)

Area of House	Recommendations	Check Here
General Household	Plants out of reach	☐
	Alcoholic beverages out of reach	☐
	Paint in good repair	☐
	Ashtrays empty and out of reach	☐
	Purses out of reach	☐
	All household and personal products out of reach	☐
Backyard	Poisonous plants fenced off	☐
	All gardening tools, pesticides, seeds, bulbs, etc., locked up	☐
	Charcoal lighter fluid and charcoal brickettes locked up	☐

Source: Adapted from Rocky Mountain Poison Center, *Checklist for poison-proofing your home.* Denver: Author, West Eighth and Cherokee, 80204, September 1978.

Table 9-7 First Aid for Poisoning

Always keep syrup of ipecac and Epsom salts at home. Ipecac causes vomiting, and Epsom salts is used as a laxative. They are sometimes used when poisons are swallowed. DO NOT use them unless the poison center or family physician has given instructions to do so.

Inhaled Poisons

If gas, fumes, or smoke have been inhaled, immediately drag or carry client to fresh air. Contact the poison center or physician.

Poisons on the Skin

If the poison has been spilled on the skin or clothing, remove clothing. Flush the involved skin areas with water for 2–3 min. Then wash gently with soap and water and rinse. Contact the poison center.

Swallowed Poisons

If *any* poison has been swallowed and the client is awake and can swallow, give the client water or milk *only* to drink. Contact the poison center or physician. *Caution:* Antidote labels on products may be incorrect. DO NOT give salt, vinegar, or lemon juice.

Poisons in the Eyes

If the poison is in the eye, flush the eye with lukewarm water from a pitcher. Hold the pitcher 1–2 in from the eye and flush the eye for 15 min. Contact the poison center.

Plant Poisons

If poisonous plants are swallowed or chewed, give one to two glasses of milk or water (if person is conscious and can swallow). Then contact poison center. For skin contact with a poisonous plant, gently wash the skin with soap and water and rinse thoroughly. Contact the poison center.

Source: Adapted from Rocky Mountain Poison Center, *First aid for poisoning.* West Eighth and Cherokee, Denver 80204, 1978.

Table 9-8 Parents' Quiz for Accident Prevention

Most serious accidents can be prevented. Parents should ask themselves these questions and take appropriate preventative measures when necessary to avoid injuries to their child.

Your Habits: do you . . .

Always have your child safely buckled in when you are driving with him or her in the car?

Put medicine away in a child-proof place after use?

Place the baby's high chair or playpen well away from stove and kitchen counters?

Turn pot and pan handles toward the back of the stove?

Keep matches and lighters away from small children?

Keep electric cords out of the reach of infants and toddlers?

Consider flammability when purchasing clothing and toys?

Make sure the baby's toys are too big to swallow?

Keep tiny things—buttons, pins, tacks, etc.—away from infants and toddlers?

Store knives and scissors well out of reach of young children?

Table 9-8 Parents' Quiz for Accident Prevention *(continued)*

Stay with your preschool child when he or she is in the bathtub or wading pool?

Have smoke alarms installed in your home?

Your Home: do you . . .

Keep potential poisons and flammable substances locked away from young children?

Have gates at stairways to keep baby or toddler from falling?

Light stairwells?

Fit stairs with treads and handrails?

Anchor scatter rugs so they won't slip?

Screen or bar high windows to keep children from falling?

Keep the telephone number of the poison control center next to your phone?

Lock or latch doors that lead to danger for a toddler?

Put dummy plugs into unused electric outlets?

Keep electric cords in good condition?

Dispose of any combustible litter in your attic and basement?

Use flame-retardant fabrics for home furnishings?

Lock up firearms?

Source: Adapted from *Your Child's Safety,* Metropolitan Life Insurance Company, New York, *Pediatric Annals* **6**:11 (1977).

Table 9-9 Car Safety for Children

In 1975, 57,000 children were injured in car crashes and 917 children under 5 yr of age were killed (National Safety Council).

A child seated on an adult's lap is not protected during a car crash; the forces generated in a crash multiply the child's weight 10 to 20 times, causing the child to be propelled into the dashboard or windshield.

Car safety belts are not safe for children who weigh less than 40 lb (abdominal injuries could result).

Children less than 55 in tall should not wear a shoulder strap (neck injuries could result).

The center of the rear seat is the safest place for a child to ride.

A safety restraint should be used every time the child is in the car. (Newborns should ride home in a safe car-restraint device, not in mother's arms.)

A car-restraint device that faces the rear or side is recommended for infants.

Car-restraint devices that have an anchoring tether are considered to be superior.

Children who can sit up without support can use one of three devices: the protective shield, the car seat with harness, or the safety harness.

Source: Adapted from Car safety restraints for children. *Consumer Reports,* **42**(6):314–317 (1977).

Table 9-10 Recommended Car Safety Restraints for Children

Restraint	For Children	Approximate Cost	Restraint	For Children	Approximate Cost
Strolee Wee Care car seat	18–43 lb 30–42 in	$45	Swyngomatic American safety seat	20–40 lb up to 40 in	37
Century Motor Toter	15–40 lb up to 40 in	35	Toddy Tot Astroseat V	up to 40 lb 15–42 in	30
GM Love Seat	20–40 lb up to 40 in	38			

Source: Adapted from Car safety restraints for children. *Consumer Reports,* **42**(6):314–317 (1977).

Table 9-11 Typical Accidents/Prevention and Normal Developmental Behavior in Childhood

Developmental Behavior	Death	Prevention
	Birth through 5 Mo	
Newborn Newborn sleeps a great deal and does little else except eat and cry Head flops, needs support Infant wriggles a lot	Falls	Never leave child unattended at any time. Carry baby firmly. Utilize car safety restraint device. Keep crib rails up when infant is in crib.

Table 9-11 Typical Accidents/Prevention and Normal Developmental Behavior in Childhood (*continued*)

Developmental Behavior	Death	Prevention
	Birth through 5 Mo (continued)	
4 Mo Infant begins to hold a rattle and puts hands in mouth Infant sucks on everything Some children able to roll over at 4 mo Moves self by pushing with feet, and may flip over Average infant can roll from side to back or back to side, hold head erect, and reach for objects; retains grasped rattle *5 Mo* Infant can pick up a toy and roll over from stomach to back Oral investigation		Keep one hand on baby while changing or reaching for equipment. Don't sit a child in an infant seat on the table or counter.
	Burns	Keep child's exposure to sun brief. Install smoke alarms. Keep child away from stove and work counters. Don't smoke or drink hot liquids while holding a baby. Use nonflammable rattles and toys. Use flame-retardant clothes. Check bath water temperature carefully before bathing baby.
	Suffocation Foreign body aspiration Inhalation/ingestion	Don't prop the baby bottle. Make sure furniture and toys are finished with lead-free paint. Keep dangerous objects out of reach (e.g., buttons, pins, beads, sharp objects, razor blades, knives, hairpins). Use firm mattress with no pillow to prevent suffocation. Crib and playpen slats should be no more than 2⅜ in apart and mattress should fit crib snugly. Keep crib free of flimsy plastics, zippered bags, pens, and plastic bags. Toys should be too big to fit in the mouth with parts that cannot be broken or removed. Toys should be tough with no sharp edges or points. Educate siblings regarding food, toys, and handling baby. Turn head to side and down when vomiting. Avoid easily aspirated foods or toys.
	Drowning	Never leave child alone in tub or sink.
	6 through 11 Mo	
6 Mo Sits with support Rolls over back to stomach and vice versa Reaches for and grasps objects Imitates *7 Mo* Sits alone	Falls	See Birth through 5 Mo above. Child still requires full-time protection. Accidents are more frequent because baby can move and grasp more. Never leave child alone on high surface or in high chair. Put gate across bottom and top of stairs.

Table 9-11 Typical Accidents/Prevention and Normal Developmental Behavior in Childhood (*continued*)

Developmental Behavior	Death	Prevention
	6 through 11 Mo (continued)	
Pushes self to hand-knee creeping position May be teething and chewing on everything Oral exploration of all objects		Remove easily-turned-over lamps and furniture.
	Burns	See Birth through 5 Mo.
8 Mo Looks for toys that have fallen from sight		Keep high chair and playpen away from cords, appliances, and stoves.
9 Mo Pulls self to knees, then to standing position Stands fairly steadily while holding onto support		Place guards around fireplaces, registers, floor furnaces, and open hearths.
		Put safety caps over electric outlets.
		Keep electric cords out of reach.
		Keep faucets out of reach.
10 Mo Is able to stand without support occasionally and walks fairly well holding onto support		Turn pot handles in.
		Don't let child play in kitchen during meal preparation.
11 Mo Stands alone but only for short periods	Suffocation	See Birth through 5 Mo.
	Foreign body aspiration Inhalation/ingestion	All poisonous materials and medicines should be locked up.
General Perfects crawling and begins walking and standing Child scares quickly Begins to climb, pulls self up and everything else down Opens drawers, cupboards, bottles, and packages		Keep foods that may choke baby out of reach (popcorn, nuts, hard candy, raw carrots, celery).
		Have syrup of ipecac and Epsom salts at home.
		Have poison center number by telephone.
	Drowning	Keep pails, pans, or tubs of water off floor so baby won't fall in them.
		Don't leave child alone or with sibling in charge of infant in bath or swimming.
	12 through 35 Mo	
12 Mo Pulls self to stand Cruises Holds cup, uses spoon May begin to walk alone	Falls	See 6 through 11 Mo.
	Cuts and lacerations	Sharp objects are an increased danger (scissors, pencils, razor blades, knives, tools).
15 Mo Walks alone Stoops to pick up objects Rolls or tosses ball Drinks from cup with little spilling		Teach child not to approach strange animals.
		Keep screens on windows, doors locked or latched, high above child's head.
		Keep garage locked and tools out of reach.
18 Mo Walks well alone Runs Climbs downstairs Uses spoon, spilling little Can turn doorknob		Never leave child alone in the car or house.
		Keep child in fenced yard.
	Burns	See 6 through 11 Mo.
		Teach child the meaning of "hot."

Table 9-11 Typical Accidents/Prevention and Normal Developmental Behavior in Childhood (*continued*)

Developmental Behavior	Death	Prevention
	12 through 35 Mo (continued)	
General Continual exploration of environment, inside and outside Imitates household tasks Has basic language development Insists on doing everything for self Often tests parent to see if limits are set and kept Critical period—Time for complete protection is past and teaching begins		Keep child away from fireplace. Teach child not to play with matches.
	Suffocation Foreign body aspiration Inhalation/ingestion	See 6 through 11 Mo. Keep houseplants and plants outdoors out of reach; many are poisonous. No area is safe from the climbing toddler; lock up all poisons or hazardous substances. Teach child not to run or walk with mouth full of food.
	Motor vehicle	Keep child away from street and driveway.
	Drowning	See 6 through 11 Mo. Never leave child alone during bathing or swimming. Be sure to empty wading pool. Child should be taught basic swimming and survival techniques. All swimming pools should be enclosed by a fence with a gate that locks.
	3 through 5 Yr	
3 Yr Jumps, pedals a tricycle Washes and dries hands Helps dress and undress self Able to understand 90% of speech Toilet trained *4 Yr* Can throw a ball overhand Buttons clothes Broad jumps Plays games with other children Runs, skips *5 Yr* Can dress and undress self Hops, can catch a ball	Falls Cuts and lacerations	See 12 through 35 Mo. Use safety glass on house, doors, shower doors. Use adhesive strips on bathtub. Keep stairways and play areas well lighted. Teach child how to handle scissors and knives.
	Burns	See 12 through 35 Mo. Teach child not to run if clothes catch fire, but to drop to the ground and roll until fire is out.
	Suffocation Foreign body inspiration Inhalation/ingestion	See 12 through 35 Mo. Child still needs supervision regarding poisons, but is past oral stage and learning limits of what can and cannot be played with. Never allow child to run or walk while eating. Continue to keep nuts, popcorn, and hard candy out of reach until 4 or 5 yr old. Check neighborhood for ditches,

Table 9-11 Typical Accidents/Prevention and Normal Developmental Behavior in Childhood (*continued*)

Developmental Behavior	Death	Prevention
	3 through 5 Yr (continued)	
		abandoned refrigerators, and ice chests.
	Motor vehicle	Instruct child in safety and pedestrian safety; wear white at night. Never allow playing near garage, driveway, or street. Teach child to refuse rides with strangers. Child should learn his or her full name, address, and phone number.
	Firearms	Keep firearms locked up. Teach child the danger of weapons and instruct never to play with them. Never keep a loaded weapon in the car or at home.
	Drowning	See 12 through 35 Mo. Continue close supervision of bathing and swimming.
	6 through 11 Yr	
General Most children have basic motor skills for running, jumping, throwing, catching, and balancing Physical growth slowed down Plays games such as tag, hide-and-seek Balancing and coordination important for hopscotch, gymnastics, jump rope, bicycling, and skating Cooperative play—baseball, tag Involved outside of home, such as time spent in school Increased independence Likes crafts, projects, and experimentation Young, school-age child clumsy Increased interest in sports, groups Children continuing to imitate parents and other adults Daring, adventurous, wanders away from home Likes to climb fences and trees Impulsive Full of energy	Motor Vehicle	See 3 through 5 Yr. Teach bike safety, emphasize avoidance of street play. Teach rules of the road, traffic signals and respect for traffic officers.
	Drowning	See 3 through 5 Yr. Teach child rules of water safety. Don't play in drainage ditch. Don't swim alone. Teach boating safety rules. Supervise ice skating and other water sports.
	Injuries/fractures Suffocation	See 3 through 5 Yr. Check yard for rusty nails and glass. Encourage children to wear shoes when playing outside. Advise parents of hazards for schoolchildren associated with sports. Teach child safety precautions, not to take chances. Give child sense of confidence and responsibility. Teach child to use kitchen implements, machines (sewing machine) correctly.

Table 9-11 Typical Accidents/Prevention and Normal Developmental Behavior in Childhood (*continued*)

Developmental Behavior	Death	Prevention
	6 through 11 Yr (continued)	
		Teach safe use of tools. Teach rules of sport and proper use and maintenance of equipment. Teach hazards of playing in excavations, old refrigerators, and deserted buildings.
	Burns	See 3 through 5 Yr. Use approved electrical toys UL (Underwriters' Laboratory). Use electrical toys under supervision. Avoid conductive kites. Supervise and teach appropriate use of matches, fires, and flammable chemicals.
	Firearms	See 3 through 5 Yr. Teach child respect for weapons. Never keep loaded weapons in the house. Don't buy firearms as gifts unless child is responsible enough to handle under close supervision.
	Inhalation/ingestion	Infrequent in this age group, but continue supervision. Child still needs reinforcement and teaching—needs to know why.
	12 through 18 Yr	
General Many physical changes and rapid growth Large muscles develop faster than small muscles; poor posture, increased clumsiness, decreased coordination Development of secondary sex characteristics Increased interest in extracurricular activities	Motor Vehicle	See 6 through 11 Yr. Have child take driver's education. Involve child in decision making regarding rules of car use. Encourage child to use responsibilities and freedom wisely. Instruct child in safety for motorscooters, motorcycles, and minibikes.
Varying degree of physical activities Increased mobility High imaginative and creative thinking Adolescents mind at point of greatest ability to acquire and utilize knowledge	Injuries/fractures	See 6 through 11 Yr. Encourage proper use of equipment and safety regulations for sports. Advise about consequences of sport injuries.
Able to problem-solve Activities include sports, dating, hobbies, dancing, and daydreaming Mood swings	Drowning	Instruct in emergency care procedures. Instruct in water safety, routine safety practices.
Increased freedom and independence	Firearms	See 6 through 11 Yr.

Table 9-11 Typical Accidents/Prevention and Normal Developmental Behavior in Childhood (*continued*)

Developmental Behavior	Death	Prevention
	12 through 18 Yr (continued)	
May get a job Learns to drive Develops adult characteristics	Inhalation/ingestion	Drug abuse prevention—give adolescent freedom to make decisions while providing information for an adequate knowledge base. Provide healthy influence for adolescent. Provide appropriate role model.

Table 9-12 Mortality from Leading Types of Accidents at Ages under 1 Year in the United States, 1972–73

Type of Accident	Average Annual Death Rate Per 100,000 Live Births		
	Both Sexes	Males	Females
Accidents—all types	54.3	61.7	46.5
Inhalation and ingestion of food and other objects	16.1	19.2	12.7
Mechanical suffocation	11.6	13.3	9.8
Motor vehicle	9.8	10.0	9.5
Fires and flames	4.8	4.8	4.7
Falls	3.3	4.2	2.2
Drowning*	2.1	2.5	1.8
All other	6.6	7.7	5.8

*Exclusive of deaths in water transportation.

Source of basic data: Reports of the Division of Vital Statistics, National Center for Health Statistics Adapted from *Statistical Bulletin,* Metropolitan Life, **56** (1975) ; *Pediatric Annals,* **6**:11 (1977).

Table 9-13 Mortality from Leading Types of Accidents Among Children Aged 1 to 4 in the United States, 1972–73

Type of Accident	Average Annual Death Rate per 100,000									
	Boys at Ages					Girls at Ages				
	1–4	1	2	3	4	1–4	1	2	3	4
Accidents—all types	38.0	44.5	40.7	36.5	30.1	25.4	32.9	27.9	21.9	18.9
Motor vehicle	13.6	12.7	13.3	14.7	13.9	10.2	10.8	11.2	9.3	9.4
Pedestrian (in traffic accidents)	6.5	3.6	6.3	7.9	8.3	3.2	2.3	3.5	3.6	4.0
Drowning*	8.3	8.8	10.2	8.4	5.6	3.6	5.1	4.6	2.8	1.8
Fire and flames	5.6	5.8	7.1	5.5	4.1	4.6	4.9	5.1	4.2	3.9
Inhalation and ingestion of food or other objects	1.8	4.1	1.8	0.9	0.5	1.4	3.2	1.2	0.7	0.6
Poisoning	1.6	3.8	1.4	0.9	0.5	1.1	2.4	1.2	0.6	0.3
Falls	1.5	2.8	1.4	1.2	0.8	1.2	2.1	1.0	1.1	0.5
Firearm missile	0.7	0.4	0.8	0.7	1.1	0.4	0.2	0.4	0.7	0.4
Accidental deaths as a percentage of all deaths	42%	34%	44%	49%	49%	36%	30%	38%	40%	41%

*Exclusive of deaths in water transportation.

Source of basic data: Reports of the Division of Vital Statistics, National Center for Health Statistics Adapted from *Statistical Bulletin,* Metropolitan Life, **56** (1975); *Pediatric Annals* **6**:11 (1977).

Table 9-14 Mortality from Leading Types of Accidents Among Children Ages 5 to 14 in the United States, 1972–1973

	Average Annual Death Rate per 100,000					
	Boys at Ages			Girl at Ages		
Type of Accident	5–9	5–14	10–14	5–9	5–14	10–14
Accidents—all types	25.9	27.8	29.5	15.0	13.4	12.1
Motor vehicle	13.1	13.3	13.5	8.9	7.9	7.1
Pedestrian (in traffic accidents)	7.3	5.2	3.3	4.7	3.3	2.1
Drowning*	5.2	5.6	6.0	1.5	1.5	1.4
Firearm missile	1.1	1.9	2.7	0.4	0.4	0.3
Fires and flames	2.1	1.5	0.9	2.1	1.5	1.0
Falls	0.6	0.6	0.7	0.3	0.2	0.2
Water transport	0.4	0.5	0.6	0.1	0.1	0.2
All other	3.4	4.4	5.1	1.7	1.8	1.9
Accidental deaths as a percentage of all deaths	54%	56%	58%	43%	42%	41%
Motor-vehicle accident deaths as a percentage of all accidental deaths	51%	48%	46%	59%	59%	59%

*Exclusive of deaths in water transportation.

Source of basic data: Reports of the Division of Vital Statistics, National Center for Health Statistics, *Pediatric Annals* **6**:11 (1977).

bibliography

American Academy of Pediatrics Accident Prevention Committee. *Poisoning prevention.* Evanston, Ill.: Author, 1960.

American Academy of Pediatrics Accident Prevention Committee. *Protect Your Baby Birth to Four Months.* Evanston, Ill.: Author, 1960.

American Academy of Pediatrics Accident Prevention Committee. *Protect Your Baby 4–7 Months.* Evanston, Ill.: Author, 1960.

American Academy of Pediatrics Accident Prevention Committee. *Protect Your Baby 7–12 Months.* Evanston, Ill.: Author, 1960.

American Academy of Pediatrics Accident Prevention Committee. *Protect Your Child 1 to 2 Years.* Evanston, Ill.: Author, 1960.

American Academy of Pediatrics Accident Prevention Committee. *Keep Your Child Safe 2 to 3 Years.* Evanston, Ill.: Author, 1960.

American Academy of Pediatrics Accident Prevention Committee. *Teach Your Child to be Safe 3 to 6 Years.* Evanston, Ill.: Author, 1960.

Arena, Jay M. *Your child and household safety.* Chemical Specialties Manufacturers Association, 50 East 41st Street, New York, NY 10017, 1970.

Borgner, Lawrence, et al. Falls from heights: A childhood epidemic in an urban area. *American Journal of Public Health,* **61**(1):90–95 (1971).

Brazelton, T. Berry. Infants and mothers—Differences in development. New York: Dell, 1969.

Brown, Marie Scott, and Murphy, Mary Alexander, *Ambulatory pediatrics for nursing.* New York: McGraw-Hill, 1975.

Colorado Department of Public Health, *Safe Toys.*

Car safety restraints for children. *Consumer Reports,* **42**(6):314–317 (1977).

Dennis, James M., and Kaiser, Albert D. Are home accidents in children preventable? *Pediatrics,* **13**:568 (1954).

Dietrich, Harry F. Accidents are preventable. *Journal of the American Medical Association,* **144**: 1175–1179 (1950).

Dietrich, Harry F. Prevention of childhood accidents—What are we waiting for? *Journal of the American Medical Association,* **156**:929–931 (1954).

Dishon, Callen. Fireproofing our children. *Today's Health,* **49**(1):39–41, 71 (1971).

Gerber Baby Foods, *A Handbook of Child Safety,* Birk & Company, Inc., 1967.

Hadden, William Jr., et al. *Accident research—Methods and approaches.* New York: Harper & Row, 1964.

Haggerty, Robert J. Home accidents in childhood. *New England Medical Journal,* **260**:1322 (1959).

Halsey, Maxwell N. *Accident prevention—The role of*

physicians and public health workers. New York: McGraw-Hill, 1961.

Harper, Paul. *Preventive pediatrics child health & development.* New York: Appleton-Century-Crofts, 1962.

Huntington, Dorothy J., et al. *Day care, serving infants 2,* 1972. Department of Health, Education, and Welfare, Office of Child Development, Superintendent of Documents, U.S. Government Printing Office, Washington, DC 20402.

Illingworth, R. S. *The development of the infant and young child, normal and abnormal.* Baltimore: Williams and Witkins, 1972.

Jacobinzer, Harold. Accidents, a major child health problem. *Journal of Pediatrics,* **46**:419–420 (1955).

Jacobs, Herbert H. *Behavioral approaches to accident research,* New York: Association for the Aid of Crippled Children, 1961.

Krogman, Welton M. *The manual of oral strengths of american white and negro children ages 3–6 years.* The Closure Committee of Glass Container Manufacturers Institute, New York, NY, 1971.

McFarland, Ross A. Epidemic logic principles applicable to the study and prevention of childhood accidents, *American Journal of Public Health,* **35**:1302–1308 (1955).

Metropolitan Life, *Your Child's Safety,* Metropolitan Life Insurance Co., 1970.

Meyer, Roger, et al. Accidental injury to the preschool child. *Journal of Pediatrics,* **63**:95–105 (1963).

Smart, Mollie S., and Smart, Russell. *Children—development and relationships,* New York: Macmillan, 1977.

U.S. Dept. of Health, Education, and Welfare, Office of Child Development. *Infant Care.* Washington: Author, 1973.

Wheatley, George M. (guest ed.). Childhood accidents: prevention and treatment. *Pediatric Annals,* **6**(11): 1–119 (1977).

Wheatley, George M. Prevention of accidents in childhood. *Advances in Pediatrics,* **8**:191–215 (1956).

World Health Organization. *Accidents in Children—Facts as Basis,* pp. 1–40, 1957.

Resources for safety literature

A handbook of child safety, Gerber Baby Foods, Freemont, MI (free).

A safe home for your children, Mead Johnson & Co., Evansville, IN 47721 (1972).

Consumer Product Safety Commission, Washington, DC 20207.

Hendrin, David, *Save your child's life.* Interprise Publications, 230 Park Avenue, New York, NY 10017. (An excellent book to have.)

Arena, Jay M., *Your child and household safety,* Chemical Specialties Manufacturer's Association, 50 East 41st, St., New York, NY 10017 (cost unknown).

Your child's safety, Metropolitan Life Insurance Company. Ask local agency. (cost unknown).

National Safety Council, 425 N. Michigan Avenue, Chicago, IL 60611. Several pamphlets available—write for list.

Office of Child Development, U.S. Dept. of Health, Education, and Welfare, Superintendent of Documents, U.S. Government Printing Office, Washington, DC 20402. Write for list. (Minimal cost—15 to 25¢)

State public health department. Several free pamphlets—call or visit their office.

Nutritional Assessment

JANE A. FOX/CHARLOTTE CRAM ELSBERRY

ALERT

1. Poor suck
2. Inappropriate weight gain
3. Signs of dehydration (poor skin turgor, sunken fontanels, etc.)
4. Infants who tire easily, change color, or consistently choke during feeding
5. Tremors
6. Infant not interested in eating
7. Signs of intolerance to a specific food
   a. Vomiting/regurgitation
   b. Diarrhea
   c. Nonconsolable and fretful infant
8. Skin rashes
9. Change in voiding or stool pattern
10. Infants/children who consume less than 16 oz or more than 32 oz of milk per day
11. Parent(s) or care giver who voices concerns

or doubts about feeding methods or nutritional well-being of infant/child
12. Parent(s) or care giver who indicates difficulty in adjusting to feeding demands
13. Infants/children with physical handicaps which affect their ability to ingest food
14. Infants/children who refuse an entire food group

I. Nutrition History—Subjective Data

A. Age

B. Concerns of parent(s)/client

C. Infant

1. Type of feeding method
2. Formula feeding
   a. Type of formula used
   b. How prepared; e.g., can rinsed or not, clean can opener
   c. When formula was started
   d. Other formulas used
   e. Number of bottles and oz consumed in 24/h period
   f. Frequency of feeding
   g. Length of time for bottle to be finished
3. Breast-feeding
   a. Length of time at each breast per feeding
   b. Number of times nursed per day
   c. Diet, medication, and fluid history of mother
   d. Problems with breasts (e.g., cracked nipples, engorgement, abscess)
   e. Notice of milk letdown in mother
4. Other fluids fed
5. Solid foods
   a. Frequency
   b. Type
   c. When introduced
6. Person(s) besides mother who feeds baby
7. Nighttime nutrition
8. Satisfaction with feeding method
9. Use of pacifier/thumbsucking
10. Baby's activity pattern after feeding
11. Siblings, other parent, and significant other's response during feeding
12. Response of parent(s) or care giver to self-feeding and inevitable mess
13. Response of parent(s) to the baby's response as new foods are introduced

D. Toddler, preschooler, adolescent, and young adult

1. Number of meals eaten per day
2. Method of feeding
3. Number of ounces of milk per day
4. Snacking habits
5. Food preferences and dislikes
6. Who plans, shops, and cooks food
7. Amount of money available for food
8. School breakfast and/or lunch
9. Other food programs, e.g., food stamps
10. Dietary recall for previous 24 hours
11. Last dental visit
12. Developmental level of behavioral eating characteristics

E. Birth weight

F. Developmental history: participation in feeding, age of weaning, pica

G. Elimination pattern, also after eating

H. Vitamin/fluoride preparations

I. Chronic problems

J. Allergies

K. Activity level

L. Sleep pattern

M. Family history

1. High blood pressure
2. Strokes
3. Heart problems
4. Diabetes
5. Obesity
6 Hyperlipidemias
7. Allergies
8. Anorexia Nervosa

II. Objective Data

A. Physical examination

1. A complete physical examination should be done on all infants.
2. The following areas should be assessed to determine nutritional status.
   a. Observe general appearance.
   b. Record height, weight, and head circumference and plot on graph.
   c. Note skin color, turgor, and subcutaneous fat.
   d. Inspect hair for luster, and inspect and palpate scalp.
   e. Inspect and palpate fontanels (infants).
   f. Inspect conjunctiva mucosa of eyes for paleness.
   g. Palpate thyroid for enlargement.
   h. Inspect mouth and teeth for caries; palpate gums, palate, and tongue.
   i. Inspect, auscultate, percuss, and palpate abdomen.
   j. Perform neurological examination appro-

priate to age: rooting and sucking reflex in infants, mental alertness, deep tendon reflexes.

k. Inspect stool, if possible.
l. Measure fat folds if obesity is suspected to determine body-fat bulk.
   (1) Use Langes's caliper.
   (2) Obtain two measurements: left triceps (limb) and left subscapular (trunk).
   (3) For single measurements on adolescents, triceps are most reliable.
   (4) Reading is done to nearest ½ mm.
   (5) Arm should be relaxed and hanging by side.
   (6) Do two readings to ensure accuracy.
m. Measure mid-upper-arm circumference.
   (1) Estimates of arm soft-tissue may be useful in determining nutritional changes.
   (2) Use metal tape with 7- to 12-mm width.
   (3) Hold arm relaxed and straight by side.
   (4) Correct tape tension is critical; the tape must go around entire arm snuggly but cause *no* skin indentation.
n. Observe parent-child interaction and feeding (infants).

B. Laboratory Data
1. Hematocrit or hemoglobin (to detect anemia)
2. Cholesterol levels in adolescents and younger children at risk
3. Routine yearly urinalysis

III. Assessment (see Table 9-15)

Table 9-15 Physical Indications of Nutritional Status of the School-Aged Child

Physical Aspect	Well-Nourished Child	Malnourished Child	Deficiency
Height and Weight	Within growth norms—steady gain and increase from year to year	Above or below growth norms—failure to gain or excessive weight gain each year	Protein, calorie, other essential nutrients
Skin	Clear, smooth, elastic and firm	Rough, dry, scaly, xerosis	Vitamin A
	Reddish-pink mucous membranes	Petechiae, ecchymoses, poor wound healing	Vitamin C
		Depigmentation of skin	Protein, calorie
		Lesions	Riboflavin
		Dermatitis, sensitivity of skin to sunlight	Niacin
		Pallor	Vitamin B_{12}, iron, folacin
Musculoskeletal	Well-developed, erect posture	Head sags, winged scapula, bowed legs, costochondral beading, cranial bossing	Calcium, Vitamin D
	Shoulder blades flat		
	Arms and legs straight	Epiphyseal enlargement of wrists	Vitamins D, C
	Skull and jaw well developed		
	Firm muscles with good tonus	Small flabby muscles, muscle weakness	Phosphorus, protein
	Moderate amount of fat	Faulty epiphyseal bone formation	Vitamin A
		Pretibial edema bilateral	Protein, calorie, thiamine
Head	Hair—smooth, good amount, lustrous	Dull, dry, depigmented, abnormal texture, easily pluckable, thin	Protein, calorie
	Eyes—clear and bright	Dull with dark circles and	Vitamin A, riboflavin

Table 9-15 Physical Indications of Nutritional Status of the School-Aged Child (*continued*)

Physical Aspect	Well-Nourished Child	Malnourished Child	Deficiency
		hollows. Bitot's spots, conjunctivitis, xerosis, night blindness (nyctalopia), light sensitivity (photophobia)	
	Mouth—pink, moist lips; pink, firm gums; full set of teeth	Cracking and scaling lips, cheilosis, fissuring of mouth corners	Riboflavin
		Spongy, swollen gums, bleed easily (gingiva)	Vitamin C
		Irregular or missing teeth with cavities; defective tooth enamel	Vitamins D, A
		Glossitis	Folacin, B_{12}, niacin, iron
		Tongue fissuring	Niacin
Neck	Normal size	Enlarged thyroid	Iodine
		Enlarged parotids	Protein, calorie
Neurological		Listless	Protein, calorie
		Loss of ankle- and knee-jerk reflexes, motor weakness, sensory loss	Thiamine
		Headache	Niacin, thiamine
		Polyneuritis, motor weakness	Thiamine
Abdomen	Flat	Distended, protrudes, hepatomegaly	Protein, calorie
Cardiac	Normal heart size and sounds	Cardiac enlargement and tachycardia	Thiamine, potassium

Source: Pearson, Gayle A. Nutrition in the middle years of childhood. *The American Journal of Maternal Child Nursing,* **2**(6):383 (1977).

IV. Promotion of Nutritional Well-Being

A. Treatments/medications

1. Vitamins (see Table 9-16)
2. Iron supplementation (see Table 9-17 and Table 9-23 for Iron: Infant Requirements)
3. Fluoride (see "Dental Health," Chap. 9)
4. Well-balanced, nutritionally sound diet (see Tables 9-16 to 9-19)

B. Counselling/prevention

1. Counselling should begin during the prenatal period with discussion of adequate maternal nutrition and selection of infant feeding method (see Table 9-20). (The American Academy of Pediatrics recommends breast-feeding, but selection should be decided by the parent(s).)
   a. Initiate feeding method—breast (see Table 9-21), bottle (see Table 9-22).
   b. Discuss infant feeding concerns (see Table 9-23).
   c. Discuss breast and bottle feeding contraindications (see Table 9-24).
   d. If the infant is to be formula-fed, discuss different types of formulas (Table 9-26) and approximate costs.
2. Discuss with parent(s) feeding capabilities of child based on his or her developmental level.
3. Counsel on calories and nutrients required by growing children. Discuss which foods contain which nutrients (Tables 9-18 and 9-19).

4. When counselling parent(s) on diet, it is important to include personal preferences and cultural food habits of parent(s), as well as economic feasibility.
5. Nutritional education is a family affair and should involve the parent(s) and client as decision maker and allow and encourage questions.
6. Teach parent(s) label reading and offer guidance in selection of most nutritious foods for least amount of money.
7. If child is at risk, suggest keeping daily food record.
8. Discuss importance of adequate nutritional intake and problems which can develop from malnourishment (mention foods.)
9. Food should *never* be used as a reward or punishment.
10. Mealtime should be a pleasant time for family members.
11. Nutritional counselling is a continual process and should be a part of every school's curriculum.
12. The practitioner should encourage and participate in public education of healthy nutritional diets.
13. Anticipatory nutritional guidance should be provided (i.e., growth spurts).
14. For special nutritional concerns, see Table 9-25.

B. Follow-up

Well-child care—more visits if problem is suspected or if reassurance and guidance are needed.

C. Consultations/referrals

1. Local school authority
   a. National School Lunch Program, Summer Food Service Program, Special Milk Program
   b. School Breakfast Program
2. Food Stamp Program—local welfare department
3. Food Distribution Program
4. Supplemental Food Program for Women, Infants, and Children (WIC)
5. Dietitian
6. Refer to local LaLeche League if breast feeding:
   LaLeche League International, Inc.
   9616 Minneapolis Avenue
   Franklin Park, IL 60131
7. Nutritionist
8. Public health nurse for home evaluation

Table 9-16 Vitamin Requirements During Infancy and Amount Contained in Milk

	Vitamins									
	A, IU	C, mg	D, IU	K, μg	E, mg	B6, mg	Thiamine, mg	Riboflavin, mg	Niacin, mg	Folacin, μg
Recommended daily dietary	1400–2000	35	400	15	4–5	0.3–0.4	0.3–0.5	0.4–0.6	5–7	50
allowances for infants 0–1 year	500	10	400	15	4	0.4	0.2	0.4	5	50
Advisable intake of vitamins during infancy (twice that required)	1898	43	22	15	1.8	0.1	0.16	0.36	1.47	31–81
1 l human milk 1 l cow's milk 16 oz evaporated milk	1025–1610	11	14 non-enriched, 400 enriched	60	0.4	0.64	0.44	1.75	0.94	37–82
1 l Enfamil	1850	5.5	400	not available	1.3	0.37	0.28	1.9	1.0	55
1 l Similac	1500	50	400	40	8.5–12.7	0.4	0.4	1.0	4.0	100
1 l SMA	2500	50	400	35	8.5–12.7	0.4	0.65	1.0	4.0	50
1 l Pro Sobee	2500	50	400	55	9.5	0.4	0.67	1.0	5.0	50
1 l Neo-Mull-Soy										
1 l Isomil	2100–2500	59–55	400–423	80–71	9–11	0.4	0.4–0.7	0.6–1.0	5.0–8.4	100

Source: Slattery, Jill S. Nutrition for the normal healthy infant. *The American Journal of Maternal Child Nursing*, **2**(2):108 (1977).

Table 9-17 Iron Content of Selected Foods Fed to Infants in the United States

Food	Essential Iron (mg/100 g of food)	Essential Iron (mg/100 kcal)
Milk or formula		
Human milk*	0.05	0.07
Cow milk*	0.05	0.07
Iron-fortified formula	0.9–1.3	1.2–1.8
Formula unfortified with iron	<0.05	<0.05
Infant cereals		
Iron-fortified (dry) mixed with milk†	7–14	7–14
Wet-packed cereal-fruit	1–6	1.3–7.5
Strained and junior foods		
Meats		
Liver and a few others	4–6	4–6
Most meats	1–2	1–2
Egg yolks	2–3	1.0–1.5
"Dinners"		
High meat	<1	<1
Vegetable-meat	<0.5	<0.5
Vegetables‡	<0.5	<0.5
Fruits‡	<0.5	<0.5

*Data reviewed by Underwood (1971).
†Assuming that one part by weight of dry cereal is mixed with six parts of milk.
‡A few varieties of vegetables and fruits provide 1 to 2 mg of iron/100 gm (1 to 3 mg/100 kcal).
Source: Foman, Samuel J. *Infant nutrition.* Philadelphia: Saunders, 1974, p. 314.

Table 9-18 Nutrients for Health*†

Nutrient	*Important Sources of Nutrients*
Protein	Meat, poultry, fish
	Dried beans and peas
	Egg
	Cheese
	Milk
Carbohydrate	Cereal
	Potatoes
	Dried beans
	Corn
	Bread
	Sugar
Fat	Shortening, oil
	Butter, margarine
	Salad dressing
	Sausages
Vitamin A (Retinol)	Liver
	Carrots
	Sweet potatoes
	Greens
	Butter, margarine
Vitamin C (Ascorbic acid)	Broccoli
	Orange
	Grapefruit
	Papaya
	Mango
	Strawberries
Thiamin(B_1)	Lean pork
	Nuts
	Fortified cereal products
Riboflavin (B_2)	Liver
	Milk
	Yogurt
	Cottage cheese
Niacin	Liver
	Meat, poultry, fish

Table 9-18 Nutrients for Health*† *(continued)*

Nutrient	*Important Sources of Nutrients*	*Nutrient*	*Important Sources of Nutrients*
	Peanuts Fortified cereal products		Collard, kale, mustard, and turnip greens
Calcium	Milk, yogurt Cheese Sardines and salmon with bones	Iron	Enriched farina Prune juice Liver Dried beans and peas Red meat

*Build and maintain body cells; regulate body processes; provide energy.
‡Table developed by Penelope S. Peckos.

Table 9-19 General Nutrition*

Dietary Recommendations	Recommended Number of Servings			
	Toddlers, Age 1–4	Preschool, Age 4–6	School, Age 7–12	Adolescent, Age 13 and over
DAIRY PRODUCTS 1 cup milk, yogurt, or calcium equivalent: 1½ slices (1½ oz) cheddar cheese 1 cup pudding 1¾ cups ice cream 2 cups cottage cheese	3 cups whole milk	3–4 cups whole milk	3–4 cups whole milk	3 cups skimmed milk (99% fat-free)
MEAT 2 oz cooked, lean meat, fish, poultry, or protein equivalent: 2 eggs 2 slices (2 oz) cheddar cheese ½ cup cottage cheese 1 cup dried beans or peas 4 T. peanut butter	2 oz	2 oz	2 oz	2–3 oz
FRUITS AND VEGETABLES ½ cup cooked fruit or citrus juice 1 cup raw or cooked vegetable Medium-sized apple, banana, or orange	4 oz	4 oz	4 oz	4 oz
GRAINS Whole grain—fortified, enriched 1 slice bread	4 oz	4 oz	4 oz	2–3 oz

Table 9-19 General Nutrition* (*continued*)

Dietary Recommendations	Recommended Number of Servings			
	Toddlers, Age 1–4	Preschool, Age 4–6	School, Age 7–12	Adolescent, Age 13 and over
GRAINS 1 cup ready-to-eat cereal ½ cup cooked cereal Pasta, grits				
OTHER† Should not replace foods from above groups Sugar Candy Cookies Desserts Soft drinks				

*Table developed by Penelope S. Peckos.

†As needed to fulfill individual caloric needs; amounts to be determined by level of activity, size, and age.

Table 9-20 Factors to be Considered When Selecting a Feeding Method

Considerations	Breast Feeding	Bottle Feeding
Preparation	Already correctly prepared	Requires exact preparation according to instructions
Temperature	Automatically correct	Bottles kept in refrigerator; need to be warmed to room temperature
Sterilization	Already sterile	Bottles and nipples carefully washed in hot, soapy water and well rinsed, air-dried
Convenience	Mother's presence necessary, or must express milk to maintain adequate milk supply	Some inconvenience in preparation; anyone can feed baby—allows father or partner participation
Mother's presence	Required	Not required
Amount of milk	Equal to sucking stimulation or how often and completely breast emptied	Easier to overfeed, dilute, or concentrate
Economy	Increased expense for mother's diet	Usually costs over $200/yr
Travel	More convenient—need to wear clothes with front zipper or buttons; only safe method if traveling in developing countries	Maximum convenience only if using commercially prepared prebottled and sealed formula
History of family allergy		More predisposed to milk and other allergies
Mother's medication	May pass into breast milk; more concentrated in breast milk, especially drugs with high lipid solubility and drugs with high alkaline pH	

Table 9-20 Factors to be Considered When Selecting a Feeding Method (*continued*)

Considerations	Breast Feeding	Bottle Feeding
	(erythromycin, antihistamines, amphetamines)	
Physical benefit to mother	Quicker postpartum involution	
Birth control pill	Contraindicated	Safe
Birth control	Not a reliable method of contraception	
Length of feeding time	Requires longer time—up to 30 min minimum	Shorter time, less sucking involved to obtain milk—varies from 10 to 30 min
Sucking	If allowed to suck on second breast for nonnutritive sucking, need will be met and pacifier may not be needed	Less sucking required; will probably need pacifier
Mother's nutrition	Diet must be high in protein and fluids	Not a direct influencing factor
Overfeeding	Difficult if only breast-fed	Easier to overfeed
Premature infant	Best suited for infant; frequently requires mother to travel to newborn special care unit	
Digestibility	More easily digested because of high fat, low ash, low casein, and high lactose	
Metabolic	Correct composition: protein, carbohydrate, and fat	Cow's milk needs to be altered; protein twice as much; carbohydrate half as much; fat approximately equal or slightly higher
Composition of milk	See Tables 9-16 and 9-26	See Tables 9-16 and 9-26
Stool composition	Higher water content, therefore softer; constipation is rare; lower feces pH—5.1, lower content of amino acids, higher content reducing sugars; cheesy smell due to fermentation	Stool more formed, therefore more likely to have constipation; pH of feces—7–10; strong odor
Stool Fora	Dominated by anaerobic *Lactobacilli,* particularly Lactobacillus; *E coli* number decreased Resistant to *Shigella* and intestinal protozoa	Flora: *Clostridium, Bacteroides, Proteus, Pseudomonas Aeruginosa; E coli* in number up to 100 times greater than in breast-fed milk
Growth	Height and weight curves equal	Gains as much, frequently more, weight than babies nursed on breast-fed milk
Mortality	No difference between breast feeding and bottle feeding in developed countries	
Morbidity		Higher in bottle-fed babies; malnutrition may be present
Allergy	Rare	Foreign proteins may be absorbed Most formula-fed infants: antibodies to cow's milk in blood—reason allergies occur Foreign proteins may predispose to

Table 9-20 Factors to be Considered When Selecting a Feeding Method (*continued*)

Considerations	Breast Feeding	Bottle Feeding
		eczema and/or ulcerative colitis If immediate family history of allergy, infant likely to develop allergic rhinitis If allergic to cow's milk, will often be allergic to other foods
Diarrhea due to lactose intolerance	None	Occurs after drinking undiluted milk
Immunoglobulins	Highest secretion concentration of all immunoglobulins in colostrum: IgG—low IgM—low IgA—high IgE	None
Antibodies	Contains antibodies to tetanus; pertussis; *Diplococcus pneumoniae;* enzymes produced by staphylococci and streptococci; diphtheria, *E. coli; Salmonella; Shigella* (GI); polio viruses; Coxsackie viruses; echoviruses; influenza viruses	None
Environmental DDT pollutants, pesticides, industrial by-products	Higher than cow's milk Frequently higher percentage in breast milk	Present
Speech	May have better speech because of better dental formation due to pushing of tongue during breast feeding	
Transfer of microorganisms	Hepatitis B antigen–RNA tumor virus cytomegalovirus	None
Sudden infant death syndrome	Breast feeding is not a guarantee against crib death	Crib death occurs *almost* exclusively in formula-fed infants
Otitis media		May increase in bottle feeding because of horizontal feeding position

Table 9-21 Guidelines for Initiation of Breast Feeding

The optimal time to initiate nursing is immediately after birth.

Reassure mother that colostrum is an important nutrient and that its utilization will provide some immunity to the newborn.

Wash hands.

Wash breasts with warm water (*no* soap) *only* if nipples are crusting or creams and/or emollients have been applied to the nipple area.

Massage breasts approximately 4 times or until skin is flushed to bring milk into the sinuses.

Roll nipples to make them erect.

Express a few drops of colostrum or milk onto baby's lips.

Root baby.

Guide nipple and areola into infant's mouth by grasping areola with index and middle finger.

Finger may need to depress breast around infant's nose to facilitate breathing.

Prior to or during feeding the infant who is excessively agitated or takes in air may need to be calmed and bubbled.

Table 9-21 Guidelines for Initiation of Breast Feeding *(continued)*

There is no one position for nursing. However, both mother and baby must be in a supported, comfortable position with the baby's head elevated.

Indications of correct placement of infant on breast
- Aereola is drawn in and out as baby sucks
- Presence of a clicking sound with swallowing

Indications that letdown reflex has occurred
- Leaking of milk from breast not being nursed
- Experiencing uterine contractions while nursing
- Experiencing a pins and needles or rushing sensation in nursed breast

Factors that promote letdown reflex
- Comfort
- Rest
- High-protein diet
- High-fluid intake

Factors that slow down or inhibit letdown reflex
- Fatigue
- Pain
- Fear and anxiety
- Embarrassment

Mother should nurse from both breasts at each feeding and begin next feeding on breast last nursed.

Gradual increments of nursing time on each breast are frequently recommended but not universally accepted. Ten minutes on the first breast is adequate. The second breast may be nursed 10 or more minutes depending on mother's time demands and infant's nonnutritional sucking needs.

Some infants may need bubbling between breasts.

Remove infant from breast by placing fifth finger into side of baby's mouth and wedging between gums to release suction.

Care of breasts after nursing
- Allow breasts to air-dry
- Wear good supportive bra

Table 9-22 Guidelines for Initiation of Bottle Feeding

Enough formula should be prepared and sufficient bottles filled to meet *that* 24-h demand.

Formula should be at room temperature in well-washed and rinsed bottles.

Nipple opening should not be enlarged.

Solid food, including cereal, should *never* be added to the bottle.

Instruct care giver in preparing formula to exact measurements.

Attention to dangers of overconcentration and dilution is advised.

Immediately prior to feeding, test temperature and flow of formula.

Mother and baby should be in a supported, comfortable position with infant's head elevated.

Baby should be held close to feeder's body and should be rotated from one arm to the other.

Root baby.

Elevate bottle to maintain a full nipple at all times.

Bubble infant every 2 oz and at end of feeding.

Never prop bottle.

Manipulation or twirling the nipple should be discouraged since it can lead to overfeeding, overstimulation, frustrated babies, and gum tissue injury.

After feeding, infant should be placed on abdomen or on right side, *never* on back.

An appropriate time to utilize a pacifier for nonnutritive sucking may occur after feeding.

Advise parent(s) or care giver to avoid excessive stimulation or physical manipulation after feeding.

Table 9-23 Infant Feeding Concerns

Problems/Concerns	Management/Counselling
Twins	
	Mother needs high-protein diet with greater fluid intake. Short frequent nursing produces more milk. Feed babies together, one on each breast. Place baby on opposite breast each feeding. Encourage hospitalization (extra 1–2 days) until there are no signs of breast engorgement.

Table 9-23 Infant Feeding Concerns (*continued*)

Problems/Concerns	Management/Counselling
	If one baby awakens to feed, wake the other baby and feed together.
	If nursing both babies is physically or psychologically too tiring, one baby can be bottle-fed, the other breast-fed and rotated for each feeding.
	Close telephone contact with mother is important.
	Refer mother to LaLeche.
Adopted child	Mother needs nursing supplementer, Woolich breast shields, breast pump (i.e., Egnell), frequent rests, fluids, and high-protein diet.
	Key concept here is frequent nipple massage and expression.
Preparation	Press warm compress to breast.
	Gently hand massage breast and express milk.
	Roll the nipple.
	Apply appropriate cream to keep nipples supple.
	Express each breast 3–5 min several times each day.
	Use breast pump several times daily once milk comes in.
	Wear breast shields (Woolich) or Nesty Cups inside bra. (Draw nipple out and stimulate.)
	Oral contraceptives may be recommended prior to baby's arrival to produce breast changes similar to pregnancy.
Arrival of baby	The more sucking the baby does, the better.
	Nurse every 2 to 3 hours for as long as baby wishes.
	Always nurse first and then supplement with bottle. (Nuk Sauger nipple or Playtex Nurser are suggested.)
	Supplements can be given by jigger, glass, spoon, eyedropper, or nursing supplementer (This allows the baby to nurse and receive formula simultaneously, prevents frustration, and allows stimulation.)
	Supplement with ¾ usual formula and ¼ water; continue to dilute formula as breast supply increases and baby is satisfied (i.e., one-half formula, one-half water).
	With frantic babies use a little formula and then breast-feed.
	Time, confidence, and reassurance are most important.
	If child is not satisfied and cries frequently, reevaluate feeding methods.
	Refer mother to LaLeche.
	Consult physician for oxytoxic nasal spray (aids letdown).
	Notify adoptive agency that mother plans to breast-feed; sometimes they can arrange for baby to be dropper-fed prior to arrival.
	Maintain close telephone contact with parents.
Sleepy or Uninterested Baby	
Prevention	Don't heavily medicate woman in labor, especially toward the end.
	Don't delay initial feeding.
	Don't let baby cry excessively before feeding; use demand feeding.
	The infant who isn't gaining enough weight frequently is sleeping 4 or 5 h at a time. Awaken and feed this baby every 2–3 h.
Counselling	Reassure mother that the infant's interest in eating will return.
	Unwrap the infant and swaddle loosely.
	Talk to infant while gently stroking the bottom of the feet.

Table 9-23 Infant Feeding Concerns (*continued*)

Problems/Concerns	Management/Counselling
	Talk to infant while rocking and eliciting the rooting reflex. Rock or bend the infant forward and backward at the waist while supporting the infant's back and chest. First, gently squeeze the cheeks together and then insert the nipple into the mouth. Second, apply upward pressure on the chin so as to hold the nipple in the mouth. Third, rhythmically stroke under the infant's chin.
Lactation-suppressing drugs	Initiate breast feeding after mother has been given a lactation-suppressing drug by recommending short, frequent nursing periods and suggesting techniques under "Adopted Child" (see beginning of this table) which may need to be used.
Jaundice	See Physiologic Jaundice, Chap. 38. Consult physician. It is now believed breast-fed babies are *not* more likely to develop physiologic jaundice than bottle-fed babies, and breast feeding does not aggravate jaundice. If phototherapy is required, see "Hospitalized Infant" (next heading).
Hospitalized Infant	Promote bonding by encouraging the mother to visit her baby frequently, and stimulate child with touch and sound. Express breast milk manually or with breast pump every 2 to 3 h during day and anytime the mother is awake during the night. Milk should be expressed into a sterile wide-mouthed bottle (freezer-stored). Mother should nurse baby as often as possible. Mother needs continual praise and encouragement.
Diet	Breast-feeding mother should have additional 600 cal and 6 g of protein per day. Drink all the liquids desired. Rarely do foods the mother eats affect the baby. Initially, eat a small amount of gas-producing foods like brussel sprouts, cabbage, chocolate, or spicy foods to see how the infant tolerates them. Gradually increase the amount ingested.
Schedule	Demand feeding is preferred. The first several months, the mother will nurse 10 times a day. Breast-fed babies eat more often because of their increased digestibility of milk. Infant should eat every 2–5 h. However, don't awaken the infant at night to feed. If a baby is placid and not gaining weight, awaken and feed more often. Also, increase the amount of sensory stimuli.

Table 9-23 Infant Feeding Concerns (*continued*)

Problems/Concerns	Management/Counselling
Collecting and Storing Breast Milk	A breast pump can be used to stimulate and initiate the letdown reflex. Do not use the milk collected in the breast pump. Once letdown reflex has occurred, milk can be rhythmically expressed by hand into a sterile wide-mouthed bottle. Store milk in refrigerator or freezer. Milk should not be refrozen. Leftover, thawed milk should not be stored in the refrigerator longer than 4 h. Milk should not be allowed to warm or thaw at room temperature. Bottle should be placed under cold running tap water. Gradually increase the warmth of the tap water. Gently rotate the bottle so that as it is being warmed the stratified layers can be homogenized. (The fat frequently rises to the top or clings to the sides.)
Flat or Inverted Nipples	Flat or inverted nipples are usually recognized in the antenatal period. The Woolich shield or Sweech's ax can be worn inside the bra as long as required for the nipples to project. Nipple rolling should be used. This same regimen may be continued or initiated after the infant's birth. The nipple may be encouraged to project by tactile stimulation and/or by placing a wet cloth on the nipple for a few seconds.
Sore or Cracked Nipples Prevention	Most clinicians advise starting with frequent but limited nursing periods. Advance the length of time as tolerated by mother. Limiting the length of nursing time for the first several days may be particularly important for the mother with red hair, fair skin, or for the first-time nursing mother. Short, frequent feedings are recommended. Correctly position the baby on breast. Rotate position of the infant on breast. Eliminate use of soap, alcohol, and astringents on nipples. Air-dry nipples after each nursing. Use of cocoa butter, etc., to keep nipple supple is not universally accepted.
Care after occurrence	Nurse for shorter times more frequently. Start nursing on least-sore breast. Encourage quicker, more successful letdown reflex Use relaxation techniques used in labor. Use oxytocin nasal spray (0.5–1.0 cm) just prior to nursing. Expose nipples to air and light after each feeding. Briefly put ice on nipple just prior to nursing. If above recommendations fail, LaLeche League states doctor may recommend use of ultraviolet lamp with the following instructions: Use an ultraviolet light bulb in any lamp socket. Sit 3 ft away from lamp.

Table 9-23 Infant Feeding Concerns (*continued*)

Problems/Concerns	Management/Counselling
	Schedule for exposing nipples: day 1, one-half min; day 2 and 3, 1 min; day 4 and 5, 2 min; day 6, until soreness is gone–3 min, as long as no reddening of skin. Never expose the baby to ultraviolet light.
Referral	Consult a physician.
Working Mother	
	Breast-feeding mother needs time at work to go to ladies room to express milk at infant's feeding time and maintain a supply. Get a supportive baby-sitter. Become skilled in massage and expression. Nurse or express milk before leaving home. Express leftover milk after feedings into a jar and freeze.
Leaky Breasts	
	This is a temporary phenomenon. It is a positive sign and means the mother has a good letdown reflex. Use commercial lactation pads, clean handkerchief, or clean, soft cloth in bra. The mother may experience a sudden letdown if a baby's cry is heard, she thinks of own baby, or normal feeding time for her baby. This condition is controlled by compressing breasts. Cross arms over breasts until the rushing sensation ceases.
Breast Feeding in Public	
	Garments which open in front or can be easily lifted from bottom should be worn. A blanket or shawl may be wrapped around the infant and draped over mother's shoulder. The mother should turn back or go to another room if in a crowded area.
Supplements	
	Sterile water can be given as needed. In warm weather, more frequent nursings will meet increased fluid demands. No solid foods are needed until infant is 6 mo of age. Nursing mother may give supplemental bottle, but the infant is required to use different sucking techniques, and mother needs sucking stimulation to maintain milk supply.
Iron: Infant Requirements	
	During the first year, 0.6 mg iron/day must reach body-iron pool. The normal term of an infant's diet must provide 1 mg/Kg per day of elemental iron by 3 mo of age. Infants with reduced iron stores (e.g., low birth weight, twins, premature infants, and those whose mothers had iron deficiency anemia during pregnancy) require about 2 mg/Kg per day elemental iron by 2 mo of age. Baby can be given iron-fortified formula or vitamins with iron. Instruct parent(s) about proper nutrition and food sources high in iron

Table 9-23 Infant Feeding Concerns (*continued*)

Problems/Concerns	Management/Counselling
	(home-blended meats, strained meats). Keep infant on formula for the first year of life.
Vitamins	The breast-fed baby needs iron, vitamin D, and fluoride (if not in water supply). The bottle-fed baby needs iron (if not in formula) and fluoride (if not in water supply).
Smoking and Alcohol Consumption	Both pass through breast milk. Moderation is advised.
Mastitis	Refer mother to physician. Antibiotics, warm soaks, excision, and drainage are usually needed. Mother may be temporarily required to stop nursing from affected breast. Maintain a milk supply through massage and expression.
Engorgement Prevention	Encourage early initial feeding. Mother should nurse around the clock including during the night. Don't wait until the milk comes in. Feed the baby on demand.
When engorgement has occurred	Place warm towels on the breast. Massage the breast until a flush is noted. Manually express milk until the areola is soft. Roll nipple and project it so that infant can latch on more easily. Express the remaining milk after feeding (may be more easily done in shower). Nurse the infant frequently. Temporarily limit fluid intake.
Increasing Milk Supply and/or Growth Spurts	The common age for growth spurts is the sixth wk and the third mo. To increase milk supply mother should Nurse more frequently. Empty breasts after each nursing. Increase fluid intake. Increase rest. Decrease other stimuli, interruptions, and responsibilities. Increase protein intake.
Nighttime bottle	Do not put milk or fruit juice in bottle during the night after the appearance of first tooth; use water instead. The young infant requires more than nutrition from a nighttime bottle. The infant cannot tolerate long periods without mother holding, cuddling, and providing a sense of security.

Table 9-23 Infant Feeding Concerns (*continued*)

Problems/Concerns	Management/Counselling
Solid Foods (Beikost)	No solid foods are necessary prior to 6 mo of age. *Never* put solid foods in bottle. Begin with 1 T rice cereal mixed with some formula fed only from spoon. As infant begins to tolerate solid food, amount can be increased to 2–4 tbsp. 1 to 2 times daily. Add one new food every 4 to 5 days to observe infant for food allergy. Begin with cereal: rice, bran, oats, and barley. Use mixed cereal only after each cereal has been given separately, and wheat cereal only *after* 6 mo. Two wk after cereal has been started, the infant can begin to be fed vegetables (green, then yellow); then fruits: bananas, applesauce. Protein foods such as chicken, fish, and eggs can also be fed to the infant, as well as citrus juices. Teach parent(s) label reading and home preparation of baby foods.
Finger Foods	Begin around 6 to 8 mo. Parent(s) should observe hand-mouth coordination. Infant should be started on pieces of crackers, soft cooked vegetables, and fruits. Counsel parent(s) about accident prevention.
Teething	Mother can teach the child not to bite breast and can utilize different conditioning techniques, such as removing the child from the breast. See Teething, Chap. 113.
Self-Feeding	Begin with finger foods. Self-feeding is important developmentally to the child. Encourage the baby to satisfy its own hunger. Place a few pieces of finger foods on a high chair, tray, or small, plastic nonbreakable plate. Replace food as it is eaten and as more is wanted.
Playing/Messy Food	Support the parent(s). This is an important developmental step. This stage will pass. Place small amounts of food on nonbreakable plates. The daily bath can be postponed until eating is completed.
Weaning Concepts to follow when weaning to cup	Go slowly. Wean when the baby gives indications of interest; i.e., when the baby plays with cup, is able to hold it, and is frequently able to put it to mouth. Try not to force the infant. Permit the child to help hold the cup.

Table 9-23 Infant Feeding Concerns (*continued*)

Problems/Concerns	Management/Counselling
Weaning from the breast to the bottle	Go slowly. The baby needs to learn and use different sucking techniques. Ideally, eliminate breast feeding, or change one feeding per wk. If necessary, this may be done every 3 or 4 days. A slow approach allows the breast to adjust to a decreased demand and maintain good skin turgor and support. The baby may refuse initially to take the bottle from the mother. In this case, have another family member or friend give the bottle to the infant.
Cesarean Section	Infant may be sleepier longer because a greater amount of analgesia and anesthesia has been administered. Infant may have secondary problems because of reasons which necessitated a cesarean section. The mother, initially, needs more care and rest. It is more difficult for the mother to find a comfortable position for holding and burping the baby. Suggest that she lie down, hold the infant on a pillow, or hold the infant in a football hold, with legs and buttocks extending toward her side rather than over her abdomen. The mother may experience difficulty in lifting the child.
Burping/Bubbling	With formula-fed infants, bubble after every 2 oz and at end of feeding. Some breast-fed infants require bubbling between breasts, and others do not. Lie the baby face down across lap and gently stroke back, *or* hold the baby up to the shoulder and gently rub or stroke back. Another method of burping is to hold the baby in a sitting position, lean baby forward onto the palm of the mother's hand, and gently rub or stroke back with the opposite hand.
Environmental Tensions and Interruptions	Feeding time should be a relaxed, enjoyable time for the baby, mother, or person feeding the infant. Suggest a private, quiet place to feed the baby. Take the phone off the hook during feeding time. Family members can and should participate, but in a relaxed, nondisruptive manner.
Nonsupporting Partner, Friends, and/or Relatives	Attempt to correct any misconceptions. Provide support to the parent(s) while helping achieve and maintain the basic goal of a content and thriving child and parent(s).
Fatigue	Assess mental vs. physical fatigue. If there is a need to determine how the parent(s) defines fatigue, do not assume it is anemia or lack of sleep. It may be caused by feelings of entrapment, selflessness, boredom, and/or resentfulness.

Table 9-23 Infant Feeding Concerns (*continued*)

Problems/Concerns	Management/Counselling
	It is necessary to achieve a consistent balance between the family's needs, the infant's needs, and the individual parent's needs. The parent(s) needs private time along with the freedom to do as he or she wishes at that time.
Refuses bottle or prefers one breast	Frequently the infant refuses the bottle when offered by the mother because he or she is able to sense and smell breast milk. Have someone besides mother feed the bottle to the infant. If the infant's refusal to take milk is related to taste, content, or suck, express breast milk into bottle. The baby's preference for one breast may be related to its feeding position, the mother's personal comfort, the milk supply in that breast, and the ease with which letdown occurs. Encourage the child to suck. One way of doing this is to place a small amount of honey on the breast. Use a correct position to maintain maximum comfort. Build up the milk supply (see "Growth Spurts" above)
Selecting Commercially Prepared Baby Foods	Read the labels. The order items are listed in indicates relative quantity; e.g., a chicken-rice dinner contains more chicken than a rice-chicken dinner. Meats contain more protein and are nutritionally better than dinner combinations. Avoid fruit juices with added sugar, tapioca or starches, baby desserts, baby foods with preservatives, coloring agents, and foods with added salt and sugar. Jars should be returned if the seal on the lid is broken or doesn't pop when opened, or if foreign debris is found on lid or on the rim of the jar. Remove food from the jar before feeding so that infant's saliva does not contaminate the remaining food.
Home Preparation of Baby Food	This type of preparation is economical and allows for creativity and utilization of a family menu. Sanitary precautions are most important. Use only fresh or frozen pure foods. Avoid additives, combinations, sugar, starches, salt, or spices. Carefully wash hands and utensils before and after using. Meat, poultry, fish, and eggs must be well cooked. Freeze food in individually wrapped packages or in ice cube containers. Prepare no more than 1-mo supply of food at one time. Avoid spinach.

Table 9-24 Breast-Feeding and Bottle-Feeding Contraindications

	Definite Contraindications	Probable Contraindications	Need to Monitor Carefully and Evaluate
	Breast-Feeding Contraindications		
Drugs	Anticancer drugs (possible exception) Methotrexate Anticoagulants Tetracyclines Metronidazole Antithyroid drugs Atropine Ergot alkaloids Cathartics (except senna) Iodides Narcotics Radio isotopes Bromides	Chloramphenicol Sulfonamides Thiazide diuretics Valium Lithium Methadone Oral contraceptives Erythromycin Antihistamines Amphetamines	Isoniazid Kanamycin Aspirin Cigarette smoking Alcohol Steroids Other diuretics Malic acid Sulfonamides Barbiturates
Maternal/ medical contraindications	Hepatitis B antigen (HAB) Active tuberculosis Currently being treated for cancer	Whooping cough RNA tumor virus Cytomegolovirus Severe epilepsy Severe psychiatric disorders	Pregnancy
Infant contraindications	G-6-PD—If a mother eats fava beans and is breast-feeding an infant with glucose 6-phosphate dehydrose deficiency (G-6-PD), infant is prone to acute hemolytic anemia.		Has neonatal jaundice, and doesn't take ready-feed formula
	Bottle-Feeding Contraindications		
Maternal/infant contraindications	Strong family history of allergies		Is handicapped, and doesn't use ready-feed formula

Table 9-25 Special Nutritional Concerns

Problem	Management
Obesity	See Obesity/Overweight, Chap. 156. Encourage breast feeding for minimum of 3 mo in infants. Carefully instruct parent(s) not to force-feed the infant. Infant does not need to finish the bottle. Encourage home preparation of baby foods. Encourage physical activity. Don't restrain the infant's arms or legs. Remove "junk food" from the house. Encourage low calorie snacks such as carrots and celery. Parent(s) must allow the child to determine when he or she is hungry and when full. Eliminate second servings; cut food into small pieces. Determine one place where eating is permitted and always eat with someone else.
Vegetarian	Counselling will depend upon classification Lacto-ovo-vegetarians eat dairy and egg products, and avoid meat, fish, poultry, and seafood. Pure vegetarians avoid foods of animal origin for health reasons. Vegans avoid foods of animal origin for philosophical reasons.
Vegetarian *(continued)*	For the infant use a soy-based formula or breast-feed for the first 6 mo. Add solid foods slowly. Vitamin B_{12} supplements are required. Follow basic principles in planning a nutritious diet. Steam rather than boil foods. Buy food that is locally grown. Avoid bruised and/or damaged fruits and vegetables. Consult or refer the client to a nutritionist.
Food faddism	Discuss the health implications of the food fad. Counsel the client about food economy. Budgeted money requires the most nutritious foods for the least amount. Avoid overpriced health food stores. Consult or refer the client to A nutritionist A public health nurse A professional counsellor Food faddism requires long-term intervention. The best method is prevention. Educate the public about a nutritional diet.

Table 9-26 Components, Effects, and Indications for Major Infant Formulas*

Formula	Company	Carbohydrate	Protein	Fat
			Milk-based	
Enfamil	Mead Johnson	Lactose	Nonfat milk	Soy and coconut oils
Similac	Ross	Lactose	Nonfat milk	Soy, coconut, and corn oils
SMA	Wyeth	Lactose	Electrodialized whey, nonfat milk	Oleo, coconut, oleic (safflower), and soybean oils
			Soy-based	
Isomil	Ross	Sucrose, corn starch, corn syrup solids	Soy protein isolate	Soy, coconut, and corn oils
Neo-Mull-Soy	Syntex	Sucrose	Soy protein isolate	Soy oil
Nursoy	Wyeth	Sucrose, corn syrup solids	Soy protein isolate	Oleo, coconut, oleic (safflower, and soybean oils)
Pro Sobee	Mead Johnson	Sucrose, corn syrup solids	Soy protein isolate	Soy oil
			Special	
Lofenalac	Mead Johnson	Corn syrup solids, tapioca starch	Specially processed hydrolyzed casein	Corn oil
Lonalac	Mead Johnson	Lactose	Casein	Coconut oil
Similac PM 60/40	Ross	Lactose	Partially demineralized whey and nonfat milk	Coconut and corn oils
Portagen	Mead Johnson	Sucrose, corn syrup solids	Sodium cascinate	Fractionated coconut oil (MCT), corn oil (trace)
Nutramigen	Mead Johnson	Sucrose, tapioca starch	Enzymically hydrolyzed 8 casein	Corn oil

*Components were obtained from product can labels, indications from the literature, and stool characteristics from clinical observations.

Table 9-26 Components, Effects, and Indications for Major Infant Formulas* *(continued)*

Stool Characteristics	Explanations
	Milk-based
Formed, greenish brown, with very little free water around the stool	Milk formulas are similar and interchangeable. An iron-supplemented formula provides the daily requirement for iron.
Similar to breast-milk stool; small volume, pasty, yellow, with some free water	SMA has a relatively low renal solute load. (Renal solute load refers to the amount of ingested protein and minerals that must be excreted by the kidneys in the form of urea and mineral salts. Fluid intake must be adequate for this excretion to take place.) It is low in sodium but supplies the daily requirement, and so is used for normal babies. (See Similac PM 60/40 for uses.)
	Soy-based
Mushy, yellow-green with more free water than cow's milk stools	Soy formulas are based on soy products. Since they do not contain milk protein or lactose, they are interchangeable in their use for milk protein hypersensitivity or lactose intolerance. (Lactose intolerance may be due to a temporary lactase deficiency following diarrhea.)
	Special
Similar to cow's-milk-formula; formed, greenish brown with very little free water around the stool	Infants with phenylketonuria are unable to convert phenylalanine to tyrosine. Unused phenylalanine accumulates in the blood causing irreversible central nervous system damage. Lofenalac is used to provide enough phenylalanine for growth while preventing excessively high levels in the blood.
Similar to cow's-milk-formula stools	Lonalac is essentially sodium free and may be used in severe renal disease or heart failure. Due to its low sodium content, it is not recommended for long-term use without sodium supplement.
Similar to cow's-milk-formula stools	This is a cow's-milk-base formula with a low renal solute load. It is low-sodium yet supplies the daily requirements of this essential nutrient. It is used in long-term management of renal or heart disease.
Similar to cow's-milk-formula stools	Pancreatic or liver disease causes interference in fat absorption. Long-chain triglycerides are absorbed through the lymphatic system, and require a certain amount of bile and pancreatic enzymes. Medium-chain triglycerides (MCT) are absorbed directly into the portal circulation, and do not require bile and pancreatic enzymes. Portagen contains MCT oil as its major fat source, and is indicated for an infant with pancreatic or liver disease.
Low volume, green stool with mucus	Nutramigen provides protein in the form of hydrolyzed casein. Protein hypersensitivity is a rare disease process, where intact proteins are not tolerated. Hydrolyzation breaks the protein structure into amino acids and polypeptides.

Source: Stokan, Rose E. The right formula for the right infant: making sense of infant nutrition. *The American Journal of Maternal Child Nursing,* **2**(2): 102–104 (1977). Copyright March/April 1977, The American Journal of Nursing Company. Reproduced with permission from *MCN: The American Journal of Maternal Child Nursing.*

bibliography

Alfin, Slater; Jelliffe, Roslyn B. and Derrick B. Nutritional requirements with special references to infancy. *Pediatric Clinics of North America* **24**:3–16 (February 1977).

Applebaum, R. M. The modern management of successful breast-feeding. *Pediatric Clinics of North America* **17**:203–225 (February 1970).

Beer, Sherry. What?! No meat!! *Pediatric Nursing* 3:16–19 (May-June, 1977).

Christophersen, Edward R., and Hall, Christine L. Eating patterns and associated problems encountered in normal children. *Issues in Comprehensive Pediatric Nursing* 3:1–16 (October 1978).

Committee on Nutrition, American Academy of Pediatrics. Iron supplementation for infants. *Pediatrics* **58**:765–768 (1976).

Countryman, Betty Ann. *How the maternity nurse can help the breast feeding mother* (Publication No. 118). Franklin Park, Ill.: LaLeche League, 1977.

DeAngelis, Catherine, et al. Introduction of new foods into the newborn and infant diet. *Issues in Comprehensive Pediatric Nursing* **2**:23–33 (January-February 1977).

Doucett, Joan S. Is breast-feeding still safe for babies? *Maternal Child Nursing* 3:345–346 (November-December 1978).

Egan, Mary C. Federal Nutrition Support Programs for Children. *Pediatric Clinics of North America* **24**:229–239 (1977).

Foman, S. *Infant nutrition* (2d ed.). Philadelphia: Saunders, 1974.

Grams, Kathryn E. Breast-feeding: A means of imparting immunity. *Maternal Child Nursing* **3**:340–344 (November-December 1978).

Grassley, Jane, and Davis, Kristine. Common concerns of mothers who breast-feed. *Maternal Child Nursing* **3**:347–351 (November-December 1978).

Habersang, Rolf, and Marsh, Alice. Iron and infant nutrition. *Issues in Comprehensive Pediatric Nursing* **2**:43–49 (January-February 1977).

Heimann, Lea Whitby. Weaning to prevent nutritional anemia. *Pediatric Nursing* **3**:8–12 (May-June 1977).

Henderson, Kathryn J., and Newton, Laura D. Helping nursing mothers maintain lactation while separated from their infants. *Maternal Child Nursing* 3:352–356 (November-December 1978).

Hormann, Elizabeth. *Relactation: A guide to breast feeding the adopted baby.* Chicago: Protection of the Unborn through Nutrition, 1971.

Kuhn, John G., Fisher, Richard G. Vitamins in pediatrics *Pediatric Nursing* **5**(2):25–31 (1979).

Mitchell, Helen S., et al. *Nutrition in health and disease,* (16th ed.). Philadelphia: Lippincott, 1976.

Neumann, Charlotte G. Obesity in pediatric practice: obesity in the preschool school-age child. *Pediatric Clinics of North America* **24**:117–122 (February 1977).

Pearson, Gayle A. Nutrition in the middle years of childhood. *Maternal Child Nursing* **2**:378–384 (November-December 1977).

Pryor, Karen. *Nursing your baby.* New York: Harper & Row, 1973.

Robson, John R. K. Food faddism. *Pediatric Clinics of North America* **24**:189–201 (February 1977).

Slattery, J. S., Pearson, G. A., and Torre, C. (eds.). *Maternal and child nutrition: assessment and counselling.* New York: Appleton-Century-Crofts, 1979.

Slattery, Jill S. Nutrition for the normal healthy infant. *Maternal Child Nursing* **2**:105–112 (March-April 1977).

Stokan, Rose E. The right formula for the right infant: making sense of infant nutrition. *Maternal Child Nursing* **2**:101–104 (March-April 1977).

Taitz, Leonard S. Obesity in pediatric practice: infantile obesity. *Pediatric Clinics of North America* **24**:107–115 (February 1977).

Vyhmeister, Irma B., et al. Safe vegetarian diets for children. *Pediatric Clinics of North America* **24**:203–210 (February 1977).

Williams, Eleanor R. Making vegetarian diets nutritious. *American Journal of Nursing* **75**:2168–2173 (December 1975).

Worthington, Patricia. Infant nutrition and feeding techniques. *Pediatric Nursing* **3**:8–12 (January-February 1977).

Zerfas, Alfred J., et al. Office assessment of nutritional status. *Pediatric Clinics of North America* **24**: 253–272 (February 1977).

Dental Health ELEANOR RUDICK

Dental decay starts early in life, and if prevention is initiated at birth it can be substantially reduced or eliminated.

ALERT

1. Bleeding
2. Inflamed, edematous gingiva
3. Delayed dentition
4. Misplaced teeth
5. Child under 3 yr with multiple caries
6. School-age child lacking previous dental care
7. Cleft palate
8. Child with braces
9. Hyperplasia (gingival)
10. Staining of teeth
11. Trauma

I. Subjective Data

A. Dentition history
1. Age of eruption of deciduous teeth
2. Teething problems
3. Age of loss of deciduous teeth
4. Age of eruption of secondary teeth

B. Diet history
1. Sugar intake
2. Between-meal eating
3. Use of fluoride
4. Bottle feeding at bedtime/naptime
   a. Duration
   b. Nature of contents

C. Medication history
1. Mother's medications during pregnancy and/or lactation (tetracycline)
2. Child's medications
   a. Iron—may cause staining
   b. Fluorides in excess and tetracyclines—may result in mottling, pitting, and staining

D. Family history
1. Dental health of parents
2. Dental health of siblings

E. Oral hygiene
1. Teeth brushing—method and equipment used; dental floss
2. Dental visits
   a. Age of first visit
   b. Frequency of visits
   c. Date of last visit
   d. Orthodonture

F. History of trauma
1. Loss of tooth/teeth
2. Replacement/reconstitution
3. Thumb-sucking

II. Objective Data

A. Physical examination
1. Complete physical examination to determine health status
2. Examination of mouth
   a. Number of teeth for age
   b. Shape of teeth: flattening—indication of bruxism
   c. Color of teeth: staining, mottling, banding
   d. Poor alignment of teeth
   e. Malocclusion
   f. Gingiva
      (1) Inflammation
      (2) Edema
      (3) Bleeding
      (4) Hyperplasia
   g. Other buccal mucosa
      (1) Inflammation
      (2) Herpetic lesions
   h. Obvious caries
      (1) "Bottle mouth"—preschool age
      (2) Rear teeth

B. Laboratory data: usually none

III. Promotion of Dental Health

A. Treatments/medications
1. Fluoridation (see Table 9-27)
   a. Begin at 6 mo of age (2 wk of age for breast-fed infants) and continue until all permanent teeth have erupted.
   b. If there is an inadequate amount of fluoride in water (less than 0.8 ppm) supplemental fluoride will be needed:
      (1) 6 mo–2 yr: 0.25 mg/day
      (2) 2–3 yr: 0.5 mg/day
      (3) 3 yr and older: 1.0 mg/day
   c. Fluoride mouthwashes are recommended from 6–16 yr of age, in addition to other fluoride therapy. Take 1 T undiluted rinse before bedtime; swish in mouth for 1–2 min, then expectorate.
2. Oral hygiene
3. Regular dental visits
4. Good eating habits
5. Prophylactic penicillin should be prescribed for any client with history of rheumatic fever

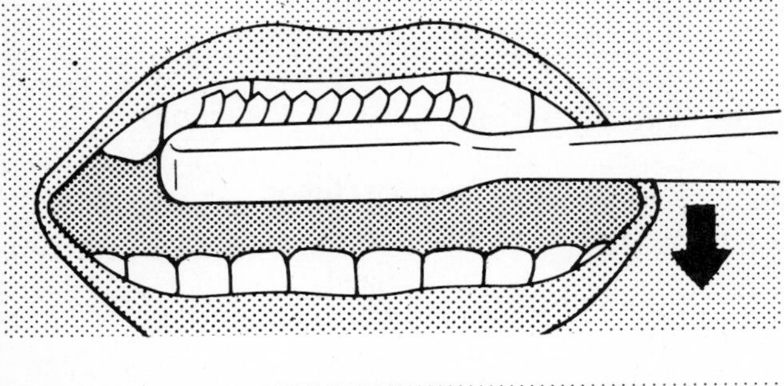

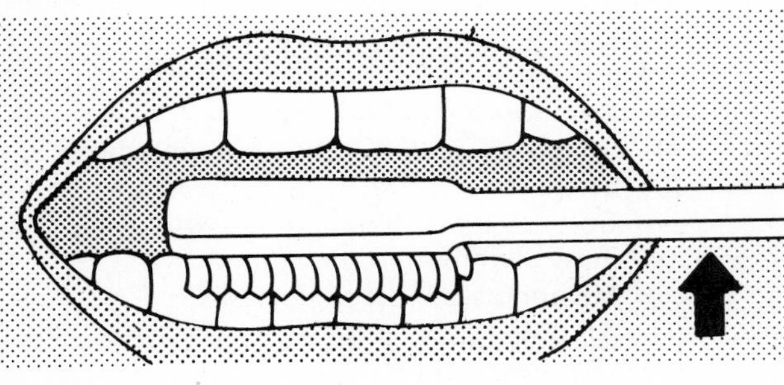

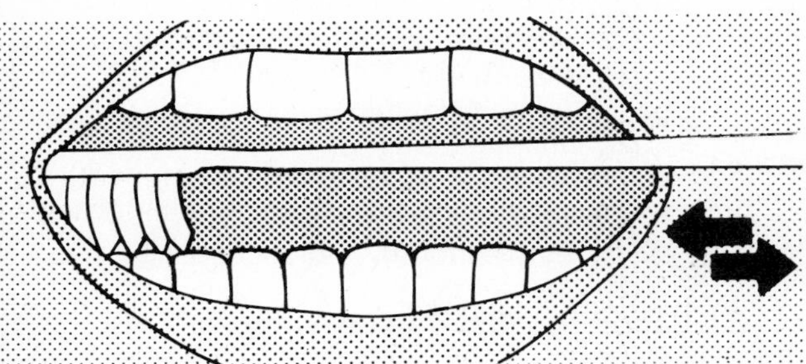

Figure 9-1 The proper method for brushing teeth. (From *Why should he have 12 cavities before high school?* The Proctor and Gamble Co., 1964)

or congenital heart disease prior to dental procedures.

6. For specific dental problems, see Table 9-28.

B. Counselling/prevention

1. Avoid bedtime bottle of milk or fruit juice. Once first tooth erupts offer water *only*, or offer bottle before putting baby in crib.
2. Avoid sucrose- or high carbohydrate-containing snacks/candies or drinks between meals.
3. Reduce frequency of eating.
4. Encourage proper oral hygiene.
   a. Brushing should be initiated once primary teeth have erupted. The parent(s) will need to assist until manual dexterity develops (see Fig. 9-1).
   b. Parent(s) can be instructed to clean baby's tooth or teeth with a gauze pad once daily.
   c. Brush teeth after every meal.
   d. Rinse mouth after snacks.
   e. Use dental floss.
   f. Use Water Pik on low pressure.

C. Follow-up

1. Begin dental visits at or before age 3.
2. Visit dentist twice yearly; more frequent visits are needed for those prone to caries.
3. Have frequent discussion of relationship between sound nutritional practices and oral hygiene.

D. Consultations/referrals

1. Dentist
2. Nutritionist
3. Social services for those with financial difficulties
4. Orthodontist as needed
5. Local water department or health department for fluoride content of local water

Table 9-27 Fluoride Preparations

Liquid (1 drop = 1 mg fluorideion)	Lozenges (½ tablet, 2–3 yr; older, 1 tablet)	Oral Rinse (0.5% sodium fluoride)
Flura-Drops	Flura-Loz	Fluorigard Dental Rinse
Fluoritab liquid	Fluoritab tablets	Aqua-Fluor One-A-Day
Luride drops	Phos-Flur chewable tablets	Janor's Sodium Fluoride Oral Rinse
Karidium liquid	Luride Lozi-Tabs	Kari Rinse
Pacemaker Nafeen solution	Nufluor chewable tablets	Pacemaker Nafeen solution
	Pacemaker Nafeen tablets	Phos-Flur oral rinse

Table 9-28 Medical Referral/Consultation*

Diagnosis	Clinical Manifestations	Management
Bottle mouth syndrome (nursing bottle caries, nursing bottle syndrome, bottle-propping caries)	Parent(s) states child takes bottle to bed at night and nap times Severe decay of primary maxillary incisors and possibly primary first molars Mandibular incisors seldom involved	Refer to dentist. Prevention is most important. Counsel parent(s) to Avoid in-crib feeding Hold infant for feeding Use only water in bottle at nap and bedtime after 12 mo of age
Caries	Obvious decay of other teeth, usually molars (much carious development seen only on x-ray)	Refer to dentist. Counsel parent(s) about efficient mouth care, diet, use of fluoride, and importance of regular dental visits every 3 mo.
Discoloration	Black to blue—primary or secondary; may be due to erythroblastosis fetalis Brownish-yellowish—primary or secondary; may be due to tetracyclines Dark banding or staining; may be due to lead ingestion or iron given orally	Refer to dentist. If client is on iron, instruct on proper administration; lead level determination may be indicated.
Malocclusion	With mouth closed, posterior mandibular teeth either behind or before maxillaries Normally interdigitation of cusps, but not in malocclusion	Refer to dentist. Inform parent(s) that problem is correctable. Counsel on importance of regular dental visits and dental hygiene.
Delayed eruption	Insufficient number of teeth for age or absence of teeth May be due to systemic or nutritional disturbances	Complete history, physical examination, and developmental assessment are needed. Refer to dentist.
Dental injury	Avulsed tooth/teeth	Immediately place tooth/teeth in saline. Immediately refer to dentist for reimplantation. Counsel parent(s) about Replacement, which is necessary for maturation of adjacent dental structures Retention—may be limited

*Follow-up by the practitioner in all instances is exceedingly important, since these conditions require long-term care and families require support to comply with dental regiments.

bibliography

Fey, Michael R. Fluoride therapy. *Nurse Practitioner,* **2**:26–27 (1977).

Filer, L. J., et. al. Fluoride as a nutrient. *Pediatrics,* **49**:456–459 (1972).

Flouride supplementation: revised dosage schedule. *Pediatrics,* **63:**150–152 (1979).

Nizel, Abraham E. Preventing dental caries: The nutritional factor. *Pediatric Clinics of North America,* **24**:141–155 (1977).

Rowe, Nathaniel H., et al. The effect of age, sex, race and economic status on dental caries experience of the permanent dentition. *Pediatrics,* **57**:457–461 (1976).

Shelton, Preston G., et al. Nursing bottle caries. *Pediatrics,* **59**:777–778 (1977).

Slattery, Jill. Dental health in children. *American Journal of Nursing,* **76**:1159–1161 (1976).

Smith, Jane Tuttle. Promoting childhood dental health. *Pediatric Nursing,* May-June (1976).

10 Assessing School Readiness

CARLA NORTH LITTLEFIELD

Over 1 million children start school for the first time each year in the United States. How well prepared these children are for the school experience is related to many variables, including the quality of health care the children received prior to school entry. The purposes of this chapter are to (1) identify those dimensions of child health and development which have a direct bearing on readiness for kindergarten, (2) provide an assessment guide for the nurse practitioner involved in the care of the preschooler who is approaching early school age, and (3) suggest means by which parents can promote their child's preschool development in the areas of socioemotional, physical-motor, and cognitive-language development.

SIGNIFICANCE OF THE PROBLEM

School readiness, for the purposes of this discussion, is defined as the child's ability to respond to and profit from the kindergarten experience in terms of total development. This readiness goes beyond chronological age and implies an age-appropriate level of maturity in all areas of development. In most states, school attendance is mandatory at 7 years and the local school boards establish the minimum age for kindergarten, often using the fifth birthday as a convenient deadline. For the child whose fifth birthday misses a specific date for kindergarten entrance, the parents may want advice from the health care professional as to whether to pursue early admission. The same principles of school readiness apply to any child who is entering kindergarten, regardless of precise age.

In many school systems the kindergarten year is no longer a play period during which the child only learns to "get along" with other children. It is evolving into an integral part of the school experience during which basic concepts related to reading, arithmetic, and language are introduced. Adjustment and achievement in kindergarten will determine how well prepared the child is for the next level of learning, in first grade. Viewed as the first step in a continuum of school learning, kindergarten then becomes a significant experience for which readiness is, sometimes wrongly, assumed.

In terms of health, the relationship between school performance and health status is, unfortunately, not always recognized by health professionals or parents. Where there have been gaps in child health supervision during the preschool years, there may be a related lag in school readiness. Viewed on a continuum, the health of the school-age child is contingent on the quality of child health supervision which began in infancy. Screening procedures during the early childhood period often reveal developmental conditions which could respond to treatment before serious deviations, disabilities, or irreversible damage occurs. Of special concern are general developmental screening, vision and hearing screening, immunizations, routine physical exams, and nutritional assessments, all of which can be performed by the knowledgeable nurse practitioner.

DEVELOPMENTAL FRAMEWORK: AN OVERVIEW

The nursing process involved in assessing and promoting school readiness is based upon scientific knowledge related to all dimensions of growth and development. This scientific base, which is continually expanding, should be very familiar to those who are providing primary health care in ambulatory pediatrics. Development follows known sequences and patterns which vary in rate from one individual to another. The unfolding of developmental stages or phases, *fairly predictable in early years,* is best viewed within a total developmental framework. The nurse's awareness of the level or stage a child is in will provide a "blueprint" for assessing the child now and also understanding the next level to be prepared for with anticipatory guidance.

Since birth or, some would argue, since conception, the child entering school has been preparing for school readiness within this developmental framework. The transition from preschooler to school-age child basically involves the completion of a series of developmental tasks which the maturing child must accomplish on the way to adulthood. The works of several theorists have contributed much to our understanding of these developmental tasks and their accomplishment, especially in psychosocial, cognitive, and social learning.

In the area of psychosocial development, Erickson (1951) has outlined eight stages which every individual normally goes through from birth to maturity. Before the school-age child can come to grips with achieving a sense of industry, which is the major psychosocial developmental task between 7 and 11 years, the foundation of trust, autonomy, and initiative must have been laid during infancy, "toddlerhood," and preschool age. Each step prepares the way for the subsequent level of development.

In the realm of cognitive development, the child has already progressed through the sensory-motor stage, according to Piaget (1950), and is now completing the preoperational tasks which lay the foundation for concrete operations to be achieved during the school-age period (7 to 11 years). The thinking of the 5-year-old is still characterized by a dominance of perceptions, centering, egocentrism, and irreversibility, with only a beginning level of deductive and inductive reasoning and abstraction.

From a social learning viewpoint (Sears, 1951; Bandura and Walters, 1963), the child entering kindergarten is moving from a parent- or family-dominated environment to one which is influenced by peers and the community. Until school age the child's behavior, attitude, and values are shaped primarily by family influences. This socialization process begins in infancy with the early parent-child relationship. Through both simple and complex social interactions the child learns which behaviors are "good" or "bad," desirable or undesirable, and appropriate or inappropriate, and also what will be rewarded or punished. External controls, especially positive social reinforcement, predominate in the preschooler's life before internal control, or self-control, is established in later childhood (McLaughlin, 1971; p. 259). Throughout school age, the child increasingly develops internal controls which effectively guide behavior toward what is socially approved, when parents or other authority figures are not there.

A developmental framework which incorporates theories related to psychosocial development, cognitive development, and the social learning process provides extremely useful concepts for assessing school readiness. Rather than conflicting with one another, these theories and their related concepts complement one another to enhance an understanding of the child's total development. For further elaboration on these theories the reader is referred to Maier's (1965) excellent discussion.

ASSESSMENT

The practitioner who is providing pediatric primary care has primary responsibility for assessing and promoting a child's school readiness. As already emphasized, this responsibility does not begin when the child is 4½ or 5 years old but rather has been an ongoing concern from the time the child was admitted to care. It is a culmination of all the efforts expended during infancy, toddlerhood, and the preschool periods by the child, the parents, and the health care providers. The commitment of the health care professional to the child's health and the identification of deviations which need evaluation and treatment will largely determine the child's readiness for school at age 5 or 6. The difficulties of providing continuing comprehensive care to the general pediatric population are well known, while solutions to problems of noncompliance, transiency, finances, motivation, and follow-up, to name a few, are not as well formulated. However, commitment to the child's health must be basic to all other considerations.

Ideally, the child has had regular physical examinations, routine serial developmental assessments with standardized instruments, and periodic evaluations of speech, vision, and hearing. For an excellent summary of the various screening and diagnostic tools available to the nurse practitioner, see Brown and Murphy (1975, Chap. 4). Screening tests are usually simple and inexpensive, performed on a population at risk for the problem for which the screening is done. According to Frankenburg (1975, p. 36), the criteria for a good screening test are:

1. Acceptability by the public and community professionals
2. Simplicity of equipment and procedures
3. Reliability in terms of the consistency or replication of results
4. Validity or the extent to which the test measures what it purports to
5. Appropriateness, especially related to the age, experience, and socioeconomic background of the population being screened and its similarity to the population on which the test was standardized
6. Costs which are reasonable

A variety of useful screening tools related specifically to school readiness are available to health professionals who have no special training in psychometrics. These have been thoroughly reviewed by Buros (1972) and Goldstein (1975, pp. 477–538) in terms of standardization, reliability, validity, and recommended use. The practitioner may wish to utilize some of these tests in conjunction with other measures indicative of school readiness.

Caution must be exercised in how the results of any one test are applied to decisions related to the individual child. Some tests are fairly good at identifying those who will succeed in kindergarten but fail to identify accurately those who are not ready. For example, one test used for prekindergarten screening accurately predicted 96 percent of the children who were subsequently successful in kindergarten, but 85 percent of the predictions were incorrect in predicting those who were not ready for kindergarten. To reduce the disadvantages imposed by a false positive, those who are shown to be "unready" on screening should be referred for further testing.

Educational specialists are especially concerned about how test scores are utilized for disadvantaged children. Although these children may enter school with lower readiness scores than advantaged children, they often "make an initial spurt when exposed to the school environment" (Lessler and Bridges, 1973, p. 39). Instead of accurately predicting success in school, for these children the tests may reflect a temporary lack of experience and training in school readiness. On the other hand, the test results probably correlate better with the readiness status of children who come from environmentally enriched backgrounds. For these reasons it is especially important to note on what kind of population a specific test was standardized and norms established. Readiness tests which have been standardized on a middle class, suburban population may not be appropriate for the child whose past environmental interactions are essentially different. In fact, it has been found that lower cutoff scores for disadvantaged children more accurately reflect school readiness and future success. In recognition of these differences some tests are now providing differential norms, adjusted cutoff scores, or separate scoring systems to compensate for socioeconomic status (Telegdy, 1974, p. 355).

The tests presented in Table 10-1 may be of some use to the nurse practitioner in screening those in need of evaluation for their level of preparation for school. These tests do not require special training, are generally easily administered by following detailed instructions, and are appropriate for testing either prekindergarten or kindergarten-age children for certain areas of development generally related to school success. The

Table 10-1 Screening Tests for Evaluating School Readiness

Test	Obtained From	Age	Purpose	Description	Standardization
ABC Inventory	Educational Studies and Development 1357 Forest Park Road Muskegon, MI 49441	Prekindergarten	Identifying children who are immature for a standard school program in kindergarten or first grade Evaluating conceptual and perceptual motor readiness	Items arranged into four groups Drawing a man Answering questions about characteristics of objects Answering questions about general topics Carrying out simple tasks related to numbers and shapes	Little information on standardization population Reliability and predictive validity criticized, particularly when used to identify individual children who were not ready for kindergarten
Denver Developmental Screening Test (DDST) (Appendix 5)	Ladoca Foundation East 51st Ave. and Lincoln St. Denver, CO 80216	Birth to 6 yr	Detecting developmental delays from infancy through preschool years Identifying children at risk for developing school problems and in need of further testing and/or referral	105 test items divided into four categories Gross motor Language Fine motor adaptive Personal/social skills	On a population which reflected socioeconomic composition of Denver
Preschool Inventory (revised 1970)	Educational Testing Service 1947 Center St. Berkeley, CA 94704	3–6 yr	Measuring achievement in areas assumed necessary for success in school Especially useful in indentifying the "degree of disadvantage" of the child from a deprived environment	Comprises 64 items divided into 4 subject areas Personal/social responsiveness Associative vocabulary Numerical concept activation Sensory concept activation Easy to administer and score Utilizes materials which are readily attainable or made	On lower and middle class children
Primary Academic Sentiment Scale (PASS)	Priority Innovations, Inc. P.O. Box 792 Skokie, IL 60076	4 yr, 4 mo to 7 yr, 3 mo	Obtaining objective information about a child's motivation for learning, level of maturity, and independence from parent	Comprises 38 items which direct child to mark a picture which reflects personal attitude or preference in a specified situation	Standardized on middle class suburban children Not recommended for disadvantaged children Some critics question if it should be used to predict

Table 10-1 Screening Tests for Evaluating School Readiness (*continued*)

Test	Obtained From	Age	Purpose	Description	Standardization
					school success; others note results correlate well with "teacher ratings of the child's academic interest"
Ready or Not? The School Readiness Checklist	Research Concepts 1368 E. Airport Rd. Muskegon, MI 49443	Prekindergarten	Providing parents with a short checklist to arrive at a rough index of the child's physical, psychological, and developmental readiness for school	43 items categorized in 7 groups related to age and growth, general activity, practical skills, memory, understanding, general knowledge, attitudes and interests	Little information provided on standardization population or reliability of the test Some demonstrated correlation with teacher ratings
Screening Test of Academic Readiness (STAR)	Priority Innovations, Inc. P.O. Box 792 Skokie, IL 60076	4 yr–6 yr, 5 mo	Measuring school readiness in groups of preschoolers and kindergarten children by identifying learning problems and those in need of individualized help	50 items divided into 8 categories: picture vocabulary, letters, copying, picture description, human figure drawing, relationships, numbers, picture completion	On middle to upper middle class suburban white population Many of the items derived from standard IQ tests; results correlate highly with IQ scores
Sprigle School Readiness Screening Test (SSRST)	Learning to Learn School, Inc. 1936 San Marco Blvd. Jacksonville, FL 32207	4 yr, 6 mo to 6 yr, 9 mo	Providing nurses and physicians with a means of making a rapid assessment of a child's cognitive readiness for school	Items comprise 9 areas: verbal comprehension, size relationships, visual discrimination, reasoning ability, understanding of numbers, analogies, information, vocabulary, spatial relationships Items similar to those on the Stanford-Binet	Lower and middle class children Relatively high reliability and validity for predicting cognitive readiness
Test of Basic Experiences	CTB/McGraw-Hill Delmonte Research Park Monterey, CA 93940	Level K: preschool and kindergarten Level L: kindergarten and grade 1	Indicating how well child's experiences have prepared him or her for scholastic activities of school Detecting deficiencies in basic experiences	Level K: 28 items divided into 5 subtests: mathematics, language, science, social studies, general concepts	On students from private and public preschools and schools

results of any one test must not be viewed as conclusive evidence of an individual's readiness for school but rather considered in conjunction with behavioral observation, a complete history, information about the family's social situation, the child's social interactions and response to previous learning experiences and the child's resourcefulness, autonomy, and coping abilities.

PARENT COUNSELLING

After the administration of a screening test focused on general development or one specifically designed to indicate school readiness, the nurse practitioner can note areas where the parent(s) and child could promote development. Clearly, children whose scores reflect abnormal or questionable development should be retested and/or referred for further diagnostic workup. But some suggestions could be useful for the child who needs assistance or encouragement in specific areas to promote readiness during the year before entering school. Such suggestions could also be useful as guidelines for anticipatory guidance as parents request ideas on enriching their child's experience prior to school entrance. These areas are conveniently divided into three major classifications of development: psychosocial emotional, physical motor, and cognitive language. The suggestions are not meant to be all-inclusive but rather starting points for both the parent(s) and the practitioner who are planning for the unique needs of the individual child.

Psychosocial and Emotional Readiness

The preschooler approaching school age becomes progressively more sociable with peers and adults, learning a great deal through play, such as taking turns, sharing, competing, cooperating, and separating from parents. Through dramatic play the child should have had the opportunity of trying out different roles which increase understanding of the adult world. Awareness of her or his own sex and identification with a parent or parent substitute of the same sex has patterned many of the preschooler's behaviors within culturally defined limitations. Where the sociocultural barriers have been exceeded, the child has been made aware of transgressions. The child is now toilet trained, has adopted the parents' table manners, can dress with minimal supervision, and has gained control over impulsive hyperactivity, temper tantrums, and aggression. Some responsibility can be taken for self away from home while at preschool or friends' homes. A firm foundation has been laid for the developing self-concept. The child's view of self as a good or bad person results largely from acceptance and approval by significant others of the child's behaviors and products. For the child entering school, the major emotional social adjustments will entail tolerating long periods away from home, adjusting to the norms of the kindergarten group, forming new friendships, and meeting new achievement demands. The child who manifests persistent negativistic behaviors, regressions, unrealistic fears, anxieties, extremes of temperament, or breath-holding spells is in need of a thorough evaluation (Gabriel, 1971).

The following are suggestions for development:

1. Facilitate social interaction with same-age peers of both sexes by means of formal preschool or Sunday school experiences, informal neighborhood groups, and supervised outings with adults (zoo, park, museum, post office, fire station, etc.).
2. Provide play materials which can be utilized for dramatic play, interactive play, and competitive games, such as old clothes, cardboard or wooden boxes, old furniture, pots, pans, nurse or doctor kits.
3. Encourage an increase in independence and initiative by letting the child make choices about games and daily activities.
4. Promote and reward self-help skills in bathing, dental care, dressing, eating, bedtime habits, and toileting.
5. Define reasonable, consistent limits and expectations within which the child can develop self-control and a sense of responsibility.
6. Promote a positive self-concept by expressing appropriate approval of behaviors and productions.
7. Promote gender identification by allowing the child to adopt appropriate sex-role behaviors.
8. Provide opportunities for separation from parents: activities away from home supervised by other responsible adults.

Physical-Motor Readiness

Physically, the child approaching school age is demonstrating changes in body proportions. The head has almost reached adult proportions, and subcutaneous fat is decreasing relative to muscle mass, which is increasing. Extremities have lengthened proportionate to trunk and have become sturdier. Because of neurological maturation both gross motor and fine motor capabilities are becoming well developed, resulting in increasing coordination and integration of bodily movements. Bowel and bladder control should now be complete, another indication of neurological maturation. Children who manifest delayed motor development, clumsiness, poor coordination, or hyperactivity are at risk for developing learning disabilities and need thorough physical and neurological evaluations.

Although not visible, dental growth and calcification are occurring within the gums. Visual acuity has reached 20/30 for the 4- and 5-year-olds, but 5 to 10 percent of this age group has one or more defects which should be identified (Charney, 1968). The child can accurately hear pure-tone frequencies ranging from 500 to 6000 Hz at 25 db, although some degree of impairment exists in 2 to 12 percent of children. Overall growth and development is greatly dependent upon a well-balanced diet which provides adequate nutrients. The child between 4 and 6 years has recommended daily allowance (RDA) needs of about 1800 cal, 30 g of protein, 800 mg of calcium, and 10 mg of iron, as well as other daily essential vitamins and minerals for optimum growth (Food and Nutrition Board, 1974). There are a variety of ways in which the essential nutrients can be included in the diet and the nurse practitioner can provide this advice.

The following are some suggestions for development:

1. Maintain regular physical, dental vision, and hearing assessments.
2. Establish a regular home dental program.
3. Provide and encourage a nutritionally balanced diet.
4. Provide opportunities for gross motor activities such as climbing, running, jumping, hopping, skipping, balancing, throwing, catching, swinging, pedaling, and pounding.
5. Provide opportunity for fine motor activities such as writing, scribbling, painting, coloring, drawing, cutting, tying, and manipulating small objects.
6. To prevent accidents, teach the child how to use toys safely and to observe traffic rules if play activities should occur near the street.

Cognitive-Language Readiness

Cognition is the process by which we gain knowledge about the world around us. It involves perception, thinking, problem solving, abstraction, and conceptualization, abilities which are related to the interaction between one's genetic inheritance and the environment in which one grows up. The importance of the environment in promoting intelligence has been indicated in studies which show a correlation between an enriching, stimulating preschool program and the measurable improvement of the child's IQ, language, and reading readiness. Approaching school age, the child is still in the preoperational stage of cognitive development and is unable to conserve quantity, length, or number. Concepts related to classification, seriation, time, space, quantity, and causality are developing but continue to be egocentric and perception-dominated.

In the realm of language, which is closely related to intelligence, the 4- to 5-year-old has mastered the basic grammar rules. Articulation continues to improve even into the first grade, where 15 to 20 percent of the children are still likely to be described as having defective articulation, which includes omissions, substitutions, distortions, or additions (Milisen, 1971, p. 624). Recent attention is focusing on children who speak a black dialect or Spanish-oriented English, nonstandard variations which have their own internal consistency, logic, and structural rules. These cross-cultural speech differences must not be confused with phonetic speech disorders in need of therapy. Children displaying these cultural differences usually belong to a speech community whose linguistic demands they do meet. Within the community they are able to communicate effectively through language, have their needs met, respond appropriately in social interchange, and generally comply with the accepted norms. In some educational systems there has been success teaching English as a second language while not ignoring or devaluing the natural dialect of the children (William, 1970, p. 410).

The following are some suggestions for development:

1. Establish an uncritical atmosphere for self-expression.
2. Introduce simple concepts related to the time of day, the day of the week, the season of the year, the dates of special holidays and birthdays.
3. Assist the child in learning mathematical concepts by analyzing daily situations in terms of classification, seriation, counting, adding, subtracting, and dividing.
4. Provide games which are intellectually stimulating and educationally appropriate for the child's age.
5. Answer questions related to causality honestly and simply in order to establish a foundation for increasing knowledge.
6. Listen to the child's accounts of happenings in daily life. Respond in a manner which provides a model for the child's expressive language skills.
7. Provide records and tapes of stories and songs which the child may listen to, sing along with, discuss, or dramatize.
8. Read to the child, utilizing the public library for an extensive variety of books and magazines.

CONCLUSION

In conclusion, school readiness is an extremely important area of pediatric development to be assessed by the nurse practitioner. Rather than including only intellectual functioning, the assessment must encompass total development as well as behavioral observations and a complete health, developmental, and social history. Specific tests have been reviewed which can be useful in providing additional information specific to school readiness. Caution must be exercised in the interpretation and application of these tests, depending on their standardization population and their reliability and validity in actually predicting readiness for school. An area of special concern is what to suggest to the parent(s) of the child who is supposedly "not ready" or who is striving toward readiness. A variety of suggestions have been posed which must be adjusted to the unique situation of the individual child. High-quality preschool programs can often overcome readiness problems. Whether the child stays at home or is enrolled in a Head Start program or a private preschool, the goal is to provide an enriched environment which promotes physical-motor, social-emotional, and cognitive-language functioning. A deficiency in any one of these areas can detract from the child's readiness for the school experience and subsequent school successes.

references

Bandura, A., and Walters, R. H. *Social learning and personality development*. New York: Holt, 1963.

Brown, Marie, and Murphy, Mary. *Ambulatory pediatrics for nurses*. New York: McGraw-Hill, 1975.

Buros, Oscar K. *The 7th mental measurements yearbook*. Highland Park, N.J.: The Gryphen Press, 1972.

Camp, B., van Doorninck, W., Frankenburg, W., and Lampe, J. Preschool development testing in prediction of school problems. *Clinical Pediatrics*, **16**(3):257–263 (1977).

Charney, Evan. Screening tests, birth to six years of age. In M. Green and R. Haggerty (ed.), *Ambulatory pediatrics*. Philadelphia: Saunders, 1968, pp. 424–435.

Erickson, Eric. *Childhood and society*. New York: Norton, 1951.

Food and Nutrition Board. *Recommended dietary allowances*. Washington, D.C.: National Academy of Sciences, National Research Council, 1974.

Frankenburg, William. Criteria in screening test selection. In W. Frankenburg and B. Camp (ed.), *Pediatric screening tests*. Springfield: Charles C Thomas, 1975, pp. 23–37.

Gabriel, H. Paul. Identification of potential emotional and cognitive disturbances in the 3 to 5 year old child. *Pediatric clinics of North America,* **18**(1): 179–189 (1971).

Goldstein, Arnold. School readiness and achievement. In W. Frankenburg and B. Camp (eds.), *Pediatric screening tests.* Springfield: Charles C Thomas, 1975, pp. 477–538.

Lessler, Ken, and Bridges, Judith. The prediction of learning problems in a rural setting. *Journal of Learning Disabilities,* **6**(2):36–40 (1973).

McLaughlin, Barry. *Learning and social behavior.* New York: The Free Press, 1971.

Maier, Henry. *Three theories of child development.* New York: Harper & Row, 1965.

Milisen, R. The incidence of speech disorders. In Lee Travis (ed.), *Handbook of speech pathology and audiology.* New York: Appleton-Century-Crofts, 1971.

Piaget, Jean. *The psychology of intelligence.* London: Routledge & Kegan Paul, Ltd., 1950.

Sears, Robert. A theoretical framework for personality and social behavior. *American Psychologist,* **6**: 476–483 (1951).

Telegdy, Gabriel. The relationship between socioeconomic status and school readiness. *Psychology in the Schools,* **11**(3):351–356 (1974).

Williams, Frederick. *Language and poverty.* Chicago: Markham Publishing Company, 1970.

PART 2

families with special needs

11 Parenting

THERESA M. ELDRIDGE

I. Basic Information

A. Parenting is a learned process whereby individuals provide for the safety and physical and emotional well-being of a child.

B. Parenting is a process by which the child is socialized to the dominant values of the parent(s)' culture.

C. Parenting is a process of child rearing accomplished, one hopes, with love, patience, and a sense of humor.

D. Knowledge of parenting and parenting skills are learned.

E. Parenting skills frequently are developed by the process of trial and error.

F. Parent(s) can develop appropriate and inappropriate parenting skills.

II. Developmental Tasks of Parenthood

A. Early parenthood: first child (Duvall, 1971)

1. Expanding and refining the communications system, mutual recognition of the involvement and emotional ties with the child, and acceptance of sharing one's mate
2. Adjusting to continuous child care, reworking patterns of responsibility and accountability
3. Meeting the increased costs of living as a child-rearing family
4. Adopting housing arrangements to accommodate a growing child
5. Reestablishing mutually satisfying sexual relationships
6. Reshaping relationships within the larger family circle
7. Adjusting to community and social life as a child-rearing family
8. Deciding to plan for further pregnancies or deciding to have no more children
9. Reworking an appropriate philosophy of family life

B. Parenthood: multiple children (Duvall, 1971)

1. Expanding and refining the communications system, acceptance and sharing between children and parent(s)
2. Adjusting to complexity of child care for more than one child, readjusting patterns of responsibility and accountability for all family members
3. Meeting the expanded costs of living for a multiple-child family
4. Adapting housing arrangements to accommodate additional family members
5. Establishing mutually satisfying sexual relationships with regard to increased demands and responsibilities of parenting more than one child
6. Reshaping relationships within the expanded family circle
7. Readjusting to community and social life as a child-rearing family
8. Deciding to plan for further pregnancies or deciding to have no more children
9. Adjusting to unique characteristics of each child
10. Reworking family structure to accommodate the needs of the new and older family members

III. Parenting Styles

A. Authoritarian

1. Stresses firm discipline and obedience to authority

2. Attempts to suppress sex role behavior that does not fit with conventional values
3. Has a hierarchic conception
4. Has more of a tendency to use physical or psychological punishment

B. Egalitarian
1. Emphasizes individual's development
2. Exerts less pressure to conform to conventional values and sex role behaviors
3. Has overlapping parental roles
4. Finds mutually acceptable alternatives

C. Overpermissive
1. Sets few or no limits
2. Punishes inconsistently or not at all
3. Places emphasis on child being the decision maker

IV. Parenting Situations

A. Extended family: multiple parenting
1. Advantages
   a. Can be helpful for inexperienced parents to have more experienced extended family members help and provide guidance.
   b. May be advantageous to child in developing trusting relationships with adults other than parent(s).
   c. Incorporates support systems.
2. Disadvantages
   a. There can be friction between parent(s) and extended family members if disagreement occurs regarding parenting issues.
   b. Parent(s) may not be able to develop full ability to parent due to family pressure or lack of opportunity.
   c. Child can be confused by the variety and possible inconsistencies of parenting from multiple sources, perhaps developing divided loyalties.

B. Nuclear family: traditional (father working, mother at home)
1. Advantages
   a. One continuous care giver may decrease inconsistency of parenting.
   b. Quantity of time available for parenting is increased.
   c. Child can develop a strong trusting relationship with at least one individual.
2. Disadvantages
   a. There may be a lack of father involvement in child care.
   b. Mother may be bored or frustrated and need relief.
   c. Quantity of time available for parenting is not necessarily positively correlated with quality.

C. Nuclear family: nontraditional (both parents working)
1. Advantages
   a. It can provide for mutual exchanging of roles between parents.
   b. It can provide for increased father involvement in child care.
   c. Child can develop trusting relationship with both parents as well as care givers at a day-care center or school.
   d. Child may be exposed to other children, which may be particularly helpful in the single-child family.
2. Disadvantages
   a. There may continue to be a lack of father involvement, thereby increasing the demands on the mother.
   b. Some parenting is transferred to the day-care center or school.
   c. Child may experience confusion with the variety of expectations and possible inconsistencies received from multiple-parenting sources.

D. Single-parent family
1. Advantages
   a. May be a more stable environment than a nuclear family experiencing difficulty and staying together only for the child's sake.
   b. May be a solution for the single men and women who do not wish to marry but do wish to have children.
   c. May have increased consistency in parenting, with decreased conflict in parenting beliefs and values.
   d. Parent may become more self-sufficient and well rounded.
2. Disadvantages
   a. Lack of either male or female sex role model
   b. Parent may work; transference of some parenting to day care or school
   c. May involve increased financial stress
   d. Limited environment for child and parent
      (1) Introduction of more variables needed, such as a grandparent providing a role model of the opposite sex
      (2) Relief needed by single parent
      (3) Variety perhaps needed by child
   e. Possible increased emotional stress for parent and child as a result of divorce, separation, death
   f. Difficulties perhaps caused by a new partner in the home
      (1) Desirable to let children know ahead of time

(2) Possible competition for the affection and attention of the parent
(3) Desirable that partner establish relationship with child
(4) Partner perhaps an outsider to the family structure; should spend time in the home, with regular routine

E. Teenage parent
1. Advantages—same as with extended or nuclear family depending on the situation, i.e., teenage girl living at home with parent(s) or living with father of child
2. Disadvantages
   a. May be single—disadvantages same as for single parent
   b. Teenager perhaps physically and emotionally immature, still a child needing parenting and not prepared to parent
   c. May have increased financial problems, i.e., may not have high school education
   d. May have negative support systems—family may be punitive if teenager pregnant out of wedlock

F. Parent utilizing day care
1. Advantages
   a. Introduces different variables in parenting—more input and experience
   b. May provide exposure to other children
      (1) Increased opportunity to develop peer relationships
      (2) Potential enhancement of child's development via imitation of peers
   c. May free parent to pursue activities which enhance financial and psychological well-being
2. Disadvantages
   a. Guilt sometimes experienced by parent for leaving child
   b. May have difficulty finding an appropriate and satisfactory facility
   c. Decreased parental involvement in child care
   d. May increase financial distress
   e. May result in beginning- and end-of-day difficulties and behavior problems, e.g., temper tantrums when parent leaves or returns to pick up child

V. Factors Affecting Parenting Skills

A. Cognitive level of parent(s) and level of understanding
B. Expectations and philosophies of parenthood
C. Temperament and personality traits of child and parent(s)
D. Parenting received by parent(s)
E. Previous experiences of parent(s)
F. Desirability of parenthood—planned or unplanned
G. Parenting readiness and ability to parent
H. Availability of support systems
I. Self-esteem of parent(s)
J. Childhood memories of parent(s)
K. Cultural, ethnic, financial background

VI. Results of Deficits in Parenting (in order of incidence)

A. Childhood behavior problems
B. Perpetual inappropriate parenting behavior (from generation to generation)
C. Child neglect; failure to thrive
D. Developmental delays in child
E. Child abuse

VII. Assessment

A. Assessment of the parent(s)
1. Readiness to parent
   a. General appearance of parent(s)
   b. Parental developmental level
      (1) Cognitive ability
      (2) Ability to read and write
      (3) Ability to follow directions
      (4) Problem-solving ability
   c. History
      (1) Child abuse of parent as a child
      (2) Type of parenting parent(s) received as children
      (3) Planned or unplanned pregnancy
   d. Steps taken to prepare for child, i.e., provision for a room, bed, clothes, time off from work, baby-sitter
   e. Philosophy and expectations of parent(s)
   f. Available support systems
      (1) Personal contacts—family, friends
      (2) Professional contacts—nurse, physician
2. Level of parenting ability: parenting behaviors-observation, and history
   a. How parent(s) meets day-to-day situations of child rearing, e.g., rivalry, toilet training, discipline
   b. Parental understanding of normal growth and development
   c. Parental flexibility in deciding on alternatives
   d. Parental willingness to respond to the child's readiness for change
   e. Parental understanding of differences in children's personalities and needs

3. Parent-child relationship
   a. Parental ability to describe child's characteristics
   b. Parental expectations of child
   c. Level of attachment: ability to touch, responses to child's actions
   d. Parental ability to describe child's typical day
   e. Child's responses to parent(s)
4. Environment
   a. Does it meet the physical needs of the child?
   b. Is it safe?
   c. Does it provide stimulation and freedom for exploration?
5. Assessment tools
   a. Broussard's Neonatal Perception Inventory (NPI): determines parental perception and expectation of an infant's behaviors
   b. Caldwell's Home Observation for Measurement of the Environment (Home): assesses the quantity and quality of social, emotional, and cognitive support available to a child in the home

B. Assessment of the child

1. Physical examination
   a. Normal growth parameters
   b. Evidence of physical trauma
2. Child-parent relationship
   a. Child's description of response to activities, including discipline—the rules of the house
   b. Child's ability to discuss concerns with parent(s)
   c. Child's ability to relate to parent(s); level of attachment
3. Assessment tools
   a. Brazelton's Neonatal Behavioral Assessment Scale: observation of the newborn's response to the environment
   b. Carey Infant Temperament Questionnaire: obtains temperament profile of infant 4 to 8 months old based on parent(s)' observations
   c. Denver Developmental Screening Test: assesses developmental ability from birth to 6 years in four areas—language, personal social, fine motor and gross motor
   d. Alpern and Boll's Developmental Profile: assesses level of functioning from birth to adolescence in five areas—fine and gross motor ability, self-help, social ability, intellectual, and communication ability

C. Potential risk factors

1. Abuse of a parent during childhood
2. Stress factors
   a. Financial
   b. Single parent
   c. Teenage parent
   d. Birth resulting from sexual assault
3. Poor parent-child bonding
4. Negative support systems or no support systems
5. Changed life-style
   a. Parent bored staying home
   b. Parent resentful of attention given child by other parent
6. New situation at home
   a. Remarried parent
   b. Single parent living with significant other
   c. New child
7. Interrelationship between parents, e.g., parent who verbally or physically assaults other parent
8. Abnormalities
   a. Child with chronic or debilitating disease
   b. Child with retarded development or physical or emotional handicap

VIII. Promotion of Appropriate Parenting

A. Role of primary health care practitioner

1. Assessment, identification, preventive counselling regarding parenting behavior and skills
2. Provision of education and counselling concerning:
   a. Normal growth and development
   b. Identification of unique characteristics and needs of each child
   c. Child-rearing practices
3. Assistance to parent(s) in identifying, developing, and modifying parenting capabilities according to own style and needs of the child
4. Demonstration of appropriate role-modeling behaviors for parent(s)

B. Education

1. High school/prenatal parenting classes
   a. Normal growth and development
   b. Current child-rearing practices
2. Literature and audiovisual aids for parent(s)
3. Parenting groups

C. Counselling

1. Identifying parental expectations of child and of parenthood
2. Identifying support systems and resources and their utilization
3. Identifying parenting skills, both strengths and weaknesses

4. Assisting parent(s) to utilize information obtained during assessment of child's physical, behavioral, and developmental status, e.g., teaching the parent of an infant who has little or no self-quieting behavior to help the infant learn such behavior, or counselling the parent of a child who is very active regarding normal expected behavior and possible alternatives for that child
5. Providing parent(s) with alternative methods of dealing with certain situations, such as discipline, sleep problems
6. Assisting parent(s) in identifying own roles

bibliography

Brazelton, T. Berry. *Infants and mothers: Differences in development.* New York: Dell, 1972.

———. Toddlers and parents—A *declaration of independence.* New York: Delacorte Press, 1974.

Callahan, Sidney. *Parenting.* New York: Doubleday, 1973.

Cannon, Rose Broechel. The development of maternal touch during early mother-infant interaction. *Journal of Obstetric, Gynecologic and Neonatal Nursing,* **6**:28–33 (1977).

Chamberlin, Robert W. Parenting styles, child behavior and the pediatrician. *Pediatric Annals,* **6**:50–63 (1977).

Chess, Stella. Temperament and the parent-child interaction. *Pediatric Annals,* **6**:26–45 (1977).

Dodson, Fitzhugh. *How to parent.* Secaucus, New Jersey: Book Sales Incorporated, 1970.

Dubois, Don R. Indications of an unhealthy relationship between parents and premature infant. *Journal of Obstetric, Gynecologic and Neonatal Nursing,* **4**:21–24 (1975).

Duvall, Evelyn. *Family development.* New York: Lippincott, 1971.

Erikson, Erik H. *Childhood and society.* New York: Norton, 1963.

Erickson, Marcene. *Assessment and management of developmental changes in children.* St. Louis: Mosby, 1976.

Farrar, Carrol Ann. A data collection procedure to assess behavioral individuality in the neonate. *Journal of Obstetric, Gynecologic and Neonatal Nursing,* **3**:15–19 (1974).

Fraiberg, Selma. *The magic years.* New York: Scribner, 1959.

Friedman, David, and Swinger, Hershel (eds.). Parenting—I: Parenting and child behavior. *Pediatric Annals,* September (1977).

———, and ——— (eds.). Parenting—II: Parenting and the behavior disorders of childhood. *Pediatric Annals,* October (1977).

Gordon, Thomas. *P.E.T. in action.* New York: Wyden Books, 1976.

Hurd, Jeanne Marie L. Assessing maternal attachment: First step toward the prevention of child abuse. *Journal of Obstetric, Gynecologic and Neonatal Nursing,* **4**:25–30 (1975).

Ilg, Frances, and Ames, Louise Bates. *Child behavior from birth to ten.* New York: Harper & Row, 1955.

Johnson, Suzanne Hall, and Grubbs, Judith Pierson. The premature infant's reflex behaviors: Effect on the maternal-child relationship. *Journal of Obstetric, Gynecologic and Neonatal Nursing,* **4**:15–24 (1975).

Kempe, C. Henry, and Helfer, Ray. *Helping the battered child and his family.* Philadelphia: Lippincott, 1972.

Klaus, Marshall H., and Kennell, John. *Maternal-infant bonding.* St. Louis: Mosby, 1976.

LeMasters, E. E. Parents in modern America. Homewood, Ill.: Dorsey, 1977.

Leonard, Susan Woolf. How first-time fathers feel toward their newborns. *Maternal Child Nursing,* November–December: 361–365 (1976).

Lewis, Michael, and Rosenblum, Leonard (eds.). *The effect of the infant on its caregiver.* New York: Wiley, 1974.

McBride, Angelo Barron. *The growth and development of mothers.* New York: Harper & Row, 1973.

Reiber, Virginia D. Is the nurturing role natural to fathers? *Maternal Child Nursing,* November–December: 366–371 (1976).

Reinhart, John B. Syndromes of deficits in parenting: Abuse, neglect and accidents. *Pediatric Annals,* **6**:7–24 (1977).

12 Adoption

MARILYN GREBIN

The primary health care practitioner is a valuable resource to the couple wishing to adopt a child. The practitioner can provide information about the adoption process and the health maintenance of the child and offer emotional support for the family unit. In this chapter some general guidelines for intervention are explored. The reader must be aware of the policies and procedures that apply within the state of origin; however, parental concerns are generally the same throughout the country.

I. Basic Information

A. The natural parent(s), adoptive parent(s), and the child have the right to obtain proper medical, legal, and social services throughout the adoption procedure.

B. Fewer children are available for adoption.
1. Birthrate is down.
2. Unmarried women are keeping their out-of-wedlock infants.

C. Children over 2 years old, nonwhite, or handicapped are difficult to place.

D. State subsidies are becoming available for adopting families.

E. Adoption agencies are simplifying procedures.
1. Older couples and single parents are being considered.
2. Adoption Resource Exchange of North America (ARENA) can provide adoption agencies with adoptable children in other states.

F. Child is placed in the home 6 to 12 months before procedure is complete.

G. "Black market" adoption procedures should be discouraged.

H. Parental rights can be terminated by the court.

II. Initial Visit with Adoptive Parent(s)

A. Gathering historical information
1. Reasons for adoption
2. Knowledge of adoption procedures
3. Parent(s) expectations of the health care provider
4. Age of the child they wish to adopt
5. Previous contact with an adoption agency
6. Willingness to adopt a handicapped or racially mixed child
7. Social history
   a. Educational preparation of the parent(s)
   b. Employment history
   c. Religion
   d. Housing situation
8. Survey of immediate family
   a. Other children
      (1) Number
      (2) Ages and sexes
      (3) Chronic or genetic problems
      (4) Any children that have recently died
   b. Medical history of adoptive parent(s) (interested in any chronic or debilitating health problems)

B. Counselling
1. Discuss emotional requirements of parent(s).
   a. Mutual acceptance that an adoption will benefit this family unit
   b. Genuine desire to give love, attention, and guidance to a child not biologically their own
   c. Maturity to accept the responsibility of being a parent
2. Encourage parent(s) to express their con-

cerns about the adoption procedures and child rearing.
3. Explain the basic adoption agency procedures
   a. Social services
   b. Legal counsel
   c. Family investigation
   d. Home survey
   e. Psychological evaluation
   f. Health assessments
4. Discuss the role of the health care provider both before and after the adoption.
5. Make yourself available to the adoptive parent(s) to answer questions during the process.

III. Arrival of the Child into the New Family Unit

A. History: The adoption agency will provide the following information for the parent(s) to serve as a data base for the health care provider.
1. Date of birth
2. Prenatal history
   a. Maternal illness
   b. Drugs taken
   c. X-rays
   d. Medical complications (high blood pressure, infection, bleeding, etc.)
   e. Gestation
3. Birth history
   a. Duration of labor
   b. Complications during delivery
   c. Apgar score
   d. Complications in infant after delivery
      (1) Respiratory distress
      (2) Cyanosis
      (3) Jaundice
   e. Birth weight and length
4. Developmental history
5. Immunizations
6. Illnesses, injuries, or diseases
7. Biological parents' medical survey

B. Preadoption physical examination is done by the adoption agency's pediatrician.

C. Within the framework of collecting a data base, the primary health care practitioner should accomplish the following.
1. A complete physical examination
2. A growth and head-circumference chart
3. A follow-up on necessary immunizations
4. Screening
   a. Vision
   b. Hearing
   c. Development
5. Laboratory testing
   a. Complete blood count
   b. Urinalysis
   c. Venereal Disease Research Laboratories (VDRL) test
   d. Tine test
6. Home visit by the primary health care practitioner or public health nurse to assist the family with any problems of child care within the home environment

D. Counselling of parent(s) should be offered.
1. Provide for assistance and support during the transition
2. Establish a good rapport with the new parent(s)
3. Promote emotional attachment process of the parent(s) and the child
4. Help to decrease anxieties in the parent(s) about child care practices which may lead to a very indulgent, overprotective attitude
5. Allow parent(s) to express fears about child rearing and growing independence
6. Educate parent(s) about the developmental process
7. Help parent(s) to anticipate and cope with normal childhood problems
8. Determine a health follow-up schedule with the parent(s)
9. Assist the parent(s) in dealing with the child's questions about origin
   a. Encourage discussions of child's background[1]
   b. Answer questions honestly, considering the child's age
   c. Encourage parent(s) to foster the child's identity by providing him or her with knowledge of origin
   d. Inform the parent(s) that a few states have provisions for opening records by the adopted child upon adulthood

E. Counselling of the older adopted child should be offered. Spend time with the older child.
1. Establish a rapport
2. Allow the child time to express problems and concerns about new parent(s), home, and school
3. Support the child's self-identity and healthy ego development

[1]Adoption should not be stressed with the child. However, the parent(s) must learn to deal with their own feelings about the child's dual identity to assist the child.

bibliography

Barnard, Martha Underwood. Supportive care for the adoptive family. *Issues in Comprehensive Pediatric Nursing,* **2**(3):22–29 (1977).

Braff, Anne M. Telling children about their adoption: New alternatives. *Maternal-Child Nursing,* July–August: 254–259 (1977).

Committee on Adoption and Dependent Care 1970–1973, American Academy of Pediatrics. *Adoption of children* (3d ed.). Evanston, Ill., 1973.

Committee on Adoption and Dependent Care. The role of the pediatrician in adoption with reference to "the right to know." *Pediatrics,* **60**(3) (1977).

Hammon, Chloe. The adoptive family. *American Journal of Nursing,* **76**:251–257 (1976).

Katz, Sanford N. The changing legal status of foster parents. *Children Today,* November–December: 12–13 (1976).

Sokoloff, Burton. Adoptive families needs for counseling. *Clinical Pediatrics,* **18**(3):184–190 (1979).

Sorosky, Arthur. On unsealing the records in adoption. *American Journal of Psychiatry,* **134**(1):95 (1977).

Walker, Lorraine Olszewski. A survey of needs of adoptive parents. *Pediatric Nursing,* **4**(2):28–31 (1978).

13 Foster Care

R. EVELYN AABEL

I. Basic Considerations

A. Placing a child in foster care is a profoundly upsetting experience for a child.

B. A child separated from those for whom strong affection has developed goes through a process of mourning.

1. Mourning is likely to become distorted, intensified, and prolonged with each subsequent separation.
2. A highly ambivalent relationship to the lost person makes it harder to complete the process of mourning.
3. Early return of the mother or prompt provision of a mother substitute helps end the mourning process.
4. Mourning may never be successfully completed because of the following.
   a. Lack of an adequate mother substitute or poor placement
   b. Unnecessary interim placement
   c. A deeply rooted problem blocking the child from forming an affectionate relationship with an adequate mother substitute
   d. Previous damage to the child when living with biologic parent(s), or from repeated separations
   e. Failure to prepare the child adequately for separation and to help work through feelings and reactions to separation
5. Long-term effects of aborted mourning are as follows.
   a. Lasting inability to become emotionally involved with people
   b. Relationships that do occur often shallow and manipulative
   c. A combination in the child of exaggerated demands for closeness and an inability to tolerate closeness
   d. Placement sometimes equally traumatic for foster parent(s)
      (1) Upset to family's life
      (2) Considerable time before foster parent(s) experiences any reward

C. Maladaptive signs often precede foster care.

1. Failure to thrive
2. Abused child (physically or sexually)
3. Psychopathic behavior
4. Personality deterioration

II. Indications for Foster Care

A. Emergency indications

1. Illness, death, or hospitalization of an immediate family member
2. Violent parent(s)
3. Fire causing destruction of the home

B. Chronic indications

1. Inadequate food, clothing, or shelter
2. Separation or divorce, with neither parent assuming child care responsibility
3. Extremely young parent(s) lacking parenting skills
4. Mentally limited parent(s) who is unable to adequately care for a child
5. Parent(s) who leaves young children unsupervised
6. Parent(s) who educationally neglects own children or fails to provide needed health care
7. Parent(s) who simply can't cope with own children

III. Subjective Data

A. Complete history on first visit of foster child

B. Areas requiring careful investigation
1. Immunizations (records often lost and frequently children overimmunized)
2. Personality history
   a. Age appropriateness and personality characteristics of playmates (especially older children)
   b. Dependent or independent behavior
   c. Temperament
   d. Ability to relate to foster parent(s) and siblings
   e. Deformities that adversely affect child's personality
3. School history
   a. Name and type of school attending
   b. Appropriate grade for age
   c. Behavior exhibited in school
   d. Need for psychological testing
4. Family history (if known)
5. Social history—foster care
   a. Reason for placement in foster care
   b. Age at first placement
   c. Number of subsequent placements and reason for being moved
   d. Frequency of caseworker visits and goals set with foster parent(s) and child
   e. Relationship of foster parent(s) with biologic parent(s)
   f. Reaction of child prior to and after visiting with biologic parent(s)
6. Habits
   a. Appetite—food dislikes and attitudes toward eating
   b. Sleeping—hours, disturbances, snoring
   c. Exercise and play
   d. Urinary and bowel (enuresis or encopresis)
   e. Disturbances—thumb-sucking and nail-biting, masturbation, breath holding, tics, temper tantrums, nervousness, etc.

IV. Objective Data

A. Physical examination
1. Complete examination including neurological exam
2. Height, weight, and head circumference (if child is under 2 years or if apparent problem with head size) plotted on growth charts
3. Observation for anxiety and other behavioral manifestations
4. Observation for general hygiene
5. If sexually active, internal exam, Pap smear, gonorrhea culture, serology, etc.
6. Child screened for growth and development using age-appropriate screening tools
7. Vision and hearing screening when indicated

B. Laboratory data dependent on age, history, and physical examination findings

V. Assessment

A. Physical evaluation

B. Developmental evaluation

C. Adjustment to foster care

VI. Management and the Role of the Primary Health Care Practitioner

A. Identify signs of unsuccessful adjustment as soon as possible, and assist with alternative plan.

B. Assess current growth and development, and counsel foster parent(s) regarding appropriate stimulation and toys.

C. When the child is extremely traumatized by separation from the mother, examine alternatives (i.e., homemaker or day care).

D. Development of security within an environment is dependent on consistency and continuity of care; therefore, assist foster parent(s) in deciding limits to be set and reasons for maintaining limits.

E. Develop a plan with the caseworker, and prepare the child for placement.
1. Explain reasons and find out how the child feels about the plan.
2. Gradually introduce the child to the new home.

F. Visit the biologic parent(s) during the child's absence to see that appropriate changes are made so that child is not returned to the same inadequate environment.

G. Moving to a new home puts a child in a vulnerable situation, so assist child and family in making the adjustment.
1. The family may find the child's behavior very confusing and upsetting. The child may exhibit rage and anxiety, which can lead to discouragement and resentment of the child.
   a. Explain to foster parent(s) the need to listen and be available to child.
   b. Don't allow the child to destroy.
   c. A child in rage may need to be restrained, but in a supportive, nonfrightening way.
   d Redirect the rage through socially acceptable channels (e.g., give a young child a

Bozo the clown or pillow to punch; an older child might use a punching bag).

e. Strenuous hikes are also good for releasing energy and provide a quiet time to be with child.

2. Explain the mourning process to foster parent(s) so that a young child's kicking, screaming, and threatening will be understood as a child's way of trying to bring back mother.
3. Help the child accept fact that someone loved is lost, and help the child reinvest feelings in a substitute.
4. Evaluate with the family the effect a foster child has on the family as a whole, as well as on individuals within the home.
5. Recommend a local foster parents association (if available).
6. If the family or the child are unable to adjust, psychiatric help should be obtained.
7. Foster parent(s) should be aware of child's prior disturbance so as not to blame self for preexisting pathology.
8. Stress the importance of the formative years and explain the difficulty in unlearning and relearning. Maybe only the progression of deterioration can be stopped.
9 Consistent, planned follow-up of children returned to biologic parent(s) is essential.
   a. Observe relationships.
   b. Sort out feelings that occur in readjustment to home.
10. Group homes or institutions may be the best plan for some children.
    a. Many disturbed children are beyond foster care.
    b. Spare child repeated failure: A complete evaluation with professional help is warranted after one or two unsuccessful placements.

---

bibliography

Geiser, Robert L., and Malinowski, M. Norberta. Realities of foster child care. *American Journal of Nursing,* **78:**430–433 (1978).

Jacobson, Elinor, and Cockerum, JoAnne. As foster children see it. *Children Today,* November–December: 32–42 (1976).

Katz, Sanford. The changing legal status of foster parents. *Children Today,* November–December: 11–13 (1976).

Redl, Fritz. *When we deal with children.* New York: Free Press, 1968.

Silver, H. K., Kempe, H. C., Bruyn, H. B. *Handbook of pediatrics.* Los Altos, Calif.: Lange, 1977.

Steinhauer, Paul D., Assistant Professor, University of Toronto. How to succeed in the business of creating psychopaths without even trying. Unpublished speech, 1974.

14 The Gifted Child

THERESA M. ELDRIDGE

I. Basic Information

A. American Association for Gifted Children definition: a child whose performance is consistently remarkable in music, art, social leadership, other forms of giftedness (Witty, 1952)

B. Gifted person—one in possession of special talents and qualities of character and temperament, i.e., drive, perseverance, determination, high energy level

C. Identified areas of giftedness[1]

1. Academic ability—does well in academic settings
2. Creativity
3. Leadership
4. Human relationships
5. Intellectual ability—conceptualization, problem solving
6. Ability in visual and performing arts, e.g., theatre
7. Psychomotor/mechanical abilities, e.g., dance

D. Giftedness not in pure form—positive correlations shown between many abilities and aptitudes

E. Early identification essential for early, special intervention

F. Giftedness sometimes cause of difficulties

1. Isolation and disassociation from peers
2. Intolerance of those less gifted
3. Increased likelihood of mental illness and emotional problems is supported by studies

G. Characteristics of gifted child

1. Generally superior physically
2. Superior intelligence—over 130 IQ
3. Quick understanding
4. Retentive memory
5. Large vocabulary, skillful use of language
6. Insatiable curiosity
7. Reading at early age
8. Sensitivity to the environment
9. Outstanding resourcefulness
10. Imagination and creativity
11. Ability to organize
12. Insightfulness

H. Characteristics of giftedness often emerge early in childhood and are reinforced or discouraged by child's experiences

I. Significant effect of early years on child's development

1. Parental understanding of normal growth and development
2. Parent-child relationship favorably or unfavorably affecting child's developmental trend

J. Gifted and talented children found in all social and ethnic groups—often found in groups placing a great emphasis on intellectual values and offering more opportunities to develop skills and talents.

K. Most gifted children endowed with exceptional heredity, propitious childhood, conducive family and community conditions

L. Health professional can help by

1. Being aware of characteristics of the gifted
2. Assisting parent(s) in identifying and manag-

[1]Adapted by Jerry Villars, Ph.D., State Coordinator, Gifted and Talented Student Programs, Colorado Department of Education, Denver, Colorado, from the Colorado State Board of Education, *The position statement on the educational programming of the gifted and talented,* June 1978.

ing special aptitudes and talents of gifted child

II. Initial History

A. Age

B. Family history

1. Learning disabilities
2. Exceptional disabilities in any of the specified areas of giftedness

C. Social history

1. Stimulation—environmental
2. Freedom for exploration
3. Home, play, and school activities

D. Developmental history—acceleration of milestones

1. Personal/social
2. Language
3. Fine motor
4. Gross motor

E. Psychosocial history

1. Interrelationships with peers, family, adults
2. Behavioral characteristics, e.g., determination, drive, high energy level
3. Emotional adjustments

F. Past history

1 Medications, e.g., medication for hyperactivity
2. IQ
3. Testing for creativity or other related testing

III. Objective Data

A. Physical examination

1. Complete physical examination
2. Psychomotor skills
3. Language skills

B. Screening or testing (appropriate to areas of giftedness and age)

1. Developmental level
   a. Denver Developmental Screening Test (DDST) (see Appendix 5)
   b. The Developmental Profile
2. Vocabulary/articulation
   a. Denver Articulation Screening Exam (DASE)
   b. Peabody Picture Vocabulary Test
3. Intellectual abilities
   a. Stanford-Binet intelligence test
   b. Wechsler Intelligence Scale for Children (WISC)
4. Creativity—standardized tests being developed for
   a. Art
   b. Music
   c. Creative arts, e.g., theater
5. Conceptualization—intelligence tests
6. Psychomotor—testing of fine and gross motor development

IV. Management of the Gifted Child and Family

A. Counselling

1. Anticipatory guidance for the expectant family
   (1) Safety
   (2) Stimulation
   (3) Freedom for exploration
2. Anticipatory guidance for child-rearing family
   a. Assistance to parent(s) in utilizing data of child's physical and behavioral status to meet the needs of child and maximize potential
   b. Instruction concerning normal growth and development so family aware of expected norms and can identify any variations
3. Early identification
   a. History and observation of child for gifted characteristics, e.g., early speech development, manual dexterity, early conceptualization
   b. Assist parent(s) in identifying unique qualities of each child and provide possible alternatives of maximizing child's best qualities
   c. Testing

B. Follow-up

1. Parent/child education regarding concept of giftedness and its impact on child and family
2. Counsel regarding emotional adjustment of family and child, to each other and to peers
3. Help child to develop healthy self-concept
4. Assist child and family in developing appropriate coping mechanisms to deal with increased emotional stressors and adjustment
5. Assist family in manipulating environment to meet needs of child and in maximizing gifted characteristics—e.g., dance class to develop psychomotor and creative skills, or space for workshop for child gifted in mechanical skills
6. Act as a resource person for special needs of family and child
   a. Parenting groups for exceptional/gifted children
   b. Groups for gifted individuals
      (1) Encourage parent(s) to provide opportunity to develop peer relationships with other gifted individuals, e.g., MENSA

(2) Can provide support for appropriate emotional adjustment

C. Consultations/referrals

1. State and federal programs for exceptional children
2. Council for Exceptional Children
3. Informal or formal parent groups, groups for gifted individuals
4. Literature: *Exceptional Child Quarterly*
5. Testing services
6. School principal, teacher, guidance counsellor, nurse

V. Behavioral Characteristics of the Gifted Child

Child may demonstrate characteristics in one or more categories and may also have a combination of qualities from each category, or may demonstrate other characteristics not identified here

A. Intellectual ability

1. Learns rapidly and easily
2. Uses a great deal of common sense and practical knowledge
3. Reasons things out; thinks clearly; recognizes relationships; comprehends meanings
4. Retains what was heard or read without much rote drill
5. Knows about many things of which most students are unaware
6. Has a large vocabulary, using it easily and accurately
7. Can read books that are 1 to 2 years in advance of the rest of the class
8. Performs difficult mental tasks
9. Asks many questions; has a wide range of interests
10. Does some academic work 1 to 2 years in advance of the class
11. Is original in thinking; uses good but unusual methods
12. Is alert, keenly observant, and quick to respond

B. Creative ability

1. Always seems to be full of new ideas pertaining to most subjects
2. Invents things or creates original stories, plays, poetry, tunes, sketches, and so on
3. Can use materials, words, or ideas in new ways
4. Is able to put two or more ideas together to get a new idea
5. Sees flaws in things, including own work, and can suggest better ways to do a job or reach an objective
6. Is willing to experiment to get answers
7. Asks many questions; shows a great deal of intellectual curiosity
8. Is flexible and open-minded, willing to try one method after another and to change mind if need be; is not afraid of new ideas and will examine them before rejecting them

C. Leadership ability

1. Is liked and respected by most class members
2. Is able to influence others to work toward desirable goals
3. Is able to influence others to work toward undesirable goals
4. Can take charge of the group
5. Can judge the abilities of other students and find a place for them in the group's activities
6. Is able to figure out what is wrong with an activity and show others how to do it better
7. Is often asked for ideas and suggestions
8. Is looked to by others when something must be decided
9. Seems to sense what others want, and helps them accomplish it
10. Is a leader in several kinds of activities
11. Enters into activities with contagious enthusiasm
12. Is elected to offices

D. Scientific ability

1. Expresses self clearly and accurately through either writing or speaking
2. Reads 1 to 2 years ahead of the class
3. Is 1 to 2 years ahead of class in mathematical ability
4. Has greater-than-average ability to grasp abstract concepts and see abstract relationships
5. Has good motor coordination, especially eye-hand coordination; can do fine, precise manipulations
6. Is willing to spend time beyond the ordinary assignments or schedule on things that are of particular interest
7. Is not easily discouraged by failure of experiments or projects
8. Wants to know the causes and reasons for things
9. Spends much time on own special projects, such as making collections, constructing a radio, making a telescope

10. Reads a good deal of scientific literature and finds satisfaction in thinking about and discussing scientific affairs

E. Writing talent
1. Can develop a story from its beginning through the buildup and climax to an interesting conclusion
2. Gives a refreshing twist, even to old ideas
3. Uses only necessary details in telling a story
4. Keeps the idea organized within the story
5. Chooses descriptive words that show perception
6. Includes important details that other youngsters miss, and still gets across the central idea
7. Enjoys writing stories and poems
8. Makes the characters seem lifelike; captures the feelings of characters in writing

F. Dramatic talent
1. Readily shifts into the role of another character
2. Shows interest in dramatic activities
3. Uses voice to reflect changes of idea and mood
4. Understands and portrays the conflict in a situation when given the opportunity to act out a dramatic event
5. Communicates feelings by means of facial expression, gestures, and bodily movements
6. Enjoys evoking emotional responses from listeners
7. Shows unusual ability to dramatize feelings and experiences
8. Moves a dramatic situation to a climax and brings it to a well-timed conclusion when telling a story
9. Gets a good deal of satisfaction and happiness from playacting or dramatizing
10. Writes original plays or makes up plays from stories
11. Can imitate others; mimics people and animals

G. Artistic talent
1. Covers a variety of subjects in drawings or paintings
2. Takes artwork seriously; seems to find much satisfaction in it
3. Shows originality in choice of subject, technique, and composition
4. Is willing to try out new materials and experiences
5. Fills extra time with drawing, painting, and sculpturing activities
6. Uses art to express own experiences and feelings
7. Is interested in other people's artwork; can appreciate, criticize, and learn from others' work
8. Likes to model with clay, carve, or work with other forms of three-dimensional art

H. Musical talent
1. Responds more than others to rhythm and melody
2. Sings well
3. Puts verve and vigor into music
4. Buys records; goes out of way to listen to music
5. Enjoys harmonizing with others or singing in groups
6. Uses music to express personal feelings and experiences
7. Makes up original tunes
8. Plays one or more musical instruments well

I. Mechanical skills
1. Does good work on craft projects
2. Is interested in mechanical gadgets and machines
3. Has a hobby involving mechanical devices, such as radios, model trains, construction sets
4. Can repair gadgets; can put together mechanical things
5. Comprehends mechanical problems, puzzles, and trick questions
6. Likes to draw plans and make sketches of mechanical objects
7. Reads *Popular Mechanics* or other magazines or books on mechanical subjects

J. Physical skills
1. Is energetic and seems to need considerable exercise to stay happy
2. Enjoys participating in highly competitive physical games
3. Is consistently outstanding in many kinds of competitive games
4. Is one of the fastest runners in the class
5. Is one of the physically best coordinated in the class
6. Likes outdoor sports, hiking, and camping
7. Is willing to spend much time practicing physical activities, such as shooting baskets, playing tennis or baseball, or swimming

bibliography

Albert, Robert. Toward a behavioral definition of genius. *American Psychologist,* **30:**140–151 (1975).

Barbe, Walter (ed.). *Psychology and education of the gifted.* New York: Appleton-Century-Crofts, 1965.

Dickinson, Rita. *Caring for the gifted child.* Boston: Christopher Publishing House, 1970.

Gallagher, James. *Teaching the gifted child.* Boston: Allyn and Bacon, 1975.

Ginsberg, Gina, and Harrison, Charles H. *How to help your gifted child: a handbook for parents and teachers.* New York: Monarch Press, 1977, from material provided by The Gifted Child Society, Inc.

Strang, Ruth. Psychology of gifted children and youth. In William Cruickshank (ed.), *Education of exceptional children and youth.* Englewood Cliffs, N.J.: Prentice-Hall, 1958.

Witty, Paul. How to identify the gifted. *Childhood Education,* **29:**313 (1953).

15 Infant Death

JOAN HAGAN ARNOLD

I. Etiology

A. Infant mortality—10 leading causes in 1977[1]

1. Congenital anomalies
2. Sudden infant death syndrome (SIDS)
3. Immaturity, unqualified
4. Respiratory distress syndrome
5. Asphyxia of newborn, unspecified
6. Hyaline membrane disease
7. Birth injury without mention of cause
8. Influenza and pneumonia
9. Accidents
10. Septicemia

B. Postneonatal mortality—10 leading causes in 1977[1]

1. Sudden infant death syndrome (SIDS)
2. Congenital anomalies
3. Influenza and pneumonia
4. Accidents
5. Meningitis
6. Respiratory distress syndrome
7. Septicemia
8. Diarrheal diseases
9. Hyaline membrane disease
10. Homicide

II. Basic Concepts

A. Information needed prior to interaction and intervention with the grieving family

1. Death—a developmental and family crisis
   a. Death is an inevitable event, but a baby is least of all expected to die. Infant death is contrary to all we are conditioned to accept in our society.
   b. The death of a child affects all family members and significant others who were attached to or made some emotional investment in the baby. No one in the family is exempt from feelings of loss and grief. The family system is changed by an infant's death.
2. Specialness of a child's death
   a. Regardless of the age or cause of a child's death, it is a devastating experience for the family.
   b. The parents must grieve the loss of a loved one and contend with the death of part of themselves. It was their child, conceived by them, part of their bodies, a result of a desire to create and form a mutual bond.
   c. At birth, a baby is a separate being, but one who continues as a part of the parents, an extension from and beyond them.
   d. When the baby dies, the parents have lost a part of themselves; part of their bodies was severed, never to be whole again.
3. Characteristics of death during infancy
   a. A baby represents many things: new life, hope, purity, wishes, dreams, fears, and fantasies. Not only is a baby part of the parents, but the parents are part of the child's self. This oneness is a critical feature of normal growth and development at this stage and a critical concept to understand when an infant's death occurs.
   b. Parents know they were responsible for creating and then sustaining their child's life through love and protection. When the baby dies, their sense of esteem as parents and care givers is shattered. Feelings of

[1]Unpublished data, Mortality Statistics Branch, Division of Vital Statistics, National Center for Health Statistics, U.S. Dept. Health, Education, and Welfare, 1977.

worthlessness and self-blame and loss of self-esteem and self-respect are paramount.

c. The parent-infant relationship is normally characterized by ambivalence and intense emotion; death strikes in the midst of the complexities of this developing relationship.

d. The meaning the baby carries for each member of the family is reflected in each person's sense of loss and means of dealing with the death: if the baby was felt to be an intruder, there is often guilt that this feeling killed the baby, as well as relief that the intruder is gone; a single adolescent mother may have welcomed her baby as a means of establishing independence, and now the baby is taken from her; a lonely parent may have wanted a baby to have somebody to love and feel important to, and now his or her life's purpose is gone.

4. Critical aspects of grief and bereavement
   a. In addition to the normal process of bereavement in which one grieves the loss of a loved one, parents must also come to terms with the loss of part of the self.
   b. Common expressions of loss after an infant's death include the following.
      (1) Aching arms wishing to hold the baby (like "phantom limb")
      (2) A hollow and empty feeling in the abdomen
      (3) Visions of the baby
      (4) Hearing the baby cry
      (5) Nightmares
      (6) Thinking of the baby in the grave
      (7) Performing simple everyday tasks for the baby as though still alive—forgetting the baby is dead
      (8) Talking to the baby
      (9) Difficulty meeting and dealing with pregnant women or families with babies
      (10) Feeling the senselessness and purposelessness of life, not caring about living, thinking how much better it would be not to live, not to feel
      (11) Confusion about sex—wanting sex to have another baby to fill the emptiness and terrified of having sex and having another baby and suffering again
      (12) Anger with God or with the world for the injustice of being selected to suffer and wondering, "Why me?"
      (13) Anger with the baby for dying and leaving
      (14) Cherishing pictures of the baby both alive and dead and being afraid to look at them but needing to keep them
      (15) Pinning something of the baby's onto one's clothing, to retain the feeling of being close
   c. Sharing memories of the child is a way to help heal oneself. There is a need to talk; frequent repetition of the same stories of events and circumstances is a way of reliving the time with the baby, and it helps in coping with the loss.
   d. Relatives, friends, and others in the community have difficulty dealing with the family who has experienced an infant's death; fear of the bereaved family is common, because of the feeling that death contaminates and tragedy will be communicated to others. There is often a feeling of helplessness, of not knowing what to say. Often the bereaved family finds they need to take the initiative and convey that it is necessary to talk about the baby.
   e. Behavioral manifestations or expressions of grief are different for each person, as each person has unique needs and ways of coping with death and the personal significance of the lost loved one. Appreciation of differences and individual strengths is essential.
   f. The process is lifelong; the family never "gets over" the death but learns to live with the loss.

B. The role of the practitioner

1. The practitioner as a facilitator
   a. Uses "self" therapeutically in the process of reaching out to families grieving the death of their infant member
   b. Conveys empathy for their pain and the intensity and differences of their feelings
   c. Expresses a desire to understand their difficulties and offers to listen with care and concern, knowing this is the most painful experience of their lives
   d. Focuses on the family, encouraging improved communication and support within the family for its individual members
   e. Needs to examine own feelings about death, personal reactions, and ways of coping with previous losses in own life and current feelings about self (this experience perhaps too painful personally, too close to

home at that point in time for practitioner to be an effective intervener)

f. Examines own behavior and avenues of intervention, recognizing that a caring professional's handicap often lies in a strong desire to help and care for others, sometimes contradicting the true nature of helping, which is to serve as facilitator so families can care for themselves

g. Recognizes that death precipitates other family problems which demand attention before the family is free to grieve the loss, e.g., money for the funeral, housing, medical problems

h. Realizes that no amount of caring on the practitioner's part can take away the family's pain, that there are no easy or speedy solutions to the experience of loss, and that involvement requires a willingness to listen and experience the pain the family will share

2. Recognizing families at risk
   a. Pathological grief responses
      (1) Early indicators
         (a) Inability to cry (*clarification:* crying in presence of others is not necessary; but it *is* important to ask if the individual can cry at some time alone and in his or her own way)
         (b) Suicide attempts
         (c) Violence—acting out
         (d) Behaving as though nothing has happened—denial
      (2) Later indicators (after 1 to 2 years)
         (a) Inability to invest self in new or reinvest self in past relationships (expected and normal for certain events which precipitate acute grief)
         (b) Depression—includes agitated depression, or psychosomatic illnesses, or poor avenues of gratification, such as alcoholism or drug abuse
         (c) Inability to carry on life in a way that resembles how it was before the death occurred
   b. Precipitation or aggravation by the death of other preexisting family problems, e.g., problems in relationships, school, behavior, previous unresolved losses

III. Information the Practitioner Should Seek from the Family through Careful Listening

A. Their understanding of the circumstances surrounding the child's death

1. The sequence of events
2. The relationships drawn upon to make sense out of what happened
3. Whether or not they had an opportunity to say "good-bye," to begin the painful process of separation
4. How they managed the funeral

B. Their understanding of what they were told happened to the child

1. Why the baby died
2. The words or phrases said by others that made the greatest impression on the family members—words they will never forget, that have significance

C. Discrepancies between what they were told and what they think really happened

D. What they perceive as their immediate problems

E. How the family feels the practitioner can be helpful to them

IV. Assessment

A. Family dynamics

1. Are there blocks in communication?
2. Are family members blaming each other or protecting each other from their own feelings or from difficult tasks?
3. Is someone in the family made to be a scapegoat or used as the focus for expressions of anger?
4. Are there other maladaptive family interactions?

B. Management of other siblings

1. Parents sense of self-esteem can begin to be restored if they are able to help their other children deal with the death of the baby.
2. The specific concerns of siblings which parents find most painful are usually unresolved areas of pain for themselves.

C. Nature of grief response and interpretation of why *their* baby died

1. They are locked into their anger and rage and have difficulty facing their sense of powerlessness and loss of esteem.
2. Rage is a normal response; expressions of grief are unique to each individual.
3. The range of normal bereavement behavior is extremely wide, particularly in the acute phase.

D. Nature and extent of support system

1. Sometimes a natural leader emerges, who takes charge and deals with the concrete issues.

2. Is there a balance in relationships: one member supporting another through the especially rough times, and is the supporter getting support?
3. Is a parent isolated and alone?

V. Management and Counselling

A. Counselling

1. The practitioner must assume the responsibility of reaching out, of taking the initiative.
2. Families *do* want to talk about their feelings after the baby dies, but so often they feel no one really wants to listen.
3. The practitioner's own reluctance to become involved, if it exists, must be examined.
4. Express understanding of how hard it must be to have lost a child—it is the most painful event in a lifetime to sustain—and concern for the survivors.
5. The practitioner's focus is on the family: how the individuals within the family unit are managing, how they relate to each other, and how they relate to the unit.
6. *Listen.*
7. Avoid offering solutions; give the family space to discover their own course of action.
8. Facilitate the expressions of grief; encourage communication between family members.
9. View the family as a vital system coping with a painful crisis—not as incapacitated and helpless.
10. Offer support and the recognition of the members' ability to make decisions; show that you believe in them, thereby fostering their ability to believe in themselves again.
11. Maximize their strengths.
12. Describe the double task of bereavement and coming to terms with part of one's self dying, too.
13. Encourage parents to help their other children come to terms with the baby's death, and appreciate the difficulty of this task.
14. Share in the memories of the baby—they soothe and help heal.

B. Follow-up

1. *Early* intervention is essential.
2. Planned follow-up is dependent upon the particular family's experiences.
   a. Experiences in preparing for the baby's death and in sharing in the time of death, in turn dependent upon support family had in beginning process of separation and recognition of the reality of the baby's dying or death
   b. Response to mobilizing in caring for the baby's body, i.e., making funeral and/or burial arrangements
   c. Particular dilemmas and desires
3. Another critical time for the practitioner to become involved is after the friends and family have left the immediate family alone and the baby is buried; suddenly there is no one to talk with; the natural support system is weakened.
4. Reaching out 4 to 8 weeks after the death is important; the shock of the death is wearing off and depression is setting in. There is usually more willingness to begin to deal with memories, to talk about the baby. This is a time when the family is expected to get back to normal living—and they are not nearly ready.
5. Other key times for interaction with the family fall around special events and times that have significance for the family, such as the anniversary of the baby's death, the baby's birthday, the subsequent medical appointment.
6. It is essential for the practitioner to remain available to the family, so family members can reach the practitioner when they feel a need.
7. The family should not be discharged from the practitioner's case load; an open door policy is preferred.

C. Referrals

1. These depend upon the family's need.
2. Community outreach is mandatory, e.g., public health nurse, visiting nurse.
3. The family may experience difficulty returning to the hospital where their infant died or was brought DOA; visiting the family in their home is preferable, since it gives them more authority, and makes the practitioner a guest.
4. Volunteer parent groups play a key role.[2] It helps enormously to talk with someone else who has lost a child. A unique bond can develop, and the volunteer serves as an example of someone who has made it, inspiring the parents to make it, too.
5. Pertinent literature is helpful.[3]

[2]For example: The National Sudden Infant Death Syndrome Foundation, Inc., 310 South Michigan Ave., Chicago; IL 60604; Council of Guilds for Infant Survival, 1800 M St., NW, Washington, DC 20037.

[3]For example: Grollman, 1976. Additional literature is available through parent organizations and USDHEW, Health Services Administration, Rockville, MD 20852.

6. Other referrals which may be appropriate include the following.
   a. Consultation with the primary physician, the medical examiner or coroner
   b. Family planning
   c. Prenatal care resources
   d. Health care referrals for parents and/or siblings
   e. Employment and school counselling
   f. Housing
   g. Public assistance
   h. Coordination with school nurse
   i. Thanatology/mental health counsellors
   j. All referrals dependent upon family needs and the problems which are felt to be critical at the time

bibliography

Blanck, Rubin, and Blanck, Gertrude. *Marriage and personal development.* New York: Columbia, 1968.

Death and children. *Journal of Clinical Child Psychology,* **3**(2):entire issue (1974).

Grollman, Earl A. *Talking about death, a dialogue between parent and child.* Boston: Beacon Press, 1976.

Hagan, Joan M. Infant death: Nursing interaction and intervention with grieving families. *Nursing Forum,* **13**(4):371–385 (1974).

Kennell, J., Slyter, H., and Klaus, M. The mourning response of parents to the death of a newborn. *New England Journal of Medicine,* **283**:344–348 (1970).

Lindemann, E. Symptomatology and management of grief. *American Journal of Psychiatry,* **101**:141–148 (1944).

Maslach, C. Burned out. *Human Behavior,* September: 16–22 (1976).

The empty cradle. *MCN, The American Journal of Maternal Child Nursing,* **2**(1):22–42 (1977).

16 The Dying Child

CLAIRE F. PETTRONE/CAROLE STONE

Care of the dying child is perhaps the greatest challenge a practitioner may have to face. Regardless of the setting, management of the dying child is most effective when carried out through the parent(s) as the primary care giver(s). The goal of the practitioner should be to develop the understanding and skills of the parent(s) and thereby the ability of the parent(s) to care for the child. This can provide a more positive death experience and a more effective resolution of the grieving process. The following is presented as a guideline for the practitioner to use in helping the parent(s) care for the child effectively. The readings suggested in the bibliography will provide more in-depth understanding of the issues addressed.

ALERT

1. Signs of severe depression and/or dysfunction in child or parent(s), i.e., severe neglect of self or child, suicidal tendencies manifested in parent(s) or child
2. Prolonged grieving state: the duration of grief is variable—the range may be 6 months to 1 year, with resolution of the acute phase in approximately 2 months
3. High-risk families, i.e., multiple recent crises, previous loss, notable disorganization of family

I. Subjective Data

A. Age of child: assessment of child's cognitive, emotional, and moral development

B. Family history/family environmental factors
   1. Family constellation
   2. Order of child in family
   3. Emotional significance of child to family
   4. Nature of marital relationship

C. Physical environmental factors
   1. Location and proximity of care
   2. Availability of transportation
   3. Physical limitations of home

D. Understanding of diagnosis and prognosis
   1. When and how child and/or family became aware of death as a possible outcome
   2. What time frame, if any, was given
   3. Whether or not information has been shared with child or other family members
   4. Parent(s)' understanding of illness
   5. Child's understanding of illness

E. Previous death experiences of child and family

F. Available support systems

G. Cultural, socioeconomic, and educational influences

H. Coping mechanisms

I. Changes in behavior patterns of child, parent(s), and siblings

J. Presence of pain and anxiety
   1. Parent(s)' description
   2. Child's description

K. Level of physical disability and disfigurement

L. Motivation and desire for knowledge and management

M. Developmental history

N. Past medical history

O. Immunization history

II. Objective Data

A. Physical examination

1. Complete physical examination
2. General physical appearance of the child and parent(s), i.e., presence of dyspnea, sighing, exhaustion, restlessness
3. Parent-child interaction

B. Laboratory data

1. As determined after consultation with physician
2. Family assessment (see Family Assessment, Chap. 1)
3. Development assessment (see Development Assessment, Chap. 6)
4. Psychological assessment (see Psychological Assessment, Chap. 2)

III. Assessment

A. Stage of parent(s) and child in grieving process

B. Sudden death with acute grief syndrome

C. Long-term illness with normal grief syndrome

D. Bereavement following death

E. Abnormal grief reaction with ineffective coping

F. Limitations of family in meeting therapeutic needs of child

IV. Management and Counselling

A. Needs of the child: guidelines for practitioner and parent(s)

1. It is important to understand the developing death concept of children (the stages in Table 16-1 are offered as a guideline; it must be recognized that the concept of death evolves gradually with many individual variations).
2. Even the very young child is able to perceive that something is terribly wrong. The child may communicate in symbolic language and the parent(s) may need help in interpreting these symbols.
3. Any question asked by a child deserves an answer in accordance with that child's developmental stage. Fears should be broken down into their tangible parts, and the child should not be overburdened with more information than he or she is able to handle.
4. Readiness for open communication may occur at night when a child's fears are most prominent.
5. The parent(s) may need help in assessing the child's readiness to discuss death; if the parent is not able to handle specific areas of discussion for which the child is ready, a significant other may fill this need.
6. It is more important that a good relationship between parent(s) and child continue than that the impending death be acknowledged by them both; if it is likely that either parent or child will become detached from the other, then it would be better not to force the awareness.
7. Asking the child to repeat what has been discussed may correct misperceptions; draw on the child's own experiences as much as possible.
8. Maintain usual family activities as long as possible.
9. Limit setting is important; negative feelings can be expressed without allowing the child to become abusive.
10. Prepare the parent(s) in advance for the child's pain; assess the emotional and physical components; differentiate pain due to illness and pain due to treatment; put a time limit on the duration of the pain, if possible.
11. Explain the character of the pain in terms of a previous experience of the child; reassure the child that everything possible will be done to help deal with the pain, such as holding, positioning.
12. Knowledge of pain medications is important; reevaluate medication needs with the parent(s) periodically.
13. Recognition of the grieving process is important (for specific guidelines, see Table 16-1).
14. It is necessary for the parent(s) to master the nursing skills necessary to care for the child at home and in the hospital setting.
15. Parental involvement in the care of the child should continue in the hospital to the extent that desire, time, and ability will allow. The practitioner should provide input to the nursing staff to ensure continuation of the care plan established at home. Providing for a primary care nurse will also ensure consistency, with the practitioner acting as a liaison and serving as an advocate for the family.

B. Needs of the parent(s)

1. The parent(s) is under stress for an indefinite period of time, which may cause vulnerability to physical and emotional dysfunc-

tion. The parent(s) must also recognize the need to prepare for more trying times ahead, i.e., by getting enough rest and proper nutrition.

2. The parent(s) should identify techniques that were effective in the past in providing rest and relaxation.
3. There is a need for the parent(s) to have time away from the terminally ill child in order to gain perspective and allow for relaxation and grieving. It is a good idea to identify and use a significant other to care for the child during this time if the parent(s) agrees. The parent(s) is better able to meet the child's needs if the parental needs are met.
4. Denial of a child's terminal illness is a protection against the shock, anguish, and intensity of feelings; it should be allowed for as long as is necessary.
5. Parents will feel they are trying to hold themselves together. The practitioner should not be discouraged if parents cannot "hear" explanations about medical diagnosis and management.
6. The desire to seek other opinions is common during the denial phase.
7. With the dawning realization of the child's impending death, the parents may feel overwhelming bitterness and anger at themselves, the child, family members, and health professionals. They should be encouraged to ventilate their feelings and participate in decision making.
8. Anger may be directed at the child, and this should be openly dealt with. There is a need for reassurance that this response is normal. The parent(s) may need guidance in expressing feelings constructively and in avoiding the assigning of blame.
9. The nearness of death often evokes a request for time through offering gifts to health professionals; rejection may stimulate withdrawal and destroy a trust relationship.
10. The imminence of death brings depression and despair. Sadness is a preparation for ultimate loss. Feelings need to be respected and encouraged. The practitioner should avoid attempts to "cheer up"; silent presence and physical touch is more helpful than words and explanations.
11. Emotional detachment may come with the awareness of the reality of death. If this stage is reached before the actual death of the child, the parent(s) may appear to be withdrawing physical and emotional support. This must not be interpreted as noncaring or neglect; perhaps a significant other can step in to meet the needs of the child. Explanations of what is taking place and encouragement to continue the care of other children will help the parent(s) reestablish self-esteem.
12. In long-term illness, with frequent remissions and exacerbations, the parent(s) may feel that the child dies many times. The practitioner should be aware that the parent(s) may not be able emotionally to reestablish a relationship with the child. Anger may be directed at the child for not dying. The reasons for this must be explained in order to allay guilt.
13. Hope is the one thread that persists throughout; it is important that this be shared between the practitioner and the family; it is an important source of nourishment for the parent(s) and the child. A sense of hope should never be totally abolished.
14. Grief work may intensify during the terminal phase. The family may be affected by high emotional overtones of those around them.
15. The need to depend on trust relationships established during previous stages is important during the terminal phase. The practitioner should be available to the family during this time.
16. The parent(s) should understand that there may be changes in the child's breathing patterns, sounds, movement, and level of consciousness during the terminal phase. The reasons for the changes must be explained.
17. Reassurance that some of the moaning may not be due to pain is needed.
18. Explanation of equipment that may become part of the child's environment is needed.
19. Patient repetition, reorientation, and reemphasis is needed during the terminal phase, talking slowly and quietly.
20. Privacy and the time for parent(s) to be alone with the child is important for the expression of grief.
21. The parent(s) should be encouraged to talk to the child. The practitioner should explain that hearing is the last sense to be lost. The feeling of things left unsaid is very difficult for the parent(s) after the child's death.
22. The practitioner should understand that after the death there may be a need to touch,

to hold, etc. The parent(s) needs time to say goodbye and may want a remembrance, such as a lock of hair. The parent(s) needs assurance that the body will be taken care of with respect.

23. The indiscriminate use of sedation for the parent(s) should be avoided; it may impede the expression of grief.
26. A date should be set for a home visit 2 to 4 weeks after the child's death; reassessment of the family's progress in grieving should be done at this time.
27. Questions pertaining to how the family members feel about themselves and the deceased child, the extent of their resumption of roles, and the return to some normal activities will help the practitioner assess the progression of the grieving process.
28. Further follow-up at 6 months and 1 year, or as desired by the family and the practitioner, is recommended.

C. Needs of siblings

1. Siblings should be told the truth simply and in accordance with their developmental understanding; often the reality is less frightening than the fantasy.
2. Open and honest communication may prevent such adverse consequences as school failure, physical complaints, and other forms of displacement.
3. The practitioner may act as a liaison between family and teachers in order to provide additional support to siblings.
4. Siblings may feel neglected or abandoned due to demands placed on the parent(s) by the terminally ill child.
5. They must grieve for the impending loss of the brother or sister and should be encouraged to visit the hospitalized child in order to match fantasy with reality and provide time to say goodbye.
6. Siblings may suffer survivor guilt. The practitioner should remember that helping parent(s) to develop the skills and confidence necessary to deal with siblings may, in turn, enable parent(s) to cope more effectively with the needs of the dying child.

D. Helping agencies

1. Candlelighters
   123 C St., SE
   Washington, DC 20003
2. PALMS (Parents Against Leukemia and Malignancies)
   American Cancer Center
   University of Kansas
   Kansas City, KA 66103
3. Leukemia Society of America
4. American Cancer Society
5. The local Red Cross
6. Church groups

E. Death at home

1. Home care is a viable alternative to hospital care when it is desired by both child and parent(s), curative treatment has been discontinued, and, most importantly, the parent(s) perceives it is possible to care for the child at home (Martinson, 1978).
2. Consideration must also be given to available coping mechanisms, the physical environment, the available resources and support systems, the nature of the disease, the complications of care, and siblings.

V. Considerations for the Practitioner

A. Continual evaluation of own concept of death needed in order to increase understanding and identify effect of death experience on self, as well as increase the ability for a therapeutic and empathetic encounter

B. Recognition of feelings of helplessness and irritability when death is prolonged and/or associated with severe distress

C. Recognition of the grieving process as it affects self

D. Utilization of own available support systems for dealing with grief

Table 16-1 Child's Concept of Death

Developmental Stage	Implications for Counselling
INFANT (see Infant Death, Chap. 15)	
No death concept; suffers only physical pain and emotional detachment from the mother	May be difficult for parent(s) to develop and maintain the parent-child bond because of the realization that fulfillment of this relationship will not be reached

Table 16-1 Child's Concept of Death (*continued*)

Developmental Stage	Implications for Counselling
	Physical comfort and relief from suffering primary to parent(s) and child
	Establishment of a parent-infant relationship encouraged; identification of child necessary in order for grieving to take place
TODDLER	
Increasingly reflects feelings of other people; no specific death concept; has not yet achieved a separate identity	Physical presence of parent(s); reassurance that "No matter what, Mommy and Daddy will always be with you"
Separation anxiety and fear of abandonment dominant	Parental feelings of concern and sadness expressible with child within limits; toddler will respond to own impending death according to the response of parent(s); further expression of strong emotional feelings with significant other adult, away from child
Anger of child toward parent(s) for failure to provide protection may produce rebellious or overly compliant behavior	Regression seen as normal and as a source of emotional comfort for the child
	Parental feelings of guilt and anger for not being able to protect the child perhaps reflected in overpermissiveness or withdrawal
PRESCHOOLER	
Death associated with sleep, not yet seen as permanent	Questions to be answered simply and truthfully on the basis of the child's reality; must listen to what the child is really asking
Illness and death sometimes viewed as punishment for real or imagined wrong; able to ask questions about death	Main concerns center on pain, isolation, and safety; assurance paramount that Mommy and Daddy will always be with child; constant reassurance that child is loved and wanted
Affective responses still influenced by parent(s) and significant others	Unconscious fears sometimes becoming manifest in an increase in nightmares; regression seen as a normal coping and comfort measure
	Play an important outlet for child's fears and anxieties; artwork a means of expression, communication, and understanding of child's thoughts
	Natural denials allowed and supported; participation in self-care indicated now
SCHOOL-AGE CHILD	
Personification of death; beginning to see death as permanent and irreversible; universality of death accepted, although death in childhood still seen as unnatural	Major fears centered on injury and mutilation; honesty and consistency in explaining procedures; participation in self-care and decision making whenever possible offering some needed mastery over environment; need for neatness and organization often apparent
Recognizes self as separate from parent(s); influence of peers and external environment now important; finiteness of time recognized	Although desperately scared and lonely, child may fear loss of learned controls; needs encouragement to express negative feelings; needs verbal and nonverbal reassurance that parent(s) will help child cope; giving illness a name helps child cope; needs
Now able to grieve own loss; does not see death as the end of physical existence, although does recognize it as the final separation from this life	

Table 16-1 Child's Concept of Death (*continued*)

Developmental Stage	Implications for Counselling
May very often come to own conclusion regarding death without being told directly; child and family able to share sadness, comfort each other, and mourn together Child able to begin to utilize supports from siblings and schoolmates Must begin to recognize more overlapping and less solidification of developing death concept now; more modified and influenced by child's experiences, training, and education	acceptance of denial, encouragement of discussion of fears, anxieties, and guilt about illness Illness and death still viewed as punishment; parent(s) no longer omnipotent; reassurance that illness is not punishment; explanation why child feels badly; child able to begin understanding diagnosis and prognosis, needing more specific information; maintenance of simplicity and honesty; recognition that apparent sophistication in using medical terminology at this age does not always connote in-depth understanding but rather a socialization process of chronic illness and an attempt to control the environment Anger may be expressed through rejection of parent(s) and peers, or increase in demands or testing; avoidance of taking anger personally; recognition that freedom to express anger can be viewed as a sign of emotional security; availability of support must continue; depression sometimes expressed in hyperactivity or new physical complaints Encouragement of visits both at home or in hospital
ADOLESCENT Universality and permanence of death understood; fascination with the idea of being and nonbeing; deeply sensitive to the meaning of death Lives in intense present, with past and future pallid by comparison; at a new starting point in life; loss of prestige, shame, and lack of fulfillment most difficult to endure Early adolescence often the most difficult period for death to occur for entire family; physical deterioration, regression and loss of control devastating	Truth and respect for individual rights of paramount importance; need for privacy; need for specific information and more in-depth understanding of illness, treatments, and procedures; preservation of body image of prime importance Support and comfort from the family sometimes rejected because of the need to express new independence; bitterness and anger often severe; may be jealous of the health of peers Availability of continued support despite rejection

bibliography

Alexander, E., and Alderstein, M. Affective responses to the concept of death in a population of children and early adolescence. *Journal of Genetic Psychology*, **93**:167–177 (1958).

Anthony, Sylvia. The child's discovery of death. New York: Harcourt, Brace & World, 1941.

Caprio, F. S. A study of some psychological reactions during prepubescence to the idea of death. *Psychiatric Quarterly*, **24**:495–505 (1950).

Chandra, R. K. A child dies. *Indian Journal of Pediatrics*, **35**:363–364 (1966).

Cook, Sarah. *Children and dying: An exploration and selective bibliographies*. New York: Health Sciences Publishing Corp., 1974.

Davoli, E., and Evers, J. C. The child's right to die at home. *Pediatrics*, **38**:925 (1966).

Easson, W. M. *The dying child*. Springfield, Ill.: Charles C Thomas, 1970.

Feifel, Herman (ed.). *The meaning of death*. New York: McGraw-Hill, 1965.

Friedman, S. B., et al. Behavioral observations of parents anticipating the death of a child. *Pediatrics*,

32:610–625 (1963).

Green, M. Care of the dying child. *Pediatrics*, **40**:492–497 (1967).

———, and Solnit, A. Reactions to the threatened loss of a child: A vulnerable child syndrome. *Pediatrics*, **34**:58–66 (1964).

Grollman, E. (ed.). *Explaining death to children.* Boston: Beacon Press, 1967.

Gyulay, Jo-Eileen. Care of the dying child. *Nursing Clinics of North America*, **11**(1):95–107 (1976).

———. *The dying child.* Philadelphia: Saunders, 1977.

Hankoff, L. D. Adolescence and the crisis of dying. *Adolescence*, **10**(39):373–389 (1975).

Hogan, R. Adolescent views of death. *Adolescence*, **5**:55–61 (1970).

Journal of Clinical Child Psychology, **3**(2):entire issue (1974).

Karon, M. The physician and the adolescent with cancer. *Pediatric Clinics of North America*, **20**:965–973 (1973).

Knudson, A., and Natterson, J. M. Participation of parents in the hospital care of fatally ill children. *Pediatrics*, **26**:482–490 (1960).

Kutscher, A. H., and Goldberg, M. R. (eds.). *Caring for the dying child and his family.* New York: Health Sciences Publishing Corp., 1973.

Langner-Bluebond, M. *The private worlds of dying children.* Princeton, N.J.: Princeton, 1978.

Lindemann, E. Symptomatology and management of acute grief. *American Journal of Psychiatry*, **101**:141 (1944).

Martinson, I. *Home care for the dying child.* New York: Appleton-Century-Crofts, 1976.

———. *Home care—A manual for implementation of home care for children dying of cancer.* Minneapolis: University of Minnesota Press, 1978.

———, et al. Home care for children dying of cancer. *Pediatrics*, **62**(1):106–113 (1978).

Maurer, A. Adolescent attitudes toward death. *Journal of Genetic Psychology*, **105**:75–90 (1964).

———. Maturation of concepts of death. *British Journal of Medical Psychology*, **39**:35–41 (1966).

Morrisey, J. R. A note on interviews with children facing imminent death. *Social Casework*, **44**:343–345 (1963).

———. Death anxiety in children with a fatal illness. *American Journal of Psychotherapy*, **18**:606–615 (1964).

Nagy, Maria. The child's theories concerning death. *Journal of Genetic Psychology*, **73**:3–27 (1948).

Ross, E. K. *On death and dying.* New York: Macmillan, 1969.

Schoenberg, B., et al. (eds.). *Loss and grief: Psychological management in medical practice.* New York: Columbia, 1971.

17 Birth Control

BARBARA TAI

Birth control has become increasingly available in recent years. However, many difficulties do exist—the attitudes of the client, the family, and society, coupled with emotions, customs, and religious beliefs, contribute to confusion and a lack of understanding.

The practitioner's function should be to provide information and educate clients about the available contraceptive methods (see Table 17-1), their side effects (see Tables 17-2 and 17-3), and the difficulties of usage and effectiveness (see Table 17-4). This is also an excellent opportunity to provide information on the anatomy and physiology of reproduction, sexually transmitted diseases, sex counselling, hygiene, and sex myths. The practitioner must be sensitive to the needs of the client. Actual birth control may not be what is needed, as in the case of the supposed contraceptive-seeking client who fears venereal disease.

Counselling on contraceptives among adolescents is a most important routine practice. It is often not requested prior to need. The confidentiality of the adolescent must be maintained. If the adolescent gives consent the parent(s) should be included in the counselling session.

The ideal method of birth control does not and perhaps never will exist. Only abstinence is 100 percent effective. The remaining methods have a multitude of inherent problems regarding their safety, effectiveness, and availability. Practitioners must be nonjudgmental; the best method is determined by the client. Since the most appropriate means of birth control varies from individual to individual, the best method is whatever most satisfies the client. The practitioner must clarify the relative advantages and disadvantages of each method in light of the client's medical and social picture. Familiarity with current effectiveness rates—both use and theoretical (see Table 17-4)—is imperative. *Theoretical effectiveness* refers to the maximum effectiveness of a method when used carefully, consistently, and according to instructions. *Use effectiveness* includes careful as well as careless use.

INITIAL VISIT

I. Subjective Data

- **A.** Reason for visit
- **B.** Medical history
  1. Significant illnesses
  2. Hospitalizations
  3. Previous medical care
- **C.** Review of systems
- **D.** Obstetric reproductive history
  1. Age of menarche
  2. Menstrual history
  3. Gravidity
  4. Parity
  5. Pregnancy outcomes
  6. Complications of any pregnancies or deliveries
  7. Last menstrual period
  8. Past/current contraception, and satisfaction with it
- **E.** Psychological background
- **F.** Diet history
- **G.** Social and economic history
- **H.** Family history

II. Objective Data

A. Physical examination, particularly

1. Height and weight
2. Blood pressure
3. Breast examination
4. Auscultation of the heart and lungs
5. Abdominal examination
6. Visualization of the cervix
7. Bimanual examination of the pelvis
8. Rectovaginal examination

B. Laboratory data

1. Hematocrit or hemoglobin
2. Urinalysis for sugar and albumin
3. Pap test
4. Other possible tests
   a. Vaginal smears and wet mounts for suspected vaginal infections
   b. Pregnancy test
   c. Serological test for syphilis and gonorrhea

III. Management

A. Treatments/medications

a. Selection of method (see Table 17-1)
b. Prescription of contraceptive method

B. Counselling/prevention

a. Assist client in selecting appropriate contraceptive method based on personal needs, medical history, and preference (see Table 17-1).
   (1) Discuss pros and cons of each method.
   (2) Note possible side effects of oral contraceptives (see Table 17-2) and IUD (see Table 17-3).
b. Discuss anatomy and physiology of reproductive system.
c. Review symptoms and prevention of sexually transmitted diseases (see Venereal Disease, Chap. 70).
d. Interpret clinical findings to client.
e. Instruct client in use of selected contraceptive method.
f. Give written instructions as a guideline.
g. Elicit from client feedback that method chosen is fully understood.
h. Emphasize backup method of contraception.

Table 17-1 Birth Control Methods

Contraindications	Effects on Menses
Pill	
Pills containing estrogens	More predictable onset of menses
Phlebitis or thromboembolic disease	Diminished menstrual pain, amount and duration of bleeding with combination pill
Possibility of pregnancy	Possible amenorrhea
Malignancy, especially of breast or reproductive system	Postpill amenorrhea
Coronary artery disease	Midcycle effects
History of impaired liver function	Eliminates pain on ovulation
History of cerebrovascular accident	Cervical secretions, nausea, and midcycle spotting are decreased
Relative contraindications—medical referral/consultation indicated	Premenstrual effects
Pregnancy within past 14 days	Increase or decrease of estrogen-related symptoms
Diagnosed migraine headaches	Weight gain
Chronic hypertension	Headaches
Diabetes, including prediabetes and strong family history	Bloating
Gallbladder disease	Breast tenderness
History of cholestasis during pregnancy	Increase or decrease of progestin-related symptoms
Acute mononucleosis	Breast tenderness
Sickle cell trait/disease	Depression
Dysfunctional uterine bleeding	Increased appetite
Elective surgery in next 4 wk	

i. Give information concerning availability of emergency services.

C. Follow-up
   a. Instruct client to telephone immediately if problems or questions arise.
   b. Do postexamination interview to determine effectiveness and satisfaction (see Table 17-7).

D. Consultations/referrals: none

SUBSEQUENT VISITS

Subsequent visits should include a complete physical with a breast and pelvic examination, urinalysis, Pap test, blood pressure, weight, and any other applicable services, as well as an evaluation of the effectiveness and satisfaction of the current birth control method (see Table 17-7).

bibliography

Hatcher, Robert A, et al. *Contraceptive technology 1978–1979* (9th ed.) New York: Irvington Publishers, 1978.

Nelson, James H. Clinical evaluation of side effects of current oral contraceptives. *Journal of Reproductive Medicine,* **6**:(1971).

Pendelton, Elaine. Family planning procedure manual for nurse-midwives. New York Department of Obstetrics and Gynecology, Downstate Medical Center, 1975.

Shapiro, Howard I. *The birth control book.* New York: St. Martin's, 1977.

Table 17-1 Birth Control Methods (*continued*)

Types Commonly Used	Other Considerations
	Pill
Combined oral contraceptive Estrogen: menstranol, ethinyl estradiol Mestranol half as potent as ethinyl estradiol when used in same milligram dose. Estrogens cannot be equated by milligrams. Least effective dose of estrogen is preferred. Progestogen: norgestrel, norethindrone, norethindrone acetate, ethynodiol diacetate, norethynodrel (see Table 17-6 for potency) Minipill (Micronor, Nor-Q.D.) Minipill contains only progestogen. Body may convert the progestogen (norethindrone) into estrogen; therefore, precautions should be taken. Pregnancy rate highest during first 6 mo of use. Backup contraceptive method should be used. Since minipills contain no estrogen, they may be choice method for adolescents. Monitor carefully any abdominal pain. Rate of ectopic pregnancies is higher while on minipill.	Particular type of oral contraceptive should be chosen on the basis of whether a person's hormonal profile is androgen- or estrogen-dominant (see Table 17-5). A pill is chosen according to its hormonal characteristics. Hormonal profile is estimated by evaluating secondary sex characteristics and the type and duration of the menstrual pattern (see Table 17-5). Discuss early danger signs. If definite complication arises, advise client to discontinue pill and obtain medical consultation. Explain common problems that occur while on pill (see Table 17-2). If problems are not severe, do not "pill hop." It is usually appropriate to continue particular pill for 3 mo before initiating change. If the condition is severe, treat immediately.

Table 17-1 Birth Control Methods (*continued*)

Contraindications	Effects on Menses
Pill (continued)	
Age 40 (age 35 if obese, hypertensive, diabetic, high-cholesterol, or heavy smoker)	
Fibrocystic breasts	
Menses established less than 1 yr	
Cardiac or renal disease	
Heavy smoker	
Lactation	
Anovular menstruation or fertility problems	
Intrauterine Device (IUD)	
Absolute contraindications	Increased amount of blood loss (not as greatly increased with Progestasert)
Active pelvic infection (acute or chronic)	Increased number of days of bleeding
Pregnancy	Increased amount of cramping (greatest with Lippes Loop and Saf-T-Coil, less with CU-7)
Dysfunctional uterine bleeding	Questionable increase in the risk of symptomatic PID, which is most likely to occur late in menses or just after cessation of menses
Relative contraindications—physician consultation indicated	Midcycle effects: increase in midcycle spotting and pain
Severe menorrhagia	Premenstrual effects: increase in premenstrual spotting
Severe dysmenorrhea	
Anemia	
History of ectopic pregnancy	
History of pelvic inflammatory disease (PID), especially if the client wishes to become pregnant	
Abnormal Pap smears	
History of endocarditis	
Rheumatic or valvular heart disease	
Allergy to copper (for copper-containing devices)	
Multiparous or grand multiparous uteri	

Table 17-1 Birth Control Methods (*continued*)

Types Commonly Used	Other Considerations
Pill (continued)	
Intrauterine Device (IUD)	
Lippes Loop (sizes A, B, C, D) Saf-T-Coil (small or large) CU-7 Progestasert	IUD may be alternative for those with contraindications to oral contraceptives. Most important factor in choosing particular IUD should be competence with its particular type of insertion. All IUDs (except Progestasert) increase the amount of blood loss, cramping, and the duration of menstrual flow. IUDs increase midcycle spotting (less with CU-7). IUDs may increase premenstrual spotting. Never insert IUD forcefully; insertion may be simpler with a small IUD, such as CU-7. Some believe IUD is not ideal choice unless client has had previous full-term pregnancy. Insertion should be done as follows. It is best if accomplished in 2 visits. First visit: examine to ensure normalcy of pelvis and absence of infection. Determine size, shape, and direction; rule out pregnancy; do laboratory work: Pap smear, GC culture; educate client. Second visit: do actual insertion (done during menses). Insertion must be done under sterile conditions. Bladder should be empty. Insert speculum and swab cervix and endocervical canal with antiseptic (Betadine). Place tenaculum on the anterior lip of the cervix at 10 and 2 o'clock, and apply slight traction to straighten the uterine axis. Uterus should be sounded, and if depth is sufficient (6 cm), insert IUD following instructions specific to the device. (If cervical spasm occurs, wait up to 2 min for it to lessen.) Trim IUD strings to $1\frac{1}{2}$-2 in. Review discomforts with client for postinsertion care. Removal done during menses is somewhat easier and ensures conception has not taken place. Discuss side effects (see Table 17-3).

Table 17-1 Birth Control Methods *(continued)*

Contraindications	Effects on Menses
Diaphragm	
Inability to achieve good fitting Inability of client to become proficient with technique Allergy to either spermatocidal preparation or latex	Possible decrease in anxiety about intercourse during menses
Foam	
Allergy to foam	None
Coitus Interruptus	
Lack of ejaculatory control (premature ejaculation)	None
Condom	
Allergy to latex	Possible decrease in anxiety about intercourse during menses
Rhythm	
Irregular intervals between menses History of anovulatory cycles Irregular temperature	None

Table 17-1 Birth Control Methods *(continued)*

Types Commonly Used	Other Considerations
	Diaphragm
Flat spring (folds flat when compressed) Coil spring (folds flat in all planes) Arcing spring (forms an arc when compressed)	Flat spring may be used with minor degree of cystocele or rectocele. Coil spring is useful for clients with good vaginal tone. Arcing is easiest to insert and is tolerated by most clients. Size range is 50–105 mm. Diaphragm must be fitted snugly between inner, lower border of symphysis pubis and posterior fornix. Diaphragm should fit against vaginal walls and cover cervix. Make sure client clearly understands the following directions. Dome must be filled with 1 tsp of spermicide. Diaphragm must remain in place 6 h after intercourse and may be inserted 6 h before. No douching is allowed during this time. If coitus is repeated, additional spermicide should be placed in the vagina. Proper care is critical: check the diaphragm carefully for holes; wash it with mild soap; dry and powder it with cornstarch.
	Foam
Many	Foam may slightly decrease the transmission of gonorrhea and trichomoniasis.
	Coitus Interruptus
	No devices are needed. No chemicals are needed. Method is available in any situation at no cost.
	Condom
Many	Decreases incidence of sexually transmitted diseases.
	Rhythm
	Client needs to keep careful chart of temperature to determine when ovulation occurs.

Table 17-2 Common Side Effects/Problems of Oral Contraceptives

Problem	Possible Etiology	Management
Nausea and/or vomiting	Excess estrogen	Decrease estrogen or prescribe minipill.
	Taking pills on empty stomach	Advise to take after a meal.
Fluid retention	Organic pathology not related to the pill	Consult physician.
	Excess estrogen	Decrease estrogen or prescribe minipill; check for edema and hypertension; consult physician.
Headaches	Excess estrogen	Decrease estrogen or discontinue pill.
	Possible social or emotional problem	Try to seek out problem. Consultation may be needed.
	Eye problems	Consult with specialist.
	Hypertension	Consult with specialist.
	Anemia	Check hematocrit; advise on nutrition; prescribe iron supplements.
	Migraine	Consult with specialist.
Breast tenderness	Excess estrogen	Decrease estrogen or prescribe minipill.
Chloasma	Excess estrogen	Decrease estrogen, prescribe minipill, or discontinue oral contraceptives.
Leukorrhea	Excess estrogen	Decrease estrogen.
	Possible trichomoniasis, moniliasis, *Hemophilus*, PID, cervicitis	Do culture, smears, and treat accordingly; advise on hygiene.
Cervical eversion	Excess estrogen	Decrease estrogen.
Elevated blood pressure	Estrogen	Monitor carefully; consult according to agency protocol; decrease estrogen. Usual level for discontinuing pills is 140/90.
Vitamin deficiencies	Estrogen	Assess dietary habits; counsel on nutrition; consult as necessary.
Vitamin C	Anemia, poor wound healing	Recommend client eat broccoli, brussels sprouts, collards, horseradish, kale, parsley, sweet peppers, turnip greens.
Vitamin B_6	Anemia, nausea, anorexia, depression	Recommend client eat liver, herring, salmon, walnuts, peanuts, wheat germ, brown rice, yeast, blackstrap molasses.

Table 17-2 Common Side Effects/Problems of Oral Contraceptives *(continued)*

Problem	Possible Etiology	Management
Folic acid	Glossitis, macrocytic and megaloblastic anemia, gastrointestinal lesions, malabsorption	Recommend client eat liver, asparagus, spinach, wheat, brans.
Vitamin B_{12}	Glossitis, peripheral neuropathy, macrocytic anemia	Recommend client eat kidney, liver, brain.
Urinary tract infection	Estrogen	Decrease estrogen; consult and treat accordingly; do urine culture and sensitivity test.
Contact lens problems	Estrogen	Decrease estrogen, prescribe minipill, or discontinue oral contraceptives.
Fatigue and depression	Progestin excess	Change to estrogen-dominant pill.
	Anemia	Test hematocrit; advise on nutrition; counsel. Give iron supplements.
	Overwork	Have patient seek practical solutions.
Decreased libido	Progestin excess	Switch to estrogen-dominant pill.
	Marital and sexual problems	Explore this subject with client.
Weight gain	Progestin	Change to estrogen dominant pill.
	Increased appetite, poor diet	Counsel on nutrition.
	Emotional factors	Explore this subject with client.
Acne, oily skin	Progestin	Increase estrogen.
Thinning of hair	Progestin	Increase estrogen.
Increased facial hair	Progestin	Increase estrogen.
Monilia, decreased vaginal secretions	Progestin	Decrease progestin and increase estrogen.
Amenorrhea	Pregnancy	Give pelvic examination, pregnancy test.
	Faulty pill taking	Review problem with client.
	Pelvic infection	Review client's history and consult physician for treatment.
	Prolonged use of oral contraceptives	Discontinue pill. Increase estrogen, decrease progestin.
Postpill amenorrhea	Improper screening of client (since related to menstrual pattern prior to oral contraceptive therapy)	Provide backup contraception, do follow-up, and refer after 3–6 mo.
	Pregnancy	Give pelvic examination, pregnancy test.

Table 17-2 Common Side Effects/Problems of Oral Contraceptives *(continued)*

Problem	Possible Etiology	Management
Spotting between menses	Faulty pill taking	Review problem with client.
	Infection, tumors, polyps, cervical lesions	Take history, give pelvic exam, and consult.
	Not enough estrogen, if early in cycle	Increase estrogen.
	Not enough progestin, if late in cycle	Increase progestin.
Excessive bleeding during menses	PID Myomas	Give pelvic exam and consult.
	High estrogen	Change to low-estrogen pill.

Table 17-3 Common Side Effects/ Problems of Intrauterine Device (IUD)

Problem	Possible Etiology	Management
Syncope (cold and clammy skin, nausea with possible vomiting, drop in pulse and blood pressure)	Vasovagal reaction on insertion	It is usually not necessary to remove device (unless perforated uterus suspected). Place and maintain client in shock position. Atropine 0.5 mg IM may be given. Repeat in 15 min if pulse less than 60 beats/min. Give oxygen as needed. Monitor pulse and blood pressure until stable. Notify physician.
Pain (from mild to severe)	Insertion	Prior to insertion explain to client that pain may be experienced. Maintain a calm and reassuring attitude Tell client that pain may be expected for a few days after insertion Analgesic *not* containing aspirin may be taken
Bleeding		Bleeding should be expected on days following insertion Menstrual flow during the first few months increases in duration and amount Intermenstrual bleeding may be experienced Diet may be supplemented with additional Vitamin C, 500 mg bid, to ensure capillary stability In the case of persistent excess bleeding beyond 3 cycles Review nutrition and concurrent medication Check for displacement of the device and other pelvic and vaginal problems Repeat hematocrit and prescribe additional iron supplements Device may be removed
Expulsion		Expulsion rate is highest during first 3 cycles Teach client how to check for strings and to report any abnormalities

Table 17-3 Common Side Effects/ Problems of Intrauterine Device (IUD) (*continued*)

Problem	Possible Etiology	Management
		Advise not to use Tampax during days of light menstrual flow
Infection	Pelvic infection Gastroenteritis Urinary tract infection, etc.	Advise client to report any signs of early pelvic infection Temperature over 99°F Vague lower-abdominal pain Foul-smelling, yellowish discharge Chills Pain during intercourse If insertion is not sterile, infection may occur within 12 h. Infection usually occurs in client with past history of pelvic infection. If future pregnancy is desired, remove IUD with onset of initial pelvic infection If no further pregnancies are desired, remove IUD with second episode of infection. Consult physician for antibiotic therapy.
Amenorrhea	Possible pregnancy (intrauterine and ectopic pregnancies must be considered)	Consult with refer to physician If pregnancy occurs, IUD should be removed (by physician) due to high risk of infection.

Table 17-4 Theoretical Effectiveness vs Use Effectiveness of Birth Control Methods

Method	Theoretical Effectiveness, %	Use Effectiveness, %
Pill (combined estrogen and progestin)	99.66	96
IUD	97–99	95
Condom	97	90
Foam	97	78
Diaphragm	97	83
Rhythm	87	79
Withdrawal	91	75–80

Table 17-5 Hormonal Profile and Type of Oral Contraceptive

Estrogen-dominant Female	Androgen-dominant Female
Hormonal Profile	
Longer and more painful periods Narrower shoulders Broader hips Larger breasts Normal female distribution of hair	Shorter periods Narrower hips Broader shoulders Smaller breasts A degree of hirsutism
Type of Oral Contraceptive	
Use of progestin-dominant pill.	Use a more estrogenic pill.
If periods are heavy, use high or intermediate progestin.	If periods are heavy, use with high or intermediate progestins.
If periods are scanty, combine with low progestin.	If periods are scanty, combine with low progestin.

Table 17-6 Relative Potency of Progestogens

Progestogen	(1 mg)
Norethindrone	1
Norethynodrel	1
Norethindrone acetate	2
Ethynodiol diacetate	15
Norgestrel	30

Table 17-7 Evaluation of Effectiveness of and Satisfaction with Current Birth Control Methods

Reevaluation	Subjective Data	Objective Data	Other Considerations
	Pill		
3-mo and 6-mo intervals	Headaches Visual problems Mood changes Weight changes Leg complaints Breast masses Menstrual irregularities Vaginal bleeding and/or discharge Pain in arms or chest	Blood pressure Weight Urinalysis Breast exam Pelvic exam Pap test (as indicated) Problem-oriented physical exam (as indicated)	Caution patients who smoke cigarettes
	IUD		
After 1 or 2 menses, then annually	Vaginal bleeding and/or discharge Fever Abdominal pain Other complaints concerning the device	Blood pressure Weight Breast and pelvic exams urinalysis	
	Diaphragm		
After 2–4 wk, then annually	Description of how diaphragm is positioned Description of function	Have client insert diaphragm, and check to determine position	

PART 3

common symptoms and problems

section 1

special senses

INTRODUCTION JANE A. FOX AND MAUREEN COLLAR

The subjective and objective data in this section deals with the eyes and ears. It should be appropriately adapted by the practitioner according to the client's presenting problem.

I. Subjective Data

A. Age and sex

B. Reason for visit and description of problem

C. Onset and surrounding circumstances

D. History of trauma, foreign body, or recent infection

E. Associated symptoms

1. Pain, tenderness
2. Discharge—odor
3. Pruritis
4. Pulling/tugging on ears
5. Headache
6. Facial asymmetry
7. Irritability
8. Swollen glands
9. Stiff neck
10. Fever
11. Tinnitus
12. Vertigo
13. Upper respiratory infection (URI)
14. Vision changes, i.e., difficulty in focusing, blurred vision
15. Hearing changes, i.e., clogged feeling in ears
16. Rash
17. Unusually large eyes
18. Photophobia
19. Excessive tearing of eyes
20. Cloudy appearance of eyes
21. Inflamed eyes
22. Abnormal eye movements
23. Constant deviation of one eye

F. Past history of

1. Eye/ear infection, disease, or trauma
2. Perforated tympanic membrane
3. Frequent URIs
4. Meningitis
5. Encephalitis
6. Head trauma
7. Mumps, Measles
8. Genetic disorders
9. Chronic diseases
10. Amblyopia
11. Vision/hearing problems

G. Prenatal history

1. Maternal infection (rubella)
2. Ototoxic drugs

H. Neonatal history

1. Birth weight
2. Neonatal problems
3. Perinatal asphyxia or infection

I. Developmental history

1. Milestones—ages when achieved
2. Social adjustment
3. Hearing/speech

a. Newborn to 4 months
(1) Quieted by parent's voice
(2) Reacts to loud and/or sudden noises
(3) Responds to social gestures with smile
b. 4 to 8 months
(1) Turns head in direction of sound
(2) Recognizes mother's voice
(3) Babbles and coos
(4) Responds to environmental sounds
c. 8 to 12 months
(1) Turns directly to sounds
(2) Makes varied noises
(3) Imitates simple sounds
(4) Responds to *no-no* and *bye-bye* and own name
d. Toddler—1 to 3 years
(1) Points to familiar objects or body parts
(2) Says single words
(3) Follows simple commands
e. Preschool—3 to 5 years
(1) Uses consonants as well as vowel sounds
(2) Speaks intelligibly to parent(s) and others
(3) Listens to radio or television at normal volume levels
f. School—5 years and over
(1) Is attentive in school
(2) Follows directions given by teacher
(3) Has good voice quality
(4) Uses clear, easily understood speech
(5) Shows normal speech pattern for age and developmental level

4. Vision
a. Infant and toddler
(1) Responsiveness to parent(s); child's behavior when parent(s) approaches crib: eye contact and motor excitation versus no eye contact and motor quieting
(2) Grasping objects and reaching out for parent(s)
(3) Visual searching for sound cue
(4) Stumbling/falling easily or knocking into things frequently
b. Preschool, school age
(1) Holding objects close to eyes
(2) Sitting close to television
(3) Difficulty seeing blackboard
(4) Reading difficulty

J. Medications

K. Allergies

L. Hospitalizations

M. Immunization history
1. Measles
2. Mumps
3. Rubella

N. Family history
1. Genetic disorders
2. Chronic diseases
3. Hearing problems
4. Vision problems
a. Amblyopia
b. Glasses
5. Allergies

O. Social history
1. Family composition
2. Interpersonal relationships
3. Living conditions
4. Economic status
5. Peer relationships
6. Emotional or behavioral problems
7. School performance
8. Constant exposure to loud noises

P. Past history and results of vision/hearing tests

II. Objective Data

A. Physical examination
1. Complete physical examination (See Chap. 7) of all infants and young children
2. Temperature
3. Eyes
a. Inspect external structures of eyes.
b. Inspect and palpate lacrimal sac.
c. Observe eyes for discharge, erythema, or lid swelling.
d. Check pupils for reaction to light and for accommodation.
e. Note facial configuration and movements.
f. Test extraocular movements (ocular rotations).
(1) Track object in all nine cardinal fields of vision.
(2) Check convergence.
g. Check Hirschberg's reflex (corneal light reflex): a beam of light from penlight should fall in exactly the same location on each cornea or pupil.
h. Give cover test: occlude one eye at a time, having client fix on object, uncover eye, and watch for movement. (There should be no movement.)
i. Screen for visual acuity.
(1) Test each eye individually.
(2) Use age-appropriate eye-screening chart.
(a) Allen chart (3- and 4-year-olds)
(b) Snellen E chart (4- and 5-year-olds)
(c) Snellen alphabet chart (5 years and up)

j. Do opthalmoscopic exam.

4. Ears
   a. Inspection of external ears for pinna formation, placement and patency of canals
   b. Otoscopic examination
   c. Pneumoscopy (air gently blown into the auditory canal through a pneumatic tube to determine mobility of the tympanic membrane)
   d. Hearing evaluation
      (1) Newborn
         (a) Hearing screen
            1. Infant in restful-sleep state
            2. Arousal response to noxious auditory stimuli
         (b) Moro reflex to loud noise
      (2) Infant
         (a) Hardy (1959): commonly used screening test
            1. Distract infant with bright toy or other visual stimuli.
            2. Administer noise 2 to 3 ft behind child.
               a. High frequency, e.g., squeaky toy, bell
               b. Medium frequency, e.g., rattle, paper
               c. Low frequency, e.g., *ba-ba*
            3. Expected response
               a. 4 months: widens eyes, ceases activity
               b. 6 months: turns head toward sound
               c. 8 months: localizes sound to side and below
               d. Over 1 year: locates source of sound precisely
         (b) Impedance audiometry
      (3) School age and older
         (a) Audiometrics
            1. Use pure-tone audiometer.
            2. Test each ear separately.
            3. Test at these frequencies: 1000, 2000, 4000 Hz.
            4. Pass if child hears all frequencies at 20 dB or 4000 Hz at 25 dB.
            5. With preschool-age child use games to elicit response.
            6. With older child instruct to raise hand when stimulus is heard.
         (b) Tuning fork (512 Hz)
            1. Weber's test
               a. Place stem on midline of scalp.
               b. Sound should be heard equally in both ears.
               c. Client will lateralize sound to the involved side in the presence of a conductive loss.
            2. Rinne's test
               a. Place stem on mastoid until sound is no longer heard.
               b. Hold fork 1 to 2 in in front of pinna.
               c. Air conduction is greater than bone conduction, and client should be able to hear fork when placed beside ear.
         (c) Impedance audiometry
            1. Monitors mobility of middle ear
            2. Differentiates sensorineural from conductive loss
5. Inspect nares for patency.
6. Inspect mouth and throat; may have referred pain.
7. Palpate and transilluminate frontal and maxillary sinuses.
8. Inspect and palpate mastoid process and cervical nodes for tenderness and swelling.
9. Give neurological examination.
   a. Cranial nerves
   b. Kernig's sign
   c. Brudzinski's sign
   d. Babinski reflex
   e. Neck rigidity
10. Assess receptive and expressive language.

B. Laboratory data

1. Give Denver Developmental Screening Test.
2. The following tests may also be utilized.
   a. Maxfield-Buchholz Scale of Social Maturity for Use with Preschool Blind Children
   b. Bayley Scales of Infant Development

bibliography

Alexander, Mary M., and Brown, Marie Scott. *Pediatric history taking and physical diagnosis for nurses.* New York: McGraw-Hill, 1979, pp. 85–126, 424–450.

Hardy, J. B., Dougherty, A., and Hardy, W. F. Hearing responses and audiometric screening in infants. *Journal of Pediatrics,* **55**:382–390 (1959).

18 Eye Deviations

MAUREEN COLLAR

ALERT
1. Sudden onset of paralytic strabismus
2. Nonparalytic strabismus in infant 6 months of age or older
3. Amblyopia (deviation of one eye)

I. Etiology

A. Strabismus
1. Developmental anomaly of the eye or orbit
2. Central nervous system disease
3. Cranial nerve impairment
4. Dysfunction of the accommodation-convergence mechanism
5. Refractive error
6. Paralysis or abnormality of the ocular muscles
7. Cataracts
8. Tumor of the retina (retinoblastoma)
9. Optic nerve atrophy
10. Ptosis

B. Amblyopia
1. Organic
   a. Chorioretinitis
   b. Macular scarring
   c. Retinoblastoma
   d. Atrophy of optic nerve
2. Functional
   a. Congenital cataracts
   b. Ptosis
   c. Corneal scarring
   d. Strabismus
   e. Refractive error

II. Assessment of Pseudostrabismus

A. Subjective data
1. Eyes appear to cross.
2. Parent(s) notes eyes are turned inward.
3. Eyes are close-set.

B. Objective data
1. Possible presence of
   a. Epicanthic folds
   b. Hypertelorism
   c. Hypotelorism
   d. Saddlenose
   e. Unequal position of eyeballs in the orbits
2. Visual acuity—normal for age
3. No movement on cover test
4. Equal light reflection in Hirschberg's test
5. Full ocular rotations without deviation
6. Ophthalmoscopic exam—within normal limits

III. Management of Pseudostrabismus

A. Treatments/medications: none

B. Counselling/prevention
1. Reassure parent(s) regarding vision and eye function.
2. Explain epicanthic folds or other facial characteristics and that they will become less apparent.
3. Explain familial traits and hereditary aspect of eyeball placement.
4. Educate parent(s) as to signs and symptoms of "true" strabismus.

C. Follow-up
1. Explore topic on successive well-child visits, to see if parent(s) has a good understanding of explanation.
2. Observe eye during routine physicals for decrease in prominence of epicanthic folds.
3. Check routine history with parent(s) for occurrence of signs or symptoms of strabismus.

D. Consultations/referrals: consult with physician (ophthalmologist) to
1. Confirm diagnosis of pseudostrabismus
2. Rule out "true" strabismus and/or ocular disease

Table 18-1 Medical Referral/Consultation

Diagnosis	Clinical Manifestations	Management
Strabismus (nonparalytic)	Onset of symptoms 6 mo or younger—neuromuscular 2–4 yr—accommodative Squinting Difficulty seeing at close range Wandering of one or both eyes Eyes not moving together Drifting of one eye when tired, ill, or exposed to bright light Eyes deviating equally in all fields of vision when tracking Movement in one or both eyes on cover test Unequal light reflection in Hirschberg's test Inability to converge to within 6 in of nose Possible failing of visual acuity screening test Possible presence of fundoscopic abnormalities	Treatment If child is 6 mo of age or older, refer immediately to physician (ophthalmologist). Treatment consists of the following methods used alone or in combination: Corrective lenses for refractive errors Surgery to correct deviations, realign eyes, and prevent amblyopia Myopic eye medication for infants too young to wear glasses and for short-term therapy Orthoptics—eye exercises, in certain cases and under the supervision of an ophthalmologist Counselling/prevention Discuss effects of strabismus on child: Self-image; personality development Social and school adjustment Explore feelings of parent(s) and child regarding required treatment procedures: Hospitalization; surgery Corrective lenses Explore financial situation: Insurance Resources for specialist's care and glasses Explain importance of early identification and treatment: Teach signs and symptoms. Stress importance of periodic vision screening. Follow-up Consult with ophthalmologist and assist in follow-up as appropriate. Continue to follow regimen for complete well-child care. Do yearly visual acuity screening and strabismus check. Consultations/referrals Refer to ophthalmologist as indicated. Refer to public health nurse if further assistance needed with transportation, community resources, or appointments. Communicate with school nurse.
Strabismus (paralytic)	Onset—after 1 yr of age Associated symptoms Headaches Uncoordinated fine or gross motor movements	Treatment Consult physician immediately. Refer client to neurologist for complete neurological evaluation.

Table 18-1 Medical Referral/Consultation (*continued*)

Diagnosis	Clinical Manifestations	Management
	Delayed growth and development Poor school performance Abnormal gait (ataxia) Personality change; mood swings Complaints of double vision History of trauma Eye injury Head injury Facial paralysis (asymmetry) Extraocular movement limited in one direction (eyes otherwise appear straight) Normal or abnormal Hirschberg's reflection (depending on position of eyes) Possible movement on cover test Possible abnormal neurological findings Abnormal deep-tendon reflexes Abnormal Babinski reflex Persistent infantile reflexes Ataxia Nystagmus Other cranial nerve impairments	Counselling/prevention Support parent(s) and child. Explain diagnostic procedures and assist in interpretation of findings. Assist parent(s) and child in working through feelings and concerns. Explore support systems. Financial needs Emotional needs Follow-up Regimen depends upon diagnosis and treatment. Follow as appropriate during and after hospitalization. Continue to follow for routine well-child care. Consultations/referrals Consult with physician. Refer to public health nurse for assistance with home care and community resources. Refer to social worker if financial aid or counselling are needed. Communicate with school nurse.
Amblyopia	Deviation of one eye Client closes one eye in order to see clearly Head tilted Resistance to occlusion of good eye Associated with monocular strabismus (paralytic or nonparalytic) Possible increased deviation of one eye on ocular rotation Unequal light reflection in Hirschberg's test Movement on cover test Greater than one line difference in score on visual acuity screening (eye chart) Ophthalmoscopic abnormality in one eye (if organic) Possible cataract, corneal scarring, or ptosis in one eye	Treatment Refer to physician (ophthalmologist) for immediate treatment. Treatment consists of one or more of the following methods: Patching or occlusion of good eye for a few weeks to several months Corrective lenses Surgery to realign eyes and restore binocular vision Pleoptics—eye exercises designed to stimulate macular vision Counselling/prevention Teach parent(s) signs and symptoms. Promote early identification and treatment. Stress importance of wearing patch at all times and complying with treatment regimen to prevent irreversible loss of vision. Discuss effects of treatment (i.e., hospitalization, surgery, eye patch) on the child. Follow-up Treat as indicated by ophthalmologist.

Table 18-1 Medical Referral/Consultation (*continued*)

Diagnosis	Clinical Manifestations	Management
		Continue to follow regimen for complete well-child care. Do periodic visual acuity screening (4 to 6 yr of age). Check for recurrence of amblyopia. Consultations/referrals Consult with ophthalmologist regarding plan of treatment. Communicate with school nurse. Refer to public health nurse if indicated.

bibliography

Kempe, C. Henry, et. al. *Current pediatric diagnosis and treatment.* Los Altos, Calif.: Lange, 1978.

O'Neill, John F. Strabismus in childhood. *Pediatric Annals,* **6**(2):10–45 (February 1977).

Rogers, Gary. Strabismus. *Pediatric Nursing,* **1**(6): 11–13 (November/December 1975).

Stager, David R. Amblyopia and the pediatrician. *Pediatric Annals,* **6**(2):46–75 (February 1977).

Taylor, D. Aspects of strabismus in children. *Nursing Times,* **72**(16):610–612 (April 1976).

19 Eye Trauma/Foreign Body

LESLIE LIETH

ALERT

1. Large laceration of globe
2. Prolapse of intraocular contents
3. Marked asymmetry of the limbal configuration
4. Suspicion of chemical burn
5. Exposure to radiation (ultraviolet or infrared light)
6. Cloudy vision
7. Double vision
8. Photophobia
9. History of blunt trauma or penetrating injury

Etiology

Trauma, chemical burns, foreign bodies, radiation burns, thermal burns

Table 19-1 Medical Referral/Consultation

Diagnosis	Clinical Manifestations	Management
Foreign body on cornea or conjunctiva	Sudden onset of pain Tearing Congestion of conjunctiva Possible irregularities on corneal surfaces Presence of foreign body in cornea or conjunctiva	For those foreign bodies not dislodged by eversion of lid, refer to physician, preferably ophthalmologist.
Corneal abrasion	Sudden onset of pain Tearing Complaint of foreign body feeling, though none visualized Congestion of conjunctiva Possible irregularity on corneal surfaces After instillation of 2% fluorescein dye, or application of moistened fluorescein strips, abrasions visualized (turn green)	Refer to physician. Usual treatment is instillation of a bacteriostatic eye ointment and application of a pressure dressing for at least 24 h. Pain medication and sedation may be necessary.
Lacerations of eyelid	Small wound on skin surface perhaps not reflection of extent of laceration of the tarsus History of trauma Possible jagged laceration of lid with profuse bleeding	Refer to surgeon, preferably ophthalmologist, for repairs. If there are no other injuries, compresses of cold tap water are effective during the first 24 h.

Table 19-1 Medical Referral/Consultation *(continued)*

Diagnosis	Clinical Manifestations	Management
Ecchymosis (black eye)	History of blunt trauma Edema of lids Ecchymosis Infection of conjunctiva Normal visual acuity and internal eye examination Negative orbital x-ray	Contusions, even if apparently mild, should be treated with suspicion. Refer to ophthalmologist or physician for examination and treatment. There may be delayed hemorrhage into the anterior chamber 1 to 3 days after injury.
Penetrating injuries	History of direct puncture by sharp object History of direct puncture by small foreign body flying at high speed History of direct puncture by blunt, forceful impact of a solid body Laceration of the globe (failure of a laceration to move suggests sclera involvement) Subconjunctival hemorrhage Persistent pain Photophobia Decreased vision Lid edema Unusual softness of the eye Vitreous hemorrhage Cataract Hyperemia Gross prolapse of intraocular contents	Refer immediately to ophthalmologist for hospital admission and treatment.
Thermal burns	History of burns to eyes, caused by direct flames, gasoline, explosions, steam, molten metal, hot air, etc. Erythema of lids Partial loss of brows and lashes Cicatricial ectropion (sagging and eversion of the lower lid) Second- and third-degree burns may produce rapid necrosis Exposure keratitis Secondary ulceration of cornea	Refer to ophthalmologist. First aid measures consist of sedation, cleansing with water, sterile ointment, and patching of both eyes.
Radiation burns	History of exposure to radiation, e.g., ultraviolet (sunlamp, snow blindness); infrared (accidental exposure to lightning, short circuit of a high-tension electrical system, eclipse of the sun) Pain Superficial punctate keratitis Conjunctivitis	Refer to ophthalmologist for treatment.

Table 19-1 Medical Referral/Consultation *(continued)*

Diagnosis	Clinical Manifestations	Management
	With infrared exposure, can have Dazzling sensation Cloudy vision Light sensitivity Chromatopsia (various color sensations such as yellow, blue, or red)	
Chemical burns	Pain History of child playing with household cleaners or accident with same Eye usually clamped shut due to spasm Irritation of sclera and conjunctiva	Apply prompt and prolonged irrigation with saline or tap water. Irrigate using several quarts of water almost continuously with short rest periods for 30 min. After or during irrigation, rush child to hospital for definitive ophthalmic care.

bibliography

Harley, R. D. Blunt trauma to the eye. *Comprehensive Therapy*, 3:29–32 (March 1977).

Liebman, Sumner, and Gellis, Sidney. *The Pediatrician's ophthalmology*. St. Louis: Mosby, 1966.

Olgesby, Richard. Eye Trauma in Children. *Pediatric Annals*, **6**:11–47 (January 1977).

Paton, D., and Goldberg, M. *Management of ocular injuries*. Philadelphia: Saunders, 1976.

Sorsby, Arnold (ed.). *Modern ophthalmology* (2d ed.). Philadelphia: Lippincott, 1972.

20 Pink Eye

M. CONSTANCE SALERNO

ALERT
1. Involvement of cornea
2. Ocular pain

I. Etiology

A. Bacterial conjunctivitis (epidemic pink eye)
1. Staphylococcus aureus
2. Diplococcus pneumoniae
3. Haemophilus influenzae
4. Haemophilus aegyptins (Koch-Weeks bacillus)
5. Streptococcus viridans

B. Viral conjunctivitis

C. Vernal conjunctivitis

D. Allergic conjunctivitis

II. Assessment

A. Bacterial conjunctivitis
1. Subjective data
   a. "Pink eye" (red swollen eyelids)
   b. Discharge prominent upon awakening
   c. Lid matting
   d. Burning
2. Objective data
   a. Generally bilateral, starting in one eye and transmitted to the other
   b. Conjunctival injection
   c. Purulent discharge
   d. Chemosis (conjunctival edema)

B. Viral conjunctivitis
1. Subjective data
   a. "Pink eye"
   b. Tender preauricular nodes
   c. Tearing (epiphora)
   d. Photophobia and blurred vision if cornea is involved
2. Objective data
   a. Conjunctival injection (red eye)
   b. Follicle formation appears as slightly pale; conjunctival elevations about 1 mm in size
   c. Watery discharge

C. Vernal conjunctivitis
1. Subjective data
   a. Pink eyes
   b. Intense itching
   c. Tearing
   d. Severe photophobia
   e. Common in the springtime
2. Objective data
   a. Bilateral
   b. Bulbar perilimbal inflammation
   c. Follicular or "cobblestone" appearing palpebral conjunctiva
   d. Long, tenacious strands of mucus
   e. Chemosis (conjunctival edema)

D. Acute simple allergic conjunctivitis
1. Subjective data
   a. Pink eyes
   b. Photophobia
   c. Foreign body sensation
   d. Itching
   e. Hypersensitivity associated with history of atopy
2. Objective data
   a. Bilateral dull red conjunctiva
   b. Chemosis
   c. Tearing

III. Management

A. Bacterial conjunctivitis (epidemic pink eye)
1. Treatments/medications
   a. Condition self-limited and lasts about 7 days
   b. 10% sodium sulfacetamide drops (Sodium

Sulamyd ophthalmic drops), 1 drop 4 times per day will shorten course

2. Counselling/prevention
   a. Highly contagious
   b. Child instructed to use own towels, etc.
   c. Compliance with medication
   d. Exclusion from school for at least 24 h after antibiotic therapy
3. Follow-up
   a. Evaluation of response to topical medication within 48 h
   b. Return visit if condition worsens or if condition persists longer than 7 days
4. Consultations/referrals
   a. Referral to ophthalmologist if condition is associated with pain or changes in vision
   b. Referral to ophthalmologist if condition persists longer than 7 days

B. Viral conjunctivitis

1. Treatments/medications

   No specific treatment
2. Counselling/prevention
   a. Highly contagious
   b. Child instructed to use own towels, etc.
   c. Exclusion from school during acute stage
   d. Expected resolution in 10 to 14 days
3. Follow-up

   Return visit if condition worsens or if purulent discharge present
4. Consultations/referrals

   If condition persists longer than 2 weeks, referral to ophthalmologist

C. Vernal conjunctivitis

1. Treatments/medications
   a. Cold packs soothing
   b. Avoidance of the allergen
   c. Oral antihistamines sometimes helpful
   d. Topical steroids sometimes necessary, but only under supervision of ophthalmologist
2. Counselling/prevention

   Chronic type, often seasonal, but symptoms usually become milder and disappear progressively with age
3. Follow-up

   As needed for symptomatic treatment
4. Consultations/referrals

   Referral to ophthalmologist for persistent condition which may need to be evaluated for short-term steroid therapy

D. Acute allergic conjunctivitis

1. Treatments/medications
   a. Avoidance of allergen
   b. Application of 0.25% phenylephrine (Neo-Synephrine) drops or 1:1000 epinephrine (Adrenalin) drops, 4 times daily
   c. Cold compresses sometimes helpful in reducing symptoms
2. Counselling/prevention
   a. Compliance with medication
   b. If symptoms are severe, identifying and desensitizing to the allergen sometimes necessary
3. Follow-up

   Return visit if condition worsens
4. Consultations/referrals

   Referral to ophthalmologist if condition worsens and/or referral to pediatric allergist for desensitization

Table 20-1 Medical Referral/Consultation

Diagnosis	Clinical Manifestations	Management
Stevens-Johnson syndrome	Mucous membranes of eyes, mouth, nose, urethrogenital organs involved (pseudomembranous conjunctivitis)	Hospitalization necessary (see Preparation for Hospitalization, Part 7)

bibliography

Frey, T. External diseases of the eye. *Pediatric Annals*, **6**:49–87 (1977).

Goscienski, P. J. Conjunctivitis. In Shirkey, H. C. *Pediatric Therapy* (5th ed.). St. Louis: Mosby, 1975, pp. 499–504.

21 Sty

M. CONSTANCE SALERNO

I. Etiology: *Staphylococcus aureus*

II. Assessment

A. Sty (hordeolum)
1. Subjective data
   a. Eyelid swelling
   b. Tenderness, pain
   c. Itch
   d. Possible drainage
2. Objective data
   a. Abscess
      (1) Points toward lid margin—internal sty
      (2) Points toward skin—external sty
   b. Erythema
   c. Lid swelling
   d. Purulent discharge

B. Chalazion
1. Subjective data
   a. Chronic nodule of lid
   b. Painless
2. Objective data
   a. Nodule in midportion of the tarsus due to obstruction of meibomian gland
   b. Nodule pointing toward conjunctival lid surface
   c. No acute inflammatory sign

C. Staphylococcal blepharitis
1. Subjective data
   a. Chronic
   b. Tiny "lump" on lower lid margin
   c. Loss of lashes
2. Objective data
   a. Inflammatory swelling of lid margin
   b. Erythema lid margin
   c. Dry, crusty scales
   d. Loss of lashes

D. Seborrheic blepharitis
1. Subjective data
   a. Chronic lid inflammation
   b. Possible history of seborrhea
2. Objective data
   a. Greasy, dandrufflike scales (scurf) on eyelashes
   b. Hyperemia of lid margins
   c. Associated seborrhea of scalp, brow, nose, and ears

III. Management

A. Sty (hordeolum)
1. Treatments/medications
   a. Warm compresses—10 to 15 min, 4 times daily
   b. Topical antibiotic therapy
      (1) Sulfacetamide ointment (Sodium Sulamyd ophthalmic ointment 10%) 3 times per day and at bedtime
      (2) Neosporin ophthalmic ointment 3 times per day and at bedtime
   c. Systemic antibiotic therapy (dicloxacillin) given in severe cases
2. Counselling/prevention
   a. Keeping hands away from eyes
   b. Compliance with treatment and medication
3. Follow-up
   Return visit if condition worsens or if not resolved in 4 to 6 days
4. Consultations/referrals
   If resolution does not occur within 1 to 2 weeks referral to ophthalmologist for possible incision and drainage

B. Chalazion
1. Treatments/medications
   a. Warm compresses—15 to 20 min, 4 times daily
   b. Topical antibiotic therapy
      (1) Sulfacetamide ointment (Sodium Sula-

myd ophthalmic ointment 10%) 3 times per day and at bedtime

(2) Neosporin ophthalmic ointment 3 times per day and at bedtime

2. Counselling/prevention
   a. Compliance with treatment and medication
   b. Chronic type of inflammation of eyelid that requires longer period for resolution
3. Follow-up
   Return visit if condition worsens or not resolved in 2 weeks
4. Consultations/referrals
   a. If resolution does not occur within 2 weeks, referral to ophthalmologist
   b. May require incision and evacuation of gelatinous material

C. Staphylococcal blepharitis

1. Treatments/medications
   a. Removal of crusts twice daily with moistened cotton swab (applying warm compresses beforehand, if necessary)
   b. Sulfacetamide or Neosporin ophthalmic ointment 3 times per day and at bedtime
   c. Hexachlorophene, containing soap—daily use for control of skin staphylococci (rub washcloth across cilia)
2. Counselling/prevention
   a. Cleanliness—attention to general hygiene
   b. Compliance with treatment and medication
   c. Review of dietary intake for appropriate nutritional status
   d. Recurrent episodes possibly occurring throughout life
3. Follow-up
   a. Return visit if condition worsens or not resolved in 2 weeks
   b. Culture and sensitivity (C and S) of lid secretion if condition not resolved
   c. Observe for corneal ulcer
4. Consultations/referrals
   a. If resolution does not occur within 2 weeks, referral to ophthalmologist
   b. Resistant cases sometimes requiring systemic antibiotic therapy or staphylococcus toxoid

D. Seborrheic blepharitis

1. Treatments/medications
   a. Removal of lid flakes with moist cotton applicators
   b. Application of 3% ammoniated mercury ointment to lids several times daily
   c. Control of scalp with selenium sulfide shampoo (Selsun Blue)
2. Counselling/prevention
   a. Long-standing problem that will require continuous attention over the years
   b. Importance of controlling the scalp and facial seborrhea through use of keratolytic agents
3. Follow-up
   Reevaluation of severe cases to rule out secondary infection with staphylococcus
4. Consultations/referrals
   If condition does not improve within 2 weeks, referral to ophthalmologist

Table 21-1 Medical Referral/Consultation

Diagnosis	Clinical Manifestations	Management
Herpes simplex	Vesicles on lid margin	Immediate referral to physician 5-iodo-2 deoxyuridine (IDU) effective in treatment of corneal lesions

bibliography

Frey, Thomas. External diseases of the eye. *Pediatric Annals*, **6**(1):49–87 (January 1977).

Raab, E. L., and Leopold, I. H. Diseases of the eye. In Shirkey, H. C. (ed.), *Pediatric therapy* (5th ed.). St. Louis: Mosby, 1975, pp. 916–917.

22 Blindness/Vision Changes

MARJORIE PECK

ALERT

1. Lack of eye contact with the primary care giver when in the alert state
2. Inability of infant to visually track an object
3. Parental report of infant's lack of responsiveness
4. Developmental delay

I. Etiology

A. Congenital

1. Genetic defects, e.g., albinism, anopthalmos, glaucoma
2. Embryopathic defects—pathogens affecting child during intrauterine life—e.g., rubella
3. Defect in fetal development without known genetic cause, e.g., glaucoma

B. Acquired

1. Infections, e.g., herpes simplex
2. Trauma—cerebral insult, birth trauma, severe asphyxia, trauma to the eye itself
3. Glaucoma secondary to trauma, tumors, infection
4. Retrolental fibroplasia

II. Assessment of the Visually Impaired

A. Subjective Data

Lack of responsiveness and lack of visual response reported by parent.

B. Objective Data

1. Significantly diminished visual acuity
2. Positive ophthalmological findings for severe visual impairment or blindness
3. Developmental delay in those areas requiring vision and in mobility

III. Management

A. Treatments/Medications

1. Treatments and medications vary widely depending upon the cause of the visual defect.
2. Glasses may be prescribed for some types of vision changes.
3. Contact lenses may be used following cataract surgery.

B. Counselling/Prevention

1. Early detection of diminished visual acuity can lead to diagnosis and treatment of those disorders that are treatable or can lead to early intervention to minimize developmental delays.
2. Parents need to understand the significance of treatment regimes if they are expected to follow through.
3. Premature infants who are treated with oxygen are at risk for retrolental fibroplasia. They should have an ophthalmological examination by an ophthalmologist skilled in working with infants and children.
4. Because of extended hospitalization, premature infants often suffer from early parent-child separation, putting them at risk for inadequate parent-child bonding. The clinician in the neonatal special care area can facilitate parent-child attachment by encouraging early parental involvement through visiting, touching, bathing, and feeding the infant (Klaus and

Kennell, 1977). The clinician should also tell the parent(s) what the risks are for the infant to be developmentally delayed or visually impaired. This is done to minimize the immobilizing shock that comes when these diagnoses are made later.

Home Management/Counselling: Infant

Affectional bonding Of primary concern is the parent-child attachment and the promotion of affectional bonds. In order to promote normal parent-child interaction it is important to evaluate and work with the parent(s) and child in the setting they are most comfortable in, i.e., their home. Support and suggestions to promote development are given to the family of a visually impaired infant or toddler through regular home visits. Blind and severely visually impaired infants lack "normal" visual, anticipatory responses. When the parent(s) approaches the crib, the sighted child turns, looks at the parent(s), and within a period of weeks to a few months after birth, smiles and displays motor excitement in anticipation of being picked up. The visually impaired infant quiets body movements, may turn the head away or toward but does not look at the parent(s); this child is listening in anticipation of being picked up. The parent(s) may interpret this as rejection rather than anticipation and may leave the child alone because "baby prefers the crib." The home visitor helps the parent(s) to interpret appropriately and to identify the child's anticipation and therefore see how important the parent(s) is to the infant.

Parental shock, fear, guilt, anger The parent(s) mourns the loss of the anticipated normal child and feels hurt and perhaps angry, depressed, frightened, or guilt-ridden with the birth of a child with visual impairment (Fraiberg, 1971). The severity and type of response varies with each family depending upon their coping patterns, feelings about the handicapped, and support systems. The home visitor may facilitate the working through of these feelings by listening, empathizing, and acknowledging these feelings as normal and understandable. When parental feelings of guilt, anger, shock, and fear are so intense and persistent or depression so severe that they interfere with parental ability to interact with the child, it is essential that the home visitor refer that parent for professional counselling.

Child development

1. *Exploration* Infants explore the world visually long before they do so with motor abilities. The primary stimulus to reach out and touch an object is visual (Fraiberg, 1977). The vision-impaired child lacks that stimulus and is not likely to reach out without assistance. Assistance can come in the following forms.

a. Crib gyms (bought or homemade) hung low so moving hands accidentally find hanging rattles that jingle when hit, soft fuzzy balls that feel good when touched, wooden spoons that clack when struck.
b. Musical mobiles, especially for the partially sighted child. Bright- and dark-colored objects against white walls attract the use of limited vision and encourage reaching out.
c. Cribs, playpens, and floors with a variety of textured, silent, and noisemaking objects within accidental reach.
d. Pillowcases filled with newspaper or plastic bags and sewn shut, to kick and find a new sound.

2. *Smiling* Smiling occurs as with the sighted child, in the first few months of life, but it does not go on to become a regular response to parental presence (Fraiberg, 1975). Parents need to be told that their visually impaired children may not smile in response to them but will demonstrate pleasure through hand and body activity. Parents often find tactile and gross motor stimulation (tickling, swinging) will elicit a laugh.

3. *Exploration with mouth* Hand-to-mouth behavior enables the child to use the tactually sensitive mouth to define dimensions, textures, and tastes of varied objects and people. If this behavior is absent, honey or applesauce on a finger, pacifier, rattle, or cube may encourage it.

4. *Sound and touch* It is most important that parents and siblings play pat-a-cake and hold the child, sing and talk constantly, clap when hands come together, and hug to help the child find trust and the beginning and ends of self. Although children are unable to localize on sound cue alone until almost the end of the first year of life, singing, talking, and sound-producing objects facilitate development of this important skill. Children will not turn toward a voice, rattle, or music box because they do not know where it is. Parents need to know this to understand why they must assist visually impaired children to search and reach with their hands. This inability to localize sound also affects mobility. The stimulus to creep is visual; children see a person or object of interest and attempt to move to it. Visually impaired children do not see the person, cannot tell where the sound comes from, and so stay put.

5. *Feeding* Like all infants, visually impaired infants require nutritional intake and the close contact of being held while fed. New textures in foods may be a bit overwhelming to visually impaired children and are often best introduced one at a time but persistently. Visually impaired children may show a reluctance to take over the task of holding their own bottles, even when they will hold other comparably shaped and weighted objects. It has proven functional to let the child be the guide for readiness to hold the bottle.

6. *Language* Early language development is like that of the sighted infant. The oohs and aahs of the early months are reinforced by parent(s) oohing and aahing back. So too with the consonants in the later half of the first year. The visually impaired child does not see the excitement of the father when "Da" is first said, and so must hear and feel through words, hugs, and kisses that this is a significant term. The home visitor encourages the parent(s) to discuss everything, to identify with words the people, body parts, objects, sounds, and smells that the infant contacts.

Home Management/Counselling: Toddler

Mobility Children do not localize to sound cue until the last quarter of their first year. The visually impaired are therefore unable to move toward sound cues. Visually impaired children may reach the readiness positions for creeping and walking within the normal developmental time frame, but they generally creep sometime after 1 year of age and walk independently from $1\frac{1}{2}$ to $2\frac{1}{2}$ years. How delayed mobility is depends upon the child, the amount of residual vision, and the presence of other handicapping conditions.

The visually impaired child who has learned to creep, cruise, and walk holding on may not walk independently for months, much to parental dismay. If parents close their eyes and try to walk, they may better understand the child's reluctance to step into the unknown. As the child becomes mobile, it is important to keep in mind that changes in the environment require that the child map out the space. Where the sighted child can take in the environment with a visual survey and then decide a course, the visually impaired child must decide to explore manually to learn what the environment contains. If furniture is moved around, the child should be physically shown the new arrangement in relationship to old landmarks, like doors and windows. Never changing the furniture is an unfair request to make of parents; changing it every week is unfair to the child. The child may be reluctant in new places, needing time to locate sensory landmarks (by touch, sound, smell, and sometimes taste). People trying to examine or test the visually impaired child may find the youngster too busy exploring the new environment to complete the examination. A second visit may be necessary for accurate results. The visually impaired child is constantly stepping into the unknown and may therefore require a parent alongside for longer periods to adjust to new places and new care givers.

Exploration and play The visually impaired child, like a sighted child, needs a safe space in which to explore and play. Cupboards with pots and pans to bang, boxes with toys, animals to touch, clothespins, and blocks are good, with breakable items out of reach until an adult can help with the exploration. Once mobile, this child too will get into everything, sometimes more slowly than the sighted child. Mouthing of objects may persist, as the mouth is still a very sensitive organ for discrimination. Handling of toys will usually vary from that of the sighted child in that the visually impaired child cannot see or enjoy the toy for its intended purpose. A push-pull toy may have its wheels spun for the sound effect; a truck may be licked for its hard, cold feeling or banged on the ground for the sound.

Language Talking parents are a must. Apples come whole, sliced, diced, cooked, smashed, and made into juice. Visually impaired children must handle, taste, and smell the fruit in all its forms while hearing the term that applies to it. Visually impaired children need to hear their names called to know someone is talking to them; they do not see people looking at them to know whom the speaker is addressing. Body part identification games and songs with motions facilitate language development.

Feeding

1. Utensils are difficult to use. It is hard to tell if the spoon is up or down, and feeling the contents may empty the spoon. Exposure to utensils and time to feel and play with them enable the child to become familiar with them.
2. Generally finger foods are easiest and the most appropriate first step toward self-feeding. Some children are reluctant to get fingers covered with food since that diminishes their sensitivity in identifying objects. Time, preferred foods, and a consistent eating place (e.g., high chair) facilitate self-feeding.
3. Nonbreakable tumblers should be used for drinking from a cup. One mother uses a coffee can (with no sharp edges) because it is easier for her son to explore the contents and measure the quantity. The cup should be placed on the table so the child knows where it came from and where to return it.
4. Self-feeding is messy at best with all children and more so for the visually impaired. Parents who are uncomfortable with the mess need encouragement to let their child be messy. Some suggestions to minimize the irritation are a plastic floor protector under the high chair, self-feeding at just one family meal per day at first, eating on the patio during nice weather so it can be hosed off.

Toilet training As with any child, *when* to toilet train depends upon the child's readiness and *how* depends upon parental preference. Few children are ready before age 2. Visually impaired children, like their sighted counterparts, need to explore the potty chair or toilet, play in it, and flush it.

Dressing Tags should be in the back of all clothes, and children need assistance with feeling the tag; the seams that mark the inside; the holes that are for arms, legs, and head; the heel or toe of socks; the buckles on the outside of the shoe to differentiate left from right. These all help to begin the process of learning self-dressing, which will continue into early school years.

Blindisms Self-stimulatory behaviors, many of which resemble autistic behaviors, usually start some time in the first year of life.

1. Hand flapping in front of eyes (try it outside on a sunny day with your eyes closed)
2. Rocking
3. Spinning self or wheels of a toy
4. Eye poking (it causes a flash of light)
5. Head banging

Blind and visually impaired children lacking a major sensory input. The attempt to make up for this is through tactile, auditory, and vestibular self-stimulation (Fraiberg, 1977). Attempts to block these behaviors may lead to intensification of the behavior or an exchange of one behavior for another (e.g., eye poking for head banging). Attempts at redirecting the child's attention to another activity may help as long as the person redirecting remains in contact with the child to provide sensory input.

As mobility increases and other developmental areas progress, allowing for increasing sensory input, the child yields most of the self-stimulatory behaviors. Some may remain and may be likened to an adult's kicking a foot or repeatedly touching lips or hair.

Management/Counselling: Age 3

Generally at age 3 or 4 preschool programs become available and appropriate for the visually impaired child. Whether the child goes into a regular preschool or a visually handicapped program will depend on the child's developmental level, adaptability, and program availability.

C. Follow-up

Routine ophthalmological examinations as indicated by the ophthalmologist are recommended. Developmental assessment should be done every 6 months up to 3 or 4 years old, and then annually. These should be done by a psychologist skilled in assessing visually impaired children. The purposes of developmental assessment are to

1. Determine developmental level, strengths, and weaknesses.
2. Determine appropriate program placement.
3. Provide countercheck and objective assistance in program planning for the home visitor.

D. Consultations/Referrals

Consultations should be made on a regular basis with the ophthalmologist and the pediatrician. Referrals for professional counselling should be made as needed.

Table 22-1 Medical Referral/Consultation

Diagnosis	Clinical Manifestations	Management
Question of blindness or visual impairment	No or poor eye contact Inability to track objects Lack of responsiveness to parent(s) Delayed development Reaching Mobility	Referral to ophthalmologist for evaluation If severe impairment or blindness is diagnosed, referral to appropriate agency for Developmental assessment Appropriate program placement for developmental facilitation
Intense and persistent parental depression, anger, fear, guilt	Inability of parent(s) to mobilize to Care for infant's basic needs Follow through with developmental program Hostility inappropriately focused on everyone and everything except for infant and/or infant's handicap Persistent (months to years) shopping for diagnosis and treatment Continual yielding of parent(s) to all of child's demands	Referral for professional counselling to enable parent(s) to work through feelings

references

Fraiberg, Selma. Intervention in infancy: A program for blind infants. *Journal of the American Academy of Psychiatry,* **10**:381–405 (1971).

———. *Insights from the blind.* New York: Basic Books, 1977, chap. 7.

———. The development of human attachments in infants blind from birth. *Merrill-Palmer Quarterly,* **21**(4):316–334 (1975).

Klaus, Marshall H., and Kennell, John H. *Maternal-infant bonding: The impact of early separation on family development.* St. Louis: Mosby, 1977, chap. 4.

bibliography

Blank, Robert. Reflections on the special senses in relation to the development of affect with special emphasis on blindness. *American Psychoanalytic Association Journal,* **23**(1):32–50 (1975).

Chase, John. Developmental assessment of handicapped infants and young children: With special attention to the visually impaired. *New Outlook,* October:341–364 (1975).

Gist, Kristen. Protocol for visually impaired infants program, Children's Hospital and Health Center. Unpublished manuscript. San Diego, 1976.

Harley, Robinson D. (ed.). *Pediatric ophthalmology.* Philadelphia: Saunders, 1975.

23 Ear Pain/Discharge

JANE A. FOX

ALERT
1. Signs of meningitis (stiff neck, severe headache, lethargy, irritability, bulging fontanel)
2. Infant less than 4 months old
3. Severe pain
4. Mastoid tenderness
5. Frequent, recurrent ear infections
6. Clients who do not improve with treatment in 48 h

I. Etiology

A. External canal
1. Bacteria
   a. *Staphylococcus aureus*
   b. *Streptococcus*
   c.. *Pseudomonas aeruginosa*
   d. *Proteus vulgaris*
2. Virus
3. Fungus
   a. *Candida*
   b. *Aspergillus*
4. Allergy
5. Trauma
6. Foreign body

B. Middle ear
1. *Streptococcus pneumoniae*
2. *Hemophilus influenzae* (under 6 years of age)
3. Beta-hemolytic streptococcus group A

II. Assessment

A. Otitis externa
1. Subjective data
   a. Ear pain or itching, especially when chewing, talking, or moving earlobe
   b. Possible decreased hearing or feeling of fullness in ear
2. Objective data
   a. Fever
   b. Possible foul-smelling, bloody, watery, purulent discharge
   c. Pain on movement of pinna or tragus
   d. External canal red, edematous
   e. Enlarged preauricular, postauricular, or anterior cervical nodes
   f. Tympanic membrane perhaps involved

B. Acute suppurative otitis media
1. Subjective data
   a. Pain which may increase with coughing or sneezing
   b. Infant or young child perhaps tugging or pulling ear
   c. Decreased hearing
   d. Occasionally asymptomatic
   e. Associated symptoms
      (1) Fever
      (2) Irritability
      (3) Disturbed sleep
      (4) Rhinorrhea or upper respiratory infection
      (5) Cough
      (6) Vomiting/diarrhea
      (7) Stiff neck
      (8) Sore throat
2. Objective data
   a. Tympanic membrane red and bulging
   b. Pneumoscopy
      (1) Movement of tympanic membrane irregular
      (2) Tympanic membrane immobile

C. Acute serous otitis media
1. Subjective data
   a. "Cold" or allergy
   b. Clogged ear
   c. Crackling sensation in ear
   d. Occasionally asymptomatic

2. Objective data
   a. Tympanic membrane
      (1) Retracted
      (2) Malleus prominent
      (3) Transparent fluid level perhaps visible
   b. Pneumoscopy
      Tympanic membrane does not move inward.

D. Chronic serous otitis media

1. Subjective data
   a. Hearing loss
   b. Ears feel plugged
   c. Little or no pain
2. Objective data
   a. Tympanic membrane
      (1) Dull, opaque
      (2) Pale or bluish tint
      (3) Retracted
      (4) Short process of malleus prominent
      (5) Bluish-grey fluid perhaps visualized
   b. Pneumoscopy
      Immobile or irregular movement of tympanic membrane
   c. Weber's test
      Lateralization to involved ear

III. Management

A. Otitis externa

1. Treatments/medications
   a. Cortisporin or VōSol otic drops—2 to 3 drops in affected ear, 3 to 4 times daily for 1 to 2 weeks
   b. Pain relief
      (1) Acetaminophen
      (2) Aspirin
      (3) Heat
   c. Systemic antibiotics if
      (1) Facial cellulitis
      (2) Furuncles
      (3) Fever
2. Counselling/prevention
   a. Keeping ear canals dry
      (1) Limited swimming until infection clears
      (2) Earplugs when showering or swimming
      (3) Two drops alcohol, Cortisporin, or VōSol otic drops during swimming season
   b. Medication
      (1) Instruct how to instill ear drops.
      (2) Stress importance of taking prescribed medication properly.
   c. Keeping foreign objects out of ears—do not clean ear canal
3. Follow-up
   a. Return visit in 3 days if not improved
   b. If symptoms reoccur, telephone and/or return visit
4. Consultations/referrals
   Note to school nurse and/or teacher if decreased hearing noted

B. Acute suppurative otitis media

1. Treatments/medications
   a. Five years of age and younger—orally for 10 days
      (1) Amoxicillin trihydrate (Amoxil)—fewer side effects than ampicillin
      (2) Or ampicillin—given 1 h before or after meals
      (3) Or penicillin V plus sulfisoxazole (Gantrisin)
   b. Over 6 years of age
      Penicillin—4 times per day, 1 h before or 2 h after meals
   c. Penicillin allergy
      Erythromycin—in 3 divided doses
   d. Injection
      Benzathine penicillin G (Bicillin)—single IM injection
2. Counselling/prevention
   a. Instruction on medications
      (1) Compliance with treament and medications
      (2) How to instill ear drops, if prescribed
   b. Aggressive early treatment of common cold to prevent otitis media
   c. Early signs of otitis media, and importance of immediate thorough treatment
   d. Explanation of position and anatomy of eustachian tube and why children are more prone to ear infections
   e. May have decreased hearing for several weeks
   f. Reminder to hold infants with head slightly elevated when feeding them
   g. Good fluid intake
   h. Importance of follow-up
   i. Instruction to observe for signs of complications
   j. Return if condition worsens
3. Follow-up
   a. Telephone call in 2 to 3 days to report progress
   b. Return visit in 10 days to 2 weeks to evaluate treatment and/or to repeat medication if not resolved
   c. Audiometric studies in 3 weeks perhaps indicated if serous otitis media results or decreased hearing noted

4. Consultations/referrals
   a. All infants less than 4 months of age should be referred to physician.
   b. Notify school nurse that hearing may be decreased for several weeks.
   c. If client or family noncompliant, notify public health nurse (PHN) for home visit.

C. Acute serous otitis media
1. Treatments/medications
   a. Saline nose drops and suction for infants
   b. Decongestants
      (1) Sudafed
      (2) Actifed
      (3) Dimetapp
2. Counselling/prevention
   Aggressive early treatment of acute suppurative otitis media (see treatment recommended under Acute suppurative otitis media, III, B)
3. Follow-up
   a. Weekly visits until tympanic membrane has normal mobility
   b. Audiometric testing when tympanic membrane appears normal
4. Consultations/referrals
   a. Refer to physician if conditions do not resolve in 1 month.
   b. Send note to school nurse.

D. Chronic serous otitis media
1. Treatments/medications
   a. Oral decongestant 3 to 4 times per day for 1 month
   b. "Pop" ears, 4 times daily
2. Counselling/prevention
   a. Aggressive early treatment of acute suppurative otitis media
   b. Importance of follow-up
   c. Instruction regarding medication
   d. Need to be supportive of client and parent(s)
      (1) Explanation of treatment plan
      (2) If myringotomy necessary,
         (a) Explain procedure.
         (b) Tubes will prevent fluid buildup by equalizing pressure in middle ear; tubes fall out spontaneously.
3. Follow-up
   a. Telephone call in 1 week
   b. Return visit in 2 weeks
   c. Audiometric testing in 3 to 4 weeks
4. Consultations/referrals
   a. Refer to physician if condition does not resolve in 1 month.
   b. Notify school nurse and teacher; child may have decreased hearing and should be seated in front row.

Table 23-1 Medical Referral/Consultation

Diagnosis	Clinical Manifestations	Management
Furuncle	Pain in external ear canal Pain when otoscope inserted Small erythematous swelling visualized in external canal	Consultation with physician Medication Cloxacillin Penicillin allergy: erythromycin Topical bacitracin ointment Warm packs for pain
Otitis media with perforation	Sudden alleviation of severe ear pain Painless serous or purulent discharge with or without odor Tympanic membrane Thick, pink, opaque Short process of malleus not visualized Perforation of tympanic membrane visualized Conductive hearing loss	Consultation with physician/referral to ear, nose, and throat specialist Medications (see Acute suppurative otitis media, III, B in outline) Counselling/prevention (see Counselling/prevention, III, B, 2) Use of earplugs when bathing, washing hair, or swimming Telephone immediately in case of Discharge reappearance Ear pain Weekly visits until discharge clears, then visits every 3 mo for evaluation Audiometric testing

Table 23-1 Medical Referral/Consultation (*continued*)

Diagnosis	Clinical Manifestations	Management
Cholesteatoma	Chronically infected ear Decreased hearing Painless discharge Perforation of tympanic membrane Visible mass at tympanic membrane	Immediate referral to physician Surgery indicated (see Preparation for Hospitalization, Part 7) After hospitalization Review of preventive measures for acute suppurative otitis media Requirement of close supervision Notification of public health nurse Notification of school nurse
Mastoiditis—chronic or acute	Follows 1 to 2 wk after untreated or improperly treated acute suppurative otitis media Pain behind affected ear Fever Draining ear Tenderness, swelling, and redness over mastoid area Signs of otitis media Irritability May have perforated tympanic membrane	Immediate referral to physician Hospitalization may be necessary (see Preparation for Hospitalization, Part 7) After hospitalization (see Cholesteatoma above)
Meningitis	Extreme irritability Severe headache Stiff neck Bulging fontanel Sudden onset of high fever Positive Kernig's sign Positive Brudzinski's sign	*Immediate* referral to physician

bibliography

Coates, H. L., and McDonald, T. J. Serous otitis media. *Postgraduate Medicine*, **57**(6):87–90 (1975).

Huber, Helen L. Draining the "fluid ear" with myringotomy and tube insertion. *Nursing 78*, **8**:28–30 (1978).

Kass, Jane Reitmann, and Beebe, Michael F. Serous otitis media. *The Nurse Practitioner*, **4**(2):25–28 (1979).

Lewin, Edward B. Middle ear disease. In Hoekelman, Robert A., et al. (eds.), *Principles of Pediatrics*. New York: McGraw-Hill, 1978, pp. 1730–1739.

Meade, Richard H. Otologic infections. In Gellis, Sydney S., and Kagan, Benjamin M., *Current Pediatric Therapy 8*. Philadelphia: Saunders, 1978, pp. 521–523.

Northern, J. L., Rock, E. H., and Frye, D. Tympanometry: a technique for identifying ear disease in children. *Pediatric Nursing*, March-April: 32–37 (1976).

Paradise, Jack L. On tympanostomy tubes: rationale, results, reservations, and recommendations. *Pediatrics*, **60**:86–90 (1970).

Tetzlaff, Thomas R., et al. Otitis media in children less than 12 weeks of age. *Pediatrics*, **59**:827–832 (1977).

24 Ear Trauma/Foreign Body

JANE A. FOX

ALERT

1. History of severe head trauma
2. Perforated tympanic membrane
3. Vertigo
4. Ataxia
5. Facial paralysis
6. Clear fluid seeping through perforated tympanic membrane
7. Blue or blue-purple tympanic membrane
8. Malodorous discharge
9. Significant hearing loss

I. Etiology

A. Trauma

B. Foreign body[1]

II. Assessment: Foreign Body in External Auditory Canal

A. Subjective data

1. Usually none
2. Parent(s)/client may report
   a. Drainage
   b. Irritation
   c. Pain
   d. Scratching ear
   e. Child constantly putting fingers in ear(s)

B. Objective data

1. Most aural foreign bodies noted during routine physical examinations
2. Foreign body visualized in external canal

[1]Any client with a self-inserted foreign body must be thoroughly examined for similar objects in other body orifices.

III. Management: Foreign Body in External Canal

A. Treatments/medications

1. Attempt removal of foreign body by flushing external canal with tap water at normal body temperature. Use either syringe or dental Water Pik set on low pressure.
2. Discontinue procedure if foreign body moves medially (may perforate tympanic membrane) or child becomes uncooperative.
3. Do not attempt removal if external canal swollen, lacerated, or bleeding.

B. Counselling/prevention

1. Reassure parent(s)/client that object can be removed.
2. Child needs a great deal of reassurance because of guilt felt about inserting foreign object. Child may become terrified over removal.
3. Discuss and explain removal procedure.
4. Counsel parent(s) about developmental level of child and appropriate accident prevention.
5. Reiterate need to keep small, dangerous objects (peanuts, peas, chewing gum, matches) away from child.
6. Parent(s) should not attempt to clean child's ear. Parent(s) can use washcloth to clean outer ear.

C. Follow-up

Return visit in 1 to 2 weeks to examine ear for residual damage

D. Consultations/referrals

Referral to physician

1. Uncooperative children
2. Clients from whom foreign object is not easily removed
3. Clients with globular objects (beads, pearls) in external canal

Table 24-1 Medical Referral/Consultation

Diagnosis	Clinical Manifestations	Management
Ear trauma (injury)	Recent history of head injury or trauma (e.g., slaps on the ear, foreign objects) Perforation of the tympanic membrane Tympanic membrane of blue or blue-purple color Facial paralysis Hearing loss Sudden onset of nystagmus	*Immediate* referral to physician and/or otologist
Sound trauma	Most common in adolescents History of constant exposure to loud noises Hearing loss noted most predominantly in high frequencies	Consultation with physician Audiometric testing Counselling on importance of eliminating exposure to loud noises

bibliography

Chasin, Werner. Foreign bodies in the ear. In Gellis, Sydney S., and Kagan, Benjamin M., *Current Pediatric Therapy 8*. Philadelphia: Saunders, 1978, p. 521.

Hoekelman, Robert A. *Principles of Pediatrics*. New York: McGraw-Hill, 1978, pp. 1767–1768.

25 Ear Wax: Excessive/ Impacted

JANE A. FOX

ALERT

1. Known or suspected perforation of the tympanic membrane
2. Purulent discharge

I. Etiology

A. Overproduction by cerumen glands

B. Overzealous attempts to remove wax

C. Narrow ear canals

D. Dermatologic disease of the periauricular skin or scalp

II. Assessment: Excessive/Impacted Cerumen

A. Subjective data

1. Ears feeling clogged
2. Decreased hearing
3. Itching

B. Objective data

1. Visualizing large plug of cerumen
2. Unable to fully visualize tympanic membrane

III. Management: Excessive/Impacted Cerumen

A. Treatments/medications

1. Removal of wax
   a. Use 2 to 3 drops of mineral oil or hydrogen peroxide 3 to 4 times a day for 2 to 3 days to soften wax.
   b. Small bits of wax can be removed by using a cotton applicator dipped in mineral oil.
   c. If the above is unsuccessful, irrigation may be necessary (may cause contamination of middle ear). *Never* irrigate if perforation of the tympanic membrane is known or suspected.
      (1) Child must be held securely.
      (2) Gently syringe ear with tap water at normal body temperature, or use a dental Water Pik on low pressure.
      (3) There is little danger of injuring the tympanic membrane provided enough space is left around the irrigating tip for the water to drain from the ear.
2. If external or acute otitis media is present, treatment as appropriate.

B. Counselling/prevention

1. Removal process is uncomfortable—not painful.
2. Client/parent(s) should not attempt to clean ears; *nothing* should be put into the ear canal.
3. Outer ear may be cleaned with a washcloth.
4. Instruct how to instill peroxide or mineral oil.
5. If hearing was decreased because of impacted wax, it will return to normal after removal.
6. Stress the importance of proper treatment, if infection is present.

C. Follow-up

None, unless pain or other complications develop

D. Consultations/referrals

None

bibliography

Capell, Peter T., and Case, David B. *Ambulatory care manual for nurse practitioners.* Philadelphia: Lippincott, 1976, p. 63.

Hoekelman, Robert A. *Principles of Pediatrics.* New York: McGraw-Hill, 1978, pp. 50–51.

Larson, George. Removing cerumen with a Water Pik. *American Journal of Nursing,* **76**:264–265 (1976).

Meyers, A. D. Practical ENT: managing cerumen impaction. *Postgraduate Medicine,* pp. 62–207 (1977).

26 Deafness/Defective Hearing/Hearing Changes[1]

MAUREEN COLLAR

ALERT

1. Lack of response to softer sounds
2. Failure in hearing screen
3. Delayed speech development
4. Persistent, frequent ear infections
5. Infants whose parent(s) suspect a hearing loss

I. Etiology

A. Conductive loss—associated with abnormality of external or middle ear, such as

1. Congenital atresia or stenosis
2. Deformity of ossicles
3. Cerumen
4. Foreign body
5. Perforated tympanic membrane
6. Serous otitis media
7. Otosclerosis
8. Acute otitis media
9. Cholesteatoma
10. Chronic otitis media

B. Sensorineural loss—involves the inner ear (organ of Corti), VIIIth cranial nerve, or midbrain

1. Birth asphyxia
2. Maternal rubella
3. Cytomegalic inclusion disease
4. Syphilis
5. Erythroblastosis
6. Hyperbilirubinemia
7. Ototoxic drugs
   a. Kanamycin
   b. Streptomycin
   c. Gentamicin
8. Mumps
9. Measles
10. Meningitis
11. Labyrinthitis
12. Tumor of acoustic nerve
13. Trauma
14. Constant exposure to high decibel noise (industrial) greater than 100 dB

[1]*Note:* This problem may be initially assessed by the practitioner. Treatment should be initiated in consultation with a physician.

II. Management of the Acoustically Handicapped Child

A. Treatments/medications

1. Initial complete evaluation
   a. Pediatric, for other abnormalities
   b. Audiologic, to determine
      (1) Degree and quality of hearing deficit
      (2) Threshold level
      (3) Decibel loss in each ear
   c. Otolaryngology—sensorineural versus conductive
   d. Etiology psychometrics—recommendations for school placement
   e. Audiometric center—fitting for hearing aid (amplification)
   f. Medication—for conductive loss
   g. Surgery—successful in only a few cases

B. Counselling/prevention

1. Parental needs
   a. Education and information
      (1) Nature of handicap
         (a) Disease process
         (b) Causes
         (c) Type of loss: sensorineural (irreversible) versus conductive (usually reversible)
      (2) Effect on child
         (a) Speech and language development

(b) Social development
(c) Learning process
(3) Interpretation of audiogram
Technical terminology
(4) Hearing aid
(a) Care and function
(b) Does not correct problem or restore normal hearing
(c) Amplifies remaining hearing (distorts sounds)
(5) Importance of parental role in child's
(a) Education
(b) Stimulation

b. Allowance for parent(s) to ventilate and work through feelings
(1) Denial and rationalization
(2) Shock
(3) Grief, despair
(4) Helplessness, guilt
(5) Anger, frustration, disappointment
(6) Realization and coping mechanisms
(7) Readiness to accept help

2. Child's needs
a. Emotional
(1) Visual and physical contact important
(2) Acceptance—positive self-image
(3) Repetition of daily routines and tasks
(4) Child first, and a child with a handicap second
b. Social
(1) Early and continuous contact with hearing children
(a) Neighbors
(b) Peers
(c) Schoolmates
(2) Age-appropriate social expectations and responsibilities
(3) Discipline
c. Educational—early and continuous education essential for development of maximum potential
(1) Must be taught to watch people's faces (lipreading, mouth and eyes)
(2) Auditory training
(3) Needs constant language stimulation and learning

3. Aids to communicating with a deaf child
a. Attract child's attention before speaking.
b. Keep your face visible to child, while talking at eye level.
c. Use simple, complete phrases; use concrete words and specific directions.
d. Talk first, then use a gesture if necessary.
e. Use good facial expression.
f. Talk in a clear, distinct voice.
g. Do not exaggerate lip movements.
h. Do not shout at child.

4. Stimulation of deaf child
a. Draw attention to all sounds in the environment and talk about them.
b. Talk *more* than usual, during all daily activities.
c. Talk to child about what is seen on TV or in picture books.
d. Encourage child to talk and make sounds, through positive reenforcement.

C. Follow-up

1. Continuation of well-child care
2. Acting as child and parent advocate
3. Acting as liaison
4. Facilitating communication with
a. School
b. Audiological staff
c. Other specialists
5. Periodic audiologic evaluation
Audiogram (threshold)
(1) Change in extent (decibels)
(2) Change in quality (frequency) of hearing deficit
6. Audiometric center reevaluation
Modification in hearing aid as child's needs change
(1) Physical growth
(2) Change in hearing deficit

D. Consultations/referrals

1. Educational placement
a. Day school for deaf
b. Residential school
c. Special class in public school
d. Manual versus oral training
2. Referral for genetic counselling and ophthalmologic evaluation if appropriate
3. Day care or sitter to provide a break for parent(s)
4. Financial assistance
National Society for Crippled Children and Adults, Inc., 11 South LaSalle St., Chicago, IL 60603
5. Referral for counselling if indicated
a. Social worker
b. Psychologist
c. Psychiatrist
6. Referral to public health nurse
a. Home care
b. Home training and stimulation
c. Community resources
7. References for parent(s)

a. *They Grow in Silence: The Deaf Child and His Family* by Eugene D. Mindel and Vernon McCay, National Association of the Deaf, Silver Spring, Md., 1971.
b. *Words from a Deaf Parent* by Elizabeth D. Spellman, Communication Research Machines, Del Mar, Calif., 1973.
c. *Volta Review* (journal, address below).

E. National and local organizations for the deaf

1. American Speech and Hearing Association
   1001 Connecticut Ave., NW
   Washington, DC 20036
2. Alexander Graham Bell Association for the Deaf (*Volta Review* and educational pamphlets)
   Volta Bureau
   1537 35th St.
   Washington, DC 20007
3. American Hearing Society
   1800 H St., NW
   Washington, DC 20001

F. Parent education and organizations

The John Tracy Clinic

a. Parent education film series
b. Correspondence course for parent of deaf children
c. *Bulletin* (publication for parent and professional)
   806 W. Adams Blvd.
   Los Angeles, Calif.

Table 26-1 Medical Referral/Consultation

Diagnosis	Clinical Manifestations	Management
Conductive hearing loss	Failure to respond to softer sounds Soft voice quality Failure to respond to name spoken softly Subtle-to-measurable delay in speech and language development Possible normal articulation High-pitched words heard better than low-pitched ones Possible abnormality of pinna or external canal Possible impacted cerumen in external canal Possible abnormality of tympanic membrane Inflammation Retraction Decreased mobility Possible enlarged adenoids Possible sinus infection Weber's test—sound lateralizes to ear with conductive loss Rinne's test—negative (bone conduction greater than air conduction) Audiometry Loss equal in all frequencies Loss less severe than sensorineural deficit (65 dB loss at the most)	Referral to audiologist for audiologic testing to determine extent of hearing deficit Referral to otolaryngologist to determine cause and rule out Middle ear disease Cholesteatoma VIIIth cranial nerve tumor Deformity of ossicles Treatment with medication perhaps indicated Surgical intervention as deemed necessary Counselling/prevention Importance of prompt treatment of ear infections and other ear complaints Early detection and prompt treatment of hearing loss essential Most conductive losses due to middle ear problems, which are treatable Routine hearing screening of all children, in preschool, kindergarten, first, third, fifth, and seventh grades Follow-up Audiometric testing following treatment for middle ear disease Then audiometric screening every 6 mo to 1 yr Consultations/referrals Referral to audiologist All children who fail hearing screen All children with frequent or chronic otitis All children with cleft palate or external ear deformity

Table 26-1 Medical Referral/Consultation *(continued)*

Diagnosis	Clinical Manifestations	Management
		All infants in which parent(s) suspect a hearing loss Consultation with physician regarding treatment of middle ear disease

Sensorineural hearing loss	Permanent/irreversible loss
	Failure to be aroused by noise when sleeping
	Failure to be startled by noise
	Failure to localize sound
	Diminished vocalizations
	Strident, loud voice
	Retarded language development
	  Uses faulty speech, "jargon"
	  Uses simple vowel sounds
	  Substitutes for consonant sounds
	Educational problems
	  Slow learner
	  Behavior problems
	  Restlessness
	  Nervousness
	Positive family history
	Positive prenatal or neonatal history
	Positive past medical history
	Otoscopic exam within normal limits
	May have abnormality of pinnas
	May have anomalies of the head, face, or neck
	Weber's test—sound lateralizes to good ear
	Rinne's test—positive (air conduction greater than bone conduction)
	Audiometry
	  Affects primarily high frequencies
	  Moderately severe to profound loss
		Referral to audiologist for complete audiometrics to determine extent of loss
		Referral to otolaryngologist to rule out middle ear disease
		Referral to audiometric center for amplification (hearing aid)
		Referral to speech or language therapist
		Referral to social worker
		Referral to local parent group
		Referral for genetic counselling
		Referral to appropriate educational program
		Counselling/prevention
		  Counselling family regarding hearing conservation
		    Avoidance of excess loud sounds
		    Avoidance of ototoxic medications
		    Prompt attention to an ear complaint
		    No self-cleaning or medication of ears
		  Counselling for parent(s)
		    Allowing ventilation of feelings
		    Educating regarding handicap
		    Guiding in parent-child interaction
		    Reviewing expected growth and development of child
		    Reviewing child's needs
		      Communications skills
		      Social contact
		      Emotional expression
		      Stimulation in home environment
		    Participation in educational program planning
		Follow-up
		  Team approach; acting as liaison and coordinator
		  Parent and client advocate
		  Following child routinely for complete well-child care
		    Reassessing hearing, language, and medical status
		    Family's adjustment
		    Child's adjustment
		    Progress in school

bibliography

Adams, Daniel, and Istre, Clifton. When the mother suspects a hearing problem. *Medical Times*, **104**(8):72–74 (1976).

Brown, Marie, and Murphy, Mary. *Ambulatory pediatrics for nurses.* New York: McGraw-Hill, 1975.

Dodds, Josephine. Testing hearing ability in the under fives. *Nursing Times*, **71**(45):1791–1792 (1975).

Jaffe, Burton F. (ed.). *Hearing loss in children.* Baltimore: University Park Press, 1977.

Kempe, C. Henry, et al. *Current pediatric diagnosis and treatment.* Los Altos, Calif.: Lange, 1978.

Northern, Jerry (ed.). *Hearing disorders.* Boston: Little, Brown, 1976.

———, and Downs, Marion. *Hearing in children.* Baltimore: Williams & Wilkins, 1978.

Spink, Diane. Crisis intervention for parents of the deaf child. *Health and Social Work*, **1**(4) (1976).

Symposium on the deaf child. *Nursing Mirror*, **143**:47 (1976).

Tsappis, Anthony. Audiological aspects of the identification of hearing impairment in early childhood. *Pediatric Nursing*, March–April:40–43 (1977).

section 2

the respiratory system

INTRODUCTION JANE A. FOX

I. Subjective Data

A. Age

B. Reason for visit and description of problem

C. Onset

D. Precipitating factors

E. Relieving factors

F. History of trauma, foreign body, recent infection

G. Associated symptoms

1. Fever
2. Nasal discharge
3. Sneezing
4. Nose bleeds
5. Watery eyes
6. Sore throat and/or difficulty swallowing
7. Hoarseness
8. Cough
9. Wheezing
10. Difficulty breathing or shortness of breath
11. Ear pain
12. Vomiting
13. Diarrhea
14. Abdominal pain
15. Tarry, black stools
16. Decreased appetite
17. Headache
18. Rash
19. Chills

H. Medications

I. Allergies

J. Immunization history—diphtheria, pertussis, tine test

K. Past medical history

1. Hospitalizations
2. Communicable diseases
3. Chronic diseases
4. Anemia
5. If history of allergies, past treatment

L. Family history

1. Cardiorespiratory diseases
2. Hematologic disorders, e.g., anemia
3. Allergies: asthma, eczema, hay fever, allergic rhinitis
4. Drug sensitivities
5. Migraine headaches
6. Epistaxis
7. Tuberculosis
8. Obesity
9. Cystic fibrosis
10. Recent illness or communicable disease in last 2 weeks

M. Social history

1. Recent change in residence
2. Pets
3. Occupation—location and type of job
4. Smoking
5. Environmental history

II. Objective Data

A. Physical examination

1. Conduct complete physical examination on all infants, young children, and those with difficulty breathing
2. Observe general appearance
3. Check vital signs, including temperature and blood pressure, character of respirations
4. Observe body position/posture
5. Inspect and palpate for sinus tenderness and facial swelling
6. Inspect eyes for swelling, tearing, appearance of conjunctiva
7. Conduct otoscopic examination
8. Inspect/palpate external nose for shape, crepitus, deviations, stability, ecchymosis, flaring
9. Inspect internal nares for patency, growths, foreign body, deviation of septum, discharge (clots, crusts). If epistaxis, check site and side of bleed, anterior or posterior blood flow, boggy inflamed mucosa, hematoma, telangiectasis, hemangioma, varicosities
10. Inspect mouth and throat for mouth breathing, excessive drooling (DO NOT use instrument examination if drooling and severe stridor), exudates, injection, postnasal drip, enlarged tonsils/adenoids, swelling of pharyngeal wall, blood
11. Inspect/palpate for enlarged lymph nodes
12. Auscultate/palpate heart
13. Inspect chest for expansion, symmetry, retractions; auscultate breath sounds; check inspiratory-expiratory ratio; palpate and percuss
14. Inspect, auscultate, palpate, and percuss abdomen
15. Inspect skin and nails for color, ecchymosis
16. Conduct neurological examination: reflexes, level of consciousness, gait, mental status

B. Laboratory data: The following may be indicated:

1. Complete blood count (CBC) and smear of peripheral blood
2. Nasal smear for eosinophil count
3. Chest x-ray (posterior-anterior and lateral)
4. Sinus x-rays
5. Nose x-rays
6. Neck x-rays (if TB is suspected)
7. Throat culture (if epiglottitis is ruled out)
8. Lateral soft tissue films of nasopharynx

27 Nasal Obstruction/ Foreign Body

JENNIFER L. PIERSMA

ALERT
1. Nasal obstruction in a newborn
2. History of head trauma followed by clear, watery rhinorrhea
3. Signs/symptoms of respiratory distress: retractions, cyanosis, tachypnea

I. Etiology

A. Congenital deformities/anomalies
B. Trauma
C. Inflammation
D. Obstruction

II. Assessment

A. Nasal obstruction due to acute rhinitis (see The Common Cold, Chap. 28)
B. Nasal obstruction due to allergic rhinitis
1. Subjective data
   a. Age: perennial usually after 3 years; seasonal usually under 2 years
   b. Precipitating factors: inhaled allergens, ingested allergens, irritants, temperature change, time of day, air pollutants, other nonspecific factors
   c. Relieving factors: mist, medication, change in weather/season/environment
   d. Associated symptoms
      (1) Watery or mucoid rhinorrhea
      (2) Persistent sneezing
      (3) Nasal pruritis
      May also include:
      (4) Ocular pruritis
      (5) Tearing
      (6) Insomnia
      (7) Irritability, moodiness
      (8) Listlessness
      (9) Headache
      (10) Earache
      (11) Anosmia
      (12) Decreased hearing
      (13) Photophobia
      (14) Pruritis of the ears, palate, and throat
   e. Family/medical history: may reveal hay fever, chronic nasal or sinus disease, asthma, eczema, migraine, irritability, allergies
   f. Nutritional history: may have intolerances, eating or feeding difficulties
   g. Environmental history may reveal any of the following—recent change in residence; contact with pets, animals, plants, weeds, trees, grasses; use of new or different soaps, deodorants, cosmetics, pillows, blankets
2. Objective data
   a. Clear or mucoid rhinorrhea
   b. Edematous turbinates, frequently pale and boggy
   May include:
   c. Conjunctival infection, edema; may demonstrate "cobblestone" appearance
   d. Allergic "shiners"
   e. Allergic "salute"
   f. Mouth breathing or gaping appearance
   g. Geographic tongue
   h. Allergic facies if chronic: mouth breathing, high-arched palate, malocclusion
   i. Nasal eosinophilia (presumptive)
   j. Positive reaction to allergy skin testing or nasal provocation testing

C. Nasal obstruction due to foreign body
1. Subjective data
   a. Age: usually toddler or preschooler
   b. History reveals insertion of object directly into nasal cavity or swallowed object vomited into nasal cavity
   c. Associated symptoms
      (1) Unilateral nasal obstruction with purulent drainage
      (2) Mouth breathing
      May include:
      (3) Coughing
      (4) Sneezing
      (5) Snoring
      (6) Nasal pain
2. Objective data
   a. Purulent nasal drainage (frequently unilateral)
   b. Foreign body generally visualized in inferior turbinate, near anterior middle turbinate

D. Nasal obstruction due to nonbacterial sinusitis
1. Subjective data
   a. Age: usually not before 8 years
   b. Recent illness: URI, allergic or vasomotor rhinitis
   c. Associated symptoms
      (1) Intermittent, profuse, clear nasal drainage
      (2) Postnasal drip on swallowing; choking on mucus at night with cough
      (3) Facial pain (corresponding to involved sinus)
      (4) Headache
      (5) Mild malaise
      (6) Toothachelike discomfort (maxillary sinusitis)
2. Objective data
   a. Clear nasal drainage
   b. Tenderness over involved sinus(es)
   c. Red, swollen nasal mucosa
   d. Postnasal drip
   e. Afebrile or low-grade fever (less than 38.4°C)
   f. Culture of discharge (nasopharyngeal) negative

E. Nasal obstruction due to bacterial sinusitis
1. Subjective data
   a. Age: usually not before 8 years
   b. Recent illness: URI, allergic rhinitis
   c. Associated symptoms may include
      (1) Mucopurulent nasal discharge
      (2) Persistent postnasal drip
      (3) Headache (usually worse in the morning and evening)
      (4) Malaise
      (5) Myalgia
      (6) Choking cough (at night)
      (7) Toothachelike discomfort
2. Objective data
   a. Yellow mucopurulent nasal discharge
   b. Tenderness over affected sinus(es)
   c. Swollen, injected nasal mucosa
   d. Postnasal drip
   e. Usually fever (38.4°C or above)
   f. Nasopharyngeal culture
   g. Sinus x-rays (consult physician): clouding of air-fluid levels

III. Management

A. Nasal obstruction due to acute rhinitis (see The Common Cold, Chap. 28)

B. Nasal obstruction due to allergic rhinitis
1. Treatments/medications
   a. Identification and avoidance (minimizing contact) of known or suspected antigen(s)
   b. Antihistamines or antihistamine-decongestants
2. Counselling/prevention
   a. Education concerning etiology, mechanism of allergy
   b. Instruction to client regarding medication
      (1) Action(s) of medication
      (2) Side effect(s) of medication, especially drowsiness with antihistamines
      (3) Importance of continuity of administration
      (4) How to give medication based on developmental age of client
   c. Importance of follow-up, especially if history of frequent serous otitis media with hearing loss
   d. Caution against use of adrenergic nasal sprays for more than 3 days due to risk of rebound edema
3. Follow-up: return visit in 7 to 10 days and then periodically as needed
4. Consultations/referrals: physician if
   a. Failure to respond or tolerate treatment
   b. Evaluation for hyposensitization if signs/symptoms remain more than mild
   c. Presence or removal of nasal polyps
   d. Psychological evaluation of parent/client, if indicated

C. Nasal obstruction due to foreign body
1. Treatments/medications
   a. General considerations

(1) Hold the head firmly to prevent movement and possible injury.
(2) Tilt the head forward or have the client lean forward to prevent aspiration.
(3) If indicated, suction nasal passage or administer topical vasoconstrictor before the removal of the object.
(4) *Reexamine* nose after the removal for the possibility of more than one foreign body.

b. Specific/alternative measures for removal
(1) Insert a large hairpin—bent to conform to the curvature of the nasal passage and hook-shaped at the end—behind the object and flick it out (other instruments which may be used are blunt forceps, wire-loop curette, alligator forceps).
(2) If the object is round, apply collodion to a cotton-tipped applicator and hold this in contact with the object for 1 to 2 min; then remove the object.
(3) Close the uninvolved nostril, place your mouth over the client's, and give a blast of air.
(4) If old enough, have the client blow his or her own nose.
(5) If it is an older client, you may insert a #8 foley catheter past the object, inflate the balloon, and withdraw the object.

2. Counselling/prevention
a. Safety education based on developmental age of client
b. Understanding of obstruction and possibility of another episode
3. Follow-up: none
4. Consultations/referrals: physician
a. If above measures unsuccessful
b. If impacted, beyond nasal vestibule, or quite large
c. If unilateral foul nasal discharge and unable to visualize foreign body

D. Nasal obstruction due to nonbacterial sinusitis

1. Treatments/medications
a. Oral decongestants or antihistamine-decongestants, to continue for 2 days after symptoms end
b. Adrenergic nose drops every 4 h
c. Increase of fluid intake to thin mucus
d. Temperature control measures for discomfort
e. Cold compresses to involved sinus(es) for discomfort
f. Mist or periodic warm showers (older client)

2. Counselling/prevention
a. Education concerning nasal hygiene
b. Instruction to client regarding medication(s)
(1) Action(s) of medications
(2) Side effects of medication, especially drowsiness with antihistamines
(3) Importance of continuity of medication
(4) How to give oral medication and nose drops based on developmental age of client
c. Instruction to client concerning signs/symptoms of secondary infection, such as increased temperature, purulent nasal drainage
d. Importance of follow-up
e. Avoidance of use of steam vaporizer; if used, emphasis on risk of scalding
f. Caution against use of adrenergic nasal sprays for more than 3 days due to risk of nasal rebound edema
g. May swim; diving permitted if nose plugs used

3. Follow-up
a. Call if there is no improvement in 2 to 3 days or if temperature goes above 38.4°C.
b. Return once a week after the treatment is initiated.

4. Consultations/referrals: refer to physician
a. If client unresponsive to above treatment
b. If chronic, recurrent sinusitis

E. Nasal obstruction due to bacterial sinusitis

1. Treatments/medications
a. See Nasal obstruction due to nonbacterial sinusitis, III, D,1.
b. Antibiotics indicated (consult physician) for 1 week.

2. Counselling/prevention
a. See Nasal obstruction due to nonbacterial sinusitis, III, D,2, above.
b. Education concerning signs and symptoms of central nervous system involvement is indicated: ataxia, increased irritability, change in mental status, lethargy, tremors, pupillary changes, meningeal signs.

3. Follow-up
a. Once a week after treatment initiated
b. Return visit in 2 days if no improvement

4. Consultations/referrals: physician if
a. No response to treatment measures
b. Client acutely ill
c. Indication of CNS or orbital involvement
d. Chronic, recurrent illness

Table 27-1 Medical Referral/Consultation

Diagnosis	Clinical Manifestations	Management
Congenital malformation (e.g., choanal atresia, cleft palate, bifid nose)	Persistent rhinorrhea in newborn Dyspnea with feeding Evidence of obstruction	Immediate referral to physician Explain diagnosis, treatment plan to family
Septal hematoma	Nasal pain Widened nasal septum Abrupt onset of nasal obstruction with history of trauma Nasal exam: tense, red swelling bilaterally	Immediate referral to physician/otolaryngologist for evacuation and packing
Septal abscess	History of septal hematoma, furuncle, dental abscess, scarlet fever, measles, or sinusitis Nasal exam: purplish swelling bilaterally Throbbing pain	Immediate referral to physician/otolaryngologist
Septal deformity	Deflected septum Mouth breathing Hypertrophy of turbinate on opposite side	Referral to physician/otolaryngologist
Nasal tumors (variable signs and symptoms)	Unilateral obstruction Nasal discharge Facial swelling Pain or pressure, worse at night Nasal exam: evidence of growth/tumor	Immediate referral to physician/otolaryngologist
Nasal fracture	History of trauma Nasal crepitus Nasal swelling Persistent nosebleed	Immediate referral to physician
Enlarged adenoids	Persistent nasal discharge Nasal speech Respiratory depression at night Persistent mouth breathing Recurrent otitis media with hearing loss	Referral to physician/otolaryngologist
Retropharyngeal abscess	Client 0-2 yr of age High fever Nuchal hyperextension Dysphagia Unilateral swelling of postpharyngeal wall Respiratory distress	*Immediate* referral; surgical emergency
Drug abuse	Chronic rhinorrhea Persistent sniffing Anosmia Hypertrophy or thickening of nasal mucosa Altered level of consciousness	Referral to physician Referral to a drug abuse prevention center

bibliography

Adams, George L., Boies, Lawrence R., and Paparella, Michael M. *Boies's fundamentals of otolaryngology* (5th ed.). Philadelphia: Saunders, 1978.

Ballenger, John J. *Diseases of the nose, throat and ear* (12th ed.). Philadelphia: Lea & Febiger, 1977.

Hinderer, Kenneth H. Nasal problems in children. *Ear, Nose, and Throat Journal* **57**:58–75 (1978).

Hoole, Axalle J., et al. (eds.). *Patient care guidelines for nurse practitioners.* Boston: Little, Brown, 1976.

Kempe, C. Henry, Silver, Henry K., and O'Brien, Donough. *Current pediatric diagnosis and treatment* (4th ed.). Los Altos, Calif.: Lange, 1976.

Miller, D., and Friday, Gilbert A. Allergic diseases of the nose and middle ear in children. *Ear, Nose, & Throat Journal,* **57**:27–52 (1978).

Pracy, R., et al. *Ear, nose, and throat.* New York: Wiley, 1977.

Wilson, T. G. *Diseases of the ear, nose, & throat in children* (2d ed.) New York: Grune & Stratton, 1962.

28 The Common Cold

JANE A. FOX

ALERT
1. Severe difficulty swallowing
2. Signs of dehydration
3. Unilateral nasal discharge
4. Green nasal discharge
5. Ear pain

I. Etiology: Numerous Viruses

II. Assessment: Nasopharyngitis (the common cold)

A. Subjective data

1. Nasal congestion/obstruction
2. Nasal discharge—mucoid or mucopurulent
3. Headache
4. Cough
5. Sneezing
6. Sore throat
7. Chills
8. Malaise
9. Watery, red eyes
10. Fever: less than 3 months of age—afebrile; more than 3 months—febrile to 104°F (38.9 to 40°C); more than 3 years—low-grade fever
11. Irritability
12. Restlessness
13. Muscle aches
14. Anorexia

B. Objective data

1. Red, swollen nasal mucosa—appears boggy
2. Nasal discharge first 2 to 3 days thin and clear and then changes to thick and mucopurulent
3. Mild erythema of pharynx and tonsils
4. Conjunctiva: watery and red
5. Tympanic membrane perhaps red; fluid may be visualized; pneumoscopy may indicate fluid present
6. Fever
7 Mild, transient leukocytosis (not exceeding 13,000 WBC/mm^3) may occur in initial stage of illness

III. Management: Nasopharyngitis (the common cold)

A. Treatments/medications

1. Fever
   - a. Aspirin or acetaminophen every 4 to 6 h for fever and irritability
   - b. Tepid baths for fever
2. Nasal congestion (only if severe or if interferes with feeding or sleeping in infant)
   - a. Infants
     - (1) 2 to 3 drops normal saline nose drops, 15 to 20 min before feeding and sleep
     - (2) Rubber bulb nasal aspiration
   - b. Older infants and children
     - (1) Nose drops
       - (a) Phenylephrine (Neo-Synephrine) 0.125 percent; over 2 years, 0.25 percent
       - (b) Xylometazoline (Otrivin pediatric nasal solution) 0.05 percent; over 2 years, 1 percent drops or spray
       - (c) Oil-base drops *contraindicated* because of possibility of aspiration, which may cause lipid pneumonia
     - (2) Oral decongestants
       - (a) Pseudoephedrine
       - (b) Dimetapp
       - (c) Actifed
3. Cough
   - a. Cough suppressants should *not* be given to children less than 3 years of age.

   b. Give glyceryl guaiacolate (expectorant) 3 times a day.
4. Cold vapor humidifier, especially at night
5. Increase fluid intake
6. Nutritious diet, but do not force
7. Bed rest only if high fever
8. Isolate, if possible, from other children
9. Vaseline around nares if excoriated
10. Vitamin C—use is controversial

B. Counselling/prevention

1. Antibiotics will not alter the course of the illness.
2. If the child is irritable, you may give a concentrated form of carbohydrate (honey, lollipop, soft drink) to treat ketoacidosis.
3. Explain treatment regimen.
4. Discuss normal course of illness.
5. Educate parent(s) on signs and symptoms of complications.
6. Counsel regarding the importance of good fluid intake and nutritious diet. Do not force the child to eat.
7. Teach how to use nasal aspirator and nose drops.
8. Do *not* use nose drops for more than 3 to 4 days because rebound swelling of the nasal mucosa may develop.
9. Counsel about the prevention of colds—proper sleep and diet, avoiding stress, drafts, etc.
10. Discuss feeding techniques—the bottle should *never* be propped; feed with the head slightly elevated to avoid fluid access, during swallowing, to eustachian tube. This helps prevent middle ear infection (otitis media).

C. Follow-up: telephone and return visit if complications develop

D. Consultations/referrals: usually none

bibliography

Boyce, W. Thomas, et al. Influence of life events and family routines on childhood respiratory tract illness. *Pediatrics* **60**:609–615 (1977).

Champoux, Suzanne, Upper respiratory tract infection—a common clinical entity for the nurse practitioner. *The Nurse Practitioner,* **2**:31–32, 35 (1977).

Gellis, Sydney S., and Kagan, Benjamin M. *Current pediatric therapy 8.* Philadelphia: Saunders, 1978, pp. 105–107.

Hoekelman, Robert A., et al. *Principles of pediatrics health care of the young.* New York: McGraw-Hill, 1978, pp. 1723–1725.

Hutchinson, Rosemary. The common cold primer. *Nursing '79,* **9**:57–61 (1979).

29 Bloody Nose

JACALYN PECK DOUGHERTY

ALERT

1. Profuse or persistent nosebleed occurring spontaneously or following trauma
2. Onset before 2 years of age
3. Family history of bleeding disorders
4. Previous history of spontaneous or easy bleeding at other sites
5. Previous history of bleeding disorder or disease
6. Presence of bleeding at other sites
7. Anemia secondary to bleed
8. Posterior bleeding
9. Presence of foreign body
10. Suspicion of nasal fracture
11. Presence of abnormal nasal vasculature
12. Hepatosplenomegaly
13. Hypertension

I. Etiology

A. Episodic minor nosebleeds
1. Traumatic
   a. Picking/rubbing
   b. External blow
   c. Blowing/sneezing
   d. Foreign body
2. Increased friability of nasal mucous membranes secondary to chronic discharge
   a. Allergic rhinitis
   b. Infection (diphtheria, congenital syphilis, chronic sinusitis, scarlet fever, etc.)
3. Salicylate-induced

B. Profuse, prolonged, or recurrent nosebleeds
1. Traumatic
   a. Picking/rubbing
   b. External blow
   c. Blowing/sneezing
   d. Foreign body
2. Polyps/tumors
   a. Nasal polyps/paranasal tumors
   b. Nasopharyngeal angiofibroma
3. Acute/chronic hematologic diseases (acute/chronic leukemia, thrombocytopenia, etc.)
4. Vascular malformations (telangiectasis, hemangiomas, varicosities)
5. Drug-related (salicylates, anticoagulants)
6. Hypertension

II. Assessment

A. Episodic minor nosebleeds
1. Subjective data
   a. Bleeding from nare(s) following trauma (picking, rubbing, external blow, blowing, sneezing, insertion of foreign body)
   b. Bleeding stopping spontaneously or easily with sustained pressure to nose for 10 min
   c. Bleeding is generally anterior (out through nares)
   d. Associated symptoms
      (1) Recent/current respiratory infection, nasal discharge
      (2) History of allergies/allergic rhinitis
      (3) Nausea and vomiting or hematemesis following bleeding
   e. Recent ingestion of aspirin
   f. Exposure to dry climate, nonhumidified air
2. Objective data
   a. If history of external blow, may have ecchymosis, swelling, malalignment, crepitus of nose
   b. Reddened site of active bleed, clot, or crust evident generally in anterior aspect of nasal septum (Kiesselbach's plexus)

c. Bleeding may be anterior (out through nares) or posterior (down pharynx)
d. May have discharge from one or both nares
e. May have inflamed boggy mucosa
f. May have foreign body

B. Profuse, prolonged, recurrent nosebleeds

1. Subjective data
   a. Profuse, prolonged, recurrent bleeding from nare(s) occurring spontaneously or following trauma (picking, rubbing, external blow, blowing, sneezing, insertion of foreign body)
   b. Bleeding does not stop spontaneously or easily with sustained pressure to nose for 10 min
   c. Bleeding may be anterior (out through nares) or posterior (down pharynx)
   d May be family history of bleeding disorders
   e. May be previous history of bleeding disorders or disease (leukemia, thrombocytopenia)
   f. May be history of bleeding at other sites
   g. May be history of hypertension
   h. May be history of aspirin or anticoagulant ingestion
2. Objective data
   a. If history of external blow, may have ecchymosis, swelling, malalignment, crepitus of nose
   b. Reddened site of active bleed, clot, or crust may be evident anteriorly or may be located posteriorly and not readily apparent
   c. Bleeding may be anterior (out through nares) or posterior (down pharynx)
   d. May be nasal discharge secondary to respiratory infection
   e. May be presence of nasal polyps, tumors
   f. May be site of nasal telangiectasis, hemangioma, or varicosities
   g. May be foreign body
   h. May be bleeding at other sites
   i. May be hepatosplenomegaly
   j. May be pallor secondary to anemia

III. Management

A. Episodic minor nosebleed

1. Treatments/medications
   a. Quiet child.
   b. Protect clothing.
   c. Place child in sitting position with head tilted forward.
   d. Instruct child to breathe through mouth.
   e. Apply firm, continuous pressure with thumb and forefinger to both sides of nose immediately superior to nasal alar cartilage for 10 min.
   f. If bleeding persists for longer than 10 min, change site where pressure is being applied.
   g. Again maintain firm, continued pressure for 10 min.
   h. If bleeding still persists, refer immediately to physician/ENT specialist (see Treatments/medications, III, B, 1, below).
   i. If suspicious of underlying allergies or allergic rhinitis, further evaluation is needed. Consider antihistamine to lessen nasal mucosa irritation.
   j. If suspicious of aspirin-related bleeding, discontinue aspirin and/or aspirin containing products.
2. Counselling/prevention
   a. Demonstration of correct method for alleviation of nosebleed
   b. Daily application of Vaseline by cotton-tipped applicator or finger to anterior nares to lessen fragility of nasal vessels
   c. Education/reassurance concerning prevalent causes of nosebleeds (trauma, picking, rubbing) and ease of occurrence
   d. Reassurance concerning amount of blood lost
   e. Humidification of air perhaps beneficial
   f. Keeping child's nails short perhaps helpful
   g. Avoidance of aspirin
   h. If suspicious of allergies as aggravating factor, counselling concerning management
   i. Hematemesis and tarry stools sometimes evident if blood swallowed by child
   j. Counselling concerning epistaxis as a sign and not a disease
   k. May be familial predisposition to epistaxis
3. Follow-up: return to clinic if nosebleeds become profuse, prolonged, or recurrent
4. Consultations/referrals:
   To physician/ENT specialist if
   (1) Nosebleed occurs in child under 2 years of age
   (2) Bleed not stopped with above treatment
   (3) Family history of bleeding disorders
   (4) Previous history of spontaneous or easy bleeding at other sites
   (5) Previous history of bleeding disorder or disease
   (6) Presence of bleeding at other sites
   (7) Decrease in hematocrit or anemia

(8) Posterior bleeding, especially in adolescent males
(9) Foreign body present
(10) Nasal polyps, tumors, telangiectasis, hemangioma, varicosities present
(11) Nasal fracture suspected
(12) Hepatosplenomegaly present
(13) Hypertension present
(14) Child on aspirin or anticoagulant therapy
(15) Significant respiratory infection (diphtheria, congenital syphilis)

B. Profuse, prolonged, recurrent nosebleeds

1. Treatments/medications by physician or ENT specialist
   a. Application of pressure (as described in Treatments/medications, III, A, 1)
   b. Nasal packing
   c. Topical anesthetic (1 percent lidocaine) and topical vasoconstrictor (1/1000 epinephrine or 1 percent cocaine)
   d. Topical thrombin
   e. Cauterization—chemical (silver nitrate) or electrocautery
2. Counselling/prevention
   a. Demonstration of correct method for alleviation of nosebleed
   b. Counselling concerning epistaxis as a sign and not a disease
   c. Cauterization may cause loss of normal nasal cilia to septal tissue, resulting in scar-tissue formation with tendency for recurrent bleeding in future
3. Follow-up: as needed by physician/ENT specialist
4. Consultation/referrals: as determined by physician/ENT specialist for further evaluation and workup

Table 29-1 Medical Referral/Consultation

Diagnosis	Clinical Manifestations	Management
Nasal trauma/nasal fracture	Profuse, prolonged, or recurrent nosebleeds May have ecchymosis, swelling, malalignment, crepitus of nose Bleeding may be anterior or posterior Bleeding may be unilateral or bilateral Septal hematoma may be present Tarry bowel movements	Immediate referral to physician/ENT specialist
Foreign body	Profuse, prolonged, or recurrent nosebleeds Presence of foreign body (most commonly beads, buttons, erasures, stones, nuts) Nasal obstruction Sneezing, discomfort, pain, nasal swelling Odor/discharge from involved side Symptoms usually unilateral Foreign body usually inserted into right nares Nausea and vomiting or hematemesis Tarry bowel movements	Immediate referral to physician/ENT specialist
Nasal polyps/paranasal tumors	Profuse, prolonged, or recurrent nosebleeds Outpouching from nasal mucosa with obstruction of airway Bleeding may be anterior or posterior May be presence of allergic signs and symptoms Nausea and vomiting or hematemesis Tarry bowel movements	Immediate referral to physician/ENT specialist

Table 29-1 Medical Referral/Consultation *(continued)*

Diagnosis	Clinical Manifestations	Management
Nasopharyngeal angiofibroma	Profuse, prolonged, or recurrent nosebleeds Posterior bleeding Occurs in adolescent males Nausea and vomiting or hematemesis Tarry bowel movements	Immediate referral to physician/ENT specialist
Acute/chronic hematologic disorders	Profuse, prolonged, or recurrent nosebleeds Signs and symptoms of systemic bleeding, bleeding at other sites May be hepatosplenomegaly May be systemic/regional lymph involvement Nausea and vomiting or hematemesis Tarry bowel movements	Immediate referral to physician/ENT specialist
Abnormal nasal vasculature	Profuse, prolonged, or recurrent nosebleeds Presence of telangiectasis, hemangioma, or varicosities in nasal mucosa Nausea and vomiting or hematemesis Tarry bowel movements	Immediate referral to physician/ENT specialist
Drug-related (aspirin, anticoagulants)	Profuse, prolonged, or recurrent nosebleeds May be other systemic signs and symptoms of increased bleeding tendency May be nausea, vomiting, hematemesis May be tarry bowel movements	Immediate referral to physician/ENT specialist
Hypertension	Profuse, prolonged, or recurrent nosebleeds Elevated blood pressure May be other systemic signs and symptoms of hypertension May be nausea and vomiting, hematemesis May be tarry bowel movements	Immediate referral to physician/ENT specialist

bibliography

Adams, George L., Boies, Lawrence, and Paparella, Michael. *Boies' fundamentals of otolaryngology* (5th ed.). Philadelphia: Saunders, 1978.

DeAngelis, Catherine. *Pediatric Primary Care* (2d ed.). Boston: Little, Brown, 1979.

Kempe, C. Henry, Silver, Henry K., and O'Brien, Donough. *Current pediatric diagnosis and treatment* (5th ed.). Philadelphia: Saunders, 1978.

Vaughan, Victor C., III, McKay, R. James, and Nelson, Waldo. *Nelson textbook of pediatrics* (10th ed.). Philadelphia: Saunders, 1975.

Table 30-1 Medical Referral/Consultation *(continued)*

Diagnosis	Clinical Manifestations	Management
	Drooling Acute airway distress with stridor Cervical adenitis Client lies with head extended	
Peritonsillar abscess	Sore throat increasingly painful on one side Dysphagia Drooling Tonsil pushed toward midline Referred pain to ear	Hospitalization IV antibiotics Tonsillectomy
Diphtheria	Sore throat Gray or white membrane forms in throat Malaise Anorexia Cervical adenitis Unimmunized or inadequately immunized	Hospitalization Intravenous and intramuscular antitoxin and large doses of penicillin Tracheostomy when airway is comprised

bibliography

Sore throat

DeWeese, D. D., and Saunders, W. H. *Textbook of otolaryngology* (4th ed.). St. Louis: Mosby, 1973. pp. 49–68.

Levy, J. S., and Lovejoy, G. S. Management of pharyngitis by nurse practitioners. *Clinical Pediatrics,* **15**:415–418 (1976).

Lipow, H. W. *Report of the committee on infectious diseases* (18th ed.). Evanston, Ill.: American Academy of Pediatrics, 1977.

———. Respiratory tract infections. In M. Green, and R. J. Haggerty (eds.), *Ambulatory pediatrics II.* Philadelphia: Saunders, 1977.

Infectious mononucleosis

Benenson, A. S. (ed.). *Control of communicable diseases in man* (12th ed.). Washington, D.C.: American Public Health Association, 1975.

Hughes, J. G. *Synopsis of pediatrics* (4th ed.). St. Louis: Mosby, 1975. pp. 778–781.

Krugman, S., Ward, R., and Katz, S. L. *Infectious diseases of children* (6th ed.). St. Louis: Mosby, 1977, pp. 170–180.

———. *Report of the committee on infectious diseases* (18th ed.). Evanston, Ill.: American Academy of Pediatrics, 1977. pp. 147–150.

Nolan, Jo Ellen W. Infectious mononucleosis. *The Nurse Practitioner,* **4**:12–14 (1979).

Scarlet fever

Benenson, A. S. *Control of communicable diseases in man* (12th ed.). Washington, D.C.: American Public Health Association, 1975. pp. 306–312.

Hughes, J. G. *Synopsis of pediatrics* (4th ed.). St. Louis: Mosby, 1975. pp. 723–726.

Krugman, S., Ward, R., and Katz, S. L. *Infectious diseases of children* (6th ed.). St. Louis: Mosby, 1977, pp. 343–351.

———. *Report of the committee on infectious diseases* (18th ed.). Evanston, Ill.: American Academy of Pediatrics, 1977. pp. 268–272.

31 Voice Changes

ELDON H. BAKER, JR.

ALERT
1. Throat clearing—excessive and/or habitual
2. Changes in vocal characteristics—hoarseness, breathiness, intensity, pitch—lasting longer than 2 weeks
3. Laryngeal stridor

I. Etiology: organic causes

A. Vocal abuse and misuse
1. Loud talking, often reaching 90 to 100 dB
2. Screaming, cheering
3. Loud, high-pitched talking to overcome ambient noise (gym, playground, high-volume music)

B. Vocal nodule, also known as singer's node
1. Prolonged vocal abuse/misuse
2. Chronic upper-respiratory problems, which may or may not be related to infection and/or allergies

C. Vocal polyps
1. Result of vocal trauma
2. Possible enlargement caused by continued vocal use
3. Generally related to single or multiple submucous hemorrhages into the vocal cords

D. Growths involving the larynx

E. Vocal cord paralysis
1. Neural lesions
2. Myopathic paralysis
3. Cord paralysis, usually unilateral (right cord)

Note: All voice changes and/or problems should be referred to a physician (otolaryngologist, laryngologist) in order to determine the etiology of the voice problem(s).

F. Functional voice problems
1. Poor speech model(s) to imitate
2. Faulty learning
3. Psychological problems

II. Assessment

A. Vocal nodule(s)
1. Subjective data
   a. Raspy and/or hoarse voice
   b. Throat clearing due to sensation of something's being caught in throat at laryngeal level
   c. Voice that tires easily
2. Objective data
   a. Possible endemic condition of vocal folds revealed by laryngoscopic examination
      (1) Growth that may be pinhead in size
      (2) Possible uni/bilateral nodule(s)
      (3) Nodule(s) that is generally located on free margin of vocal cords (anterior to middle third of cord)
   b. Raspy and/or hoarse voice

B. Polyps
1. Subjective data
   a. Hoarseness
   b. Respiratory difficulty
2. Objective data
   a. Dyspnea and stridor that indicate enlarged and possibly subglottic polyp
   b. Laryngoscopic examination to determine presence and type (pedunculated or sessile) of polyp

C. Chronic laryngitis, hoarseness
1. Subjective data
   a. Hoarseness
   b. Allergies
   c. Chronic pharyngitis/sinusitis

d. Vocal misuse, if possible infection and/or chronic irritation are ruled out
2. Objective data
a. Juvenile papillomatosis
b. Carcinoma
c. Possible thickened and inflamed vocal cord
d. Glandular involvement

D. Vocal abuse and misuse
1. Subjective data
a. Hoarseness
b. Dysphonia
c. Excessive throat clearing and/or coughing
2. Objective data
a. Nodules
b. Polyps
c. Visible neck tension

III. Management

A. Vocal nodule(s)
1. Treatments/medications: none
2. Counselling/prevention
a. Modification of vocal use
b. Motivation of need for correct vocal use
c. Family involvement in monitoring vocal use
3. Follow-up
a. Periodic laryngoscopic inspection by otolaryngologist
b. Motivation through classmates, teacher, home, environment
c. Ongoing speech therapy
4. Consultations/referrals
a. Advise school personnel of specific needs for child.
b. Counsel family as to needs of child and how to facilitate good vocal habits.
c. Consult physician.

B. Polyps
1. Treatments/medications
a. Surgical intervention and/or speech therapy
b. Speech therapy following surgery
2. Counselling/prevention
a. Instruction as to proper use of voice.
b. Stressing how and how not to abuse/misuse voice.
c. Counselling about hard vocal attack and initiation of soft vocal initiation.
3. Follow-up
a. Periodic laryngoscopic inspection by otolaryngologist
b. Speech therapy for child
4. Consultations/referrals
a. Consult with school personnel regarding child's vocal problem and/or needs.
b. Involve family member(s) in child's speech therapy program.

C. Chronic laryngitis/laryngosis
1. Treatments/medications
a. Antibiotics, if laryngitis is associated with infection
b. Reduced vocal use
c. Oral prednisolones, 5 mg twice daily (usually prescribed for professional singers in emergency situations)
2. Counselling/prevention
a. Instructions as to proper voice use
b. Conducting school in-service programs for children and teachers
c. Conferring with parent(s) regarding vocal use and needs of seeking proper medical attention
3. Follow-up
a. Periodic laryngoscopic inspection
b. Speech therapy for child
4. Consultations/referrals
a. Consult with school personnel regarding child's vocal problem(s).
b. Consult and involve parent(s), teachers, and child's peers in helping to change the child's vocal habits.
c. Consult physician.

D. Vocal abuse and misuse
1. Treatments/medications
a. Professional counselling
b. Speech therapy
2. Counselling/prevention
a. Auditory training to teach vocal awareness
b. Relaxed voice production
c. New voice use
3. Follow-up
a. Rechecking at 1-month intervals after termination of voice therapy
b. Checking with parent(s)/guardian to see if carry-over is stabilized at play and at home
4. Consultations/referrals
a. Consult with school personnel regarding needs as outlined by speech therapist.
b. Obtain assistance from school personnel (teachers, custodians, cafeteria workers) in helping the child to monitor and change speech habits.
c. If there is no improvement, refer to laryngologist/physician.
d. Consult and obtain help from parent(s)/guardian in helping the child to modify speech habits.

Table 31-1 Medical Referral/Consultation

Diagnosis	Clinical Manifestations	Management
Papilloma	Respiratory obstruction Hoarseness Aphonia Dyspnea Possible recurring growths	Immediate referral to physician Removal of growths (surgical) Voice therapy as indicated Further management according to Preparation for Hospitalization, Part 7
Malignant neoplasms	Hoarseness (early symptom if locus is on true cords) Extrinsic larynx-lump in the neck Pain during deglutition of hot or citric liquids Ulceration and/or appearance of leukoplakia-like condition (specifically of true cords) revealed during laryngoscopic exam	Immediate referral to physician Surgical management Speech therapy
Psychological disturbances	Hoarseness Aphonia Breathiness Loudness Hypertense voice Hyperactivity	Referral to physician/psychologist/laryngologist Counselling for family/parent(s)/guardian Referral to school psychologist/counselor Speech therapy

bibliography

Brodnitz, Friedrich S. *Vocal rehabilitation* (4th ed.). Rochester: American Academy of Ophthalmology and Otolaryngology, 1971.

Caccamo, James M. Speech and language problems: how you can help. *Issues in Comprehensive Pediatric Nursing*, 3:15–20 (1978).

DeGowin, Elmer L., and DeGowin, Richard L. *Bedside diagnostic examination* (3d ed.). New York: Macmillan, 1976.

Fairbanks, Grant. *Voice and articulation drill book* (2d ed.). New York: Harper & Row, 1960.

Johnson, Wendell et al. *Diagnostic methods in speech pathology*. New York: Harper & Row, 1963.

———. *Speech handicapped school children* (3d ed.). New York: Harper & Row, 1967.

Murphy, Albert T. *Functional voice disorders*. Englewood Cliffs, N.J.: Prentice-Hall, 1964.

Saunders, William H. *The larynx*. Summit, N.J.: Ciba Pharmaceutical Co., 1964.

Wilson, Kenneth D. *Voice problems of children*. Baltimore: Williams & Wilkins, 1972.

32 Airway Obstruction/ Breathing Difficulty

JENNIFER L. PIERSMA

Airway obstruction and breathing difficulty may accompany many disorders affecting respiratory function. The focus of the following chapter is on disorders of the respiratory system. The practitioner must carefully assess the client in relation to his or her past medical history, family/home environment, severity of illness, and degree of pulmonary dysfunction.

ALERT

1. Signs/symptoms of moderate to severe respiratory distress
2. Stridor at rest
3. Excessive drooling
4. Chronic bronchitis
5. History of aspiration
6. Unimmunized child, especially against diphtheria and pertussis

I. Etiology

A. Airway obstruction
1. Inspiratory obstruction (upper airway)
2. Expiratory obstruction (lower airway)

B. Parenchyma
1. Reduction in parenchyma
2. Disorders affecting the interstitium

C. Chest wall and mediastinum
1. Respiratory musculature
2. Neuromuscular disease
3. Structural abnormalities
4. Pleural disease

D. Anxiety: hyperventilation

II. Assessment

A. Laryngotracheobronchitis
1. Subjective data
   a. Age (most common): 6 months to 3 years
   b. Onset: gradual; client usually worse at night
   c. Recent illness: prior upper-respiratory infection
   d. Aggravating factors: low humidity
   e. Associated symptoms
      (1) Barking cough
      (2) Hoarseness
      (3) Wheezing
      (4) Stridor
      (5) Mild fever
   f. Medical history: possible prior incidence of viral croup
2. Objective data
   a. Healthy appearance
   b. Barking cough
   c. Hoarseness
   d. Stridor
   e. Wheezing, inspiratory and/or expiratory if lower respiratory tract involved
   f. Retractions, sternal, subcostal, and/or abdominal
   g. Mild fever
   h. White blood cell count usually elevated (less than 15,000)

B. Acute bronchitis
1. Subjective data
   a. Recent illness: associated with upper- or lower-respiratory infection, measles, whooping cough
   b. Aggravating factors: infection, allergies
   c. Associated signs/symptoms
      (1) Low-grade fever

(2) Initially dry, hacking, nonproductive cough
(3) Gagging on secretions (younger client)
(4) Chest pain

2. Objective data
   a. Cough, productive or nonproductive
   b. Coarse rales and rhonchi
   c. Possible increased respiratory rate
   d. Leukocytosis (with bacteria)
   e. Normal chest x-ray (with possible increased bronchial markings)

C. Asthma, mild or moderate attack *(known asthmatic)*

1. Subjective data
   a. Onset: episodic, acute, or gradual
   b. Allergies: any exposures
   c. Aggravating factors: anxiety-producing event, upper-respiratory infection, allergic reaction, physical activity, chronic infection, weather change(s), environmental irritants (e.g., pollution, tobacco smoke)
   d. Associated signs/symptoms
      (1) Mild respiratory distress
      (2) Coughing
      (3) Wheezing
      (4) Tightness in chest
   e. Medical history: recurrent (chronic) bronchitis, bronchiolitis (infant)
   f. Family history: asthma, lung problems, allergies
   g. Past treatments: bronchodilators, mist, or other
2. Objective data
   a. General: anxiousness, diaphoresis, sitting position
   b. Sneezing, nasal congestion
   c. Coarse rales
   d. Hyperresonant chest on percussion
   e. Wheezing most prominent on expiration
   f. Suppressed breath sounds, prolonged expiratory phase
   g. Mild to moderate respiratory distress
   h. Tachycardia
   i. Eosinophilic accumulation in nose or in sputum
   j. Peripheral-blood eosinphilia
   k. Hyperinflation, indicated by chest x-ray

D. Bronchiolitis

1. Subjective data
   a. Age: under 2 years
   b. Recent illness: minor upper-respiratory infection prior to onset
   c. Associated symptoms
      (1) Nasal drainage
      (2) Irritating cough
      (3) Decreased appetite (difficulty feeding)
      (4) Low-grade fever
      (5) Increased respiratory distress
      (6) Difficulty sleeping
2. Objective data
   a. Anxious appearance
   b. Cyanosis
   c. Nasal flaring
   d. Respiratory rate: 60 to 80 breaths per min
   e. Expiratory wheezing, increased expiratory phase
   f. Inspiratory rales
   g. Possible palpable liver and/or spleen
   h. Retractions, intercostal, subcostal
   i. Usually normal white blood cell count
   j. Chest x-ray: possible hyperinflation, flattened diaphragm, areas of collapse

E. Mild viral pneumonia

1. Subjective data
   a. Onset: gradual
   b. Recent illness: prior upper-respiratory infection
   c. Associated symptoms
      (1) Dry, hacking, usually nonproductive cough
      (2) Mild increase in respiratory rate
      (3) Abdominal distention
      (4) Marked variation in clinical manifestations
2. Objective data
   a. General: mildly ill client
   b. Inspiratory crepitant rales, scattered or localized
   c. Coarse expiratory rhonchi (few)
   d. Adequate air exchange to periphery
   e. Elevated or normal white blood cell count
   f. Chest x-ray: increased perihilar/peribronchial markings; possible patchy areas of infiltration (in some cases, absent findings)

F. Bacterial pneumonia

1. Subjective data
   a. Onset: sudden
   b. Recent illness: mild upper-respiratory infection
   c. Associated symptoms
      (1) Cough
      (2) Increased respiratory rate
      (3) Abdominal distention
      (4) High fever
      (5) Older client may complain of chest pain with cough or splint affected side on deep inspiration
2. Objective data

a. General: fretful, splinting of affected side
b. Stiffness of neck
c. Chest dullness
d. Tachypnea
e. Depressed breath sounds
f. Inspiratory rales
g. Abdominal distention, tenderness
h. White blood cell count elevated (18,000 to 40,000)
i. Sputum/blood cultures to identify etiological agent
j. Chest x-ray: lobar or segmental consolidation, patchy infiltration

G. Bronchiectasis

1. Subjective data
   a. Age: usually under 5 years
   b. Onset: after recurrent infection
   c. Recent illness: pneumonia, measles, foreign body reaction, tuberculosis
   d. Associated symptoms
      (1) Cough (worse in morning)
      (2) Increased amount of sputum (white-gray)
      (3) Low-grade, intermittent fever
2. Objective data
   a. Healthy appearance
   b. Productive cough
   c. Possible clubbing of fingers
   d. Dullness on percussion; possibility of decreased air entry
   e. Positive sputum culture
   f. Chest x-ray: variable—increased pulmonary markings, chronic pneumonia, displacement of heart and mediastinum

H. Hyperventilation

1. Subjective data
   a. Age: usually over 6 years
   b. Onset: acute, possibly following anxiety-producing event
   c. Associated symptoms
      (1) Numbness in the hands
      (2) Perioral paresthesia
      (3) Faintness, light-headedness
   d. Medical history: prior "attacks"
2. Objective data
   a. Anxious client
   b. Marked tachypnea, signing respirations
   c. Other findings normal
   d. Normal physical examination between attacks

III. Management

A. Laryngotracheobronchitis

1. Treatments/medications
   a. Use cool-mist vaporizer or steam up the bathroom by running hot water in the shower/bath.
   b. Encourage intake of fluids.
   c. Keep client calm and quiet.
   d. Control temperature if fever is present.
2. Counselling/prevention
   a. Watch for signs/symptoms of increased respiratory distress.
   b. Use temperature-control measures: sponging, giving antipyretics (dose for age and frequency of administration), taking a temperature.
   c. DO NOT use medications containing a sedative, since they may depress respiratory center and mask anxiety and restlessness.
   d. Avoid use of steam vaporizers; if used, emphasize risk of scalding child.
3. Follow-up: call in 20 min to assess child's response to above measure(s).
4. Consultations/referrals: notify physician if child develops stridor at rest or develops other signs/symptoms of increased respiratory distress.

B. Acute bronchitis

1. Treatments/medications
   a. Supply mist or high humidity.
   b. Use postural drainage (see Figs. 144–1 to 144–10).
   c. Administer cough expectorant for 5 days.
2. Counselling/prevention
   a. Discuss signs/symptoms of increased respiratory distress.
   b. Instruct parent(s) with demonstration on postural drainage.
   c. DO NOT use cough suppressants, since coughing clears secretions.
   d. DO NOT use medications with antihistamines, since they tend to dry secretions.
   e. Avoid use of steam vaporizers due to risk of scalding child.
3. Follow-up
   a. Recommend return visit if signs/symptoms worsen or fail to improve in 48 h, or if cough does not disappear in 7 to 10 days.
   b. Recommend return visit in 7 to 10 days for very young infant.
4. Consultations/referrals: consult physician if condition worsens, fails to improve in 48 h, or becomes chronic.

C. Asthma, mild or moderate attack *(known asthmatic)*

1. Treatments/medications

a. Promptly administer oral bronchodilator or inhalant.
b. If this is unsuccessful, consult physician, give epinephrine (adrenaline 1:1000), 0.01 to 0.3 mL/kg subcutaneously every 20 min up to 3 doses.
c. Encourage intake of fluids.
d. Keep client calm and quiet.

2. Counselling/prevention
   a. Attempt environmental control of allergies.
   b. Stress importance of prompt administration of bronchodilators at onset of respiratory difficulty.
   c. Investigate presence of excessive parental anxiety/overprotection.
   d. Assist the client to openly discuss illness and possible solutions to problems encountered.
3. Follow-up
   a. Client may return home if chest is clear to auscultation.
   b. Return visit in 24 h is necessary if chest is not completely clear to auscultation.
4. Consultations/referrals: refer to physician if client fails to respond to treatment or persists in wheezing.

D. Bronchiolitis, acute

1. Treatments/medications
   a. Use postural drainage.
   b. Encourage intake of fluids.
   c. Maintain body warmth.
   d. Administer antibiotics if secondary infection occurs. (If antibiotics are indicated, consult physician.)
   e. If client is febrile, treat appropriately for age.
2. Counselling/prevention
   a. Instruct parent(s) with demonstration on postural drainage.
   b. Discuss signs/symptoms of increased respiratory distress.
   c. Discuss temperature-control measures: sponging, giving antipyretics(dose for age and frequency of administration), taking a temperature.
   d. Discuss other supportive measures: encouraging fluids, positioning of small infant (on abdomen or in semi-Fowler's position), maintaining body warmth.
   e. DO NOT use medications with a sedative action.
3. Follow-up
   a. Return visit is necessary if client continues to be symptomatic after 7 to 10 days.
   b. Return visit in 2 days if client has elevated temperature (101°F) unresponsive to supportive treatment.
4. Consultations/referrals: refer to physician if respiratory distress continues or for child under 4 months of age.

E. Mild viral pneumonia

1. Treatments/medications
   a. Keep humidity high.
   b. Use postural drainage, if necessary.
   c. Encourage adequate fluid intake.
   d. Encourage bed rest; client can be on feet as tolerated.
   e. If client is febrile, treat appropriately for age.
2. Counselling/prevention (see Acute bronchitis, III, B)
3. Follow-up
   a. Call daily until client is afebrile and has no symptoms of respiratory distress.
   b. Recommend return visit for repeat chest x-ray in 72 h (until clear); consult physician for necessity/timing of follow-up films.
   c. If condition worsens, client should return immediately.
   d. Return visit in 3 weeks.
4. Consultations/referrals: consult physician for all pneumonias or if condition fails to improve in 48 h or to resolve in 3 weeks.

F. Bacterial pneumonia

1. Treatments/medications
   a. Follow treatment in Mild viral pneumonia, III, E, above.
   b. Give antibiotic as indicated for etiologic agent (consult physician).
2. Counselling/prevention
   a. Follow procedure for Acute bronchitis, III, B.
   b. Educate parent(s) regarding medication.
      (1) Importance of giving prescribed amounts at the times indicated
      (2) Method of giving medications based on developmental age of the client
3. Follow-up (see Mild viral pneumonia, III, E)
4. Consultations/referrals: consult physician.

G. Bronchiectasis

1. Treatments/medications
   a. Postural drainage (aerosol or systemic bronchodilator, if indicated)
   b. Mist
   c. Antibiotic therapy, 10 to 14 days or as indicated for etiologic agent in sputum culture (consult physician)
2. Counselling/prevention

See Bacterial pneumonia, III, F

3. Follow-up:
   Return visit is necessary in 10 to 14 days for recheck and repeat chest x-ray.
4. Consultations/referrals: consult physician.

H. Hyperventilation

1. Treatments/medications
   Rebreathe into paper bag.
2. Counselling/prevention
   a. Investigate etiology of hyperventilation episodes with parent and client.
   b. Discuss ways to handle anxiety.
   c. Discuss physiologic mechanism of hyperventilation and purpose of rebreathing.
3. Follow-up: none is indicated.
4. Consultations/referrals: if hyperventilation persists as coping mechanism, consider psychological consultation.

Table 32-1 Medical Referral/Consultation

Diagnosis	Clinical Manifestations	Management
Foreign Body Aspiration	Sudden onset of gagging, coughing, choking Mild to severe respiratory distress; tachypnea, stridor, cyanosis Hoarseness Other: dependent on level of lodgment	Immediate referral to physician Immediate endoscopy if severe distress Treatment according to Preparation for Hospitalization, Part 7 Safety education of family, client, as indicated
Epiglottitis	3–7 years of age Sudden onset of high fever Excessive drooling Difficulty in swallowing Severe sore throat Muffled phonation Respiratory distress	Immediate referral to physician Visualization of epiglottis, tracheostomy tube present (only by physician) Intubation or tracheostomy Treatment according to Preparation for Hospitalization, Part 7 Explanation of diagnosis, treatment plan, and prognosis to family, client
Pneumothorax	Unilateral hyperresonance Decreased chest movement Decreased breath sounds Muffled heart sounds Sudden, sharp pain (older client) Shifting of trachea, heart, mediastinum to unaffected side	Immediate referral to physician Treatment depending on degree of pneumothorax Treatment according to Preparation for Hospitalization, Part 7
Chronic diseases Respiratory or cardiac	Failure to thrive Cyanosis Marked intolerance to exercise Feeding difficulties (newborn) Attacks of shortness of breath Recurrent respiratory infections Tachypnea Tachycardia Murmurs Clubbing	Referral to physician
Other	Chronic bronchitis Weight loss	Referral to physician

Table 32-1 Medical Referral/Consultation *(continued)*

Diagnosis	Clinical Manifestations	Management
	Recurrent pulmonary Infections Recurrent tonsillitis Persistent fever Recurrent foul sputum Possibly normal chest exam	

bibliography

DeAngelis, Catherine. *Pediatric primary care* (2d ed.). Boston: Little, Brown, 1979.

Green, Morris, and Haggerty, Robert J. (eds.). *Ambulatory pediatrics II.* Philadelphia: Saunders, 1977.

Illingsworth, R. S. *Common symptoms of diseases in children* (5th ed.). London: Blackwell, 1975.

Kempe, C. Henry, Silver, Henry K., and O'Brien, Donough. *Current pediatric diagnosis and treatment* (4th ed.). Los Altos, Calif.: Lange, 1976.

Kravath, Richard E., Pollak, Charles P., and Borowiecki, Bernard. Hypoventilation during sleep in children who have lymphoid airway obstruction treated by nasopharyngeal tube and t and a. *Pediatrics* 59(6):865–871 (1977).

Nelson, Waldo, E. et al. (eds.). *Textbook of pediatrics* (10th ed.). Philadelphia: Saunders, 1975.

Rudolph, Abraham M. (ed.). *Pediatrics* (16th ed.). New York: Appleton-Century-Crofts, 1977.

Thorn, George W. et al. (eds.). *Harrison's principles of internal medicine* (8th ed.). New York: McGraw-Hill, 1977.

Wasson, John, Walsh, B. Timothy, Thompkins, Richard, and Sox, Harold. *The common symptom guide.* New York: McGraw-Hill, 1975.

33 Wheezing

DIAN NORTON CHIAMULERA

ALERT

1. Respiratory distress
2. Children under 5 mo of age
3. Suspicion of foreign-body aspiration
4. First time wheezing
5. Failure of acute attack to respond to treatment
6. Persistent wheezing despite therapy
7. No response to epinephrine
8. Frequent, repeated attacks
9. Fever 101°F and over
10. Tachycardia
11. Signs of respiratory failure

I. Etiology

A. Narrowing of bronchioles
B. Partial obstruction of large bronchi
C. Alveolar fluid accumulation

II. Assessment

A. Acute tracheobronchitis

1. Subjective data
   a. Dry cough, which increases at night time
   b. Restlessness and irritability
   c. Mild tachypnea
   d. History of URI of several days duration
   e. Dyspnea
   f. Systemic symptoms, e.g., headache, lethargy
2. Objective data
   a. Fever—extends from low-grade to a high of 103°F
   b. Wheezes—inspiratory and/or expiratory; improves with coughing

B. Acute laryngotracheobronchitis

1. Subjective data
   a. URI symptoms, which usually precedes onset
   b. Laryngospasm at night
   c. Dyspnea and restlessness
   d. Barking cough
   e. Marked hoarseness
2. Objective data
   a. Inspiratory stridor
   b. Minimal fever
   c. Dyspnea
   d. Inspiratory or expiratory wheezes
   e. Lower rib retraction

C. Bronchiolitis

1. Subjective data
   a. Age: under 2 yr; peak age 6 mo
   b. History of URI
   c. Abrupt onset of dyspnea
   d. Difficulty sleeping and eating
   e. Restlessness
   f. Hacking cough
2. Objective data
   a. Tachypnea
   b. Tachycardia
   c. Respiratory distress, flaring nostrils, rib retractions
   d. Fever—usually low-grade
   e. Wheezing, grunting, sometimes rales
   f. Decreased-breath sounds

g. Prolonged expiration
h. Percussion—hyperresonant

D. Acute bronchial asthma

1. Subjective data
   a. Cough
   b. Tightness in chest, dyspnea
   c. Anxiety, restlessness, apprehension
   d. Vomiting after severe coughing
   e. Wheezing
   f. History of allergies
   g. Family history of allergies
2. Objective data
   a. Wheezing—expiratory and/or inspiratory
   b. Prolonged expiration
   c. Occasionally rales
   d. Tachypnea
   e. Nasal flaring, intercostal retractions, use of accessory muscles for breathing
   f. Decreased-breath sounds
   g. Tachycardia

III. Management

A. Acute tracheobronchitis

1. Treatments/medications
   a. Cool-mist vaporizer for moisture
   b. Increase fluid intake
   c. Acetaminophen for fever
2. Counselling/prevention
   a. Increase humidity.
      (1) Cool-mist vaporizer reduces chances of steam burning ill child or other young children in family.
      (2) If vaporizer is not available, provide steam by turning on hot water taps in closed bathroom.
   b. Instruct parent(s) to watch for
      (1) Increased restlessness
      (2) Fever
      (3) Dyspnea
      (4) Retractions
   c. Increase fluid intake.
      (1) Give child clear fluids.
      (2) Offer fluids frequently in small quantities.
   d. Instruct parents on how to administer acetaminophen depending on age of child and how supplied.
3. Follow-up
   a. Return visit immediately if there are signs of respiratory distress
   b. Return visit if no improvement in 7 days
4. Consultations/referrals—refer to physician all clients with
   a. Chronic cardiorespiratory disease
   b. Respiratory distress
   c. Failure to respond to treatment within 48 h

B. Acute laryngotracheobronchitis

1. Treatments/medications
   a. Increase humidity. Advise treatment with cool-mist vaporizer or steam-filled bathroom.
   b. Increase fluid intake.
2. Counselling/prevention
   Instruct on use of vaporizer or increasing humidity with steam.
3. Follow-up
   Return visit if symptoms increase or client does not respond to treatment
4. Consultations/referrals: refer to physician all clients with
   a. Signs of epiglottitis
   b. Respiratory distress

C. Bronchiolitis

1. Treatments/medications
   a. Use cool-mist vaporizer.
   b. Increase fluid intake to ensure adequate hydration.
2. Counselling/prevention
   See Acute tracheobronchitis, III, A, 2 (above).
3. Follow-up
   Return visit in 24 h if no improvement
4. Consultations/referrals: refer client to physician when
   a. Client is under 3 mo of age.
   b. There is respiratory distress.
   c. There have been repeated episodes.

D. Acute bronchial asthma

1. Treatments/medications
   a. Acute therapy
      (1) Treat with epinephrine 1:1000: subcutaneous injection, 0.01 mL/kg, with maximum dose of 0.3 mL/kg.
      (2) If chest is not clear, repeat dose every 20 min for a maximum of 3 doses.
      (3) Monitor apical heart rate.
      (4) Increase oral fluid intake.
      (5) Begin postural drainage (see Cystic Fibrosis, Chap. 144, Figs. 1 to 10).
      (6) When chest is clear, give one dose Sus-

Phrine (oil base epinephrine; 0.005 mL/kg subcutaneously for prolonged bronchodilatation, 8–10 hours).

b. Maintenance therapy
  (1) Give theophylline elixir, 4–6 mg/kg every 6 h. This is recommended for children less than 40 kg. Continue for 2 wk *after* symptoms have disappeared.
  (2) Give aminophylline tablets, 200 mg every 6 h. This is recommended for children over 40 kg. Continue for 2 wk *after* symptoms have disappeared.
  (3) The medications recommended in (1) and (2) may avert a severe attack if taken when the client begins to experience respiratory difficulty.
  (4) Increase fluid intake.

2. Counselling/prevention
  a. Give instruction regarding medication, percussion, and postural drainage.
  b. Discuss possible precipitating factors and ways of avoiding these factors.
  c. Advise environmental control of allergies.
  d. Be supportive to child and parent(s). Openly discuss the illness and associated problems.

3. Follow-up
  a. Return visit in 2 wk for evaluation
  b. Return visit sooner if no improvement

4. Consultations/referrals
  a. Refer client to physician if
    (1) Acute attack does not respond to treatment.
    (2) Wheezing persists despite maintenance therapy.
  b. Refer client to allergy clinic for workup.
  c. Refer client for professional counselling as needed.

Table 33-1 Medical Referral/Consultation

Diagnosis	Clinical Manifestations	Management
Status asthmaticus	Failure of child to respond to treatment for acute asthma Decreased or absent breath sounds Severe retractions and use of accessory muscles Cyanosis Decreased level of consciousness	*Immediate* referral to physician Hospitalization—see Preparation for Hospitalization, Part 7 Emotional support to parents and child
Foreign body—incomplete obstruction	Sudden gasp, gag, or cough Tachypnea, stridor, localized wheezing, decreased-breath sounds	*Immediate* referral to physician Removal of foreign body Hospitalization—see Preparation for Hospitalization, Part 7
Cystic fibrosis	Varies depending on age the diagnosis is made Pulmonary Infant—tachypnea, retractions, tympanitic abdomen, nasal flaring, wheezes and rales, decreased-breath sounds Later childhood—isolated pulmonary disease, diffuse wheezes, and rales Meconium ileus Pancreatic insufficiency Cirrhosis of the liver Progressive chronic lung disease Obstructive overinflation Irreversible bronchial damage Pulmonary insufficiency	Consultation with physician Chest x-ray Pulmonary function tests Sweat test See Cystic Fibrosis, Chap. 144.

Table 33-1 Medical Referral/Consultation *(continued)*

Diagnosis	Clinical Manifestations	Management
Pulmonary edema	Tachypnea, dyspnea, and orthopnea Chronic hacking cough Productive cough with pink, frothy sputum Diffuse wheezes, rales Tachycardia Marked perspiration; skin cool and clammy; sometimes cyanotic	*Immediate* referral to physician Hospitalization—see Preparation for Hospitalization, Part 7

bibliography

Buckley, Rebecca. Advances in asthma/allergy. *Pediatric Nursing,* **5**(2):40B–42D (1979).

Eichenwald, H. F. Respiratory infections in children. *Hospital Practice,* 11:81–90 (1976).

Fisher, L. New frontiers in the treatment of asthma in children, *American Lung Association Bulletin,* **62**:2–5 (1976).

Gellis, S. S., and Kagan, B. M. *Current Pediatric Therapy.* Philadelphia: Saunders, 1976.

Glezen, W. P. Pathogenesis of bronchiolitis-epidemiologic considerations. *Pediatric Research,* **11**:239–43 (1977).

Illingsworth, R. S. *Common Symptoms of Disease in Children* (5th ed.). London: Blackwell Scientific Publications, 1975, pp. 157–159.

McGeady, Stephen J., and Sherman, Brock V. Management of the child with recurrent asthma. *Pediatric Annals,* **6**(8):11–23 (1977).

The Philadelphia Regional Pediatric Pulmonary Disease Program. Emergency room treatment of acute asthma. *Pediatric Annals,* **6**(8):7–10 (1977).

Waechter, E., Blake, F. *Nursing Care of Children.* Philadelphia: Lippincott, 1976, pp. 548–552.

34 Cough LESLIE LIETH

ALERT
1. Dyspnea
2. Retractions
3. Cyanosis
4. Past history of asthma
5. Tachypnea
6. Productive cough
7. Wheezing
8. Rales
9. Croupy cough
10. Hemoptysis
11. Limited chest expansion
12. Chronic cough
13. Paroxysmal cough with whoop

I. Etiology

A. Viral
B. Bacterial
C. Inhalants
D. Food allergies

II. Assessment

A. Common cold (acute nasopharyngitis)
1. Subjective data
   a. Runny nose
   b. Sneezing
   c. Periodic dry cough
   d. Normal temperature, or minimally elevated
   e. Anorexia
   f. Headache
2. Objective data
   a. Febrile or afebrile
   b. Inflamed, swollen mucous membranes of nose
   c. Nasal discharge
   d. Lungs clear, or referred sounds auscultated
   e. No signs of respiratory distress
   f. May have mild cervical lymphadenopathy

B. Laryngitis
1. Subjective data
   a. Nasal congestion
   b. Sore throat
   c. Croupy cough
   d. Hoarseness
   e. Afebrile
2. Objective data
   a. Croupy cough
   b. Pharyngeal inflammation
   c. No signs of respiratory distress
   d. Hoarse voice
   e. Afebrile

C. Viral pharyngitis
1. Subjective data
   a. Gradual onset
   b. Mild malaise
   c. Sore throat
   d. Dry cough
   e. Low-grade fever
   f. Hoarseness
   g. Nasal congestion
2. Objective data
   a. Low-grade fever
   b. Dry cough
   c. Nasal congestion
   d. Conjunctivitis
   e. Mild tonsillar erythema
   f. None or small amount of exudate
   g. Mild anterior cervical lymphadenopathy

D. Acute bacterial sinusitis
1. Subjective data
   a. Usually occurs after acute phase of nasopharyngitis

b. Thick nasal discharge
c. Periodic bouts of coughing—worse at night
d. Sinus pain, headache
e. Febrile

2. Objective data
a. Mucopurulent nasal discharge
b. Fever
c. Local tenderness
d. Dry cough

III. Management

A. Common cold (acute nasopharyngitis)

1. Treatments/medications
a. Antipyretics for fever
b. Vaporizer
c. Nose drops (normal saline, or for older children ephedrine or epinephrine in isotonic salt solutions) 2 drops in each nostril 4 or 5 times per day for 3–4 days
d. Use of nasal aspirator 15 min after instillation of nose drops

2. Counselling/prevention
a. Encourage increased intake of fluids.
b. Discuss accident prevention when using vaporizer.
c. For instillation of nose drops, have client lie on back with head hyperextended.
d. Instill nose drops 15 min before feeding.
e. Use bottle of nose drops for only one person and only one illness.
f. Parent(s)/client should expect illness to last about 1 wk and appetite to decrease.

3. Follow-up
a. Telephone call in 1–3 days to discuss progress
b. No return visit necessary unless condition worsens or not resolved in 2 wk

4. Consultations/referrals: none

B. Laryngitis

1. Treatments/medications
a. Chloraseptic mouthwash—gargling when necessary
b. Vaporizer
c. Antipyretics (aspirin or acetaminophen) for fever and/or discomfort
d. Increased fluid intake

2. Counselling/prevention
a. Speak softly, do not scream.
b. Parent(s)/client should expect illness to last about 1 wk.

3. Follow-up
a. Return immediately or phone call if any respiratory distress, trouble breathing
b. Return visit not necessary unless not resolved in 2 wk

4. Consultations/referrals: consult with physician if signs of airway obstruction

C. Viral pharyngitis

1. Treatments/medications
a. Throat culture to rule out group A beta-hemolytic streptococcal infection
b. Chloraseptic mouthwash—gargling when necessary
c. Vaporizer when necessary
d. Antipyretics (aspirin or acetaminophen) for fever and/or discomfort
e. Increased fluid intake

2. Counselling/prevention
a. Advise that illness will last about 1 wk.
b. Explain importance of calling for results of throat culture.

3. Follow-up
a. Parent(s)/client to call in 24–48 h for results of throat culture
b. Return visit if symptoms worsen or not resolved after 2 wk

4. Consultations/referrals: none

D. Acute bacterial sinusitis

1. Treatments/medications
a. Culture—posterior nasal cavity with wire applicator
b. Antibiotic therapy—drug of choice ampicillin—given for 10–14 days
c. Phenylephrine hydrochloride, 0.25%, nose drops every 4 h for 3–4 days
d. Analgesics as needed
e. Vaporizer as needed

2. Counselling/prevention
a. Nose drops should be instilled 15 min before feeding, with head hyperextended.
b. Nose drop bottle should be used for one person for one illness.
c. Stress importance of continuing antibiotic therapy for prescribed time period.
d. Give side effects of medications prescribed.

3. Follow-up
a. Return visit 10–14 days
b. Phone call if culture and sensitivity doesn't correlate with prescribed antibiotic

4. Consultations/referrals
a. Consult physician for treatment.
b. Refer to physician if not resolved after antibiotic course.

Table 34-1 Medical Referral/Consultation

Diagnosis	Clinical Manifestations	Management
Aspiration—foreign body	Sudden onset of cough in a client previously well; choking, gagging, wheezing Dysphagia Hoarseness Hemoptysis Dyspnea Cyanosis Limited chest expansion Decreased vocal fremitus Impaired or hyperresonant percussion note Diminished-breath sounds distal to foreign body X-ray positive for presence of foreign body	Refer client immediately to physician and/or emergency room for hospital admission. Counselling/prevention See Preparation for Hospitalization, Part 7. Remove small objects from young child's environment. Do not give large pieces of food to young child. Check toys for loose parts (e.g., stuffed animals with plastic "pull-off" eyes).
Croup	Usually complaint of URI for several days before cough and respiratory distress develop Occurs most frequently at night Barking cough Retractions Respiratory distress Inspiratory stridor Bilaterally diminished-breath sounds Rhonchi and scattered rales Anxious and frightened child Pharyngeal inflammation	Refer client to physician and/or emergency room for hospital admission. Treatment—do not use tongue blade to examine throat if croupy, barking cough is present. Counselling/prevention See Preparation for Hospitalization, Part 7. If treated at home, explain Use of vaporizer Need to force fluids Importance of not upsetting child That condition may worsen at night Observing for signs of increased respiratory distress
Epiglottitis	Sudden onset Within hours of onset, respiratory distress is present High fever Dyspnea Severe sore throat Drooling Fever Inspiratory stridor Pallor or cyanosis Nasal flaring Retractions Hyperextension of neck Inflamed pharynx; large, edematous, cherry-red epiglottis White blood cells usually markedly	Refer client immediately to physician and/or emergency room for prompt care and admission. With signs of epiglottitis present, perform no examination of pharynx with tongue depressor unless tracheostomy equipment is present. Call ahead to hospital in case of need for emergency tracheotomy. Counselling Support family with seriously ill child. See Preparation for Hospitalization, Part 7.

Table 34-1 Medical Referral/Consultation *(continued)*

Diagnosis	Clinical Manifestations	Management
	elevated with striking polymorphonuclear leukocytosis Child in sitting position, leaning forward with mouth open and tongue protruding X-ray of neck showing swollen epiglottis, ballooning hypopharynx	
Asthma	Can have past history of asthma Family history of asthma Cough Dyspnea History of allergies Usually preceded by mild URI Wheezing Prolonged expiratory phase	Treatments/medications Promptly administer bronchodilators by inhalation of aerosols or by oral, subcutaneous, or intravenous routes. Following attack, client is maintained on oral bronchodilator for 3 or more days. Encourage intake of large amount of fluids. Refer client to physician for treatment of acute attack; hospitalization may be needed. See Allergies, Chap. 137, and Wheezing, Chap. 33.
Cystic fibrosis	Chronic cough or recurrent symptoms in the upper or lower respiratory tract History of meconium ileus or meconium plug syndrome in nursery Ravenous appetite with poor weight gain Frequent, large, foul-smelling, poorly formed bowel movements Can have family history of disease Positive sweat test	Refer client to physician for diagnostic workup and treatment. See Cystic Fibrosis, Chap. 144.
Tuberculosis	Young child Slight cough, fever, fatigability, or High fever, frequent cough, respiratory distress Adolescent to adult Low-grade fever, chronic cough, anorexia, or Chronic cough, large amount of sputum, high fever, weight loss History of contact with disease If acute, moist rales, dullness to percussion, respiratory distress, fever Positive skin testing for tuberculosis Positive chest x-ray Positive sputum specimen for acid-fast bacilli	Refer client to physician. Advise appropriate chemotherapy for prolonged period of 12–24 mo. If client is acutely ill, hospitalization is necessary. Prevent disease by early detection with routine skin testing yearly or biyearly. Prophylactic administration of medications is usually given to all household members of person with active disease. Skin testing and chest x-rays of all who have close contact with person with active disease is recommended; and repeat skin testing every 6 mo. Report active disease to dept. of communicable diseases. Refer client to public health nurse for tracing close contacts and supervising family treatment.

Table 34-1 Medical Referral/Consultation *(continued)*

Diagnosis	Clinical Manifestations	Management
Pertussis	Initially dry cough and nasal discharge for 1–2 wk Severe cough occurring in bursts or paroxysms Cough more severe at night Expiratory cough may persist for 15–30 s Typical "whoop" heard between paroxysms Decreased appetite Difficulty breathing Vomiting Mucous plug expelled after paroxysm Face very red during paroxysm with veins of scalp prominent Watery, puffy eyes with subconjunctival hemorrhages White blood cell count markedly elevated, usually between 15,000 to 30,000 with 80–90% lymphocytes.	Refer client to physician. Report case to dept. of communicable diseases. Most cases need hospitalization. Adequate immunization can prevent disease. See Preparation for Hospitalization, Part 7. For those treated at home Maintain nutrition. Advise that client may be more comfortable outdoors (isolated in back yard). Refeed client after vomiting.
Viral pneumonia	Nasal congestion Dry, hacking, usually nonproductive cough Gradual onset Mild tachypnea Fever 100–104°F In severe cases, may complain of dyspnea Inspiratory crepitant rales Coarse expiratory rhonchi Restlessness White blood cell count normal or mildly elevated Chest x-ray diagnostic of infiltrate	Refer client to physician. Take chest x-ray. Get complete blood count. Admit client to hospital if a young child or if toxic symptoms occur. Advise use of vaporizer. Administer antipyretics for fever when necessary. If necessary, teach parent(s) how to administer postural drainage. Encourage fluid intake and advise that appetite may be decreased. Assure parent(s) if child is not initially hospitalized that course of condition will be followed closely. Parent/client should call or return if there is any respiratory distress. If not hospitalized, client should return every 1–3 days until improvement is noted.
Mycoplasma pneumonia	Usually gradual onset Primarily children 5–15 y of age Malaise Headache Anorexia Fever Sore Throat Nonproductive, paroxysmal cough	Consult and/or refer client to physician. Give client tuberculin skin test. Advise use of vaporizer. If necessary, teach parent(s) how to administer postural drainage. Administer antipyretics for fever. Have client take erythromycin orally for 10 days.

Table 34-1 Medical Referral/Consultation *(continued)*

Diagnosis	Clinical Manifestations	Management
	Scattered, fine crepitant rales Rarely severely ill looking Positive test for cold agglutins Chest x-ray reveals infiltrate	Ask client to return every 1–3 days until improvement noted.
Bacterial pneumonia	Can have prodrome of mild URI for several days or a week Fever Poor feeding, anorexia Irritating cough Headache Drowsiness Abdominal pain Tachypnea Mild to severe respiratory difficulty Rales (infants may not have) Retractions Grunting Mild cyanosis Elevated white blood cell count Chest x-ray diagnostic	Refer client to physician. Refer client for hospitalization when necessary (see Preparation for Hospitalization, Part 7). Treat client with antibiotics. Counselling/prevention See "Viral Pneumonia," sec. 2 of this table. Follow-up If not hospitalized, client should visit every 1–3 days until improvement is noted.
Bronchiolitis	Disease of infants and young children Common in winter and spring Prodrome of URI for 1 to several days Abrupt onset of tachypnea, respiratory distress Retractions Tachypnea Tachycardia Nasal flaring Expiratory wheezing Normal white cell count	Refer client to physician. Admission to hospital for infants may be needed. Give symptomatic treatment, using bronchodilators in older infants. Use oxygen and vaporizer. Treat with antibiotics if indicated.
Bronchitis	Usually prodrome of URI Gradual onset of dry, hacking cough Afebrile or low-grade fever Cough becomes productive Purulent sputum Vomiting Nasal, pharyngeal, and conjunctival infection Roughening of breath sounds, rhonchi	Consult with physician. Administer antipyretics when necessary. Advise use of vaporizer. Teach parent(s) how to administer postural drainage. Maintain adequate fluid intake. Young infants may need hospitalization. Advise that disease should last 7–10 days. Telephone daily.

Table 34-1 Medical Referral/Consultation *(continued)*

Diagnosis	Clinical Manifestations	Management
Bronchitis	May have coarse and fine rales Leukocytosis	Have client return every 2–4 days until improvement is noted.
Congestive heart failure	Dyspnea on exertion Respiratory difficulty Difficulty in feeding, with small frequent feedings Relief of dyspnea in sitting position Sweating Chronic, hacking cough Retractions Hepatomegaly Neck vein distention Increasing rales	Refer client to physician for hospital admission. If heart disease is chronic, refer client to social worker where necessary. Give emotional support to family with acutely ill child.

bibliography

Anastasiades, Anastiasios. Tuberculosis in children: Current concepts. *Pediatric Annals* **6**(12):797–819 (1977).

Dewey, J. Eighteen ways to live with asthma. *Nursing '75,* April:48–51 (1975).

Green, Morris, and Haggerty, Robert. *Ambulatory Pediatrics II.* Philadelphia: Saunders, 1977.

Holsclaw, Douglas. Recognition and management of patients with cystic fibrosis. *Pediatric Annals,* **7**(1):9–27 (1978).

Letter: Management of asthma in children. *Journal of the American Medical Association,* **230**(7):962–963 (1974).

Nelson, John, et al. *Pediatrics (10th ed.).* Philadelphia: Saunders, 1975.

Rudolph, A., Barnett, H. L., and Einhorn, A. *Pediatrics (16th ed.).* New York: Appleton-Century-Crofts, 1977.

section 3

the cardiovascular system

INTRODUCTION JANE A. FOX

I Subjective Data

A. Age and race

B. Reason for visit and description of problem

C. Prenatal history

D. Neonatal history

E. Past medical history

1. Childhood diseases
2. Rheumatic fever
3. Heart murmur
4. Congenital heart disease
5. Urinary tract infections
6. Acute glomerulonephritis
7. Pyelonephritis
8. Emotional instability
9. Hypertension

F. Recent history of

1. Trauma to abdomen or flank
2. Fractures
3. Infections: skin and upper respiratory, especially streptococcal

G. Associated symptoms

1. Dizziness
2. Headache (especially on awakening)
3. Blurred vision
4. Chest pain, palpitations or shortness of breath
5. Weakness, easy fatigability
6. Polyuria
7. Muscle cramps
8. Excessive diaphoresis (perspiring)
9. Recent weight gain or loss
10. Chronic cough

H. Medications

1. Vasopressors
2. Corticosteroids
3. Antihypertensives
4. Nonproprietary drugs
5. Street drugs
6. Contraceptives

I. Allergies

J. Hospitalizations/surgery

K. Immunization history

L. Diet history

M. Developmental history

N. Patterns and habits

1. Reaction to physical activity
2. Smoking
3. Sleep/activity

O. Family history

1. Congenital cardiac disease
2. Premature deaths from coronary disease
3. Myocardial infarctions
4. Hypertension
5. Stroke
6. Heart failure
7. Diabetes
8. Uremia of unknown origin

9. Polycystic kidneys
10. Other renal problems
11. Emotional instability
12. Allergies
13. Obesity
14. Elevated cholesterol levels
15. Rheumatic fever

P. Social history

1. Living conditions
2. Family constellation
3. Financial status

II. Objective Data

A. Physical examination

1. Complete physical examination if cardiac condition suspected
2. General appearance—note gait, coordination, speech, physical deformity
3. Height, weight, head circumference—plot on graph
4. Blood pressure readings
   a. With client quiet and relaxed
   b. Using appropriate size cuff (Table 36-2) (covering two-thirds of the extremity)
   c. Supine, in all extremities to detect differences
   d. Sitting, in right arm
   e. Standing (after 3 min), for possible postural changes
   f. Using mercury manometer, placed at the level of the client
   g. Record on percentile charts (Fig. 37-1)
   h. In some infants, the flush or Doppler method perhaps necessary
5. Skin—color, condition, edema, digital clubbing
6. Fundoscopic examination
7. Neck—note prominence or distention of jugular veins
8. Heart—palpate point of maximum impulse (PMI), auscultate for rhythm and murmurs
9. Chest and lungs—chest configuration, auscultate for rales or wheezing
10. Abdomen—inspect and palpate for enlarged kidneys and liver tenderness, hepatojugular reflex
11. Pulses (radial, brachial, femoral, popliteal, dorsal pedal)—palpate bilaterally for character, symmetry, rate, rhythm
12. Neurological examination for signs of cerebral vascular disease (defects in mentation or motor function)

B. Laboratory data

1. The following may be indicated and ordered by the practitioner.
   a. Complete blood count
   b. Urinalysis and culture
   c. Blood chemistries
   d. Blood gases
   e. Blood urea/nitrogen
   f. Serum creatinine
   g. Antistreptolysin titer
   h. Chest x-ray
   i. Electrocardiogram
2. The following may be ordered by the physician.
   a. Intravenous pyelogram
   b. Photocardiogram
   c. Cardiac catheterization and angiography

35 Heart Beat/Rate Changes/ Murmurs

JANE ELLEN MEAD

All pediatric clients suspected of having a cardiac problem must be referred to a physician for evaluation, primary diagnosis, and treatment. The practitioner's involvement is in the initial screening and eventual follow-up, and in the maintenance of an active interest during the treatment phase.

I. Etiology

A. Congenital heart disease
1. Premature birth
2. Intrauterine aberrations
3. Chromosomal aberrations
4. Anatomical structural deformity
5. Environmental stimuli during intrauterine development
6. Genetic inheritance

B. Acquired heart disease
1. Anatomical
   a. Stenosis
   b. Weakening of musculature
2. Drug-induced
   a. Overdosage
   b. Hypersensitivity
3. Gas exchange (O_2–CO_2 imbalance)
4. Traumatic: surgical intervention
5. Infectious: group A beta-hemolytic streptococcus
6. Neoplastic: cardiac tumors

Table 35-1 Medical Referral/Consultation

Diagnosis	Clinical Manifestations	Management
Congenital heart disease	Cyanosis more pronounced after exertion	Referral to physician/pediatric cardiologist
Shunts:		
Left-right	Edema, especially periorbital or scrotal	Medications: Digoxin/Lanoxin, diuretics
Ventricular septal defect	Tachypnea/dyspnea	Increased rest
Atrial septal defect	Tachycardia/bradycardia	Nutrition in well-balanced proportions
Patent ductus arteriosus	Variation in quality of pulses	Hospitalization if necessary (see Preparation for Hospitalization, Part 7)
Endocardial cushion defect	Positive hepatojugular reflux	
Right-left	Variation in blood pressure in extremities	Parental instruction and counselling of diagnosis, treatment, and prognosis
Transposition of great vessels		Surgical correction sometimes necessary
Total anomalous venous return	Digital clubbing	
	Poor skin turgor	Follow-up at weekly/monthly visits
Truncus arteriosus	Decreased weight and development for age	
Tetrology of Fallot		Notification of school nurse
Tricuspid atresia	Chest deformity or predominance	Notification of community nursing service
Ebstein's anomaly		
Obstructive	Headaches	
Coarctation of aorta	Dizziness	

Table 35-1 Medical Referral/Consultation *(continued)*

Diagnosis	Clinical Manifestations	Management
Aortic stenosis Pulmonary stenosis	Sudden nasal hemorrhaging Visual disturbances Tired after eating or exertion Increased sweating Decreased appetite Frequent "coldlike" symptoms, upper respiratory infections Possibly asymptomatic	
Acquired heart disease	Cyanosis/pallor Tachycardia/bradycardia Tachypnea/dyspnea Respiratory retractions and nasal flaring Diaphoresis Edema Precordial bulge or predominance ECG irregularity Deviation of point of maximum impulse Presence of gallop rhythm Lethargy/fatigue Evidence of weight loss or decreased rate of development Digital clubbing Palpitations Dizziness Nausea, vomiting Anxiety Visual disturbances Fainting	Referral to physician/cardiologist Medications: antiarrhythmics, diuretics, antibiotics Surgery not indicated Hospitalization if necessary (see Preparation for Hospitalization, Part 7) Follow-up at weekly/monthly visits
Congestive heart failure	Dyspnea/tachypnea/orthopnea Cyanosis Edema Cough Rales Diaphoresis Liver enlargement Gallop rhythm Tachycardia Lethargy	Immediate referral to physician/cardiologist Medications: Digoxin/Lanoxin, diuretics Hospitalization as necessary (see Preparation for Hospitalization, Part 7)
Rheumatic fever	Recent streptococcal infection Fever Murmur	Refer to physician/cardiologist. See Acute Rheumatic Fever, Chap. 145. Refer to public health nurse (PHN) for throat cultures of family members.

Table 35-1 Medical Referral/Consultation *(continued)*

Diagnosis	Clinical Manifestations	Management
	Migratory polyarthritis with swelling, warmth, tenderness of joints Chorea Erythema on trunk Nodules over joint processes	
Bacterial endocarditis	Fever of unknown origin Diaphoresis, chills, especially at night Mild respiratory infection Anorexia Weight loss Murmur Enlarged spleen Anemia Petechiae	Refer to physician/cardiologist. See Preparation for Hospitalization, Part 7. Treatment is long-term antibiotic therapy.

bibliography

Congenital cardiac defects. *The American Journal of Nursing,* **78**(2):255–278 (1978).

Gottesfeld, Ilene Burson. The family of the child with congenital heart disease. *MCN: The American Journal of Maternal Child Nursing,* **4**(2):101–104 (1979).

Jackson, Patricia Ludder. Digoxin therapy at home: keeping the child safe. *MCN: The American Journal of Maternal Child Nursing,* **4**(2):105–109 (1979).

Kupst, Mary Jo, et al. Helping parents cope with the diagnosis of congenital heart defect: an experimental study. *Pediatrics,* **50**(1):266–271 (1977).

Naddas, Alexander S., and Fyler, Donoly C. *Pediatric Cardiology.* Philadelphia: Saunders, 1972.

Smith, Kathleen Moreau. Recognizing cardiac failure in neonates. *MCN: The American Journal of Maternal Child Nursing,* **4**(2):98–100 (1979).

The University of Cincinnati Symposium. The infant and child with cardiovascular disease. *Heart and Lungs* **3**(3):390–428 (1974).

36 Pediatric Hypertension

KATHLEEN M. BUCKLEY

ALERT

1. Fundoscopic changes
2. Left ventricular hypertrophy based on ECG or chest x-ray findings
3. Signs of cardiac decompensation
4. Signs of increased intracranial pressure
5. Systolic blood pressure > 90 mmHg

I. Etiology

A. Primary (essential) hypertension

B. Secondary hypertension (Table 36-1)

1. Renal causes
2. Vascular causes
3. Adrenal causes
4. Neurogenic causes
5. Miscellaneous causes

II. Assessment: Primary Hypertension

A. Subjective data—nonspecific

B. Objective data

1. Sustained sitting diastolic blood pressure > 90 mmHg (Table 36–2)
2. Ocular fundi changes of hypertensive retinopathy
3. Auscultation of apical heave, murmurs reflecting dilation, a prominent aortic component of second and fourth heart sound; signs of cardiac decompensation
4. X-ray or ECG evidence of left ventricular hypertrophy
5. No evidence of other secondary causes of renal disease

III. Management: Primary Hypertension

A. Treatments/medications: to be prescribed only after consultation with a physician (see Tables 36-3 and 36-4)

B. Counselling/prevention

1. Instruct the parent(s) on medications.
   a. Compliance with treatment and medications
      (1) The regime should be simple and interfere as little as possible with normal activities.
      (2) Awareness of the cost of various hypotensive agents and the family's ability to meet this cost is important.
   b. Common side effects (Table 36-3)
      (1) Explain the anatomy and physiology of hypertension.
      (2) Instruct the parent(s) about the probable cause of hypertension, the disease process, and why it must be treated (refer to major complications).
      (3) Identify and evaluate with the parent(s) the "predisposing factors" of hypertension.
         (a) Heredity—encourage at least yearly blood pressure checks for the family.
         (b) Race—hypertension is more common among black than among white individuals.
         (c) Nutritional considerations—excess consumption of saturated fats, cholesterol, sodium, and calories causes nutritional risks with hypertension.
2. Explain *systolic* and *diastolic* blood pressure.
3. Encourage ordinary physical exercise, including physical education, and adequate rest (isotonic exercises such as weight lifting or wrestling should be avoided).

4. Encourage weight reduction in the obese client, and place the client on a moderate salt-restricted diet if sodium intake is greater than 8 g/day.
5. Keep dietary and physical restrictions to a minimum, since they tend to single out the child as being abnormal.
6. Encourage the parent(s) to allow the child to lead as normal a life as possible and to discipline the child in the same manner they do the siblings.
7. Demonstrate the technique of blood pressure measurement for monitoring at home to parent(s) able to accept the responsibility.
8. Tell the parent(s) and child to return to the clinic or office if the condition worsens.

C. Follow-up

Arrange a return visit in 1 to 4 weeks to evaluate treatment and/or adjust medication.

D. Consultations/referrals

1. Refer clients with obesity or high salt ingestion to a dietician for instructions in weight reduction or a moderate salt-restricted diet.
2. Notify the public health nurse for reinforcing information about weight reduction, diet, exercise, and drug therapy if client or family is noncompliant.
3. Refer to social worker for problems with living conditions or family's ability to comply with treatment regimen.
4. Notify the school nurse for routine follow-up and blood pressure measurements.

Table 36-1 Causes of Secondary Hypertension

Renal Causes	*Adrenal Causes*
Glomerulonephritis	Adrenogenital syndrome
Pyelonephritis	Neuroblastoma
Hydronephrosis	Pheochromocytoma
Trauma	Cushing's disease
Hypoplastic kidney	Primary aldosteronism
Polycystic kidney	Secondary aldosteronism
Wilms' tumor (other renal tumors)	Adrenal hyperplasia
Collagen diseases, e.g., polyarteritis nodosa, systemic lupus, erythematosus	Adrenal adenoma
Hemolytic uremic syndrome	*Neurogenic Causes*
Renal transplant rejection	Trauma
Vascular Causes	Inflammatory disease
Coarctation of the aorta	Tumors
Renal artery abnormalities	Encephalitis
Aortic arteritis	Increased intracranial pressure
Generalized hypoplasia of the aorta	*Miscellaneous Causes*
Thrombosis of a renal artery	Renal parenchymal damage from irradiation
	Use of corticosteroids, vasopressor drugs
	Burns
	Poliomyelitis
	Lead nephropathy

Table 36-2 Dimensions for Appropriate Size Cuff

Cuff Name	Range of Dimensions of Bladder, cm	
	Width	Length
Newborn	2.5–4	5–10
Infant	6–8	12–13.5
Child	9–10	17–22.5
Adult	12–13	22–23.5
Large adult arm	15.5	30
Adult thigh	18	36

Source: Blumenthal, Sidney. Report of the task force on blood pressure control in children. *Pediatrics,* **59:**(suppl.):797–820 (1977).

Table 36-3 Antihypertensive Drugs for Ambulatory Treatment

Drug	Oral Dose	Major Side Effects
Chlorothiazide (Diuril)	Infants < 6 mo: 20–30 mg/kg per day in one dose Children > 6 mo: 20 mg/kg per day in two divided doses	Hypokalemia Hyperuricemia
Reserpine (Serpasil)	Clients weighing < 25 kg: 0.02 mg/kg per day one dose or two divided doses Clients weighing > 25 kg: 0.25–0.5 mg/kg per day in one dose or two divided doses	Nasal stuffiness Depression Sedation Irritability Nausea Bradycardia
Hydralazine (Apresoline)	0.75 mg/kg per day in four to six divided doses	Headache Tachycardia Nausea and vomiting Lupus syndrome
Methyldopa (Aldomet)	10–40 mg/kg per day in three divided doses	Sedation Postural hypotension False positive Coombs test Hemolytic anemia Leukopenia Diarrhea
Guanethidine (Ismelin)	0.2 mg/kg per day as a single dose	Postural hypotension Bradycardia Generalized muscle weakness on rising Diarrhea Nausea and vomiting

Table 36-4 Medical Referral/Consultation: Secondary Hypertension

Diagnosis	Clinical Manifestations	Management
Renal hypertension	History of nephritis, urinary tract infections, urinary abnormalities Unilateral or bilateral enlargement of the kidneys Costovertebral angle tenderness with acute infection Presence of casts in urinalysis Impaired renal function* Postive urine cultures Pyelogram showing deformed renal pelvis	Referral to physician Medications for urinary tract infection (UTI) Sulfonamide Ampicillin Analgesic and antipyretic drugs Counselling/prevention Teach client and family signs and symptoms of UTI. Encourage intake of fluids. Explain disease process and its therapy. Culture for UTI 24–48 h after initiation of therapy Every 3 mo × 3 cultures Every 6 mo × 2 cultures
Renovascular disease	History of trauma to abdomen or flank Pain (aneurysm) Hematuria Presence of bruit in the left or right epigastrium or flank* Murmurs over abdominal aorta or renal arteries Inequality in size of kidneys Impaired renal function	Refer to physician. See Preparation for Hospitalization, Part 7.
Coarctation of the aorta	Nonspecific subjective findings Absence, weakness, or delay of femoral pulses in comparison with radial pulses* Basal systolic murmur Difference between arm and leg pressures Chest x-ray evidence of rib notching and small aortic knob as a late finding	Refer to physician. See Preparation for Hospitalization, Part 7.
Pheochromocytoma	Attacks of acute anxiety, headaches, nausea and vomiting, pallor, profuse perspiration, palpitation, tremors, dizziness, weakness, and tachycardia* Symptoms sometimes sustained producing papilledema, retinopathy, and enlargement of heart Abdominal and precordial pain Dilated pupils with blurring of vision	Refer immediately to a physician. See Preparation for Hospitalization, Part 7.

*Primary Clinical Manifestation

Table 36-4 Medical Referral/Consultation: Secondary Hypertension *(continued)*

Diagnosis	Clinical Manifestations	Management
	Sharp rise in blood pressure induced by palpation of tumor Increased urinary excretion of vanillylmandelic acid X-ray studies to localize tumor	
Primary aldosteronism	Episodes of general muscle weakness or paralysis, paresthesia Polyuria and nocturia Hypokalemia* Hypoactive or absent tendon reflexes	Refer to physician.
Cushing's disease	History of gain in weight, bruising, and weakness Cushingoid features: truncal obesity, purple striae, and hirsutism* Acne, finely grained skin, and bruises X-ray evidence of osteoporosis Adrenocortical steroid excretion under a variety of conditions Polycythemia X-ray studies to localize tumor	Refer to physician.

*Primary Clinical Manifestation

bibliography

Blumenthal, Sidney. Report on the task force on blood pressure control in children. *Pediatrics,* **59**(suppl.): 797–820 (1977).

Kempe, C. Henry et al. *Current pediatric diagnosis and treatment* (4th ed.). Los Altos, Calif.: Lange, 1976.

Loggie, Jennifer M.H. Hypertension in children and adolescents. *Hospital Practice,* **10**:81–92 (1975).

37 Adolescent Hypertension

MARILYN GREBIN

I. Etiology

The causes of primary hypertension are unknown; however, genetic and environmental factors may contribute.

II. Assessment

A. Subjective data

1. History of obesity
2. Poor dietary habits
3. Black (more prevalent in blacks)
4. Use of birth control pill
5. Smoking
6. Family history of hypertension, heart attack, stroke, renal disease
7. Lack of exercise

B. Objective data

1. Obesity may be a symptom of hypertension.
2. All other findings should be normal.
3. Diastolic pressure should be less than 100 mmHg for an adolescent 13 to 18 years of age.
4. If the client's blood pressure is plotted on the percentile chart (Fig. 37-1) at the 95th percentile, further investigation is required.

Note: Screening, evaluation, counselling, and follow-up may be done by the primary health care practitioner; however, treatment with medication should be determined by the physician.

III. Management

A. Treatments/medications

Antihypertensive medications will be prescribed by the physician after an examination of the findings.

B. Counselling/prevention

1. Reduce sodium intake by a moderately restricted salt diet.
2. Plan a balanced, low-calorie diet.
   a. Avoid fast foods and sweets.
   b. Keep a diet diary, counting calories.
3. Avoid smoking.
4. Gradually increase physical activity.
5. Have adequate rest periods.
6. Avoid stressful situations.
7. Discontinue birth control pills.
8. The practitioner should counsel the client/parent on drug therapy (see Table 36-3).
   a. Encourage compliance with the therapeutic regimen and the necessary follow-up visits.
   b. The client/parent should alert the practitioner to any unpleasant side effects, such as light-headedness, dizziness, urinary frequency, sedation, altered bowel habits, orthostatic hypotension.

C. Follow-up

Blood pressure measurement and recording at 1- to 4-week intervals

D. Consultations/referrals

1. Consult physician if blood pressure is sustained in the 95th percentile.
2. Refer to dietician for low-calorie, sodium-restricted diet.

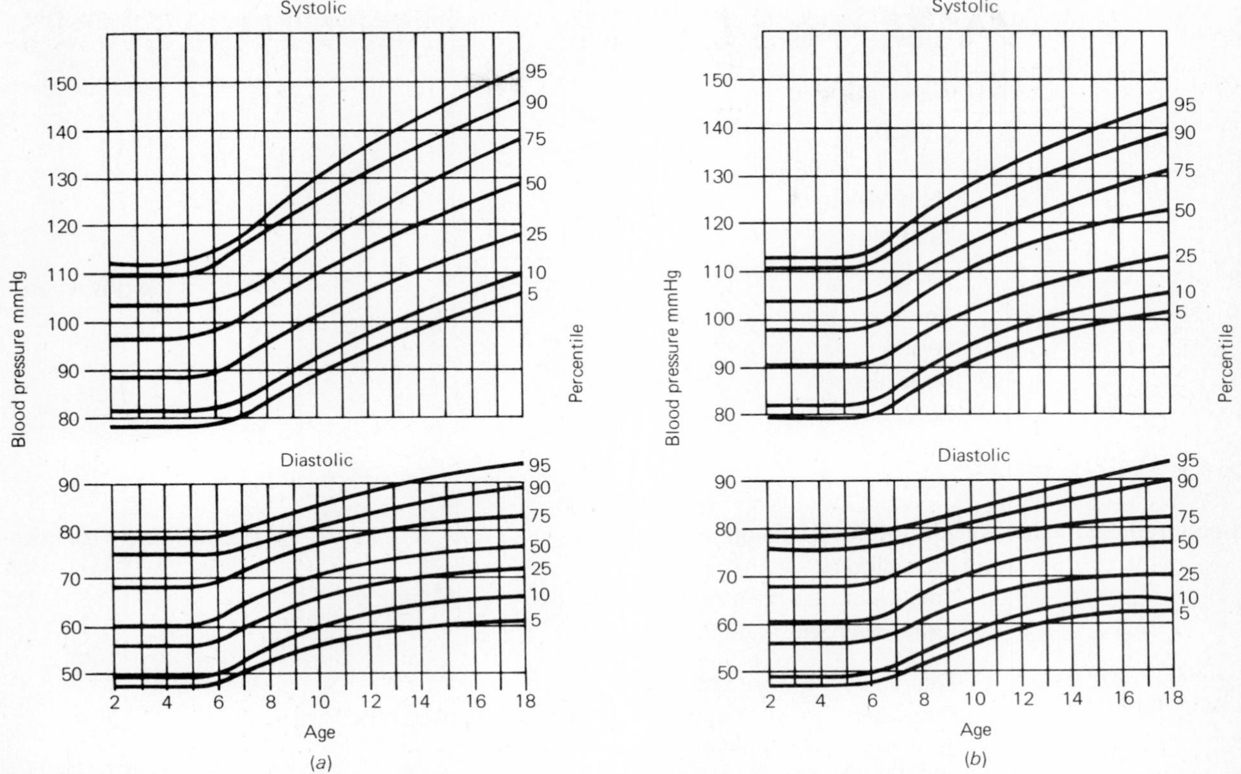

Figure 37-1 Blood pressure percentile charts for boys *(a)* and girls *(b)* between 2 and 18 years of age. Blood pressure percentile charts should not be used to evaluate specific blood pressure measurements but rather to plot *over a period of time* a child's blood pressure pattern as the child grows and matures. (From Report of the Task Force on Blood Pressure Control in Children. *Pediatrics,* **59** (suppl.):803, 1977. Used with permission.)

Table 37-1 Medical Referral/Consultation: Identifiable or Secondary Hypertension

Diagnosis	Clinical Manifestations	Management
Renal artery stenosis	Hypertension Congestive heart failure (Found on arteriography)	Referral to physician
Wilms' tumor	Abdominal distention and pain Fever Abdominal mass which does not cross the midline (firm and nontender in the renal area) Hypertension	Referral to physician
Glomerulonephritis	Occurs 1–3 wk after infectious process Fever > 101°F (>38.3°C) Anorexia Nausea Vomiting	Referral to physician

Table 37-1 Medical Referral/Consultation: Identifiable or Secondary Hypertension *(continued)*

Diagnosis	Clinical Manifestations	Management
	Hematuria Oliguria Edema Hypertension Albuminuria	
Chronic pyelonephritis	Fever Pain Pyuria Hypertension Polyuria Nocturia Uremia	Referral to physician
Pheochromocytoma	Abrupt hypertension Pounding headache Feeling of vasoconstruction of the extremities Exhaustion after attack	Referral to physician
Adrenal hyperplasia (congenital)	Tall, muscular, wiry body build Pubic hair 2–4 yr of age followed by axillary hair, acne Female: failure of development of secondary sex characteristics Male: testes remaining small Sustained hypertension at age 2–3 yr	Referral to endocrinologist
Coarctation of the aorta	Persistent hypertension Weakness and numbness of the legs Headaches Abdominal murmurs Unequal pulses in the upper and lower extremities Unequal blood pressures in upper and lower extremities	Referral to cardiologist
Systemic lupus erythematosus	Fever Anorexia Weight loss Arthralgia Skin lesions Hypertension Hepatosplenomegaly	Referral to physician
Drugs Sympathomimetics Corticosteroids Nephrotoxic agents Oral contraceptives	Possible hypertension	Referral to physician

bibliography

Berenson, G. S., Voors, A. W., Webber, L. S., and Frerichs, R. R. Blood pressure in children and its interpretation. *Pediatrics*, **61**(2):333–335 (1978).

de Castro, Fernando, et al. Hypertension in adolescents. *Pediatric Nursing*, **1**(4):30–31 (1975).

Devices for measuring blood pressure. *The Medical Letter*, **19**(13):55–56 (1977).

Heavenrich, Robert, M., Cinque, and Thomas J. Childhood high blood pressure: a new emphasis. *Pediatric Annals*, **6**(6):7–13 (1977).

Kilcoyne, Margaret M. Natural history of hypertension in adolescence. *The Pediatric Clinics of North America*, **25**(1):47–54 (1978).

———. Adolescent Hypertension. *The American Journal of Medicine*, **58**(6):735–739 (1975).

Lieberman, Ellin. Diagnostic evaluation of hypertensive children. *Pediatric Annals*, **6**(6):41–56 (1977).

McEnery, Paul T., and Davis, Charles A. Nonpharmacological interventions in hypertension. *The Pediatric Clinics of North America*, **25**(1):127–136 (1978).

Moss, Arthur J. Indirect methods of blood pressure measurement. *The Pediatric Clinics of North America*, **25**(1):3–14 (1978).

National Heart, Lung and Blood Institute's Task Force on Blood Pressure Control in Children. Report of the task force on blood pressure control in children. *Pediatrics*, **59**(5):797–820 (1977).

Rames, Linda, et al. Normal blood pressures and evaluation of sustained blood pressure evaluation in childhood: the Muscatine study. *Pediatrics*, **61**(2):245–250 (1978).

Sinaiko, Alan R., and Mirkin, Bernard L. Therapeutic agents for pediatric hypertension. *Pediatric Annals*, **6**(6):58–71 (1977).

section 4

the hemopoietic system

INTRODUCTION JANE A. FOX

I. Subjective Data

A. Age, sex, race

B. Reason for visit and description of problem

C. Onset

D. Associated symptoms

1. Lethargy/apathy
2. Irritability
3. Easy fatigability
4. Shortness of breath on exertion
5. Paleness of skin
6. Weight loss
7. Sleep problems
8. Headache
9. Muscle weakness
10. Vomiting
11. Diarrhea
12. Constipation
13. Swollen hands/feet
14. Painful joints
15. Fever
16. Easy bruising or petechiae
17. Behavior or personality changes

E. Prenatal history—iron pills, anemia

F. Birth history—Apgar score

G. Neonatal history

1. Number of days in hospital—mother and child
2. ABO incompatibility
3. Rh negative
4. Type of feeding and difficulty feeding
5. Drug administration—vitamin K
6. Presence of cephalohematoma
7. Sepsis
8. History of icterus—day began and treatment
9. History of use of phenol disinfectant in nursery

H. Developmental history

I. Nutritional history (complete)

1. Appetite changes
2. Infant
   a. Iron-fortified formula, milk, or cereal
   b. Iron supplementation in medicinal form
   c. Daily intake of cow's milk—if in excess of 32 oz per day, possible refusal of other food groups
   d. Solid foods
3. Older child—24-h diet recall

J. Immunization history

K. Elimination history

L. Past medical history and hospitalizations

1. Congenital disorders or chronic problems (convulsions, sickle cell disease, other blood disorders)
2. Iron deficiency anemia
3. Lead poisoning
4. Past screening for sickle cell disease/trait, other anemias
5. Recurrent infections

M. Allergies

N. Family history

1. Sickle cell disease/trait
2. Thalassemia
3. Iron deficiency anemia
4. Lead poisoning
5. Maternal blood type and Rh factor

O. Social history

II. Objective Data

A. Physical examination

1. Conduct complete physical examination (see Chap. 7, Health History and Physical Examination).
2. Measure height, weight, temperature, pulse, blood pressure.
3. Inspect/palpate skin for color, edema, turgor.
4. Inspect and palpate all joints for tenderness/swelling.
5. Inspect conjunctiva and mucous membranes for color.
6. Auscultate heart for murmurs.
7. Palpate abdomen for organomegaly.

B. Laboratory data

1. Complete blood count, including hematocrit, hemoglobin, reticulocyte count
2. Peripheral smear
3. Sickle cell preparation on all blacks, Orientals
4. Urinalysis
5. Hemoglobin electrophoresis if sickle cell disease suspected
6. Bilirubin level on icteric neonates
7. Denver Developmental Screening Test

38 Physiologic Jaundice in the Newborn[1]

MARILYN GREBIN

ALERT
1. Jaundice at birth or within the first 24 h
2. Jaundice appearing after the third day and within the first week
3. Jaundice noted after the first week
4. Persistent jaundice during the first month

I. Etiology

A. Imbalance between formation and elimination of bilirubin—immature glucuronide conjugation system in the liver

B. Breast-feeding

C. Nursery cleansing with phenol disinfectant

II. Assessment

A. Physiologic jaundice

1. Subjective data
   a. Mother and family history negative for chronic diseases
   b. Infant difficult to feed
2. Objective data
   a. Physical examination normal except for icteric sclera and skin noted on third day of life
   b. Bilirubin levels less than 10 mg per 100 mL in the full-term infant, less than 15 mg per 100 mL in the premature infant

B. Physiologic breast milk jaundice

1. Subjective data
   a. Breast-feeding
   b. Infant 1 to 8 weeks of age
   c. Familial history of breast milk jaundice
   d. Slow development of jaundice
   e. Good appetite
2. Objective data
   a. Growth and development normal
   b. Abnormal neurological signs absent
   c. Possible rise of bilirubin to 20 mg per 100 mL (glucuronyl transferase activity inhibited by breast milk)
   d. Bilirubin decreases when breast-feeding discontinued

C. Physiologic jaundice from use of phenol disinfectant

1. Subjective data
   a. Infants are well.
   b. Icteric skin and/or sclera may be noted on third day by nursery staff.
   c. Phenol disinfectant used to clean nursery bassinets.
2. Objective data
   a. Bilirubin (unconjugated) elevated on third or fourth day (phenol disinfectant inhibits glucuronyl transferase activity)
   b. Physical examination normal except for icteric sclera and skin

III. Management

A. Treatments/medications: daily bilirubin determinations

B. Counselling/prevention

1. Small frequent feedings for the infant who feeds poorly (i.e., 1 to 2 oz of formula every 1 to 2 h)
2. Discontinuance of phenol disinfectants for nursery cleaning
3. Reassurance to parent(s) that icterus will disappear by the seventh day of life
4. Discontinuance of breast-feeding in the infant with breast milk jaundice for 3 to 5 days, then resumption when level drops
5. Nursery observation daily for

[1]Physiologic jaundice often appears on the third day and regresses between the fifth to seventh day. All infants with jaundice must be evaluated by a physician.

a. Increase in icterus, increase in bilirubin
b. Signs of hypoglycemia
c. Respiratory distress
d. Diarrhea
e. Seizures
f. Lethargy
g. Poor feeding

C. Follow-up

1. Return visit 7 to 10 days after hospital discharge
2. Regular 6-week check
3. Telephone communication with the parent(s) between visits to discuss infant's status

D. Consultations/referrals

All icteric infants must be examined by a physician.

Table 38-1 Medical Referral/Consultation

Diagnosis	Clinical Manifestations	Management
JAUNDICE AT BIRTH OR WITHIN THE FIRST 24 h*		
Hemolytic disease of the newborn	Palpable spleen Enlarged liver Fourth day jaundice and organomegaly regress Moderate pallor on fourth day Poor feeding Regurgitation or vomiting Generalized edema	Immediate referral to physician
Cytomegalic inclusion disease (CID)	Premature, infected infant Petechiae and ecchymosis Jaundice a few hours after birth Hepatosplenomegaly Fever 102–103°F (38.9–39.4°C) Tachypnea Dyspnea	Immediate referral to physician
Congenital toxoplasmosis	Skin hemorrhages Hepatosplenomegaly Jaundice	Immediate referral to physician
JAUNDICE APPEARING AFTER THE THIRD DAY*		
Sepsis	Fever Abdominal distention Jaundice Hepatomegaly Vomiting and diarrhea sometimes occurring Pustules on the skin Erythema multiforme	Immediate referral to physician
Glucose-6-phosphate dehydrogenase (G-6-PD) deficiency	Anemia Jaundice Hepatosplenomegaly Mediterranean or Oriental origin	Immediate referral to physician See Anemia, Chap. 39
Hemolytic disease of the newborn Cytomegalic inclusion disease (CID)	See Jaundice at Birth or within the First 24 h, above	Immediate referral to physician
Congenital toxoplasmosis	See Jaundice at Birth or within the First 24 h, above	

*These disorders may appear anytime but are more likely to appear during these times.

Table 38-1 Medical Referral/Consultation *(continued)*

Diagnosis	Clinical Manifestations	Management
	See Jaundice at Birth or within the First 24 h, above	
JAUNDICE AFTER THE FIRST WEEK OF LIFE*		
Biliary atresia	Jaundice at 2–3 wk of age Dark urine Acholic stools Small degree of failure to thrive Hepatomegaly Irritability (probably from pruritus of the skin	Immediate referral to surgeon
Hepatitis	Jaundice a few weeks after birth Abdominal distention Hepatomegaly Poor appetite, vomiting Dark urine Sometimes exhibition of signs of genetic disease such as Down's syndrome (trisomy 17–18 E)	Immediate referral to physician
Herpetic hepatitis	Toxic infant Jaundice Skin vesicles	Immediate referral to physician
Hypothyroidism	Subnormal temperature Circulatory mottling Poor feeding Inactivity Constipation Persistent jaundice	Immediate referral to physician
Galactosemia	Jaundice within first 2 wk Poor weight gain Irritability Vomiting Cataracts Proteinuria	Immediate referral to physician
PERSISTENT JAUNDICE AFTER THE FIRST MONTH*		
Inspissated bile syndrome	Jaundice, from any previously described disorders which have upset the conjugating, excretory capacity of the hepatocytes, may endure for 2–3 mo of life. Bilirubin levels may be as high as 50 mg/100 mL.	Immediate referral to physician

*These disorders may appear anytime but are more likely to appear during these times.

bibliography

Gellis, Sydney. Phenol disinfectant and neonatal hyperbilirubinemia. *Pediatric Notes*, **2**:35 (1978).

Schuman, Harriot. Understanding neonatal jaundice-that darn yellow baby. *Pediatric Nursing*, July-August:38–40 (1976).

Shaeffer, Alexander, and Avery, Mary Ellen. *Diseases of the newborn* (4th ed.). Philadelphia: Saunders, 1977.

Silverman, Arnold, Roy, Claude, and Cozetto, Frank. *Pediatric clinical gastroenterology*. St. Louis: Mosby, 1975.

Thaler, Michael. Jaundice in early infancy. *Pediatric Annals*, **6**:8–27 (1977).

39 Anemia

ALERT
1. Jaundice
2. Shortness of breath
3. Stupor
4. Paleness
5. Persistent high fever
6. Chest pain—dyspnea
7. Painful joints
8. Unexplained abdominal or skeletal pain
9. Present/past history of swollen hands/feet
10. Frequent fatigue
11. Known sickle cell disease or positive family history

Iron Deficiency Anemia[1] JULIE COWAN NOVAK

I. Etiology

A. Inadequate supply of iron in diet

B. Inadequate supply of iron at birth

1. There is no replacement of fetal or perinatal blood loss.
2. Prematurity: Iron stores are laid down at the end of gestation so that a decreased amount of iron is received by a premature infant. It is recommended that normal-term infants receive 1 mg/kg per day of elemental iron, not to exceed 15 mg/day, while the premature infant should receive 2 mg/kg per day.
3. Twinning
4. Severely iron deficient mother

C. Blood loss without replacement

1. Occult blood loss from the gastrointestinal tract; either drug induced, caused by pathologic states, or sensitivity to the protein component of whole non-heat-treated cow's milk
2. Obvious blood loss (i.e., trauma)
3. Menses (additional 1 to 2 mg of iron lost per day)

D. Increased demand for iron due to accelerated growth or energy expenditure

1. Prematurity
2. Peak incidence during 6 months to 3 years of age
3. Adolescence
4. Pregnancy, parturition, lactation (additional 1 mg of iron lost per day)
5. Athlete

II. Assessment

A. Subjective data—possible complaint of one or more of the following

1. Decreased activity level
2. Lethargy
3. Easy fatigability
4. Shortness of breath on exertion
5. Pallor of skin
6. Poor iron intake in diet—takes more than 32 oz of milk per day, resulting in refusal of other foods
7. Appetite decrease

[1]*Note:* If iron deficiency anemia is mild, it is usually asymptomatic and is picked up on routine screening.

Table 39-1 Anemia Present If Hemoglobin and Hematocrit Levels Are below These Values

Age	Sex	Hemoglobin Concentration, g/100 mL	Hematocrit
6 mo–10 yr	Male and female	11	34
10–14 yr	Male and female	12	37
Over 14	Male	13	41
Over 14	Female	12	37

Source: Fomon, Samuel, et al. *Nutritional disorders of children.* Washington, D.C.: Dept. of HEW, 1976, p. 97.

8. Premature birth, lacking iron-fortified formula or supplemental iron during the first year of life
9. Weight loss
10. Irritability
11. Sleep problems
12. Neuromuscular symptoms—headache, tinnitus, faintness, muscle weakness, decreased attention span
13. Pica behavior

B. Objective data

1. If the anemia is mild, the physical examination may be normal.
2. If more severe, the following may be noted.
   a. Pallor of skin and conjunctiva
   b. Angular stomatitis
   c. Atrophic changes of tongue
   d. Koilonychia—flat or concave, brittle fingernails
   e. Poor weight gain
   f. Systolic murmurs
   g. Splenomegaly
   h. Poor muscle tone
3. Laboratory values will be below the designated limits in Table 39-1.
4. The red blood cell morphology will be hypochromic, microcytic erythrocytes, with some variety of size and shape.
5. Stools perhaps positive for occult blood.

III. Management

A. Treatments/medications

1. Decrease total milk intake to no more than 16 oz/day, and increase intake of foods high in iron content (see Methods of increasing dietary intake of iron, III, B, 2, below).
2. Substitute iron-fortified formula for whole cow's milk in infant less than 18 months of age.
3. For medications, see Table 39-2.

Table 39-2 Dosage of Ferrous Sulfate (Fer-In-Sol) for Treatment of Iron Deficiency Anemia*

Drug	Weight	Dose
Fer-In-Sol drops 0.6 mL=15 mg elemental iron (The most commonly used form in young children)	8–10 kg 10–12 kg	0.6 mL tid 0.9 mL tid
Fer-In-Sol syrup 0.5 mL=30 mg elemental iron (Usually given by the teaspoon)	12–16 kg 16–22 kg 22–30 kg	1¼ tsp tid 1¾ tsp tid 2½ tsp tid
Ferrous sulfate capsules 60 mg elemental iron per capsule (Enteric-coated and sustained-release are not recommended, as they transport iron past the duodenum and upper jejunum where 90% of iron absorption occurs. Robinson, 1978, p. 11.)	over 30 kg	1 capsule tid

*6 mg elemental iron per kilogram per day in divided doses (tid).
Note: Correct dose should be given tid for 2 to 3 mo. Iron is best absorbed when given between meals, but to minimize GI upset it may be given 20 to 30 min before or after meals. Offer with fruit juice, vegetable juice, or water. Avoid giving with milk.

B. Counselling/prevention

1. Prevention of iron deficiency anemia is very important.
   a. Iron requirements

Age	Dosage
6 mo–10 yr	10–15 mg iron/day
Adolescent male	18 mg iron/day; after growth spurt, 10 mg iron/day
Adolescent female	18 mg iron/day

   b. Medicinal iron supplement from 3 to 18 months of age[2]
      (1) 0.3 mL Fer-In-Sol once a day for infant weighing 4 to 7 kg (9 to 15 lb)
      (2) 6 mL Fer-In-Sol once a day for infant weighing over 7 kg (15 lb)
2. Explain methods of increasing dietary intake of iron. Nutrition education is the best preventive measure.
   a. Iron-fortified milk
   b. Red meat, pork, liver
   c. Iron-fortified cereals
   d. Egg yolk
   e. Dried fruit, dark green leafy vegetables, kidney beans, chick-peas, split peas
   f. Peanut butter
   g. Nuts (for child over age 4 years)
3. Explain that stools may be black because of sulfide salt formation.
4. Explain that teeth may be discolored during therapy. Offer iron with juice to decrease incidence of staining. To remove stains, brush teeth with sodium bicarbonate or hydrogen peroxide. Rinse well with water.
5. Gastrointestinal upset, particularly nausea, is the most frequent side effect of iron therapy. Other side effects include constipation, diarrhea, and epigastric pain. Although iron is best absorbed when given between meals, it may be given with juice 20 to 30 min before or after meals to minimize GI upset.
6. Give adequate explanation to client and parent(s) and write out instructions.

C. Follow-up

1. Repeat hemoglobin, hematocrit, and reticulocyte count in 1 to 2 weeks. All values should increase. Peak reticulocyte count is achieved on the fifth to tenth day of treatment. Hematocrit should return to normal within 1 month.
2. Reassess monthly until the anemia has corrected.
3. Continue treatment for 2 to 3 months. Explain importance of this measure to client and parent(s).
4. Evaluate compliance of client and/or parent(s).
5. Elicit information concerning stool color and bowel pattern.

D. Consultations/referrals—refer to physician those clients who have

1. Abnormality on physical examination
2. History of unexplained blood loss
3. Age less than 9 months
4. Family history of anemia unrelated to nutrition
5. Hematocrit less than 25 percent
6. Abnormal red blood cell (RBC) morphology
7. Low hematocrit despite 1 month of iron therapy
8. Anemia which returns after treatment

[2]Accidental ingestion of medicinal iron may result in iron intoxication. Like all medications, it should be kept in a locked container out of the reach of children.

Thalassemia Minor (Cooley's trait)

JULIE COWAN NOVAK

I. Etiology

Genetic defect in which there is a mild deficiency in the production of the beta chain of hemoglobin

II. Assessment

A. Subjective data

Usually asymptomatic, but parent(s) may describe signs of mild anemia

A. Objective data

1. Mediterranean, black, or Oriental ancestry
2. Slight splenomegaly
3. Mild anemia—hemoglobin (Hgb) rarely under 9 g/100 mL, and may be within the normal range
4. Red cells small and hypocromic; mean corpuscular volume (MCV) low

5. Target cells and basophilic strippling perhaps present on peripheral smear
6. Elevation of Hgb A_2 and/or Hgb f on electrophoresis
7. Bone marrow may show excessive iron deposition in the older child

III. Management

A. Treatments/medications

1. No therapy is indicated.
2. Iron should definitely NOT be administered.

B. Counselling/prevention

1. Genetic counselling is of utmost importance.
2. Explain what thalassemia minor is and answer any questions.
3. Prevention is through identification of carriers.

C. Follow-up

As needed for well-child visits

D. Consultations/referrals

Consult with physician for confirmation of diagnosis.

Beta Thalassemia Major[3] (Mediterranean anemia, Cooley's anemia) JULIE COWAN NOVAK

I. Etiology

A. Thalassemia major is transmitted when both parents have thalassemia minor; 25 percent of their children may be homozygous for the trait.

B. Abnormally shaped cells are produced, which are deficient in hemoglobin and destroyed more quickly than normal cells would be. These cells are incapable of normal incorporation of hemoglobin. To compensate, the hematopoietic tissue produces more fetal hemoglobin than is normal, but the amount is inadequate for the effective transportation of oxygen. Rapid destruction of immature and defective erythrocytes takes place.

Table 39-3 Medical Referral/Consultation: Thalassemia Major

Clinical Manifestations	Management
May be of Mediterranean, African, or Chinese ancestry	*Immediate* referral to a physician
Parent(s) with thalassemia minor	Frequent transfusions to maintain the hemoglobin above 8–11 g/100 mL
Severe anemia present by 1 yr of age	Chelation to treat iron overload is used under research protocol
Hepatosplenomegaly	
Mongoloid facies	Folic acid 5–10 mg daily
Protrusion of teeth	
Broad, heavy-appearing hands	Splenectomy possibly indicated
Lymphadenopathy	Genetic counselling is of the utmost importance
Laboratory data reveals Microcytic anemia Low erythrocyte count Decreased hemoglobin level Increased nucleated RBC precursors Increased reticulocyte count Basophilic stippling and target cells on peripheral smear	Assist parent(s) in understanding the child's condition, with its poor prognosis Provide emotional support of child and parent(s) and help them to live as normal a life as is possible and to cope with their anxiety and deal with their fears.
Roentgenographic studies show abnormal skull x-ray Widening of medullary spaces Thinning of the cortices Decrease in the size of the bony trabeculae	

[3]This condition is chronic and should be managed by a physician.

Sickle Cell Anemia M. CONSTANCE SALERNO

I. Etiology

A. Inherited recessive disorder

B. Every person possesses a pair of genes that control the synthesis of hemoglobin. One gene is inherited from each parent. The gene for sickle hemoglobin (hemoglobin S) is present in about 8 percent of American blacks. Inheritance of the hemoglobin S gene from both parents results in sickle cell anemia and is present in about 0.2 percent of black children. The offspring of two parents with sickle cell trait (hemoglobin AS) have a 1 in 4 (25 percent) chance of having sickle cell anemia (hemoglobin SS). Each child has a 1 in 2 (50 percent) chance of carrying the sickle cell trait (hemoglobin AS) and each child has a 1 in 4 (25 percent) chance of receiving normal hemoglobin (hemoglobin AA).

II. Assessment

A. Subjective data

1. Both parents carry sickle cell gene (hemoglobin AS)
2. May have present or past history of
   a. Pain, swelling, tenderness of hands and feet
   b. Anorexia
   c. Weakness
   d. Painful joints
   e. Abdominal pain
   f. Low back pain
   g. Priapism (persistent erection of penis)
   h. Cough
   i. Chest pain
   j. Shortness of breath

B. Objective data

1. Physical examination may show
   a. Irritability
   b. Pallor and/or jaundice
   c. Fever
   d. Puffy hands and feet, painful to touch
   e. Increased pulse and respiration
   f. Splenomegaly
   g. Hematuria
   h. Thin and small for age
2. Laboratory data indicates
   a. Blood smear positive for hemoglobin S
   b. Hemoglobin electrophoresis confirms diagnosis of sickle cell anemia

III. Management

A. Treatments/medications (no specific therapy)

1. Minor episodes of pain
   a. Adequate fluids
   b. Analgesics: aspirin/acetaminophen
   c. Assurance of rest
2. Proper nutrition: well-balanced meals
3. Supplemental vitamins first 18 months
4. Supplemental iron first 12 months
5. Encouragement of normal activity after pain has subsided

B. Counselling/prevention

1. Sickle cell trait (SCT)
   a. All blacks should be screened for SCT.
   b. Genetic counselling should be provided for those who carry SCT. Each carrier should know that if he or she marries another person with SCT their children may have sickle cell anemia. A complete explanation of sickle cell anemia and its clinical manifestations should be included.
2. Sickle cell anemia (SCA)
   a. Be aware of signs of impending crisis.
      (1) Pain in back or abdomen, arms, hands, legs, feet
      (2) Pallor
      (3) Lethargy, listlessness
      (4) Sleepiness
      (5) Irritability
      (6) High fever
   b. Avoid areas of low oxygen concentration, e.g., air travel and mountains.
   c. Avoid exposure to infections.
   d. Cuts and sores should be cleansed properly and evaluated frequently while healing.
   e. Immunizations should be kept up to date.
   f. Polyvalent vaccine against pneumococcal infection is recommended at age 1 year.
   g. Adequate fluids should be taken during hot weather and exercise.
   h. Avoid fatigue.
   i. Avoid drugs that cause acidosis or constriction of blood vessels.
   j. Prepare an emergency treatment plan when away from home.

(1) Name and telephone number of physician
(2) Name of facility child should be taken to
(3) Identification card stating the diagnosis, blood type, medicines being taken, and list of any allergies

k. Care between crises should include the following.
(1) Recommend activity appropriate to the child's needs.
(2) Treat the child in as normal a manner as possible, including setting limits on behavior.
(3) Avoid overindulgence in toys, etc.
(4) Encourage well-balanced meals and plenty of fluids.
(5) Stress the importance of compliance with medications.

l. Dental supervision is imperative.

C. Follow-up
1. Continuity of child and family care
2. Anticipatory guidance
3. Availability for continued psychological support

D. Consultations/referrals
1. School nurse
2. Schoolteacher

Table 39-4 Medical Referral/Consultation

Diagnosis	Clinical Manifestations	Management
Aplastic crises (decreased production of RBCs)	Pale Lethargic Sleeping excessively Stuporous Dyspneic	Immediate referral to physician Hospitalization See Preparation for Hospitalization, Part 7 Laboratory work includes complete blood count (CBC), reticulocyte count and serum electrolytes, blood pH, blood cultures Intravenous (IV) antibiotic therapy Oxygenation Hydration Blood transfusions Analgesics
Hyperhemolytic crises (increased rate of RBC destruction)	Same as for aplastic crises Jaundice	
Acute sequestration (massive collection of sickle RBCs in spleen)	Hypovolemic shock	
Sepsis (pneumococcal or other infection)	Persistent high fever Same as for aplastic crises	

Note: Sickle cell anemia should be managed in consultation with a physician. Any client in sickle cell crisis should be referred *immediately* to a physician and prepared for hospitalization.

Glucose 6-Phosphate Dehydrogenase (G-6-PD) Deficiency

JULIE COWAN NOVAK

I. Etiology

A. Transmitted as a sex-linked trait and of intermediate dominance; full expression in males and in rare homozygous females

B. Most common drug offenders (clinical picture characterized by an acute hemolytic episode due to defiency of G-6-PD enzyme in the erythrocytes following exposure to one of these substances)

1. Antimalarials
2. Sulfonamides, sulfones
3. Nitrofurans
4. Antipyretics
5. Analgesics
6. Synthetic vitamin K
7. Uncooked fava beans
8. Other less common offenders: ascorbic acid, chloramphenicol, methylene blue, quinidine

II. Assessment

A. Subjective data

1. Exposure to drug
2. Parent notes color change (24 h after exposure)
   a. Pallor
   b. Jaundice

B. Objective data

1. Incidence of 2 to 25 percent in blacks, Italians, Greeks, Middle Easterners, and Orientals.
2. Skin may show pallor or jaundice.
3. Laboratory data reveals normochromic erythrocytes with Heinz bodies formation.
4. There is an elevated reticulocyte count.

III. Management

A. Treatment/medications

1. Discontinue exposure to the offending agent.
2. It may be necessary to treat anemia.

B. Counselling/prevention

1. Explain the importance of avoiding exposure to specific drugs (list drugs to be avoided).
2. Genetic counselling is of the utmost importance.
3. A screening blood test should be administered to ethnic groups mentioned above.

C. Follow-up: as needed

D. Consultations/referrals

1. Refer to a physician any client in an acute hemolytic episode.
2. Consult with a physician if there is no crisis but the suspicion of G-6-PD.

bibliography

Committee on Nutrition of the Mother and Preschool Child. *Iron nutrition in adolescence.* Washington D.C.: National Academy of Sciences, 1976.

Dallman, P. R. Iron, vitamin E, and folate in the preterm infant. *Journal of Pediatrics,* **85**:742 (1974).

Desforges, J. F. Sickle cell anemia. In S. S. Gellis and B. M. Kagan (eds.), *Current pediatric therapy.* Philadelphia: Saunders, 1978, pp. 267–270.

Doswell, W. M. Sickle cell anemia. *Nursing 78,* **8**:65–68 (1978).

Duckett, C. L. Caring for children with sickle cell anemia. *Children,* **18**:227–231 (1971).

Duffy, Thomas P. Anemia in adolescence. *Medical Clinics of North America,* **59**:1488 (1975).

Fomon, Samuel J. *Infant nutrition.* Philadelphia: Saunders, 1974, pp. 267 and 298.

———. *Nutritional disorders of children: Prevention, screening, follow-up.* Washington D.C.: U.S. Government Printing Office, 1976.

Kellaher, T. I., and Fischer, J. M. A review of iron therapy. *U.S. Pharmacist,* January:36–44 (1978).

Kempe, H. C., Silver, H. K., and O'Brien, D. *Current pediatric diagnosis and treatment.* Los Altos, Calif.: Lange, 1979.

Marlow, Dorothy R. *Textbook of pediatric nursing.* Philadelphia: Saunders, 1977, pp. 459–464.

McFarlane, J. M. Everyday care of the child with sickle cell anemia. *Pediatric Nursing,* **2**:9–11 (1976).

Piomelli, S., Brickman, A., and Carlos, E. Rapid diagnosis of iron deficiency by measurement of free erythrocyte porphyrins and hemoglobin: The FEP-hemoglobin ratio. *Pediatrics,* **57**:136 (1976).

Rios, E., Lipschitz, D. A., Cook, J. D., and Smith, N. J. Relationship of maternal and infant iron stores as assessed by determination of plasma ferritin. *Pediatrics,* **55**:694 (1975).

Robinson, L. A., Brown, A. L., and Underwood, T. Iron therapy, helps and hazards. *Pediatric Nursing,* November-December:9–13 (1978).

Scipien, G. M., Barnard, M., Chard, M., Howe, J., and Phillips, P. *Comprehensive pediatric nursing* (2d ed.). New York: McGraw-Hill, 1979.

Shirkey, H. C. *Pediatric drug handbook.* Philadelphia: Saunders, 1977, p. 163.

Wood, Camilla. Iron deficiency anemia. *Nurse Practitioner,* May–June:24–29 (1977).

section 5

the gastrointestinal system

INTRODUCTION JANE A. FOX

I. Subjective Data

- **A.** Age, sex, race
- **B.** Reason for visit and description of problem
- **C.** Onset
- **D.** Parental definition of diarrhea/vomiting
- **E.** Associated symptoms
  1. Nausea/vomiting
  2. Diarrhea
  3. Constipation
  4. Abdominal pain/cramping
  5. Fever
  6. Chills
  7. Blood in stool or rectal bleeding
  8. Painful bowel movements
  9. Rectal itch
  10. Flatus
  11. Blood in vomitus
  12. Nasal congestion
  13. Sore throat
  14. Ear pain
  15. Cough
  16. Chest pain
  17. Dysuria
  18. Frequency of urination
  19. Change in urine or stool color
  20. Painful or sore gums
  21. Bleeding gums
  22. Mouth sores
  23. Halitosis
  24. Irritability/disturbed sleep
  25. Anorexia
  26. Weight gain or loss
  27. Abdominal distention
- **F.** Elimination history
  1. Normal stool pattern
  2. Voiding pattern
  3. History of enuresis or encopresis
  4. Bathroom habits
- **G.** Nutritional history
  1. Food and fluid intake in past 24 h
  2. Feeding methods and techniques
     - a. Breast/bottle
     - b. How infant is fed: held, in bed
     - c. Bubbling
     - d. Who feeds infant
  3. Interruption in dietary habits
     - a. Formula changes
     - b. Introduction of new baby foods
     - c. Introduction of whole milk
     - d. Change from baby to table foods
- **H.** Prenatal history
- **I.** Birth history
- **J.** Neonatal history
- **K.** Developmental history
  1. Milestones
  2. Age at which toilet training was completed
     - a. Difficult training

   b. Family disturbances or birth of sibling during training period
   c. Punishments given during training period

L. Immunization history

M. Allergies

N. Current medications

O. Present/past history

1. Recent infections: viral, streptococcal
2. Congenital anomalies
3. Seizure disorder
4. Pica
5. Vitamin C deficiency
6. Leukemia
7. Diabetes
8. Pregnancy
9. Pneumonia
10. Anemia
11. Liver disease, i.e., hepatitis
12. Recent dental surgery
13. Ingestion of foreign body
14. Poison ingestion
15. Colic
16. Hernia
17. Hemorrhoids

P. Hospitalizations

Q. School performance and attention span

R. Behavior and temperament

S. Recent travel outside country by family with or without client

T. Sleep history

U. Family history

V. Social history

1. Relationships with family members and peers
2. Alcohol use
3. Smoking
4. Sexual activity and contraception

W. Careful, thorough review of systems

II. Objective Data

A. Physical examination

1. A complete physical examination should be performed on all infants and young children (see Health History and Physical Examination, Chap. 7).
2. Naked weight and height should be plotted on a graph.
3. Obtain vital signs and blood pressure.
4. Determine state of hydration.
   a. Dehydrated client
      (1) Unwell appearance
      (2) Lethargic or irritable
      (3) Poor skin turgor, especially on abdomen and calves of legs
      (4) Skin that feels dry
      (5) Rapid, weak pulse
      (6) In infancy, depressed anterior fontanel, palpate sitting up
      (7) Sunken eyes and dark surrounding skin
      (8) Low intraocular pressure
      (9) Absence of tears—severe dehydration
      (10) Dry mucous membranes of mouth
   b. State of hydration
      (1) Presence of tears and saliva—adequately hydrated
      (2) Absence of tears and dry mouth—5 percent dehydration
      (3) Absence of tears, dry mouth, sunken eyes, depressed fontanel, and poor skin turgor—10 percent dehydration
5. Inspect and palpate for lymphadenopathy.
6. Inspect mouth for the following.
   a. Moisture, inflammation
   b. Condition of gingiva
   c. Presence of plaque adhering to tooth surfaces
   d. Lesions
   e. Bleeding
7. Inspect nose, throat, ears for signs of infection and/or bleeding.
8. Determine cardiac and respiratory status.
9. Inspect abdomen for visible peristalsis, striae, symmetry, distention, bowel loops, masses, abdominal respirations.
10. Auscultate abdomen for frequency and quality of bowel sounds, bruits.
11. Lightly palpate abdomen for skin turgor, nodules, tenderness, rigidity, guarding, inguinal node enlargement.
12. Deeply palpate abdomen for tenderness, rebound pain, masses, or organomegaly.
13. Measure abdomen if you suspect abdominal distention.
14. Inspect genitalia.
15. Inspect anus and rectal area for signs of redness, excoriation, tears, fistulae, bleeding, or hemorrhoids.
16. Rectal exam may be indicated.
17. Inspect skin for color, turgor, texture, rash.
18. Inspect and palpate joints for redness, swelling, tenderness.

B. Laboratory data

1. The following tests may be indicated.
   a. Complete blood count (CBC) with differential
   b. Urinalysis
   c. Urine culture

d. Stool specimen for occult blood, ova, and parasites
e. Erythrocyte sedimentation rate
f. Stool culture
g. Pregnancy test
h. X-ray—flat plate of the abdomen
i. Scotch tape perianal impression to examine for enterobius eggs
j. Electrolytes
k. Throat culture
l. Culture of oral lesions
m. Chest x-ray

2. The following tests may be indicated after physician consultation.
   a. Barium enema
   b. Intravenous pyelogram (IVP)
   c. Bone age
   d. Supine and upright x-rays of the abdomen
   e. Upper GI series
   f. Stool pH and reducing substances
   g. Serum amylase
   h. Blood culture
   i. Sweat test

40 Difficulty with Sucking/Eating/Swallowing

ELEANOR RUDICK

ALERT
1. Cyanosis
2. Excessive, frothy mucus
3. Barking cough (croup)
4. Signs of airway obstruction

I. Etiology

A. Developmental delayed maturation
B. Emotional
C. Neurological insult
  1. Birth injury
  2. Infection
    a. Meningitis
    b. Encephalitis
D. Trauma (accidents)
E. Allergy

II. Assessment: Ankyloglossia (tongue-tie)

A. Subjective data
  1. Parent(s) report infant has difficulty sucking.
  2. Parent(s) or client report speech problem.
B. Objective data
  1. Infant
    a. Short frenulum
    b. Tight band of muscle under tongue on palpation
    c. Poor suck
  2. Child
    a. Inability to protrude tongue beyond the lips
    b. Tight band of muscle under tongue on bimanual palpation
    c. Inability to repeat "ta-ta-ta" with incisor teeth separated $\frac{1}{4}$ to $\frac{1}{2}$ in

III. Management: Ankyloglossia

A. Treatments/medications
  1. Surgical repair may be indicated.
  2. Speech therapy may be indicated.
B. Counselling/prevention
  1. Importance of treatment
  2. Reassurance treatment will improve speech
  3. Instruction to parent(s)
    a. How to support muscle under chin during feedings
    b. Frenulum expected to stretch with time
C. Follow-up: as needed to reassure parent(s)
D. Consultations/referrals
  1. Refer to physician if necessary—surgical correction after 8 to 10 months.
  2. Refer for speech evaluation and therapy.

bibliography

Hoekelman, Robert A., et al. (eds.). *Principles of pediatrics: health care of the young.* New York: McGraw-Hill, 1978, pp. 747–752.

Vaughan, Victor C. and McKay, R. James (eds.). *Nelson textbook of pediatrics* (10th ed.). Philadelphia: Saunders, 1975, pp. 800, 803–809.

Table 40-1 Medical Referral/Consultation

Diagnosis	Clinical Manifestations	Management
Esophageal atresia and fistula	Excessive salivation Choking with feedings Cyanosis with feedings Regurgitation Abdominal distention	Immediate referral to physician Radiologic study Surgery indicated—determined by type of lesion See Preparation for Hospitalization, Part 7 Postsurgery Review of feeding techniques Well-child supervision
Esophageal stenosis	Those of esophageal obstruction when infant starts solid or semisolid foods	Immediate referral to physician Radiologic and esophagoscopic examinations Esophagoscopic dilatation
Esophageal spasm	Severe, sudden symptoms of obstruction	Referral to physician Infant—as in esophageal stenosis Older child—may be emotional cause (see Family Assessment, Chap. 1)
Esophageal foreign body	History of coughing, gagging, choking, dyspnea, dysphagia, drooling, pain	Immediate referral to physician Counsel parent(s) regarding Radiographic studies Surgical removal Teaching about accident prevention For repeaters See Family Assessment, Chap. 1. See "Accident Prevention" in Chap. 9.
Epiglottitis (ages 2–7)	High fever Sore throat Rapidly progressing respiratory obstruction Respiratory stridor Hoarseness Brassy cough Dysphagia and drooling Irritability and restlessness Hyperextension of neck in young child Sitting position, leaning forward in older child	*Immediately* refer client to a physician. If epiglottitis is suspected, avoid depressing the tongue unless tracheotomy can be performed at once. Hospitalization is indicated—see Preparation for Hospitalization, Part 7. Posthospitalization—counsel concerning the prevention of respiratory infection.
Brain damage (see Cerebral Palsy, Chap. 151)	Poor sucking High-pitched cry Other abnormal reflexes Failure to gain weight Seizure activity	Referral to physician—to multiprofessional diagnostic and evaluative service Well-child supervision Periodic reevaluation by multiprofessional service Referral to public health nurse (PHN) These children require long-term supervision and constant reevaluation as they grow and develop; consequently, families require support, understanding, and encouragement to cope.

41 Blood in Vomitus

MARILYN GREBIN

I. Etiology (see Assessment)

II. Assessment[1]

Entity	Age	Amount	Clinical Features	Etiology	Diagnosis
Swallowed maternal blood	Newborn	Variable	Appears well	Delivery	Apt-Downey test
Stress ulcer	Newborn and older child	Large	Sick, pale appearance; shock	CNS disease, sepsis, difficult perinatal period	Upper GI series, nasogastric tube
Hemorrhagic gastritis	Newborn	Large	Sick, pale appearance; shock	CNS disease, sepsis, difficult perinatal period	Nasogastric tube, endoscopy
Hemorrhagic disease of the newborn	Newborn	Variable	Melena; skin or umbilical bleeding	Vitamin K deficiency, clotting disorders, liver disease	Coagulation studies
Peptic disease	Any age	Large	Appears well; vomiting, pain, anemia	Duodenal or antral ulcer	Upper GI series, endoscopy
Esophageal varices	Any age	Large	Well or ill appearance	Portal hypertension	Esophagography, esophagoscopy
Peptic esophagitis	Any age	Small	Vomiting, dysphagia, failure to thrive	Hiatal hernia, severe chalasia	Esophagography, esophagoscopy
Gastric outlet obstruction	Any age	Small	Vomiting, failure to thrive	Hypertrophic pyloric stenosis, antral ulcers, pyloric webs or diaphragm	Upper GI series
Erosive gastritis or esophagitis	Any age	Small	Vomiting, pain, dysphagia	Acids, alkalis, iron, aspirin	History of ingestion, endoscopy

[1]*Note:* The primary health care practitioner should be aware of the conditions causing hematemesis and may assist the physician in the work-up, but the diagnosis will be assigned by the physician.

Entity	Age	Amount	Clinical Features	Etiology	Diagnosis
Gastritis	Any age	Small	Protracted vomiting	Gastroenteritis	History, endoscopy
Swallowed blood	Any age	Moderate to large	Nausea, nasal bleeding	Ear, nose, throat, or dental bleeding	History

Source: Roy, C. C., Silverman, A., and Cozzetto, F. J. *Pediatric clinical gastroenterology* (2d ed.). St. Louis: Mosby, 1975, p. 24.

III. Management

A. Counselling/prevention: The practitioner may assist the client and parent(s) in understanding the illness and the treatment regimen.

1. Explain the necessary tests done by the physician.
   a. Upper GI series
   b. Endoscopy
   c. Blood tests
   d. Esophagoscopy
2. See Preparation for Hospitalization, Part 7.
3. Explain the importance of compliance with medical/nursing home care.
4. Give guidance for follow-up after client's discharge from the hospital.

42 Nausea/Vomiting

HARRIETT S. CHANEY/JANE A. FOX

ALERT
1. Bulging fontanel
2. Hematemesis
3. Poison ingestions
4. Bile in vomitus
5. Tarry and/or bloody stools
6. Evidence of salicylate abuse
7. Acute, localized, or diffuse abdominal pain —moderate to severe
8. Projectile vomiting
9. Persistent vomiting
10. Jaundice
11. Abdominal mass
12. Visible peristalsis
13. Dehydration
14. Abdominal distension
15. History of anemia
16. Recent head trauma
17. Drowsiness
18. Poor suck
19. Failure to gain weight or weight loss
20. Psychological disturbances

I. Etiology (see Table 42-1)

Table 42-1 Etiology of Vomiting

Gastrointestinal Tract

Congenital
- Chalasia—hiatal hernia (regurgitation)
- Atresia—stenosis (tracheoesophageal fistula, prepyloric diaphragm, ileal atresia)
- Duplication
- Volvulus (errors in rotation and fixation, Meckel's diverticulum)

Table 42-1 Etiology of Vomiting *(continued)*

Gastrointestinal Tract (continued)

- Congenital bands
- Hirschsprung's disease
- Meconium ileus (CF), meconium plug
- Celiac disease

Acquired
- Acute infectious gastroenteritis, food poisoning (staphylococcal, clostridial)
- Gastritis, duodenitis
- Peptic ulcer—common presentation in child less than 6 yr
- Intussusception
- Incarcerated hernia—inguinal, internal secondary to old adhesions
- Trauma—duodenal hematoma, traumatic pancreatitis, perforated bowel
- Pancreatitis—mumps, trauma, cystic fibrosis, hyperparathyroidism, hyperlipidemia
- Cow's milk protein intolerance, food allergy, eosinophilic gastroenteritis
- Disaccharidase deficiency
- Adynamic ileus—the mediator for many non-GI etiologies
- Crohn's disease
- Neonatal necrotizing enterocolitis
- Chronic granulomatous disease with gastric outlet obstruction

Nongastrointestinal Tract

Infectious—otitis, UTI, pneumonia, upper respiratory infection, sepsis, meningitis

Metabolic—amino and organic acidurias, galactosemia, fructosemia, adrenogenital

Table 42-1 Etiology of Vomiting *(continued)*

Nongastrointestinal Tract (continued)
syndrome, renal tubular acidosis, diabetic ketoacidosis, Reye's syndrome
Central nervous system (CNS)—trauma, tumor, infection, diencephalic syndrome, supratentorial (migraine, cyclic vomiting, rumination), autonomic (pain, shock)
Medications—anticholinergics, aspirin, alcohol, idiosyncratic reaction (e.g., codeine)

Source: Hoekelman, Robert A., et al. *Principles of pediatrics: health care of the young.* New York: McGraw-Hill, 1978, p. 711. Used with permission.

II. Assessment

A. Spitting up/regurgitation

1. Subjective data
   a. Infant is usually less than 7 months old.
   b. Parent(s) reports infant "spits up" milk/formula immediately or soon after feeding.
   c. History may reveal inadequate/improper feeding and/or feeding techniques, i.e., formula improperly prepared, inadequate bubbling after feeding, inadequate nipple hole in feeding bottle.
   d. The parent(s) may prop the bottle for feedings, lie the infant down after feeding without bubbling, and/or provide excessive stimulation following feeding.
   e. Social/family history may indicate recent tension/stress.
2. Objective data
   a. The infant appears well.
   b. Weight gain is normal.
   c. There are no abnormal physical findings.

B. Overfeeding (see "Nutritional Assessment," in Chap. 9)

1. Subjective data
   History reveals overfeeding for current weight and age.
2. Objective data
   a. Client is of normal height and weight or is overweight for the present height. The growth chart may indicate a sudden increase in weight.
   b. Head circumference is normal.

C. Acute gastroenteritis (see Diarrhea/Loose Stools, Chap. 47)

1. Subjective data
   a. Acute onset of nausea/vomiting
   b. Headache
   c. Low-grade fever and malaise
   d. Abdominal pain/cramping
   e. May have ear pain, sore throat, urinary frequency, or pain on urination
   f. May have diarrhea
2. Objective data
   a. Fever common
   b. Mild to moderate dehydration
   c. Minimal to moderate abdominal tenderness
   d. Hyperactive bowel sounds
   e. Physical exam may reveal upper respiratory infection (URI), tonsillitis, or otitis media
   f. Complete blood count (CBC)—usually normal, occasionally slight leukopenia
   g. Stool positive for occult blood

D. Acute gastritis

1. Subjective data
   a. Acute onset of nausea/vomiting
   b. Possible excessive consumption of spicy foods, alcohol, carbonated and/or caffeinated beverages, or aspirin, or psychological stress/crisis
   c. Food intolerance between episodes of nausea and vomiting
   d. Possible report by parent(s) that child ingested aspirin or ferrous sulfate
   e. Abdominal pain
   f. Tarry stools
2. Objective data
   a. Minimal or no dehydration
   b. Minimal to moderate epigastric tenderness
   c. Physical examination sometimes normal or indicating signs of bleeding
      (1) Hypotension
      (2) Pallor
      (3) Tachycardia
   d. Stool guaiac test positive
   e. Hyperactive bowel sounds

E. Nausea/vomiting/upset stomach in absence of mucosal disturbance

1. Subjective data
   a. Gradual onset resulting from overeating, physical or mental fatigue
   b. Early pregnancy
2. Objective data
   a. Sporadic episodes
   b. Temperature, CBC—normal
   c. Minimal to no dehydration
   d. Abdominal musculature soreness due to vomiting and retching

III. Management

A. Spitting up/regurgitation

1. Treatments/medications

a. Use proper formula and feeding techniques.
b. Decrease stress/tensions.
c. Try changing type of formula; offer feedings which are thickened.
d. Hold infant in upright position during feeding and maintain sitting position for 30 min after feeding.

2. Counselling/prevention
a. Reassure parent(s) this usually disappears before the infant is 8 months of age and some spitting up is normal.
b. Educate regarding proper formula preparation and breast- and bottle-feeding techniques.
c. Assist parent(s) in alleviating stress and making mealtime relaxing, i.e., take phone off hook, use rocking chair.
d. Teach how to avoid aspiration.

3. Follow-up: as needed
4. Consultations/referrals
Referral to physician
Infants over 8 months of age
Infants who fail to maintain growth parameters

B. Overfeeding (see "Nutritional Assessment" in Chap. 9)

1. Treatments/medications
Proper nutrition for age and weight
2. Counselling/prevention
a. Parent education should begin during the prenatal period.
b. Discuss with parent(s) the child's nutritional needs and diet.
c. Do *not* use food as a reward.
d. Do *not* put cereal or other solid food in the bottle.
e. Educate parent(s) in proper formula/food preparation and feeding techniques.
3. Follow-up: as needed
4. Consultations/referrals: usually none

C. Acute gastroenteritis (see Diarrhea/Loose Stools, Chap. 47)

1. Treatments/medications
a. Antiemetics and sedatives should *not* be used for infants.
b. Restrict diet.
(1) Stop all oral intake for 3 to 4 h in infants, and 6 h in older children.
(2) Then begin clear fluids in frequent small amounts; progress in quantity as tolerated.
(a) Infants—give sugar water, as tolerated; progress to half-strength and then full-strength formula.
(b) Older children (½ to 1 oz every hour)—give Jell-O water, flat coke, sweetened tea, bouillon soup; introduce dry toast and crackers, progressing to soft, bland food and then to a normal diet, as tolerated.
2. Counselling/prevention
a. Acute gastroenteritis is of limited duration, usually 24 h to 3 days.
b. Maintain adequate fluid intake.
c. Avoid carbonated beverages (shake to remove bubbles), milk, and milk products.
d. Instruct on signs of dehydration.
e. Rest, gradually resuming normal activity.
3. Follow-up
a. Telephone in 24 h to report progress.
b. If condition worsens or there are signs of dehydration, telephone immediately.
4. Consultations/referrals
a. Consult/refer to physician.
(1) Infants/children with signs of dehydration
(2) Clients with persistent symptoms
b. If there is bacterial food poisoning, report it to the health department.

D. Acute gastritis

1. Treatments/medications
a. Liquid antacid frequently for 5 to 10 days, then 2 h after meals (p.c.) and at bedtime (h.s.)
b. Diet restrictions
2. Counselling/prevention
a. Illness is usually of limited duration, 24 h to 3 days.
b. Discontinue use of gastric irritants.
c. Identify situation stresses.
d. Counsel on diet restrictions: small amounts of crushed ice, then clear, bland liquids, advancing to soft, bland diet to be maintained for several weeks.
e. Client should chew food well and avoid mealtime stress.
f. Client should maintain adequate fluid intake.
g. Advise parent(s) that client should rest during acute phase, and then gradually resume normal activity.
h. Counsel parent(s) on accident prevention and proper administration of medication.
3. Follow-up
a. Telephone call in 24 h to report progress
b. Return visit in 3 days if not improved
4. Consultations/referrals
a. Immediate referral to physician of clients with

(1) Hematemesis
(2) History of poison ingestion

b. Consult physician on all
(1) Infants and young children
(2) Clients who show no improvement within 3 days

E. Nausea, vomiting, upset stomach in absence of mucosal disturbance

1. Treatments/medications: none
2. Counselling/prevention
   a. Discontinue overindulgence; if indicated, small feedings should take place 6 times per day.
   b. Identify the sources of depression, anxiety, fatigue.
   c. Discuss the importance of adequate sleep and ways to decrease anxiety.
3. Follow-up
   a. Return visit in 1 week if not improved.
   b. Telephone immediately if symptoms increase in severity.
4. Consultations/referrals
   a. Obstetrical services if pregnant
   b. Professional counselling for testing and/or for individual or group treatment programs

Table 42-2 Medical Referral/Consultation

Diagnosis	Clinical Manifestations	Management
Chalasia (gastroesophageal incompetence)	Symptoms start between third and tenth day of life. Infant regurgitates when laid down. Infant appears hungry, feeds eagerly. There is slow weight gain or weight loss. Diagnosis is confirmed by fluoroscopic examination.	Refer to physician. Symptoms usually disappear within weeks or a few months. Reassure parent(s). Hold infant in upright position for 30–60 min after feeding.
Intestinal atresia and stenosis	Vomiting No bowel movements Abdominal distention Usually begins first day or week of life May visualize peristalsis X-ray shows no air in small intestine	Immediately refer to a physician. Surgery is indicated. See Preparation for Hospitalization, Part 7, and Newborn Assessment, Chap. 8.
Meconium ileus	Associated with cystic fibrosis Symptoms beginning soon after birth Vomiting Abdominal distention Abdominal palpation revealing firm, rubberlike loops of bowel Barium enema showing microcolon	Immediately refer to a physician. Surgery is indicated. See Preparation for Hospitalization, Part 7. Sweat test should be ordered. See Cystic Fibrosis, Chap. 144.
Imperforate anus	Beginning 24–36 h after birth No meconium passed in first 24–48 h of life Abdominal distention Vomiting Anal opening malpositioned	Immediately refer to a physician. Surgery is indicated. See Preparation for Hospitalization, Part 7.
Congenital megacolon or Hirschsprung's disease	Usually Caucasian male Abdominal distention No bowel movements Nausea	Immediately refer to a physician. Surgery is necessary. See Preparation for Hospitalization, Part 7.

Table 42-2 Medical Referral/Consultation *(continued)*

Diagnosis	Clinical Manifestations	Management
	Malnutrition Foul odor of breath and stool Diagnosis may be rectal biopsy	This disease is a congenital anomaly, and familial incidence is about 10%. Teach colostomy care and other procedures to parent(s).
Intussusception	Rare in infants under 6 mo Usually 6 mo to 2 yr of age Sudden onset Vomiting Abdominal pain "Currant jelly" stool Abdominal palpation revealing sausage-shaped mass Abdominal x-ray confirming diagnosis	Immediately refer to a physician.
Intestinal malrotation	Bile-stained vomitus Decrease in or lack of stool Abdominal pain	Immediately refer to a physician. Surgery is indicated. See Preparation for Hospitalization, Part 7.
Pyloric stenosis	Most common in male infants Onset usually at 3–4 wk but may begin from first week of life through 4 mo Vomiting progressing to projectile vomiting Weight loss Peristaltic waves left to right visualized during or immediately following feeding Enlarged, firm pylorus on palpation (upper right quadrant)	Same as for Intestinal malrotation, above.
Hiatal hernia	Onset of symptoms between 1 wk and 1 mo of age Forceful vomiting Elimination patterns unchanged May be family history of vomiting Diagnosis made by barium x-ray	Refer to physician. Hospitalization may be required. Treatment may include postural therapy, i.e., maintaining the infant in a sitting position of at least 60° for 24 h/day. Nurse with the baby in an infant-sized chair or harness. The position is maintained during the night. Parent(s) should keep a record of the vomiting episodes. Feedings should be small and frequent—either by breast or bottle— with thickener (Nestargel) added to the formula.
Ulcers Duodenal/peptic	May occur at any age May have strong familial history	Refer to physician. Discuss diet therapy.

Table 42-2 Medical Referral/Consultation *(continued)*

Diagnosis	Clinical Manifestations	Management
	Infant Vomiting GI bleeding Poor feeder Abdominal distention Failure to thrive Irritability Age 1–6 yr Vomiting Hemorrhage Vague abdominal pains Poor eating habits Over 6 yr Abdominal pain Vomiting GI blood loss	Antacids are helpful. Professional counselling may be indicated.
Acute appendicitis	Mild to severe pain, initially periumbilical, then right lower quadrant Contralateral rebound tenderness Possible anorexia Vomiting *following* periumbilical pain Leukocytosis	Immediately refer to a physician. Surgery is indicated. See Preparation for Hospitalization, Part 7.
Acute pyelonephritis	Toxic appearance Vomiting Abdominal pain High fever Frequency of urination Pain on urination	Consult a physician. See Pain and Burning during Urination, Chap. 76.
Metabolic disorders	May begin immediately after birth or later when specific foods introduced Vomiting Poor feeding Lethargy	Refer to a physician.
Intestinal obstruction	Colicky pain, nausea, vomiting, distention; if strangulation occurred, pain severe and constant Progressive, rapid dehydration Early shock	Immediate physician referral Abdominal decompression Medical or surgical approach to release obstruction
Acute cholecystitis	Severe right upper quadrant pain with local guarding Minimal icterus Fever Leukocytosis, low-grade hyperbilirubinemia	Immediate physician referral Conservative management (75%), bed rest Analgesics

Table 42-2 Medical Referral/Consultation *(continued)*

Diagnosis	Clinical Manifestations	Management
Viral hepatitis	Jaundice, anorexia, fatigue Abnormalities of olfaction and taste Fever between 100 and 104°F Right upper quadrant or epigastric pain Cough, coryza Dark urine, light stools Pruritis	Immediate physician referral
Increased intracranial pressure	Projectile vomiting Headache Altered level of responsiveness Bradycardia or tachycardia Elevated blood pressure Abnormal pupillary response Bulging fontanel	Immediate physician referral
Severe dehydration	Occurs easily in infants, young children, and the chronically ill, or after prolonged episodes of nausea and vomiting Poor skin turgor Dry mucous membranes of nose and mouth; dry axillary beds Decrease in ocular tension Rapid weak pulse, hypotension Muscle weakness Diminished or absent deep tendon reflexes Hemoconcentration, electrolyte imbalance	Immediate physician referral Fluid and electrolyte replacement
Labyrinthitis	Nausea, vomiting associated with vertigo, tinnitus, staggering Nystagmus either horizontal, vertical, or rotary Usually secondary to an upper respiratory infection	Physician consultation Medications: antiemetic, tranquilizer, antivertigo Bed rest with activity as tolerated
Anemia	In moderate to severe anemia: anorexia, headache, palpitations, dyspnea, ankle edema, numbness and tingling, increasing fatigability Sore tongue, angular stomatitis, thinning or spooning of nails Pale, dry, brownish skin Dry, scanty hair Pearly white sclera	Refer to a physician. Replace iron. See Anemia, Chap. 39.
Diabetic acidosis	Nausea and vomiting associated with abdominal pain and tenderness Kussmaul's respiration	Immediately refer to a physician. Replace insulin. Replace fluids and electrolytes.

Table 42-2 Medical Referral/Consultation *(continued)*

Diagnosis	Clinical Manifestations	Management
	Dehydration: dry skin, decreased ocular tension, poor urinary output, hypotension Glucose and ketonuria	See Diabetes, Chap. 147.
Carcinoma	Anorexia, abdominal discomfort, anemia, weight loss, rapid filling upon eating Mild, intermittent to constant, severe boring pain Anemia Palpable mass, enlarged nodular liver	Refer to a physician. Surgical resection is indicated. Chemotherapy is indicated. See Neoplastic Disease, Chap. 148.
Heavy metal poisoning	Accidental or intentional poisoning with antimony, arsenic, cadmium, copper, mercury, silver, thallium Nausea and vomiting, usually intense and with rapid onset	Immediate physician referral British antilewisite (BAL) treatments
Anorexia nervosa	Self-induced vomiting Profound weight loss Severe psychological disturbance: withdrawal, obsessions, depressions, delusions Vitamin deficiencies Subnormal blood pressure, temperature Delayed sexual maturity	Refer to a physician. Parental or nasogastric feeding may be indicated. Psychotherapy is indicated. Consider operant conditioning approaches. See Malnutrition, Chap. 43.
Hyperemesis gravidarum	Exaggerated nausea and vomiting during pregnancy Weight loss and dehydration Acid base imbalance Hypokalemia Hemoconcentration Oliguria	Obstetrical services referral Antiemetic Hydration

bibliography

DeAngelis, Catherine. *Pediatric primary care* (2d ed.). Boston: Little, Brown, 1979.

Gellis, Sydney S., and Kagan, Benjamin M. *Current pediatric therapy 8.* Philadelphia: Saunders, 1978.

Green, Morris, and Richmond, Julius B. *Pediatric diagnosis* (2d ed.). Philadelphia: Saunders, 1962.

Hoekelman, Robert A., et al. *Principles of pediatrics: Health care of the young.* New York: McGraw-Hill, 1978.

Illingworth, R. S. *Common symptoms of disease in children.* London: Blackwell Scientific Publications, 1975.

Thorn, G. W., et al. (eds.). *Harrison's principles of internal medicine.* New York: McGraw-Hill, 1977.

Wallach, Jacques. *Interpretation of diagnostic tests.* Boston: Little, Brown, 1974.

43 Malnutrition ELEANOR RUDICK

ALERT
Obvious extremes

I. Etiology
- **A.** Improper or inadequate food intake
- **B.** Inadequate absorption of food
- **C.** Inadequate food supply
- **D.** Poor dietary habits
- **E.** Food faddism
- **F.** Emotional factors
- **G.** Drugs
- **H.** Illness

II. Assessment: Iron Deficiency Anemia (see Anemia, Chap. 39)
- **A.** Subjective data
  1. Usually none
  2. May complain of
     - a. Pallor
     - b. Pica
     - c. Anorexia
     - d. Irritability
- **B.** Objective data
  1. Pallor
  2. Tachycardia, cardiac enlargement
  3. Systolic murmur (often)
  4. Enlarged spleen (10 to 15 percent of cases)
  5. Obesity or underweight
  6. Hematocrit less than 33; hemoglobin less than 11
  7. Occult blood in stool

Table 43-1 Medical Referral/Consultation

Diagnosis	Clinical Manifestations	Management
Malabsorption syndromes* Lactase deficiency Congenital (rare) Developmental Secondary (common)	Watery diarrhea, abdominal distention, dehydration, vomiting within hours of feeding of human or cow's milk (congenital) Symptoms developing in adolescents or young adults; high incidence in blacks and Orientals (developmental) May develop following disease which damages gastrointestinal epithelium or gastroenteritis; Stools perhaps not watery and perhaps containing fat and nitrogenous material; symptoms similar to those in congenital; may last from days to weeks—the more severe the gastroenteritis the longer the intolerance (secondary)	Refer to physician Test stool for pH (6 or less), and reducing substance (greater than + 1 = malabsorption) Blood/lactose tolerance test May biopsy small intestine Elimination of all sources of lactose Caution: prepared foods sometimes containing lactose Counsel: removal of lactose from diet Follow-up to assess chronicity Referral to public health nurse (PHN)

*See Cystic Fibrosis, Chap 144.

Table 43-1 Medical Referral/Consultation *(continued)*

Diagnosis	Clinical Manifestations	Management
Celiac sprue (childhood celiac disease of gluten-induced enteropathy)	Onset commonly in first 2 yr Chronic diarrhea Irritability Vomiting Failure to grow and to gain weight† Stools—rancid, bulky, and poorly formed	Refer to physician. See Preparation for Hospitalization, Part 7. Demonstration of impaired intestinal absorption Characteristic changes in intestinal mucosa (peroral biopsy) Beneficial response to strict gluten-free diet Refer to nutritionist for counselling on diet, care in shopping (prepared foods), and food preparation. Follow up with well-child supervision and measurements of improvement; gluten-free diet continues for the life of the individual.
Marasmus (infantile atrophy)	Failure to gain, then loss of weight, then emaciation Loss of skin turgor and subcutaneous tissue Abdomen distended or thin muscle atrophy Lowered basal metabolic rate (BMR) and blood pressure Temperature subnormal Pulse slow May be fretful, then listless Appetite diminishes Diminished responses	Immediately refer to physician. See Preparation for Hospitalization, Part 7. Rehabilitation is prolonged. Refer to PHN for home assessment and education of parent(s).
Kwashiorkor (inadequate protein intake following weaning)	Reduce physical activity Muscular weakness Apathy Irritability Gross or slight edema May have skin changes Sparse, grayish hair, pulls out easily Chronic diarrhea Anorexia	Refer immediately to physician. See Preparation for Hospitalization, Part 7. Rehabilitation is prolonged. Refer to PHN for home assessment and education of parent.
Anorexia nervosa (now seen in girls 9–14 yr of age)	Weight loss—at least 25–30 percent of body weight without evident organic basis Distortion of body image or appetite Increase of body hair Decreased temperature, pulse, blood pressure Decreased leukocyte count, amenorrhea, or delayed menses	Immediately refer to a physician. See Preparation for Hospitalization, Part 7 (as long as 3 mo). Avoid risk of circulatory collapse. Increase food intake. Separate from environment in which symptoms developed. Management is based on understanding, firmness, consistency,

†See Failure to Thrive, Chap. 134.

Table 43-1 Medical Referral/Consultation *(continued)*

Diagnosis	Clinical Manifestations	Management
	Hyperactivity—excessive energy output	low pressure for eating, and extreme patience.
	Family setting—usually emotional unavailability of mother, and warm, close relationship with father which becomes difficult at puberty	Psychotherapy for child and family may be indicated. Decision for discharge is based on all factors, not on weight gain alone. Follow up with psychiatrist. Follow up with practitioner for nutritional status.

bibliography

Baisley, Marie, et al. Nutrition in disease and stress. *Nursing Digest*, March–April:27–29 (1975).

Barnes, H. Verdain, and Berger, Ruth. An approach to the obese adolescent. *Medical Clinics of North America*, **59**(6):1507–1516 (1975).

Beal, Virginia A. Nutrition in children. In Helen M. Wallace, et al. (eds.), *Maternal and child health practices*. Springfield, Ill.: Charles C Thomas, 1973.

Birch, Herbert G. Malnutrition, learning and intelligence. *American Journal of Public Health*, **62**(6):773–784 (1972).

Center for Disease Control. *Nutrition surveillance*. Atlantic: Author, 1975.

Committee on Nutrition (AAP). Commentary on breast-feeding and infant formulas, including proposed standards for formulas. *Pediatrics*, **57**(2):278–285 (1976).

———. Nutritional aspects of vegetarianism, health foods, and fad diets. *Pediatrics*, **59**(3):460–464 (1977).

———. Special diets for infants with inborn errors of amino acid metabolism. *Pediatrics*, **57**(5):783–792 (1976).

Duffy, Thomas P. Anemia in adolescence. *The Medical Clinics of North America*, **59**(6):1481–1496 (1975).

Heald, Felix P. Adolescent nutrition. *The Medical Clinics of North America*, **59**(6):1329–1336 (1975).

McMillan, Julia A., et al. Iron sufficiency in breast-fed infants and the availability of iron from human milk. *Pediatrics*, **58**:(5):686–690 (1976).

Mauer, Alvin M. Malnutrition—Still a common problem for children in the United States. *Clinical Pediatrics*, **14**(1):23–24 (1975).

Neumann, Charlotte G., and Jelliffe, Derrick B. (eds.). Nutrition in pediatrics. *The Pediatric Clinics of North America*, **24**(1) (1977).

Pisacano, John C., et al. An attempt at prevention of obesity in infancy. *Pediatrics*, **61**(3):360–364 (1978).

Rios, Ernesto, et al. The absorption of iron as supplements in infant cereal and infant formula. *Pediatrics*, **55**(5):686–692 (1975).

Williams, Eleanor R. Making vegetarian diets nutritious. *American Journal of Nursing*, **75**(12):2168–2173 (1975).

Winick, Myron. Cellular growth during early malnutrition. *Pediatrics*, **47**(6):773–784 (1972).

44 Mouth Sores LESLIE LIETH

ALERT
1. Sudden onset of fever
2. Malaise with painful erosions involving mucous membranes
3. "Bulls-eye" lesions on dorsa of the hands, palms, extremities

I. Etiology

A. Viral
1. Herpes simplex
2. Vaccinia
3. Adenovirus
4. Varicella—zoster
5. ECHO
6. Coxsackie types

B. Fungal
1. *Candida albicans*
2. *Histoplasma capsulatum*

C. Bacterial
1. Group A beta hemolytic streptococcus
2. *Mycoplasma pneumoniae*

D. Drug reaction, side effect
1. Sulfonamides
2. Barbiturates
3. Butazones

E. Susceptibility to infection due to local traumatic factors accompanied by acute stress

F. In many cases etiology unknown

II. Assessment

A. Oral moniliasis (oral thrush)
1. Subjective data
   a. Parent(s) notes white lesions in mouth or a coated tongue.
   b. Client may have decreased appetite.
   c. Client may have increased irritability.
   d. Disease usually occurs in newborns or young infants.
2. Objective data
   a. Many times the disease is accompanied by red, inflamed diaper rash.
   b. Lesions are small white flakes or larger patches appearing on the tongue, buccal mucosa, gum margins, or lips.
   c. Culture of lesions is positive for *Candida albicans* on Nickerson's media

B. Canker sores (aphthous ulcers)
1. Subjective data
   a. Follows situations of stress
   b. Painful lesions
   c. Trouble taking food
2. Objective data
   a. Localized ulcers occurring singly and then multiplying
   b. Found on oral mucosa

C. Herpetic gingivostomatitis
1. Subjective data
   a. Headache
   b. Fever
   c. Pain or sore gums
   d. Irritability
   e. Drooling
   f. Sores on gums or in mouth
   g. Malaise
2. Objective data
   a. Documented fever
   b. Regional lymphadenopathy
   c. Red oral mucosa
   d. Lesions, usually vesicles, which progress to shallow ulcers with an erythematous halo
      (1) May involve only the gingiva, or all of the oral mucosa
      (2) Lasts 7 to 10 days

D. Streptococcal gingivitis/stomatitis
1. Subjective data
   a. Sudden onset of symptoms
   b. Localized pain on gums and/or throat
   c. Fever
   d. Anorexia
   e. Nausea and/or vomiting
   f. Headache
   g. May have history of contact with infected person
2. Objective data
   a. Throat culture positive for group A beta strep
   b. Gingiva very red, swollen, painful
   c. Inflammation (with or without exudate) usually extending to the mucosa and pharynx
   d. Localized lymphadenopathy
   e. Fever

E. Varicella
1. Subjective data
   a. Exposure to disease
   b. Usually no prodrome
   c. Fever
   d. Rash—usually starting on trunk, scalp, or face
   e. Pruritis
   f. Can have painful mouth sores
2. Objective data
   a. Lesions usually occurring in different stages at same time
   b. Lesions change from macule to papule, to vesicle with surrounding erythema, to crusted papule
   c. Distribution usually limited to trunk, scalp, face, and extremities
   d. Lesions can be seen in genital area and as ulcers in mucous membranes of the mouth, most commonly over the palate

F. Herpangina
1. Subjective data
   a. Acute onset
   b. High fever
   c. Anorexia
   d. Sore throat
   e. Headache
2. Objective data
   a. Hyperemic pharynx
   b. Lesions initially white or gray papules, later shallow ulcers 1 to 5 mm in size with red areola
   c. Lesions located on anterior pillars of the fauces, and less frequently on the palate, tonsils, uvula, and tongue

G. White-sponge nevus
1. Subjective data
   a. Chronic condition
   b. Family history of same
2. Objective data
   a. Mucosa appears white, thickened, and parboiled, and is soft and spongy to touch.
   b. Lesions involve entire oral mucosa or are distributed in patches.

III. Management

A. Oral moniliasis (thrush)
1. Treatments/medications
   a. Oral nystatin suspension (1 mL/100,000 units): Dosage is 1 to 2 mL qid administered with a dropper, slowly instilled onto the lesions before swallowing. Continue medication for 2 to 3 days after the lesions resolve or until the next visit.
   b. Less commonly used is topical application of 1% gentian violet, also placed onto lesions, tid.
2. Counselling/prevention
   a. Counsel parents of newborns about correct method of sterilization of bottles and formula.
   b. Advise that gentian violet is temporarily disfiguring and stains clothes and bed linens.
   c. Care should be taken that an excess of the gentian violet is not swallowed.
   d. Instruct regarding medication, giving written instruction if indicated.
3. Follow-up: return visit in 2 weeks
4. Consultations/referrals
   a. Refer to physician if not resolved after initial treatment.
   b. Refer to the public health nurse (PHN), if the problem is not resolving with treatment, to supervise treatment at home.

B. Canker sores (aphthous ulcers)
1. Treatments/medications
   a. Topical application of tincture of benzoin, or
   b. Topical application of gentian violet 1% solution
   c. Mouthwash with anesthetic component
2. Counselling/prevention
   a. Advise client that pain will last 5 to 10 days.
   b. Advise a bland diet.
3. Follow-up: none
4. Consultations/referrals: none

C. Herpetic gingivostomatitis
1. Treatments/medications

a. Antipyretics for fever and/or pain (aspirin or acetaminophen every 4 h as needed)
b. Bland diet
c. Encouragement of fluid intake
d. Nonprescription local anesthetics for temporary pain relief
e. Rinsing of mouth every 2 h (with mouthwash, e.g., Chloraseptic)

2. Counselling/prevention
a. Instruct on symptomatic treatment.
b. Advise that client's appetite will return when pain lessens.
c. Advise that disease is self-limiting, and lesions will last 7 to 14 days.

3. Follow-up
a. Telephone call in 2 to 3 days to report progress
b. Telephone call in 2 weeks if not resolved

4. Consultations/referrals
Physician if not resolved after 2 weeks

D. Streptococcal gingivitis/stomatitis

1. Treatments/medications
a. Oral penicillin G: Children and adults are given 200,000 or 250,000 units tid or qid for a full 10 days, or
b. Benzethine penicillin (intramuscular injection):
(1) Children—single injection of 600,000 to 900,000 units;
(2) Adults—1.2 million units,
c. For clients with penicillin allergy, oral erythromycin for 10 full days
d. Good oral hygiene (including frequent brushing and rinsing with mouthwash)
e. Encouragement of fluid intake
f. Throat cultures indicated for symptomatic family members

2. Counselling/prevention
a. Instruct on medications.
(1) Importance of giving antibiotic for 10 full days
(2) Observation for penicillin allergy
b. Explain complication of strep infection and give written explanation if available.
c. Instruct to call for results of throat cultures of those family members involved.
d. Client can return to school after 24 h if feeling better.

3. Follow-up
a. Telephone call in 1 to 3 days to report progress
b. Visit in 3 weeks to include
(1) Physical examination: skin; lymph; ear, nose, and throat (ENT); heart; blood pressure; musculoskeletal; abdomen
(2) Urinalysis and microscopic examination
(3) Throat culture

4. Consultations/referrals
a. Refer to physician for any complications
(1) Allergy to penicillin
(2) Positive culture after finishing treatment
(3) Abnormal urinalysis
(4) Signs/symptoms of urinary tract involvement
(5) Increase in blood pressure
(6) Heart murmur
(7) Complaints of painful, tender joints
b. Send letter to school nurse that the child can return to school

E. Varicella

1. Treatments/medications
a. Antipyretics for fever
b. May use oral antihistamine for itching
c. Soothing baths with oatmeal/colloidal bath powder
d. Local application of calamine lotion sometimes used for itching

2. Counselling/prevention
a. Trim the child's fingernails.
b. Soothing baths help pruritis and prevent secondary infection of lesions.
c. Advise that other children in the household not previously infected will probably contract the disease.

3. Follow-up: appointment 10 days to 2 weeks or earlier if necessary

4. Consultations/referrals
a. Reportable disease form sent to department of communicable diseases
b. Letter or phone call to school advising of diagnosis, and later, letter to school clearing child to return to classes when resolved

F. Herpangina

1. Treatments/medications
a. Antipyretics for fever
b. Mouthwashes with anesthetic if necessary

2. Counselling/prevention: Advise parent(s)/client that the fever will last 1 to 4 days and the ulcers will heal within a week.

3. Follow-up: return visit if condition worsens

4. Consultations/referrals: none

G. White-sponge nevus

1. Treatments/medications: none

2. Counselling/prevention: Advise client that condition may spread or change until adolescence and then stop.

3. Consultations/referrals: consultation with oral surgeon to confirm diagnosis

Table 44–1 Medical Referral/Consultation

Diagnosis	Clinical Manifestations	Management
Mononucleosis	Insidious or acute onset Malaise Sore throat Pharyngitis Fever Lymphadenopathy Splenomegaly Lesions, anywhere on oral mucosa, consisting of numerous small ulcers, which appear before generalized manifestation of disease Macular, generalized skin rash, most prominent on the trunk Changes in lymphocytes Positive heterophil antibody test	Referral to physician for treatment May need hospitalization (see Preparation for Hospitalization, Part 7) See Sore Throat, Chap. 30
Erythema multiforme (Stevens-Johnson syndrome)	Sudden onset of symptoms History reveals evidence of a recognized precipitant (see etiology) Lesions may be Painful erosions with hemmorrhagic crusts (can involve mucous membranes of the mouth, lips, nose, eyes, urethra, vagina, anus) Erythematous plaques, 1 to 2 cm in diameter with blue or purplish center ("bulls-eye" or "target" lesions), that may become bullous; lesions appearing on the dorsa of the hands, palms, wrists, forearms, feet, and legs Other signs and symptoms can include Malaise Fever, chills Cough Conjunctivitis Rhinitis	Refer to physician immediately (most cases need hospitalization). Treatment is symptomatic. Will include therapy for underlying cause, if known Steroid therapy used for severe cases See Preparation for Hospitalization, Part 7. Mucous membrane lesions may persist for weeks or months; advise about the importance of a bland diet and mouthwashes, as needed.

bibliography

Bhaskar, S. N. *Synopsis of oral pathology.* St. Louis: Mosby, 1965.

Gellis, Sydney, and Kagin, Benjamin. *Current pediatric therapy 8.* Philadelphia: Saunders, 1978.

Goldberg, Marshall P. The oral mucosa in children. *Pediatric Clinics of North America,* **25**:239–262 (1978).

Jones, J. H. Healthy and diseased gingiva. *Practitioner,* **214**:356–364 (1975).

Kerr, D., Ash, M. M., and Millard, H. D. *Oral diagnosis.* St. Louis: Mosby, 1974.

Rudolph, A., Barnett, H. L., and Einhorn, A. *Pediatrics* (16th ed.). New York: Appleton-Century-Crofts, 1977.

45 Gum Problems

LESLIE LIETH

ALERT

1. Necrosis of gingival margins and interdental papillae, leaving craterlike depressions
2. Sudden onset of mucous membrane lesions, accompanied by "bulls-eye" lesions on dorsa of the hands, palms, wrists, or extremities, with fever, conjunctivitis, and rhinitis
3. Chronic gingival bleeding and erythema
4. Dilantin ingestion and gingival enlargement
5. Massive hemorrhages into the skin, muscles, joints
6. Petechiae and ecchymosis in mucous membranes
7. Small, solitary, soft, red, circumscribed enlargement of gingiva

I. Etiology

A. Viral
   1. Herpes simplex
   2. Vaccinia
   3. Adenovirus

B. Fungal
   1. *Candida albicans*
   2. *Histoplasma capsulatum*

C. Bacterial
   1. Group A beta hemolytic streptococcus
   2. *Mycoplasma pneumoniae*

D. Drug reaction, side effect
   1. Dilantin
   2. Sulfonamides
   3. Barbiturates
   4. Butazones

E. Susceptibility to infection due to
   1. Chronic diseases (i.e., diabetes mellitus, etc.)
   2. Hormonal changes (pregnancy, puberty)
   3. Bacterial plaque adhering to teeth
   4. Local traumatic factors accompanied by acute stress

II. Assessment

A. Herpetic gingivostomatitis
   1. Subjective data
      a. Headache
      b. Fever
      c. Pain or sore gums
      d. Irritability
      e. Drooling
      f. Sores on gums or in mouth
      g. Malaise
   2. Objective data
      a. Documented fever
      b. Regional lymphadenopathy
      c. Red oral mucosa
      d. Lesions, usually vesicles, which progress to shallow ulcers with an erythematous halo
         (1) May involve only the gingiva, or all of the oral mucosa
         (2) Lasts 7 to 10 days

B. Streptococcal gingivitis/stomatitis
   1. Subjective data
      a. Sudden onset of symptoms
      b. Localized pain on gums and/or throat
      c. Fever
      d. Anorexia
      e. Nausea and/or vomiting
      f. Headache
      g. May have history of contact with infected person
   2. Objective data
      a. Throat culture positive for group A beta streptococcus

b. Gingiva very red, swollen, painful
c. Inflammation (with or without exudate) usually extending to the mucosa and pharynx
d. Localized lymphadenopathy
f. Fever

C. Eruption gingivitis
1. Subjective data
a. Localized gingival pain or soreness
b. Drooling
c. Irritability
d. Decreased appetite
2. Objective data
Localized inflammatory reaction occurring about an erupting tooth

D. Oral moniliasis (oral thrush)
1. Subjective data
a. White lesions in mouth or coated tongue
b. May have decreased appetite
c. May have increased irritability
d. Usually occurs in newborns or young infants
2. Objective data
a. Many times the disease is accompanied by red, inflamed diaper rash.
b. Lesions are small white flakes or larger patches appearing on the tongue, buccal mucosa, gum margins, or lips.
c. Culture of lesions is positive for *C. albicans* on Nicherson's media.

III. Management

A. Herpetic gingivostomatitis
1. Treatments/medications
a. Antipyretics for fever and/or pain (aspirin or acetaminophen q4h, prn)
b. Bland diet
c. Encourage fluid intake
d. Nonprescription local anesthetics for temporary pain relief
f. Rinsing of mouth every 2 h (with mouthwash, e.g., Chloraseptic)
2. Counselling/prevention
a. Instruct on symptomatic treatment.
b. Advise that the client's appetite will return when the pain lessens.
c. Advise that the disease is self-limiting and lesions will last 7 to 14 days.
3. Follow-up
a. Telephone call in 2 to 3 days to report progress
b. Telephone call in 2 weeks if not resolved
4. Consultations/referrals
Physician if not resolved after 2 weeks

B. Streptococcal gingivitis/stomatitis
1. Treatments/medications
a. Oral penicillin G for 10 full days, or
b. Benzathine penicillin (intramuscular injection), or
c. For clients with penicillin allergy, oral erythromycin for 10 full days
d. Good oral hygiene (including frequent brushing and rinsing with mouthwash)
e. Encouragement of fluid intake
f. Throat cultures indicated for symptomatic family members
2. Counselling/prevention
a. Instruct on medications.
(1) Importance of giving antibiotic for 10 full days
(2) Observation for penicillin allergy
b. Explain complication of strep infection and give written explanation if available.
c. Instruct to call for results of throat cultures of those family members involved.
d. Client can return to school after 24 h if feeling better.
3. Follow-up
a. Telephone call in 1 to 3 days to report progress
b. Visit in 3 weeks to include
(1) Physical examination: skin; lymph; ear, nose, and throat; heart; blood pressure; musculoskeletal; abdomen
(2) Urinalysis and microscopic examination
(3) Throat culture
4. Consultations/referrals
a. Refer to physician for any complications
(1) Allergy to penicillin
(2) Positive culture after finishing treatment
(3) Abnormal urinalysis
(4) Increase in blood pressure
(5) Heart murmur
(6) Signs or symptoms of urinary tract involvement
(7) Complaints of painful, tender joints
b. Send letter to the school nurse that the child can return to school.

C. Eruption gingivitis
1. Treatments/medications
a. For nonmolars: local anesthetics (nonprescription) applied to gum; teething ring
b. For molars: frequent mouthwashes for food particles under skin
2. Counselling/prevention
Advise that appetite will decrease until resolved.
3. Follow-up

Client/parent should telephone if situation not resolved after 5 to 7 days.

4. Consultations/referrals

If molar: Refer to dentist if infected or inflamed.

D. Oral moniliasis (thrush)

1. Treatments/medications
   a. Oral nystatin suspension (1 mL/100,000 units). Dosage is 1 to 2 mL qid administered with a dropper, slowly instilled onto lesions before swallowing. Continue medication for 2 to 3 days after the lesions resolve or until the next visit.
   b. Less commonly used is topical application of 1% gentian violet, also placed onto lesions, tid.
2. Counselling/prevention
   a. Counsel parents of newborns about the correct method of sterilizing bottles and formula.
   b. Advise that gentian violet is temporarily disfiguring and stains clothes and bed linens.
   c. Care should be taken that an excess of the gentian violet is not swallowed.
   d. Instruct regarding medication, giving written instruction if indicated.
3. Follow-up: visit in 2 weeks
4. Consultations/referrals
   a. Refer to physician if not resolved after initial treatment.
   b. Refer to the public health nurse (PHN), if the problem is not resolving with treatment, to supervise treatment at home.

Table 45–1 Medical Referral/Consultation

Diagnosis	Clinical Manifestations	Management
Vincent's infection (trench mouth)	Necrosis of gingival margins and interdental papillae, leaving craterlike depressions Lesions covered with gray or grayish-yellow pseudomembrane, which is easily removed leaving bleeding ulcer Erythematous appearance of lesion margins Lesions involving either a small area or all of the teeth Other signs and symptoms Pain of varying degrees Excessive salivation Wedging sensation of teeth Foul breath odor Local lymphadenopathy Fever Malaise Anorexia Other systemic manifestations	Referral to physician and/or dentist Counselling Bland diet Mouthwashes every 2 h and as needed, with Chloraseptic or half-strength peroxide
Erythema multiforme (Stevens-Johnson syndrome)	Sudden onset of symptoms History reveals evidence of a recognized precipitant (see etiology) Lesions may be Painful erosions with hemmorrhagic crusts Can involve mucous membranes of the mouth, lips, nose, eyes, urethra, vagina, anus Erythematous plaques, 1 to 2 cm	Referral to physician immediately (most cases needing hospitalization) Treatment is symptomatic Will include therapy for underlying cause if known Steroid therapy for severe cases Counselling/prevention See Preparation for Hospitalization, Part 7. Mucous membrane lesions may persist for weeks or months;

Table 45-1 Medical Referral/Consultation *(continued)*

Diagnosis	Clinical Manifestations	Management
	in diameter with blue or purplish center ("bulls-eye" or "target" lesions), that may become bullous Lesions appear on the dorsa of the hands, palms, wrists, forearms, feet, legs Other signs and symptoms can include Malaise Fever, chills Cough Conjunctivitis Rhinitis	advise concerning the importance of a bland diet and mouthwashes as needed.
Periodontitis	Chronic condition Red swollen gingiva Pressure to gums may cause bleeding or exudation of pus Recession of gingiva Teeth sometimes loose and/or separating from the gum	Referral to dentist Counselling/prevention Good dental hygiene, with frequent tooth brushing Follow-up at dentist at least every 6 mo
Gingival hyperplasia	History of ingestion of Dilantin Generalized enlargement of gingiva Pale, firm, granular appearance of gingiva Can have some bleeding of gums	Referral to dentist Counselling/prevention Same as for periodontitis, but, also Support to client and family because it is a chronic condition
Hormonal gingivitis	Enlargement of gingival tissues Tissue soft, spongy, bluish-red Tendency for tissues to bleed Presence of predisposing hormonal changes (puberty or pregnancy)	Treatment and management same as for periodontitis, except can assure client this is usually a temporary condition
Scurvy (vitamin C deficiency)	Petechial or massive hemorrhages into the skin, muscles, joints, etc. Osteoporosity Slow wound healing Reduction in resistance to infection Digestive disturbances with loss of appetite Low-grade fever Vague symptoms of irritability which become progressively worse Pseudoparalysis of legs sometimes occurring with edema	Referral to physician for treatment of disease Referral to dentist Treatment with ascorbic acid, either oral or parenterally, or foods high in same Counselling/prevention Prevent by maintaining infants and children on vitamin C, either in vitamin supplements or in orange or tomato juice. A breast-feeding woman should take a minimum of 150 mg of vitamin C per day. Advise not to boil juices.

Table 45-1 Medical Referral/Consultation *(continued)*

Diagnosis	Clinical Manifestations	Management
	Depression of the sternum Anemia usually present Oral changes include Petechiae and ecchymoses in the mucous membranes Hyperemia, edema, and enlargement of gingiva Increased bleeding tendency of gingiva Loosening of teeth Loss of teeth Secondary infections, i.e., Vincent's infection	Follow-up visits depend on the severity of the symptoms.
Gingivitis as a side effect of chronic disease	History of or suspicion of systemic chronic disease, i.e., diabetes, leukemia Generalized enlargement of gingiva Painful gingiva Increased bleeding tendency of gingiva Loosening of teeth Increased susceptibility to ulcerations, infections	Management same as for periodontitis
Gumboil (parulis or periodontal abscess)	Small, solitary, soft, red, circumscribed enlargement of gingiva Minimal gingival discomfort May be history of similar episode in same area which ruptured and exuded pus	Referral to dentist Drainage and correction of periodontal disease is indicated. See also management for periodontitis.

bibliography

Bhaskar, S. N. *Synopsis of oral pathology.* St. Louis: Mosby, 1965.

Gellis, Sydney, and Kagin, Benjamin. *Current pediatric therapy 8.* Philadelphia: Saunders, 1978.

Jones, J. H. Healthy and diseased gingiva. *Practitioner,* **214**:356–364(1975).

Kerr, D., Ash, M. M., and Millard, H. D. *Oral diagnosis.* St. Louis: Mosby, 1974.

Rudolph, A., Barnett, H. L., and Einhorn, A. *Pediatrics* (16th ed.). New York: Appleton-Century-Crofts, 1977.

46 Abdominal Distention

MARILYN GREBIN

The causes of abdominal distention are listed in this chapter. The practitioner should be concerned with recognizing the signs and symptoms of the diagnosis, eliciting a history, and performing a physical examination on the client who does not appear critically ill. The final diagnosis will be assigned after the physician examines and tests the client.

ALERT

1. Toxic appearance
2. Rectal bleeding
3. Blood in vomitus
4. Hematuria
5. High fever
6. Dehydration
7. Recent trauma
8. Dyspnea
9. Cyanosis
10. Severe abdominal pain
11. Signs of shock

I. Etiology

A. Congenital disorders
B. Infection
C. Neoplastic disease
D. Metabolic disorders
E. Obstructive disorders
F. Trauma
G. Emotional disorders

II. Management

A. Explain to client/parent(s).
1. Medications and treatments
2. Specific medical procedures
3. Specific surgical intervention as determined by the physician

B. See Preparation for Hospitalization, Part 7.

Table 46-1 Medical Referral/Consultation

Diagnosis	Clinical Manifestations	Management
Megacolon (Hirschsprung's disease) (congenital)	*First week of life* Failure to pass meconium Anorexia Vomiting of bile Abdominal distention Rapid breathing Irritability Appearance—failure to thrive *Infancy* Severe diarrhea Abdominal distention Vomiting	Immediate referral to the physician

Table 46-1 Medical Referral/Consultation *(continued)*

Diagnosis	Clinical Manifestations	Management
	Childhood Obstipation—stool has offensive odor, ribbonlike appearance Prominent abdominal vasculature Peristaltic waves Palpable fecal masses	
Prune-belly syndrome (congenital)*	Deficiency of the abdominal musculature with bulging of abdominal structures Cryptorchidism Urinary tract anomalies (found on x-ray) Megaloureter Cystic renal dysplasia Urethral obstruction Megacysts Patent urachus Meatal stenosis More prevalent in males than females by 5%	Referral to urologist Abdominal binder
Fetal ascites (congenital)	Abdominal distention Flattening of the umbilicus Fluid wave present	Immediate referral to the physician
Intestinal duplication (congenital)	Abdominal distention Colicky pain Rectal bleeding Partial or total obstruction Palpable masses may be present	Immediate referral to surgeon
Malrotation and volvulus (congenital)	High obstruction within first 3 wk of life Vomiting of bile Upper abdominal distention Visible peristalsis Melena or currant-jelly stools	Immediate referral to surgeon
Colonic stenosis or atresia (congenital)	Absence of meconium Obstipation Abdominal distention Vomiting With stenosis—failure to thrive and diarrhea are present	Immediate referral to surgeon
Imperforate anus (congenital)	Failure to pass meconium Abdominal distention Bulging of the anal membrane	Referral to surgeon
Appendiceal abscess (infection)	Abdominal distention	Immediate referral to surgeon

*Usually occurs only once in a family

Table 46-1 Medical Referral/Consultation *(continued)*

Diagnosis	Clinical Manifestations	Management
	Palpable mass in the right lower quadrant of the abdomen High fever Generalized or localized peritonitis White cell count may be elevated	
Peritonitis (infection)	Rapid onset of Abdominal distention Severe abdominal pain Absence of bowel sounds Vomiting Abdominal tenderness High fever Toxic appearance Rapid pulse Abdominal rigidity or soft resistance Tenderness on rectal exam	Immediate referral to physician
Pancreatitis (infection)	Abdominal distention slight Abdominal pain and tenderness Nausea and vomiting Pale color to skin Mild scleral icterus Diminished bowel sounds Palpable epigastric mass Positive Cullen's sign (bluish discoloration around umbilicus) Signs of parotitis in 50% of cases	Immediate referral to physician
Glomerulonephritis (infection)	Positive history of pharyngitis or impetigo Darkly colored urine Facial edema or periorbital edema Decreased urinary output Flank or midline abdominal pain Irritability Low-grade fever Acute hypertension Enlarged liver	Refer to the physician after the results of complete blood count (CBC), urinalysis, chest x-ray, and electrolytes are obtained.
Gastroenteritis (nonspecific) (infection)	Abdominal distention Vomiting (6–24 h) Fever Diarrhea Tympanic sound on abdominal percussion Cramping pain	Refer to the physician all infants and children who appear dehydrated See Diarrhea/Loose Stools, Chap. 47

Table 46-1 Medical Referral/Consultation *(continued)*

Diagnosis	Clinical Manifestations	Management
	Increased bowel sounds Possible signs of dehydration (may or may not be present)	
Necrotizing enterocolitis (infection)	Neonatal age group History of fever in the mother History of early ruptured membranes Abdominal distention Vomiting Blood-streaked diarrhea Shock and sepsis	Immediate referral to physician
Wilms' tumor (neoplastic)	Abdominal distention and pain Fever Abdominal mass which does not cross the midline (firm and nontender in the renal area) Possible hypertension	Immediate referral to physician
Neuroblastoma (neoplastic)	Abdominal distention Palpable mass which crosses the midline	Immediate referral to physician
Ovarian cysts and tumors (neoplastic)	Abdominal pain Gradual abdominal enlargement Functional tumors may precipitate precocity	Immediate referral to gynecologist
Mesenteric cyst (neoplastic)	Rare in infants and children Most cases are asymptomatic Increasing abdominal distention Palpable, smooth, round, nontender mobile masses	Referral to physician
Pancreatic cyst (neoplastic)	Asymptomatic Abdominal distention May appear after abdominal trauma	Immediate referral to physician
Liver tumor, primary or metastatic (neoplastic)	$>$ boys than girls Abdominal pain or discomfort Abdominal distention Palpable abdominal mass Anorexia and weight loss Fatigue Pallor Signs of hypoglycemia	Immediate referral to physician

Table 46-1 Medical Referral/Consultation *(continued)*

Diagnosis	Clinical Manifestations	Management
Malabsorption (general presentation of all or some of the findings depending on the causative agent) (metabolic)	Onset of symptoms with food intake History of abdominal surgery History of infections Visits out of the country Failure to thrive Weight loss and anorexia Fever Peripheral edema Alterations of texture in skin and hair Clubbed fingers Abdominal tenderness and distention Evidence of bony deformities Anemia Muscle weakness Irritability	Refer to physician for workup. The practitioner may assist the physician in the counselling of the parent(s) and in the follow-up once the diagnosis is assigned.
Constipation (obstruction)	See Constipation/Fecal Impaction, Chap. 49.	See Constipation/Fecal Impaction, Chap. 49.
Air or fluid distention in the bowel (obstruction)	Abdominal distention Irritability Abnormal feeding habits Increased flatus	Observe parent and child during feeding. Counsel regarding Quiet, happy environment during feeding to decrease anxieties Small, frequent feedings Frequent burping of infants Avoidance of gassy foods for children
Perforated viscus (obstruction)	Anorexia Vomiting Abdominal distention Dyspnea and cyanosis	Immediate referral to physician
Hydronephrosis (obstruction)	Infants Abdominal mass Abdominal distention Children Abdominal cramping Hematuria	Referral to physician
Intestinal obstruction (obstruction)	History of maternal hydramnios Vomiting of bile Abdominal distention Failure to pass meconium Obstipation	Immediate referral to surgeon

Table 46-1 Medical Referral/Consultation *(continued)*

Diagnosis	Clinical Manifestations	Management
	Family history of congenital anomalies Aspiration of feedings	
Paralytic ileus (obstruction)	Abdominal distention Absence of bowel sounds Minimum pain Obstipation	Immediate referral to surgeon
Cystic fibrosis (obstruction)	Respiratory findings Cough with thick mucus Noisy respirations (rhonchi, wheezing) History of recurrent upper respiratory infections Increased respiratory rate Digital clubbing Cyanosis Positive sweat test Gastrointestinal findings Intestinal obstruction Malabsorption and failure to thrive (despite a large appetite) Abdominal distention and ascites Abdominal pain Steatorrhea with mild diarrhea	Refer to the physician. See Cystic Fibrosis, Chap. 144.
Meckel's diverticulum (obstruction)	Painless rectal bleeding Anemia Abdominal pain and distention	Immediate referral to surgeon
Intussusception (obstruction)	Abdominal pain Vomiting Currant-jelly stools Prostration and fever Abdominal tenderness and distention Palpable sausage-shaped mass in the abdomen Diarrhea or constipation	Immediate referral to surgeon
Herniae (obstruction)	Inguinal Swelling of the inguinal area Tenderness and pain Nausea and vomiting Abdominal distention	Refer to the surgeon for evaluation and timing of repair. See Herniae, Chap. 55.
	Umbilical Protrusion of the umbilicus	Refer to the surgeon. Repair is done after age 2 yr. See Herniae, Chap. 55.
Ulcer (obstruction)	Irritability	Referral to surgeon

Table 46-1 Medical Referral/Consultation *(continued)*

Diagnosis	Clinical Manifestations	Management
	Hematemesis Abdominal distention Tarry stools Excessive hunger pains in children Abdominal pain	Management by the practitioner for diet counselling, as recommended by physician
Pyloric stenosis (obstruction)	Distention of the upper abdomen Projectile vomiting Constipation Poor weight gain Gastric peristaltic waves Olive-size mass palpated to the right of the umbilicus	Referral to surgeon
Bezoar (obstruction)	History of tricophagy (habit of eating hair) Pain and distention of the upper abdomen Anorexia and weight loss Occasional vomiting	Referral to surgeon
Ruptured spleen (trauma)	History of trauma Abdominal pain Vomiting Abdominal tenderness Abdominal rigidity and distention Pallor Rapid circulatory collapse	Immediate referral to surgeon
Lacerated liver (trauma)	History of trauma Abdominal distention Right flank tenderness Dullness to percussion of the abdomen Signs of acute abdomen shock Signs of shock	Immediate referral to surgeon
Hematoma of the abdominal wall (trauma)	History of trauma Abdominal distention Discoloration of injured area Palpable tender mass Area of trauma sometimes feels warm	Immediate referral to physician
Psychogenic constipation (emotional)	See Constipation/Fecal Impaction, Chap. 49.	See Constipation/Fecal Impaction, Chap. 49.

Table 46-1 Medical Referral/Consultation *(continued)*

Diagnosis	Clinical Manifestations	Management
Urinary retention (emotional)	Observation of parent-child relationship History of poor urinary output Dull percussion over bladder area Evidence of positive urine culture Pain or tenderness over the bladder area	Urine culture Examination for anomalies of external genitalia Referral to physician Parent/client counselling to decrease anxieties Psychological evaluation

bibliography

Gellis, Sydney. Prune Belly Syndrome: Report of 20 cases and description of Lethal variant. In *The 1975 yearbook of pediatrics*. Chicago: Year Book, 1975, pp. 254–255. (Presented by Rogers, L. W., and Ostrow, P. T., in *Journal of Pediatrics*, 83:786–793, 1973.)

Silverman, A., Roy, C., Cozzetto, F. *Pediatric clinical gastroenterology* (2d ed.). St. Louis: Mosby, 1975.

Vaughn, Victor C., McKay, James R. *Nelson textbook of pediatrics* (10th ed.). Philadelphia: Saunders, 1975.

47 Diarrhea/Loose Stools

JANE A. FOX

ALERT
1. Bloody diarrhea
2. Prolonged and persistent diarrhea
3. Infants less than 4 months of age
4. Signs of dehydration

I. Etiology

A. Acute diarrhea
  1. Infectious
    a. Viral (nonspecific gastroenteritis)
    b. Bacterial gastroenteritis
    c. Parenteral infections
    d. Parasites
  2. Noninfectious
    a. Food intolerance/dietary indiscretion
    b. Antibiotics (antibacterial agents)
    c. Poison ingestion/laxatives
    d. Constipation—pseudodiarrhea

B. Chronic diarrhea
  1. Food/milk allergy
  2. Irritable colon syndrome
  3. Inflammatory bowel disease
  4. Malabsorption syndromes
  5. Genetic disorders
  6. Anatomical/mechanical disorders
  7. Malnutrition

II. Assessment

A. Viral (nonspecific) gastroenteritis
  1. Subjective data
    a. Acute onset
    b. Vomiting followed by diarrhea
    c. Abdominal pain
    d. May be associated with upper respiratory infection (URI) or otitis media
    e. Other family members perhaps having similar symptoms
  2. Objective data
    a. Afebrile, or low-grade fever
    b. Generalized abdominal tenderness
    c. Hyperactive bowel sounds
    d. May be dehydrated

B. Food intolerance/dietary factors
  1. Subjective data
    a. History revealing overfeeding or underfeeding or addition of new foods to diet
    b. Improper formula or formula preparation
    c. Frequent loose or watery stools
    d. Slight abdominal cramps immediately before bowel movement
  2. Objective data
    a. Usually afebrile
    b. No localized abdominal tenderness
    c. Hyperactive bowel sounds

C. Food/milk allergy (allergic gastroenteritis)
  1. Subjective data
    a. Most frequently first year of life
    b. Food allergy
      (1) Can be related to any portion of gastrointestinal tract
      (2) Diarrhea with increased mucus; possibly streaked with blood
    c. Milk allergy
      (1) Diarrhea only when whole milk given
      (2) Milk substitutes—no diarrhea
      (3) Diarrhea reoccurring when milk reintroduced
    d. Vomiting
    e. Abdominal pain/cramping
    f. Systemic manifestations or history of
      (1) Eczema
      (2) Rhinitis

(3) Asthma
(4) Headache
(5) Behavioral changes

2. Objective data
   a. Generalized abdominal tenderness
   b. Hyperactive bowel sounds
   c. Possible fever
   d. Weight loss or no weight gain
   e. Eosinophilia

D. Diarrhea from antibacterial therapy

1. Subjective data
   a. Currently receiving antibiotics
   b. Most commonly involved drugs
      (1) Ampicillin
      (2) Neomycin
      (3) Tetracycline
   c. Mild abdominal cramps
2. Objective data
   a. Generalized abdominal tenderness
   b. Hyperactive bowel sounds

E. Parenteral infections

1. Subjective data
   a. Current illness
      (1) Upper respiratory infection
      (2) Otitis media
      (3) Urinary tract infection
2. Objective data
   a. Physical findings concurring with present illness
   b. Hyperactive bowel sounds

F. Pinworms

1. Subjective data
   a. Anal itching
   b. Restlessness
   c. Insomnia
   d. Hyperactivity
2. Objective data
   Cellophane tape perianal impression taken first thing in the morning on consecutive days: positive for ova

G. Constipation/pseudodiarrhea

1. Subjective data—encopresis with diarrhea
2. Objective data—rectal examination revealing rectum containing large masses of feces

III. Management

A. Viral (nonspecific) gastroenteritis

1. Treatments/medications—diet modification and restriction
   a. Initial 24 h
      (1) Clear fluids should be given, i.e., water, flat soda, Jello-O, Jell-O water, Kool-Aid, Hi-C, Hawaiian Punch, tea without sugar.
      (2) Avoid milk and fruit juices.
      (3) Offer child 2 oz of clear fluid every 1 to 2 h as tolerated; gradually increase to 4 or 5 oz every 4 to 6 h.
      (4) Clear fluids should not be continued for more than 48 h; reactive loose stools may occur.
   b. Second 24 h
      (1) Infant
         (a) Dilute usual formula to half strength, or dilute skim milk with half water.
         (b) Increase formula volume slowly over 18 h.
         (c) After 18 h, return to regular formula.
      (2) Older child/adolescent/young adult. Begin bland solids, i.e., bananas, rice, cereal, saltines, Ritz crackers, dry cereal, apples/apple puree, pears, boiled eggs, lean meats, chicken, custard, pudding, toast with jelly
   c. Third day: regular diet, as tolerated
2. Counselling/prevention
   a. Instruction on signs of dehydration
   b. Review of diet restrictions
   c. Importance of good fluid intake
   d. Telephone call or return visit if
      (1) Symptoms persisting for more than 24 h after treatment initiated
      (2) High or prolonged fever
      (3) Decrease in urinary output
      (4) Blood or mucus in stool
      (5) Currant-jelly-type stool with severe abdominal pain (intussusception, complication in children 3 months to 2 years of age)
      (6) Unable to retain fluids
      (7) Stomach becomes distended
      (8) Excessive water loss in stool (diaper soaked)
      (9) Child refusing bottle
   e. Telephone call for laboratory results
3. Follow-up
   a. Close follow-up important
   b. Daily weights
4. Consultations/referrals: usually none

B. Food intolerance/dietary factors

1. Treatments/medications
   a. Decrease sugar in the formula.
   b. Eliminate the causative agent from the diet.
2. Counselling/prevention
   a. Proper formula preparation and feeding techniques
   b. Instruction to client/parent to keep food diary if happens again

3. Follow-up: telephone call regarding progress
4. Consultations/referrals: none

C. Food/milk allergy

1. Treatments/medications
   a. Eliminate causative food.
   b. Eliminate cow's milk from diet and begin soy bean formula.
2. Counselling/prevention
   a. Have client/parent keep a food diary, recording
      (1) Time and type of food intake
      (2) Type of gastrointestinal symptoms experienced
3. Follow-up
   a. Telephone contact as needed
   b. Return visit in 2 weeks
4. Consultations/referrals: refer to an allergist

D. Diarrhea from antibacterial therapy

1. Treatments/medications
   a. Stop oral administration of the causative drug.
   b. Begin a lactose-free diet.
2. Counselling/prevention: see III, A, 2 above
3. Follow-up: see III, A, 3 above
4. Consultations/referrals: none

E. Parenteral infections: see Viral (nonspecific) gastroenteritis, III, A

F. Pinworms *(Enterobius vermicularis)*: see Pinworms, Chap. 53

1. Treatments/medications—Mebendazole 100 mg, chewable tablet, single dose for all ages
2. Counselling/prevention
   a. Life cycle of parasite
   b. Probability of reinfection
   c. Normal hygiene and cleanliness
   d. Hand washing and fingernail cleanliness
   e. Animals not responsible for transmission of pinworm infection
3. Follow-up
   a. Symptoms commonly reoccur.
   b. If there is frequent reinfection, simultaneously treat all family members every 2 weeks for a total of three doses.
4. Consultations/referrals: public health nurse (PHN) for those with frequent reinfection

G. Constipation/pseudodiarrhea

1. Treatments/medications
   a. Digital removal of ampullary impaction
   b. Followed by two to four consecutive isotonic enemas in a 24- to 36-h period, until clear return
   c. Retraining program to establish regular bowel pattern
      (1) Ingestion of bulk foodstuffs
      (2) Mineral oil—5 mL in morning and evening
      (3) Regular, relaxed visits to the toilet
2. Counselling/prevention
   a. The cooperation and patience of motivated parent(s) and child are needed.
   b. Review all procedures and medications.
   c. Outline the goals of the "retraining" program.
   d. Offer support and praise.
3. Follow-up: weekly visits to offer support and examine for constipation
4. Consultations/referrals: consultation with physician

Table 47-1 Medical Referral/Consultation

Diagnosis	Clinical Manifestations	Management
Escherichia coli gastroenteritis	Most common in children less than 18 mo Produces two types of presenting symptoms Type I Fever Sudden onset of explosive, watery stools Stools perhaps containing mucus, pus, blood Type II Gradual onset Afebrile Foul-smelling, green, slimy, loose stools Stool culture and rectal swab positive for *E. coli*	Neomycin 100 mg/kg per day orally in three divided doses for 3–5 days Counselling Stool precautions Hospitalization sometimes indicated See Viral (nonspecific) gastroenteritis Daily follow-up, more frequently depending on condition Consultation with physician Referral to public health nurse (PHN)

Table 47-1 Medical Referral/Consultation *(continued)*

Diagnosis	Clinical Manifestations	Management
Salmonellosis	Follows ingestion of contaminated food Nausea, vomiting Headache Abdominal pain Fever Green, loose stools with odor of spoiling eggs Hyperactive peristalsis Mild abdominal tenderness Stool culture positive for *Salmonella*	Consultation with physician Diet restrictions—see Treatments/medications, III, A, 1 Counselling Careful hand washing/hygiene techniques Organism excreted for several weeks Stool precautions Follow-up: as needed Referral to PHN and report to health department
Shigellosis	Abrupt onset Abdominal cramps Fever and chills Cloudy sensorium Severe forms: frequent, explosive, watery, yellow-green stools, may contain blood-specked mucus Stool culture positive for shigellosis	Referral to physician Severe forms: ampicillin the drug of choice Counselling Stool precautions See, Counselling/prevention, III, A, 2 Close follow-up—telephone and return visits as needed Referral to PHN and report to health department
Staphylococcus aureus	Follows ingestion of contaminated food Suspect if entire family or large group of people have similar symptoms Severe nausea Vomiting with retching Abdominal pain Low-grade fever or afebrile Watery, loose stool Stool sometimes containing blood and mucus Stool culture positive for *Staphylococcus*	For diet restrictions, see Treatments/medications, III, A, 1 above. Refer severe cases to a physician.
Amebiasis (parasites)	Intermittent episodes of four to six liquid, bloody, mucoid stools per day Constipation present between diarrhea episodes Abdominal pain Nausea Low-grade fever Possibly asymptomatic Culture of freshly passed, warm stool positive for specific organism	Refer to physician Medication should be prescribed only by a physician See Pinworms, III, F, above, and Chap. 53. Follow-up with two or more fecal examinations at weekly intervals after completion of treatment. Refer to PHN.
Poison ingestion/laxatives	History confirming ingestion of poison Iron Arsenic (ant poison) Insecticides	Refer immediately to a physician. See Poisoning, Chap. 170

Table 47-1 Medical Referral/Consultation *(continued)*

Diagnosis	Clinical Manifestations	Management
	Abrupt onset Generalized abdominal cramps Nausea/vomiting Large, nonbloody, explosive stools	Laxatives are to be used in children only when prescribed. Refer to PHN.
Irritable colon syndrome	Family history of irritable colon	
	Pediatric client: 6 mo to 4 yr	
	Loose, foul-smelling, mucus-streaked stools, 3–5 times daily, usually in the morning Normal growth and development	Consultation with physician Therapeutic intervention not beneficial Normal diet: 90% cured by 3–4 yr of age *No* laxatives or iced or chilled foods Offer reassurance and support to parent(s) Follow-up—every 4–8 wks to plot height and weight and continue offering reassurance to parent(s)
	Adolescent/young adult	
	Alternating constipation and diarrhea Abdominal pain, especially when constipated Mucus accompanying hard bowel movements History most important in revealing factors which exacerbate or alleviate symptoms	Consultation with physician Diagnostic procedures: sigmoidoscopy and barium enema sometimes indicated Recommendations of good sleep patterns and good diet For constipation: large amounts of cooked or raw fruits and vegetables; bran Large amounts of fluid No laxatives or enemas Follow-up—as needed every 3–6 wk Notification of school nurse
Inflammatory bowel disease	Acute or chronic diarrhea Weight loss Abdominal pain Fever Blood in stool Anemia Other systemic signs may be present	Referral to physician Hospitalization sometimes necessary High-protein, high-carbohydrate, normal fat, high-vitamin diet Small, frequent meals Activity according to ability Combination of drugs sometimes effective Antidiarrheal agents Opiates (acute attacks) Anticholinergic agents to decrease rectal spasm Aspirin Psychotherapy Counselling/prevention Description of disease Compliance with treatment regimen Support and reassurance

Table 47-1 Medical Referral/Consultation *(continued)*

Diagnosis	Clinical Manifestations	Management
		Follow-up—telephone call daily in exacerbation period Notification of school nurse, school teacher, PHN
Malabsorption syndrome	Failure to thrive Height and weight not increasing Abdominal distention Foul-smelling, pale, greasy, bulky stools, which contain large amounts of fat Abdominal pain Vomiting	Referral to a physician

bibliography

Gangarosa, Eugene J. Recent developments in diarrheal diseases, *Postgraduate Medicine,* **62**:113 (1977).

Gellis, Sydney S., and Kagan, Benjamine M. *Current Pediatric Therapy 8*. Philadelphia: Saunders 1978, pp. 185–196, 203, 239, 574–576, 591.

Ling, Syllis, and McCammon, Sarah P. Dietary treatment of diarrhea and constipation in infants and children, *Issues in Comprehensive Pediatric Nursing* 3:17–28 (October 1978).

Silverman, A. Roy, C., and Cozetto, F. *Pediatric clinical gastroenterology*. St. Louis: Mosby 1975.

Tallett, Susan, et. al. Clinical, laboratory and epidemiological features of a viral gastroenteritis in infants and children. *Pediatrics,* **60**:217–222, (August 1977).

48 Infantile Colic

THERESA M. ELDRIDGE

Infantile colic is a symptom complex characterized by paroxysmal abdominal pain, presumably of intestinal origin, and severe crying. Colic attacks 11 to 23 percent of full-term and low-birth-weight infants. It is equally divided between male and female, breast-fed and bottle-fed babies, and it is seen primarily in Caucasians.

ALERT
1. Projectile vomiting
2. Signs and symptoms of dehydration
3. Signs and symptoms of shock
4. Bloody stools

I. Etiology

A. Gastrointestinal
1. Air swallowing
2. Hunger
3. Food allergy
4. Immaturity of gastrointestinal tract
5. Fat malabsorption
6. Lactose intolerance
7. Gastroesophogeal reflux
8. Hypermobility of gastrointestinal system

B. Environmental
1. Parental attitudes
2. Fatigue
3. Reaction to environmental stimuli

C. Central nervous system immaturity

II. Assessment

A. Subjective data
1. Age: Birth to 6 months
2. Onset usually late afternoon/evening (6 to 10 p.m.), sudden, occurring same time every day
3. Parent(s) reporting loud, continuous paroxysms of crying lasting one-half to several hours; distended, firm abdomen; legs drawn up to abdomen; flushed face or circumoral pallor; flatulence; rhythmic cry or scream; symptoms frequently following feeding
4. Possible history of gastroenteritis or other illness
5. May have history of allergies to milk, other foods

B. Objective data
1. Legs drawn up to abdomen; distress
2. Abdomen: firm, distended; flatulence
3. Laboratory data normal

III. Management

A. Treatments/medications (when supportive treatment not successful)
1. Antispasmodics
2. Sedatives
3. Antihistamines

B. Counselling/prevention
1. Encourage parent(s) to relax.
2. Reassure parent(s) that the child is essentially healthy, although in pain.
3. Encourage parent(s) to discuss feelings and anxieties.
4. Encourage parent(s) to feed and care for the child in a quiet, unhurried, relaxed atmosphere, to sit in a comfortable chair while feeding, and to put on quiet music.
5. Advise parent(s) to decrease extraneous stimuli, such as television, radio, and the telephone.
6. Encourage parent(s) to get out of the house and have outside activities.
7. Focus on the positive characteristics and aspects of the child.

8. Encourage parent(s) to call for support and reinforcement.
9. Advise parent(s) on frequent, thorough burping.
10. Suggest rhythmic motions, like swinging and rocking the baby.
11. Warm baths may relax the baby.
12. Advise parent(s) to apply a hot-water bottle or heating pad to the child's abdomen.
13. The insertion of a rectal thermometer or glycerine suppository can aid the expulsion of gas.
14. Advise parent(s) to feed as soon as the child indicates hunger.
15. Encourage parent(s) to talk with other parents of colicky infants.

C. Follow-up

1. Parent(s) should call, as needed.
2. Parent(s) should return to the clinic if there are any signs or symptoms of illness.

D. Consultations/referrals: usually none

Table 48-1 Medical Referral/Consultation

Diagnosis	Clinical Manifestations	Management
Appendicitis	Constant abdominal pain Abdominal guarding Fever	Immediate referral to physician
Intussusception	Currant-jelly stools Pallor, sweating Lassitude Low-grade fever Vomiting	Immediate referral to physician
Meckel's diverticulum	Bright-red blood from rectum Signs and symptoms of shock Signs and symptoms of intestinal obstruction	Immediate referral to physician
Acute enteritis	Fever Watery, frequent stools Bloody stools	Referral to physician

bibliography

Bakwin, Ruth M. Psychosomatic factors with particular reference to the parents of the colicky infant. *Pediatrics*, **18**(5):833–835 (1956).

Brazelton, T. Berry. Crying in infancy. *Pediatrics*, **29**:579–588 (1962).

Breslow, Lawrence. An analysis of etiology of colic in infants. *Pediatrics*, **18**(5):838–839 (1956).

———. A clinical approach to infantile colic. *The Journal of Pediatrics*, **50**:196–206 (1957).

Carey, William B. Maternal anxiety and infantile colic. *Clinical Pediatrics*, **7**(10):590–595 (1968).

Glaser, Jerome. Introduction to colic in infants. *Pediatrics*, **18**(5):828–832 (1956).

Harley, Louis M. Fussing and crying in young infants. *Clinical Pediatrics*, **8**(3):138–141 (1969).

Holmes, Carl A. Infantile colic. *Clinical Pediatrics*, **8**(10):566–569 (1969).

Illingworth, R. S. Three months' colic. *Archives of Diseases in Childhood*, **29**:165–174 (1954).

Neff, Frank C. The treatment of colic in infants. *Journal of the American Medical Association*, **114**(18):1745–1748 (1940).

Nelson, Waldo E. (ed.). *Textbook of pediatrics* (10th ed.). Philadelphia: Saunders, 1975.

Rowell, Patricia. Infantile colic: Reviewing the situation. *Pediatric Nursing*, May–June:20–21(1978).

Wessel, Morris, et al. Paroxysmal fussing in infancy, sometimes called "colic." *Pediatrics*, **14**(5):421–434(1954).

49 Constipation/Fecal Impaction

LESLIE LIETH

I. Etiology

A. Colonic stasis

B. Increased water absorption from stool in colon

C. Disturbances in propulsion of material into the lower colon due to

1. Neuromuscular disorders
2. Prolonged bed rest
3. Hypothyroidism

II. Assessment

A. Functional constipation

1. Subjective data
   a. Chronic condition
   b. Family history of constipation
   c. Pain on defecation
   d. Hard stools
   e. Infrequent bowel movements
   f. Huge bowel movements
   g. Soiling
   h. Vague complaints of abdominal pain
2. Objective data
   a. Usually normal growth
   b. Variable abdominal distention and masses
   c. Cavernous rectum, often filled with feces
   d. Normal blood work
   e. X-ray findings reveal colon dilated to anus

B. Anal fissure

1. Subjective data
   a. Acute or chronic condition
   b. Blood-streaked stool or toilet paper
   c. Hard bowel movements
   d. Pain on defecation
2. Objective data
   With client in knee-chest position, tear visualized in anal canal at the mucocutaneous junction

C. Faulty infant feeding

1. Subjective data—parent(s) reveals by history
   a. Improper preparation of formula
   b. Infrequent, hard bowel movements
   c. Straining to pass stool
2. Objective data
   Physical examination can show child with delayed growth or normal development.

III. Management

A. Functional constipation

1. Treatments/medications
   a. Remove impaction (if present) with hypertonic phosphate enemas (3 mg/kg), to be held for 45 to 60 min if possible.
   b. Pairs of enemas may be given morning and night until impaction is alleviated.
   c. Give light mineral oil (cold), 3 to 5 mL/kg per day divided into two doses, increased by 15 to 30 mL/day, until multiple, spontaneous bowel movements are achieved.
   d. The client is maintained for 2 to 3 months on same large doses of mineral oil.
   e. In addition to the episodes when the child responds to the urge to defecate, the child should also be seated on a comfortable commode at regular periods each day for 15 min.
   f. At the end of this period, the bowel movements become predictable and the client can be having one or two bowel movements during these regular periods, even with a large intake of mineral oil.
   g. The child who is not toilet trained does not have to have the bowel movements at regular periods. Once the stools are soft and the bleeding has stopped, these children can be maintained on small doses of min-

eral oil to keep bowel movements normal.

h. After the 2 to 3 months of regimen, withdraw the oil slowly, decreasing the amounts taken over a period of 4 to 6 weeks.

i. Encourage the continuance of the established conditioned pattern, using a comfortable commode.

j. Manipulate the diet by limiting the amount of milk and by encourầging the use of laxative foods, such as prunes, and those with roughage and bran.

k. Occasional use of enemas, with periods of illness, can be expected.

2. Counselling/prevention
   a. The parent(s) can give the child sweetened fluids or hard candy to suck on after the oil. Also, mineral oil should never be forced, due to the seriousness of its aspiration.
   b. Oil leakage indicates the dose is too low to soften the stool, and parent(s) should not cut the amount.
   c. Once the stools are soft, the child gains reassurance that the passing of stool does not have to be a painful experience.
   d. Discourage the use of laxatives by the client or the family.
3. Follow-up
   a. Appointments during therapy should be every 2 to 3 weeks.
   b. Availability for telephone consultation is essential.
4. Consultations/referrals
   a. Consult with physician for therapy.
   b. Refer to physician for further workup if oil regimen does not produce spontaneous bowel movements after 3 to 4 weeks.
   c. Evaluate children for resistance to therapy due to severe emotional problems, and refer them for psychiatric consultation.
   d. Send letters to the school nurse and the teacher regarding frequent bowel movements: They should let the child out of class when necessary.

   e. The client may be referred to a nutritionist for diet counselling.

B. Anal fissure

1. Treatments/medications
   a. High intake of stool softeners, such as fruits, juices, prunes, and bran
   b. Mineral oil regimen if necessary (see treatment for Functional constipation, III, A above)
2. Counselling/prevention
   a. Counsel about diet.
   b. Cleanse anal area well.
   c. Recommend sitz baths, if necessary.
   d. Keep anal area lubricated with Vaseline.
3. Follow-up: appointment 1 to 2 weeks
4. Consultations/referrals
   a. Refer to a physician if the problem is not resolved with the diet change.
   b. Refer to a nutritionist if necessary.

C. Faulty infant feeding

1. Treatments/medications: none
2. Counselling/prevention
   a. Written explanations with proper formula dilution and preparation
   b. Formulas commonly used today
      (1) Enfamil, Similac, SMA, etc.
         (a) A ready-to-feed formula should never be diluted or have sugar added.
         (b) Instructions on cans of concentrated or powdered forms are to be followed exactly.
      (2) Evaporated milk formulas (EVM)
         (a) For infants up to 1 month
             10 oz EVM
             20 oz water
             2 tablespoons dark Karo syrup
         (b) For infants over 1 month
             13 oz EVM
             19 oz water
             3 tablespoons dark Karo syrup
3. Follow-up: as for well-child care
4. Consultations/referrals: Notify visiting nurse for supervision of formula preparation at home.

Table 49-1 Medical Referral/Consultation

Diagnosis	Clinical Manifestations	Management
Hirschsprung's disease	No meconium passed for first few days of life Chronic constipation Distended, tympanitic	Referral to surgeon Counselling Teach colostomy care (if surgery is done in stages

Table 49-1 Medical Referral/Consultation *(continued)*

Diagnosis	Clinical Manifestations	Management
	abdomen with flaring costal margins Small extremities Lack of urge to defecate Rectal examination revealing empty ampulla, and on withdrawing the finger, the escape of gas, with or without a small amount of liquid fecal material Barium enema is diagnostic of condition	and colostomy is present). See Preparation for Hospitalization, Part 7.
Hemorrhoids	Rare in children Chronic or acute constipation Painful bowel movements Rectal bleeding External skin tags, hemorrhoids seen on rectal examination	Referral to physician for treatment See Hemorrhoids, Chap. 54 Methods of treatment differing according to the severity of the case; various treatments include Injection Dilitation of anus under general anesthesia Strangulation by rubberbands Excision and ligation Cryosurgery Client education Reinforce need to keep stools soft with intake of prunes, high fiber, bran, etc. Recommend sitz baths as needed for pain or discomfort.
Hypothyroidism	Congenital Present from birth to 2 yr Constipation; feeding problems; lethargy; respiratory problems; umbilical hernia; enlarged, protruding tongue; abnormal facies; hoarse cry; subnormal temperature; mental and developmental retardation; delayed dentition Anemia; T_3, T_4 levels low or borderline; x-rays of long bones showing retardation of osseous	Referral to physician for treatment Daily sodium levothyroxine (L-thyroxine)—dosage depending on age Counselling Weight loss and hair loss are common side effects. Medications are not to be stopped without consulting a physician. Medications are to be taken for the entire life. Necessary support or referrals provided if the child is retarded.

Table 49-1 Medical Referral/Consultation *(continued)*

Diagnosis	Clinical Manifestations	Management
	development; x-rays of skull showing large fontanels with wide sutures Acquired Myxedematous changes in the skin; constipation; sleepiness; mental decline; cessation or retardation of growth in a previously normal child; obesity with below normal height for age; T_3 and T_4 below normal	
Lead poisoning	History of Paint/plaster ingestion Pica Poor appetite Infrequent, hard bowel movements Lethargy Elevated blood lead level Elevated free erythrocyte protoporphyrin (FEP) test Elevated FEP Anemia sometimes present Physical examination can reveal Pale color Hepatosplenomegaly Abdominal masses	Refer to a physician See Lead Poisoning, Chap. 155 Screen the family for lead poisoning. Refer to the department of health for detection of the source of lead. Familiarize the family with the sources of lead, and inform them about the prevention of lead poisoning and possible signs and symptoms of intoxication.

bibliography

Benson, J. A. Simple chronic constipation: Pathophysiology and management. *Postgraduate Medicine*, **57**(1):55–60 (1975).

Fleisher, David R. Diagnosis and treatment of disorders of defecation in children. *Pediatric Annals*, **5**:70–101 (1976).

Green, Morris, and Haggarty, Robert. *Ambulatory Pediatrics II*. Philadelphia: Saunders, 1977.

Ling, Syllis, and McCammon, Sarah P. Dietary treatment of diarrhea and constipation in infants and children. *Issues in Comprehensive Pediatric Nursing*, **3**:17–28 (October 1978).

Partridge, J. P. Treatment of hemorrhoids. *Nursing Times*, **71**:928–929 (1975).

Rudolph, Abraham, Barnett, Henry L., and Einhorn, Arnold. *Pediatrics* (16th ed.). New York: Appleton-Century-Crofts, 1977.

Shirkey, Harry C. *Pediatric therapy*. St. Louis: Mosby, 1975.

50 Stool Incontinence (Encopresis)

MARILYN GREBIN

I. Etiology

A. Primary encopresis

Due to incomplete toilet training

B. Secondary encopresis

1. Organic—Hirschsprung's disease
2. Toilet phobia—remembering a painful bowel evacuation; anal fissure
3. Chronic constipation and/or impaction causing megacolon
4. Stress reaction—to home or school situations
5. Neurodevelopmental—hyperkinesis, poor neuromuscular coordination

II. Assessment

A. Primary encopresis

1. Subjective data
   a. Age below 4 years
   b. Regimented toilet training
   c. Punishments given for lack of performance on the toilet
   d. New sibling may have been born during training period
   e. Hyperactive behavior
   f. Poor eating habits coupled with constipation
   g. Difficult or painful bowel evacuation
2. Objective data
   a. Physical examination normal except for possible palpable fecal masses on abdominal examination
   b. Developmental delays
   c. Hyperactive behavior

B. Secondary encopresis (nonorganic)

Note: All children with encopresis must be seen by the physician to rule out a possible organic cause.

1. Subjective data
   a. Age greater than 4 years
   b. Passage of stool into clothing
   c. Excessive punishment for accidents
   d. Gastrointestinal upsets
   e. Poor school performance
   f. Possible enuresis
   g. Chronic constipation
   h. Episode of rectal bleeding
   i. Hyperactivity
   j. Irregular eating habits
2. Objective data

   Physical examination—normal, except for possible palpable fecal masses on abdominal examination

III. Management (same management for both primary and secondary encopresis)

A. Treatments/medications: none

B. Counselling/prevention

1. Personalized parent counselling and information concerning the treatment regimen should be given.
2. Parent(s) should be informed about emotional disturbances that may affect the child.
3. Parent(s) should be instructed not to punish the child for soiling.
4. The child should use the toilet with feet on the floor, or an adaption should be constructed for smaller children.
5. Counsel about diet.
   a. Avoidance of more than 12 to 16 oz of milk
   b. Increase of roughage with bran, prunes, vegetables
6. Discuss with the child how the bowel works and how waste has to pass out.
7. Encourage the child to visit the bathroom at least twice per day.

8. Diagram the normal bowel and the bowel stretched with stool. (Levine, 1976)
9. Encourage children to clean themselves after an accident without blaming them for the accident.
10. Many physicians order enemas and laxatives to begin the bowel training.
11. After the initial catharsis, 30 mL of mineral oil twice daily (for a 7-year-old) plus two multivitamins per day may be used. (Levine, 1976)
12. Allow the child to express fears, problems, or concerns.

C. Follow-up

Monthly visits with supportive counselling for both parent(s) and child

D. Consultations/referrals

1. Consultation with the pediatrician must occur before any treatment is begun.
2. Professional counselling may be recommended in cases where the child has difficulty coping with stress and feelings.

bibliography

Fitzgerald, Joseph. Encopresis, soiling, constipation: What's to be done. *Pediatrics,* **56**(3):348–349 (1975).

Gellis, Sidney S., Kagen, B. *Current pediatric therapy 8.* Philadelphia: Saunders, 1978.

Hein, Herman A., Beerends, Jerold J. Who should accept primary responsiblility for the encopretic child? *Clinical Pediatrics,* **17**(1):67–70 (1978).

Levine, Melvin D. Children with encopresis: A descriptive analysis. *Pediatrics,* **56**(3):412–416 (1975).

Levine, Melvin D., Bakow, Harry. Children with encopresis: A study of treatment outcomes. *Pediatrics,* **58**(6):845–852 (1976).

Wright, Logan, Walker, Eugene C. Treatment of the child with psychogenic encopresis. *Clinical Pediatrics,* **16**(11) (1977).

51 Abdominal Pain

MARILYN GREBIN

ALERT

1. Severe testicular pain
2. Frank rectal bleeding, tarry stool
3. Trauma
4. Currant-jelly stool
5. Palpable abdominal mass
6. Cyanosis
7. Shock
8. Rebound abdominal tenderness
9. Oliguria
10. High fever and pain
11. Hepatosplenomegaly
12. Pregnancy and pain
13. Flank tenderness
14. Toxic appearance
15. Vomiting, dehydration
16. Jaundice
17. Purpura

I. Etiology

A. Congenital
B. Infectious
C. Metabolic
D. Obstructive
E. Traumatic
F. Toxic
G. Emotional
H. Idiopathic
I. Hematologic
J. Allergic

Note: All children with chronic abdominal pain must be examined by a physician.

II. Management

A. Treatments/medications

The physician will determine the need for treatments and medication.

B. Counselling/prevention

1. Encourage parent(s) to support the hospitalized child, by being available and understanding the child's fears of the experience.
2. Make time available each day to allow the parent(s) to express parental fears and concerns about the child.
3. Identify adolescent health care needs, and participate in group sessions designed to share information.
4. Anticipate parent/child needs, to assist in preparing coping mechanisms for stressful times.
5. Assist parent(s) in maintaining normal growth and development skills for the ill child.
6. Teach the importance of discipline for the ill child.
7. Counsel regarding special nutritional needs and feeding techniques.
8. Encourage client and parent compliance with the medical/nursing management, and follow up.
9. Assist in the preparation of the child and parent(s) for outcomes to chronic disease processes.
10. Encourage the establishment of the parental bond with the hospitalized newborn.
11. Assist in the explanation of treatments.
12. Encourage awareness of the process of infections and the need for early intervention.
13. Assist in explaining side effects and complications and the need to notify the physician.
14. Encourage participation in school and activities as soon as the physician determines the condition is stable.

15. Spend time with the client discussing his or her expectations and perceptions of illness and treatment.

C. Follow-up

1. Medical—as indicated by the physician
2. Nursing determined after assessing the counselling needs of the client and parent

D. Consultations/referrals

1. School nurse—for clients with chronic diseases
2. Public health nurse—to assist the new mother in handling the newborn at home and to identify toxic sources within the home
3. Physician as indicated in Table 51-1

Table 51-1 Medical Referral/Consultation

Diagnosis	Clinical Manifestations	Management
	Newborn—Infant	
Colic (idiopathic)	Crying with flexing of legs Irritability Improvement with expulsion of flatus	See Infantile Colic, Chap. 48.
Herniae* (obstruction)	Swelling of inguinal or umbilical area Vomiting Abdominal distention Pain and/or tenderness	Refer to surgeon for evaluation and timing of repair procedure. See Herniae, Chap. 55.
Testicular torsion* (obstruction)	Sudden onset Severe pain reflected to abdomen Swelling of the testicle	Immediate surgical referral
Anal fissures* (trauma)	Crying during defecation Irritability Bright-red blood or streaking after defecation	Referral to surgeon
Viral gastroenteritis* (infection)	Abdominal distention Vomiting (6–24 h) Fever Diarrhea Cramping pain Tympanic sound on abdominal percussion Increased bowel sounds Possible signs of dehydration	Referral to the physician for hospitalization of all infants exhibiting these symptoms
Trauma during delivery (trauma)	Listlessness Rapid respirations Abdominal distention Pain Rapidly progressive anemia	Immediate referral to surgeon
Volvulus (obstruction)	High obstruction within first 3 wk of life	Immediate referral to surgeon

*These disorders may occur in any other age group but are more common within the age range in which they are placed.

Table 51-1 Medical Referral/Consultation *(continued)*

Diagnosis	Clinical Manifestations	Management
	Newborn—Infant (continued)	
	Bilious vomiting Abdominal distention and pain Visible peristalsis Melena or currant-jelly stools	
Intussusception* (obstruction)	Abdominal pain Vomiting Currant-jelly stools Fever Abdominal tenderness and distention Palpable sausage-shaped mass in the abdomen Diarrhea or constipation	Immediate referral to surgeon
Intestinal obstruction* (obstruction)	History of maternal hydramnios Vomiting of bile Abdominal distention Failure to pass meconium Obstipation Family history of congenital anomalies Abdominal pain—crying, irritability Aspiration of feedings	Immediate referral to surgeon
Intestinal duplication (congenital)	Abdominal distention Colicky pain—irritability, crying Rectal bleeding Partial or total obstruction Palpable mass perhaps present	Immediate referral to surgeon
Pyloric stenosis (obstruction)	Full-term infant—most often male Nonbilious projectile vomiting Weight loss Colicky pain—irregular crying Constipation Abdominal distention (upper) Hungry baby—irritable Olive-size mass perhaps palpable to the right of the umbilicus	Referral to surgeon
Perforated viscus (obstruction)	Normal appearance at birth Refusal to feed Vomiting Irritability, crying, pain	Immediate referral to surgeon

*These disorders may occur in any other age group but are more common within the age range in which they are placed.

Table 51-1 Medical Referral/Consultation *(continued)*

Diagnosis	Clinical Manifestations	Management
	Newborn—Infant (continued)	
	Abdominal distention Dyspnea Cyanosis Shock	
Necrotizing enterocolitis (infection)	Premature infant History of fever in the mother History of early ruptured membranes Abdominal distention Irritability, crying, pain Vomiting Blood-streaked diarrhea Sepsis and shock	Immediate referral to surgeon
	Preschool age group, 2–5 yr	
Appendicitis* (infection)	Fever Anorexia Abdominal pain Rebound abdominal tenderness Abdominal auscultation Absence of sounds, or High-pitched sounds White blood count not higher than 15,000	Immediate referral to surgeon
Hydronephrosis* (obstruction)	Abdominal distention Palpable abdominal mass Flank/abdominal pain Hematuria Pyuria Oliguria	Referral to physician
Pyelonephritis* (infection)	Chills High fever Abdominal and flank pain Vomiting Malaise	Urinalysis Urine culture Complete blood count Antibiotics after consultation with physician Acetaminophen or aspirin for fever Increased fluid intake
Lead poisoning* (toxic)	Constipation Abdominal pain Anorexia Sporadic vomiting	Refer to the physician. See Lead Poisoning, Chap. 155.

*These disorders may occur in any other age group but are more common within the age range in which they are placed.

Table 51-1 Medical Referral/Consultation *(continued)*

Diagnosis	Clinical Manifestations	Management
	Preschool age group, 2–5 yr (continued)	
	Apathy Anemia Irritability Coordination difficulties	
Constipation* (obstruction or emotional)	See Constipation/Fecal Impaction, Chap. 49.	See Constipation/Fecal Impaction, Chap. 49.
Meckel's diverticulum (obstruction)	Painless rectal bleeding Anemia Abdominal distention Abdominal pain	Immediate referral to surgeon
Acute and chronic* pancreatitis (infection)	Sudden onset of mild to severe abdominal pain, localized in the epigastrium radiating to the back Nausea and vomiting Pallor Prefers lying on side with knees flexed Abdominal distention Abdominal tenderness Hepatosplenomegaly Diminished bowel sounds Positive Cullen's sign—bluish discoloration around the umbilicus Clinical mumps in > 50% cases	Referral to physician
Juvenile diabetes* (metabolic)	See Diabetes, Chap. 147.	See Diabetes, Chap. 147.
Rheumatic fever* (infection)	Abdominal pain may present before any of the cardinal symptoms Carditis Polyarthritis Chorea Erythema marginatum Subcutaneous nodules	Referral to physician See Acute Rheumatic Fever, Chap. 145
Acute intermittent porphyria attack (hematologic)	Severe, poorly localized abdominal pain Vomiting Constipation Tachycardia Hypertension Emotionally labile	Immediate referral to physician

*These disorders may occur in any other age group but are more common within the age range in which they are placed.

Table 51-1 Medical Referral/Consultation *(continued)*

Diagnosis	Clinical Manifestations	Management
	Preschool age group, 2–5 yr (continued)	
	Urine perhaps normal in color but containing high levels of porphobilinogen	
	School-age group, 6–18 yr	
Mittelschmerz (idiopathic)	Cramping abdominal pain Present at the time of ovulation	See Puberty/Menarche, Chap. 60.
Ectopic pregnancy (obstructive)	Missed one or two periods Slight vaginal bleeding Sudden severe unilateral abdominal pain Vertigo, fainting, or shock Vaginal examination Motion of cervix causes severe pain. Palpable tender boggy mass on one side.	Immediate referral to physician
Renal calculi (obstructive)	Tenderness in the renal area Pyuria Hematuria Renal colic radiating to the lower abdomen Vomiting	Referral to physician
Peptic ulcer*, gastric or duodenal (metabolic)	Abdominal (upper) pain after eating Rectal bleeding (perforation common) Tarry stools	Referral to physician Encouragement of compliance with treatment regime Diet counselling
Asthma* (allergy or infection)	Abdominal pain See Wheezing, Chap. 33.	See Wheezing, Chap. 33, and Allergies, Chap. 137.
Ulcerative colitis (infectious)	Bloody diarrhea Abdominal pain and tenesmus Anorexia Nausea and vomiting Dehydration Weight loss Retarded growth Low-grade fever in the evening	Immediate referral to physician
Crohn's disease* (congenital)	Arthritis Uveitis Stomatitis	Immediate referral to physician

*These disorders may occur in any other age group but are more common within the age range in which they are placed.

Table 51-1 Medical Referral/Consultation *(continued)*

Diagnosis	Clinical Manifestations	Management
School-age group, 6–18 yr (continued)		
	Erythema nodosum Growth retardation Crampy abdominal pain—begins with eating Anorexia Nausea Vomiting Diarrhea Abdominal guarding	
Sickle cell anemia* (hematologic)	See "Sickle cell anemia" in Chap. 39.	See "Sickle Cell Anemia" in Chap. 39.
Pneumonia, bacterial* (infection)	High fever Increased respiratory rate Increased pulse rate Cough—progresses from dry to moist Thoracic and abdominal pain Vomiting Headache	Immediate referral to physician
Hiatal hernia* (congenital)	Vomiting, coffee-ground or frank blood; night vomiting Malnutrition Aspiration pneumonia Chronic cough Bronchitis Asthmalike attacks Substernal pain Heartburn Nausea Bloaty or full feeling	Referral to physician
Abdominal epilepsy* (congenital)	History positive for familial epilepsy Other causes of abdominal pain ruled out Sudden onset and termination of abdominal pain EEG abnormalities Improvement of symptoms with anticonvulsant medication	Referral to physician
Gilbert's disease (idiopathic)	> 18 yr of age Mild fluctuating jaundice Malaise	Referral to physician

*These disorders may occur in any other age group but are more common within the age range in which they are placed.

Table 51-1 Medical Referral/Consultation *(continued)*

Diagnosis	Clinical Manifestations	Management
	School-age group, 6–18 yr (continued)	
	Fatigue Abdominal pain	
Dubin-Johnson syndrome (congenital)	> 18 yr of age Mild icterus Nonspecific abdominal pain Palpable, tender liver Elevated bilirubin (2–8 mg/100 mL)	Referral to physician
Henoch-Schönlein syndrome* (hematologic)	Rash Urticarial lesions Erythematous maculopapules Hemorrhage Leaves brownish discoloration Joints Edematous Erythematous Warm Painful and tender Colicky abdominal pain Vomiting Melena	Immediate referral to physician
Psychosocial* (emotional)	Superachiever—very intelligent No tolerance for failure Obsessive-compulsive personality Harbors fears Psychosomatic abdominal pains Expresses anger poorly May be immature Learning disabilities Phobias	Thorough examination by the physician to rule out pathologic causes of abdominal pain Supportive counselling for the client and the parent(s) on a regular basis Referral to psychologist for evaluation and counselling Explanation that the client's pain is real
Mesenteric adenitis* (infection)	Abdominal pain—diffuse Nausea and vomiting Positive streptococcus culture Fever	Referral to physician
Mononucleosis* (infection)	Anorexia General malaise Fever Lymphadenopathy Pharyngitis Splenomegaly Abdominal pain Liver sometimes palpable	Referral to physician

*These disorders may occur in any other age group but are more common within the age range in which they are placed.

bibliography

Apley, J. *The child with abdominal pain* (2d ed.). Philadelphia:Lippincott, 1975.

Arney, William Ray, Nagy, Jill N., and Little, George A. Caring for parents of sick newborns. *Clinical Pediatrics*, **17**:35–39 (1978).

Bain, Harry W. Chronic vague abdominal pain in children. *Pediatric Clinics of North America*, **21**:991–999 (1974).

Berger, Henry, Honig, Paul, and Lieberman, Ronald, Recurrent abdominal pain. *American Journal of Diseases of Children*, **131**:1340–1344 (1977).

Byrn, James, et al. Unusual manifestations of Henoch-Schönlein syndrome. *American Journal of Diseases of Children*, **130**:1335–1337 (1976).

Hardgrove, Carol, and Rutledge, Ann. Parenting during hospitalization. *American Journal of Nursing*, **75**:836–838 (1975).

Silverman, Arnold, Roy, C., and Cozzetto, Frank. *Pediatric clinical gastroenterology* (2d ed.). St. Louis: Mosby, 1975, pp. 30–33, 237–238.

Stapleton, F. Bruder, and Lindshaw, Michael A. Urinary tract infections in children: diagnosis and management. *Issues in Comprehensive Pediatric Nursing*, **2**:1–10 (March-April 1978).

Winter, S. T. Recurrent abdominal pain in children. *Clinical Pediatrics*, **15**:771–773 (1976).

52 Rectal Bleeding

MARILYN GREBIN

I. Etiology: see Table 52–1

II. Assessment: see Table 52–1

III. Management

Counselling/prevention—The practitioner may assist the parent(s) and the client in understanding the illness and the treatment regimen.

1. Explanation of the necessary tests done by the physican
2. Guidance for follow-up after discharge from the hospital
3. Explanations that will lead to compliance with medical/nursing home care
   a. Dietary alterations
   b. Removal of objects in the environment that are harmful if ingested by a small child
4. See Preparation for Hospitalization, Part 7

Note: The primary health care practitioner should be aware of the conditions causing rectal bleeding and may assist the physician in the work-up, but the diagnosis will be assigned by the physician.

Table 52-1 Clinical Clues to Causes of Rectal Bleeding

Entity	Age	Amount; Appearance	Clinical Features	Etiology	Diagnostic Means
Swallowed blood	Newborn	Variable; tarry to dark red	Appears well	Delivery	Apt-Downey test
Hemorrhagic disease of newborn	Newborn	Large; red to tarry	Hemorrhages elsewhere	Clotting disorders, vitamin K deficiency, others	Coagulation studies; prothrombin time and PTT, platelet count, others
Stress ulcer	Newborn to any age	Large; red to black	Shocklike, pale, sickly appearance	Difficult labor and delivery, CNS injury, sepsis	Nasogastric tube; upper gastrointestinal series normal or abnormal
Hemorrhagic gastritis	Newborn	Large; red to black	Shocklike, pale, sickly appearance	Stressful labor and delivery	Nasogastric tube; normal upper gastrointestinal series
Necrotizing enterocolitis	Newborn	Variable; red to currant jelly	Prematurity, diarrhea, sickly appearance	Hirschsprung's disease, prematurity, Shwartzman phenomenon	Palpation of abdomen, scout films of abdomen
Actue colitis	Any age	Variable; red	Sickly, toxic appearance, diarrhea, abdominal pain	Infection, allergy, isosensitization, chronic ulcerative colitis, chronic active hepatitis, ischemia	Proctoscopy, biopsy, barium enema
Infectious diarrhea	Any age	Small; red	Diarrhea, fever	Bacterial (*Salmonella, Shigella,* pathogenic *Escherichia coli*), viral, or parasitic infection	Stool cultures
Milk allergy	Neonate and infant	Occult to small; red	Colic, diarrhea, vomiting, edema, rhinitis, asthma, atopic dermatitis	Bovine milk protein allergy	Dietary changes, administration of steroids
Midgut volvulus	Neonate	Variable; red to tarry	Shock, bile-stained vomitus, pain, obstruction	Malrotation with malfixation of mesentery	Upper gastrointestinal series
Anal fissure	Infant	Small; red	Constipation, rectal pain	Constipation	Inspection of anus, anoscopy

Table 52-1 Clinical Clues to Causes of Rectal Bleeding *(continued)*

Entity	Age	Amount; Appearance	Clinical Features	Etiology	Diagnostic Means
Cryptitis, proctitis	Any age	Small; red	Colicky episodes, rectal pain, diarrhea	Gastroenteritis, ulcerative colitis, regional ileitis	Stool culture, proctoscopy
Polyps	Any age	Small to moderate; red	Absence of pain; mucus, intermittent diarrhea	Idiopathic, genetic, or familial	Proctoscopy, barium enema, upper gastrointestinal series
Intussusception	Usually less than 2 yr	Variable; red, currant jelly, tarry	Colicky pain, abdominal distention, vomiting	Idiopathic; polyps, Meckel's diverticulum, lymphonodular hyperplasia, tumors	Barium enema
Intestinal parasites	Any age	Occult to small; red	Diarrhea, cramps, weight loss	Amebiasis, *Trichuris*, hookworms, others	Proctoscopy and biopsy; stool examination for eggs; barium enema
Meckel's diverticulum	Usually less than 2 yr	Large; red to tarry	Usually absence of pain; pale, shocklike appearance; anemia	Congenital	Laparotomy, radioactive scan
Duplications	Usually less than 2 yr	Variable to large; red to tarry	Mass, intestinal obstruction, absence of pain	Congenital	Upper gastrointestinal series, barium enema, radioactive scan, laparotomy
Nodular, lymphoid hyperplasia	Usually less than 2 yr	Small; red	Appears well, postinfectious diarrhea	Disrupted mucosa, idiopathic	Proctoscopy, barium enema
Hemangiomas and telangiectasia	Any age	Occult to large	Absence of pain; mucocutaneous lesions	Congenital	Physical examination, selective angiography, laparotomy
Peptic ulcer	Any age (most 5–15 yr)	Occult to large; tarry	Epigastric pain	Idiopathic; CNS disease, steroids, burns, sepsis	Physical examination, upper gastrointestinal series, endoscopy
Henoch-Schönlein purpura	3–10 yr	Small to large; red to tarry	Abdominal pain, vomiting, arthritis, purpura, hematuria	Idiopathic	Physical examination, upper gastrointestinal series, barium enema

Table 52-1 Clinical Clues to Causes of Rectal Bleeding *(continued)*

Entity	Age	Amount; Appearance	Clinical Features	Etiology	Diagnostic Means
Chronic ulcerative colitis	Any age (most 10–19 yr)	Small to occult; red	Abdominal pain, tenesmus, diarrhea	Idiopathic	Proctoscopy, rectal biopsy, barium enema
Regional enteritis (Crohn's disease)	Most 10–19 yr	Occult to small, sometimes large; red	Abdominal pain, diarrhea, anorexia, weight loss	Idiopathic	Proctoscopy, upper gastrointestinal series, barium enema
Esophagitis	Any age	Occult to small	Dysphagia, vomiting, heartburn	Hiatal hernia, pyloric outlet obstruction	Esophagography, esophagoscopy, upper gastrointestinal series
Esophageal varices	Any age (most 3–5 yr)	Large; tarry	Hematemesis, signs of portal hypertension	Cirrhosis or portal vein obstruction	Esophagography, esophagoscopy
Hemorrhoids	Adolescent	Small; red	Pain on defecation	Constipation, perianal disease, portal hypertension, Crohn's disease	Anoscopy, digital examination
Foreign body	Toddler to school age	Variable; red	Rectal pain	Irritation effect of foreign body	Digital examination, proctoscopy, radiography
Hemolytic-uremic syndrome	Usually under 5	Small to large; red	Postdiarrhea, edema, hematuria	Postgastroenteritis(?), platelet thrombi(?)	Laboratory studies, barium enema, rectal biopsy

From Roy, C. C., Silverman, A., and Cozzetto, F. J. *Pediatric clinical gastroenterology* (2d ed.). St. Louis: Mosby, 1975, pp. 27–29.

53 Pinworms

M. CONSTANCE SALERNO

I. Etiology: *Enterobius vermicularis*

II. Assessment

A. Subjective data

1. Rectal itch (intense and pruritis at night)
2. Restlessness
3. Decreased appetite
4. Pinworms visualized by parent(s)
5. History revealing other family members with similar symptoms

B. Objective data

1. View of pinworms as they emerge from anus, especially at night
2. Perianal rash
3. Vaginitis with leukorrhea rarely present in girls
4. Microscopic identification of eggs on clear cellophane tape (applied over the anus in early morning)

III. Management

A. Treatments/medications

1. Treat client and other family members who have symptoms.
2. Enterobiocide—one dose
   a. Vermox (Mebendazole) chewable tablet—children over 2 years
   b. Povan (pyrvinium pamoate) tablet
   c. Antiminth (pyrantel pamoate) suspension
3. Medication possibly repeated once, 10 to 14 days after initial dose

B. Counselling/prevention

1. Instruct client and parent(s) regarding personal hygiene: hands should be washed *before* and *after* toileting and *before* eating.
2. Instruct parent(s) in the procedure for identification of worms.
   a. Spread buttocks and view anus with flashlight at night or in the early morning.
   b. Cellophane tape may be applied with the sticky side pressed against the anus. Microscopic identification of eggs adhering to the cellophane tape confirms the diagnosis.
3. Infection is usually present in other family members, especially children. Family members who manifest symptoms should be treated concurrently.
4. Povan colors the stools red, and if the client has an emesis, it, too, may be reddish.
5. Wearing tight underpants prevents direct finger contact with the anus.

C. Follow-up: return visit if recurrence of symptoms

D. Consultations/referrals: none

bibliography

Ingalls, A. J., and Salerno, M. C. *Maternal and child health nursing* (4th ed.). St. Louis: Mosby, 1979, pp. 655–656.

Turner, J. A., and Seidel, J. Parasitic infections. In Gellis, S. S., and Kagan, B. M. (eds.), *Current pediatric therapy 8*. Philadelphia: Saunders, 1978, p. 652.

54 Hemorrhoids

HARRIETT S. CHANEY

ALERT

1. Intense anal or rectal pain
2. Anemia
3. Purulent anal discharge
4. Other sources of colon bleeding: polyp, enteric colitis, ulcer
5. Occurrence of symptoms before adolescence

I. Etiology—Internal and External Hemorrhoids

A. Varicose dilation of the superior and inferior hemorrhoidal plexus
B. Portal hypertension
C. Congestive heart failure
D. Straining at stool
E. Pregnancy

II. Assessment

A. Internal hemorrhoid
1. Subjective data—straining on stool
2. Objective data
    a. Painless, bright-red rectal bleeding
    b. Soft bluish mass above pectinate line
    c. No-to-minimal anemia

B. External hemorrhoid
1. Subjective data
    a. Perianal pruritis, pain
    b. Straining on stool
    c. Pain in anal area upon defecation, sitting
2. Objective data
    a. Perianal or anal canal bulging of bluish, tender mass
    b. Prolapsing of hemorrhoid to outside of the anal sphincter
    c. Bleeding upon defecation
    d. No-to-minimal anemia

III. Management

A. Internal hemorrhoid
1. Treatments/medications
    a. Nupercaine hydrochloride ointment application
    b. Analgesic—aspirin or acetaminophen
    c. Frequent sitz baths
2. Counselling/prevention
    a. Sit as little as possible.
    b. A recumbent position will relieve varicosity distention.
    c. Include stool-softening elements in the diet, such as fresh fruits, juices, and fresh vegetables.
    d. Drink an adequate amount of fluids each day.
    e. Report acute severe pain, because it may indicate thrombosis of varicosity.
    f. Report any sign of ulceration or infection.
3. Follow-up: return visit in 1 week if not improved
4. Consultations/referrals: consultation with physician if anemia progresses or thrombosis or infection are apparent.

B. External hemorrhoid
1. Treatments/medications
    a. Nupercaine hydrochloride ointment application
    b. Analgesic—aspirin
    c. Frequent sitz baths
    d. Application of astringent lotion or solution to hemorrhoid
2. Counselling/prevention
    a. Sit as little as possible.
    b. A recumbent position will relieve varicosity distention.
    c. If varicosity has prolapsed through the anal sphincter, carefully attempt to reinsert it into the anal canal.

d. Include stool-softening elements in the diet, such as fresh fruits, juices, and fresh vegetables.
e. Drink an adequate amount of fluids each day.
f. Report acute severe pain, because it may indicate thrombosis of varicosity.
g. Report any sign of ulceration or infection.

3. Follow-up: return visit if no improvement in 1 week
4. Consultations/referrals: consultation with physician if anemia progresses or thrombosis or infection are apparent.

Table 54-1 Medical Referral/Consultation·

Diagnosis	Clinical Manifestations	Management
Rectal fistula	A tract that goes from the anal canal to skin outside the anus, or from an abscess to either the anal canal or perianal area Drainage of pus Pain	Physician referral Surgical excision Meticulous rectal cleanliness See Preparation for Hospitalization, Part 7
Rectal fissure	Longitudinal crack of the skin along the anal canal to the outside Local tenderness Intense burning and sphincter muscle spasm upon defecation	Physician referral Surgical excision Meticulous rectal cleanliness See Preparation for Hospitalization, Part 7.
Polyps	Occasional rectal bleeding Painless Occasional abdominal cramping, abdominal mass, or bloody exudate if partial intussusception has occurred Polyps visualized upon proctoscopy	Physician referral Surgical excision See Preparation for Hospitalization, Part 7

bibliography

Bergerson, Betty S. *Pharmacology in nursing.* St. Louis: Mosby, 1976.

Buls, John G., and Goldberg, Stanley M. Modern management of hemorrhoids. *Surgical Clinics of North America,* **58**(3):469–475 (1978).

Hoole, A. J., Greenberg, R. A., and Pickard, C. G. *Patient care guidelines for family nurse practitioners.* Boston: Little, Brown, 1976.

55 Herniae

ELEANOR RUDICK

ALERT
1. Signs of intestinal obstruction. An irreducible incarcerated hernia is a surgical emergency.
2. Signs of respiratory distress
3. Umbilical hernia past age 3 years

I. Etiology

A. Umbilical—imperfect closure or weakness of umbilical ring

B. Inguinal—persistence of processus vaginalis

C. Diaphragmatic

1. In posterolateral segments—failure of pleuroperitoneal canal to close during embryonic development
2. In anterior portion—failure of midline fusion of the two anlagen of the diaphragm
3. Hiatal—shortened esophagus with portion of stomach displaced upward through diaphragm into thoracic cavity

II. Assessment: Umbilical Hernia

A. Subjective data

1. Usually present at birth
2. May or may not change in size with age

B. Objective data

1. Soft swelling, covered by skin
2. Protrusion during crying, coughing, straining
3. Easily reduced through fibrous ring
4. Size varies between 1 and 5+ cm
5. Most frequent in blacks and girls

III. Management: Umbilical Hernia

A. Treatments/medications

Surgery may be indicated in children over 2 years or in large (over 6 cm) herniae.

B. Counselling/prevention

Need to reassure parent(s)

a. Most umbilical herniae disappear spontaneously by 1 year of age.
b. Strapping is ineffective.
c. Surgery is usually unnecessary.

C. Follow-up: Measure palpable opening at each well-child visit.

D. Consultations/referrals: Consult physician if condition persists or palpable opening increases in size.

Table 55-1 Medical Referral/Consultation

Diagnosis	Clinical Manifestations	Management
Inguinal hernia	Mass appears intermittently in inguinal region. Hernial sac can be emptied by gentle compression. Hernial sac can be made to fill with crying or straining in infant. Hernial sac can be made to fill when older child stands, coughs, or lifts.	Referral to physician Surgery when diagnosed, to prevent Incarceration Obstruction Testicular atrophy Enlargement of ring Truss not recommended See Preparation for Hospitalization, Part 7

Table 55-1 Medical Referral/Consultation *(continued)*

Diagnosis	Clinical Manifestations	Management
	Hydrocele may be present; it is not reducible. The symptoms may be those of incomplete obstruction.	Usually hospitalized 1 day or less May do routine bilateral exploration in children under 2 yr Check for recurrence
Incarcerated inguinal hernia	Occurs most often under 6 mo Child fretful, vomiting Firm, tender, globular, irreducible swelling below external ring Possible bloody stool Unless relieved, progresses to Abdominal distension Cessation of bowel movements Persistent vomiting Fever	Immediate referral to physician Manipulative reduction (if present less than 12 h and no bloody stool) Gentle, firm pressure while infant sucks strongly on pacifier Sedation Trendelenburg's position—elevation of buttocks, ice bag to area Hospitalization perhaps necessary (see Preparation for Hospitalization, Part 7) Parent should remain to prevent child from crying excessively Observation for signs of peritoneal irritation Surgery within 24–48 h, after correction of any metabolic imbalance If irreducible—emergency surgery
Diaphragmatic hernia	Congenital or acquired (through trauma) Respiratory distress in neonatal period Vomiting Severe, colicky pain Discomfort with eating Constipation Dyspnea Possible scaphoid abdomen Changes in percussion note and breath sounds over chest containing abdominal contents Newborn symptoms varying from very slight to severe, depending on the degree of displacement	Immediate referral to physician—hospitalization Resuscitation needed Positioning of infant so that head and thorax are higher than abdomen and feet In hospital X-ray study Nasogastric intubation Correction of acidosis Surgical correction indicated Postsurgery Follow-up—attention to hypoplastic lung Well-child supervision See Preparation for Hospitalization, Part 7

bibliography

Gellis, Sydney S., and Kagan, Benjamin M. *Current pediatric therapy 8*. Philadelphia: Saunders, 1978, pp. 195–196, 417–419, 779.

Hoekelman, Robert A. The pediatric physical examination. In Barbara Bates, *A guide to physical examination* (2d ed.). Philadelphia: Lippincott, 1979, pp. 407–413.

Vaughan, Victor C., and McKay, R. James. (eds.). *Nelson textbook of pediatrics* (10th ed.). Philadelphia: Saunders, 1975, pp. 868–871.

Young, Daniel G., and Weller, Barbara F. *Baby surgery*. Baltimore: University Park Press, 1971, pp. 144–154.

56 Stool Color/Odor Changes

HARRIETT S. CHANEY

ALERT

1. Weight loss
2. Stool colors of gray, clay, bright red, tarry black
3. Anemia
4. Change in stool consistency, frequency
5. Stool color change, associated with abnormal skin color; jaundice

I. Etiology

A. Stool color changes

1. Nonpathological
   a. Dark brown—meat protein, cocoa
   b. Dark green—spinach, iron, mercurous chloride
   c. Red—beets, phenolphthalein, tetracycline in syrup
   d. Yellow—senna, santonin, rhubarb
   e. Black—medications with bismuth, iron
2. Pathological
   a. Tarry black—upper GI bleeding
   b. Bright-red blood—lower GI bleeding
   c. Gray with silvery sheen—steatorrhea
   d. Clay—biliary obstruction

B. Odor changes in stool

1. Normal variations due to diet
2. Foul odor associated with bulky, greasy stool, gray in color with a silvery sheen, is due to steatorrhea

II. Assessment

A. Nonpathological stool color changes

1. Subjective data
   a. Ingestion of agent known to alter normal stool color, e.g., spinach, iron, beets, cocoa, bismuth
   b. History negative for pain, other stool changes
2. Objective data
   a. Physical exam within normal limits
   b. Stool negative for occult blood

B. Odor changes in stool due to normal variation

1. Subjective data
   a. Change gradual or acute in onset
   b. Change not associated with bulky, greasy stools, gray in color with a silver sheen
   c. Diet change
2. Objective data
   a. Normal physical findings
   b. Stool negative for occult blood
   c. Stool analysis within normal limits

III. Management

A. Nonpathological stool color change

1. Treatments/medications: none
2. Counselling/prevention
   a. Inform client/parent(s) of etiology and normal laboratory values.
   b. Reassure client and parent(s).
3. Follow-up: return visit or phone call if client discontinues suspected ingestant and symptoms remain.
4. Consultations/referrals: refer to a physician all complaints of gray, clay, tarry-black stools and instances of bright-red bleeding in the absence of overt hemorrhoidal bleeding.

B. Odor changes in stool

1. Treatments/medications: none
2. Counselling/prevention: Inform client of normal variation due to diet.

3. Follow-up: none
4. Consultations/referrals
   a. Refer to a physician if the complaint is associated with bulky, greasy stools, gray with a silver sheen.
   b. Consider psychological consultation if symptoms reflect a preoccupation with excreta.

Table 56-1 Medical Referral/Consultation

Diagnosis	Clinical Manifestations	Management
Malabsorption steatorrhea	Stool with foul odor, bulky, foamy, gray with silvery sheen, and floating	Referral to physician
	Can be associated with weight loss, edema, tetany, bleeding, anemia, arthritis	
	Peripheral neuropathy, night blindness, nocturia	
	Associated with numerous diseases: pancreatic insufficiency, liver disease, lymphatic obstruction, Whipple's disease, inflammatory disorders, sprue, endocrine disorders	

bibliography

Melasanos, Lois, et al. *Health assessment.* St. Louis: Mosby, 1977.

section 6

the reproductive system

INTRODUCTION JANE A. FOX

I. Subjective Data

A. Age and sex

B. Reason for visit and description of problem

C. Onset

D. Associated symptoms

1. Nausea/vomiting
2. Fever
3. Abdominal pain
4. Pain and/or burning on urination
5. Headache
6. Fatigue
7. Irritability
8. Rash
9. Genital lesions
10. Vaginal discharge
11. Genital itching and burning
12. Penile discharge
13. Menstrual cramps
14. Vaginal bleeding
15. Breast lumps and/or changes
16. Nipple discharge
17. Visual changes
18. Conjunctivitis
19. Painful joints
20. Height and/or weight changes

E. Prenatal history—maternal ingestion of diethylstilbestrol or estradiol

F. Birth history—number of weeks gestation, testes in scrotum

G. Diet history

H. Current medications and/or opportunity for drug ingestion by child of

1. Estrogen or diethylstilbestrol
2. Androgens
3. Anabolic steroids
4. Use of cosmetic creams containing estrogen

I. Sexuality

1. Feelings and attitudes of parent(s) about discussing sex and answering child's questions regarding sexuality
2. Parental attitudes toward nudity, masturbation, homosexuality
3. Child's knowledge and understanding of body changes occurring during puberty
4. Sex education received (school, home)
5. Age at onset of
   a. Areola pigmentation
   b. Breast development
   c. Pubic hair strands
   d. Axillary and facial hair
   e. Acne
   f. Voice changes
   g. Nocturnal emissions
   h. Ejaculation
6. Sexual activity

J. Menstrual history

1. Age of menarche
2. Frequency/regularity of menses

3. Character, duration, amount of flow
4. Premenstrual symptoms
5. Associated pain—relation to menstrual cycle (time of occurrence and duration)
6. Last menstrual period (LMP)
7. Presence of abnormal bleeding at any time during cycle

K. Contraceptive history

1. Method(s) used
2. Frequency of use
3. Satisfaction with method
4. Date(s) and reasons if method(s) discontinued
5. Desire for birth control information

L. Obstetrical history (see Table 71-4)

1. Prior pregnancies—dates, problems, type of delivery or of termination
2. Current pregnancy
   a. First day of last normal menstrual period
   b. Date of conception, if known
   c. Date of quickening (first perception of fetal movement), if relevant
   d. Common pregnancy-related discomforts
   e. Danger signs (See Pregnancy, Chap. 71, Alert)
   f. Psychosocial
      (1) Pregnancy planned/unplanned
      (2) Desire to keep pregnancy or abort
      (3) Feelings about pregnancy (client, family, father of baby)
      (4) Presence or absence of significant supportive others
   g. Prepregnant weight

M. Past/present history of

1. Hospitalizations
2. Allergies
3. Venereal disease or exposure
4. Encephalitis
5. Meningitis
6. Head trauma
7. Skeletal fractures
8. Cardiac disease
9. Diabetes
10. Hypertension
11. Renal disease/urinary tract infections
12. Cancer
13. Thyroid disease
14. Liver disease
15. Seizure disorders
16. Anemia
17. Severe varicosities
18. Rheumatic fever
19. Rubella/rubella vaccination
20. Psychiatric problems
21. Testes in scrotum at birth or any time since
22. Breast lumps

N. Family history

1. Sexual development (precocious/delayed puberty)
2. Chronic conditions
3. Toxemia of pregnancy
4. Congenital anomalies
5. Repeated spontaneous abortions
6. Multiple gestations
7. Cryptorchidism
8. Cancer
9. Fibrocystic disease or breast lumps

O. Social history

1. Marital status
2. Education
3. Vocational status
4. Economic status
5. Cultural and religious background
6. Sleeping and living conditions
7. Drug/nicotine/alcohol intake

II. Objective data

A. Physical examination

1. Complete physical examination usually indicated
2. Height and weight
3. Vital signs
4. Inspection and palpation of breasts and axillae
5. Abdominal examination
6. Inspection of external genitalia
7. Males: palpation of testes to determine presence bilaterally
   a. Test cremasteric reflexes.
   b. Apply manual pressure behind testes and "milk" into scrotal sac.
   c. If the testes are not palpated, have the client cough or strain (sitting in a chair with knees flexed against the chest and feet on the chair seat).
8. Females: pelvic examination
   a. Speculum examination
   b. Bimanual examination
9. Neurological examination
10. If foreign body discovered, careful examination of all body orifices

B. Laboratory data

1. The following tests may be indicated
   a. Papanicolaou smear
   b. Complete blood count (CBC)
   c. Erythrocyte sedimentation rate (ESR)

d. Urinalysis
e. 24-h urinalysis for gonadotropins, gonadal hormones, and 17-ketosteroids
f. Plasma luteinizing hormone (LH), follicle-stimulating hormone (FSH), testosterone or estradiol levels including free estradiol level
g. Stained vaginal smear for estrogen effect
h. Confirmation of pregnancy
   (1) Urinary immunological tests (from 6 weeks after last menses)
   (2) Serum radioimmunoassay tests (from 8 days after conception)
   (3) Ultrasonography to determine gestational age (from 6 weeks after last menses)
i. Pregnancy
   (1) Clean catch urine
   (2) Blood group and Rh factor
   (3) Venereal Disease Research Laboratory (VDRL) test
   (4) CBC
   (5) Rubella titer
   (6) Hemoglobin electrophoresis (if client black or of Mediterranean origin)
   (7) Papanicolaou smear
   (8) Cervical cultures
j. Exposure to venereal disease
   (1) VDRL for syphilis
   (2) If syphilis suspected—treponemal antibody tests (rough estimate of immunity status)
      (a) Treponema pallidum immobilization (TPI) test
      (b) Fluorescent treponemal antibody (FTA) test
      (c) Fluorescent treponemal antibody absorption (FTA-ABS) test
   (3) Gram strain of urethral discharge, including cervical in female; anorectal and pharyngeal cultures needed dependent on sexual practices
   (4) Microscopic dark-field examination of tissue fluid from lesions (washing first with saline) or aspirate from enlarged lymph node (by physician)
k. Wet mount for causative organism (vaginal discharge)

2. The following tests may be indicated and ordered after consultation with the physician.
   a. Kidney function tests
   b. Buccal smear to determine sex
   c. Brain scan
   d. Electroencephalogram (EEG)
   e. Skull x-rays
   f. Bone age
   g. Mammography (usually not indicated)

57 Undescended Testes

JANE COOPER EVANS

ALERT

1. Testes less than 2.5 cm below pubic crest in male infants weighing less than 2500 g at birth
2. Testes less than 4 cm below pubic crest in term infant
3. Male with undescended testicle over gestational age of 46 weeks
4. Male past puberty with undescended testes
5. Concommitant hypospadias with undescended testes

I. Etiology (basically unknown)

A. Mechanical

1. Small inguinal canal
2. Inadequate superficial inguinal ring
3. Short vas deferens or spermatic vessels
4. Adhesions

B. Genetic

1. Familial tendency (congenital)
2. Testicular dysgenesis
3. Hypogonadism or intersexuality (very rare)
4. Associated with upper urinary tract abnormalities (10 percent)

C. Other

1. Estrogen (estradiol) therapy of mother without human chorionic gonadotropin during pregnancy
2. Premature birth

II. Assessment (Retractile testes)

1. Subjective data
   a. Family history of retractile testes
   b. History of occasional descent
2. Objective data
   a. Elevation of testes with cremasteric reflex
   b. Testicular descent in warm water, with pressure or in tailor position
   c. Palpable intermittently in scrotum

III. Management (Retractile testes)

1. Treatments/medications: none
2. Counselling/prevention: Instruct client and family to report any complaint of pain and/or to return for another visit.
3. Follow-up: Return visit every 6 months to compare size of (right) and (left) testes and to check for complete descent
4. Consultations/referrals: None unless bilateral testes growth differs

Table 57-1 Medical Referral/Consultation

Diagnosis	Clinical Manifestations	Management
Undescended (cryptorchid) testes	Testes nonpalpable, or palpable outside scrotum in male over 46 wk gestation Undescended testes smaller in size than descended testes	Consult physician; refer for surgery. Medication: Some physicians will try human chorionic gonadotropin (HCG) IM 500 to 1000 units twice weekly for 6 wk (50% effective). Surgery is indicated in second year of life.

Table 57-1 Medical Referral/Consultation *(continued)*

Diagnosis	Clinical Manifestations	Management
		See Preparation for Hospitalization, Part 7. Prepare parent(s) and child for "rubber band" attached to the child's thigh postoperatively. Reassure the child that his penis will not be cut in any way. Instruct the parent(s) how to keep the suture line clean and free of fecal material. Instruct the parent(s) about the need for postoperative therapeutic play.
Ectopic testes	Testes nonpalpable Testes palpable in pubic, perineal, or femoral position, or in superficial inguinal area lateral to superficial ring Undescended testes appreciably smaller than descended testes	Refer to physician. Evaluate kidney function. Surgery is indicated with histological changes. See Preparation for Hospitalization, Part 7. Prepare parent(s)/client for prosthesis if one is to be inserted. Reassure the child, regardless of age, that the penis will not be cut in any way. Instruct the parent(s) how to keep the suture line clean and free of fecal material. Instruct the parent(s) about the need for postoperative therapeutic play.

bibliography

Attanasio, A., Rager, K., and Eupta, D. Plasma testosterone in prepubertal cryptorcial boys under long-term HCG therapy. *Hormone Research,* **7**:77–82 (1976).

Gardner, Lytt I. *Endocrine and genetic diseases of childhood.* Philadelphia: Saunders, 1969, pp. 564, 572–575.

Hadzisel, N. F., Herzog, B., and Seguchi, H. Surgical correction of cryptorchidism at 2 years: Electron microscopic and morphometric investigations. *Journal of Pediatric Surgery,* **10**:19–26 (1975).

Lipshultz, L. I. Cryptorchidism in the subfertile male. *Fertility and Sterility,* **27**:609–620 (1976).

McMillan, J. A., Nieburg, P. I., and Oski, F. A. *The whole pediatrician catalog.* Philadelphia: Saunders, 1977, pp. 315–316.

Raifen, J., and Walsh, P. C. The incidence of intersexuality in patients with hypospadias and cryptorchidism. *Journal of Urology,* **116**:769–770 (1976).

Vaughan, Victor C., III, and McKay, R. James. *Nelson's textbook of pediatrics* (10th ed.). Saunders, 1975, pp. 1368–1369.

58 Sexual Concerns/Myths

CHRISTINA M. GRAF

ALERT
1. Symptoms of organic disturbance
2. Indications of significant emotional/psychological disturbance
3. Behavior inappropriate for level of development or age group
4. Indications of significantly disordered family

I. Concerns Related to Children Prior to Adolescence

A. General information
1. Concerns usually expressed by parent(s)
2. Specific behaviors usually related to development level and normal for age group

B. Contributing factors
1. Inadequate or incomplete information on development, including sexual development
2. Parental constraints or feelings of inadequacy in discussing sexuality
3. Lack of availability of educational and counselling services for parent(s)
4. Feelings of inadequacy among health care professionals in discussing sexuality and sexual concerns

C. Guidelines for counselling parent(s)
1. Assess parental understanding of development and reproduction, and provide necessary information.
2. Provide the opportunity for parent(s) to discuss his or her own feelings about sexuality, sex education, and sexual discussions.
3. Review growth and development relative to the age of the child.
4. Relate activities to normal sexual interests of the specific age group.
5. Emphasize the importance of parental reaction to activities.
6. Emphasize that sexual curiosity in children is normal, that repeated questioning indicates a need to assimilate information and not an abnormal preoccupation, and that appropriate discussion of sexual development and activity does not lead to inappropriate behavior.
7. Review points to be considered in approaching a child's questions about sex.
   a. Determine specifically what the child is asking.
   b. Answer questions in an open and matter-of-fact manner.
   c. Use the correct terms.
   d. Avoid plant and animal illustrations when discussing human reproduction.

D. Expressed concerns (Table 58-1)

II. Concerns Related to Adolescents

A. General information
1. Concerns usually expressed by the adolescent
2. Specific behaviors usually related to developmental level and normal for age group

B. Contributing factors
1. Inadequate and incomplete sex information
2. Lack of availability of counselling and health care services
3. Constraints within families on discussion of sexuality
4. Influence of peer group in conveying information, setting group standards, etc.
5. Societal pressure, including exposure to sexual stimuli and information through communications and entertainment media
6. Feelings of inadequacy among health care professionals in discussing sexuality and sexual concerns

C. Guidelines for counselling adolescents

1. Determine understanding of development, reproduction, and sexuality, and provide necessary accurate information.
2. Use correct terminology.
3. Provide privacy and confidentiality.
4. Approach in an open and nonjudgmental manner.
5. Utilize appropriate communication skills to promote discussion.

D. Expressed concerns (Table 58-2)

Table 58-1 Expressed Concerns Related to Children Prior to Adolescence

Age Group	Expressed Concern	Points for Counselling
Infant/toddler	Handling genitals	This reflects normal interest in the body; distract with activity involving the use of hands.
	Showing interest in watching others in bathroom	This reflects normal curiosity about self and others.
	Nudity	Nudity has no moral connotation for the child, who will often persist because the parent(s) demonstrates concern or embarrassment.
Preschooler	Masturbation	This activity is normal for the age group and is pleasurable without being sexual stimulation. A boy may hold his penis to reassure himself that it is there rather than for a pleasurable response. Emphasize to the child that there is an appropriate time and place for this activity.
	Interest in babies, where they come from, etc.	This is a normal interest for this age group, but detailed discussion will mean little. Explore fantasies, correct misconceptions, and answer questions simply.
	Increasing interest in observing or touching genitalia of others and women's breasts	It is related to establishing the child's own body image and to identifying and confirming differences in sexes.
School-age child	Increased interest in reproduction	Discuss in increasing detail as the child shows interest and understanding; repeated questions reflect the need to assimilate increasingly complex information.
	Use of "dirty" words	The child generally does not understand their meaning but uses them to shock parent(s).
	Precocious puberty	Review normal development and emphasize normal variations in development. If signs of true precocious puberty are present, refer for medical evaluation and treatment (see Precocious Puberty, Chap. 61).

Table 58-2 Expressed Concerns/Myths Related to Adolescents

Category	Expressed Concern/Myth	Points for Counselling
	Physical Changes	
Body image	Differences in development from peers indicates abnormality.	Emphasize individual variation as normal; review sequence of development; identify for individual what has occurred and what can be expected.

Table 58-2 Expressed Concerns/Myths Related to Adolescents *(continued)*

Category	Expressed Concern/Myth	Points for Counselling
	Physical Changes (continued)	
	Size of breast or penis relates to sexual ability.	Breast and penis size are not indicators of sexuality.
Menarche/ menstruation (See Puberty/ Menarche, Chap. 60)	Menarche is considered "the curse," as evidence of injury or illness.	Review the physiology of menstruation and its relationship to reproduction.
	Physical activity must be restricted during menstruation.	Menstruation is a normal process and usual activities can be continued and are recommended.
	Bathing, showering, or shampooing hair during menstruation can cause illness.	Review hygiene during menstruation; water cannot enter the vagina during bathing or showering.
Nocturnal emissions ("wet dreams")	Nocturnal emissions indicate sexual disturbance.	Review normal development and physiology of adolescence. Nocturnal emissions occur without sexual stimuli and are a normal response, especially during adolescence.
	Sexual Activity	
Masturbation	Masturbation leads to blindness, insanity, impotency, acne, etc.	Masturbation commonly occurs in adolescence, especially among boys. It is a physical release for sexual tension. It does not injure the body. Excessive masturbation may contribute to interpersonal isolation.
Sexual fantasies	Sexual fantasies indicate sexual abnormality.	These are normal during adolescence. There is rarely any basis in fact.
Homosexuality	Attraction to the same sex or a few homosexual experiences with pleasurable results indicate the individual is homosexual.	Adolescent homosexual experiences tend to be exploratory and transient. Pleasurable responses to homosexual experiences can be consistent with heterosexual development.
Intercourse	Initial inability to have intercourse indicates permanent impotence.	Various stresses may affect the ability to have intercourse at any given time; difficulties do not necessarily indicate impotence and can be resolved between two people who are concerned and work with patience and understanding.
	Sexual ability is increased with use of alcohol or drugs.	Small amounts may release inhibitions; larger amounts usually decrease sexual appetite and interfere with sexual functioning.
	Sexual activity adversely affects athletic performance.	Athletic ability is not decreased—or increased—by sexual activity.
	Intercourse is not safe during menstruation.	Intercourse during menstruation is not harmful.
	Making out, necking, petting, and intercourse are expected, and are necessary as proof of masculinity, femininity, affection, popularity, etc.	The decision to engage in sexual activity is the prerogative of the individual and should not be dictated by social custom or group pressure. Discussion of individual values, reasons for sexual activity, degrees of commitment, and

Table 58-2 Expressed Concerns/Myths Related to Adolescents *(continued)*

Category	Expressed Concern/Myth	Points for Counselling
	Sexual Activity (continued)	
		attendant responsibilities can assist the individual in making the decision.
Conception/ contraception	Conception cannot occur The first time a girl has intercourse During the first year after menarche If menstrual cycles are irregular During the "safe" period If the couple is standing during intercourse If the male withdraws prior to ejaculation If the female douches following intercourse	Review the physiology of conception and methods of contraception. Although there are times when pregnancy is less likely to occur, unprotected intercourse makes pregnancy possible. The only means of avoiding pregnancy are abstinence and adequate contraception.
	Contraception is the responsibility of the female.	Avoiding unwanted pregnancies is the responsibility of both partners.
Venereal disease	Spread of venereal disease is prevented by withdrawal, douching, or use of oral contraceptives.	Review venereal disease: contact, treatment, effects. Venereal disease can be contracted from any infected individual. The possibility of spread can be decreased by the correct use of a condom, but other approaches to prevention are valueless.
	Venereal disease is not spread if the act is pleasurable, during homosexual acts, or during oral-genital or anal-genital contact.	Venereal disease can be contracted from any infected individual and can be spread through contact with mouth or rectum; spread is not related to the degree of pleasure experienced during the act.
	Treatment for one type of venereal disease cures other types and prevents recurrence.	Treatment for venereal disease is specific for each type and does not prevent reinfection. In addition, initial treatment for venereal disease may not be totally effective; therefore, follow-up examination for test of cure is important. Untreated or inadequately treated venereal disease can lead to severe physical problems.

bibliography

Brown, Fred. Sexual problems of the adolescent girl. *Pediatric Clinics of North America,* **19**:759–764 (1972).

Brown, Jacqueline T., and Clancy, Barbara J. Meeting the needs of teens regarding their sexuality. *Issues in Comprehensive Pediatric Nursing,* **1**:29–44 (1976).

Duncan, Jane Watson. An essay on adolescent girls. *Medical Clinics of North America,* **58**:847–856 (1974).

Graft, Christina M. Sex and the adolescent. *Issues in Comprehensive Pediatric Nursing,* **1**:31–41 (1976).

McCary, James Leslie. *Sexual myths and fallacies.* New York: Schocken Books, 1973.

Rybicki, Laura L. Preparing parents to teach their children about human sexuality. *Maternal Child Nursing,* **1**:182–185 (1976).

Satterfield, Sharon. Common sexual problems of children and adolescents. *Pediatric Clinics of North America,* **22**:643–654 (1975).

59 Vagina: Foreign Body

BARBARA J. CHOPLIN / MARY ANN KASPER

ALERT
1. Vaginal discharge
2. Malodorous vaginal discharge
3. Blood-tinged vaginal discharge
4. Low pelvic pain (with large object)
5. Dysuria (child)

I. Etiology

A. Inflammatory reaction to foreign body

B. Inflammatory reaction to foreign body and erosion of vaginal mucosa

C. Inflammatory reaction to foreign body and size of object

D. Child curiosity and exploration

E. Evidenced in adolescents and young adults as a result of
1. Mental disturbance
2. Masturbation
3. Contraception
4. Correction of prolapse

F. Types of foreign bodies
1. Children
   a. Lipstick
   b. Crayon
   c. Pencil
   d. Paper
   e. Stone
   f. Nut
   g. Coin
   h. Button
   i. Bean
   j. Seed
2. Adults
   a. Vaginal tampon
   b. Diaphragm
   c. Vaginal pessary
   d. Bottle
   e. Glass (small drinking or highball)

II. Assessment

A. Subjective data
1. Difficulty and burning with urination
2. Vaginal discharge
3. Foul-smelling vaginal discharge
4. Blood-tinged discharge
5. Difficulty with bowel movements
6. Low abdominal pain
7. Parent(s) reports child manipulates and explores vagina
8. Previous history of foreign body in the vagina
9. Adolescent, young adult
   a. Inability to insert vaginal tampon
   b. Painful intercourse

B. Objective data
1. Vaginal discharge
2. Malodorous vaginal discharge
3. Bloody vaginal discharge
4. Edema of vaginal introitus
5. Visualization of foreign object by vaginoscopy (using nasal or ear speculum)
6. Visualization of protrusion or abnormality of vaginal vault by vaginoscopy
7. Bladder distention

III. Management

A. Treatments/medications
1. Examine using speculum.
2. Remove foreign object if not entrapped.
3. Take culture of discharge.
4. Do vaginal irrigation with small catheter and gravity flow (child).
5. Do vaginal irrigation with gravity flow (adult).
6. Cleanse perineum, using a front to back motion with castile soap, rinse, and pat dry.

B. Counselling/prevention

1. Discuss plan of treatment.
2. Support and reassure the child and adult.
3. Support parent(s) of the child; explain that exploration and manipulation is normal and the child is not a "bad girl."
4. Instruct on perineal hygiene, sitz bath, and proper underclothing (cotton and loose-fitting).
5. Educate client and parent(s) to prevent reoccurrence.

C. Follow-up

1. Do reexamination if
   a. Discharge does not disappear rapidly.
   b. Inflammation does not subside in 3 days.
   c. Secondary irritation does not subside in 3 weeks.
2. If condition reoccurs, consider referral to rule out emotional disorders.

D. Consultations/referrals

1. Refer to physician if unable to remove the entrapped object, or if further treatment is needed.
2. Refer for professional counselling if reoccurrence or if inordinate masturbation.

Table 59-1 Medical Referral/Consultation

Diagnosis	Clinical Manifestations	Management
Vaginal foreign body (entrapped)	Vaginal discharge Malodorous vaginal discharge Blood-tinged vaginal discharge Dysuria (child) Edema of vaginal introitus Entrapped foreign body Bladder distention Enlarged and tender inguinal nodes Abdominal tenderness Firm mass felt upon rectal examination	Refer to physician. Obtain medical history. Have physician remove entrapped object (under anesthesia if necessary). Use pharmacological intervention. Administer analgesics. Do vaginal irrigation. Recommend perineal hygiene. Use sitz bath. Refer for professional counselling.

bibliography

Given, F. T., and Mattox, H. E. Large foreign body in the vagina. *North Carolina Medical Journal* **31**:91—92 (1970).

Huffman, John. Premenarchal vulvovaginitis. *Clinical Obstetrics and Gynecology* **3**:581–593 (1977).

McAllister, D., and Gusdon, John. Vaginal foreign body of long duration in a child. *American Journal of Obstetrics and Gynecology* **115**(2):278 (1973).

Romney, Seymour, et al. *Gynecology and obstetrics: The health care of women.* New York: McGraw-Hill, 1975, pp. 122, 230–231.

Schneider, G. T. Vaginitis in adolescent girls. *Clinical Obstetrics and Gynecology,* **14**:1057–1079 (1971).

Scipien, Gladys, et al. *Comprehensive pediatric nursing* (2d ed.). New York: McGraw-Hill, 1979, pp. 806–807.

60 Puberty/Menarche

CHRISTINA M. GRAF

ALERT

1. Onset of pubertal development prior to 8 years of age in females and 10 years of age in males (see Precocious Puberty, Chap. 61)
2. Onset of pubertal development delayed beyond 13.4 years of age in females and 13.7 years of age in males (see Delayed Puberty, Chap. 62)
3. Failure of pubertal changes to progress (see Delayed Puberty, Chap. 62)
4. Absence of menarche in females over 17 years of age whose sexual development has otherwise been normal

I. Etiology

A. Hypothalamus stimulation of the anterior pituitary causes release of gonadotropic hormones (primarily the follicle-stimulating hormone [FSH]).

B. Stimulated by gonadotropic hormones, gonadal hormones are released.

1. Androgens
   a. Action in males: development of testes, scrotum, penis; voice changes; growth of pubic and axillary hair; skeletal and muscular growth
   b. Action in females: development of clitoris and labia majora, growth of pubic and axillary hair, skeletal and muscular growth
2. Estrogens
   a. Action in males: osteogenesis
   b. Action in females: development of uterus, tubes, cervix, vagina, external genitalia; breast development; distribution of body fat; osteogenesis
3. Progesterone
   a. action in males: acne
   b. action in females: endometrial secretions, breast development, voice changes, acne

II. Assessment

A. Sequence of pubertal development in males

1. Genital development
   a. Enlarged testes and scrotum
   b. Elongated penis
   c. Adult genitalia in size and shape
   d. Genital development beginning between 9.5 and 15.5 years of age (mean 11.6 years), usually reaching adult stage within 2 to 5 years of onset
2. Pubic hair development
   a. Sparse growth at base of penis
   b. Darker, coarser growth
   c. Growth spreading upward from base of penis in diamond-shaped pattern
   d. Thickening and spreading to thighs
   e. Onset between 9 and 12 years of age, with complete development by late teens
3. Growth spurt
   a. Average age at onset 13.5 years
   b. Follows typical pattern: hands and feet, calves and forearms, hips, chest, shoulders, trunk
   c. Height increasing 7 to 12 cm at peak of spurt
   d. Maximum height reached in late teens
   e. Weight almost doubling between 12 and 16 years of age
4. Axillary hair development—occurs between 12.5 and 16.5 years of age
5. Facial and body hair development—occurs between 14.5 and 17.5 years of age

6. Nocturnal emissions, ejaculations
   a. Usually occur 1 year after onset of genital development.
   b. Mature sperm production occurs between 14.5 and 17.5 years of age.

B. Sequence of pubertal development in females
1. Breast development
   a. Budding of breasts
   b. Enlargement of breasts and areola
   c. Growth to mature breasts
   d. Development begins with budding between 8 and 13 years of age (mean 11.5 years) and usually reaches mature stage in 4.5 years from onset.
2. Pubic hair
   a. Sparse, slightly pigmented hair along labia
   b. Darker, coarser hair
   c. Growth across mons veneris in triangular-shaped pattern
   d. Thickening and spreading to thighs
   e. Onset usually coincides with breast budding; development completed in late teens
3. Growth spurt
   a. Average age of onset 10.5 years
   b. Follows typical pattern: hands and feet, calves and forearms, hips, chest, shoulders, trunk
   c. Height increases 6 to 11 cm at peak of spurt
   d. Maximum height usually reached by 16 years
4. Axillary hair—occurs between 12 and 15 years of age
5. Menarche
   a. Average age of onset 12.5 to 13.5 years, with range from 9 to 17 years
   b. Usually occurs 0.5 to 5.8 years (average 2.3 years) following breast budding; occurs following maximum growth rate
   c. Initial cycles usually anovulatory and irregular
   d. Ovulatory cycles usually established within 2 years following menarche

III. Management

A. Counselling
1. Emphasize variations among individuals in growth and development.
2. Review developmental sequence.
   a. Identify development which has occurred.
   b. Explain what can be expected according to normal sequence.
3. Clarify misconceptions related to pubertal changes, sexual myths, etc.
4. Provide opportunity for client/family to express concerns or ask questions about puberty, sexual development, etc.
5. Review physiology of menarche and discuss hygiene, activity, and relief of attendant discomforts.
6. Provide information where needed on sexual activity, contraception, venereal disease, and pregnancy.

B. Follow-up: the frequency of return visits determined by the need for counselling

C. Consultations/referrals
Referral to a physician is required if there is any indication of abnormal development or pathology.

bibliography

Goldfarb, Alvin F. Puberty and menarche. *Clinical Obstetrics and Gynecology*, **20**:625–632 (1977).

Kagut, Maurice D. Growth and development in adolescence. *Pediatric Clinics of North America*, **20**:789–806 (1973).

Millar, Hilary E. C. *Approaches to adolescent health care in the 1970s*. Washington, D.C.: U.S. Department of Health, Education, and Welfare, 1975.

Scipien, G. M., Bernard, M. U., Chard, M. A., Howe, J., and Phillips, P. J. *Comprehensive pediatric nursing* (2d ed.). New York: McGraw-Hill, 1979.

61 Precocious Puberty

JANE COOPER EVANS

ALERT

1. Sexual development in female less than 8 years of age
2. Sexual development in male less than 10 years of age
3. Disproportionate enlargement of genitalia
4. Lack of gonadal development with presence of secondary sex characteristics

I. Etiology

A. Idiopathic, constitutional, or cryptogenic (9 times more common in females)

1. Premature thelarche
2. Premature pubarche
3. True precocious puberty

Note: All cases of early sexual development should be referred to a physician for diagnosis of cause.

B. Central nervous system (CNS) disorder (50 percent more common in males)

1. Brain tumor (granuloma, hamartoma)
2. Benign tumor hypothalamus
3. Albright's syndrome (pigmentation and bone dysplasia)
4. Neurofibromatosis
5. Following encephalitis or meningitis
6. Head trauma
7. Degenerative lesions of midbrain and hypothalamus
8. Tuberous sclerosis
9. Toxoplasmosis
10. Congenital syphilis

C. Tumors (other than CNS)

1. Adrenal (most common)
2. Ovarian/testicular cyst or neoplasm
3. Pineal
4. Pituitary

D. Hypothyroidism

Table 61-1 Medical Referral/Consultation

Diagnosis	Clinical Manifestations	Management
Premature thelarche	Unilateral or bilateral breast development without any other pubertal changes (most often between ages 1 and 3) No areolar changes and usually no nipple enlargement No development of labia minora, vagina, or uterus Growth and ossification normal (no rapid growth) Laboratory work negative for cornification of vaginal epithelium and urinary estrogens	Consult physician to reinforce diagnosis. Instruct parent(s) and child about condition—puberty will occur at normal time. Schedule follow-up visits every 3–6 mo, depending on development. No treatment is necessary—condition may be transient or persist for years.

Table 61-1 Medical Referral/Consultation *(continued)*

Diagnosis	Clinical Manifestations	Management
	Only free estradiol elevated—estrone and estradiol normal Plasma levels of gonadotropins and urinary 17-ketosteroids normal, as is bone age	
Premature pubarche (adrenarche)	Growth of pubic hair (occasionally axillary hair also) in female under 8 or male under 10 yr No other evidence of sexual development Normal height and ossification for age Normal 17-ketosteroids, and gonadotropins,	Consult physician—may refer to rule out other causes. No treatment required. Follow-up every 6 mo. Complete neurological and physical exam Repetition of EEG and skull series because of high incidence of CNS lesions after further maturation
True precocious puberty	Penis and testes increase in size simultaneously. Development of labia minora, vagina, or uterus, as well as breasts, occurs. Ovulation or spermatogenesis occurs. Bone age moderately increased. Urinary gonadotropins are elevated to adolescent levels. Urinary 17-ketosteroids are elevated to adolescent levels.	Consult physician and refer to rule out other causes. Assess child's understanding of sex and educate accordingly. Assist parent(s) to understand Precocious sexual development does not necessarily mean precocious mental development. Sexual drive is not abnormal. Sterility or aberrant sexual behavior is atypical. Assist child in dealing with sexual advances from others. Help parent(s) understand that child needs to be shielded against sexual abuses. Reassure parent(s) that the only long-term result of precocious puberty is shorter-than-average height. Increase intake of vitamin D, calcium, and protein. Explore possibilities of accelerating academic development, if the child's IQ is high enough. Medications, possibly prescribed by the physician, are cyproterone or medroxyprogesterone acetate Follow-up. Complete physical examination, including abdominal, genital, and rectal, every 4–6 mo, to detect adrenal tumor, ovarian neoplasm, abdominal mass, or testicular tumor Complete neurological examination, including eyes, visual fields, EEG, and skull x-rays (if possible), every 6 mo
CNS lesion	Premature pubarche in males without other signs of sexual maturation	Immediately refer to a physician.

Table 61-1 Medical Referral/Consultation *(continued)*

Diagnosis	Clinical Manifestations	Management
	Sexual development in males between 6 and 10 yr Sexual development in females between 6 and 8 yr Onset within 2 yr of birth usually indicative of hamartoma Neurologic signs and symptoms Urinary gonadotropins elevated *only* with chorionepithelioma	After lesion is identified, surgery may be indicated. See Preparation for Hospitalization, Part 7. After hospitalization assist the child to ventilate feelings, and counsel accordingly.
Tumors (other than CNS lesion)	Acne, hirsutism, and/or clitoral enlargement Unilateral enlargement of the testes Unilateral enlargement of the ovary Masculinization in females Feminization in males Adrenal mass Circulating estrogen/testosterone levels elevated above that of other gonadal hormones Vaginal smear positive for estrogen, with excess squamous epithelium (some keratinization) Elevated pregnanediol Elevated 17-ketosteroids, especially with adrenal tumors and hepatomas	Immediately refer to a physician. Surgery is indicated to remove tumor after identification. See Preparation for Hospitalization, Part 7. After hospitalization assist child to ventilate feelings, and counsel accordingly.
Hypothyroidism	Development of secondary sex characteristics—especially breast development in females and testicular enlargement in males Prepubertal bone age Growth retardation Sparse or absent pubic hair and axillary hair Estrogenized vaginal mucosa and menstrual bleeding—especially with minimal breast development Excessive pigmentation, galactorrhea, and papilledema Enlargement of sella turcica Plasma levels of prolactin and thyroid-stimulating hormone (TSH) are elevated Follicle-stimulating hormone (FSH) and luteinizing hormone (LH) elevated to adult levels Protein-bound iodine (PBI) level below 2.5 μg per 100 mL of serum	Immediately refer to a physician. Treatment with thyroid hormones Follow-up Counselling for any psychological problems or adjustment problems Checking on compliance with drug regimen

bibliography

Gardner, Lytt I. *Endocrine and genetic diseases of childhood.* Philadelphia: Saunders, 1969, pp. 544–562.

Kauli, R., Pertzelan, A., Prager-Lewin, R., et al. Cyproterone acetate in treatment of precocious puberty. *Archives of Diseases in Childhood,* **51**:202–208 (1976).

Radfar, N., Ansusingha, K., and Kenny, F. M. Circulating bound and free estradiol and estrone during normal growth and development and in premature thelarche and isosexual precocity. *Journal of Pediatrics,* **89**:719–723 (1976).

Silver, H. K., Kempe, C. H., and Bruyn, H. B. *Handbook of pediatrics* (11th ed.). Los Altos, Calif.: Lange, 1975, pp. 183, 405–407.

Vaughan, Victor C., III, and McKay, R. James. *Nelson's textbook of pediatrics* (10th ed.). Philadelphia: Saunders, 1975, pp. 1294–1299, 1354–1358.

62 Delayed Puberty

JANE COOPER EVANS

ALERT

1. Lack of breast buds and pubic hair strands in a female 13.4 years of age
2. Failure of female to progress from breast bud to larger and more elevated breast with a wide areola in 1 year
3. Absence of menarche in female within 5 years of development of breast buds
4. No growth of external genitalia or pubic hair strands in a male 13.7 years of age
5. Failure of male to progress from reddening and enlargement of scrotum to enlargement of penis in 2.2 years

Etiology

A. Constitutional/idiopathic (90 percent cases)

B. Congenital disorders

1. Chromosomal disorders
   a. Turner's syndrome (common cause)
   b. Klinefelter's syndrome (common cause)
   c. Testicular feminization
   d. Gonadal agenesis
2. Malabsorption syndromes
3. Congenital hypothalamic disorders
   a. Laurence-Moon-Biedl syndrome
   b. Prader-Willi syndrome
4. Congenital pituitary gonadotropin deficiency
5. Hypothyroidism or hyperthyroidism

C. Malnutrition

1. Socioeconomic
2. Anorexia nervosa
3. Pica

D. Infections or neoplasms of hypothalamus, pituitary, or gonads

E. Systemic disease

1. Chronic heart, renal, hepatic, or lung disease
2. Anemias
3. Collagen diseases
4. Inflammatory bowel disease (increased sedimentation rate)
5. Diabetes mellitus

Table 62-1 Medical Referral/Consultation*

Diagnosis	Clinical Manifestations	Management
Constitutional/idiopathic delayed puberty	Short stature for age Below 3 standard deviations of mean height for age Linear growth rate 3.75–5 cm/yr Bone age retarded by 1.5–4 yr Absence of sexual development Plasma gonadotropin levels below normal for age	Consultation with physician Laboratory tests Blood: CBC, LH, FSH, gonadal hormones, and growth hormone study Chromosomal analysis Urinary gonadotropins Bone age x-rays

*All clients require physician consultation or referral to rule out pathology.

Table 62-1 Medical Referral/Consultation *(continued)*

Diagnosis	Clinical Manifestations	Management
	Growth hormone below normal in some males	Medication: *none* unless severe psychological or social disability exists Spironolactone 5 mg/kg daily for 1 wk (boys only) In males: fluoxymesterone 10 mg daily by mouth for 4–6 mo (larger doses or longer treatment not recommended because of early epiphyseal closure) In females: none, but in severe cases, low-dose cyclic estrogens given for 3 mo Counselling Alleviate anxiety about masculinity or femininity. Give estimate of approximate adult height from the Greulich and Pyle tables. Weekly psychological counselling may be necessary with severe social or psychological disability. Follow-up visit every 6 mo
Turner's syndrome (XO syndrome)	Female Height below 3rd percentile for age Absence of sexual development, or no more than stage 3 pubic hair Chromosomal XO karyotype or mosaic karyotype (buccal smear perhaps normal) Coarctation of aorta perhaps present Elevation of serum LH and FSH sometimes to postmenopausal range Sometimes short or webbed neck, shieldlike chest, cubitus valgus, lymphedema of hands or feet present	Referral to physician Laboratory tests Serum LH and FSH determination Chromosomal analysis Cyclic medication Conjugated estrogen tablets 2.5 mg daily for first 25 days of the month Medroxyprogesterone acetate tablets 10 mg daily for days 18 through 25 of the month Counselling Reassure girls about femininity. Psychological counselling may be necessary.
Klinefelter's syndrome	Eunuchoid body build No growth of testes (small, firm) or penis Gynecomastia perhaps present bilaterally Mental subnormality *possibly* present Chromosomal karyotype of XXY with 47 chromosomes Elevated urinary FSH level Low plasma testosterone Height at or greater than 50th percentile, but a decreased upper-to-lower body segment ratio	Consultation with physician Chromosomal and urinary FSH studies Medication: methyltestosterone 20–40 mg daily by mouth for 3–6 mo to reduce gynecomastia Plastic surgery perhaps indicated for gynecomastia Counselling Explain diagnosis and ramifications to parent(s) and child. Psychological counselling may be necessary should antisocial personality or schizophrenia develop.

Table 62-1 Medical Referral/Consultation *(continued)*

Diagnosis	Clinical Manifestations	Management
	Arm span exceeding height by more than 2.5 cm Males below 3rd percentile in height possibly having male Turner's syndrome	Follow-up: yearly visits to pick up developing antisocial personality or schizophrenia

bibliography

Barnes, H. V. The problem of delayed puberty. *Medical Clinics of North America,* **59**:1337–1347 (1975).

Barnes, H. V. The teenager with pubertal delay. *Primary Care,* **3**:215–229 (1976).

Gruelich, W. W., and Pyle, S. I. *Radiographic atlas of skeletal development of hand and wrist* (2d ed.). Stanford, Calif.: Stanford, 1959.

Kogut, M. D. Growth and development in adolescence. *Pediatric Clinics of North America,* **20**:794–795 (1973).

Prader, A. Delayed adolescence. *Journal of Clinical Endocrinology & Metabolism,* **4**:143–155 (1975).

Root, A. W., and Reiter, E. O. Evaluation and management of the child with delayed pubertal development. *Fertility Sterility,* **27**:745–755 (1976).

Santen, R. J., Kulin, H. E., Loriaux, D. L., and Friend, J. Spironolactone stimulation of gonadotropin secretion in boys with delayed adolescence. *Journal of Clinical Endocrinology & Metabolism,* **43**:1386–1390 (1976).

Vaughan, Victor C., III, and McKay, R. James. *Nelson's textbook of pediatrics* (10th ed.). Philadelphia: Saunders, 1975.

63 DES Daughters/Sons

BARBARA J. CHOPLIN/ MARY ANN KASPER

ALERT[1]

1. Young female or male (7 to 27 years of age) with maternal history of diethylstilbestrol (DES) ingestion during pregnancy
2. Abnormal vaginal bleeding
3. Vaginal discharge
4. Infertility (female and male)
5. Dysuria (male)

I. Etiology

A. DES or chemically related nonsteroid synthetic-estrogen ingestion

B. Known teratogenic effect, i.e., exposure is harmful first 18 weeks of gestation

II. Assessment

A. DES daughters

1. Subjective data
   - a. Irregular frequency, amount, and duration of menstrual flow
   - b. Vaginal discharge
   - c. Infertility
   - d. Fear of cancer
   - e. History of maternal DES ingestion
     - (1) Mother of affected daughter—received a "drug" to treat high-risk pregnancy between 1940 and 1971
     - (2) DES used to control miscarriage, vaginal bleeding, diabetes, and toxemia
2. Objective data
   - a. Nonheoplastic changes in the female genital tract
     - (1) Vaginal adenosis (tiny cysts, ulcers, or papillary lesions)
     - (2) Cervical ectropion, or eversion
     - (3) Vaginal and cervical ridges; collars, rims, cockscomb cervix, pseudopolyp
     - (4) Red granular mucosa on cervix and vaginal wall
   - b. Clear-cell adenocarcinoma of the vagina and cervix

B. DES sons

1. Subjective data
   - a. Difficulty passing urine
   - b. Infertility
2. Objective data
   - a. Epididymal cysts
   - b. Hypotrophic testes
   - c. Induration of the testicular capsule
   - d. Semen analysis
     - (1) Abnormalities in the appearance of the sperm
     - (2) Marked reductions in sperm count
     - (3) Decreased sperm mobility

III. Management

A. DES daughters

1. Treatments/medications: treatment is by physician; see Medical Referral/Consultation, Table 63-1.
   - a. Do screening exam once client begins to menstruate or reaches age of 14.
   - b. Record mother's history, obtain medical records.
2. Counselling/prevention
   - a. Offer reassurance and support.
     - (1) Recognize client's anxiety regarding examination and possible findings.
     - (2) Be honest and empathetic in approach.

[1]Any client whose mother is reported to have taken diethylstilbestrol during pregnancy should be referred to a physician.

(3) Support the mother due to her possible feelings of guilt.
(4) Enhance mother/child relationship through communication; i.e., suggest mother inform daughter of findings.

b. Explain tests and procedures for initial examination.

c. Provide anticipatory guidance about medical intervention and preventive treatment.
(1) Use photographs and printed instructions in explaining tests and procedures to be used during medical intervention.
(2) Give appropriate and correct information.
(3) Stress importance of follow-up with explanation of possible risks.
(a) Girls with history of DES exposure should not take oral contraceptives or "morning-after pill."
(b) Presence of adenosis is not a contraindication to future pregnancy.
(c) Infertility can occur but is not common; successful pregnancy and delivery have been achieved.
(d) Risk of clear-cell carcinoma is small.

3. Follow-up
a. Client will need follow-up throughout life.
(1) Frequency is dependent upon severity of findings.
(2) Suggest examinations every 6 months as adenosis can progress to neoplastic changes.
(3) Include pelvic examination with cervical vaginal cytology and iodine staining.
b. Strive to establish a trust relationship with client.

4. Consultations/referrals:
Refer to physician, as it is difficult without colposcopic evaluation to identify difference between vaginal and cervical effects of DES and simple erosion, benign cyst, or irritation.

B. DES sons

1. Treatments/medications: treatment is by physician; see Medical Referral/Consultation, Table 63-1.
2. Counselling/prevention
a. Record mother's history; obtain medical records.
b. Give reassurance and support.
(1) Recognize client's anxiety regarding examination and possible findings.
(2) Be honest and empathetic in approach.
(3) Help mother deal with possible feelings of guilt.
(4) Enhance mother/child relationship through communication; i.e., suggest mother inform son of findings.
c. Explain tests and procedures for initial examination.
d. Provide anticipatory guidance about medical intervention and preventive treatment.
(1) Use photographs and printed instructions in explaining tests and procedures to be used during medical intervention.
(2) Give appropriate and correct information.
(3) Stress importance of follow-up with explanation of possible risks.
(a) Subinfertility and infertility can occur.
(b) Research to date has not demonstrated development of malignant lesions.
3. Follow-up: frequency is dependent upon findings.
4. Consultations/referrals: consult physician and refer if necessary.

Table 63-1 Medical Referral/Consultation

Diagnosis	Clinical Manifestations	Management
FEMALE		
Abnormal changes in vagina and/or cervix Abnormal pap smear Abnormal iodine test	Young female with maternal history of DES ingestion during pregnancy Abnormal vaginal bleeding Vaginal discharge Infertility Nonneoplastic changes in the female tract	Referral to physician Management contingent upon findings: Biopsy of lesion, then histopathologic diagnosis Cryosurgery Cautery Hysterosalpinography Pharmacological intervention

Table 63-1 Medical Referral/Consultation *(continued)*

Diagnosis	Clinical Manifestations	Management
	Vaginal adenosis (tiny cysts, ulcers, or papillary lesions) Cervical ectropion, or eversion Vaginal and cervical ridges; collars, rims, cockscomb cervix, pseudopolyp Red granular mucosa on cervix and vaginal wall Clear-cell adenocarcinoma of the vagina and cervix	Progesterone vaginal suppositories Acidification of vagina with creams, jellies Treatment for clear-cell carcinoma Surgery Radical hysterectomy Vaginectomy Radiation
MALE		
Dysuria Infertility	Young male with maternal history of DES ingestion during pregnancy Epididymal cysts Hypotrophic tests Induration of the testicular capsule Semen analysis Abnormalities in the appearance of the sperm Marked reduction in sperm count Decreased sperm mobility	Referral to physican Laboratory studies Urine cytology Prostatic fluid cytology Semen analysis

bibliography

Auclair, Carolyn. Consequences of prenatal exposure to diethylstilbestrol. *Journal of Obstetric, Gynecologic and Neonatal Nursing* 8(1):35–39 (1979).

Bibbo, M., et al. Follow-up study of male and female offspring of DES-exposed mothers. *American Journal of Obstetrics and Gynecology* 1:1–8 (1977).

Emans, S., and Goldstein, D. *Pediatric and adolescent gynecology*. Boston: Little, Brown, 1977, pp. 123–126.

Hajj, Samir, and Herbst, Arthur. Evaluation and management of diethylstilbestrol-exposed offspring. *Surgical Clinics of North America* 1:87–96 (1978).

Herbst, A., Scully, R., and Robboy, S. Diethylstilbestrol-exposed females. In *Office gynecology*. Baltimore: Williams & Wilkins, 1976, pp. 133–143.

Schwartz, R., and Stewart, N. Psychological effects of Diethylstilbestrol exposure. *Journal of the American Medical Association* 3:252–254 (1977).

Weiss, Kay, and Elkin, Sandra. DES daughters and sons. *Woman*, Program Part I, 432, and Part II, 433. Buffalo: Public Television WNED.

64 Vaginal Spotting/Bleeding

MARY ANN KASPER/BARBARA J. CHOPLIN

ALERT

1. Suspicion of physical and/or sexual abuse
2. Neonate
   a. Vaginal bleeding in first few days of life (rare)
   b. Vaginal bleeding associated with gynecomastia
3. Child: vaginal spotting or bleeding due to
   a. Foreign body in the vagina (see Vagina: Foreign Body, Chap. 59)
   b. Ingestion of exogenous hormones
   c. Precocious sexual development before age 8 (see Precocious Puberty, Chap. 61)
   d. DES daughter with premenarcheal vaginal bleeding (see DES Daughters/Sons, Chap. 63)
4. Adolescent
   a. Menstruation
      (1) Menorrhagia (excessive menstrual flow)
      (2) Oligomenorrhea (infrequent menses)
   b. Abortion
   c. Foreign bodies
5. Young adult
   a. Pregnancy
   b. Contraception
      (1) Breakthrough bleeding or spotting due to oral contraceptive
      (2) IUD cramping
         (a) Menorrhagia
         (b) Intermenstrual spotting
   c. Dysfunctional menstrual disorders
      (1) Menorrhagia
      (2) Oligomenorrhea
   d. Intermenstrual disorders
      (1) Menorrhagia
      (2) Metrorrhagia
      (3) Menometrorrhagia
   e. Foreign body
   f. Vaginal lacerations (see Common Genital Lesions, Chap. 69)
   g. Vaginal infection (see Vaginal Discharge, Chap. 66)

I. Etiology

A. Neonate

Endometrial sloughing due to postdelivery maternal estrogen withdrawal

B. Child

1. Inflammatory reaction and erosion of vaginal mucosa due to foreign body
2. Hormone ingestion
3. CNS, pituitary or ovarian lesions; adrenal tumor; or iatrogenic ingestion of estrogen or birth control pills
4. Maternal history of DES ingestion during pregnancy

C. Adolescent

Cyclic sloughing of the endometrium due to

a. Menorrhagia: organic lesions, endocrine disturbances, emotional disturbances, or presence of IUD
b. Oligomenorrhea: cyclic ovulation that has not been established, result of birth control pills, or emotional disturbances

D. Young adult

1. Pregnancy
   a. Abortion
      (1) Abnormalities of ovum and sperm
      (2) Abnormalities of the female generative tract
      (3) Maternal host factors
      (4) Decreased production of progesterone
      (5) Incompetent cervix
   b. Hydatidiform mole: unknown, degenerative process in chorionic villi

c. Ectopic pregnancy: gestational implant outside uterine cavity
d. Premature separation of the placenta: unknown, contributing factors
(1) Pregnancy-induced hypertension (Toxemia)
(2) Chronic hypertension
(3) Multigravida
(4) History of reproductive wastage
(5) Uterine manipulation and trauma
(6) Low socioeconomic status
e. Placenta previa: unknown, reduced vascularity of upper-uterine segment due to scarring or tumor
2. Contraception
a. Oral contraceptives
(1) Failure of synthetic sex steroids to provide adequate stimulus to the endometrium
(2) Failure to maintain endometrium until end of pill cycle
b. IUD: unknown, reaction to foreign body
3. Dysfunctional menstrual disorders
4. Intermenstrual disorders
a. Uterine fibroids
b. Endometrial hyperplasia
c. Chronic cervicitis
d. Cervical erosion
e. Cervical polyps
f. Endometriosis
g. Ovulation/anovulation
h. Uterine cancer
5. Foreign body
6. Vaginal lacerations
7. Vaginal infection

II. Assessment

A. Neonate: Vaginal bleeding
1. Subjective data: none
2. Objective data
a. Small amount of bleeding on diaper or tissue
b. Edema of vulva

B. Child: see Table 64-1, Medical Referral/ Consultation

C. Adolescent/young adult
1. Menstruation
a. Subjective data
(1) Irregular- or regular-cyclic, dark-red vaginal bleeding
(2) Vaginal bleeding for 2 to 7 days
(3) Scanty or heavy menstrual periods
(4) Cramping with vaginal bleeding
(5) Heavy, dull backache
(6) Nausea and vomiting
(7) Heachache
(8) Bloating and weight gain
(9) Irritability and mood swings
b. Objective data
(1) Development of secondary sex characteristics commensurate with age
(2) Pelvic examination findings related to
(a) Age (puberty/adult cycle)
(b) Sexual activity (pregnancy/abortion)
(c) Type of contraception (pills/IUD)
(d) Pathology
2. Contraception
a. Oral contraceptives
(1) Subjective data
(a) History of taking oral contraceptives
(b) Bleeding early in pill cycle (before day 10)
(c) Bleeding that never ceases completely after menstruation
(d) Bleeding of the eleventh cycle day
(2) Objective data: none
b. IUD
(1) Subjective data
(a) History that reveals IUD being used
(b) Heavy menstruation
(c) Incomplete relief of menstrual cramps
(2) Objective data: none

III. Management

A. Neonate: vaginal bleeding
1. Treatments/medications: none
2. Counselling/prevention
a. Explain and discuss with parent(s) the condition and its cause. Condition is usually self-limited.
b. Allay undue concern.
c. Stress that discharge and edema beyond neonatal period is abnormal and requires prompt attention.
d. Teach proper perineal hygienic measures.
3. Follow-up: usually none
4. Consultations/referrals: none

B. Child: see Table 64-1, Medical Referral/ Consultation

C. Adolescent/young adult
1. Menstruation
a. Treatments/medications
(1) Usually none
(2) Comfort measures
(3) See Menstrual Cramps, Chap. 65
(4) Pelvic examination to rule out pathology
(5) Pap smear and cervical culture
(6) Pregnancy test if indicated

(7) Reevaluation of contraception, e.g., remove IUD, adjust birth control pill dosage

b. Counselling/prevention

(1) Reassure and support client.

(a) Teaching client about

1. Cause of menstrual cramps

2. Comfort measures

a. Heating pad or hot water bottle applied to the abdomen

b. Exercise and activity as tolerated

c. Knee-chest position

d. Warm liquids

e. Warm bath

f. High calcium and protein intake

g. Nonprescription drugs

3. Hygiene

4. Dispelling myths

5. Contraceptive counselling

(b) Convey positive attitude.

(2) Explain examination procedures and preliminary findings.

(3) Provide anticipatory guidance about medical follow-up.

c. Follow-up: frequency depends on findings.

d. Consultations/referrals: refer to physician those with

(1) Excessive menstrual flow

(2) Severe, incapacitating cramps unresponsive to comfort measures

2. Contraception

a. Oral contraceptives

(1) Treatments/medications

(a) Examine for other causes of bleeding.

(b) Observe for one more cycle, then reassess.

(c) Change medication to one with greater androgen and progestin potency.

(d) If that fails, change medication to one with greater estrogen content.

(e) Discontinue oral contraceptive and choose an alternative method of contraception.

(f) See Birth Control, Chap. 17.

(2) Counselling/prevention

(a) Reassure and support client.

1. Recognize client's anxiety regarding examination and possible findings.

2. Be honest and empathetic in approach.

3. Provide emotional support.

(b) Explain procedures of examination.

(c) Provide anticipatory guidance about intervention and treatment.

1. Give appropriate and correct information about

a. Breakthrough bleeding and spotting

b. Follow-up during three cycles

c. Backup method of contraception

d. Proper method of pill taking

2. Stress importance of follow-up.

(3) Follow-up: frequency depends on findings.

(4) Consultations/referrals: consult physician.

b. IUD

(1) Treatments/medications

(a) Vaginal examination to confirm cause of bleeding and presence of IUD.

(b) Assess for signs and symptoms of infection.

(c) Assess for pregnancy (i.e., spontaneous abortion or ectopic pregnancy).

(d) See Birth Control, Chap. 17.

(2) Counselling/prevention

(a) Reassure and support client.

1. Recognize client's anxiety regarding examination and possible findings.

2. Be honest and empathetic in approach

3. Provide emotional support.

(b) Explain procedures used in examination.

(c) Provide anticipatory guidance about intervention and treatment.

1. Give appropriate and correct information about

a. Expulsions, most of which occur within 3 months

b. Methods and time to check for string

c. Alternate method of contraception

2. Stress importance of follow-up.

(3) Follow-up: frequency depends on findings.

(4) Consultations/referrals: consult physician.

Table 64-1 Medical Referral/Consultation

Diagnosis	Clinical Manifestations	Management
CHILD		
Ingestion of exogenous hormones	History of taking estrogen or birth control pills Menstruation Early development of secondary sex characteristics	Consult with/refer to physician. Symptoms are usually self-limited. Reassure parent(s). Counsel regarding accident prevention (see Chap.9).
Precocious sexual development	Possible history of ingestion of estrogen tablets Early development of secondary sex characteristics Acne Hirsutism Voice change Increased muscle mass Clitoromegaly Menstruation before age 8 Early breast development Taller than average 8–10-year-old child Ovarian masses easily palpable when present	Refer to physician/endocrinologist. See Precocious Puberty, Chap. 61. Reassure child and parent(s). Recognize child's anxiety regarding examination and findings. Assist child and parent(s) to understand their reactions. Be honest, calm, and empathetic in approach. Explain examination procedures and preliminary findings to parent(s) and child.
ADOLESCENT		
Menorrhagia Oligomenorrhea	Development of secondary sex characteristics commensurate with age Pelvic examination findings related to Age Sexual activity Type of contraception Pathology	Refer to physician. Treat according to findings. Follow for several cycles to assess flow. Reevaluate contraception; i.e., remove IUD, adjust birth control pill dosage. Recommend medical or surgical treatment of pathological conditions.
YOUNG ADULT		
Abortion	Missed period Spotting Cramping backache Dark, bright-red vaginal bleeding Cervix closed and noneffaced or open and effaced Soft, enlarged uterus Possible presence of Hegar's and Chadwick's signs Persistent vaginal bleeding Observation of tissue Weak positive pregnancy test Decreased hemoglobin and hematocrit	Refer to physician. Obtain history. Assess for signs of shock. Assess blood loss. Save all tissues and clots passed. Observe for signs of cramping. Give RhoGAM within 72 h, if appropriate. Discuss Recovery time Danger signs Signs of infection Provide contraceptive information. Suggest home treatment. Modified activity Avoidance of stress Avoidance of orgasm

Table 64-1 Medical Referral/Consultation *(continued)*

Diagnosis	Clinical Manifestations	Management
		Avoidance of straining at stool Saving any clots, tissues Support through grief process.
Hydatidiform mole	Prior treatment with Clomid Excessive nausea and vomiting Pregnancy test (strongly positive in early pregnancy) Uterus larger than expected gestational size No fetal heart rate No fetal parts noted on abdominal palpation Signs and symptoms of preeclampsia before or by 20 wk gestation Dark brown and watery bleeding Passage of grapelike tissue	Refer to physician. Auscultate fetal heart rate. Do ultrasonography amniography. Determine HCG level. Evacuation of uterine contents (by physician) Supervise follow-up for 1 yr. Monitor HCG levels. Advise against conception for 1 yr. Discuss low incidence of reoccurrence in young female. Discuss risk, treatment, and cure rate of choriocarcinoma. Use chemotherapy for choriocarcinoma.
Ectopic pregnancy	History of Pelvic inflammatory disease Gonorrhea Abdominal surgeries Spontaneous or elective abortions Previous ectopic pregnancy Shock Bloody vaginal discharge Lower-abdominal tenderness upon pelvic examination Enlarged adnexal mass and/or cul-de-sac mass Elevated temperature	Refer *immediately* to physician. Monitor vital signs. Type and cross-match blood. Have blood transfusion available. Culdotomy Culdocentesis Laparoscopy Laparotomy Sedate client. Prevent infection. Prevent hemorrhage.
Premature separation of the placenta	Female in third trimester Sudden, severe abdominal pain Excessive movement of baby with onset of pain History may include Abdominal, uterine surgery or trauma Chronic hypertension Pregnancy-induced hypertension Multiparity Fetal wastage Sickle cell disease Shock Irritable uterus	Refer *immediately* to physician. No rectal or vaginal examinations. Monitor vital signs; assess for shock. Position client on left side and elevate legs. Give nothing by mouth. Type and cross-match blood. Check hemoglobin, hematocrit, and fibrinogen levels. Auscultate fetal heart rate.

Table 64-1 Medical Referral/Consultation *(continued)*

Diagnosis	Clinical Manifestations	Management
	Dark red vaginal bleeding Fetal distress Enlargement of uterus Laboratory findings Hemoconcentration Anemia, particularly in concealed hemorrhage Hypofibrinogenemia	Have blood available. Pelvic exam under double setup (by physician). Prepare for abdominal surgery.
Placenta previa	Female in late-second or third trimester Multigravida with history of rapid successive pregnancies Bright-red vaginal bleeding Soft uterus Abnormal fetal presentation upon palpation Fetal heart rate within normal limits	Refer *immediately* to physician. No rectal or vaginal examinations. Monitor vital signs and evaluate for shock. Auscultate fetal heart rate. Put client in semi-fowlers position. Give nothing by mouth. Type and cross-match, blood; determine hemoglobin, hematocrit, and fibrinogen levels. Sonography to locate placenta (diagnostic).
Intermenstrual disorders	Frequent, excessive and/or, prolonged vaginal bleeding Difficult and painful vaginal bleeding Intermittent vaginal bleeding Bleeding with intercourse or douching Lower-abdominal discomfort Dyspareunia Low-back pain Burning and itching Vaginal bleeding which is dark, bright-red, scanty or in large clots Malodorous vaginal discharge Edematous, excoriated perineal area Mucopurulent cervical discharge Cervical abnormalities, i.e., edema, lesion, erosion Large, boggy, friable cervix Tenderness and pain upon pelvic examination Retroversion of uterus with tender uterosacral ligaments Uterine enlargement and irregularities Signs of anemia	Refer to physician. Do laboratory screening as indicated. Treatment may consist of any of the following Hormone therapy Antibiotic therapy Endometrial or cervical biopsy Dilatation and curettage Removal of polyp(s) Conization Cautery Removal of foreign body Laparoscopy Laparotomy Pharmacological therapy

bibliography

Beazley, J. Inevitable antepartum hemorrhage. *Nursing Times*, August: 985–987 (1971).

Clark, A., Affonso, D. *Childbearing—A nursing perspective*. Philadelphia: Davis, 1976, pp. 623–631.

Goodrich, F. Obstetric hemorrhage. *American Journal of Nursing* **11**:96–97 (1962).

Halstead, Lois. The use of crisis intervention in obstetrical nursing. *Nursing Clinics of North America,* March:69–76 (1974).

Jensen, M., Benson, R., and Bobak, I. *Maternity care—The nurse and the family*. St. Louis: Mosby, 1977, pp. 223–246.

Kitay, David. Bleeding disorders in pregnancy. *Contemporary OB/Gyn,* January:87–94 (1976).

Pritchard, Jack, and MacDonald, Paul. *Williams obstetrics* (15th ed.). New York: Appleton-Century-Crofts, 1976, pp. 398–515.

Romney, Seymour, et al. *Gynecology and obstetrics: The health care of women*. New York: McGraw-Hill, 1975, pp. 737–746.

Tucker, J. Nursing care in obstetric hemorrhage. *American Journal of Nursing*, **11**:98–101 (1962).

Turbeville, J. Nurses' role in hospital care. *Hospital Topics*, June:85–88 (1972).

65 Menstrual Cramps

CHRISTINA M. GRAF

ALERT
1. Constant, severe pain
2. Moderate pain unrelieved by conservative treatment

I. Etiology

A. Primary dysmenorrhea
1. The specific etiology is unknown.
2. Emotional stress may exacerbate symptoms, but the etiology is rarely psychogenic.
3. Possibly it is initiated by the release of excessive amounts of prostaglandin.

B. Secondary dysmenorrhea—symptom of organic disturbance, including
1. Congenital anomalies of the genitalia
2. Pelvic inflammatory disease
3. Endometriosis

II. Assessment

A. Primary dysmenorrhea
1. Subjective data
   a. Pain
      (1) Onset following establishment of anovulatory cycle, usually 2 to 5 years after menarche
      (2) Occurs with menstruation, lasting 12 to 24 h after flow commences
      (3) Character and location of pain perhaps varying, but usually cramping in the lower abdomen
   b. Nausea and vomiting sometimes present
   c. Frequently associated with anxiety symptoms
   d. Others in family sometimes experiencing similar problems
2. Objective data
   a. Physical examination normal
   b. Absence of symptoms of pelvic pathology

B. Secondary dysmenorrhea: see Table 65-1

III. Management

A. Primary dysmenorrhea
1. Treatments/medications
   a. Analgesics—aspirin, Darvon, or Empirin every 3 to 4 h for two to three doses
   b. If dysmenorrhea severe, establishment of several initial anovulatory cycles with hormonal therapy
   c. Surgical intervention by physician
      (1) Cervical dilatation
      (2) Presacral neurectomy
2. Counselling/prevention
   a. Continue normal activities, including exercise.
   b. Warm baths and short periods of rest may help.
   c. Use analgesics before pain becomes too severe.
   d. Emphasize that the condition is self-limiting and benign and that normal sexual activity and fertility can be expected.
   e. The condition is frequently resolved following pregnancy.
3. Follow-up
   a. Telephone call following next menstrual cycle to report progress
   b. Return visit if pain increases or occurs outside of menstruation, or if additional menstrual disorders occur
4. Consultations/referrals
   a. Psychiatric evaluation if severe emotional problems are present
   b. Referral to physician for consistent, severe pain, or for moderate pain unrelieved by conservative treatment

B. Secondary dysmenorrhea: see Table 65-1

Table 65-1 Medical Referral/Consultation

Diagnosis	Clinical Manifestations	Management
Primary dysmenorrhea (unrelieved by conservative treatment)	See Primary dysmenorrhea, II, A Moderate to severe pain	Referral to physician Treatments/medications Estrogen/progesterone preparations to induce anovulatory cycles Cervical dilatation perhaps providing relief for several months, but pain usually returning Presacral neurectomy (infrequent) Counselling Side effects of hormonal treatment may include nausea, fluid retention, midcycle bleeding; report if persistent or severe. Be alert for symptoms of thrombophlebitis. If surgical intervention is planned, explain procedure and expected effects. Follow-up Report results following the next several menstrual cycles. Persistent pain following establishment of anovulatory cycles must be reported; it usually indicates organic disorder.
Secondary dysmenorrhea with congenital anomalies	Menstrual discharge may be dark brown or black in color and reduced in amount. Character and duration of pain are variable. Disease may be associated with dyspareunia or infertility, or repeated abortions, miscarriages, or premature delivery. Anomalies may be detected on physical examination, by x-ray visualization, or by surgical exposure.	Referral to physician Management will depend on the nature of the anomaly. Explain all procedures for diagnosis or treatment thoroughly. Review the anticipated effects of the treatment, including effect on sexual activity and fertility.
Secondary dysmenorrhea with pelvic inflammatory disease	Pain occurring either with menstruation or throughout cycle; may be very mild Vaginal discharge noted prior to menstruation Associated symptoms perhaps including elevated temperature, dysuria, gastrointestinal symptoms History of sexual activity, pregnancy, or abortion	Immediate referral to physician Treatments/medications Probenecid 1 g po followed in 30 min with aqueous penicillin G 4.8 million units IM If allergic—tetracycline 1.5 g po then 0.5 g qid for 4 days Analgesics and antipyretics as indicated Hospitalization usually necessary if

Table 65-1 Medical Referral/Consultation *(continued)*

Diagnosis	Clinical Manifestations	Management
	Pelvic examination—cervix tender on motion Abdominal examination—adnexal mass present Endocervical culture positive for gonorrhea	Diagnosis uncertain and surgical emergencies must be excluded Pelvic abscess suspected Client pregnant Client unable to tolerate or follow outpatient regime Counselling/prevention Emphasize the importance of the treatment regime. Instruct in the transmission and prevention of venereal disease. Follow-up Report to the health department for contact screening. Repeat endocervical culture 7–14 days after the completion of treatment for test of cure. Schedule a return visit if symptoms reappear.
Secondary dysmenorrhea with endometriosis	Pain–onset most frequent in ages 20–30; deep-seated aching or bearing down in lower abdomen or back; radiation to rectal or perineal area; begins 1–2 days prior to menstruation, subsides at end of period; later, duration increasing Associated symptoms—dyspareunia, cyclic bowel disturbance, infertility Hard, fixed fibrotic nodules in uterosacral ligaments, cul-de-sac, posterior surface of lower uterine wall, or cervix Visualization with culdoscopy or laparoscopy Microscopic examination of resected lesions	Referral to physician Treatments/medications With minimal symptoms—analgesics for discomfort, continued observation for progression With mild symptoms—administration of estrogen/progesterone combinations for 6–12 mo Surgical intervention if conservative hormonal therapy fails; type and extent dependent on progression of disease, age of client, and degree of concern for preserving childbearing functions Supervening pregnancy frequently interrupts course of disease in earlier stages Counselling/prevention Explain course of disease and beneficial effects of childbearing. Review treatment selected, including expected effects and possible side effects. Emphasize importance of regular follow-up. Follow-up: regular examination at least every 6–12 mo

bibliography

Ballard, Phyllis. Menstrual disorders in adolescence. *Issues in Comprehensive Pediatric Nursing*, **2**:21–33 (1978).

Bryner, James R., and Greenblatt, Robert B. Diagnosing and treating endometriosis. *Contemporary OB/Gyn,* **8**:81–88 (1976).

Green, Thomas H. *Gynecology: essentials of clinical practice*. Boston: Little, Brown, 1978.

Huffman, John W. Gynecologic problems that beset the adolescent. *Contemporary OB/Gyn*, **6**:81–89 (1976).

66 Vaginal Discharge

CHARLOTTE CRAM ELSBERRY

ALERT
1. Persistent, nonresponsive vaginitis or vaginal discharge
2. Unusual vaginal discharge
3. Vaginal discharge with fecal particles or fecal odor

I. Etiology

A. Specific organism
B. Foreign object or agent
C. Allergic reaction
D. Normal physiological response

II. Assessment (see Tables 66-1 and 66-2)

III. Management

A. Treatments/medications

1. Return the vagina to a normal pH (slightly acid, 6.5 to 7).
2. Promote normal vaginal epithelial proliferation.
3. Eradicate implicated etiology.
4. Remove any foreign bodies.

B. Counselling/prevention

1. Take the medication for the full length of time prescribed. Don't stop when the discharge gets better, or when menstruating. Finish all the medication.
2. If the symptoms get worse, telephone immediately.
3. The other sexual partner(s) should seek treatment (even if asymptomatic). The implicated organism will be transmitted back and forth. Legally, it may be inappropriate to send home medication for the treatment of a partner without a direct diagnosis.
4. Refrain from sexual intercourse until both partners have finished treatment, or utilize condoms while under treatment.
5. Keep vulva and perineal area dry and free from moisture and heat. This may necessitate more frequent changes of underwear; rinse the genitalia and perineal area with lukewarm water after urinating and defecating; wear either no panty hose or only hose with mesh inserts, which allow for air circulation, and wear slacks less often.
6. Do not apply powder to genitalia or the perineal area.
7. Wear cotton underpants or underpants with a cotton crotch insert.
8. When bathing, wash genitalia with a mild soap. Soaps such as Dial and Lifebuoy may aggravate the condition by killing normal flora or changing the pH.
9. After urinating or defecating, wipe from the front to the back so that organisms or fecal material are not brought near the vagina.
10. Clients with large thighs or chapped or excoriated thighs frequently profit from wearing protective thigh guards, which may be purchased in the notions section of a store.
11. Eat yogurt or drink acidophilous milk to promote or maintain normal flora, including *Lactobacillus.*
12. Do not scratch area if possible; scratching will further irritate the area and spread the infection.
13. Vaginal medication is frequently prescribed for use morning and evening. Leaking of medication onto the vulva is good and necessary but may feel uncomfortable. This is not as much a problem if the medication is inserted before retiring for the night; how-

ever, some women like to protect the bed with an object such as a Pamper under the sheet. During the day, some women wish to wear a sanitary pad, or clean dry handkerchief. Regardless, the woman should be encouraged to allow some air circulation and not allow the area to become warm.

14. Do not wear tight clothing (slacks, girdles, panty hose).
15. Wash all clothes that have come in contact with the vulva before reusing.
16. Do not walk around in a wet bathing suit; change into dry clothing.
17. Do not douche before coming in for a health visit and/or pelvic exam.
18. When bathing in a common facility, the tub should be washed out well with a cleansing agent prior to use.
19. Vaginal douching is usually not necessary. Frequent douching can lead to a vaginal environment conducive to infections and/or cause an increase in the production of normal leukorrhea. If an occasional douche is desired, it may be prepared by adding 1 tablespoon of white vinegar to 1 qt warm water.
20. If a vaginal infection occurs while using a diaphragm for contraception, it is advisable to obtain and use a new one.
21. Don't wear underpants or such to bed.

C. Follow-up

Schedule a return visit 1 to 2 weeks after treatment. The infection is gone when the organism is eliminated, not when the symptoms are gone.

D. Consultations/referrals

1. Notify the health department if cultures prove positive for venereal disease.
2. Refer to a physician and/or nurse-midwife
   a. Clients with persistent, nonresponsive vaginal discharge
   b. Clients with a vaginal discharge either stained with fecal material or with a fecal odor
   c. All young women who have not had a previous internal exam or who have had trouble during previous exams

bibliography

Monif, Gilles R. G. *Infectious diseases in obstetrics and gynecology.* New York: Harper & Row, 1974.

Nofziger, Margaret. *A cooperative method of natural birth control* (2d ed.). Summertown, Tenn.: Book Publishing Co., 1978.

Rein, Michael F., and Chapel, Thomas A. Trichomoniasis, candidiasis, and the minor venereal diseases. *Clinical Obstetrics and Gynecology,* **18**(1):73–88 (1975).

Table 66-1 Normal Physiological Vaginal Discharge (Leukorrhea)

Type	Etiology	Subjective Data	Objective Data	Treatments/ Medications	Counselling/ Prevention	Follow-Up	Consultations/ Referrals
Premenstrual leukorrhea	Change in hormone balance with decrease of estrogen and progesterone	Not noticed in all women Occurs 2 wk to several days prior to onset of menses May be slightly pruritic with slight odor May decrease in amount	Discharge is white, yellow, or opaque; sticky, thick, and pasty.	None	Reassurance of its normalcy Normal hygiene	None	None
Leukorrhea of sexual arousal	Probably occurs as a result of vaginal sweating Some of the discharge may be produced by the cervical and Bartholin's glands	Occurs when sexually aroused (either mentally or physically)	Like normal physiological leukorrhea, however, greater in amount and more mucoid	None	Explain its benefit and use as a lubricant. Without its occurrence, dyspareunia might be present. If so, sexual counselling may be indicated.	None	None
Leukorrhea of pregnancy	Change in hormone balance	Client notices an increase in the amount of vaginal discharge.	The discharge is more acidic, due to lactic acid. The discharge is thick, white, crumbly.	None	Explain its relationship to pregnancy. Explain normal hygiene. Emphasize it is a factor that can prevent vaginitis, to which pregnant women are more prone.	None	None

Table 66-1 Normal Physiological Vaginal Discharge (Leukorrhea) *(continued)*

Type	Etiology	Subjective Data	Objective Data	Treatments/ Medications	Counselling/ Prevention	Follow-Up	Consultations/ Referrals
Puerperal discharge	Sloughing of endomentrial and endocervical cells	It occurs after a woman has had a baby. It usually lasts 1–4 wk. It is nonirritating.	Initially, it is mixed with blood. The color goes from red to pink to brown. Later, it is whitish yellow in color.	None	Normal hygiene Usually the use of vaginal tampons not recommended	None	None
Birth control pill leukorrhea	Due to alterations caused by birth control pills	Client notices a decrease in the amount of vaginal discharge. Client notices that her discharge is always the same.	Discharge is milky thin, and less in amount.	None	Explain its relationship to birth control pills	None	None
Normal female leukorrhea	Secretions from the vagina and cervix	None	Amount variable Little odor May be cloudy white, transparent, or filmy Nonirritating	None	It is normal for women to have this vaginal discharge. Recommend normal hygiene. Refer to Counselling/ prevention, III, B.	None	None

Table 66-1 Normal Physiological Vaginal Discharge (Leukorrhea) *(continued)*

Type	Etiology	Subjective Data	Objective Data	Treatments/ Medications	Counselling/ Prevention	Follow-Up	Consultations/ Referrals
Newborn leukorrhea	High levels of estrogen and progesterone are transferred via the placenta.	None	Thick mucoid discharge at introitus Discharge sometimes tinged with pink (blood)	None	Reassure parent(s) that it is normal. The discharge may be washed away with warm water.	None	None
Puberty leukorrhea	Change in hormone balance with onset of estrogen production	None	Clear, mucoid discharge	None	Reassure that it is normal. Explain its positive value and function. Discuss basic vaginal hygiene.	None	None
Leukorrhea associated with ovulation	Change in the hormone balance with a peak level of estrogen	It starts to occur several days prior to ovulation. With a 28-day menstrual cycle, it starts to occur between day 10 and 13.	Discharge is clear, thick, tenacious, mucoid, nonirritating. Discharge is more alkaline.	None	Explain the relationship of its occurrence to ovulation. Explain how the alkaline and tenacious discharge aids the transport of the sperm. The occurrence of the discharge may be used as an aid to indicate "unsafe days" if pregnancy is not desired.	None	None

Table 66-2 Abnormal Vaginal Discharge

Etiology	Subjective Data	Objective Data	Treatments/ Medications	Counselling/ Prevention	Follow-up	Consultations/ Referrals
			Physiochemical Agents			
An allergic response is often associated with the use of vaginal douches, sprays, and contraceptives; of cleansing agents; and of corrosive chemicals applied externally.	Client will complain of a hot, heavy, painful vulva sensation. Client may complain of a malodorous discharge that is yellow, perhaps streaked with blood or pus, and watery. Client may complain of symptoms associated with previously described infectious vaginal discharges that are secondary.	The vulva is red with white patches. It may be swollen. The vagina is inflamed and may be ulcerated. The vaginal discharge is due to secondary infection (refer to other vaginal discharges).	Stop utilizing the agent. Sitz baths and/or cold compresses may relieve the symptoms.	Warn the client of possible allergic reactions to the common offenders.	None, unless symptoms persist or reappear	None
			Presence of a Foreign Object			
Any foreign agent present at the introitus or in the vagina, or blocking a gland	Complains of a long-standing, purulent, malodorous discharge	Visualization or palpation of a foreign object Purulent, malodorous vaginal discharge that may be streaked with pus or blood	Remove the object if it can be easily seen, if it doesn't appear to be embedded, and if it can be removed with minimal trauma to the client. Recommend warm saline soaks or baths. The physician may prescribe estrogen vaginal cream or an antibiotic.	Discuss with the client the need to come for medical help immediately when a foreign body becomes lodged. Client should call if a fever develops, if the symptoms don't subside, or if the condition gets worse.	Telephone follow-up in 48 h Return visit in 1–2 wk for reexamination	Refer to the physician if the object is embedded, if the client is febrile, if the object does not come out easily after the initial trial, if the object cannot be visualized, or if the client is young and has not had previous pelvic examination. Professional

Table 66-2 Abnormal Vaginal Discharge *(continued)*

Etiology	Subjective Data	Objective Data	Treatments/ Medications	Counselling/ Prevention	Follow-up	Consultations/ Referrals
			Presence of a Foreign Object (continued)			
			The foreign object should be cultured.			counselling may be indicated.
			Trichomonas			
Trichomonas vaginalis, a protozoa (pear-shaped with four flagella)	Foul odor and copious vaginal discharge Pruritis Dysuria and/or urinary frequency Dyspareunia Postcoital spotting Swelling	Discharge is yellow, green, or grayish; frothy or foamy; and bubbly, thin, and profuse. It has a foul odor. Reddening and excoriation of the vulva may occur if the infection is severe. The urethral meatus may be prominent and red. The vaginocervical mucosa may be swollen or friable. The vagina may have a strawberry or measlelike appearance.	Flagyl 250 mg (should not be given in first trimester of pregnancy, and controversy exists whether it should be given at all during pregnancy) 8 pills orally at once (2 g) 1 pill orally tid for 10 days Other trichomonicidal vaginal suppositories or tablets Acidic vaginal douche (white vinegar and water), but not during pregnancy	Usually transmitted by Intercourse Washcloths Towels Bathing suits Moist objects See Counselling prevention, III, B Seeking of methods to correct concurring environmental upsets or changes	See Follow-up, III, C.	Consultation with physician For treatment during pregnancy, if you have no medically approved standing orders to cover treatment during pregnancy If condition persists or doesn't respond to treatment If condition frequently recurs Referral of other sexual partner(s) for treatment
			Monilia			
Candida albicans, a fungus	Pruritis (intense) Dysuria Swollen feeling around vulva Rarely occurring in premenarchal or postmenopausal women Frequently client either pregnant	Discharge is white, thick, floculent, patchy, cheesy (similar to cottage or cream cheese). Odor is strong but not malodorous. Reddening and swelling of the vulva and vagina occur.	Monistat 7 vaginal cream—one application daily for 7 days, or other antifungal vaginal tablets, suppositories, or creams For vulvar discomfort, witch hazel compresses and/or antifungal ointments	Client should be aware of predisposing factors. See Counselling/ prevention, III, B.	See Follow-up, III, C.	Consult physician if discharge Persists. Doesn't respond to treatment. Frequently recurs.

Table 66-2 Abnormal Vaginal Discharge *(continued)*

Etiology	Subjective Data	Objective Data	Treatments/ Medications	Counselling/ Prevention	Follow-up	Consultations/ Referrals
			Monilia (continued)			
	or diabetic; using birth control pills; has been taking an antibiotic, corticosteroid hormones, or anticancer drugs; or has glycosuria	There is evidence of scratching. Wet smear with potassium hydroxide (KOH) is positive for yeast cells with hypha and buds. Use Nickersons culture media to determine fungal growth. Use Gram-Claudius stain for presence of yeast cells. Do a Pap smear for presence of yeast cells.	Alkaline vaginal douche (baking soda and water), but not during pregnancy Eating yogurt, drinking acidophilous milk			
			Nonspecific Vaginitis			
Most often due to *homophilus vaginalis,* bacteria	Client complains frequently of leukorrhea, pruritis. Client may complain of vaginal odor. Disease occurs in all age groups.	Vagina is reddened and may have the strawberry or measlelike appearance found with *Trichomonas*. The discharge is usually gray, strong in odor, and hemogenous. Wet smear indicates presence of clue cells and neutrophilis. Culture the discharge to isolate the organism.	Tripple sulfa vaginal creams. The optimum time to start the above is on the last day of menses. Reinfection may require the use of a systemic antibiotic (ampicillin). If the sexual partner(s) has positive culture, the partner should be treated with a systemic antibiotic.	See Counselling/ prevention, III, B.	See Follow-up, III, C.	If no symptomatic relief occurs after treatment, consult and probably refer the client to a physician.

67 Penile Discharge

HARRIETT S. CHANEY

ALERT

1. Papular, petechial, or hemorrhagic pustular skin lesions
2. Chancre of syphilis
3. Fever
4. Pain and/or swelling of joints
5. Conjunctivitis

I. Etiology

A. *Neisseria gonorrhoeae*
B. *Chlamydia* species
C. *Trichomonas vaginalis*
D. *Escherichia coli*
E. Unknown

II. Assessment

A. Gonorrhea

1. Subjective data
   a. Known exposure 2 to 6 days prior to onset
   b. Profuse, purulent urethral discharge
   c. Associated with dysuria and frequency
   d. Homosexual male may complain of sore throat, rectal burning, pruritis, tenseness, and rectal discharge
2. Objective data
   a. Gram-positive smear
   b. Culture: *N. gonorrhoeae*

B. Nongonococcal urethritis (NGU)

1. Subjective data
   a. Usually milky, early morning discharge; may also mimic gonococcal discharge, i.e., purulent, profuse
   b. Dysuria, frequency
2. Objective data: Gonococcal organisms cannot be identified.

C. Trichomoniasis

1. Subjective data
   a. Acute purulent discharge
   b. Associated with itching, dysuria
   c. May be asymptomatic
2. Objective data: culture: *T. vaginalis*

D. Prostatitis

1. Subjective data
   a. Pain in lower back, testes, perineum
   b. Tenesmus
   c. Discharge murky white although may be purulent
   d. Fever, nausea, malaise, loss of libido
2. Objective data
   a. Culture: negative or *E. coli*
   b. Enlarged tender prostate

III. Management

A. Gonorrhea

1. Treatments/medications
   a. Probenecid, 1 g orally, followed in 30 min by aqueous procaine penicillin, 4.8 million units IM, *or*
   b. Ampicillin, 3.5 g orally, and probenecid, 1 g, at the same time, *or*
   c. Tetracycline HCl, 1.5 g orally initially, then 0.5 g qid for 4 days, *or*
   d. Spectinomycin HCl, 2 g IM for one injection
2. Counselling/prevention
   a. Avoid sexual activity for 2 days.
   b. Force fluids, and temporarily discontinue the use of alcohol.
   c. Encourage the client to inform sexual contacts so they can seek treatment.
   d. Prevention includes avoidance of sexual contact with individuals known to have a

venereal disease, and the utilization of a condom will give partial protection.

3. Follow-up
   a. Return office visit in 7 to 10 days for repeat urethral culture
   b. Return visit if symptoms repeat
4. Consultations/referrals
   Report case to health department.

B. Nongonococcal urethritis (NGU)

1. Treatments/medications: tetracycline, 500 mg every 6 h for 7 days
2. Counselling/prevention
   a. Avoid sexual activity for 2 days.
   b. Force fluids, and temporarily discontinue the use of alcohol.
   c. Encourage the client to inform sexual contacts so they can seek treatment.
   d. Do not take tetracycline with milk, milk products, antacids, or iron.
   e. Utilization of a condom can provide partial protection.
3. Follow-up: return visit if symptoms repeat or if not improved after 7 days
4. Consultations/referrals: none

C. Prostatitis

1. Treatments/medications
   a. Begin treatment immediately
   b. Tetracycline, 250 to 500 mg orally every 6 h for 10 days, or
   c. Ampicillin, 500 mg orally every 6 h for 10 days
   d. Analgesic: aspirin or acetaminophen
2. Counselling/prevention
   a. Take sitz baths tid.
   b. Symptoms will be improved after 3 to 5 days, and sexual activity may be resumed.
   c. Do not take tetracycline with milk, milk products, antacids, or iron.
3. Follow-up
   a. Return office visit if no improvement after 3 days
   b. Return office visit if symptoms recur
4. Consultations/referrals
   a. Refer to the physician if there is no improvement or if the client has tenderness of the epididymis or diabetes.
   b. Refer to the physician if episodes recur.

Table 67-1 Medical Referral/Consultation

Diagnosis	Clinical Manifestations	Management
Disseminated gonnococcal infection	Fever and polyarthralgias of the wrists, fingers, knees, ankles; purulent synovial fluid accumulating Papular, petechial, or hemorrhagic pustular skin lesions on distal extremities Myopericarditis, endocarditis, meningitis, toxic hepatitis	Immediate physician referral Massive systemic antibiotics
Lymphogranuloma venereum (LGV)	Majority of cases involving travelers, sailors, servicemen returning from abroad; male homosexuals; or individuals of low socioeconomic status Painless vesicle, papule, or ulcer on penis which occurs 3 days to 3 wk after exposure and heals within several days Inguinal, deep iliac, peripectal, or femoral lyphadenopathy Adenopathy may be unilateral and initially discrete, but it advances to extensive enlargement of the nodal chains. If the client is homosexual, there may be a mucopurulent or bloody anal discharge, tenesmus, diarrhea, perirectal abscess, or anal fistula.	Physician referral Antibiotics: tetracycline or triple sulfonamide

Table 67-1 Medical Referral/Consultation *(continued)*

Diagnosis	Clinical Manifestations	Management
Reiter's syndrome	Mucopurulent discharge	Physician referral
	Dysuria, hematuria, edema of meatus	Antibiotics—tetracycline
	2 days to 4 wk following exposure, development of conjunctivitis, mucocutaneous lesions, and arthritis	Salicylates
	Ankles, knees, and toe joints becoming warm, erythematous, and painful; multiple or single joints involved	
	Remission after 2–4 mo with recurrent attacks after sexual exposure	

bibliography

Fowkes, William C., and Hunn, Virginia K. *Clinical assessment for the nurse practitioner.* St Louis: Mosby, 1973.

Graf, Christina. Sexually-transmitted disease: a new look at an old problem. *Issues in Comprehensive Pediatric Nursing,* March-April:11–20 (1975).

Harvey, A., Johns, R. J., Owens, A. H., and Ross, R. S. (eds.). *The principles and practices of medicine.* New York: Appleton-Century-Crofts, 1976.

Hoole, A. J., Greenberg, R. A., and Pickard, C. G. *Patient care guidelines for family nurse practitioners.* Boston: Little, Brown, 1976.

Hudak, C. M., Redstone, P. M., Hokanson, N. L., and Suzuki, I. E. *Clinical protocols: a guide for nurses and physicians.* Philadelphia: Lippincott, 1976.

Mahoney, J. D., Bevan, J., and Wall, B. Default patterns of patients attending clinics for sexually transmitted diseases. *British Journal of Venereal Disease,* **54**(2):124–127 (1978).

Terho, Pertli. Chlamydia trachomatis in nonspecific urethritis. *British Journal of Venereal Disease,* **54**(3):251–256 (1975).

Thorn, G. W., Adams, R. D., Braunwald, E., Isselbacker, K. J., and Petersdorf, R. B. (eds.). *Harrison's principles of internal medicine.* New York: McGraw-Hill, 1977.

68 Breast Lumps/Changes

MARY ANN KASPER/BARBARA J. CHOPLIN

ALERT
1. Mass
2. Nipple changes
3. Nipple discharge
4. Pain and/or tenderness
5. Skin changes
6. Increased temperature
7. Family history of breast cancer

I. Etiology

A. Fibrocystic disease most common lesion (seen in the age group between 20 and 45)

B. Cancer (most common in women over 40 years)

C. Fibroadenoma (common in women 15 to 60 years)

D. Intraductal papilloma (common in women 35 to 43 years)

E. Estrogen hormone imbalance in male during puberty

II. Management

A. Treatments/medications: see Table 68-1

B. Counselling/prevention

1. Provide reassurance and support.
   a. Recognize the client's anxiety regarding examination and findings.
   b. Be honest, calm, and empathetic in approach.
   c. Support the client, recognizing that the client may feel guilty, perhaps because of a delay in seeking health care.
   d. Enhance the client's self-esteem and self-worth.
2. Explain examination procedures and preliminary findings.
3. Provide anticipatory guidance about medical intervention and preventive treatment.
   a. Give appropriate and correct information.
      (1) Identify clients with high risk for cancer
         (a) Those with a family history of breast cancer
         (b) Those who have never been pregnant
         (c) Those with a history of early menarche or late menopause
         (d) Those who have not breast-fed
         (e) Those with history of breast lesions
      (2) Listen to the client's concerns and dispel misconceptions.
      (3) Emphasize the importance of breast self-examination on a regular basis.
      (4) Teach breast self-examination, breast hygiene, and proper breast support.
      (5) Use photographs and printed instructions in explaining tests and procedures to be used during medical intervention.

C. Follow-up

1. Dependent upon medical findings
2. Plan of treatment documented
   a. Postsurgery
   b. Rehabilitation
3. Reassurance and support regarding psychological adjustment
4. Encouragement of women to talk with other women regarding regular breast self-examination and health care

D. Consultations/referrals

1. Referral to physician for further diagnostic evaluation and treatment
2. Referral to lay support groups, such as Reach for Recovery

Table 68-1 Medical Referral/Consultation

Diagnosis	Clinical Manifestations	Management
Fibrocystic disease	Mass(es) in one or both breasts Pain and tenderness, particularly prior to menstruation Firm, smooth, round, mobile mass, unilateral or bilateral Tenderness on palpation or pressure Females 20–45 yr of age	Referral to and/or consultation with a physician Treatment dependent upon medical diagnosis Laboratory screening as indicated Treatment may consist of any of the following Mammography Xerography Thermography Biopsy Mastectomy Pharmacological therapy Chemotherapy Hormone therapy
Cancer	Unilateral mass, most frequently in upper, outer quadrant of breast Solid Irregular Poorly delineated Nonmobile Discharge from nipple Nipple retraction Edema, creating orange-peel appearance of breast Skin retraction or dimpling of breast Breasts asymmetrical with body movement Weight loss History: client usually denies pain Females 40 yr old and over	
Fibroadenoma	Unilateral or bilateral mass Mobile Firm Solid Well-delineated Multiple tumors History: client denies pain Females 15–16 yr of age	
Intraductal papilloma	Soft, poorly delineated mass Small mass, difficult to palpate Moderate pain and discomfort Serous, serosanguineous, or bloody discharge from nipple Females 35–43 yr of age	
Gynecomastia	Young adolescent males Breast enlargement, unilateral or bilateral Possible slight tenderness	Consult a physician. Reassure client and parent(s) that condition is temporary; it usually disappears within 1 yr.

bibliography

Cameron, C. T., and Adair, F. E. The clinical features and diagnosis of the common breast tumors. *Medical Journal of Australia*, **2**:651–654 (1965).

Malasano, L., et al. *Health assessment*. St. Louis: Mosby, 1977, pp. 182–194.

Martin, Leonide. *Health care of women*. Philadelphia: Lippincott, 1978, pp. 302–333.

Regenie, Sandra, et al. The self-instructional package: An educational resource breast disease. *Journal of Nurse-Midwifery*, **4**:8–15 (1975).

Rosen, Yale, et al. Fibromatosis of the breast. *Cancer*, **4**:1409–1413 (1978).

69 Common Genital Lesions

CHARLOTTE CRAM ELSBERRY

ALERT
1. Teeth marks or broken skin
2. Abscess or cyst on or near genitalia
3. Hematoma on or near genitalia
4. Pregnant woman
5. Persistent lesion(s)

I. Etiology

A. Condyloma acuminatum
1. Interaction between latent virus and/or *Trichomonas* and host tissue
2. Probably strong endocrine dependency

B. Bartholin's duct cyst
1. Can be caused by several organisms
2. Most commonly, *Neisseria gonorrhoeae*, streptococci, staphylococci, *Escherichia coli*

C. Sexual trauma
1. Bites
2. Trauma leading to tissue injury swelling and hematoma

II. Assessment

A. Condyloma acuminatum
1. Subjective data
   a. Rarely occurs prior to puberty or after menopause
   b. Warts growing on or near genitalia
   c. Fetid-smelling discharge and/or pain, caused by secondary infection of lesion(s) or wart(s)
2. Objective data
   a. Initially lesions or warts are multiple, small, and discretely defined.
   b. As the lesions grow larger, they resemble cauliflower or raspberries.
   c. Lesions are found on the
      (1) Female
         (a) Perineum (vulva, labial folds, vestibule)
         (b) Vagina
         (c) Cervix
         (d) Mons pubis
      (2) Male
         (a) Penis
         (b) Pubic hair (mons)
         (c) Scrotum
   d. A foul, fetid-smelling discharge is present if there is a secondary infection. If no ulceration is present, the agent is probably *Trichomonas.*
   e. Wet mount to identify the causative agent.

B. Sexual trauma
1. Subjective data
   a. Open cut/sore
   b. Heavy dragging sensation
   c. Pain (frequently increasing)
   d. Feels like sitting on eggs
   e. Pressure sensation
   f. Bleeding
2. Objective data
   a. Bite
      1. Visualization of teeth marks
      2. Hanging or missing piece of tissue
      3. Bleeding
      4. Discharge or exudate at sore
   b. Hematoma
      1. Firm or soft swelling of varying size
      2. Bluish discoloration
      3. Tender to touch
      4. Visualized on external genitalia and/or near introitus

III. Management

A. Condyloma acuminatum
1. Treatments/medications

a. 20 to 25 percent podophyllin in tincture of benzoin
   (1) Paint lesion(s) weekly.
   (2) Paint lesion(s) less than 2 cm in size.
   (3) Do not use on cauliflowerlike lesion(s).
   (4) Apply petroleum jelly to the surrounding area to protect it.
   (5) It is often not successful on lesion(s) on the mons pubis.
   (6) Do not use during pregnancy.
b. Electrocautery
c. Surgical excision
d. Treatment of causative agent and/or concomitant vaginitis

2. Counselling/prevention
   a. Wash and rinse the area treated with podophyllin thoroughly, 4 to 6 h after treatment to prevent burning.
   b. See Vaginal Discharge, Chap. 66, "Counselling/prevention," III, B.
   c. Reassure pregnant client that lesion(s) will recede and can be treated.
3. Follow-up
   a. 1 to 2 weeks after treatment
   b. Repetition of wet mount examination 1 to 2 weeks after treatment
4. Consultations/referrals: referral to physician
   a. Pregnant women with large growing lesion(s)
   b. Lesion(s) larger than 2 cm
   c. Lesion(s) resistant to treatment

B. Sexual trauma

1. Treatments/medications
   a. Bite
      (1) Cleansing of debris area
      (2) Antibiotics
      (3) Sitz baths or compresses
      (4) Use of sutures if bleeding can't be stopped by pressure
   b. Hematoma
      (1) Small—sitz baths or warm compresses
      (2) Increasing in size, large, or dropping hematocrit (Hct)
         (a) Evacuate, pack, and/or suture.
         (b) Use antibiotics.
         (c) Use warm compresses.
2. Counselling/prevention
   a. Educate to prevent reoccurrence.
   b. Educate public about need for treatment after human bites.
   c. Discuss treatment plan.
   d. Support and counsel because of possible sexual abuse.
3. Follow-up
   a. Telephone contact within 24 h
   b. Reexamination 1 week later
4. Consultations/referrals
   a. Consult immediately with a physician about the bite.
   b. Refer to a physician immediately when suturing is required.
   c. Refer to a physician immediately any individual with a large hematoma, a hematoma increasing in size, or dropping Hct.

Table 69-1 Medical Referral/Consultation

Diagnosis	Clinical Manifestations	Management
Bartholin duct cyst	Soft swelling in the middle or lower third of the labia minora and/or distortion of the introitus Heavy dragging sensation (Usually) only one duct affected Pain Dyspareunia Tenderness Swelling; edematous, turgid Overlying skin reddened and very tender Pressure over gland leading to expression of pus Laboratory White blood count (WBC) with shift to left Erythrocyte sedimentation rate (ESR) elevated Smears or cultures from duct positive for causative organism	Referral to physician Excision and drainage of duct Antibiotic therapy Bed rest Moist and dry heat Analgesics

bibliography

Benson, Ralph C. *Handbook of obstetrics and gynecology* (7th ed.). Los Altos, Calif.: Lange, 1976.

Lukacs, Janet and Corey, Lawrence. Genital herpes simplex virus infection: An overview. *The Nurse Practitioner*, **2**:7–10 (1977).

Monif, Gilles R. G. *Infectious diseases in obstetrics and gynecology*. New York: Harper & Row, 1974.

Novak, Edmund R., and Woodruff, J. Donald. *Novak's gynecologic and obstetric pathology* (7th ed.). Philadelphia: Saunders, 1974.

70 Venereal Disease

CHARLOTTE CRAM ELSBERRY

ALERT

1. Young and sexually active
2. Previous history of venereal disease
3. Pregnant woman and/or pregnant woman with little or no prenatal care
4. Discharge from penis or vagina
5. Sexual contact with someone who has venereal disease
6. Abscess or cyst of the Skene's or Bartholin's glands
7. Lower quadrant abdominal pain
8. Individual living in an institution
9. Painful, stiff joints
10. Sore or lesion on genitalia
11. Flat warts on genitalia
12. Small, raised, maculopapular skin lesion(s) at wrists or near joints
13. Placenta that is
    a. Dull in color
    b. Greasy feeling and very heavy
14. A genital sore or lesion with systemic symptoms

I. Etiology

A. *Neisseria gonorrhoeae* bacteria
1. Incubation period short
    a. Average onset fifth day
    b. Range of days prior to onset: 2 to 10
2. No immunity
3. Majority of females and males asymptomatic

B. *Treponema pallidum,* spirochete
1. Sexually transmitted
2. Transmitted to fetus via placenta after 18th week of gestation
3. Incubation period usually 10 to 14 days; longest 60 days

C. Herpesvirus hominis type II
1. Transmitted sexually or through close personal contact
2. Incubation period usually 2 to 7 days
3. After infection the virus dormant, but can be reactivated by
    a. Cold
    b. Fever
    c. Intense sunlight
    d. Emotional stress
4. Controversy whether an oncogenic agent

II. Assessment

A. Gonorrhea in infant and prepubescent female (see Table 70-1)

B. Gonnorrhea in adolescent and adult
1. Subjective data
    a. Onset of symptoms 3 to 5 days after exposure
    b. Dysuria
    c. Discharge from genitalia
    d. Urinary frequency
    e. Anal symptoms
        (1) Usually asymptomatic
        (2) Sore, cracked, itching, burning
        (3) History of anal coitus
        (4) Pain on defecation
        (5) Blood or pus in stool
    f. Pharyngeal symptoms
        (1) Usually asymptomatic
        (2) Sore throat
        (3) Hoarse voice
        (4) Bleeding, sore gums
2. Objective data
    a. Purulent discharge from genitalia
    b. Afebrile
    c. For the female

(1) Cervicitis
(2) Hyperemic, tender cervix (no pain on motion)
(3) Green or green-yellow discharge from cervical os or vagina
(4) No adnexal tenderness
(5) Bartholin's or Skene's glands
(a) Local redness
(b) Tenderness
(c) Swelling/edema
(d) Obstruction of ducts (cyst/abscess)

d. For the male
(1) Whitish discharge from penis
(2) Redness/swelling of urethra
(3) No adenopathy

e. Anal (male/female)
(1) Reddening and excoriation around anus
(2) Tears, cracks, or fistulas

f. Pharyngeal (male/female)
(1) Local adenopathy
(2) Red and inflamed
(3) Enlarged tonsils

g. Gonococcal growth on Thayer-Martin selective medium

h. Positive oxidase reaction

i. Gram-negative diplococcal morphology on smear from culture

C. Primary syphilis in adolescent and adult

1. Subjective data
a. Sore or ulcer on genitalia, anus, eyelid, fingers, lip, mouth, or nipple lasting 1 to 6 weeks
b. Sore heals spontaneously

2. Objective data
a. Small, papular breaks which look like an ulcer that is
(1) Superficial
(2) Painless (unless secondarily infected or extragenital)
(3) With a clean, granular base
(4) With margins that are scrolled or rolled and well defined

b. Ulcer or chancre can be visualized on
(1) Penis
(2) Labia
(3) Vaginal wall
(4) Cervix
(5) Lip
(6) Mouth
(7) Tongue
(8) About the anus
(9) Within the rectum
(10) Tonsils
(11) Eyelid
(12) Breast or nipple
(13) Fingers

c. Regional lymphadenopathy
(1) Enlarged
(2) Firm
(3) Tender

d. *T. pallidum* on dark-field examination

e. Rapid plasma reagin (RPR) test reactive

f. If the VDRL test is positive, a fluorescent treponemal-antibody absorption (FTA-ABS) test is done; if positive, treatment is necessary.

g. Dark-field examination of oral lesions positive for *T. pallidum*

D. Herpesvirus type II in adolescent and adult

1. Subjective data
a. Painful and sore lesion(s) or blister(s) on genitalia
b. Sudden increase in vaginal discharge
c. Dysuria
d. Dyspareunia
e. Fever
f. Myalgia
g. Malaise

2. Objective data
a. Inguinal adenopathy tender to touch
b. Lesion
(1) Site of lesion (common)
(a) Male—penis, scrotum
(b) Female—cervix, vulva, vagina (labia usually type I)
(2) Initially, multiple vesiculoulcerative lesions
(3) After rupture and secondary infection—painful, eroded, shallow ulcer covered with shaggy-white membrane
(4) Lesion(s) larger and greater in number in primary infection and occurring on one or more common sites
(5) Lesions are smaller and fewer and localized or confined to one site in recurrent infections
(6) Pap smear positive for herpes type II
(7) Positive serological analysis for herpes
(8) A positive culture

II. Management

A. Gonorrhea in infant and prepubescent female (see Table 70-1)

B. Gonorrhea in adolescent and adult

1. Treatments/medications for uncomplicated gonorrhea
a. Aqueous procaine penicillin G 4.8 million units IM divided in two doses administered

at the same time plus 1 g probenecid po 1 h prior to penicillin injection
 b. Ampicillin 3.5 g po with 1 g probenecid po
 c. Penicillin allergy
  (1) Erythromycin 1.5 g po then 0.5 g po 4 times a day for 4 days
  (2) Tetracycline 1.5 g po initially then 0.5 g po 4 times a day for 4 days (not used in pregnancy)
 d. Screening for syphilis
2. Counselling/prevention
 a. Educate to prevent reoccurrence.
  (1) Encourage treatment for contacts.
  (2) Abstain from intercourse until 10 days after both client and partner(s) have both finished treatment.
  (3) Use condoms during coitus until 2 weeks after treatment.
  (4) This is a good opportunity to discuss sexuality, contraception, and gynecological and genitourinary care, and to screen for coexistent health problems.
 b. Discuss the treatment plan with the client.
 c. Reassure that the diagnosis will not be shared with other family member(s).
 d. Initiate community programs for screening and dissemination of knowledge, including epidemic nature and need for follow-up to determine care.
 e. Double-glove when examining or performing procedures on client.
 f. Stress the need for consistent, careful hand washing.
 g. Stress the importance of seeking immediate treatment if the client suspects or actually has had exposure.
3. Follow-up
 a. Repeat (GC) gonorrheal cultures (GC) 2 weeks after the treatment.
 b. Repeat cultures are particularly important due to the increasing resistance of gonorrhea to penicillin, and also since the level of treatment hasn't been determined for anal and pharyngeal gonorrhea.
 c. Follow up the reported contacts.
4. Consultations/referrals
 a. A report to the local health department
 b. Consultation with physician for
  (1) Treatment of pharyngeal or anal gonorrhea
  (2) Pregnant woman with penicillin allergy
 c. Referal to physician
  (1) Client with positive cultures after treatment
  (2) Prepubescent child with gonorrhea
  (3) Client with positive culture and joint pain and/or skin lesions on wrist or near joints
  (4) Client with symptoms of pelvic inflammatory disease (see Table 70-2)

C. Primary syphilis in adolescent and adult

1. Treatments/medications
 a. Benzathine penicillin G 2.4 million units IM at single session (1.2 million units in each buttock to equal 2.4 million units)
 b. Aqueous procaine penicillin G 4.8 million units total: 600,000 U IM daily for 8 days
 c. Allergy to penicillin
  (1) Tetracycline hydrochloride 500 mg 4 times a day po 1 or 2 h after meal for 15 days
  (2) Erythromycin 500 mg 4 times a day po for 15 days (Steorate, ethylsuccinate, or base)
 d. Erythromycin estolate and tetracycline not recommended in pregnancy
 e. Erythromycin efficacy in pregnancy not well established; therefore, allergy documentation to penicillin very important
 f. Each positive nontreponemal (VDRL, Wassermann, Kolmer) serologic test should be confirmed with a treponemal (FTA-ABS, *T. pallidum* immobilization (TPI) test, FTA) serologic test
 g. Diagnosis of the stage of the disease necessary, since treatment based on the stage
 h. Serologic detection tests not positive until the late primary stage
 i. Stable or rising titers during year after treatment indicating inadequate therapy, reinfection, or false positive serology
2. Counselling/prevention
 a. Refer to counselling/prevention under gonorrhea.
 b. Mark and dispose of needles carefully and appropriately.
 c. Warn about Jarisch-Herxheimer reaction after first penicillin injection.
  (1) Chills
  (2) Fever
  (3) Headaches
  (4) Myalgia
  (5) Arthralgia
  (6) Lesions more prominent, edematous, brilliant
3. Follow-up
 a. Follow up on reported contacts.
 b. Repeat VDRL or RPR test 1 or 2 weeks later

if the initial test is negative and there is suspected clinical evidence of syphilis.

c. Follow clinically and serologically every 3 months for 1 year.
   (1) Nontreponemal test usually reverts within 3 months or decreases by at least two dilutions.
   (2) 97 percent will be seronegative 2 years after treatment.

4. Consultations/referrals
   a. Report to local health department.
   b. Consult with physician for
      (1) Pregnant woman with penicillin allergy
      (2) A titer that is not negative 9 months after treatment for primary syphilis
   c. Refer to physician
      (1) Positive nontreponemal test and a negative treponemal test
      (2) Pregnant woman with positive serologic titer for syphilis and no clinical evidence of syphilis
      (3) Client with serological titer that is stable or rising during first year of treatment

D. Herpes virus hominis type II

1. Treatments/medications
   a. Symptomatic relief
      (1) Local analgesic ointment
      (2) Witch hazel compresses or Tucks
      (3) Individual, portable, disposable sitz bath
   b. Treatment of secondary bacteria or mycotitic infected ulcers
      (1) Bacterial—local or systemic sulfonamides
      (2) Mycotitic—mycostatin or mycostatin ointment
   c. Protection of skin from maceration and abrasion
   d. Photoinactivation—questionable oncogenic effect
   e. Internal/external povidone-iodine solution—still experimental
   f. Cytosine arabinoside—Adenosine arabinoside
      (1) Use only if the infection threatens life.
      (2) It causes bone marrow supression.
   g. GC culture before initiating systemic therapy
2. Counselling/prevention
   a. No sexual intercourse or oral-genital sex until lesion(s) abated (if must, use condoms)
   b. Inactivated herpesvirus vaccine still under investigation
   c. Strong association with cervical cancer and need for at least yearly gynecological examination and Pap smear
   d. Culture negative before attempting pregnancy
   e. If pregnant, immediate medical attention if lesion(s) occur
3. Follow-up
   a. Repeat gynecological exam and Pap smear at least once a year.
   b. Repeat cultures until negative if pregnancy is desired.
4. Consultations/referrals
   a. Consult with a physician for a nonpregnant individual with recurrent herpesvirus type II.
   b. Inform the pediatrician prior to the birth of a fetus exposed to herpesvirus type II.
   c. Refer to a physician
      (1) Pregnant woman with herpesvirus type II—either primary or recurrent
      (2) Primary herpesvirus type II

Table 70-1 Pediatric Gonorrhea

Infant	Prepuberty (female)
Etiology	
N. gonorrhoeae	*N. gonorrhoeae*
Transmitted to eyes of newborn by birth, through an infected birth canal	Transmission Sexual Nonsexual Bedclothes, towels, common bathtubs Hands of infected individual
Subjective Data	
Discharge from eye	Vaginal discharge
Blots over eye	
Mother with a positive GC culture and not treated prior to giving birth	
Objective Data	
Conjunctivitis Discharge intially watery Discharge later purulent	Vaginal discharge profuse, purulent, and irritating
Opacity of cornea	Vulva (erythema, edema, excoriation)
Ulcerated cornea	Signs of acute pelvic inflammatory disease rare
Culture of discharge positive for *N. gonorrhoeae*	Culture of discharge positive for *N. gonorrhoeae*

Table 70-1 Pediatric Gonorrhea *(continued)*

Infant	Prepuberty (female)
Treatments/Medications	
1% silver nitrate solution to eyes (do not irrigate with saline or ophthalmic ointments like tetracycline, erythromycin, or neomycin combined with silver nitrate therapy) Aqueous crystalline penicillin G 50,000 units/kg daily in 2 or 3 doses Frequent saline irrigations Penicillin, tetracycline, or chloramphenicol eye drops	Aqueous procaine penicillin G 75,000–100,000 units/kg 1% plus probenecid 25 mg/kg po
Counselling/Prevention	
Treatment of mother or infected carrier Prophylactic instillation of silver nitrate to eyes	Prevention of child abuse
Follow-up	
Reculture 14 days after treatment	Reculture 14 days after treatment
Consultations/Referrals	
Immediate referral to physician, report to health department	Immediate referral to physician,report to health department

Table 70-2 Medical Referral/Consultation

Diagnosis	Clinical Manifestations	Management
Pelvic inflammatory disease	General symptoms Chills Fever 101–103° F and tachycardia or Nausea Vomiting Malaise Anorexia Pelvic findings Pain with motion of cervix or uterus Uterus: size, position, and consistency normal but may be fixed Adnexa: tender, may feel thick and full, may be fixed Masses and abscesses may be palpated in cul-de-sac Vaginal staining or discharge Abdominal exam Involuntary muscle guarding If infection severe or long in duration Distension Tympany Decreased or absent bowel sounds Severe bilateral abdominal pain Rebound percussion and tenderness Laboratory Positive gonorrheal culture Cervical culture possibly revealing gonococci Increased white blood count (WBC) and shift to left Increased sedimentation rate	Referral to physician Antibiotic therapy May require hospitalization See Preparation for Hospitalization, Part 7

Table 70-2 Medical Referral/Consultation *(continued)*

Diagnosis	Clinical Manifestations	Management
Syphilis Secondary—occurs usually 6–8 wk after primary chancre	Generalized, nonpruritic, transitory rash Macular lesions of a pinkish color on thorax and reddish brown on palms and soles Papular lesions perhaps changing to form a ring or arciform lesions—"annular syphilids" on the face "Split papules" under the breast, between the toes, at corners of mouth, behind ears, and at nasolabial folds Highly infectious condyloma lata (large, pale, moist, flat, confluent, circumscribed papules) found in anal, genital, and axillary areas Mucus patches (painless, dull, erythematous or greyish white erosions) on the lips, mouth, tongue, palate, throat, and genitalia Temporary alopecia Tenderness when pressure applied to bones Iritis—rarely Generalized lymphadenopathy History of malaise, anorexia, arthralgias, headache, sore throat, low-grade temperature	Referral to physician Report to health department Antibiotic therapy After treatment titer initially rising and usually falling—76% negative 2 yr after treatment
Tertiary	During early latent phase (less than 4 yr duration) relapses to secondary-type symptoms 4 yr after initial symptoms, client not infectious Late latent phase (infection greater than 4 yr is asymptomatic except for reactive serologic tests) Late syphilis Nodular or squamous skin lesions that are Destructive Spread peripherally Subcutaneous infiltrate and perforate skin leaving a round, cut-out ulcer Nervous system Deafness Diplopia General paresis Tabes dorsalis Meningitis Cardiovascular—aortic insufficiency aneurysm and arterial occlusion Positive cerebral spinal fluid for *T. pallidum*	Referral to physician A report to health department Antibiotic therapy After treatment, follow-up with cerebrospinal fluid analysis for cure
Acquired	Symptoms perhaps present at birth or emerging later Alopecia Pneumonia Adenopathy Enlarged liver—jaundice Enlarged spleen Inflammation of kidney	Refer to the physician. Report to the health department. Antibiotic therapy is indicated. Treat if at birth the maternal

Table 70-2 Medical Referral/Consultation *(continued)*

Diagnosis	Clinical Manifestations	Management
	Skin eruptions (blisters with yellow discharge), thrombocytopenia Meningitis Conjunctivitis Rhinitis Progressive emaciation of face with mucus patches on lips or in mouth Inflammation of fingers and toes including nail deformities Abdominal distension Pseudoparalysis Hemolytic anemia	treatment was inadequate, unknown, with drugs other than penicillin, or inadequately followed up. A cerebrospinal fluid examination should be done prior to treatment.

bibliography

Blount, J. H., Darrow, W. W., and Johnson, R. E. Venereal disease in adolescents. *Pediatric Clinics of North America*, **20**(4):1021–1033 (1973).

Hart, Gavin. *Chancroid, Donovanosis, lymphogranuloma venerum.*(DHEW Publication No. (CDC) 75-8302). Atlanta: Public Health Service Center for Disease Control, Bureau of State Service, Venereal Disease Control Division.

Jaffe, Harold W. The laboratory diagnosis of syphilis: New concepts. *Annals of Internal Medicine*, **83**(6):846–849 (1975).

Mead Johnson Laboratories. Herpes genitalis: Diagnosis. *The Overview Series and Management.* Evansville, Ind. Author, 1976, (47721, Serial No. P661754107).

Monif, Gilles R. G. *Infectious diseases in obstetrics and gynecology.* New York: Harper & Row, 1974.

Rudolph, Andrew H., and Duncan, W. Christopher. Syphilis—Diagnosis and treatment. *Clinical Obstetrics and Gynecology*, **18**(1):163–182 (1975).

U.S. Dept. Health, Education, and Welfare, Public Health Service Center for Disease Control, Bureau of State Services, Venereal Disease Control Division. Atlanta: Author. *Criteria and Techniques for the diagnosis of gonorrhea*, 1978.

________Criteria and techniques for the diagnosis of early syphilis. Atlanta: Author, 1976.

________Recommended treatment schedules for syphilis. Atlanta: Author, 1976.

71 Pregnancy and Labor

LOIS KOPP DANIELS

Pregnancy

ALERT

1. Presenting symptoms of pregnancy
   a. Missed menstrual period/irregular menses
   b. Fatigue/dizziness
   c. Nausea and/or vomiting
   d. Urinary frequency
   e. Breast tingling/tenderness
2. Preexisting conditions requiring medical supervision
   a. Cardiac disease
   b. Diabetes mellitus
   c. Hypertension
   d. Renal disease/recurrent urinary tract infections
   e. Cancer
   f. Thyroid disease
   g. Liver disease
   h. Seizure disorders
   i. Anemias/hemoglobinopathies
   j. Severe varicosities/thromboembolic problems
3. Danger signs in pregnancy
   a. Vaginal bleeding
   b. Persistent/severe nausea and vomiting
   c. Chills and/or fever
   d. Dysuria
   e. Severe unremitting frontal headaches
   f. Visual disturbances
   g. Persistent edema of hands and face
   h. Rupture of membranes prior to term
4. See also Table 71-1, Medical Referral/Consultation

I. Assessment

A. Obstetrical history (see Table 71-2)

B. Calculate estimated date of confinement (EDC).

1. Last menstrual period (LMP) minus 3 months plus 7 days.
2. Use gestational wheel.

C. Calculate current week of pregnancy (starting from 1 week post-LMP).

1. Use gestational wheel.
2. Compare calculation with other findings for consistency.
   a. See Table 71-3, Guide to Antepartal Management.
   b. See Table 71-4, Size/Date Discrepancy.

D. Assessment should include

1. Intrauterine pregnancy
   a. _____ weeks by dates (from LMP)
   b. _____ weeks by other findings (size, pregnancy test)
2. Normalcy of course (or specific problems)

II. Management

A. Treatments/medications

1. Ferrous sulfate, 325 mg twice daily, 2 h after meals, with orange juice
2. Prenatal vitamins with folic acid

B. Client counselling

1. Nutrition
   a. Consult Table 71-5 for client's ideal weight and compare to prepregnant weight.
   b. Consult Table 71-6 for client's caloric and protein requirements.

c. If there is more than a 10-lb deficit between the prepregnant and ideal weights, plan for weight gain beyond 24 lb for pregnancy by adding 20 g protein daily per pound of desired gain, prorated over the remaining weeks of pregnancy.
d. If the client was overweight, use the ideal weight for calculating needs; protein can be added if the client fails to gain.
e. Add 25 g protein and 250 cal daily after the twentieth week of pregnancy.
f. For the following stress factors, add 20 g protein and at least 200 cal daily
   (1) Poor obstetrical history (e.g., repeated spontaneous abortions/prematures)
   (2) Weight loss/failure to gain
   (3) Pregnancies spaced less than 1 year apart
   (4) Emotional stress
   (5) Twin gestation
g. Use 24-h diet history to assess adequacy.
h. Use the following sample as an outline of the essentials
   (1) 1 qt milk or exchanges
   (2) 2 eggs
   (3) 1 orange or other citrus fruit
   (4) 1 additional fruit
   (5) 2 servings meat/fish/poultry/rice and beans
   (6) 2 servings vegetables
   (7) 3 to 4 servings bread/cereals
i. Encourage high-protein snacks and ways to camouflage disliked foods (e.g., milk).
j. Tell client reasons for high-protein diet.
   (1) Minimum 24-lb weight gain accounted for by changes due to pregnancy and growth of fetus
   (2) Weight gain in pregnancy directly related to infant's birth weight
   (3) Larger (7.5 to 8.5 lb) infants having more brain cells than smaller infants
   (4) Weight loss/failure to gain resulting in ketosis, which is harmful to fetal brains

2. General hygiene/activity
   a. Bathing
      (1) Throughout pregnancy unless membranes ruptured or client having vaginal bleeding
      (2) As long as client comfortable getting into and out of bathtub/shower
   b. Sexual intercourse
      (1) Throughout pregnancy unless membranes ruptured, vaginal bleeding, placenta previa, or low-lying placenta
      (2) Position changes necessitated by enlarging uterus
      (3) Orgasm causes uterine contractions but these unrelated to premature labor
   c. Exercise
      (1) Maintain any which the client does regularly.
      (2) Walking is excellent for the prevention of thromboembolic problems and constipation.
   d. Travel
      (1) Automobile travel is safe, providing the client walks around at least every 1 to 2 h to avoid thromboembolic problems.
      (2) Seat belts should be worn both under the abdomen and across the chest.
      (3) Air travel is safe.
3. Normalcy of emotional changes
4. Danger signs (see Alert)
   a. Client should report them immediately.
   b. Provide client with access to you between visits.
5. Common pregnancy-related discomforts
   a. See Table 71-7, Common Pregnancy-Related Complaints.
   b. Emphasize physiologic causes.
6. Preparation for childbirth
   a. Refer the client to an organized series of classes.
   b. If there is no program available, see the bibliography for references.
   c. Discuss local hospital policies; arrange for a hospital tour if desired.

C. Follow-up

1. See Table 71-3, Guide to Antepartal Management, for a schedule of routine return visits.
2. Follow up specific laboratory findings.
   a. Rubella titer less than 1:8
      (1) Counsel client regarding exposure during first trimester.
      (2) Schedule postpartum vaccination.
      (3) Counsel client that she should not get pregnant for at least 3 months after vaccination.
   b. Hemoglobin AS (sickle cell trait)
      (1) Observe for borderline anemia.
      (2) Repeat urine cultures at least once a trimester, since these clients have increased susceptibility to urinary tract infections.
      (3) Try to obtain blood from the father of the baby for electrophoresis.
      (4) Counsel the client accordingly.

c. Rh negative (also Duffy negative) with negative antibody screen
   (1) If Duffy is positive, treat the client as Rh positive; no further follow-up is needed.
   (2) Try to obtain the blood type of the father of the baby.
   (3) Repeat antibody screen once per trimester.
   (4) Explain reasons to the client.

d. Positive Venereal Disease Research Laboratory (VDRL) test
   (1) Question the client for history of syphilis (even if treated) within past 2 years.
   (2) Counsel the client that pregnancy, use of marijuana, collagen disorders, mononucleosis, and other factors can cause a positive VDRL.
   (3) Obtain a blood specimen for a fluorescent treponemal-antibody absorption (FTA-ABS) test.
   (4) If the FTA-ABS is positive, consult the physician regarding treatment.

e. Positive gonorrhea culture
   (1) Treat with 4.8 million units of aqueous procaine penicillin G (IM) preceded by 1 g probenecid po 20 to 30 min before the penicillin.
   (2) If allergic to penicillin, consult regarding treatment.
   (3) Repeat culture in 2 weeks.
   (4) Counsel client regarding implications and importance of contacts receiving treatment.
   (5) Report, as required by law.

f. Proteinuria on Dipstix examination of urine
   (1) Obtain clean-catch specimen and recheck.
   (2) Question the client regarding vaginal discharge, symptoms of urinary tract infection, and symptoms of toxemia.
   (3) If 1+ or greater, on clean-catch specimen, consult regarding management.

g. Glycosuria on Dipstix examination of urine
   (1) Question client to determine if fasting specimen versus specimen 2 h postprandial
   (2) Obtain fasting specimen
   (3) If specimen is fasting, refer client for glucose testing

D. Consultations/referrals

1. Women, Infants and Children (WIC) program or other source of aid for food
2. Social services
3. Preparation for childbirth classes
4. La Leche League (for breast-feeding)
5. See Table 71-1

III. Subsequent Visits

A. See Table 71-1

B. See Table 71-3

Labor

ALERT

1. Premature labor (prior to 37 weeks gestation)
2. Presence of vaginal bleeding
3. Rupture of membranes with no labor
4. Meconium-stained amniotic fluid (yellow-green color)
5. Fetal heart rate less than 120 beats/minute, during, after, or between contractions
6. Fetal malpresentation (see Figs. 71-1 to 71-4)
7. Superimposed complications (see Table 71-1)

I. Assessment

A. True versus false labor (see Table 71-9)

B. Stage/phase of labor

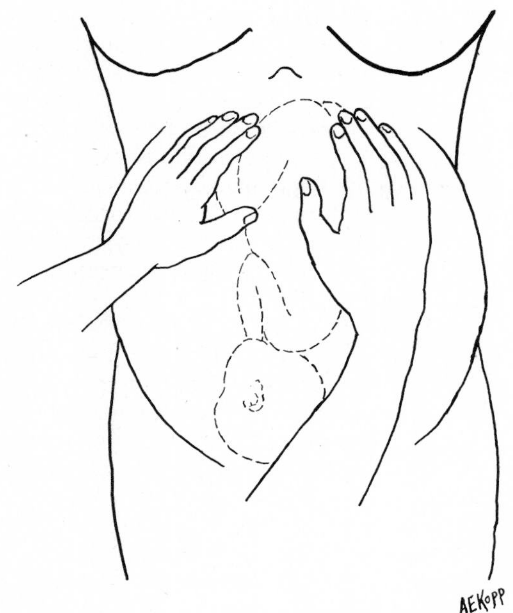

Figure 71-1 Abdominal palpation, first maneuver. While standing at client's side, facing her head, place hands on sides of uterine fundus. If, as in most cases, the breech is there, it will be an irregular mass which is less hard than the head. When it is ballotted, the entire fetal body will move. Finding fetal small parts in the fundus strengthens the diagnosis. *(Drawing by A. E. Kopp.)*

1. Early (0 to 4 cm dilatation) first stage
2. Active (4 to 10 cm dilatation) first stage
3. Second stage (completely dilated)

C. Term versus premature labor

D. Superimposed complications

1. See Alert.
2. See Table 71-1.

II. Management

A. False labor (see Table 71-9, no pelvic changes)

1. Seconal, 200 mg po, stat.
2. Client returns home.
3. Have client maintain the regular diet.
4. Have client call to report danger signs or true labor.

B. Early labor

1. Returns home
2. Clear liquid diet
3. Ambulation at will (if membranes intact or ruptured with fetus engaged)
4. Slow, deep breathing and relaxation with contractions
5. Comes to hospital when contractions are uncomfortable and 5 min (nullipara) or 10 min (multipara) apart, or danger signs appear

C. Active labor

1. Vistaril, 50 to 100 mg IM, may be given to help the client relax.
2. The client should go to the hospital.
3. A clear liquid diet should be maintained.
4. The client should practice slow, deep breathing and relaxation with contractions.

D. Delivery imminent

1. The cervix is dilated fully and the client is pushing (nullipara), or the cervix is more than 8 cm dilated (multipara).
2. Keep the client and prepare for emergency delivery and ultimate transfer to the hospital.

E. Referrals

1. See Alert.
2. See Table 71-1.
3. Notify the hospital of the client's arrival, and include relevant data, including pregnancy course.

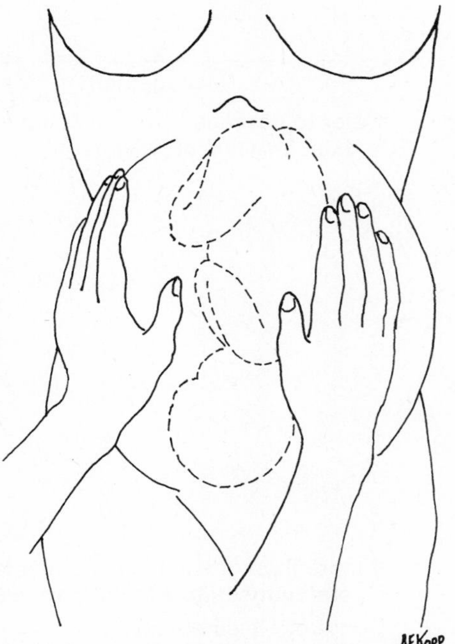

Figure 71-2 Abdominal palpation, second maneuver. While standing at client's side, facing her head, move hands from uterine fundus down to sides of abdomen. Use one hand to steady the uterus while the opposite one palpates fetal parts. Feel for the firm, smooth, convex area of the fetal back as opposed to the uneven, "lumpy," perhaps moving fetal limbs (small parts). *(Drawing by A. E. Kopp.)*

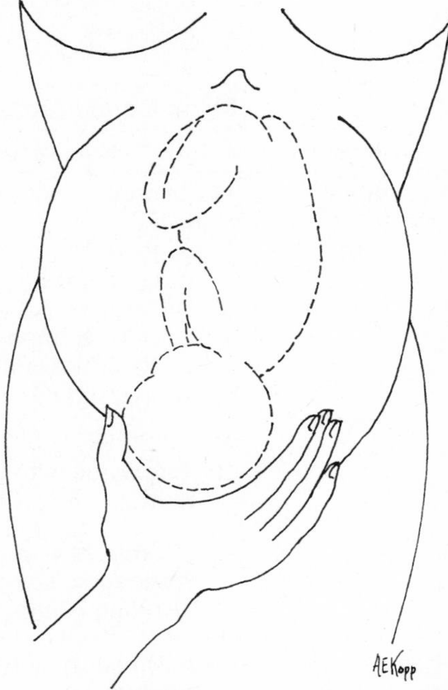

Figure 71-3 Abdominal palpation, third maneuver. While standing at client's side, facing her head, grasp the lower uterine segment, directly above the symphysis pubis, between the thumb and fingers of one hand while the other hand is on the uterine fundus to provide stability. In most cases the head will be over the pelvic inlet and will be felt as a hard, globular, smooth part which is easily ballotted. When it is moved, the entire fetal body does not move. *(Drawing by A. E. Kopp.)*

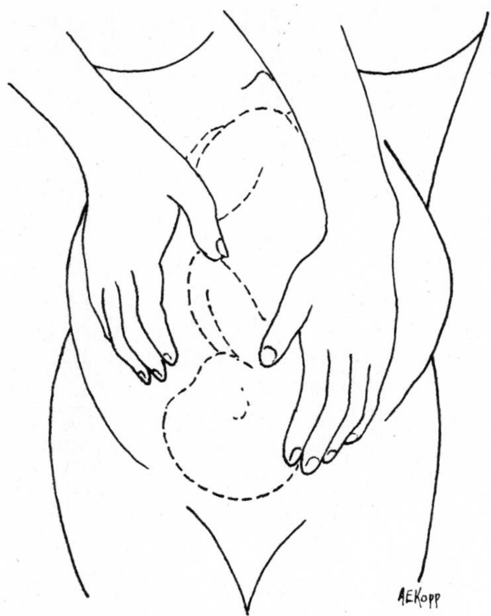

Figure 71-4 Abdominal palpation, fourth maneuver. Turn to face the client's feet and ask her to flex her hips and her knees. As she inhales and exhales deeply and slowly, perform this maneuver during exhalation. Gently but firmly press the fingers of both hands toward the symphysis pubis. One hand will meet resistance (cephalic prominence) before the other. The prominence is most often the fetal forehead and is opposite the fetal back when the head is flexed. This maneuver can also assess whether the presenting part is dipping into the pelvic inlet or remains floating above the symphysis pubis. If the presenting part is deep (engaged) in the pelvis, it will be difficult to palpate and will be "fixed" (unable to be ballotted). This maneuver can often be diagnostic of a breech presentation when no cephalic prominence is palpated and the examining hands converge above the pubis. Moving fetal limbs helps confirm the diagnosis in some cases. *(Drawing by A. E. Kopp.)*

Table 71-1 Medical Referral/Consultation

Diagnosis/Problem	Clinical Manifestations	Management
Potential inadequate pelvic capacity	Primigravida with previously untested pelvis History of Difficult forceps or vacuum extraction deliveries with maternal or fetal trauma Long, difficult labors Height under 5 ft Large fetus Primigravida with unengaged fetus, at term	Refer to physician, with accompanying data, for clinical pelvimetry
Vaginal bleeding	See Table 71-8 Vaginal Bleeding in Pregnancy, see Vaginal Spotting/ Bleeding, Chap. 64	
Potential gestational diabetes	Family history of diabetes in parents, siblings Obesity (greater than 20% for height) Over age 25 History of/current episode of glycosuria in fasting urine specimen Polyhydramnios (excess amniotic fluid) History of Infants weighing more than 4000 g (8 lb 13 oz)	If more than one clinical manifestation, refer immediately to the physician. Conduct 1-h screen. Counsel the client to fast from midnight to the morning of the test. Draw fasting blood sugar specimen. Give the client 50 g commercial oral glucose preparation. Draw 1-h blood specimen. If fasting (whole blood) sugar is $>$ 95

Table 71-1 Medical Referral/Consultation *(continued)*

Diagnosis/Problem	Clinical Manifestations	Management
	Term size infants (over 2500 g) with respiratory distress syndrome Unexplained stillborns, repeated spontaneous abortions, repeated premature infants	mg% or 1-h value > 130 mg%, refer client to the physician. Counsel client about the importance of the test; fetus can be compromised and need careful surveillance during last 6–8 wk of pregnancy and during labor.
Potential intrauterine growth retardation	See Table 71-4, Size/Date Discrepancy.	
Multiple gestation	See Table 71-4, Size/Date Discrepancy.	
Toxemia of pregnancy (preeclampsia)	Hypertension after twenty-fourth week of pregnancy Systolic 140 or 30 mmHg rise above baseline, *or* Diastolic 90 or 15 mmHg rise above baseline Persistent edema of hands, face; perhaps abdomen and sacrum Significant proteinuria (greater than 1+ on clean-catch specimen) Excessive weight gain (greater than 2 lb/week) If severe, may include all of the above plus Hyperreflexia with clonus Oliguria Hypertension of 160/110 Epigastric pain from liver enlargement If eclamptic, convulsions and/or coma sometimes accompanying above symptoms	Check fetal heart tones. Refer immediately to the physician with the accompanying data. Explain to the client the severity of her condition. If severe, or eclamptic, refer the client to the hospital immediately.
Anemia (see Chap. 39)	Usually due to iron or folic acid deficiency in pregnancy May also be due to pica (starch, clay, ice) Physiologic drop in hematocrit peaks at 28–32 wk, but should not exceed 10% drop	Counsel about nutrition, as indicated. Increase iron intake to 3 times daily. Explain the importance to the client of the following The baby may deplete the mother's own stores. The mother is predisposed to poor labor, lacerations, hemorrhage, and infection. If anemia persists after documented adequate iron intake, refer to the physician with the accompanying data.
Urinary tract infection (see also Pain and Burning during Urination, Chap. 76)	Bacteriuria (> 100,000 colonies in a clean-catch specimen) May be asymptomatic	DO NOT use Tetracycline Sulfonamides

Table 71-1 Medical Referral/Consultation *(continued)*

Diagnosis/Problem	Clinical Manifestations	Management
		Consult or refer to a physician; even asymptomatic bacteriuria should be treated in pregnancy.
Hyperemesis gravidarum	Nausea and vomiting severe enough to cause weight loss and/or dehydration May accompany hydatidiform mole or multiple gestation May be psychogenic	Refer to a physician with the accompanying data.
Rh negative with positive antibody screen (sensitized)	May have history of Transfusions Therapeutic abortions not followed by RhoGAM injection Previous delivery without follow-up RhoGAM injection Previously affected (jaundiced) infant	Refer to a physician with the accompanying data.
Cervical culture positive for beta-hemolytic Streptococcus group B	None	Consult with the physician for treatment during pregnancy and/or intensive observation of neonate for sepsis.
Premature rupture of membranes (prior to onset of labor)	Gush or uncontrolled trickle of fluid from vagina May be clear or stained yellow *(a sign of fetal distress)* Sterile speculum examination Pooling of fluid in posterior vaginal fornix with fundal pressure Fluid turning Nitrazine paper vivid blue Fluid forming "fern" pattern upon microscopic examination if air-dried on glass slide	DO NOT do a digital exam; perform a sterile speculum exam. Check fetal heart tones. Check for uterine contractions. Check temperature. Refer client to the physician with the accompanying data since ascending infection is possible.
Fetal malpresentation (other than cephalic) at term (36 wk)	See Fig. 71–1 through 71–4, on abdominal palpation.	Refer to the physician with the accompanying data.
Postdatism	Client is beyond EDC, or "overdue."	Begin workup and consultation at 41 wk to allow time for scheduling tests, etc. Document week of pregnancy by all available parameters. Counsel client to report decreased fetal movement (less than 15 movements/h; 70 movements/12 h). Check for cervical "ripening" (dilatation, effacement, softening, anterior position, engagement of presenting part). Consult at 41 elapsed weeks for medical follow-up with accompanying data.

Table 71-2 Obstetrical History Information

Each Pregnancy
Year
Type of Termination of Pregnancy

Spontaneous Abortion	Therapeutic Abortion	Premature Labor	Term Labor
Length of pregnancy Complications: transfusions, dilatation and curettage (D and C) afterward, infection Did client receive RhoGAM if Rh negative?	Length of pregnancy Type of procedure: D&C, suction, saline, prostaglandin, other Complications: transfusions; follow-up D&C, hemorrhage; infection Did client receive RhoGAM if Rh negative?	Length of pregnancy Events immediately preceding Type of labor: painful, painless, premature rupture of membranes Condition and weight of baby; is baby still alive? Did client receive RhoGAM if Rh negative?	Length of pregnancy Length of labor; induction Type delivery: spontaneous vaginal delivery, forceps delivery, vacuum extraction, Cesarean section Type of episiotomy; other lacerations Anesthesia/analgesia used Weight of baby; condition of baby then and now Complications of pregnancy, labor, postpartum period; hypertension, anemia, hemorrhage, infection, other Did client receive RhoGAM if Rh negative and baby Rh positive?

Table 71-3 Guide to Antepartal Management

Week Post-LMP	Essential Data	Management
0–12	*Diagnosis and dating of pregnancy* Subjective data Date and normalcy of LMP Signs and symptoms of early pregnancy: nausea, vomiting, fatigue, urinary frequency, breast tingling or tenderness Date of positive/negative pregnancy test Objective data Breast changes: increased size, more erectile nipples, pigmentation changes, Montgomery's follicles on areola, prominent venous pattern Uterine changes: Goodell's sign (approximately 6 wk), Hegar's sign (6–10 wk), Chadwick's sign (8–12 wk) Uterine size changes: 6–8 wk = small lemon; 8–10 wk = medium orange; 10–12 wk = approaching grapefruit size Other changes: listen for fetal heart with Doppler instrument (first audible at 12 wk) Pregnancy test positive at 6 wk. *General Progress* Weight gain Blood pressure	Refer for a therapeutic abortion, if indicated. Initiate or reinforce diet counselling. Initiate or reinforce iron and vitamin therapy. Treat common discomforts of pregnancy. Discuss normal emotional changes. Request the client to Return to clinic in 4 wk unless indicated sooner. Bring a 7-day diet history. Report danger signs immediately. Report the date of quickening, if it occurs prior to the next visit.

Table 71-3 Guide to Antepartal Management *(continued)*

Week Post-LMP	Essential Data	Management
	24-h diet recall Urine for Dipstix examination for glucose, protein, and ketones (if severe nausea and vomiting and/or weight loss), pregnancy test, if indicated Laboratory data from previous visits, if available Data related to specific discomforts *Danger Signs* (See Alert and Table 71-1) *Emotional Changes* May include: ambivalence, disbelief/denial of reality of pregnancy, emotional liability, panic at being in uncontrollable situation, more frequent dreams	
12–20	*Dating of Pregnancy* Subjective data Same as above, as necessary Signs of resolution of nausea, fatigue, urinary frequency Braxton Hicks contractions may appear as early as 16 wk Quickening, felt as a "flutter" suprapubically, 16–18 wk in multipara, 18–20 wk in nullipara Objective data Breast changes: colostrum perhaps present at 16 wk, especially in multipara Uterine changes Palpable as abdominal organ at 12 wk Halfway between symphysis pubis and umbilicus at 16 wk Three-fourths way up from symphysis pubis to umbilicus at 18 wk At the umbilicus or approaching 20 cm above the symphysis pubis at 20 wk Fetal heart tones audible by fetoscope at 18–20 wk; often suprapubically Fetal movement audible by fetoscope around 20 wk Fetus ballottable upon bimanual examination *General progress* Weight/gain: at least 4–5 lb by 20 wk Blood pressure/urine/laboratory data Data related to specific discomforts *Danger Signs* (see Alert and Table 71-1) *Emotional Changes* May include increasing impatience for baby's first move and for pregnancy to "show"; relief or excitement at quickening, continued dreams/nightmares, surfacing of	Same as above Particular emphasis upon steady weight gain Request the client to Report the date of quickening, if it has not yet occurred. Return weekly for fetal heart tone checks if not yet heard and near 20 wk.

Table 71-3 Guide to Antepartal Management *(continued)*

Week Post-LMP	Essential Data	Management
	old conflicts (particularly regarding client's mother), increasing introspection	
20–28	*Dating of Pregnancy* Subjective data Same as above, as necessary Increasing fetal movement; beginning patterns of movement Objective data Uterine changes: Height of uterus above pubis, measured in cm, corresponds roughly to week of gestation; each fingerbreadth above umbilicus = 2 wk. Other changes: Fetal lie and fetal parts begin to be palpable at 26–28 wk; fetal movements are definitely palpable; fetal heart tones are clearly heard with fetoscope. *General Progress* Weight increase 1 lb/week Blood pressure/urine/laboratory (see above) Data related to specific discomforts *Danger signs* (see Alert and Table 71-1) *Emotional Changes* Client may begin to relate to the baby as a person and may call the baby a name. Plays with baby to provoke movement *Other* May make plans for preparation for labor	Same as above Increase of 20 g protein and 200 cal each day after 20 wk
28–36	*Dating of Pregnancy* Subjective data: same as above, as necessary Objective data Uterus continuing to grow at relatively constant rate (see above for measurement above symphysis pubis in cm or above umbilicus in fingerbreadths) Fetal lie, presentation, parts easily palpable by examiner (see Figs. 71-1 through 71-4) Fetal heart tones easily auscultated with fetoscope *General Progress* Weight, urine (see above) Laboratory; hematocrit showing physiologic drop; should not exceed 10% Diastolic blood pressure showing slight drop *Danger Signs* (see Alert and Table 71-1)	Same as above, as necessary Repeat of hematocrit 28–32 wk when greatest physiologic drop evident Repeat of cervical culture for beta-hemolytic streptococcus Referral to preparation for childbirth classes at 30 wk, or initiation of the teaching of breathing and relaxation techniques for labor Request client to Practice breathing and relaxation techniques daily. Return to clinic in 2 wk if progress is normal.

Table 71-3 Guide to Antepartal Management *(continued)*

Week Post-LMP	Essential Data	Management
	Emotional Changes See above; increasing concern with labor, possible fear of labor, dreams of death or injury, other threatening themes	
36–40	*Dating of Pregnancy* Subjective data Same as above, as necessary Frequent Braxton-Hicks contractions Lightening perhaps occurring, particularly in nulliparas Objective data Digital pelvic examination reveals progressive changes in cervical dilatation, effacement, movement of cervix from posterior to anterior position, softening of cervix, and descent of the fetus. *General Progress* (see above) *Danger Signs* (see Alert, Table 71-1 and Labor Alert) *Emotional Changes* May include increasing impatience for labor to start, boredom with being pregnant, difficulty sleeping; may want induction to "get it over with"	See management above. Refer client for clinical pelvimetry if indicated (see Table 71-1) at 36 wk. Repeat VDRL, hematrocrit, and cervical cultures for gonorrhea and beta-hemolytic streptococcus, at 36 wk. Discuss with client Signs of labor When to call/come to the hospital How to get to the hospital Request client to Continue practicing breathing and relaxation techniques. Return to clinic in 1 wk.

Table 71-4 Size/Date Discrepancy

Problem	Possible Etiology	Management
Uterine size at least 3 cm less than expected for stage of gestation	Inaccurate dating from last menstrual period Hydatidiform mole (⅓ of uteri are smaller, especially later in pregnancy) Intrauterine growth retardation Missed spontaneous abortion Pseudocyesis Fetal demise	Clarify date and normalcy of last menstrual period. Early, middle, late in month Near holidays/special days Normal in terms of length and character of flow, premenstrual symptoms Pinpoint date of conception, if possible. Times of sexual activity or abstinence Times of contraceptive use/nonuse Ascertain other signs of pregnancy. Early signs (nausea, breast changes, etc.) Positive pregnancy test, if at 6 wk after last menstrual period Date of quickening, first audible fetal heart tones Assess for additional factors contributing to poor fetal growth. Substance abuse (drug, alcohol, nicotine) Superimposed medical problems (e.g., hypertension) Poor nutritional status (weight loss, failure to gain, anemia) Assess for factors relating to hydatidiform mole (see Table 71–8).

Table 71-4 Size/Date Discrepancy *(continued)*

Problem	Possible Etiology	Management
		Assess for factors relating to missed abortion, fetal demise, pseudocyesis. Repetition of pregnancy test (may remain positive up to 2 wk after pregnancy terminates) History of vaginal spotting/bleeding during first 12 wk No fetal heart tones at expected times (12–14 wk with Doppler instrument, 20 wk with fetoscope) Refer to physician with accompanying data.
Uterine size at least 3 cm larger than expected for stage of gestation	Inaccurate dating from last menstrual period Hydatidiform mole (⅓ of uteri are larger, especially in early pregnancy) Multiple pregnancy Polyhydramnios (excess amniotic fluid)	Clarify date and normalcy of last menstrual period. Pinpoint time of conception, if possible. Ascertain other signs of early pregnancy. Assess for factors relating to multiple pregnancy. Family history (maternal) of fraternal twins History of use of ovulation-inducing drugs (e.g., Clomid) or birth control pills within 2 mo prior to conception Excessive or persistent nausea and vomiting Excessive weight gain Excessive fetal movement perceived by the client or examiner Palpation of more than one fetus or auscultation of more than one fetal heart Anemia Assess for amount of amniotic fluid in relation to fetal size. Difficulty in palpating fetal parts Difficulty in auscultating fetal heart tones Presence of "fluid thrill" (examiner's hand on one side of abdomen feels motion of fluid when opposite side is tapped) Refer to physician with accompanying data.

Table 71-5 Ideal Weight for Height

	Weight*		
Height	Small Build	Medium Build	Large Build
4′11″	103	110	120
5′0″	106	113	123
5′1″	109	116	126
5′2″	112	120	130
5′3″	115	123	134
5′4″	119	128	138
5′5″	123	132	142
5′6″	127	136	146
5′7″	131	140	149
5′8″	135	144	154
5′9″	139	148	159
5′10″	143	152	163
5′11″	147	156	167
6′0″	151	160	171

*Subtract 1 lb for every year below age 25.

Table 71-6 Caloric and Protein Requirements

	Sedentary		Moderate	
Body Weight	Calories	Protein (g)	Calories	Protein (g)
80	1600	40	1900	40
85	1650	43	1950	43
90	1700	45	2000	45
95	1750	48	2050	48
100	1800	50	2100	50
105	1875	52	2175	52
110	1950	53	2250	53
115	2025	54	2325	54
120	2100	55	2400	55
125	2150	57	2450	57
130	2200	58	2500	58
135	2250	59	2550	59
140	2300	60	2600	60
145	2350	63	2650	63
150	2400	65	2700	65
155	2450	68	2750	68
160	2500	70	2800	70
Teenagers 13–15 yr old:			2600	80
Teenagers 16–19 yr old:			2400	75

Table 71-7 Common Pregnancy-Related Complaints

Problem	Etiology	Clinical Manifestations	Management
Nausea and/or vomiting	Increased levels of estrogen and human chorionic gonadotropin (HCG); occasionally psychogenic if persistent or severe	Most severe in first trimester Usually occurs at same time(s) each day; not always in morning May take form of intolerance to certain foods/odors Can cause weight loss or failure to gain	Medications Bendectin, two tablets at bedtime, one during the day (6 h before nausea tends to occur) Beminal Forte, or other high-potency B complex vitamin, one capsule daily Counselling Explain the physiologic basis and probable duration. Avoid high-protein and fatty foods, an empty stomach, and specific foods which cause nausea. Increase carbohydrate intake and keep food in stomach (toast and jam before arising; Coke or Coke syrup). Referral to physician If persists beyond 14 wk If severe enough to cause weight loss/dehydration
Heartburn	Hormonal relaxation of cardiac sphincter; reflux of gastric contents into esophagus; later in pregnancy, may be due to pressure on stomach from enlarging uterus	Sharp epigastric pain sometimes radiating to back May be related to specific foods or occur at specific times	Medications Give Maalox, 30 mL 1 h after eating, as needed. Do not give antacids containing sodium bicarbonate (e.g., Rolaids).

Table 71-7 Common Pregnancy-Related Complaints *(continued)*

Problem	Etiology	Clinical Manifestations	Management
			Recommend the avoidance of spicy or fatty foods, lying down after meals, allowing stomach to become empty. Recommend the drinking of milk.
Round ligament pain	Stretching and contraction of uterine round ligaments which insert into inguinal canal and top of labia majora	Sharp, pulling twinge in inguinal area, radiating down into labia Exaggerated by activities such as walking or turning in bed	Medications Give acetaminophen, 325 mg every 4 h, as needed. Do not give aspirin in third trimester of pregnancy. Counselling Explain the physiologic basis. Decrease activities which initiate or exacerbate the problem. Stop activity when the pain occurs, and flex the hip on the affected side. Apply local heat or take warm baths.
Constipation	Relaxation of large intestine due to hormonal effects; increased water absorption; exaggerated by oral iron intake, poor dietary intake of fluids and roughage, inadequate exercise	Hard, difficult-to-pass stools Must be differentiated from mere change in bowel habits	Medications Milk of magnesia, 30 mL at bedtime Colace, 100 mg at bedtime Fermalox perhaps a less constipating form of oral iron, but expensive Counselling Explain the physiologic basis. Increase exercise. Increase fluid intake and dietary roughage. Establish a relaxed, regular toilet routine.
Low backache	Muscle fatigue from accentuated lordosis of pregnancy; exaggerated by poor posture and poor body mechanics when bending or lifting; accentuated by wearing high-heeled or platform shoes	Dragging backache in lumbosacral area Frequently more severe in multiparas with poor abdominal muscle tone or who lift child or other objects Differentiate from pyelonephritis and labor	Medications Give acetaminophen, 325 mg every 4 h, as needed. Do not give aspirin in third trimester of pregnancy. Counselling Explain the physiologic basis. Show client how to use the legs for leverage when bending to pick up something. Rest one foot on a stool or box when standing for long periods (ironing). Teach pelvic rock.
Sciatica	Pressure on sciatic nerve from increased mobility of sacroiliac joint due to hormonal effect on connective tissue	Sharp, shooting pain down posterior thigh frequently initiated or exaggerated by exercise (walking, vacuuming, etc.)	Medications Acetaminophen, 325 mg every 4 h, as needed Counselling Explain the physiologic basis. Avoid activities which initiate or exaggerate the problem.

Table 71-7 Common Pregnancy-Related Complaints *(continued)*

Problem	Etiology	Clinical Manifestations	Management
			Apply heat locally or take warm baths. A maternity girdle will immobilize the pelvic joints, but it is expensive.
Dependent edema	Mechanical obstruction of venous return by enlarging uterus	Usually increases as day goes on rather than being present in morning upon awakening May occur after long periods of standing or in hot weather Usually in lower extremities but can occur in hands Must be differentiated from more severe, generalized edema of toxemia	Medications None: DO NOT GIVE DIURETICS IN PREGNANCY. DO NOT RESTRICT SODIUM. Counselling Explain the physiologic basis. Have the client rest on left side, flat in bed, at least 2 h/day. Maintain a diet high in protein, and supplement it with high-protein milkshakes (1 cup milk, ½ cup yogurt or ice cream, flavoring, banana, 1–2 eggs, ¼ cup dry powdered milk). Increase fluid intake to 2–3 L daily. Elevate legs when sitting. Report danger signs of toxemia.
Vaginal discharge	Normal leukorrhea of pregnancy due to increased vascularization and mucosal proliferation from hormonal effects	Profuse, white, creamy discharge Nonirritating and nonodorous Must be differentiated from infections, i.e., moniliasis, trichomoniasis, bacterial infections (see Vaginal Discharge, Chap. 66)	Medications See Vaginal Discharge, Chap. 66, for treatment of specific infections. DO NOT use Flagyl or Betadine Vaginal Gel during pregnancy. Counselling Explain the physiologic basis. Keep perineal area clean and dry; expose it to the air. Wear cotton underwear. Avoid nylon underwear, pantyhose, tight pants, douching, feminine hygiene products, and water softeners in the bath water.

Table 71-8 Vaginal Bleeding in Pregnancy

Problem	Clinical Manifestations	Management
Hydatidiform mole	Intermittent or continuous bleeding prior to 12 wk post-LMP May be profuse and red or scant and brownish in color May have severe or persistent nausea and vomiting In early pregnancy, uterus perhaps larger than expected for stage of gestation; later, is smaller Absence of fetal heart tones at expected times (12–14 wk with Doppler instrument, 20 wk with fetoscope)	Referral to physician with accompanying data

Table 71-8 Vaginal Bleeding in Pregnancy *(continued)*

Problem	Clinical Manifestations	Management
	Positive pregnancy test Bimanual examination: uterus feeling soft, no fetus ballottable, ovaries perhaps slightly enlarged and tender Client perhaps showing hypertension/toxemia prior to 24 wk	
Spontaneous abortion	Occurs during first trimester Dark-red vaginal spotting; may increase to bright-red, heavy bleeding Suprapubic cramping or lower backache usually present	See Vaginal Spotting/Bleeding, Chap. 64
Ectopic pregnancy	Pain is the most common symptom (90% of the cases); it is often stabbing, sudden; it may be crampy and intermittent. Pain frequently radiates to the shoulder. An acute episode may be precipitated by straining at stool, coitus, coughing, sneezing. Bleeding is usually scant and dark in color. An ectopic pregnancy may occur as early as 14 days after conception; therefore, amenorrhea may *not* be part of the history. It often occurs 6–12 wk after the last menstrual period. Client may have a history of previous tubal infection/surgery. Pelvic examination may cause pain on lateral motion of the cervix; the exam may reveal increased uterine size and softening; adnexal mass and tenderness.	Immediate referral to physician See Vaginal Spotting/Bleeding, Chap. 64 See also Abdominal Pain, Chap. 51
Cervicitis (or other cervical pathology)	Bright-red bleeding; painless; frequently postcoital May have history of long-standing or recurrent vaginal infection or gonorrhea Can occur at any time in pregnancy	Check fetal heart tones. *Do not examine any client with painless, bright-red bleeding in pregnancy* Counsel client regarding pelvic precautions (i.e., no douching, no intercourse, no tampons). Refer with accompanying data for ultrasound location of placenta.
Placenta previa/ low-lying placenta	Bright-red, painless bleeding May be profuse and occur without warning (client may awaken in a pool of blood) May be postcoital May cease spontaneously Usually occurs near end of second trimester	Check fetal heart tones. *Do not examine any client with painless, bright-red bleeding in pregnancy*. Counsel client regarding accurate assessment of amount of bleeding (pad count) and pelvic precautions (no douching, no intercourse, no tampons).

Table 71-8 Vaginal Bleeding in Pregnancy *(continued)*

Problem	Clinical Manifestations	Management
		If bleeding stops, refer client for ultrasound localization of placenta. If bleeding continues, refer by ambulance to hospital.
Abruptio placentae (premature separation of the placenta)	Variable amount of red bleeding Localized or generalized abdominal pain which may be severe Uterus perhaps tender upon palpation; hypertonus perhaps present, to the point of rigidity Client sometimes complaining of contractions but with pain unremitting between contractions Fetal heart tones perhaps absent or at abnormal rate (< 120, > 160 beats/min) Client sometimes hypertensive	Check fetal heart tones. Palpate uterus for tone, contractions, tenderness. Place pen mark at height of fundus to observe for continuing uterine enlargement with growing retroplacental clot. Refer, by ambulance, to the hospital and include accompanying data.

Table 71-9 True versus False Labor

True Labor	False Labor
Contractions perceived in lower back radiating to front	Contractions often limited to lower abdomen
Contractions increase in frequency, intensity, and duration	Contractions remain the same or become irregular
Contractions unrelieved by position change, ambulation, alcohol ingestion, or warm bath	Contractions relieved by position change ambulation, alcohol ingestion or warm bath

bibliography

Abbott, M. I. Teens having babies. *Pediatric Nursing*, **4**:23 (1978).

Bahr, J. E. Herpesvirus hominis type 2 in women and newborns. *Maternal and Child Nursing*, **3**:16 (1978).

Beazley, J. M. Fallacy of fundal height. *British Medical Journal*, **4**:404 (1970).

Benirschke, K., and Kim, C. K. Multiple pregnancy: I. *New England Journal of Medicine*, **288**:1276 (1973).

Bing, E., and Colman, L. *Making love during pregnancy*. New York: Bantam, 1977.

Bracken, M. D., et al. Abortion, adoption or motherhood; An empirical study of decision-making during pregnancy. *American Journal of Obstetrics and Gynecology* **130**:251 (1978).

Burrow, G. N., and Ferris, T. F. *Medical complications during pregnancy*. Philadelphia: Saunders, 1975.

Clark, A., and Affonso, D. *Childbearing, a nursing perspective*. Philadelphia: Davis, 1976.

Colman, A., and Colman, L. *Pregnancy: The psychological experience*. New York: Herder and Herder, 1971.

Connaughton, J. F., et al. Perinatal addiction: Outcome

and management. *American Journal of Obstetrics and Gynecology* **129**:679 (1978).

Corrinet, Ann Malley and Elsberry, Charlotte Cram. Nine months is not enough. In Suzanne Hall Johnson (ed.), *High risk parenting,* Philadelphia: Lippincott, 1979, p. 193.

Crosby, W. M. Automotive trauma and the pregnant patient. *Contemporary OB/GYN,* **8**:115 (1976).

Curda, L. R. What about pica? *Journal of Nurse-Midwifery,* **22**:7 (1977).

Fielding, J. E. Smoking and pregnancy. *New England Journal of Medicine,* **298**:337 (1978).

Fitzhugh, M., and Newton, M. Posture in pregnancy. *American Journal of Obstetrics and Gynecology,* **85**:1091 (1963).

Frigoletto, F. D., and Rothchild, S. B. Altered fetal growth: An overview. *Clinical Obstetrics and Gynecology,* **20**:915 (1977).

Gohari, P., et al. Immediate and long-term risks to IUGR children. *Contemporary OB/GYN* **8**:79 (1976).

Goodlin, R. C., and Haesslein, H. C. When is it fetal distress? *American Journal of Obstetrics and Gynecology,* **128**:440 (1977).

Goodner, D. M. Teratology for the obstetrician. *Clinical Obstetrics and Gynecology,* **18**:245 (1975).

Grant, H., and Murray, R. *Emergency care* (2d ed.). Bowie, Md.: Robert J. Brady, 1978, p. 391.

Greenhill, J. P., and Friedman, E. A. *Biological principles and modern practice of obstetrics.* Philadelphia: Saunders, 1974.

Hazlett, B. E., and Kenshole, A. B. Pregnancy and diabetes. *Primary Care,* **4**:643 (1977).

Hill, R. M., et al. Utilization of over-the-counter drugs during pregnancy. *Clinical Obstetrics and Gynecology,* **20**:381 (1977).

Holtzman, L. C. Sexual practices during pregnancy. *Journal of Nurse-Midwifery,* **21**:29 (1976).

Houde, C., and Conway, C. E. Teen-age mothers: A clinical profile. *Contemporary OB/GYN,* **7**:71 (1976).

Jacobson, H. N. Current concepts in nutrition: Diet in pregnancy. *New England Journal of Medicine,* **297**:1051(1977).

Kieval, J. Gestational diabetes: Diagnosis and management. *Journal of Reproductive Medicine,* **14**:70 (1975).

Lappe, F. *Diet for a small planet.* New York: Ballantine Books, 1975.

Little, R. E. Moderate alchohol use during pregnancy and decreased infant birth weight. *American Journal of Public Health,* **67**:1154 (1977).

Lugo, G., et al. Intrauterine growth retardation, clinicopathology and findings in 233 consecutive infants. *American Journal of Obstetrics and Gynecology,* **109**:615 (1971).

Luke, B. Maternal alcoholism and fetal alcohol syndrome. *American Journal of Nursing,* **77**:1924 (1977).

Marquart, R. K. Expectant fathers: What are their needs? *Maternal and Child Nursing,* **1**:32 (1976).

Mercer, R. Becoming a mother at sixteen. *Maternal and Child Nursing,* **1**:44 (1976).

Meyer, M. B., and Tonascia, J. A. Maternal smoking, pregnancy complications and perinatal mortality. *American Journal of Obstetrics and Gynecology,* **128**:494 (1977).

Nesbitt, R. E. L. Prenatal identification of the fetus at risk. *Clinics in Perinatology,* **1**:213 (1974).

Noble, E. *Essential exercises for the childbearing years.* Boston:Houghton Mifflin, 1976.

Nutrition during pregnancy and lactation (Rev. ed.). Sacramento: California Department of Health, Maternal and Child Health Unit, 1975.

Oxorn, H., and Foote, W. R. *Human labor and birth* (3rd ed.). New York:Appleton-Century-Crofts, 1975.

Pitkin, R. M. Nutritional support in obstetrics and gynecology. *Clinical Obstetrics and Gynecology,* **19**:489 (1976).

Prenatal Diet Counselling in the Prenatal Clinic. Prepared by members of the faculty, Maternal-Newborn Nursing Program, Yale University School of Nursing, under a grant from the National Foundation for the March of Dimes, New Haven, 1976.

Primrose, T., and Higgins, A. A study in antepartum nutrition. *Journal of Reproductive Medicine,* **7**:256 (1971).

Reed, D. M., and Stanley, F. J. (eds.). *The epidemiology of prematurity.* Munich: Urban and Schwarzenberg, 1977.

Rubin, R. Cognitive style in pregnancy. *American Journal of Nursing,* **70**:502 (1970).

Sadovsky, E., Correlation between electromagnetic recording and maternal assessment of fetal movement. *Lancet,* **1**:1141 (1973).

Smith, P. B., et al. The medical impact of an antepartum program for pregnant adolescents: A statistical analysis. *American Journal of Public Health,* **68**:169 (1978).

Streissguth, A. P. Maternal drinking and the outcome of pregnancy: Implications for child mental health. *American Journal of Orthopsychiatry,* **47**:422 (1977).

Tejani, N., and Mann, L. I. Diagnosis and management of the small-for-gestational-age fetus. *Clinical Obstetrics and Gynecology,* **20**:943 (1977).

Breathing/relaxation techniques for preparation for childbirth[1]

Ewy, Donna, and Ewy, Roger. *Preparation for childbirth: A LaMaze guide*. New York: Signet, 1972. An illustrated, step-by-step guide which includes comfort measures during pregnancy, husband's role, and techniques for various phases of labor.

Hartman, Rhonda E. *Exercises for true natural childbirth*. New York: Harper & Row, 1975. Based upon the "husband-coached" method of childbirth preparation, this book emphasizes practical ways to prepare for and relief of pregnancy discomforts; it includes excellent photographs.

Maternity Center Association. *Preparation for childbearing* (4th ed.). New York: Author, 1973. This brief, illustrated manual describes comfort measures during pregnancy and techniques for use during labor.

[1]All these publications are available for order through International Childbirth Education Association, Supplies Center, P.O. Box 70258, Seattle, WA 98107.

72 Postpartum Checkup

BARBARA TAI

ALERT
1. Poor adaptation by either mother or father to infant
2. Breast problems
3. Positive Homans' sign
4. Enlarged thyroid
5. Poorly healing episiotomy or lacerations

I. Assessment

A. Subjective data—6 weeks postpartum

1. The parent(s) describes the adjustment to the infant as satisfactory.
2. If breast-feeding, the mother states that milk is adequate and nipples are in good condition.
3. The chosen feeding method is satisfactory to the parent(s) and infant.
4. There is no lochia or lochia alba.
5. There is no leg pain.
6. Contraception has been initiated.
7. Menses may have begun.

B. Objective data—6 weeks postpartum

1. Weight—12 to 15 lb loss, possibly more since birth
2. Blood pressure within normal limits
3. Breasts, if not breast-feeding, returned to prepregnant state
4. Good abdominal muscle tone and no diastasis
5. Negative Homans' sign
6. Thyroid not enlarged
7. Uterus involuted
8. Episiotomy and/or lacerations well healed
9. Urine showing no albumin
10. Mother/father adjusting to infant (see Neonatal Perception Inventory, Appendix 5)

Note: The postpartum examination is most frequently conducted at 6 weeks, but much anticipatory guidance could be given at a 2-week postdelivery examination.

II. Management

A. Treatments/medications

1. Birth control (see Birth Control, Chap. 17)
   a. If lactating, the mother may be best advised to select a method other than the oral contraceptive.
   b. It is believed that the mini-pill has no detrimental effect on lactation, but it may be best to avoid it.
   c. Foam and condoms may have been prescribed after delivery.
   d. If the examination reveals complete involution and the absence of pathology, any birth control method may be instituted.
   e. Some practitioners recommend waiting 3 months after a Cesarean section before inserting an intrauterine device (IUD).
2. Exercise to overcome muscular weakness, and Kegal exercises to increase muscle tone of the pelvic floor.

B. Counselling/prevention

1. Encourage parent(s) to verbalize concerns.
2. Reassure parent(s) that every parent does have some negative feelings.
3. Discuss birth control methods (see Birth Control, Chap. 17).
4. If the client is not lactating, remind her not to express any residual milk, as this will only increase the problem.
5. If breast-feeding, discuss breast care and

specific concerns (see "Nutritional Assessment" in Chap. 9).

6. Instruct on exercises (sit-ups, leg raises, etc.) to strengthen abdominal muscles.
7. Instruct on Kegal exercises.
8. Stress that amenorrhea is not a reliable indicator of anovulation.
9. Discuss return of ovulation and menses.
   a. Nonnursing mother—return of ovulation in 2 to 3 weeks, return of menses in 4 to 6 weeks postpartum
   b. Nursing mother—return of ovulation by 9 weeks, return of menses in 4 to 18 months postpartum
10. Help parent(s) deal with sibling adaptation.

C. Follow-up

1. As needed for specific concerns
2. 6 months to 1 year for Pap test
3. Depending on birth control method selected (see Chap. 17)

D. Consultations/referrals

1. Refer to physician all clients with
   a. Positive Homans' sign
   b. Poorly healing episiotomy or lacerations
2. Consult physician on all clients with
   a. Enlarged thyroid
   b. Breast infections
   c. Subinvolution of the uterus
3. Professional counselling may be indicated for families with difficulty adjusting to the infant.
4. Refer to the public health nurse if there are feeding or adjustment problems.

bibliography

Clark, Ann L., and Dyonne, D. Alfonso. *Childbearing: a nursing perspective.* Philadelphia: Davis, 1976.

Noble, Elizabeth. *Essential exercises for the childbearing years.* Boston: Houghton Mifflin, 1976.

Pritchard, Jack A., and Macdonald, Paul C. (eds.). *Williams obstetrics* (15th ed.). New York: Appleton-Century-Crofts, 1976.

73 Unwanted Pregnancy

NANCY E. DEVORE

ALERT
1. Moderate to severe depression
2. Psychosis
3. "Acting out" behavior, including recidivism
4. Mental retardation or severe emotional immaturity
5. Any significant medical or obstetrical problems in the client

I. Etiology

A. Medical factors
1. Genetic, metabolic, or anatomic disorders confirmed by amniocentesis or other tests
2. Exposure to teratogenic agents in early pregnancy
3. Severe medical conditions in the client
4. Ignorance of sexual activity or contraception
5. Contraceptive failure

B. Social factors
1. Rape
2. Intrafamilial forces
   a. Encouragement from parent or mate
   b. Incest
   c. Replacement for self (an aid in separation from an intolerable family situation)
3. Acquisition of status among friends and peers
4. Manipulation of a relationship or situation
5. Social situation (age, marital status, finances)

C. Psychological factors
1. Neurotic characteristics
2. Attempt to "prove" sexual adequacy
3. Attempt to ward off depression
4. Expression of anger toward self or another
5. Magical thinking—denial that own sexual behavior will lead to pregnancy

II. Assessment

A. Subjective data
1. Report of not wanting the pregnancy
2. Report of excessive physical discomforts of pregnancy
3. Report of high ambivalence about the pregnancy persisting past the first trimester
4. Lack of fantasies about the fetus
5. Report of lack of feeling or negative feeling for the fetus or infant
6. Failure to make necessary preparations for the new baby

B. Objective data
1. Attempt at self-abortion
2. Persistent nausea and vomiting past the first trimester
3. Exclusive reference to the baby as "it" in late pregnancy and postpartum
4. Lack of warm mother-infant interaction and mothering activities
5. Distancing feeding postures
6. Overt rejection of or hostility toward the infant
7. Signs of postpartum depression or psychosis
8. Eating and sleeping problems in the infant

III. Management

A. Treatments/medications
1. Termination techniques (see Table 73-1)
2. Techniques for enhancing mother-infant relationship (if client elects to keep the infant)
   a. Childbirth education classes
   b. Encouragement of a support person to participate in antepartum visits and in labor and delivery
   c. Encouragement of bonding with the infant at birth
   d. Encouragement of breast-feeding, unless client is strongly opposed

e. Utilization of social services to help with other problems
f. Anticipatory guidance on infant care and the parental role

3. Contraceptive information and methods

B. Counselling/prevention

1. Immediate goals
   a. Accept the reality of the situation.
      (1) Confront any denial (the lack of early objective signs of pregnancy makes the event seem unreal).
         (a) Stress evident body changes.
         (b) Show results of pregnancy tests.
         (c) Show blueness of cervix (with mirror).
         (d) Describe the size of the uterus in concrete terms, e.g., "It is the size of an orange," instead of "It is 8-week size".
      (2) Explore ambivalence toward the pregnancy.
         (a) Discuss maternal feelings versus individual or family plans and aspirations.
         (b) Explore feelings of anger, depression, shame, guilt, anxiety.
         (c) Discuss doubts about the capacity to be a parent.
         (d) Discuss stresses caused by physical and emotional changes.
   b. Regain control of own body and life.
      (1) Such an unwanted physical event implies the loss of control of one's own bodily functions.
      (2) Client can regain self-direction by making an active decision concerning the pregnancy.
         (a) Discuss how by waiting and not actively deciding, the client is making a passive decision.
         (b) If the client agrees, involve the mate and the family in the discussion, but the decision rests with the client.
      (3) Use a structured interview to provide a sense of security—avoid a nondirective approach.
   c. Explore the available options.
      (1) Provide information on the options.
         (a) Carry pregnancy and keep the infant
         (b) Carry pregnancy and give up the infant
            1. Temporary placement—foster care
            2. Permanent placement—adoption
         (c) Abortion
      (2) Discuss anxieties about labor and delivery or about the abortion procedure—provide needed information.
   d. Help the family develop its own problem-solving skills.
2. Long-term goals
   a. Explore etiological factors.
   b. Explore the feelings of the client and mate about childbearing and child rearing.
   c. Help the client to accept the loss if abortion or adoption is selected.
      (1) Identify and aid the mourning process.
      (2) Encourage the client to see the infant who is to be adopted.
   d. Prevent a disturbed family system if the client keeps the infant.
      (1) Stress the individuality of the infant.
         (a) Encourage fantasy construction during the pregnancy.
         (b) Encourage choosing names for the infant.
         (c) Encourage identification of unique features of the infant.
      (2) Aid the acceptance of the mothering role.
         (a) Utilize role playing.
         (b) Encourage the client to make things for the infant.
      (3) Explore any signs of a disturbed mother-infant relationship.
   e. Prevent future unwanted pregnancies through sex education and contraceptive counselling.

C. Follow-up

1. Physical checkup
   a. Vaginal delivery or termination: return visit in 6 weeks
   b. Abdominal delivery or termination: return visit in 2 weeks to check suture line and then at 6 weeks for full examination
2. Contraceptive method checkup
3. Ongoing psychological counselling as indicated

D. Consultations/referrals

1. Social service for vocational, educational, financial, environmental needs
2. Planned Parenthood, United Community Services, Birthright, local department of public welfare for assistance with carrying the pregnancy
3. National Organization of Women, Planned Parenthood, Clergy Consultation Service, Zero Population Growth for assistance with abortion
4. Professional counselling
5. Parent self-help groups and social service, if evidence of hostility toward infant.

Table 73-1 Termination Techniques

Abortion Method	Procedure	Disadvantages
Menstrual extraction (done 4–6 wk after last menses)	Office procedure Soft, flexible tube used to suction endometrium under local anesthesia or sedation	Mild brief cramping May be done unnecessarily as difficult to establish early pregnancy Occasional cervical tear May be incomplete Associated hemorrhage or infection Requires repeat
Suction abortion (done 6–12 wk after last menses)	Office or hospital procedure Cervical dilation under local or general anesthesia Suction of endometrium through nonflexible catheter	Moderate cramping Occasional cervical tear or uterine perforation May be incomplete Associated hemorrhage or infection Requires repeat
Dilation and curettage (done 6–12 wk after last menses)	Usually hospital procedure Cervical dilation under general anesthesia Scraping of the endometrium with a sharp curet	Possible uterine perforation or cervical tears Occasional retained tissue with hemorrhage or infection
Dilation and evacuation (done 13–20 wk after last menses)	Usually hospital procedure Cervical dilation with laminaria or cervical dilators Uterus emptied under paracervical or general anesthesia with instruments to extract the fetal parts. Suction or sharp curettage concludes the procedure.	Possible uterine perforation or cervical tears Occasional hemorrhage or infection Very rarely retained tissue Perhaps cervical incompetence in subsequent pregnancies
Hypertonic saline infusion (done 16–24 wk after last menses)	Usually hospital procedure Solution instilled in amniotic sac through abdomen under local anesthesia Causes uterine contractions Occasionally need oxytocin for stimulation of labor Causes fetal death	May cause fluid and electrolyte imbalance, coagulopathy hypernatremia with associated CVA, atony, retained placenta with hemorrhage and infection Psychological effect of delivering a fully formed infant Contraindicated with liver or kidney problems, cardiac failure, hypertension.
Prostaglandin infusion (done 16–24 wk after last menses)	Hospital procedure Same technique as for saline May work faster than saline May not cause fetal death For hypertensive client, vaginal suppositories must be used instead of infusion (a different form of prostaglandin)	Causes nausea, vomiting, fever, diarrhea, hypertension May cause cervical perforation, uterine rupture, retained placenta with hemorrhage or infection, anaphylactic reaction Psychological effect of delivering a fully formed and possibly alive infant Contraindicated for client with history of convulsions, epilepsy, asthma, hypertension

Table 73-1 Termination Techniques *(continued)*

Abortion Method	Procedure	Disadvantages
Hysterotomy (done at 16–24 weeks after last menses)	Hospital procedure Fetus extracted through small abdominal incision under general anesthesia Rarely used at present	Major surgery with highest complication and mortality rate of all abortion methods May limit a woman to future cesarean section Psychological effect of delivering a formed and possibly alive infant

Table 73-2 Medical Referral/Consultation

Diagnosis	Clinical Manifestations	Management
Moderate to severe depression (Rosenthal, 1975)	Suicidal or infanticidal thoughts or gestures Depressed affect Serious attempts at self-abortion Severe self-depreciatory thoughts Obsessive rumination about the crisis Social withdrawal Inability to carry on daily activities Sleep disturbances Anorexia	Place client under constant supervision for protection Referral to professional counsellor for evaluation, medication, therapy, and possible hospitalization Referral to social service
Psychosis	Impairment of capacity to test reality Disturbance in mood, behavior, or thinking Deficits in perception, language, or memory	Referral to professional counsellor for evaluation, medication, therapy, and possible hospitalization Referral to social service
"Acting out" behavior	Truancy Running away Promiscuity Abuse of drugs or alcohol Recidivism	Referral for professional counselling Coordinate care with any social welfare agencies to which the client is known
Mental retardation or severe emotional immaturity	Deficit in mothering or child-rearing capacity Lack of socialization skills Poor judgment Poor impulse control Intellectual functions slowed	Referral for professional counselling Referral to social service
Any significant medical or obstetrical problems in the client	History of habitual spontaneous abortions Numerous previous induced abortions Hypertension or other serious medical conditions	Consult with obstetrician for plan of management or transfer care Referral to professional counsellor or social service personnel as need arises

bibliography

Boston Women's Health Book Collective. *Our bodies, ourselves* (2d ed.). New York: Simon and Schuster, 1976.

Bracken, Michael, Klerman, Lorraine, and Bracken, Maryann. Abortion, adoption or motherhood: an empirical study of decision-making during pregnancy. *American Journal of Obstetrics and Gynecology*, **130**:251–262 (1978).

Grimes, David, et al. Mid-trimester abortion by dilatation and evacuation. *The New England Journal of Medicine*, **296**:1141–1145 (1977).

Hatcher, Robert, et al. *Contraceptive technology 1978–1979* (9th ed.). New York: Irvington Publishers, 1978.

Palomaki, Jacob F. Abortion techniques: what are their risks and complications? *Contemporary Ob/Gyn*, **9**:73–77 (1977).

Rosenthal, Miriam, and Rothchild, Ellen. Some psychological considerations in adolescent pregnancy and abortion. *Advances in Planned Parenthood*, **9**:60–69 (1975).

section 7

the urinary system

INTRODUCTION JANE A. FOX

I. Subjective Data

A. Age and sex
B. Reason for visit and description of problem
C. Time of onset
D. History of trauma to abdomen, lower back, or urethra
E. Color of urine
F. Blood noted on underclothing
G. Associated symptoms
1. Polyuria
2. Strong odor to urine
3. Oliguria
4. Frequency
5. Hematuria
6. Urgency and/or incontinence
7. Nocturia
8. Dysuria
9. Lower abdominal pain
10. Back or flank pain
11. Fever or chills
12. Malaise
13. Joint pain
14. Anal itching
15. Urethral or vaginal discharge
16. Skin lesions or rashes
17. Conjunctivitis
18. Passing gravel in urine
19. Polydipsia

H. History of enuresis
I. Toilet training
1. Age began
2. Method used
3. Use of punishments or rewards
4. Household changes during toilet training
5. Age completely trained
6. Age bed-wetting began again

J. Past medical history
1. Previous urinary tract infection (UTI)—any urine testing done and results
2. Kidney disease—especially acute glomerulonephritis or kidney stones
3. With child, especially if mentally retarded, note history of putting foreign objects into body orifices

K. Hospitalizations
L. Injuries or illnesses—especially venereal disease; seizures, allergies, mental retardation, liver disease, blood dyscrasias, sickle cell anemia, congenital anomalies, diabetes
M. Patterns and habits—elimination, sleep, sexually active (contraception)
N. Diet history—change in usual diet
O. Developmental history
P. Social history—interpersonal relationships with
1. Parent(s)

2. Siblings
3. Schoolmates
4. Teachers

Q. School performance

R. Family history
1. Kidney disease
2. UTI
3. Pinworms
4. Varicella
5. Scabies
6. Anemia
7. Blood disease
8. Renal disease
9. Enuresis
10. Congenital anomalies
11. Juvenile diabetes

II. Objective Data

A. Physical examination
1. Complete physical examination for any child under 4 years of age or being seen for the first time
2. Older child
   a. Height, weight, head circumference
   b. Temperature, pulse, blood pressure
   c. General appearance and nutritional status
   d. Inspection of skin for jaundice, petechiae and ecchymoses, rashes, hematomas, edema (especially around eyes)
   e. Auscultation for heart murmurs
   f. Bimanual examination of both kidneys for enlargement
   g. Palpation of abdomen for abdominal masses, tenderness, or organomegaly
   h. Check for costovertebral angle (CVA) tenderness
   i. Inspection of external genitalia and, in males, palpation of prostate for tenderness and palpation of testes
   j. Palpation of lymph nodes
   k. Observation of joint mobility
   l. Neurological exam for mental status, abnormal movements, cranial nerves
   m. Observe client in act of voiding for
      (1) Quality of stream
      (2) Hesitancy or difficulty initiating stream
      (3) Dribbling
      (4) Straining
      (5) Active bleeding
      (6) Pain (observe facial expression)

B. Laboratory data: any of the following tests may be indicated
1. Ordered by practitioner
   a. Urinalysis
   b. Midstream urine for culture and sensitivity
   c. Complete blood count
   d. Tine test
   e. Blood urea, nitrogen, and creatinine
   f. Vaginal or urethral smear for gonorrhea
   g. Vaginal swab for *Monilia* or microscopic examination for *Trichomonas*
   h. Stool for ova and parasites
   i. Cellophane tape perianal impression
   j. VDRL
   k. 2-hr-postprandial blood sugar (if diabetes suspected)
   l. Residual urine testing
2. Ordered after physician consultation
   a. Intravenous pyelogram (IVP)
   b. Voiding cystourethrogram (VCUG)
   c. EEG with sleep tracing
   d. Blood culture
   e. Glucose tolerance test
   f. Toxicology blood levels (if nephrotoxic drug ingestion suspected)
   g. Bone marrow
   h. Partial thromboplastin time
   i. Factor VIII level

74 Blood in Urine

MARILYN GREBIN

ALERT
1. Gross hematuria
2. Flank pain
3. Blood at the urethral meatus

I. Etiology

A. Hematologic disorders
B. Infectious disorders
C. Metabolic disorders
D. Obstructive disorders
E. Traumatic disorders
F. Toxic disorders

II. Assessment

A. Urinary tract infection
1. Subjective data
   a. Higher incidence in females
   b. A child who was completely toilet trained now exhibits nocturia and enuresis
   c. Dysuria and/or frequency
   d. Urinary retention
   e. Hematuria
   f. Strong odor to urine
   g. Fever
2. Objective data
   a. Bladder distention—with history of retention
   b. Dysuria while observing urination
   c. Fever
   d. Urine culture greater than 100,000 colonies of one specific bacteria

B. Cystitis (viral)
1. Subjective data
   All the above symptoms except fever
2. Objective data
   a. Sudden onset of gross hematuria
   b. Sterile urine culture

C. Self-inflicted trauma
1. Subjective data
   a. Allergies precipitating scratching
   b. Skin rash
   c. Disturbed social situation causing anxiety
2. Objective data
   a. Evidence of bleeding at the meatus
   b. Scratch marks around genitalia
   c. Evidence of local infection

D. Ulceration of the urethra from diaper dermatitis and/or meatitis
1. Subjective data
   a. History of chronic diaper dermatitis
   b. Allergies to disposable diapers
   c. Use of strong detergents to clean cloth diapers
   d. Poor dietary intake including insufficient fluids
2. Objective data
   a. Severe diaper dermatitis
   b. Open weeping or bleeding ulcers around the meatus
   c. Poor parent-child relationship

III. Management

A. Urinary tract infection
1. Treatments/medications
   a. Gantrisin 150 mg/kg per day for 10 to 14 days *or*
   b. Ampicillin 100 to 200 mg/kg per day for 10 to 14 days *or*
   c. Bactrim 100 mg/kg per day for 10 to 14 days
2. Counselling/prevention
   a. Encourage compliance with prescribed medical regimen and follow-up.
   b. Discuss toilet habits and cleansing after bowel movements and urination to prevent

bacterial contamination of the urinary meatus.
   c. Advise the client to avoid bubble baths.
   d. Advise the client to avoid tight clothing such as bodysuits and nylon underpants.
3. Follow-up
   a. A urine culture follow-up should be done at 48–72 h after treatment is initiated, 3 months after treatment, at 6 months, and at 1 year.
   b. If the history suggests that this infection may not be the first an intravenous pyelogram (IVP) and voiding cystourethrogram (VCU) to determine structural anomaly should be done after the treatment is completed.
4. Consultations/referrals: urologist
   a. Treatment failure
   b. To evaluate IVP and VCU

B. Viral cystitis
1. Treatments/medications: none
2. Counselling/prevention: symptoms last for 4 days
3. Consultations/referrals: urologist (after obtaining urinalysis)

C. Self-inflicted trauma
1. Treatments/medications
   a. Local cleaning
   b. Keeping client's fingernails short and clean
2. Counselling/prevention
   a. Avoid snug underclothing.
   b. Observe the child's behavior.
   c. Increase parent-child activities.
3. Follow-up: return visit in 1 week
4. Consultations/referrals: none

D. Ulceration of the urethra from diaper dermatitis
1. Treatments/medications
   a. Soap and water cleansing at each diaper change
   b. Application of bacitracin ointment
2. Counselling/prevention
   a. Encourage proper food and fluid intake.
   b. Encourage the use of a fabric softener or fine detergents in the wash water of diapers and clothing.
3. Follow-up: 1 week to evaluate healing process and obtain urine culture
4. Consultations/referrals
   a. Urologist
   b. Public health nurse for home visit in severe cases

Table 74-1 Medical Referral/Consultation

Diagnosis	Clinical Manifestations	Management
Acute glomerulonephritis	Hematuria (smoky or dark appearance in urine) Oliguria Slight edema in the early stage Hypertension Positive laboratory data Proteinuria Azotemia Electrolyte imbalance	Referral to physician immediately after return of positive laboratory results
Renal tuberculosis	Rarely found in children Fever Emaciation Local pain, tenderness, and enlargement of the kidneys Frequency Dysuria Hematuria	Referral to physician
Renal calculi	More common in boys than girls Hematuria Colicky flank pain Repeated urinary tract infections	Referral to physician

Table 74-1 Medical Referral/Consultation *(continued)*

Diagnosis	Clinical Manifestations	Management
Renal trauma	Gross hematuria Colicky flank pain History of trauma	Referral to physician
Poisoning with nephrotoxic agents	Hematuria Hemaglobinuria History of ingestion of nephrotoxic agent	Referral to physician. See Poisoning, Chap. 170.
Trauma (urethral and bladder)	Failure to pass urine or dysuria History of injury of fractured pelvis Blood at the urethral meatus	Consult with the physician.
Sickle cell disease	See Anemia, Chap. 39.	Consult with the physician. See Anemia, Chap. 39.
Hemophilia (Factor VIII deficiency)	Excessive bruising or hematoma after minor injury Evidence of hemarthrosis or spontaneous hematuria	Consult with the physician. See Hemophilia, Chap. 143.

bibliography

Dodge, W., West, E. Smith, E. and Brunce, H. Proteinuria and hematuria in school children: Epidemiology and early natural history. *Journal of Pediatrics,* **88**(2):327–347 (1976).

Urinary tract infections. *The Medical Letter,* **20**(1):3 (1978).

Treatment of urinary tract infections. *The Medical Letter,* **19**(21):87 (1977).

West, Clark. Asymptomatic hematuria and proteinuria in children: Causes and appropriate diagnostic studies. *Journal of Pediatrics,* **89**(2):173–183 (1976).

75 Urine Color/Odor Changes

KATHLEEN M. BUCKLEY

ALERT
1. Severe pain
2. Frequent, recurrent urinary tract infections (UTI) (greater than three per year)
3. Hypertension—blood pressure greater than 140/90 mmHg
4. Protein in urine—greater than 1+ or 2+
5. Casts in the urine
6. Hematuria

I. Etiology

A. Discolored urine (see Table 75-1)

1. Colorless—urine of low concentration
   a. Excessive fluid intake
   b. Chronic glomerulonephritis
   c. Diabetes mellitus
   d. Diabetes insipidus
2. Cloudy white
   a. Phosphates in an alkaline urine (disappears with addition of acid)
   b. Epithelial cells from lower genitourinary tract
   c. Bacteria
   d. Pus
   e. Chyle
3. Dark color
   a. Concentration, as in fever
   b. Urobilin or bilirubin
4. Dark yellow
   a. Highly concentrated, normal urine
   b. Bile
   c. Carotene-containing foods
   d. Vitamin B complex
5. Red
   a. Beets, blackberries, aniline dyes from candy, rhodamine B in foodstuffs
   b. Blood as red cells or hemoglobin (See Hematuria, I, B, below)
   c. Favism
   d. Drugs—phenolphthalein
   e. Serratia marcescens
6. Red-brown
   a. Myoglobinuria
   b. Urates
   c. Porphyria
7. Green or blue
   a. Hypercalcemia
   b. Biliverdin (chronic obstructive jaundice)
8. Dark brown–black
   a. Alkaptonuria
   b. Tyrosinosis
   c. Melanosis
   d. Acid hematin (hemoglobin standing in acid urine)

B. Hematuria

1. Nonrenal bleeding
   a. UTI
   b. Renal calculi (rare)
   c. Foreign body in urethra or bladder
   d. Bladder tumors (rare)
   e. Congenital urinary tract anomalies
2. Extraglomerular renal bleeding
   a. Hydronephrosis
   b. Polycystic kidney disease
   c. Sickle cell trait
   d. Wilms' tumor
   e. Renal hemangioma
   f. Renal tuberculosis (rare)
   g. Acute pyelonephritis
   h. Trauma
3. Glomerular bleeding
   a. Glomerulonephritis (most common—acute poststreptococcal)

b. Hereditary nephropathy (Alport's syndrome)
c. Benign familial hematuria

C. Foul-smelling urine: UTI

II. Assessment—UTI

A. Subjective data
1. History of UTI
2. Flank or abdominal pain
3. Dysuria
4. Frequency (nocturia)
5. Urgency

B. Objective data
1. Fever and chills
2. Foul-smelling urine
3. Cloudy urine
4. Hematuria (usually gross)
5. Pyuria
6. Bacteriuria

III. Management—UTI

A. Treatments/medications
1. Sulfonamide
2. Ampicillin
3. Analgesic and antipyretic drug

B. Counselling/prevention
1. Teach client and family signs and symptoms of UTIs.
2. Encourage fluids.
3. Explain disease process and its therapy.

C. Follow-up—culture for UTI
1. 24 to 48 h after initiation of therapy
2. 1 week after completion of therapy
3. Every 3 months for 9 months
4. Every 6 months for 1 year

D. Consultations/referrals: refer frequent, recurrent UTIs to a urologist.

Table 75-1 Drugs that Color the Urine

Urine Color	Associated Drug or Chemical
Blue	Methylene blue
Brown–black	Aniline dyes
	Cascara
	Chlorinated hydrocarbons
	Hydroxyquinone
	Melanin
	Methocarbamol (Robaxin)
	Naphthalene
	Napthol
	Nitrites
	Phenol
	Phenyl salicylate (Salol)
	Pyrogallol
	Quinine
	Resorcinol (Resorcin)
	Rhubarb
	Santonin
	Senna
	Thymol
Green (blue + yellow)	Anthraquinone
	Arbutin
	Bile pigments
	Eosins
	Methocarbamol (Robaxin)

Table 75-1 Drugs that Color the Urine *(continued)*

Urine Color	Associated Drug or Chemical
	Methylene blue Resorcinol (Resorcin) Tetrahydronaphthalene Thymol
Magenta–purple	Fuchsin Phenolphthalein
Orange–orange-red	Phenazopyridine (Pyridium)
Orange–red-brown	Combinations of phenazopyridine (Pyridium) and other drugs used as urinary antiseptics Santonin
Pink and red–red-brown	Aminopyrine Anthraquinone and its dyes Antipyrine (Pyrazoline) Chrysarobin (alkaline urine) Cinchophen Danthron (Dorbane) (pink to violet—alkaline urine) Diphenylhydantoin (Dilantin) Emodin (alkaline urine) Eosins (red with green fluorescence) Hematuria producers (mercuric salts, irritants, etc.) Hemolysis producers Phenindione (Danilone, Hedulin, Indon) Phenolic metabolites (glucuronides) Phenolphthalein (alkaline urine) Phensuximide (Milontin) Porphyrins Santonin (alkaline urine) Thiazolsulfone (Promizole) Urates (especially newborn infants and during tumor lysis)
Rust	Chlorzoxazone (Paraflex)
Yellow or brownish	Danthrone (Dorbane) (acid urine) Heavy metals (bismuth, mercury) Liver poisons (jaundice) Alcohol Arsenicals Carbon tetrachloride Chloral hydrate Chlorinated hydrocarbon Chlorobutanol (chlorbutol, Chloretone) Chloroform Cinchophen

Table 75-1 Drugs that Color the Urine *(continued)*

Urine Color	Associated Drug or Chemical
	Naphthalene Neocinchophen Nitrofurantoins Pamaquine (Aminoquin, Béprochine, Gamefar, Plasmoquine, Praequine, Quipenyl) Sulfonamides Tribromomethanol with amylene hydrate (Avertin)
Yellow or green	Carotene-containing foods Methylene blue Riboflavin Vitamin B complex Yeast concentrate

Source: Shirkey, Harry C. Drugs that discolor the urine. In Shirkey, Harry C. (ed.), *Pediatric therapy* (5th ed.), St. Louis: Mosby, 1975.

Table 75-2 Medical Referral/Consultation

Diagnosis	Clinical Manifestations	Management
Acute glomerulonephritis	History of recent upper respiratory or skin infections (streptococcal) Evidence of nephrotic syndrome Impaired renal function Hypertension Urinalysis with red blood cells, white blood cells, and various casts Proteinuria (3+ or 4+)	Refer to the physician. See Preparation for Hospitalization, Part 7.
Traumatic hematuria	History of trauma to abdomen, lower back, or urethra Gross bright-red blood in urine with or without casts (may be microscopic hematuria) Abdominal or flank pain	Refer to the physician. Obtain intravenous pyelogram on client.
Foreign body in bladder or urethra	Extreme frequency Urgency Local pain	Refer to the physician. Obtain an abdominal x-ray. See Preparation for Hospitalization, Part 7.

bibliography

DeGowin, Elmer L., and DeGowin, Richard L. *Beside diagnostic examination* (3d ed.). New York: Macmillan, 1976.

Green, Morris, and Richmond, Julius B. *Pediatric diagnosis*. Philadelphia: Saunders, 1962.

Illingworth, R. S. *Common symptoms of diseases in children* (5th ed.). Oxford: Blackwell Scientific Publications, 1975.

Northway, James D. Hematuria in children. *Journal of Pediatrics*, **78**:381–396 (1971).

Rubin, Mitchell I., and Barratt, T. Martin (eds.). *Pediatric nephrology*. Baltimore: Williams & Wilkins, 1975.

Wasson, John, et al. *The common symptom guide*. New York: McGraw-Hill, 1975.

76 Pain and Burning during Urination

LESLIE LIETH

ALERT

1. Fever, vomiting, irritability, poor weight gain in infant
2. Recurrent urinary tract infections
3. Gross hematuria
4. Enuresis
5. Acute lower-abdominal pain
6. Triad of dysuria, joint pain, and burning, itching eyes
7. Foul-smelling vaginal discharge in young child
8. Decreased urinary stream
9. Straining to void

I. Etiology

A. Bacterial
B. Viral
C. Fungal
D. Parasitic
E. Mechanical

II. Assessment

A. Urinary tract infection
  1. Acute pyelonephritis
    a. Infants
      (1) Subjective data
        (a) Fever
        (b) Loss of appetite
        (c) Vomiting
        (d) Diarrhea or constipation
      (2) Objective data
        (a) Fever
        (b) Irritability
        (c) Jaundice
        (d) Anemia
        (e) Poor weight gain
        (f) Leukocyturia
        (g) Microscopic hematuria
        (h) Clean-catch midstream urine revealing greater than 100,000 colonies of an isolated organism
    b. All others
      (1) Subjective data
        (a) Fever, chills
        (b) Abdominal pain
        (c) Vomiting
        (d) Malaise
        (e) Dysuria
      (2) Objective data
        (a) Fever
        (b) Suprapubic, abdominal, or flank pain
        (c) CNS signs, i.e., meningism, stupor, delirium, or convulsion
        (d) See Infants, II., A., I., a. above
  2. Infections of the lower tract
    a. Subjective data
      (1) Fever
      (2) Dysuria
      (3) Burning on urination
      (4) Frequency
      (5) Urgency
      (6) Abdominal pain
      (7) Less frequently can have
        (a) Enuresis
        (b) Gross hematuria
        (c) Foul-smelling urine
    b. Objective data
      (1) Fever
      (2) Abdominal pain
      (3) Gross hematuria
      (4) Foul-smelling urine
      (5) See Acute pyelonephritis, II, A, 1 above

B. Hemorrhagic cystitis

1. Subjective data
   a. Fever, chills
   b. Acute lower-abdominal pain
   c. Dysuria
   d. Frequency
   e. Gross hematuria
2. Objective data
   a. Fever
   b. Suprapubic tenderness
   c. Gross hematuria
   d. Anemia

C. Urethritis

1. Subjective data
   a. Dysuria
   b. Frequency
   c. Urethral discharge
   d. Foul-smelling urine
2. Objective data
   a. Inflammation of the distal two-thirds of the urethra
   b. Leukocyturia
   c. Urethral discharge
   d. Foul-smelling urine
   e. Fever (rare)
   f. Can have negative urine culture or positive culture with greater than 100,000 colonies of an isolated organism
   g. Microscopic hematuria and proteinuria

D. Reiter's syndrome

1. Subjective data
   a. Usually history of sexual activity
   b. Dysuria
   c. Joint pain
   d. Eye discharge
   e. Reddened, burning, itching eyes
   f. May have urethral discharge
2. Objective data
   a. Most frequently found in young men
   b. Warm, erythematous, tender joints (usually two or more joints involved)
   c. Urethral meatus perhaps edematous and reddened
   d. May have urethral discharge
   e. Conjunctivitis
   f. Mucotaneous lesions—anywhere on the body, usually in genital area, palms and soles, and mouth
   g. Proteinuria
   h. Microscopic hematuria
   i. Negative eye, urine cultures
   j. Elevated erythrocyte sedimentation rate (ESR)
   k. Mild leukocytosis

E. Prostatitis

1. Subjective data
   a. Low-back pain
   b. Perineal or testicular discomfort
   c. Fever, chills
   d. Dysuria
2. Objective data
   a. Low-back pain
   b. Perineal or testicular discomfort
   c. A tense, extremely tender prostate on examination
   d. Fever
   e. Microscopic pyuria, hematuria

F. Balanitis and balanoposthitis

1. Subjective data
   a. Usually found in circumsized males
   b. Dysuria
2. Objective data
   a. Inflammation of glans (balanitis), or
   b. Inflammation of glans with inflammation of the prepuce (pothitis)
   c. Microscopic hematuria

G. Vaginitis/vulvovaginitis (see Vaginal Discharge, Chap. 66)

1. Monilial vaginitis
   a. Subjective data
      (1) Local pain
      (2) Itch
      (3) Possibly dysuria
      (4) White cheesy discharge
   b. Objective data
      (1) Inflammation of vulva
      (2) White cheesy discharge
      (3) Vaginal swab positive nickerson's media
2. Trichomonas vaginitis
   a. Subjective data
      (1) See II, G, 1, a above
      (2) Yellow-green, frothy discharge with a fetid odor
   b. Objective data
      (1) Inflammation of vulva
      (2) Yellow-green, frothy discharge with a fetid odor
      (3) Observation of trophozoites in vaginal secretions under microscope
3. Hemophilus vaginalis
   a. Subjective data
      (1) See II, G, 1, a above
      (2) Milky, viscid discharge
   b. Objective data
      (1) Inflammation of vulva
      (2) Milky, viscid discharge
4. Gonorrhea (see Venereal Disease, Chap. 70)
   a. Subjective data
      (1) See II, G, 1, a above

(2) Frequency
(3) Urgency
(4) Foul-smelling, purulent discharge
(5) Can have history of contact with infected person

b. Objective data
(1) Purulent vaginal discharge
(2) Vaginitis
(3) Cervicitis
(4) Inflammation of vulva
(5) Positive culture for Neisseria gonorrhoeae

5. Pinworms (See Pinworms, Chap. 53)
a. Subjective data
(1) Perianal itching
(2) See II, G, 1, a above

b. Objective data
(1) Vulvovaginitis
(2) Stool specimen showing presence of *enterobius vermicularis,* or positive cellophane tape test

6. Scabies (see Scabies, Chap. 101)
a. Subjective data
(1) Complaint of lesions on body, as described in objective findings
(2) See II, G, 1, a above

b. Objective data
(1) Inflammation of vulva
(2) For description of lesions, see Scabies, Chap. 101

H. Vaginal foreign body (see Vagina: Foreign Body, Chap. 59)

1. Subjective data
a. Foul-smelling discharge
b. Burning on urination
c. History of child putting objects into body orifices

2. Objective data
a. Foul-smelling discharge
b. Presence of foreign body
c. Vulvovaginitis

I. Meatal ulcer/meatal stenosis

1. Ulcer
a. Subjective data
(1) Dysuria
(2) Inflammation and ulceration of meatus

b. Objective data
(1) Inflammation and ulceration of meatus
(2) Can have microscopic hematuria

2. Repeated inflammation possibly leading to meatal stenosis
a. Subjective data
(1) Decreased urinary stream
(2) Dysuria
(3) Frequency
(4) Straining to void

b. Objective data
(1) Decreased urinary stream
(2) Straining to void
(3) Dribbling

III. Management

A. Asymptomatic bacteriuria

1. Treatments/medications
a. Treatment of first episode (by history) can be by primary care practitioner according to medical protocol
b. Antibiotic therapy, per sensitivity results of urine culture, for 14 days
c. Increase in fluid intake
d. Bed rest
e. Intravenous pyelogram (IVP) and voiding cystourethrogram (VCU) to rule out structural abnormalities; to be scheduled after acute episode is resolved

2. Counselling/prevention
a. Alert the client to the signs and symptoms of urinary tract problems, i.e., nocturia, frequency, flank pain, dysuria, suprapubic pain, etc.
b. For females: reinforce the importance of good feminine hygiene.
c. Recommend voiding after sexual intercourse.
d. Stress compliance with the treatment regimen.

3. Follow-up
a. Repeat urine culture 48 to 72 h after starting treatment.
b. Repeat urine culture 1 week after stopping treatment, and at 3, 6, 9, 15, and 36 months after treatment.

4. Consultations/referrals
Refer to the physician if there are any complications (hypertension, subsequent infections, abnormal IVP or VCU, etc.).

B. Symptomatic bacteriuria

1. Treatments/medications
a. Antibiotic therapy started immediately before results of urine culture (ampicillin or cephalexin)
b. Change in antibiotic therapy per sensitivity results if necessary
c. Antibiotic therapy for longer period, usually for 6 to 8 weeks
d. IVP and VCU (see III., A., 1., e. above)
e. Bed rest
f. Increase in fluid intake

2. Counselling/prevention: see III, A, 2 above
3. Follow-up: see III, A, 3 above
4. Consultations/referrals
   a. Consult with or refer to physician for treatment.
   b. Client may have to be hospitalized.

C. Urethritis: see III, A, 1 through 4 above

D. Hemorrhagic cystitis

1. Treatments/medications
   a. Bed rest
   b. Increase in fluid intake
   c. Pain helped with analgesics, and hot or cold compresses over bladder area
   d. If bacterial (positive urine culture), see III, A, 1 above
2. Counselling/prevention: see III, A, 2 above
3. Follow-up
   a. If bacterial, see, III, A, 3 above
   b. If two negative urine cultures, follow-up visits every 4 to 7 days until resolved
4. Consultations/referrals: refer to or consult with a physician for treatment.

E. Reiter's syndrome

1. Treatments/medications: salicylate therapy
2. Counselling/prevention: for salicylate therapy
   a. Advise client of signs and symptoms of salicylate poisoning.
   b. Aspirin should be taken with milk to avoid gastric upset.
3. Follow-up
   The frequency of the visits depends on the client's response to therapy and the severity of the symptoms.
4. Consultations/referrals: refer to the physician for treatment

F. Prostatitis

1. Treatments/medications
   a. Without documented bacteriuria, treatment is symptomatic, including prostatic massage and warm sitz baths
   b. With documented bacteriuria, appropriate antibiotic therapy, see III, A, 1 above
   c. If positive gonorrheal culture, see III, G, 1 below and Venereal Disease, Chap. 70
2. Counselling/prevention
   a. Reinforce and explain treatments: sitz baths, etc.
   b. See III, G, 2 if gonorrhea.
3. Follow-up: weekly visits until resolved
4. Consultations/referrals: refer to a physician if complications arise or if treatment is unsuccessful.

G. Gonorrhea (see Venereal Disease, Chap. 70)

1. Treatments/medications
   a. Aqueous procaine penicillin G, 4.8 million units divided into at least two injections given at different sites at one visit, intramuscularly, together with 1 g oral probenecid, 30 min prior to the injections
   b. Alternate regimen: ampicillin 3.5 g given as a single oral dose with 1 g oral probenecid simultaneously
   c. Serologic test for syphilis at the time of diagnosis
2. Counselling/prevention
   a. Thorough explanation of disease and treatment
   b. Sex education and counselling as needed
   c. Case contact finding
3. Follow-up
   a. Cervical or urethral smears should be obtained 7 and 14 days after treatment.
   b. At-risk clients should have tests for syphilis and gonorrhea every 6 months.
4. Consultations/referrals: report to the local health department.

H. Balantitis/balanoposthitis

1. Treatments/medications
   a. Possibility of foreign body in urethra should be ruled out
   b. Adequate hygienic measures: retracting foreskin, sitz baths at least 2 or 3 times per day
   c. Application of local antibiotic ointment (bacitracin, etc.)
   d. Systemic broad-spectrum antibiotics for secondary infection or to prevent same
   e. Can apply cold compresses for comfort
2. Counselling/prevention
   a. Explain good hygienic measures.
   b. Explain medications and side effects, if any.
3. Follow-up: weekly appointments until resolved
4. Consultations/referrals
   a. If recurrent, refer to a surgeon for circumcision.
   b. If infected, refer to or consult with a physician.

I. Meatal ulcer or stenosis

1. Treatments/medications
   a. Exposure to air
   b. Local antibiotic ointment
2. Counselling/prevention
   a. Proper cleansing with soap and water
   b. Avoidance of rubber pants
3. Follow-up: appointment in 1 or 2 weeks

4. Consultations/referrals: if stenosis, refer to physician for urethral meatotomy.

J. Vaginal foreign body (see Vagina: Foreign Body, Chap. 59)

K. Vulvovaginitis/vaginitis (see Vaginal Discharge, Chap. 66)

1. Nonspecific vaginitis or vulvovaginitis
   a. Treatments/medications
      (1) Local cleansing with mild soap and an abundance of water
      (2) If not responding to this treatment, can use topical estrogen cream to the vagina, at night for 2 weeks, then every 3 to 4 days for 6 weeks
   b. Counselling/prevention
      (1) Advise wearing cotton underpants
      (2) No douching with any of the treatments
      (3) No bubble baths; showers preferred
   c. Follow-up: appointments weekly until resolved
   d. Consultations/referrals: consultation with or referral to physician if not responding to treatment
2. Monilial vaginitis
   a. Treatments/medications
      (1) Nystatin suppositories (one-half or one) morning and night or once at bedtime for 2 weeks
      (2) Local cleansing with mild soap and an abundance of water
   b. Counselling/prevention: see III, K, 1, b above
   c. Follow-up: appointment 2 weeks after starting treatment
   d. Consultations/referrals: consultation with physician if not responding to treatment
3. Trichomonas vaginitis
   a. Treatments/medications
      (1) Flagyl 250 mg, one tablet once or twice daily for 5 days (dose depending on age)
      (2) Partner to be treated at same time
      (3) Local cleansing with soap and water
   b. Counselling/prevention: see III, K, 1, b above
   c. Follow-up: weekly appointment until resolved
   d. Consultations/referrals: consultation with physician if not responding to treatment
4. Hemophilus vaginalis
   a. Treatments/medications
      (1) Ampicillin, orally for 5 days (see Oral Medications, Appendix 2 for common dosages)
      (2) Local cleansing with soap and water
   b. Counselling/prevention: see III, K, 1, b above
   c. Follow-up: weekly appointments until resolved
   d. Consultations/referrals: consultation with a physician if not responding to treatment
5. Gonorrhea: see III, G above
6. Pinworms (see Pinworms, Chap. 53)
   a. Treatments/medications
      (1) Pyrvinium pamoate (Povan), 5 mg/kg, orally in single dose, *or*
      (2) Piperazine citrate (Antepar), 65 mg/kg, orally, daily, in mornings, for 7 to 10 days, *or*
      (3) Thiabendazole, 25 mg/kg, orally, twice daily, for 2 days
      (4) Re-treat with medication (especially single-dose treatment) 1 to 2 weeks later
      (5) All infected persons in household to be treated at same time
      (6) If recurrent infection, can treat all members of household (whether documented as infected or not); treatment of all persons at same time
      (7) For perianal irritation or vulvovaginitis, can use soothing ointment, such as A and D Ointment, applied to perineum
   b. Counselling/prevention
      (1) Meticulous hygiene: to include careful cleansing of perineum, hands, and the nails at least 3 times a day to reduce transmission
      (2) Daily changing of underclothes, night clothing, and bed linen
      (3) Importance of proper group treatment and follow-up visits to ensure eradication of infection
      (4) Stools, vomitus, and underclothes stained bright red in clients taking Povan
   c. Follow-up
      (1) Appointment 1 week after treatment
      (2) All infected persons having at least three negative early-morning cellophane tape tests for pinworm
   d. Consultations/referrals
      (1) Consult with physician or medical protocol for treatment.
      (2) Advise visiting nurse or public health nurse of recurrent infection; they may supervise group treatment.
7. Scabies (see Scabies, Chap. 101)

bibliography

Gellis, Sydney, and Kagin, Benjamin M. *Current pediatric therapy 8.* Philadelphia: Saunders, 1978.

James, John. *Renal disease in childhood.* St. Louis: Mosby, 1976.

Kelolis, P. P., King, L. R., and Belman, A. B. *Clinical pediatric urology.* Philadelphia: Saunders, 1976.

Kunn, C. M. New development in the diagnosis of urinary tract infections. *Journal of Urology,* **113**:585–594 (1975).

Pearson, Linda B. Urinary tract infections. *The Nurse Practitioner,* **3**:33–38 (1978).

Rapkin, Richard H. Urinary tract infections in childhood. *Pediatrics,* **60**:508–511 (1977).

Stapleton, F. Bruder, and Linshaw, Michael A. Urinary tract infections in children: Diagnosis and mangement. *Issues in Comprehensive Pediatric Nursing,* **2**:1–10 (1978).

Winterborn, M. H. The management of urinary infections in children. *British Journal of Hospital Medicine,* **17**:453–461 (1977).

77 Bed-wetting MARILYN GREBIN

ALERT

1. Hyperglycemia
2. Abnormal intravenous pyelogram (IVP) findings
3. Lower spinal cord defect
4. Polyuria
5. Abnormal EEG

I. Etiology

A. Psychological (emotional disturbances)

B. Toilet training

1. Primary enuresis
   a. Toilet trained too early
   b. Incomplete toilet training
2. Secondary
   Enuresis beyond age 5 years

C. Physical disorders (see Table 77–1)

II. Assessment—Primary and Secondary Enuresis (in the absence of structural anomalies)

A. Subjective data

1. Toilet training
   a. Too early
   b. Incomplete
   c. Completed but the child began to wet after age 5 years
2. Parent/sibling/child relationship abnormal
3. Recent psychological trauma within the family
   a. Death
   b. Divorce
   c. Poor school performance
   d. Recent hospitalization
   e. Sleep disturbances

B. Objective data

1. Physical examination normal
2. Absence of positive laboratory data

III. Management—Primary and Secondary Enuresis (in the absence of structural anomalies)

A. Treatments/medications

1. Bladder exercises: Encourage the child to hold urine in the bladder for as long as possible during the day.
2. Record intake and output for 1 week.
3. The physician may prescribe Tofranil[1] under 12 years 25 mg at bedtime; over 12 years 50 mg at bedtime.
4. Restrict fluids 3 to 4 h before bedtime.
5. Void before going to bed.
6. Awaken 3 h after sleep to void.
7. Have the child care for his or her own wet clothing and bed linen.

B. Counselling/prevention

1. Allow the child to visit alone with the health care practitioner or psychologist to discuss anxiety-producing situations.
2. Discuss the psychological basis for this problem with the parent(s).
   a. Allow them to vent any problems.
   b. Educate them in dealing with the child.
3. Parent(s) and siblings should not ridicule or be punitive.
4. Discuss and explain treatment regimen with the child and the parent(s).

C. Follow-up

1. Visit with the parent(s) bimonthly.

[1]The physician must determine the need for medication after all other methods have been tried.

2. Visit with the child either weekly or biweekly, depending upon the magnitude of the problems within the family.

D. Consultations/referrals

1. The physician will prescribe any medications.
2. Recommend professional counselling if psychological problems exist.

Table 77-1 Medical Referral/Consultation

Diagnosis	Clinical Manifestations	Management
Spina bifida occulta	Loss of urinary sphincter control during day and night Weakness or paralysis of lower extremities Neurosensory changes	Refer to a neurologist.
Meningomyelocele	Loss of urinary and anal sphincter control during the day and night Flaccid paralysis of the lower extremities Enlarged sac on the lower back Transillumination of the sac	Refer to a neurologist.
Ectopic ureteral insertion Urethral stricture Urethral stenosis	Findings of IVP	Refer to a urologist.
Epispadias Hypospadias	Intermittent loss of urinary control Abnormal urinary stream Urethral opening abnormally placed	Refer to a urologist.
Diabetes mellitus	Polyuria Polydipsia Polyphagia Weight loss Vomiting Enuresis Possible dehydration Urinalysis positive for glucose Elevated postprandial blood sugar	Refer to a physician. See Juvenile Diabetes, Chap. 147.
Diabetes insipidus	Polyuria 300–400 mL/kg per day Enuresis Polydipsia Sleep disturbance Fatigue Infants—excessive irritability Urine specific gravity 1.001–1.005	Refer to a pediatrician. See Juvenile Diabetes, Chap. 147.
Urinary tract infection	Young children Fever Abdominal pain Thirst Dysuria Enuresis	See Pain and Burning during Urination, Chap. 76.

Table 77-1 Medical Referral/Consultation *(continued)*

Diagnosis	Clinical Manifestations	Management
	Older children Fever Dysuria Frequency Enuresis Flank or abdominal pain	
	Urine culture (done on urine with specific gravity of 1.005) > 100,000 colonies of one specific bacteria	
Nocturnal epilepsy	Seizure activity recorded on the EEG during sleep Enuresis	Refer to a neurologist

bibliography

Christophersen, Edward R., and Rapoff, Michael A. Enuresis treatment. *Issues in Comprehensive Pediatric Nursing,* **2**:34–52 (March-April 1978).

De Angelis, Catherine. *Pediatric primary care* (2d ed.). Boston: Little, Brown, 1979.

Impramine for enuresis. *The Medical Letter,* **16**(5), (1974).

Kennell, Carol. Outpatient management of the juvenile diabetic. *Pediatric Nursing,* **2**(6):19–23 (1976).

Simonds, John F. Enuresis. *Clinical Pediatrics,* **16**(1): 79–82 (1977).

section 8

the neuropsychiatric system

INTRODUCTION JANE A. FOX

I. Subjective Data

A. Age and sex

B. Reason for visit

C. Description of problem

1. First symptom
2. Exact date and time of onset of first symptom and date of onset of additional symptoms
3. Description of onset—sudden or gradual
4. Has condition improved, worsened, or remained unchanged
5. Precipitating and/or alleviating factors
6. Previous diagnosis and treatment
7. Current medications

D. Date client was last completely well

E. Associated symptoms

1. Headache
2. Convulsions
3. Loss of consciousness
4. Anxiety
5. Nervousness
6. Hyperactivity
7. Appetite changes
8. Sleep changes
9. Vision changes
10. Delayed growth and development
11. Poor school performance
12. Vertigo
13. Mood changes
14. Personality changes
15. Speech difficulty or changes
16. Clumsiness
17. Ataxia
18. Weakness
19. Tremors
20. Tics
21. Paresthesia
22. Hallucinations
23. Memory changes and/or loss
24. Depression

F. Past/present medical history

1. Illness
2. Seizures, "spells," "fits"
   a. Date of first attack
   b. Description of seizure
      (1) Events preceding attack
      (2) Detailed description of attack—incontinence, loss of consciousness, etc.
      (3) Description of behavior following attack
   c. Frequency of attacks
   d. Date of last attack
   e. Past/current treatments, medications
3. Injuries/accidents (especially head injury)
   a. Loss of consciousness—length of time
   b. Seizures
   c. Bleeding from mouth, nose, eyes, ears
   d. Loss of memory
   e. Confusion
   f. Personality changes
   g. Headache
   h. Dizziness
   i. Incontinence—bowel and/or bladder
4. Psychiatric disorders

5. Hospitalizations
6. Chronic diseases
7. Previous record of head circumference, height, and weight
8. Last vision and hearing test—results

G. Prenatal history

H. Birth history
1. Type of delivery
2. Was mother awake?
3. Apgar score
4. Gestational age
5. Birth weight
6. Difficulties with infant
   a. Breathing
   b. Color
   c. Muscle tone

I. Neonatal history
1. Length of hospitalization
   a. Mother
   b. Infant
2. Feeding method—problems
3. Illnesses

J. Developmental history
1. Developmental milestones—dates achieved
2. Personality development
3. School progress

K. Immunization history

L. Diet history

M. Family history
1. Epilepsy/seizures ("spells")
2. Headaches
3. Neurological diseases
4. Psychiatric disorders
5. Congenital anomalies
6. Chronic disorders
7. School problems/failure
8. Genetic disorders
9. Mental retardation
10. Family members institutionalized

N. Social history
1. Living conditions
2. Relationships with family members, friends, significant others
3. School attending
   a. Satisfaction/dissatisfaction
   b. Performance
   c. Educational level
4. Employment status—satisfaction with current job
5. Economic status
6. Hobbies
7. Exercise
8. Recent changes in living conditions, school, job
9. Stresses in family/personal life—death, loss, financial
10. Habits
   a. Tobacco
   b. Drugs
   c. Alcohol

II. Objective Data

A. Physical examination
1. Complete physical examination (see Health History and Physical Examination, Chap. 7)
2. Height, weight, head circumference
3. Vital signs
4. General appearance and behavior (dress, posture, eye contact, voice quality, etc.)
5. Carefully inspect for any signs of physical abuse (self-inflicted or other)
6. Neurological examination
   a. In all clients six years of age and under a Denver Developmental Screening Test (see Appendix 5) should be done and can be used to evaluate many of the areas below.
   b. Evaluate cerebral function
      (1) General behavior
      (2) Level of consciousness (alert, lethargic, drowsy, irritable, stuporous)
      (3) Orientation (name, date, place, time) (difficult to determine in infant and young child; note response to mother's face)
      (4) Memory—recent, remote
      (5) Emotional status/mood
      (6) Attention span
      (7) Intellectual capacity—testing depends on client's age and may include
         (a) Repeating groups of numbers
         (b) Adding or subtracting two digits
         (c) Understanding and communicating effectively
         (d) Ability to repeat phrases verbatim
         (e) Comprehending and carrying out verbal commands
         (f) Reading ability and comprehension
         (g) Ability to draw, write, and copy shapes
            1. At 3 to 4 years can copy cross
            2. At 4 to 5 years can copy square
            3. At 5 to 6 years can copy triangle
            4. At 6 to 7 years can copy diamond
      (8) Ability to recognize familiar sounds with eyes closed
      (9) Visual recognition of familiar objects
   c. Test cranial nerve function (see Table 1)
   d. Test cerebellar function
      (1) Observe fine motor skills—undressing,

dressing, putting raisin in bottle, drawing, unbuttoning clothes, playing with and ability to manipulate toys

(2) After 5 years of age—test rapid alternating movements, i.e. finger to nose with eyes opened and closed; touch fingers to thumb in quick succession; pat knees with palm of hand and then with back of hand

(3) Balance and gait
  (a) Walks with eyes open, then closed
  (b) Tandem walk—heel to toe
  (c) Romberg test
    1. Client stands erect with feet together
    2. Client walks first with eyes opened, then with eyes closed
    3. Only minimal swaying should be observed
  (d) Stand on one foot
    1. 4-year-old—5 s with arms extended
    2. 6-year-old—5 s with arms closed
    3. 7-year-old—5 s with eyes closed
  (e) Hops in place on each foot

e. Test motor system
  (1) With client at rest, inspect and palpate muscles for size and consistency. If a discrepancy in muscle size is suspected, use tape measure and measure corresponding muscles at same position on both limbs.
  (2) Muscle tone
    (a) Passive range of motion
    (b) Active range of motion
  (3) Muscle strength
  (4) Inspect for abnormal muscle movements

f. Test sensory system
  (1) Limited benefit in children under 5 years of age
  (2) With client's eyes closed, determine his or her perception of sensation being tested. Compare both sides of body and corresponding extremities.
  (3) Primary forms of sensation
    (a) Superficial tactile sensation: stroke corresponding body parts with cotton; note response.
    (b) Pain—response to light pinprick
    (c) Temperature—response as various body parts are touched with test tubes of hot and cold water
    (d) Vibration—ability to feel when vibration stops as bony prominences are touched with vibrating tuning fork
    (e) Deep pain (usually not done) sensitivity as Achilles tendon and calf and forearm muscles are squeezed
    (f) Motion and position—ability to state direction as fingers and toes are moved
  (4) Cortical and discriminatory forms of sensation
    (a) Two point discrimination—ability to determine if being touched on one or two points as various body parts are touched simultaneously with sharp object
    (b) Point localization—ability to point to spot just touched, only one spot is touched
    (c) Stereognosis—ability to identify familiar objects (key, coin, comb) placed in hand
    (d) Graphesthesia—ability to identify numbers and letters drawn on palm of hand

g. Test reflex function
  (1) Deep tendon reflexes (see Table 2)
  (2) Superficial reflexes (see Table 2)
  (3) Infant reflexes (see Table 3)

h. Determine handedness

i. Meningeal signs
  (1) Stiff neck
  (2) Kernig's sign
  (3) Brudzinski's sign

j. Evaluate for "soft" neurological signs (see Table 4)

B. Laboratory data

1. CBC
2. Urinalysis
3. Vision testing
4. Audiometric studies
5. Electroencephalogram (EEG)
6. Skull x-rays
7. Lumbar puncture (ordered by physician)
8. Psychological testing

Table 1 Cranial Nerves

Number and Name		Function	Test
I	Olfactory	Smell	Client, with eyes closed, identifies familiar odors (peanut butter, oranges, alcohol) bilaterally
II	Optic	Vision	Visual activity (test with and without glasses) Visual fields Opthalmoscopic examination
III	Oculomotor	Eye movement: upward, downward, elevation of eyelids Pupillary constriction	Extraocular movements Ptosis Pupillary reactions Nystagmus } Cranial nerves III, IV, VI are tested together
IV	Trochlear	Eye movement: downward, medial	
V	Trigeminal	Motor—masseter and temporal muscles, lateral jaw movement Sensory—face, anterior half of scalp	Facial (forehead, cheeks, jaw) sensation to light touch, pain, temperature Clench jaw—palpate masseter and temporal muscles for strength of muscle contraction Corneal reflex bilateral
VI	Abducens	Eye movement: lateral	
VII	Facial	Motor—facial expressions, secretion of saliva Taste—anterior two-thirds of tongue	Is able to raise eyebrows, frown, smile, wrinkle forehead, puff out cheeks Closes eyes tightly, cannot be opened by examiner Identifies salt and sugar placed on both sides of anterior surface of tongue
VIII	Acoustic	Hearing and balance	Audiometry Weber test Rinne test
IX	Glossopharyngeal	Motor—pharynx Sensory—posterior one-third of tongue and pharynx	Client drinks—observe swallowing Gag reflex Movement of uvula when either side stroked with tongue blade Ability to speak clearly without hoarseness } Cranial nerves IX, X are tested together
X	Vagus	Sensory—external auditory meatus, pharynx, heart, lungs, abdomen Motor—soft palate, pharynx, larynx	
XI	Spinal accessory	Innervates sternocleidomastoid and trapezius muscles	Client shrugs shoulders—trapezius muscle strength symmetrical Strength of sternocleidomastoid muscle—resists attempts to turn head in opposite direction
XII	Hypoglossal	Innervates tongue muscles	Client sticks out tongue—note asymmetry, deviations, tremors, fasciculations Client presses tongue against tongue blade—note tongue strength

Table 2 Deep and Superficial Reflexes

Reflexes: Deep	Reflexes: Superficial	Stimulus	Normal Results	Involved Segment
Biceps muscle	—	Tap biceps tendon.	Forearm flexes at elbow.	C5–C6
Forearm pronator muscles	—	Tap palmar side of forearm medial to styloid process of radius.	Forearm pronates.	C6
Triceps muscle	—	Tap triceps tendon.	Forearm extends at elbow.	C6–C7
Brachioradial muscle	—	While holding forearm in semipronated position, tap styloid process.	Forearm flexes at elbow.	C7–C8
Finger (flexion)	—	Tap palm at tip of fingers.	Fingers flex.	C7–T1
Abdominal muscles	—	Tap inferior thorax, abdominal wall, and symphysis pubis.	Abdominal wall contracts; leg adducts when symphysis pubis is tapped.	T8–T12
—	Abdominal muscles	Stroke upper, middle, and lower skin on abdomen.	Abdominal muscles contract with retraction of umbilicus toward stimulated side.	T8–T12
—	Cremasteric muscle	Stroke medial upper leg in adductor region.	Testicles move up.	L1–L2
Adductor muscle	—	Tap medial condyle of tibia.	Leg adducts.	L2–L4
Quadriceps muscle (knee jerk)	—	Tap tendon of quadriceps femoris muscle.	Lower leg extends.	L2–L4
Triceps sural muscle (ankle jerk)	—	Tap Achilles tendon.	Plantar flexion of foot occurs.	L5–S2
—	Plantar area	Stroke lateral side on sole of foot.	Plantar flexion of toes occurs.	S1–S2

Source: From Conway, B. L. *Pediatric neurological nursing.* St. Louis: Mosby, 1977, p. 139.

Table 3 Common Infant Reflexes*

Reflex	How to Elicit	Infant's Response	Clinical Significance	Remarks
Acoustic blink (blinking in response to sound)	Clap hands loudly, approximately 30 cm from infant's head.	By 3 days old infant can blink both eyes.	If no response, repeat in 2–3 days; if no response again, there may be a hearing deficit.	Do not repeat more than 3 times.

*All infants and children with abnormal responses or reflexes present beyond the expected age should be evaluated by a physician.

Table 3 Common Infant Reflexes* *(continued)*

Reflex	How to Elicit	Infant's Response	Clinical Significance	Remarks
Ankle clonus	Press thumbs sharply against infant's feet; quickly release and observe for clonus.	Dorsiflexion of foot Minor clonus normal	More than 10 beats in infant less than 3 mo old or more than 3 beats in infant more than 3 mo old may indicate upper motor neuron damage.	Refer to physician if ankle clonus is noted.
Babinski	Using a blunt object, stroke lateral sole of infant's foot from heel across to below the toes.	Fanning of toes, especially great toe. When child begins to walk, normal response: toes curve downward toward stimulus.	Positive response in child of more than 2 years old may indicate upper motor neuron lesion.	Refer to physician if there is a positive response in child over 2 years old.
Bauer's (spontaneous crawling)	With infant in prone position, gently press soles of infant's feet.	Infant should attempt to make crawling movements forward.	Response is absent in a weak or depressed infant.	Response is difficult to elicit during first 3 days of life.
Galant's	Gently scratch with finger along sides of infant's spinal column approximately 3 cm from midline from shoulder to buttocks.	Infant curves trunk to side scratched.	If there is a spinal cord lesion, there is a lack of response below level of lesion.	Best response is obtained at 5–6 days of age. It disappears by 2 mo.
Glabella	Briskly tap bridge of the infant's nose (glabella).	Infant closes eyes tightly.	Asymmetry may indicate paralysis.	
Landau	Support the infant's abdomen with your hand and place other hand on infant's back. Infant's head and legs should extend on either side of your hand.	Infant should lift head and extend spine and legs.	Response can be elicited between 3–18 mo of age. Lack of or poor response may indicate cerebral palsy.	

*All infants and children with abnormal responses or reflexes present beyond the expected age should be evaluated by a physician.

Table 3 Common Infant Reflexes* *(continued)*

Reflex	How to Elicit	Infant's Response	Clinical Significance	Remarks
Magnet	Exert light pressure on soles of infant's feet.	Infant extends legs toward pressure.	Absence of response may indicate lower spinal cord damage. Weak response may indicate breech delivery or sciatic nerve damage.	There may be difficulty eliciting response during first 2 days of infant's life.
Moro (startle response)	With infant in supine position, support infant's trunk with one of your hands and the head and neck with your other hand. With infant's head in midline position and neck muscles relaxed, lightly drop the head backwards a few centimeters.	Abduction of arms and shoulders. Extension of arm at elbow. Extension of fingers; thumb and index finger form a C Later, arm abducts at shoulder.	Response is present at birth and disappears at about 3 mo. Asymmetry may indicate fractured clavicle or paralysis. Presence beyond 6 mo indicates neurological disease.	Elicit response 3 or 4 times to obtain all responses.
Neck righting	With infant supine, turn infant's head to one side.	Infant's body turns in same direction as head.	Response present between 3 mo and 2–3 years of age. Absence indicates spasticity, e.g., cerebral palsy.	
Optical blink	Suddenly shine bright light in infant's open eyes.	Infant closes both eyes quickly.	Lack of response may indicate blindness or poor or no light perception.	Response usually disappears by 1 year of age.
Palmer grasp	Infant supine with head midline, press your fingers into infant's palms from ulnar side; do not touch dorsal side.	Infant's hands grasp examiner's fingers; grasp should be strong and symmetrical.	Response suggests cerebral dysfunction if it persists beyond 4 mo of age.	If response is asymmetrical, check head position. If response is weak, get infant to suck, which enhances grasp.

*All infants and children with abnormal responses or reflexes present beyond the expected age should be evaluated by a physician.

Table 3 Common Infant Reflexes* *(continued)*

Reflex	How to Elicit	Infant's Response	Clinical Significance	Remarks
Parachute	Hold infant in prone position and descend infant toward surface (examining table).	Infant's fingers and upper limbs abduct and extend to protect head.	Lack of response or asymmetry by 5–6 mo is abnormal.	There should be a partial reaction by 4–5 mo, a fully developed reaction by 9 mo.
Placing	Hold infant erect with dorsal side of one of the infant's feet touching table edge.	Infant's knees and hips flex; foot rises and is placed on table.	Response is absent in paralysis or in infant of breech delivery.	Response is present at birth but difficult to elicit before 4 days of age. Response disappears around 6 wk of age.
Plantar grasp	Place your fingers across base of infant's toes, or place thumbs against balls of infant's feet and press.	Infant's toes turn downward and curl around fingers.	Absence of response may indicate lower spinal column defect.	Response is present at birth; disappears between 8–15 mo. Infant unable to walk until reflex disappears.
Protective side turning	Infant in prone position with head midline.	Infant should turn head to side.	Absence of response may be early sign of cerebral palsy.	
Recoil of the arm	Extend both of infant's arms simultaneously by pulling out at the wrists, then let go quickly.	Both arms flex at the elbows.	Lack of response may indicate apathetic or hypotonic infant.	Strongest response occurs during first 2 days of life, but reflex is present throughout neonate period.
Rooting	Infant supine, head midline, hands against chest. With your finger stroke skin at corners of infant's mouth, upper lip, and lower lip.	Infant's head turns to side stimulated. Lower lip stimulated—mouth opens, lower jaw drops. Upper lip stimulated—mouth opens, head bends backwards. Infant attempts to suck finger in each instance.	Absence of response may indicate depressed infant or severe CNS disease.	Response is present at birth and usually disappears before 12 mo of age. Infant may turn in opposite direction when not hungry.

*All infants and children with abnormal responses or reflexes present beyond the expected age should be evaluated by a physician.

Table 3 Common Infant Reflexes* *(continued)*

Reflex	How to Elicit	Infant's Response	Clinical Significance	Remarks
Stepping	Hold infant upright with feet touching hard surface.	Infant makes alternating stepping movements—"walks."	Response is absent in depressed infant, with breech delivery, or in paralysis.	Response is difficult to elicit during first 4 days of life. Response fades before 6 mo of age.
Sucking	With infant supine, place your index finger about 4 cm into infant's mouth.	Vigorous, rhythmic sucking should occur. Note tongue action, rate, amount of suction (strength), pattern of grouping of sucks.	Poor suck may indicate maternal barbiturate use (passed in breast milk), CNS depression, or apathetic infant.	Poor suck leads to feeding problems and failure to thrive. May be weak first 2–3 days of life.
Tonic neck	With infant supine, turn infant's head to extreme right or left.	Infant's arm and leg extend on side head is turned to; arm and leg flex on opposite side (fencer's position).	Presence beyond 6 mo indicates central motor lesion.	Response may be present at birth but usually not until 2–3 mo of age. Disappears by 5–6 mo of age.

*All infants and children with abnormal responses or reflexes present beyond the expected age should be evaluated by a physician.

Sources: Adapted from Alexander, Mary M., and Brown, Marie Scott. *Pediatric history taking and physical diagnosis for nurses.* New York: McGraw-Hill, 1979, pp. 355–362; and Erickson, M. L. *Assessment and management of developmental changes in children.* St. Louis: Mosby, 1976, pp. 62–66.

(Table 4 is located on pages 518 and 519.)

bibliography

Alexander, Mary M., and Brown, Marie Scott. *Pediatric history taking and physical diagnosis for nurses* (2d ed.). New York: McGraw-Hill, 1979.

Bates, Barbara. *A guide to physical examination.* Philadelphia: Lippincott, 1974, pp. 263–313.

Conway, B. L. *Pediatric neurological nursing.* St. Louis: Mosby, 1977.

Erickson, Marcene L. *Assessment and management of developmental changes in children.* St. Louis: Mosby, 1976.

Essentials of the neurological examination. Philadelphia: Smith Kline Corp., 1974 (revised Jan. 1976).

Gofman, H. F., and Allmond, B. W., Jr. Learning and language disòrders in children, Part II: the school-age child. In Gluck, L., et al. (eds.), *Current problems in pediatrics.* Chicago: Yearbook, 1971, pp. 53–54.

Malasanos, Lois, et al. *Health assessment.* St. Louis: Mosby, 1977, pp. 379–418.

Table 4 Evaluation of Soft Neurological Signs in the School-Age Child

Evaluation of Fine-Motor Coordination	
Observe the child: 1. Undressing, unbuttoning 2. Tying shoes	*Note:* The child's general facility and coordination with these small muscle tasks.
3. Rapidly alternating touching fingertips with thumb 4. Rattling an imaginary doorknob 5. Unscrewing an imaginary light bulb	On items 3, 4, 5, 8, and 9, any marked movement of other parts of the body that mirror or duplicate movements of the test side. Such movements are called associated motor movements, mirror movements, adventitious overflow movements, or synkinesia. When marked they are felt to represent, particularly after 8 to 10 years, a lack of normal cortical inhibition.
6. Grasping and using a pencil; penmanship 7. Rapidly moving tongue 8. Gripping with hand 9. Inverting both feet (Look for similar movements of the hands. See below.)	Excessive pressure on the pencil point or a pencil held too lightly. Fingers placed directly over the point or fingers placed too far (greater than 1 inch) from the point may all indicate difficulty with the coordination of fine musculature within the hands.
10. Repeating several times rapidly: kitty, kitty, kitty; pa, ta, ka (Accurate reproduction of these sounds generally indicates adequate articulatory coordination.)	Presence of dysdiadochokinesia, noting speed, accuracy, and sequencing of maneuvers.
Evaluation of Special Sensory Skills	
Dual Simultaneous Sensory Tests (face-hand testing) With the client's eyes closed (but first demonstrating items 1 and 2 below with client's eyes open), simultaneously: 1. Touch both cheeks 2. Touch both hands 3. Touch right check and contralateral hand 4. Touch right cheek and homolateral hand 5. Touch left cheek and contralateral hand 6. Touch left cheek and homolateral hand	*Note:* Rostral dominance: failure to perceive hand stimulus when the face is simultaneously touched. Approximately 80 percent of normal children are able to perform this test without rostral dominance by age 8 years.
Finger Localization Test (finger agnosia test) Touch two fingers or two spots on one finger simultaneously with the client's eyes closed, after demonstrating first with eyes open. Ask the client: "How many fingers am I touching—one or two?"	*Note:* The number of correct responses in four trials for each hand; six correct answers out of eight are accepted as a "pass." Half of all children pass this test by age 6 years, 90 percent by age 7½ years. This test reflects a child's orientation in space, concept of body image, praxic ability, and sensation to touch and position sense.

Table 4 Evaluation of Soft Neurological Signs in the School-Age Child *(continued)*

Evaluation of Child's Laterality and Orientation in Space	
Imitation of Gestures Have the child imitate the following gestures performed by the examiner, emphasizing first that the child must use the same hand as the examiner: 1. Extend index finger 2. Extend little and index finger 3. Extend index and middle finger 4. Touch two thumbs and two index fingers together simultaneously 5. Form two interlocking rings, thumb and index finger of one hand with thumb and index finger of other hand 6. Point index finger of one hand down toward the cupped fingers of the opposite hand held below	*Note:* Difficulty with fine finger movements, manipulation, and/or reproduction of correct gesture. After approximately age 8 years, marked right-left confusion with regard to examiner's right and left. This test reflects a child's ability with finger discrimination, postural praxis, awareness of self-image, and right-left, front-back, up-down orientation.
Following Directions Ask the child to: 1. Show me your left hand 2. Show me your right ear 3. Show me your right eye 4. Show me your left elbow. 5. Touch your left knee with your left hand 6. Touch your right ear with your left hand 7. Touch your left elbow with your right hand 8. Touch your right cheek with your right hand 9. Point to my left ear 10. Point to my right eye 11. Point to my right hand 12. Point to my left knee	*Note:* Items 1 through 8 are mastered by approximately age 6 years; items 9 through 12 are mastered by approximately age 8 years. Aside from correct versus incorrect responses, any difficulty with following the sequence of directions.

Reproduced with permission from Gofman, H. F., and Allmond, B. W., Jr. (1971).

78 Large Head/Small Head

ELEANOR RUDICK

ALERT
1. Abnormal increase in head size in infancy
2. Signs of increased intracranial pressure

I. Etiology
- **A.** Familial characteristic
- **B.** Intrauterine infection
- **C.** Birth trauma
- **D.** Congenital defect (aqueductal stenosis)
- **E.** Extrinsic lesion (as aneurysm, tumor)
- **F.** Recessive inheritance

Table 78-1 Medical Referral/Consultation

Diagnosis	Clinical Manifestations	Management
Caput succedaneum	Diffuse edematous swelling of soft tissue of scalp Possible extension across midline and suture lines Possible presence of ecchymosis Possible presence of molding Area of edema determined by presenting part of head	Consultation with physician Counselling Disappearance of edema in a few days No treatment necessary Disappearance of molding in a few weeks Follow-up: well-child supervision
Cephalohematoma	Subperiosteal hemorrhage (limited to surface of one cranial bone) No discoloration of overlying scalp Pulsation indicative of cranial meningocele	Referral to physician to rule out underlying fracture or meningocele Counselling No treatment required Resolution of most cases in 2–3 wk, depending on size of head Aspiration contraindicated Follow-up: well-child supervision
Hydrocephaly	Onset in infancy Rapid increase in head size Bulging fontanels Separation of cranial sutures Dilated scalp veins Thin and shiny scalp skin High-pitched cry	Immediate referral to physician Continued observation and hospitalization for cerebrospinal fluid (CSF) examination and neuroradiologic studies to determine cause Obstructive

Table 78-1 Medical Referral/Consultation *(continued)*

Diagnosis	Clinical Manifestations	Management
	If severe, setting-sun sign (eyes deviated downward) Poor growth and development, depending on severity of condition Onset later in childhood Possibly no appreciable head enlargement Signs of increased intracranial pressure Papilledema Commonly Spasticity and ataxia—especially of the legs Urinary incontinence Progressive decline in higher-cortical functioning	Communicating Individualized treatment determined by Type of lesion Rate of head enlargement Spontaneous arrest Meningomyelocele Shunt procedure for infant Revision with growth Observation for blockage; infection Shunt procedure for older child Shunt failure—signs of increased intracranial pressure, headache, vomiting, stupor Repeated intelligence tests for early detection of decline in mental function Follow-up Well-child supervision, nutrition Assistance to family based on assessment of ability to cope Referral of family to social service agency/parent group Referral to orthopedist and nephrologist
Megalocephaly	Rare Excessive brain growth Often unknown etiology Large head size Developmental delay No signs of increased intracranial pressure	Immediate referral to physician Hospitalization for neuroradiological studies to differentiate from hydrocephaly Guarded prognosis: severe mental deficiency common Assistance to family based on ability to cope; social service assistance/institutionalization if required
Microcephaly	Defect in growth of brain Head size > 3 SD below norm In recessively inherited form Backward sloping of forehead Large ears Mental retardation Possibly good motor development	Referral to physician Hospitalization Mother's urine tested for PKU Skull x-rays CSF study Serologic tests of mother and child Correct diagnosis—important for genetic counselling Not treatable—chronic-care managment and special education necessary Assistance to family determined by its ability to cope; social service referral
Craniosynostosis (premature closure of sagittal suture)	Long, narrow head Bony ridge over obliterated suture Associated complications rare	Referral to physician Counselling Surgery for isolated sagittal craniosynostosis questionable, except for cosmetic or psychological reasons

Table 78-1 Medical Referral/Consultation *(continued)*

Diagnosis	Clinical Manifestations	Management
Craniosynostosis (premature closure of coronal suture)	Severe deformity of face and orbits Possible exophthalmos, strabismus, nystagmus Possible papilledema, optic atrophy, and loss of vision More severe complications with involvement of both coronals and other bones Other malformations (cardiac, choanal atresia) possible, most frequently syndactylism	Immediate referral to physician Surgical intervention early in infancy to lessen or avoid cerebral or visual damage possibly caused by lesion Hospitalization Radiologic studies Some forms are of genetic origin: important for genetic counselling Family assessment for ability to cope; possible long-term social service; guarded outcome

bibliography

Bates, Barbara. *A guide to physical examination* (2d ed). Philadelphia: Lippincott, 1979, pp. 383–388.

Braney, Marie Louise. The child with hydrocephalus. *American Journal of Nursing*, **72**:828–831 (1973).

Fields, Grace. Social implications of long-term illness in children. In John A. Downey and Niels L. Low (eds.), *The child with disabling illness*. Philadelphia: Saunders, 1974, pp. 541–557.

Gomez, Manuel R., and Reese, David F. Computed tomography of the head in infants and children. *The Pediatric Clinics of North America*, **23**:473–498 (1976).

Green, Morris, and Haggerty, Robert J. (eds.). *Ambulatory pediatrics II*. Philadelphia: Saunders,

McCullough, David C., et al. Computerized axial tomography in clinical pediatrics. *Pediatrics*, **59**:173–181 (1977).

Steele, Shirley (ed.). *Nursing care of the child with long-term illness*. New York: Appleton Century Crofts, 1971, pp. 390–401.

Vaughan, Victor C., and McKay, R. James (eds.). *Nelson textbook of pediatrics* (10th ed.). Philadelphia: Saunders, 1975, pp. 38, 352, 1417–1482.

79 Blackout Spells/Seizures

MICHAELINE KELLEY/JOHN WALLACH

ALERT

1. Continued, uninterrupted seizures (status epilepticus)
2. Signs of meningitis
3. First-time seizure
4. Familial history suggestive of epilepsy
5. Familial history of sickle cell disease
6. Brief lapses or total loss of consciousness associated with convulsion(s)
7. Children presenting with high fever with a past history of febrile convulsions
8. Child presenting with first-time seizure and history of pertussis vaccine in the past 24 h
9. Head trauma (recent or past history)
10. Chronic illness, i.e., diabetes, mental retardation
11. Hematocrit (Hct) below normal
12. Any neurological abnormality
13. Sensitivity to penicillin or aspirin
14. Drug abuse
15. Recent ingestion of toxic material(s)

I. Etiology

A. See Table 79–1

B. Syncope

1. Transient loss of consciousness is due to inadequate blood flow to the brain.
2. Predisposing factors include emotional stress, poor ventilation, fatigue, pain, dehydration, etc.

C. Breath-holding attacks

Temporary loss of consciousness coupled with a brief, generalized seizure following an emotional or physical upset

II. Assessment

A. Syncope (simple faint)

1. Subjective data
   a. Witnessed report of loss of consciousness and muscle tone for less than 1 min
   b. Precipitating factors including emotional stress, fatigue, compromised nutritional status, prolonged standing, etc.
   c. May be history of previous breath-holding attacks in early childhood
2. Objective data
   a. Physical examination normal
   b. Laboratory data within normal limits

B. Breath-holding attacks

1. Subjective data
   a. Witnessed report of loss of consciousness coupled with brief, generalized muscular twitching
   b. Precipitating factors include emotional or physical trauma
   c. Attacks perhaps characterized by cyanotic or pallid effect
   d. Attacks most common between 1 and 5 years of age; onset usually before 18 months of age
   e. Attacks perhaps occurring several times a day or once every few months
   f. History of previous aggressive behavior
2. Objective data
   a. Practitioner may witness attack during physical examination.
      (1) Child cries out 2 to 3 times
      (2) Child holds breath on expiration
      (3) Period of apnea 5 to 10 s
      (4) Child may be cyanotic; slight twitching may or may not be observed
      (5) Child recovers in 2 to 3 min
      (6) If precipitating event is pain, the child may become pallid instead of cyanotic and lose consciousness without crying out

(7) Heart rate slows
(8) Blood pressure drops acutely

b. Physical examination is normal.
c. Laboratory data may be within normal limits, or Hct and hemoglobin (Hgb) may reveal a concurrent iron deficiency anemia.
d. It appears to be more common in white, male children.

III. Management

A. General management of seizures

1. Treatments/medications
   a. Medications—see Table 79–2
   b. Acute care of seizures—see Table 79–3
   c. Temperature control if needed
2. Counselling/prevention
   a. Carefully explain seizures and seizure management to client, parent(s), siblings, and other care givers (baby-sitters, grandparents, teachers).
   b. Instruct in what to do when seizure occurs (Table 79-3).
   c. Allay any misconceptions.
   d. Instruct parent(s)/care givers on temperature control.
   e. Educate and provide with written instructions regarding medications, compliance, and toxic side effects (Table 79–2).
   f. Instruct parent(s) and care givers to document frequency of seizures, duration, time of occurrence, and descriptions of preictal, ictal, and postictal phases (incontinence, level of consciousness, type of activity, etc.).
   g. Stress that the child is not to be treated as "special." It is important to both love and set limits. Overprotectiveness must be avoided.
   h. If hospitalization is needed, see Preparation for Hospitalization, Part 7.
   i. Hazardous activities should be avoided (e.g., swimming, horseback riding, working with sharp tools, etc.) unless supervised.
   j. Client should wear a Medic-Alert bracelet at *all* times—disease, medication, dosage should be included.
   k. Adolescents often rebel against the treatment regimen—parent(s) should be aware of this and help to understand and support the child during this difficult time before acceptance of the disease is accomplished.
   l. Public education to teach others about seizures and correct misconceptions is important.
3. Follow-up
   a. Telephone contact as needed
   b. Support for client, parent(s), and care givers—should be main focus
   c. Return visits as determined by neurologist and for well-child care
4. Consultations/referrals
   a. Refer to neurologist/physician for medication regimen.
   b. Notify school nurse and teachers.
   c. Consult with employers (if client so desires).
   d. Refer to public health nurse to assess the family's ability to deal with chronic illness and comply with the treatment regimen.
   e. Refer to a dentist for regular visits if anticonvulsants are prescribed.
   f. May wish to refer for group counselling.

B. Syncope (simple faint)

1. Treatments/medications
   a. Medication not usually recommended
   b. Sitting position with head lowered between knees or supine position with elevation of lower extremities
   c. Spirits of ammonia
2. Counselling/prevention
   a. Nutritional counselling
   b. Avoidance of stressful situations when possible
   c. Instruction to parent(s) on management of attack (see above)
   d. Reassurance to client that condition is not chronic
   e. If attacks recurrent, documentation regarding precipitating factors and frequency
3. Follow-up
   a. Telephone call within 24 h to report condition
   b. Return visit as needed for reassurance and reevaluation
4. Consultations/referrals
   a. Usually none indicated
   b. Professional counselling if attacks frequent and precipitated by severe emotional stress

C. Breath-holding attacks—see Breath-Holding, Chap. 118

Table 79-1 Etiologic Factors Associated with Epilepsy

I. Prenatal Factors
- A. Genetic
  1. Genetic epilepsy
  2. Inborn errors of metabolism
     - a. Carbohydrate: glycogen storage disease, hypoglycemia
     - b. Protein: phenylketonuria, maple syrup urine disease
     - c. Fat: cerebral lipidoses, leukodystrophies
  3. Heredofamilial diseases: myoclonus epilepsy
- B. Congenital structural anomalies
  1. Porencephaly
  2. Vascular malformations
  3. Neurocutaneous syndrome
  4. Developmental defects of brain
- C. Fetal infections
  1. Viral encephalopathy: rubella, cytomegalic inclusion disease
  2. Protozoan meningoencephalitis: toxoplasmosis
- D. Maternal disease
  1. Toxemia of pregnancy
  2. Chronic renal disease
  3. Diabetes mellitus
  4. Radiation during pregnancy
  5. Drug usage and drug intoxication
  6. Trauma

II. Perinatal Factors
- A. Trauma
- B. Hypoxia
- C. Jaundice
- D. Infection
- E. Prematurity
- F. Drug withdrawal

III. Postnatal Factors
- A. Primary infection of central nervous system
- B. Infectious diseases of childhood with encephalopathy (e.g., measles, mumps)
- C. Head trauma
- D. Circulatory diseases
  1. Vascular anomalies
  2. Occlusive diseases: arterial, venous
  3. Hemorrhage
  4. Hypertensive encephalopathy
- E. Toxic encephalopathy
  1. Thallium
  2. Lead
  3. Convulsogenic drugs: INH, steroids
- F. Allergic encephalopathy
  1. Immunization reactions
  2. Drug reactions
- G. Physical and metabolic encephalopathies
  1. Fever and febrile convulsions
  2. Anoxia and hypoxia
  3. Prolonged convulsions with cyanosis
  4. Electrolyte disturbance
  5. Acute porphyria
  6. Hypoglycemia
  7. Hypocalcemia
  8. Hypomagnesemia
  9. Hyponatremia and hypernatremia and others
  10. Pyridoxine deficiency or dependency
- H. Degenerative diseases of the brain

  Tumors

Source: Rudolph, Abraham (ed.). *Pediatrics 16.* New York: Appleton-Century-Crofts, 1977, p. 1842.

Table 79-2 Antiepileptic Medications

Drugs	Dosage
BARBITURATES	
Phenobarbital (Luminal) (grand mal, focal, psychomotor)	1–6 mg/kg body weight per day
Mephobarbital (Mebaral) (minor motor)	Under 5 years old: 16–32 mg 3 or 4 times a day Over 5 years old: 32–64 mg 3 or 4 times a day
Metharbital (Gemonil) (minor motor)	Initial pediatric dose: one-half of a 100-mg tablet 1 to 3 times daily depending on age and weight of the client 5–15 mg/kg per day recommended for children
HYDANTOINS	
Phenytoin (Dilantin) (grand mal, focal, psychomotor)	5 mg/kg per day in 2 or 3 equally divided doses to 300 mg per day Daily maintenance dose:4–8 mg/kg
Mephenytoin (Mesantoin) (grand mal, focal, psychomotor)	4–10 mg/kg per day, usually requiring 1–4 tabs per day (0.1 to 0.4 g) Maintenance after starting with ½ or 1 tab per day for 1 week: daily dose increased by ½ or 1 tab weekly
SUCCINIMIDES	
Phensuximide (Milontin) (petit mal, minor motor)	20–40 mg/kg per day Average: 1.5 g per day
Ethosuximide (Zarontin) (petit mal)	Under 6 years old: 250 mg per day in divided doses to start Over 6 years: 500 mg per day Dosage increased by 250 mg once a week until 1 g per day is reached in children under 6 yr or 1.5 g per day in children over 6 yr
Methsuximide (Celontin) (petit mal)	Individualized according to responses of each client; suggested dose: 300 mg per day for first week
OXAZOLIDINEDIONES	
Trimethadione (Tridione) (petit mal, minor motor)	150 mg to start, gradually raised to amounts that are effective and well tolerated (10–25 mg/kg per day)
Paramethadione (Paradione) (petit mal, minor motor)	300–900 mg daily in 3 or 4 equally divided doses

Side Effects	Remarks
Drowsiness, skin rash, fever, increased irritability, ataxia	Contraindicated for clients with porphyria or nephritis
Dizziness, headache, confusion, nausea, vomiting, epigastric pain, hypotension, allergic reactions, anemia, agranulocytosis, thrombocytopenia	Contraindicated for clients with past history of barbiturate hypersensitivity Porphyria may result May be habit forming
Mild gastric distress, dizziness, increased irritability, skin rash, drowsiness	Contraindicated for clients with past history of barbiturate hypersensitivity May be habit forming Porphyria may result
Gastric distress, diplopia, ataxia, dysarthria, mental confusion, dizziness, headache, rash, blood dyscrasias, liver damage	Hyperplasia of the gums (50% of the cases) Known to increase frequency of petit mal attacks
Blood dyscrasias, rashes, ataxia, epigastric distress, diplopia	Contraindicated for clients with past history of hypersensitivity to hydantoin products Should be used only after less toxic anticonvulsants have failed to control seizures
Anorexia, hiccoughs, nausea, vomiting, drowsiness, skin eruptions, dizziness	Blood dyscrasias reported; caution advised if client has known liver or renal disease Contraindicated for clients with past history of hypersensitivity to succinimides Known to increase frequency of grand mal seizures
Anorexia, hiccoughs, nausea, vomiting, drowsiness, motor incoordination, blood dyscrasias	Hypersensitivity reactions rare In long-term therapy, blood studies and liver function tests periodically Known to increase frequency of grand mal seizures
Nausea, vomiting, anorexia, diarrhea, ataxia, irritability, drowsiness, dizziness, skin rash	Contraindicated for clients with past history of hypersensitivity to succinimides Blood dyscrasias reported Caution if client has known liver or renal disease
Drowsiness, upset stomach, photophobia, (day blindness), rash	Under long-term therapy, hypersensitivity reactions involving bone marrow, liver, skin and kidneys
Drowsiness, nausea, vomiting, ataxia, diplopia, vertigo, hiccoughs, anorexia, possible precipitation of a grand mal seizure	Should be discontinued in the event of skin rash or depression of blood count Clients should immediately report sore throat, fever, easy bruising, petechiae and epistaxis. Contraindicated in clients with liver or renal disease

Table 79-2 Antiepileptic Medications *(continued)*

Drugs	Dosage
MISCELLANEOUS	
Primidone (Mysoline) (grand mal, focal, psychomotor)	10–20 mg/kg per day
Clonazepam (Clonopin) (petit mal, myoclonic)	Maintenance dose: 0.1–0.2 mg/kg per day in children
Carbamazepine (Tegretol) (grand mal, focal, psychomotor)	7–20 mg/kg per day
Diazepam (Valium) (minor motor, status epilepticus)	1 mg–2.5 mg 3 or 4 times daily, increased gradually as needed for status epilepticus 0–1 year old: 1–2 mg IV 5 years old: 5 mg IV 12 years and above: 10 mg IV
Valproic acid (Depakene) (absence seizures)	15 mg/kg per day initially to 30 mg/kg per day maximum

Table 79-3 Acute Care of Witnessed Seizures

1. Remain calm.
2. Remain with the person until the seizure has passed.
3. Do not move the person unless absolutely necessary.
4. Do not force anything between the teeth. If the mouth is open, place a soft object between the side teeth, e. g., a handkerchief.
5. Remove or loosen tight clothing, especially around the neck.
6. Turn the head to the side and check for patent airway.
7. Clear the surrounding area of objects that might pose a threat of injury.
8. Place a pillow or rolled-up jacket under the head.
9. Do not attempt to restrain during the attack. This might result in increased muscular movements leading to fractures and dislocations.
10. *Do not* be alarmed over brief periods of apnea or cyanosis. *Do be concerned* if the person passes from one seizure to another without regaining consciousness. This is status epilepticus and constitutes a medical emergency.
11. Carefully note preictal, ictal, and postictal behaviors (before, during, and after seizure).
12. Note any incontinence associated with the attack.
13. Reassure and reorient the person after an attack.

Table 79-4 Medical Referral/Consultation

Diagnosis	Clinical Manifestations	Management
Febrile convulsions	Age between 6 mo and 8 yr Sudden rise in fever usually over 102.2°F or 39°C or above Witnessed convulsion usually occurring within 24 h after onset of fever; convulsion described as follows	Refer to neurologist for all first-time seizures. Instruct parent(s)/care givers on temperature taking and temperature control. Offer support and reassurance to

Side Effects	Remarks
Skin rash, ataxia, anorexia, drowsiness, nausea, vomiting, emotional disturbances, megaloblastic anemia	Contraindicated for clients with past history of hypersensitivity to phenobarbital In long term therapy, blood studies necessary periodically
Drowsiness, ataxia, irritability, hyperactivity, anorexia, hypersalivation, behavior changes	Contraindicated for clients with past history of hypersensitivity to benzodiazepines, liver disease, or acute narrow-angle glaucoma
Lethargy, ataxia, slurred speech, nystagmus, diplopia, nausea, vomiting, liver toxicity, leukopenia	May lead to aplastic anemia; not to be used in clients with previous bone marrow depression and sensitivity to any tricyclic compound.
Drowsiness, fatigue, ataxia, rash, venous thrombosis, phlebitis at injection site	Contraindicated with narrow-angle glaucoma Danger of respiratory depression with IV use
Drowsiness, gastrointestinal disturbances, alopecia	Possible hepatic toxicity and thrombocytopenia

Table 79-4 Medical Referral/Consultation *(continued)*

Diagnosis	Clinical Manifestations	Management
	A loss of consciousness May be coupled with tonic and clonic movements, body stiffness, ocular deviations, or general loss of muscle tone Usually lasting less than 5 min and not exceeding 20 min History sometimes revealing recent episode of nausea, vomiting, and diarrhea History sometimes revealing recent episode of acute illness, e. g., urinary tract infection (UTI), upper respiratory infection (URI), or otitis media History sometimes revealing generalized rash, tinnitus, dizziness, and gastrointestinal upsets Family history of febrile convulsions Family history of sensitivity to aspirin or penicillin Developmental history normal for age Physical exam perhaps normal or revealing signs of dehydration, UTI, URI, otitis media, salicylate poisoning, or penicillin sensitivity Normal EEG following the attack	parent(s)/care givers. Stress that convulsions of this type usually end by 6 yr of age. See Preparation for Hospitalization, Part 7. See General management of seizures, III, A.

Table 79-4 Medical Referral/Consultation *(continued)*

Diagnosis	Clinical Manifestations	Management
Epilepsy (types of seizures) Grand mal (major motor, generalized, tonic/clonic epilepsy)	Usually associated with an "aura" Always associated with loss of consciousness and complete loss of postural muscle tone Most common type of seizure in childhood Actual attack (ictal phase) lasting approximately 60 s; entire grand mal seizure lasting 5–15 min Attack characterized by tonic/clonic movements, brief periods of apnea and cyanosis, followed by stertorous breathing, increased salivation, vomiting, and incontinence Following attack, autonomic functions return to normal; client may complain of confusion, dizziness, headache, or sleepiness Usually experiences amnesia about attack EEG usually normal between seizures Physical exam normal Possible family history of epilepsy	Refer to a neurologist. Refer to a physician for medication regimen. See General management of seizures, III, A.
Petit mal (absence of attacks)	Onset with aura Occur in childhood; tend to decrease and disappear with age Attacks characterized by brief "daydreaming" episode, where person becomes pale and stares into space (usually 5–10 s) No complete loss of postural muscle tone Eyes may roll back into head; possible twitching of face, head, or upper extremities Recovers immediately after attack May experience many attacks in one day; most common time of attack is upon awakening EEG normal between attacks Physical exam normal Possible family history of epilepsy	Refer to a neurologist. Refer to a physician for medication regimen. Alert teacher to presence of attacks. Provide education and support.
Minor motor (petit mal variance)	Occurs in young children; usually intellectually impaired with history of prenatal, perinatal, or postnatal complication May present with following types of seizures Akinetic Sudden loss of postural muscle tone and consciousness	Refer to a neurologist. Refer to a physician for medication regimen. See General management of seizures, III, A. Seizures of akinetic type may warrant use of protective headgear.

Table 79-4 Medical Referral/Consultation *(continued)*

Diagnosis	Clinical Manifestations	Management
	Brief period of confusion sometimes following attack May sustain traumatic injury due to fall EEG abnormal Usually developmentally delayed Myoclonic Brief contractions or spasms of single muscle or muscle group; usually affecting trunk muscles and extremities Attacks often precipitated by increased sensory stimulation EEG variable depending upon severity	
Psychomotor (temporal lobe epilepsy)	Usually occurs in adults Symptoms and duration extremely varied Attacks usually characterized by Automatisms (repetitious acts) Stare or blank expression May present with incoherent speech Sometimes rages, tantrums, and psychoticlike behavior Amnesia usually present EEG helpful in diagnosis because difficult to differentiate this from childhood temper tantrums Physical exam normal Possible family history of epilepsy	Refer to a neurologist. Refer to a physician for medication regimen. Alert teacher, care givers, and employer (if client desires) that seizure is not a manifestation of psychotic disturbance. Provide education and support.
Focal motor (partial seizures)	Occur in children and adults; onset in adulthood indicative of underlying pathology Most common type, Jacksonian seizure, characterized by Attack limited to one part of body, i.e., foot or hand Convulsive movements spreading up the extremities toward the trunk Total loss of consciousness rare Usually lapse of awareness Physical exam for children normal; for adults, may indicate lesion or vascular pathology Abnormal EEG pattern sometimes present	Refer to a neurologist. Refer to a physician for medication regimen. Provide education and support.
Status epilepticus	Usually seen with grand mal seizures, but may occur with any type of seizure Characterized by rapid, continuous seizures without regaining consciousness; may last for hours or days Presence constituting medical emergency	*Immediately* refer to a physician. Prepare client for immediate transport to the hospital.

Table 79-4 Medical Referral/Consultation *(continued)*

Diagnosis	Clinical Manifestations	Management
	Failure to intervene perhaps leading to irreversible brain damage Frequent side effect of rapid withdrawal or change in anticonvulsant medication History of previous status attacks Physical exam reveals client in acute distress Hypoxia Diaphoresis Tonic/clonic movements Incontinence Elevated blood pressure	
Pertussis vaccine-induced encephalopathy	Generalized convulsions High fever History of recent pertussis vaccine	Refer to a physician. See "Immunizations" in Chap. 9.
Meningitis	Convulsions, possibly opisthotonus High fever Nuchal rigidity Bulging fontanels in infants Positive Kernig's sign Dyspnea Irritability Headache	Immediate referral to physician
Lead encephalopathy	Vomiting Constipation Irritability Lethargy Convulsions Anemia Blue "lead line" along gums Lead level elevated	Refer to a physician. See Lead Poisoning, Chap. 155.
Drug abuse-induced seizures (salicylate intoxication, Valium abuse)	Convulsions Respiratory and cardiovascular failure Increased respiratory rate followed by respiratory alkalosis Metabolic acidosis Hyper- or hypoglycemia Bleeding disorders sometimes developing	Immediately refer to a physician. See Drug Abuse, Chap. 157. See "Accident Prevention" in Chap. 9.
Head injury	History of recent trauma to head followed by loss of consciousness History of past head trauma	Refer to a physician. See Head Injury, Chap. 166. See "Accident Prevention" in Chap. 9.

Table 79-4 Medical Referral/Consultation *(continued)*

Diagnosis	Clinical Manifestations	Management
	May exhibit personality changes, confusion, or amnesia Presence of clear drainage (cerebrospinal fluid) from nose or ears	

bibliography

Binder, Ruth McGillis, and Howry, Linda Berner. Nursing care of children with febrile seizures. *Maternal Child Nursing* **3**:270–273 (1978).

Gellis, Sydney S., and Kagan, Benjamin M. *Current pediatric therapy 8*. Philadelphia: Saunders, 1978.

Green, Morris, and Richmond, Julius B. *Pediatric diagnosis* (2d ed.). Philadelphia: Saunders, 1962.

Hoole, Axalla J., et al. *Patient care guidelines for family nurse practitioners*. Boston: Little, Brown, 1976.

Livingston, Samuel, et al. Epilepsy: diagnosis and treatment. *Pediatric Nursing* **2**:23–27 (1976).

Livingston, Samuel, et al. Antiepileptic drug interactions and teratogenicity. *Pediatric Annals,* **8**(4): 103–113 (April 1979).

———. Initiation of drug therapy. *Pediatric Annals,* **8**(4):15–43 (1979).

———. Maintenance of drug therapy. *Pediatric Annals,* **8**(4):47–84 (1979).

———. Managing side effects of antiepileptic drugs. *Pediatric Annals,* **8**(4):97–102 (1979).

———. The medical treatment of epilepsy: an introduction. *Pediatric Annals,* **8**(4):10–14 (1979).

Rudolph, Abraham M. (ed.). *Pediatrics 16*. New York: Appleton-Century-Crofts, 1977.

Swift, Nancy. Helping patients live with seizures. *Nursing 78* **8**:24–31 (1978).

Willis, John K., and Oppenheimer, Edgar Y. Children's seizures and their management. *Issues in Comprehensive Pediatric Nursing* **2**:56–66 (1977).

80 Hyperactivity

KAREN A. BALLARD

Hyperactivity can be a primary or secondary symptom for a variety of physical and psychological disturbances. If an underlying illness is identified, it should be treated and the client reevaluated.

I. Etiology

A. Biochemical, genetic base

B. Environmental factors

C. Social factors

II. Assessment

A. Subjective data

1. Pure hyperactivity is
   a. A single, functional disturbance
   b. A consistent high level of inappropriate activity which is not under child's direct control
   c. In various manifestations, present at all developmental stages
   d. Usually manifested by the time child is 3 to 4 years old
   e. Characterized primarily by restlessness and inattentiveness
2. Diagnosis—dependent on a detailed, accurate history
   a. Parent(s) describes child as
      (1) Being very active—wearing out clothes and shoes at an accelerated rate
      (2) Lagging developmentally
      (3) Having frequent temper outbursts
      (4) Being a disciplinary, management problem
      (5) Having poor peer, sibling relationships
      (6) Having aberrant eating and sleeping behaviors
      (7) Having disturbed prenatal and birth history
         (a) Toxemia, eclampsia, or hypertension
         (b) Low birth weight
         (c) Low Apgar score
         (d) Evidence of respiratory distress
   b. Teacher(s) description may indicate
      (1) Peer isolation
      (2) Frequent fighting
      (3) Physical incapability of sitting still
      (4) Inability to complete assignments
      (5) Preference for playing with younger children
      (6) Daydreams
      (7) Child's being very active in playground activities

B. Objective data

1. Physical examination—can indicate soft, neurological signs
   a. Impaired fine-motor coordination
   b. Nonpersistence in motor activities
   c. Choreiform movements (irregular, jerky limb movements)
2. Laboratory data
   a. Normal CBC and urinalysis
   b. EEG results may indicate irregularities in about 50 percent of hyperactive children; other data may
      (1) Indicate a high verbal IQ with a low performance IQ
      (2) Support impression that learning and performance problems stem from the inability to focus and sustain attention

III. Management

A. Treatments/medications: sedatives contraindicated; most commonly used drugs,

Ritalin (methylphenidate), Dexedrine (dextroamphetamine), and Cylert (magnesium pemoline) (see Table 80-1), are

1. Used primarily on school days and given before meals
2. Titrated in dosage until there is either a clinical improvement in behavior or side effects
3. Given a trial period of 1 to 3 weeks; if side effects occur, drug is decreased or discontinued.

B. Counselling/prevention

1. Advise parent(s) that correlating functional hyperactivity with minimal brain damage is an unfortunate confusion of terms and a disservice to the child.
2. Parent(s) should be instructed in the multifaceted causality and told to focus on developing a harmonious, cooperative treatment plan for the child.
3. Counsel parent(s) to
   a. Make expectations clear to child.
   b. Keep verbal responses and instructions clear and brief.
   c. Utilize behavioral time-limited discipline (see Discipline, Chap. 117).
   d. Avoid physical punishment.
   e. Separate child from situation when he or she is physically disruptive.
   f. Provide close supervision in sibling/peer play to promote acceptance into group.
   g. Anticipate stressful situations (bad weather, long trips) and provide diversions.
4. Parent(s) and teacher should form a therapeutic alliance in caring for child.
   a. Meet frequently.
   b. Compare results of interventions.
   c. Avoid criticizing.

C. Follow-up

1. Monitor closely if child is on pharmacological therapy.
2. Provide supportive counselling and guidance according to changes in child's behavior.

D. Consultations/referrals

1. Professional counselling.
2. Teacher and school nurse.
3. Parent support groups.
4. The Association for Children with Learning Disabilities, 5225 Grace St., Pittsburgh, PA 15236; National Special Education Information Center, Box 1492, Washington, DC 20013.
5. Consultation with physician for medications.

Table 80-1 Medications

Drug	Dosage	Side Effects	Remarks
Diphenhydramine (Benadryl)	Orally; 5 mg/kg per 24 h divided into four doses; dosage should not exceed 300 mg/day	Drowsiness Dryness of mouth, nose, and throat Confusion Nervousness and restlessness Nausea and vomiting Diarrhea or constipation Tightness of chest Thickening of bronchial secretions	Drug is basically a potent antihistamine with anticholinergic, antitussive, antiemetic, and sedative effects. Drug can be used in very young children except in premature or newborn infants. Drug can be taken with food. Drug is one of the safest psychoactive drugs.
Dextroamphetamine sulfate (Dexedrine)	Orally; in children 3–5 yr, 2.5 mg/day, with weekly increments of 2.5 mg; in children 6 yr and older, 5 mg/day, with weekly increments of 5 mg; total dosage should not exceed 40 mg/day	Insomnia Anorexia Irritability Headache Dryness of mouth Gastrointestinal distress	Drug is contraindicated in Children under 3 yr Hypertensive clients Drug should be used with caution in presence of diabetes. Give 1 h before meals.

Table 80-1 Medications *(continued)*

Drug	Dosage	Side Effects	Remarks
		Paradoxical reactions High potential for abuse	If administered twice daily, give before breakfast and lunch. Check BP and pulse. Weigh client twice weekly. May lead to drug dependence. Instruct parent(s) on signs of overdose. Restlessness Tremor Rapid respiration Confusion Assaultiveness Panic states Nausea, vomiting Abdominal cramps Convulsions Coma
Pemoline (Cylert)	Orally; over 6 yr, 37.5 mg/day, with weekly increments of 18.75 mg to average dose of 56.25–75 mg/day; dosage should not exceed 112.5 mg/day	Insomnia Anorexia Weight loss Irritability Headache Drowsiness Mild depression Skin rashes Temporary suppression of growth rate	Drug should be administered in single, morning dose. Drug is not recommended for children under 6 yr. Clinical improvement is gradual and may take 3–4 wk. Drug should be interrupted once or twice a year in order to test continued need.
Methylphenidate (Ritalin)	Orally; over 6 yr, 5 mg/day, with weekly increments of 5–10 mg until average dose of 20–30 mg/day; dosage should not exceed 60 mg/day	Growth retardation Anorexia Weight loss Lowered seizure threshold Irritability Insomnia Dizziness Headache Skin rashes Blood dyscrasias (anemia, leukopenia, thrombocytopenia)	Administer before breakfast and lunch. Drug is contraindicated in Children under 6 Hypertension Convulsive disorder Agitation Drug can cause psychological dependency. Check BP and pulse. Weigh client twice weekly. Instruct parent(s) on signs of overdose. High BP Cardiac arrhythmias Tachycardia Agitation Nausea and vomiting Personality changes

Table 80-2 Medical Referral/Consultation

Diagnosis/Problem	Clinical Manifestations	Management
Severe emotional symptoms; psychosis	Hyperactivity accompanied by Mutism Severe regression Self-destructive behavior	Refer for professional counselling.

bibliography

Barkley, Russell. Do stimulant drugs improve the academic performance of hyperkinetic children? A review of outcome studies. *Clinical Pediatrics* **17**:85–92 (1978).

Conrad, P. Situational hyperactivity: A social system approach. *Journal of School Health* **47**:280–285 (1977).

DeAngelis, Catherine. *Pediatric primary care* (2d ed.). Boston: Little, Brown, 1979.

Eissler, R., Freud, A. Kris, M. and Solnit, A. (eds.). *An anthology of the psychoanalytic study of the child.* New Haven, Conn.: Yale, 1977.

Fremost, T. S., et al. What you should know about hyperactivity. *Mental Hygiene* **60**:10–13 (1976).

Greenberg, J. S. Hyperkinesis and the schools. *Journal of School Health* **46**:91–97 (1976).

Gross, Mortimer. Growth of hyperkinetic children taking methylphenidate, dextroamphetamine, or imipramine/desipramine. *Pediatrics* **58**:423–431 (1976).

Gross, Mortimer, and Wilson, W. C. *Minimal brain dysfunction.* New York: Brunner Mazel, 1974.

Johnson, Charles, and Prinz, Robert. Hyperactivity is in the eyes of the beholder. *Clinical Pediatrics* **15**:222–238 (1976).

Millichap, J. G. The hyperactive child. *Practitioner* **217**:61–65 (1976).

Pratt, Sandra, and Fischer, Joel. Behavior modification: Changing hyperactive behavior in a children's group. *Perspectives in Psychiatric Care* **13**:37–42 (1975).

Ross, Dorothea, and Ross, Sheila. *Hyperactivity: Research, theory and action.* New York: Wiley, 1976.

Rutter, Michael. *Helping troubled children.* New York: Plenum, 1975.

———, and Hersov, Lionel (eds.). *Child psychiatry—Modern approaches.* London: Blackwell, 1977.

Safer, Daniel, and Allen, Richard. *Hyperactive children—Diagnosis and management.* Baltimore: University Park Press, 1976.

Schmitt, B. Guidelines for living with a hyperactive child. *Pediatrics* **60**:387 (1977).

Shaw, Dr. Charles. *When your child needs help.* New York: Morrow, 1972.

Wolraich, Mark. Stimulant drug therapy in hyperactive children: Research and clinical implications. *Pediatrics* **60**:512–517 (1977).

81 Speech Changes/ Articulation Disorders

ELDON H. BAKER, JR.

ALERT

1. Cleft palate
2. Cerebral palsy
3. Impaired hearing
4. Dental anomalies
5. Obvious oral/structural anomalies, which include tongue and soft-tissue structures—general paralysis, flaccid and spastic

I. Etiology

A. Organic factors

1. Dentition
   a. Spaces between teeth
   b. Malocclusion
2. Palatal vault size/shape
   a. High palatal vault
   b. Narrow palatal vault
3. Tongue size/shape
   a. Tongue too large in relation to dental arch size
   b. Tongue unable to make rapid muscular movements for production of certain phonetic combinations
   c. Tongue-tie
4. Auditory proficiency
   a. Sound discrimination
   b. Pitch discrimination

B. Faculty learning

1. Disruption of normal learning process
2. Lack of stimulation and/or motivation

C. Developmental factors

1. Physical development
2. Illnesses
   a. Deprivation of socialization
   b. Trauma to oral structures
3. Intelligence and social maturity

II. Assessment[1,2]

A. Defective pronunciation of *s* and *z*, interdental lisp

1. Subjective data
   a. Disorder calls attention (negative) to speaker.
   b. Mouth fails to close sufficiently
2. Objective data
   a. Tongue tip approximates the edges of the front teeth.
   b. Often portion of tongue tip is visible during production of *s*.
   c. Resultant sound is [θ] (unvoiced *th*) with words like *sum* sounding like *thumb.*

B. Lateral lisp

1. Subjective data
   a. Speech may be unintelligible.
   b. Speech is perhaps uncomfortable for the listener.
   c. Disorder may call attention (negative) to speaker.
2. Objective data
   a. Tongue fails to maintain tight contact with the upper teeth and alveolar ridge.
   b. Breath stream allowed to escape uni- or bilaterally over the blade portion(s) of the tongue.
   c. Air escapes at point adjacent to lingual surface of cuspid(s) and/or bicuspid(s).
   d. Breath stream may be heard as emitted striking buccal surface.

[1]Space limitations prevent the inclusion of the differential diagnosis of all speech sounds. Most common consonant articulation errors are covered. The reader is referred to the bibliography for additional sources.

[2]Clients with articulation disorders should be referred to a speech therapist for evaluation and treatment.

C. Defective pronunciation of *r*

1. Subjective data
   a. Pronunciation sounds like "Bostonian" accent.
   b. Speech is infantile.
2. Objective data
   a. Hearing loss may be indicated, as fine discrimination is necessary for exact articulatory placement/production.
   b. Client has lack of motor control of tongue.
      (1) Paralysis
      (2) Poor oral motor kinesthesia (awareness)
   c. Foreign language background may result in variation of *r* production.
      (1) Rolling *r* sound
      (2) Trilled *r* sound
      (3) Client substitutes *w* for *r*, *w/r.*

D. Defects in pronunciation of [ð] and [θ], voiced and unvoiced *th*

1. Subjective data
   a. Speech may be unintelligible.
   b. Speech is perhaps uncomfortable for the listener.
   c. Disorder may call attention (negative) to speaker.
2. Objective data
   a. Sounds are not related to *t* or *h*.
   b. Common infantile substitution is *f* for [θ], *f/θ*.
   c. Auditory-discrimination abilities are often depressed.
   d. Both sounds are easily taught because of high visibility in production.

III. Management

A. Articulation disorders

1. Treatments/therapy
   a. Eliminate or minimize affecting factors.
   b. Teach auditory discrimination to assist the child in self-monitoring.
   c. Have child learn correct production of sound in isolation.
      (1) Oral motor exercises
      (2) Developing better oral awareness (teeth, lips, tongue, voice, and velum)
   d. Strengthen correct production of target sound.
   e. Have child transfer use of correct sound to nonsense syllables and short commonly used words.
   f. Increase the use of the correct sound in words, sentences, and spontaneous connected speech.
   g. Encourage carry-over to nontherapy situations.
2. Counselling/prevention
   a. Provide children with good speech models.
   b. Seek assistance of teachers in obtaining information about the child's classroom speech.
   c. Provide opportunities for child to express self freely without interruption and/or criticism.
3. Follow-up
   a. Give periodic diagnostic testing to chart progress.
   b. Communicate with other specialists to share information and seek new ideas or methods of remediation of specific problems.
   c. Hold phone conversations with parent(s).
4. Consultations/referrals
   a. Share therapy results, rationale, and procedures with all persons who work with the child in the school setting—principal, teacher, cafeteria personnel, custodians, etc.
   b. In the case of any suspect changes in child's physical well-being, refer child to proper medical authority—dentist, school nurse, otolaryngologist, psychologist, audiologist, marriage and family counselor for parent(s)/guardians.

Table 81-1 Medical Referral/Consultation

Diagnosis	Clinical Manifestations	Management
CLEFT PALATE Unilateral, bilateral, partial, or complete Submucous cleft Acquired cleft due to trauma	Incomplete closure of lip, alveolus, palate(s) Bifid uvula, which may indicate submucous cleft Cleftlike wound, which is evidence of oral trauma	Refer to physician. See Cleft Lip/Cleft Palate, Chap. 154.

Table 81-1 Medical Referral /Consultation *(continued)*

Diagnosis	Clinical Manifestations	Management
	Any combination of cleft conditions	
	Repaired-cleft situations, including repaired lip	Consult parent(s) as to history and any related problems that should be noted for future reference and/or management of existing condition.
CEREBRAL PALSY	Clinical manifestations of cerebral palsy (CP) are too numerous to include in this section. (Assume that the severely palsied child would be in a special school or program.) CP can cause all speech pathologies and even pathologies of speech that are as yet unknown, since it affects the neural mechanisms involved in speech and support systems (respiration, cranial nerves). Refer to bibliographic entries for additional information.	Consult with parent(s)/care giver as to any special medications and/or specific needs of child. Speech pathologist can help determine method of communication if child is unable to verbalize needs. Contact allied personnel regarding needs and assessment of child for optimum educational and health development. See Cerebral Palsy, Chap. 151.
IMPAIRED HEARING	Obstruction in external ear Excessive cerumen Foreign bodies Middle ear infection	Refer to otolaryngologist/audiologist for complete audiometric evaluation and assessment.
	Decrease in vocal intensity Increase in vocal intensity Short attention span Difficulties in following directions	Confer with parent(s)/care giver regarding history and/or previous medical treatments. See Deafness/Defective Hearing/Hearing Changes, Chap. 26, and Ear Pain/Discharge, Chap. 23.
DENTAL ANOMALIES AND IRREGULARITIES	Dull, continuous, throbbing pain. Possibly loose, carious, and raised tooth Possibly visible parulis on both lingual and/or buccal sides of tooth Edema—nasolabial fold, angle of jaw, eye, lips	Refer immediately to physician and dentist. Use cold packs for pain. Recommend saline mouthwashes. For counselling/prevention Instruct client in oral hygiene. Do follow-up.
	Deformation of teeth Rotated, tilted, incompletely erupted teeth Partial/incomplete eruption of supernumerary teeth Absence of dentition	Refer to oral specialists—orthodontist, otolaryngologist. Refer to speech pathologist. Refer to prosthodontist.
PARALYSIS OF ORAL-SOFT-TISSUE STRUCTURE(S)	Inability to voluntarily position tongue or lips on command	Consult physician: refer to otolaryngologist and/or neurologist.

Table 81-1 Medical Referral/Consultation *(continued)*

Diagnosis	Clinical Manifestations	Management
	Asymmetry of oral/facial structures—smiling, expressions	
	Asymmetry of velar tensors and levators during phonation of nonnasal sounds	

bibliography

Anderson, Virgil A. *Improving the child's speech.* New York: Oxford, 1953.

Fairbanks, Grant. *Voice and articulation drill book* (2d ed.). New York: Harper & Row, 1960.

Fisher, Hilda B. *Improving voice and articulation.* Boston: Houghton Mifflin, 1966.

Johnson, Wendell, et al. *Diagnostic methods in speech pathology.* New York: Harper & Row, 1963.

——— *Speech-handicapped school children* (3d ed.). New York: Harper & Row, 1967.

Travis, Lee E. *Handbook of speech pathology and audiology.* New York: Appleton Century Crofts, 1971.

Van Riper, Charles. *Speech correction, principles and methods.* Englewood Cliffs, N.J.: Prentice-Hall, 1963.

82 Headaches ELEANOR RUDICK

ALERT
1. Headache in young child
2. Vision changes

I. Etiology

A. Vascular
1. Migraine
2. Secondary to fever
3. Hypertensive

B. Related to epilepsy

C. Secondary to changes in intracranial pressure
1. Brain tumor
2. Low cerebrospinal fluid (CSF) pressure

D. Tension

E. Related to psychiatric disease

F. Eyestrain (refractive error)

G. Nasal sinus pain

H. Trauma

I. Referred pain from teeth or ear

II. Assessment: Tension Headache, Eyestrain

A. Subjective data
1. Pain
   a. Usually precipitated by emotional stress
   b. Does not start suddenly
   c. Radiates from neck to frontal region bilaterally; sometimes frontally predominant; dull, steady; increases with time
   d. Relieved by sleep and medication
   e. May cause vomiting
2. Social history may reveal
   a. Strained family relationships
   b. Strained peer relationships
   c. Poor scholastic standing

B. Objective data: physical examination and laboratory data that are essentially negative

III. Management Tension Headache, Eyestrain

A. Treatments/medications
1. Give aspirin or acetaminophen for pain.
2. Apply warm packs to back of neck.
3. Apply warm or cool packs to forehead.
4. Correct refractive error.

B. Counselling/prevention
1. Discuss with parent(s) and client the emotional nature of the symptoms.
2. See child alone and encourage ventilation.
3. Keep diary of headache activity—precipitating factors, character, duration and relief of pain.

C. Follow-up
1. See client weekly.
2. Provide individual counselling.

D. Consultations/referrals
1. If client is depressed, refer for professional counselling.
2. Contact guidance counsellor and teacher at school.
3. If refractive error is evident, refer client to ophthalmologist.

bibliography

Batzdorf, Ulrich. The management of cerebral edema in pediatric practice. *Pediatrics,* **58**(1):78–87 (1976).

Pearson, Linda Buck. A protocol for the chief complaint of headache. *The Nurse Practitioner,* **2**(1):12–16, 37 (1976).

Prensky, Arthur L. Migraine and migrainous variants in pediatric patients. *Pediatric Clinics of North America,* **23**(3):461–471 (1976).

Table 82-1 Medical Referral/Consultation

Assessment	Clinical Manifestations	Management
Classic migraine	Onset in late childhood/early adolescence Preceded by visual aura Positive family history History of repeated vomiting in infancy Throbbing, unilateral head pain Nausea and vomiting Usually terminated by sleep Frequency (appears to be) increased by stress Absence of findings on funduscopic, physical, and neurological examinations	Refer to neurologist. Laboratory data may include Skull x-rays. EEG. Brain scan to ensure benign condition. Therapy may include Vasoconstrictors: Cafergot—1 tablet (over 10 yr of age) at first sign of attack; repeat 4 times at 30-min intervals as needed (used in clients whose attacks occur once per month or less). Aspirin. Assess family to determine possible sources of tension.
Headache as a symptom of epilepsy	Part of aura preceding grand mal seizure Postictal event Part of autonomic seizure	Refer to neurologist for Possible change in dosage of anticonvulsant medication Change in or addition to medication Reevaluation of seizure status
Headache secondary to intracranial pressure change Increased Decreased	Increased intracranial pressure Pain that follows change in head position Morning headache suspicious of brain tumor Vomiting (with nausea) followed by feeling of well-being Occipital pain indicative of posterior fossa tumor Presence of funduscopic changes Decreased intracranial pressure Usually due to persistent CSF leak after spinal tap Occurs after traumatic meningeal tears Appears on assumption of upright position; relieved by lying down	Refer immediately to physician for Diagnostic procedures Skull x-rays. Brain scan. EEG. Possible surgery. Possible chemotherapy. Possible radiation. See Preparation for Hospitalization, Part 7.
Headache related to psychiatric disease	Described as continuously present Symptoms of depression Appearance of suffering Depressed speech Poor appetite; constipation Insomnia	Refer for professional counselling. See Family Assessment, Chap. 1. Medication possibly tranquilizer, determined by client's age.

83 Anxiety

KAREN A. BALLARD

ALERT
1. Shortness of breath
2. Edema
3. Diastolic heart murmur
4. Systolic heart murmur greater than grade II/VI

I. Etiology of Childhood Anxiety

A. Contagion—close contact with anxious people

B. Experience—people and sudden, upsetting events

C. Intrapsychic—specific problems in parent-child relationship

II. Assessment

A. Subjective data

1. Anxiety is normal, is usually perceived by the client as diffuse and undirected, and may noticeably increase in preadolescence, especially in girls.
2. Events precipitating anxiety should be seen as trigger phenomena, not as the main cause.
   a. New experiences
   b. Darkness
   c. Examinations
   d. Separation
3. Episodes occur with the following frequency
   a. Usually 2 to 3 times per week
   b. Duration—from several minutes to 30 minutes
4. Client is described as
   a. Hyperactive—restless and fidgety
   b. Having short attention span
   c. Performing tasks and play activities rapidly
   d. Having difficulty maintaining peer relationships
   e. Having disturbed sleep pattern
   f. Showing physical symptoms and complaining
   g. Performing poorly in school
   h. Performing poorly at work
5. Mild anxiety may be perceived as a general fearfulness, and may present as
   a. Changes in skin color
   b. Sweating palms
   c. Dry mouth
   d. Increased heart rate
   e. General muscle tenseness
6. Severe anxiety (anxiety attack) can be very upsetting, especially when accompanied by terror episodes, and may present as
   a. Cardiac complaints
      (1) Rapid heart rate
      (2) Chest pains—"I have pain around my heart."
   b. Respiratory complaints
      (1) Fear of dying
      (2) Shortness of breath—"I'm afraid I can't breathe."
   c. Digestive complaints—vomiting, stomach ache
   d. Dizziness
   e. Shaking, trembling, panic stare
   f. Profuse sweating
   g. Frequent urinating
   h. Pleas for reassurance and comfort
7. Normal anxiety is differentiated from severe abnormal anxiety by quantitative/qualitative evaluation.
   a. Difference in frequency
   b. Severity and persistence
   c. The client's own ability to tolerate the anxiety

8. Anxiety in children frequently occurs in the evening, either just prior to bedtime or during sleeping period and is more frequent in boys than in girls.

B. Objective data

1. Physical examination—should be normal; some or all of the physical symptoms associated with anxiety (see above) may be present.
2. Laboratory data—normal

III. Management

A. Treatments/medications

1. Severe anxiety—although debatable, it may be necessary to administer low doses of phenothiazine tranquilizers, diazepam, or chlordiazepoxide.
2. Medication therapy should be short-term, concurrent with counselling or psychotherapy, and used only after consultation with a physician.

B. Counselling/prevention

1. Explain to parent(s) that apparent event-related anxiety in children is often the trigger of more serious difficulties.
2. Parent(s) and client should be engaged in family/individual psychotherapy.
3. Specific parent-child problems should be explored and identified.
4. Often a calm and authoritative, reassuring manner in the practitioner will effectively reduce and/or alleviate the presenting anxiety; however, additional counselling should always be planned.

C. Follow-up

1. Number of visits depends on severity of anxiety; visits are usually weekly for 3 to 6 months, and can be tapered if symptoms are alleviated.
2. Focus should be on any parent-child relationship problems and/or on the client's responses and tolerance to anxiety-stimulating environments.

D. Consultations/referrals

1. Professional counselling
2. Teacher and school nurse

Table 83-1 Medical Referral/Consultation

Diagnosis/Problem	Manifestations	Management
Cardiac problems	Any abnormal cardiac findings upon physical examination Shortness of breath Edema Diastolic heart murmur Systolic heart murmur greater than grade II/VI	Immediate referral to pediatric cardiologist

bibliography

Barnett, Henry. *Pediatrics* (16th ed.). New York: Appleton Century Crofts, 1977.

Elliot, Raymond. Influencing the behavior of children in emotional conflict. *The Nurse Practitioner* **2**:18–19 (1977).

Kanner, Leo. *Child psychiatry* (4th ed.). Springfield, Ill.: Charles C Thomas, 1972.

Padilla, E. R., Rohsenow, D. J., and Bergman, A. B. Predicting accident frequency in children. *Pediatrics* **58**:223–226 (1976).

Rutter, Michael, and Hersor, Lionel (eds.). *Child psychiatry—Modern approaches.* London: Blackwell, 1977.

Scipien, Gladys, et al. *Comprehensive pediatric nursing* (2d ed.). New York: McGraw-Hill, 1979.

Shaw, Charles. *When your child needs help.* New York: Morrow, 1972.

84 Depression

PAULENE S. JOHNSON

ALERT
1. Behavior which interferes with activities of daily living
2. Suicidal thoughts or behavior (see Suicide, Chap. 85)

I. Etiology

A. Core factors of depression
1. External loss
   a. Death of a loved one
   b. Illness that changes the client's ability to function
   c. Parental separation or divorce
   d. Additions or deletions in family constellation
   e. Change in family's place of residence
   f. Graduation from school
2. Internal loss
   a. Encountering personal attitudes and actions which violate the client's beliefs and values
   b. Interpersonal conflicts that threaten to disrupt the client's sense of security and self-esteem

B. Although the onset of depression is almost always a response to loss, the maintenance of depressive behaviors may be a result of operant conditioning. For example, concern and sympathy from others may serve to reinforce symptoms.

II. Assessment

A. Subjective data
1. Vague physical complaints, particularly those involving the GI tract, constipation, loss of appetite
2. Pain which increases in the morning and lessens toward noon
3. History of multiple illnesses over prolonged period of time in either client or family
4. History of insomnia, nightmares
5. Fatigue
6. Inability to concentrate
7. Decision-making difficulty
8. Irritability
9. Recent weight loss/gain
10. Loss of significant person through death or separation
11. Loss of pet
12. Difficulty with school work
13. Graduation from school
14. Expressed feelings of hopelessness, helplessness, guilt
15. Depreciatory self-description

B. Objective data
1. Physical examination within normal limits
2. Laboratory data within normal limits
3. Evidence of self-inflicted abuse
4. Slow walking
5. Slumping rather than sitting straight
6. Talking slowly and with difficulty
7. Affect: flat, hostile, or cries easily
8. Lack of eye contact

III. Management[1]

A. Treatments/medications
1. Supportive therapy
2. Medications
   a. Use only when client is managed in consultation with physician/psychiatrist.

[1]*Note:* Moderate and severe depression should be managed in consultation with a physician and/or professional counsellor.

b. Most antidepressant medications achieve optimum effectiveness in 10 to 14 days. This is important information to convey to the client/family who may be tempted to discontinue the medication before the results of the drug therapy become apparent.

3. Antidepressant drug therapy is initiated in the lower end of the therapeutic-dosage range, and is gradually increased if necessary only after careful evaluation
   a. Nortriptyline HCl (Aventyl)—adolescents, 30 to 50 mg/day in divided doses; not recommended for children under 12 years
   b. Amitriptyline HCl (Elavil)—adolescents, 10 mg 3 times per day, with 20 mg at night; not recommended for children under 12 years
   c. Imipramine HCl (Tofranil)—adolescents, initially 30 to 40 mg daily in divided doses; children over 6 years, initially 25 mg daily in divided doses; not recommended for children under 6 years
   d. Doxepin HCl (Sinequan)—adolescents, 25 mg 3 times per day; not recommended for children under 12 years

B. Counselling/prevention—provide supportive therapy.

1. Establish an empathetic, sensitive, and stable relationship.
2. If depression is due to loss of a loved one, a cathartic experience enabling the client to work through anger and guilt usually facilitates the healthy expression of sorrow and diminishes the depression. As losses are acknowledged, the client needs to sense others care.
3. Involve family members early in the treatment regime, and encourage their assessment of relationships and communication patterns. If communication appears to be a problem, identify the maladaptive modes of communication and assist the client and family in developing more adaptive methods of relating to each other. When working with the family of a depressed child, it is important to avoid placing blame or creating guilt feelings among family members. If the problem appears to be conditioned depressive behavior rather than primary depression, encourage family members to acknowledge the client's positive behavior with frequent and immediate attention and decrease the amount of attention focused on the "sick" behavior.
4. The client who expresses feelings of helplessness and hopelessness needs to gain a sense of control and self-worth. Increasing coping abilities often promotes this development. Coping abilities can be strengthened by
   a. Assisting the client in redefining personal assets and liabilities and in establishing goals congruent with own strengths
   b. Helping to identify and develop alternate ways of functioning
   c. Aiding development of the ability to anticipate and plan for difficult situations
   d. Encouraging healthy self-interest
   e. Involving the depressed client in appropriate task performances, since recognition and approval of the performance by those significant to the client is crucial

C. Follow-up—encourage frequent visits for supportive therapy and evaluation during initial stages of treatment, and thereafter, well-child-care visits.

D. Consultations/referrals

1. Client with any depressive syndromes should be referred to physician and/or professional counsellor.
2. Evaluation of school environment sometimes reveals sources of stress.
3. Family therapy often has a high success rate in the treatment of depressed families.

bibliography

Arieti, Silvano. *Severe and mild depression: a psychotherapeutic approach.* New York: Basic Books, 1978.

Kiev, Ari. Management of depressed and suicidal patients. *American Journal of Psychotherapy* **25:** 345–354 (1975).

Kovacs, Maria, et al. The use of motives in the psychotherapy of attempted suicides. *American Journal of Psychotherapy* **29:**363–368 (1975).

Liberman, R., and Raskin, D. Depression: A behavioral formulation. *Archives of General Psychiatry* **24:** 515–523 (1971).

Spiegle R. Anger and acting out; Masks of depression. *American Journal of Orthopsychiatry* **21:**597–606 (1976).

Wicks, Robert J. *Counseling strategies and intervention techniques for human services.* Philadelphia: Lippincott, 1977.

Table 84-1 Medical Referral/Consultation

Diagnosis/Problem	Clinical Manifestations	Management
Depression, severe, with suicide proneness	Walks in almost paralyzed fashion; talks with great difficulty Expresses wish to die ("No reason to live.") Makes bizarre statements Fears suicidal thoughts or actions are uncontrollable Is extremely agitated Is obsessed by guilt States loved ones would be better off if he or she were dead Has history of suicide attempt(s) Has history of suicide in the family	Refer immediately to psychiatrist. Take action to ensure safe environment.

85 Suicide

NANCY ANN CALLAND HART

ALERT

1. Giving away of prized possessions
2. Increasing moroseness and isolation from others
3. Statements such as, "My family would be better off without me."
4. A sudden elevation of mood
5. Frequent self-destructive acts

I. Etiology: Theories of Suicide

A. *No one comprehensive theory*

B. Constellation of feelings common to both those who attempt and those who complete suicide

1. Deprivation
2. Guilt
3. Helplessness, hopelessness, worthlessness
4. Impulsive rejection

C. Developmentally related theories

1. Infancy
   a. Maternal-infant bond is not established.
   b. Formation of basic trust is disrupted.
      (1) Loss of parent(s)
      (2) Inability of parent to provide warm, trusting relationship
2. Childhood
   a. Child 8 years or younger may not understand the finality of death.
   b. Heaven may seem a temporary place where there are no frustrations.
   c. Completed suicide is extremely uncommon for children under 12 years of age.
      (1) Inability to develop an effective plan
      (2) Inability to procure means to complete the act
      (3) Close adult supervision
      (4) Depressions not as overwhelming as those of adolescents
3. Adolescence
   a. This is normally a time of rapid change and high stress.
   b. Coping mechanisms are severely tested.
      (1) Intensified feelings of self-awareness
      (2) Possible feelings of inferiority to peers
      (3) Struggle with independence versus dependence
      (4) Rapid physical changes
      (5) Emerging sexual feelings that may cause confusion, frustration, guilt
      (6) Concerns over future vocation
      (7) Struggle to establish personal identity
      (8) Very idealistic attitudes which may lead to discouragement with existing realities
   c. There are relatively few places where children/adolescents can seek out help.

D. Long-standing history of multiple problems which seem to escalate

1. Wide range of problems have beem implicated.
   a. Chronic illness
   b. Intrafamily tensions
   c. Frequent residential moves
   d. School failure; dropping out of school
   e. Parental loss, especially by desertion, divorce, or separation
   f. Relatives and/or friends who committed suicide
   g. Circumscribed social life; lack of close, personal friend
   h. Alcoholic parent(s)
   i. Parental feelings of ambivalence; actual physical and/or emotional abuse

j. Economic problems
k. Lack of environmental control
l. Lack of warm, loving parent(s)

2. Long-standing problems plus developmental tensions create explosive situation.
3. Severing of meaningful relationships or failure of boyfriend/girlfriend to fill the void may lead to suicide attempt.

E. Sociological theories

1. Rapid social change
2. Rising divorce rate with subsequent family alienation
3. Availability of cars, drugs, alcohol
4. Inability of society to provide integrating mechanisms for adolescents

F. Freudian theory

1. Individual's ego identifies itself with beloved person.
2. Individual is denied this person through loss by death or rejection.
3. Instead of destroying loved one, the angered individual destroys the representation of that object within himself or herself, i.e., the self.

G. Suicide is not necessarily associated with mental illness; the relationship between depression and suicide is not clarified by research.

H. Aggression/impulsiveness in preadolescents and younger children

1. Child may turn aggression towards self as punishment for guilt because of death wishes or masturbatory activities.
2. Aggression often represents elements of revenge or spite toward parent(s) or whole family.
3. Childhood suicide is marked by impulsiveness, i.e., little or no planning or premeditation.

II. Assessment: Potential Suicide

A. Subjective data

1. Feelings of helplessness, hopelessness, and worthlessness
2. Apathy, boredom
3. Feelings of rejection, isolation
4. Deflated self-image
5. Feelings of anger, aggression
6. Sexual anxieties
7. Excessive worry over academic success
8. Sleep disturbances
   a. Nightmares
   b. Difficulty falling asleep
   c. Early-morning awakening
9. Loss of appetite, excessive eating
10. Feelings of depression
11. Decrease in or lack of ability to tolerate frustration
12. History of acting out behaviors
    a. Truancy
    b. Delinquent acts
       (1) Stealing
       (2) Vandalism
    c. Running away from home
    d. Promiscuity
    e. Excessive use of addictive substances
    f. Reckless driving
    g. Aggressive acts toward family and/or peers
13. Accident proneness
14. School difficulties
    a. Declining grades
    b. Disrupting classroom behavior
15. Withdrawal from peers, usual activities
16. Inactivity; decrease in verbal communications
17. Excessive crying
18. Increased intrafamily tensions
19. Possible history of past loss with prolonged grief reaction

B. Objective data

1. Little or no eye contact
2. Possible happy or jovial appearance
3. Crying
4. Low voice; not very verbal
5. Usually normal physical examination, possibly with signs of self-inflicted wounds (scars on wrists) and other signs of physical abuse, signs of drug-induced toxicity, or pregnancy
6. Physical appearance that may reveal poor personal hygiene

III. Management: Potential Suicide

A. General

1. Practitioners need to identify and resolve their own feelings.
   a. Possible anger toward client
   b. Possible ambivalent feelings about life, death, and death by suicide
2. Treatments/medications
   a. Short-term management
      (1) Do psychological evaluation of client and family.
      (2) Determine if suicide is still a possibility.
      (3) Show empathetic acknowledgment of pain; adolescent may feel there is someone who understands.
      (4) Be sensitive to subtle changes in mood, behavior.

(5) Mutually attempt to find solutions to any immediate problems, e.g., overloaded school schedule.

b. Long-term management

(1) Demonstrate a caring, concerned attitude.

(a) Adolescent may test this by calling to talk at inconvenient times.

(b) Adolescent needs to feel someone cares.

(c) Practitioner must recognize own limitations; i.e., he or she cannot be "all-loving."

(2) Determine individual's personality strengths and emphasize them.

(a) Enlist family/friends to provide information about past and present strengths.

1. Child or adolescent may be incapable of seeing any good in self ("tunnel vision").

2. Past strengths may be an important resource which could affect present ability to cope.

(b) Be aware of client's potentialities; this awareness can be very supportive and offer hope.

(c) Explore these areas with client.

1. Interest and/or participation in sports

2. Hobbies

3. Interest and/or participation in the expressive arts

4. Health status

5. Job experiences

6. Special aptitudes, e.g., typing

7. Intellectual strengths

8. Appreciation of beauty, aesthetic strengths

9. Organizational strengths

10. Creativeness

11. Relationship strengths, i.e., capacity to get along with others

12. Spiritual strengths

13. Emotional strengths, i.e., ability to give love

(3) Frequently assess client's ability to function.

(4) Allow ventilation of feelings.

(a) Client may not be very verbal, especially if depressed.

(b) In the beginning, short frequent contacts are effective.

(c) Decide mutually on frequency, length of sessions.

(d) Talk about actual suicide attempt and events preceding it.

(5) Explore alternative, constructive ways of coping.

(6) Establish what in life is meaningful to the client.

(a) Find out what the individual values or loves most.

(b) Suggest a book that deals with this theme (e.g., Frankl, 1963).

(7) Help client determine immediate goals.

(a) To regain emotional balance

(b) To learn to utilize adaptive behaviors as solutions to life's problems

3. Counselling/prevention

a. Primary prevention

(1) Promote health education courses that include instruction on emotional health in elementary and junior and senior high schools.

(2) Establish and promote hotlines.

(3) Sponsor conferences for health professionals about suicide.

(4) Work along with school nurse to screen for emotionally distressed students.

(5) Act as consultant for agencies which work with youths, such as runaway houses, church youth groups.

b. Secondary prevention

(1) Be active in case finding, remembering *anyone can be suicidal*.

(2) Initiate prompt treatment.

c. Tertiary prevention

(1) Continue relationship with client until a high level of wellness is reached.

(2) Act as liason with community mental health centers and schools in this effort.

4. Postvention—care of the survivors

a. Recognize reactions of survivors.

(1) Shame

(2) Guilt

(3) Anger

(4) Hatred

(5) Confusion

(6) Obsessive thoughts about the suicide

(7) Possible long-term physical and emotional sequelae

b. Survivors often feel isolated.

(1) Friends may avoid them; it is an awkward situation.

(2) Survivors become absorbed in own thoughts.

c. Provide opportunities for ventilation of feelings.

(1) One-to-one
(2) Small groups
(3) Be accessible as a compassionate, caring person

5. Follow-up
   a. Keep in constant contact; be available to individual if situation escalates.
   b. Be alert to any physical or psychological changes.
6. Consultations/referrals
   a. Refer for professional counselling as necessary following psychological assessment.
   b. If referral is made, personally escort client to decrease feelings of rejection.

B. Potential suicide: very depressed person

1. Treatments/medications
   a. Ask directly whether client is contemplating suicide.
   b. This will not "cause" a suicide.
2. Counselling/prevention (see General management, III, A)
3. Follow-up (see General management, III, A)
4. Consultations/referrals (see General management, III, A)

C. Potential suicide: threatening suicide

1. Treatments/medications
   a. Document the degree of suicidal ideation.
      (1) Less serious: "Sometimes I wish I were dead."
      (2) More serious: "I constantly think about suicide, and I have a plan."
   b. Determine cause of suicidal feelings.
      (1) Precipitating event
      (2) Chronic problems
   c. Find out if there are specific plans, and determine lethality of plans.
   d. Determine duration of threat.
   e. Determine if there have been any previous attempts.
   f. Determine if adolescent has recently been using drugs/alcohol.
      (1) If alcohol use is heavy, client is at greater risk and may need hospitalization.
      (2) Encourage teenager not to drink or use drugs.
2. Counselling/prevention (see General management, III, A)
3. Follow-up (see General management, III, A)
4. Consultations/referrals—refer to physician/psychiatrist any client who
   a. Is severely depressed
   b. Has serious suicidal ideation
   c. Has specific plans
   d. Has attempted suicide
   e. Has a sudden elation of mood

references

Frankl, Viktor. *Man's search for meaning.* New York: Washington Square Press, 1963.

bibliography

Aguilera, Donna. *Crisis intervention.* St. Louis: Mosby, 1974.

Copel, Sidney. *Behavior pathology of childhood and adolescence.* New York: Basic Books, 1973.

Draper, Edgar. A developmental theory of suicide. *Comprehensive Psychiatry* **17**:63–80 (1976).

Duncan, Jane W. The immediate management of suicide attempts in children and adolescents. *The Journal of Family Practice* **4**:77–80 (1977).

Grollman, Earl. *Suicide.* Boston: Beacon Press, 1971.

Haim, Andre. *Adolescent suicide.* New York: International Universities Press, 1974.

Hart, Nancy A., and Keidel, Gladys. The suicidal adolescent. *American Journal of Nursing* **79**(1): 80–84 (1979).

Hofmann, Adele D. Adolescents in distress: Suicide and out-of-control behaviors. *Medical Clinics of North America* **59**:1429–1437 (1975).

Marks, Philip A., and Haller, Deborah L. Now I lay me down for keeps: A study of adolescent suicide attempts. *Journal of Clinical Psychology* **33**:390–400 (1977),

McAnarney, Elizabeth R. Suicidal behavior of children and youth. *Pediatric Clinics of North America* **22**:595–604 (1975).

Prentice, Glen. Evaluating suicide potential. *The Nurse Practitioner* **2**:30–31 (1977).

Table 85-1 Medical Referral/Consultation

Diagnosis	Clinical Manifestations	Management
Immediately following an attempt	Depend on Method utilized Success of attempt	Physical protection If possible, prevent any physical harm. Remove pills, firearms, etc. Use physical containment, if necessary. Protect others from injury. If any harm has occurred, transport client to hospital. Psychological intervention Set goals. Restore calm atmosphere. Establish more rational thought processes. Presence of helping person may have tranquilizing effect. Tension is reduced. Client can hand over responsiblity of coping to practitioner. Establish "lifeline." Calmly reassure client to promote feelings of safety. Show that actions will be taken to preserve life. Quality of relationship between practitioner and client is important. Be sincere, warm. Use firm, positive manner. Avoid judgmental or moralistic attitude, as that will only alienate adolescent. Avoid bargaining or threatening. Psychotherapeutic agents may be necessary. Give chlorpromazine 10 mg IM to an average-sized adolescent or $^1/_4$ mg/lb. Dose may be repeated in 30–45 min. Monitor blood pressure for hypotensive effects. Determine if client has recently taken another drug.

section 9

the musculoskeletal system

INTRODUCTION JANE A FOX

I. **Subjective Data**

A. Age

B. Reason for visit and description of problem

1. Onset
2. Present history of trauma, injury
3. Association with pain
   a. Precise time of onset
   b. Specific location of pain
   c. Progression and severity
   d. Alteration by activity
      (1) Worse in early morning or late in day
      (2) Relieved by rest

C. Birth history

1. Trauma
2. Breech delivery

D. Past/present history of and treatment received

1. Fractures/dislocations
2. Sprains/strains
3. Deformities
4. Joint swelling/pain/redness
5. Joint laxity/hypermotility
6. Muscle weakness/cramps
7. Paralysis
8. Limp
9. Back pain or other pain
10. Limitation of movement
11. Swelling
12. Bleeding tendency
13. Severe illness/infection
14. Clumsiness
15. Other trauma

E. Recent history of minor infections or contact with infectious illness

1. Skin
2. Respiratory system

F. Alteration in normal behavior

1. Activity pattern and ease of fatigue
2. Appetite
3. Sleep

G. Developmental history

H. Immunization history

1. Polio
2. Tetanus

I. Congenital anomalies

J. Onset of puberty

K. Family history

1. Height characteristics
2. Toe-walking
3. Rheumatoid arthritis
4. Genetic disorders
5. Back deformity/other skeletal deformities
6. Recent infectious diseases
7. Joint laxity or hypermotility
8. Bleeding tendency
9. Limp

L. Social history

1. School, occupational, and recreational activities
2. Exercise interests and tolerance

3. Living conditions and financial capability to comply with treatment regimen

II. Objective Data

A. Physical examination

1. Take temperature, height, and weight.
2. Observe general body configuration for signs of scoliosis; leg-length discrepancy; hip, leg, or foot deformities; and determine range of motion (hip–Ortolani's sign).
3. Note the following.
   a. Leg lengths
   b. Measurements of calf and thigh circumference bilaterally
   c. Position of patellae
   d. Intermalleoli interval, with knees together (knock-knee interval)
   e. Intercondylar interval, with ankles together (bowleg interval)
   f. Position of feet
   g. Presence of joint contractures
4. Examine gait.
   a. With child undressed
   b. For distance of 20 to 30 ft
   c. Observing back, hip, knee, foot
   d. Noting step length; rate; if antalgic (associated with pain); gluteus medial lurch; knee flexion; degree of asymmetry (unilateral/bilateral); and degree of discrepancy
5. If leg-length inequality is suspected
   a. Measure height of lift needed under short side to level pelvis.
   b. Measure length from anterior superior iliac spine to medial malleolus.
   c. Recognize that results provide good clinical guide, not exact measurement.
6. Palpate every inch of spine and extremities. If foot deformity is noted, attempt passive correction to the midline.
7. Perform neurological examination.
   a. Muscle groups: size, tone, strength
   b. Sensory exam
   c. Reflexes
8. Inspect and palpate spine for scoliosis.
   a. Spine and chest must be exposed.
   b. Have client bend forward at waist with feet together, knees unbent, both arms hanging freely, and back parallel to floor.
   c. Examine from the front and rear. Note any
      (1) Lateral spinal curvature
      (2) Unilateral prominence or projection of the rib cage.
   d. Have client stand erect with feet together; inspect and palpate spinous process for asymmetry.
      (1) Difference in shoulder or scapula height
      (2) Prominence of one scapula or one hip
      (3) Difference in size of spaces between trunk and arms
      (4) Curve in the alignment of the vertebral spinous process
9. Examine injured part.
   a. Swelling
   b. Area/point of maximum tenderness
   c. Instability and comparison with opposite side
   d. Drainage
   e. Voluntary function
   f. Range of motion

B. Laboratory data: the following may be indicated.

1. Complete blood count and erythrocyte sedimentation rate if active infection is suspected.
2. Do urinalysis.
3. Take x-ray (bilateral for comparison) for
   a. Suspected bone or joint abnormality
   b. Suspected foreign body
   c. Significant or progressive deformity
   d. Suspected abnormality of bone (fracture, dislocation); rupture of ligament; or soft-tissue abnormality
   e. Significant swelling and no bony abnormality; in this case, stress films.
4. Do culture of joint fluid if aspiration is indicated.

86 Foot Deformities

ELEANOR RUDICK

ALERT
Fixed position

I. Etiology (often unknown)

A. Flatfoot (pes planus)
1. Fat distribution in infant's foot resembles flat foot
2. Familial/ethnic
3. Compensatory
   a. Position of preference in crib
   b. Short first metatarsal
   c. Genu valgum (knock-knee)
   d. Increased pelvic inclination
4. Connective tissue laxity
5. Tightness of calf muscle
6. Component of more serious disease, e.g., cerebral palsy, Marfan's syndrome

B. Metatarsus adductus
1. Possible genetic factor
2. Intrauterine position
3. Crib position

C. Clubfoot
1. Genetic
2. Possible intrauterine environmental factors
3. Part of larger pathological problem
   a. Hydrocephalus
   b. Myelomeningocele
   c. Cerebral palsy

II. Assessment: Flatfoot

A. Subjective data
1. Complaints of foot pain/fatigue
2. No noticeable arch in foot

B. Objective data
1. Valgus heel
2. Lateral displacement of anterior foot
3. No arch visible when client stands on toes
4. Inability to stand on heels
5. Shoes worn on inner side

III. Management: Flatfoot

A. Treatments/medications
1. "Cookies" in shoes
2. Shoe lifts
3. Improving muscle strength by walking on tiptoes 5 to 10 min/day.

B. Counselling/prevention
1. Reassure parent(s) that infant's feet normally appear flat and that it is difficult to make a definite diagnosis until child is about 9 years of age.
2. Some pain may be relieved by using "cookies" in shoes.
3. Instruct parent(s) that best treatment is probably exercises to strengthen the foot-supporting muscles.

C. Follow-up: see client as needed and for well-child care.

D. Consultations/referrals: consult physician/orthopedist if child still has no arch by the age of 4.

Table 86-1 Medical Referral/Consultation

Diagnosis	Clinical Manifestations	Management
Metatarsus adductus (6–8 wk of age)	Forefoot adduction; possible valgus heel, ankle; cushion unaffected; pigeon-toe frequently associated with congenital dysplasia of hip	Refer to orthopedist. Counsel regarding treatment. The earlier the treatment, the better the results. For young infant use simple splint, if passive correction is easily achieved. For older infant use Denis-Browne splint to prevent internal rotation in sleep. When passive correction and active eversion cannot be elicited, use serial casting, then splinting for maintenance. If untreated, condition may persist for life. Client requires long-term follow-up, hospitalization for recasting. Consider social service referral based on family assessment.
Clubfoot	Foot Varus forefoot; varus heel Fixed equine position Smaller affected foot Neonate: hind foot possibly red and shiny with paucity of soft tissue about heel Single deep transverse crease at heel: almost pathognomonic of severe deformity requiring surgery Ankle: axis of cushion altered Knee: possible genu valgum; patella directed laterally Leg: length discrepancy Back: possible scoliosis Other foot: possibly flat	Refer immediately to orthopedist. Treat as follows. Start serial casting on first day of life if possible. After that use splinting. Then use corrective shoes. Use night splinting (until client is 5 yr). Surgery may be indicated for residual problems. Parents and children can be assured a good result with immediate, diligent, and long-term treatment. Social service referral should be based on family assessment.

bibliography

Bunch, Wilton H. Common deformities of the lower limb. *Pediatric Nursing,* **5**(4):18–22 (1979).

Clarren, Sterling K., and Smith, David W. Congenital deformities. *Pediatric Clinics of North America,* **24**(4):665–677 (1977).

Kane, Rosamond, and Krom, Wilfred. Deformities of the foot. In John Downey and Niels L. Low (eds.), *The child with disabling illness.* Philadelphia: Saunders, 1974, pp. 389–407.

Stabeli, Lynn T. Torsional deformities. *Pediatric Clinics of North America,* **24**(4):799–811 (1977).

Vaughan, Victor C., and McKay, R. James (eds.). *Nelson textbook of pediatrics* (10th ed.). Philadelphia: Saunders, 1975, pp. 1492–1493.

87 Leg Deformities

CAROLYN B. COLWELL

ALERT
1. Obvious deformity where correct alignment cannot be achieved passively
2. Generalized neurological dysfunction or muscular weakness
3. Unilateral or asymmetrical involvement

I. Etiology

A. Congenital abnormalities
1. Abnormal intrauterine position
2. Hereditary abnormalities
   a. Joint laxity
   b. Dwarfism
3. Myelodysplasia
4. Cerebral palsy

B. Trauma
1. Fractures
2. Epiphyseal plate disturbances

C. Infection
1. Bone: osteomyelitis
2. Joint: septic hip
3. Neurogenic: poliomyelitis

D. Acquired diseases
1. Blount's disease (tibia vara)
2. Rickets
3. Persistent malposture

E. Tumors

II. Assessment

A. Femoral anteversion
1. Subjective data: client or parent(s) complains of pigeon-toed or knock-kneed appearance
2. Objective data
   a. More frequent in girls
   b. In-toeing
   c. Possible bowlegged appearance
   d. Possible clumsy gait with patellae facing inward
   e. Excessive internal rotation of hips
      (1) Usually beyond 90°
      (2) Tested with client prone, hips extended, and knees flexed
   f. Possible limited external rotation of hips, with client in above position

B. Genu varum (bowleg)
1. Subjective data
   a. Age range, 1 to 3 years
   b. Normal growth and development
2. Objective data
   a. Presence of bowleg interval
   b. Rolling gait
   c. Possible in-toeing

C. Genu valgum (knock-knee)
1. Subjective data
   a. Common age range, 3 to 7 years
   b. Possible inactivity or obesity
   c. Normal growth and development
2. Objective data
   a. Presence of knock-knee interval
   b. Awkward gait
      (1) Knees rubbing
      (2) Legs swinging out
   c. Possible pronated feet
   d. Possible in-toeing or out-toeing

D. Internal tibial torsion
1. Subjective data
   Possible familial history of abnormal internal tibial torsion
2. Objective data
   a. In-toeing gait
   b. Line drawn from proximal tibial tubercle through midpoint between the medial and lateral malleoli intersects fourth or fifth toe

III. Management

A. Femoral anteversion

1. Treatments/medications: none
2. Counselling/prevention
   a. Spontaneous correction will probably occur at age 7 or 8.
   b. Recommend positional changes.
      (1) No sitting on feet
      (2) Encouragement of cross-legged tailor's position
   c. Recommend passive stretching exercises if muscle contracture exists in internal rotation.
3. Follow-up: client should make return visit in 3 to 6 months.
   a. Observe for change.
   b. Verify original diagnosis.
4. Consultations/referrals: client should see orthopedist if
   a. Client is over age 8.
   b. There is no spontaneous improvement in gait, appearance, or range of motion.

B. Genu varum

1. Treatments/medications
   a. There is no treatment.
   b. If client has significant problem of hyperelastic flatfeet, order Thomas heel with longitudinal arch support.
2. Counselling/prevention: condition follows normal developmental pattern.
   a. Spontaneous correction will occur with weight bearing and growth.
   b. Client may develop knock-knee at age 3, which then corrects by age 7.
   c. Encourage patience in allowing for normal growth.
3. Follow-up
   a. Reexamine in 3 to 6 months.
   b. Do sooner if there is significant parental anxiety.
4. Consultations/referrals: client should see orthopedist if
   a. Problem persists beyond age 3.
   b. Condition is progressive.

C. Genu valgum

1. Treatments/medications: none
2. Counselling/prevention
   a. Spontaneous correction occurs in most all children between ages 2 and 6.
   b. Normal growth pattern shows that from ages 1 to 7
      (1) Child may have bowleg ages 1 to 3.
      (2) Child may have knock-knee ages 3 to 7.
3. Follow-up
   a. In 3 to 6 months recheck diagnosis.
   b. Examine sooner if deformity appears to be increasing.
4. Consultations/referrals: client should see orthopedist if
   a. Intermalleolar interval is greater than 10 cm.
   b. Gait is seriously affected.
   c. Condition is progressive.

D. Internal tibial torsion

1. Treatments/medications: none
2. Counselling/prevention
   a. Recommend no sitting on feet.
   b. Spontaneous correction will probably occur with growth.
3. Follow-up
   a. In 3 to 6 months recheck diagnosis.
   b. Examine if deformity increases.
4. Consultations/referrals: client should see orthopedist if
   a. Deformity is excessive.
   b. Condition persists after age 3.
   c. Condition is progressive.

bibliography

Ferguson, Albert Barnett, Jr. *Orthopedic surgery in infancy and childhood* (4th ed.). Baltimore: Williams & Wilkins, 1975.

Gellis, Sydney S., and Kagan, Benjamin M. *Current pediatric therapy 8:* Philadelphia: Saunders, 1978.

Hughes, James G. *Synopsis of pediatrics (4th ed.).* St. Louis: Mosby, 1975.

Sharrard, W. J. W. *Pediatric orthopaedics and fractures.* Oxford: Blackwell, 1971.

Tachdjian, Mihran O. *Pediatric orthopedics.* Philadelphia: Saunders, 1972.

Table 87-1 Medical Referral/Consultation

Diagnosis	Clinical Manifestations	Management
CONGENITAL ABNORMALITIES		
Achondroplasia (hereditary generalized skeletal dysplasia)	Extremities disproportionately short in relation to head and trunk Cranial deformities Prominent forehead Depressed base of nose Marked lumbar lordosis Height rarely exceeding 55 in	No specific treatment known Orthopedic correction of deformities (may improve appearance)
TRAUMA	History of trauma Asymmetrical deformity	Dependent on severity of deformity Possible Osteotomy Lengthening procedures Shortening procedures
INFECTION		
Poliomyelitis (acute infectious viral disease)	History of acute infection Presence of atrophic muscles Probable asymmetry Possible impaired growth of involved lower extremity	Comprehensive rehabilitation program Multiple surgical procedures Prevention: oral trivalent-attenuated polio vaccine
ACQUIRED DISEASES		
Blount's disease (also called tibia vara—growth disturbance of medial aspect of proximal tibial epiphysis)	Bowleg interval Progressive curvature Abrupt angulation just below knee Possibility of pronated feet and obesity	Bracing If established deformity, probable need for osteotomy
Rickets (inadequate calcification of bone matrix caused by disturbance in calcium and phosphorus metabolism)	Generalized muscle weakness and lethargy Delay in sitting, standing, and walking Possible genu varum or genu valgum deformity Possibly familial	Dependent on cause and whether rickets are vitamin D-refractory or non-vitamin D-refractory Possible osteotomy
TUMORS	Most commonly unilateral Diagnosed with x-ray and biopsy	Dependent on type and extent of tumor Possible radical surgery

88 Joint Pain/Swelling

CAROLYN B. COLWELL

ALERT
1. Acute pain and/or symptoms of systemic infection
2. Open, draining wound
3. Significant muscle contracture

I. Etiology

A. Congenital diseases
1. Joint dislocations
   a. Hip
   b. Knee
2. Hemophilia
3. Sickle cell anemia
4. Syphilis

B. Trauma
1. Soft-tissue injuries
2. Fractures
3. Dislocations
4. Foreign body

C. Infection
1. Bacterial or suppurative arthritis
2. Tuberculosis
3. Rheumatic fever

D. Acquired Diseases
1. Hip
   a. Legg-Calvé-Perthes disease
   b. Acute transient synovitis
   c. Slipped femoral capital epiphysis
2. Knee
   a. Osgood-Schlatter disease
   b. Monarticular arthritis
   c. Osteochondritis dissecans
   d. Popliteal cyst
3. Foot
   a. Kóhler's disease
   b. Freiberg's disease
4. Juvenile rheumatoid arthritis
5. Scurvy

E. Tumors
1. Benign
2. Malignant
3. Leukemia

F. Nocturnal pains ("growing pains")

G. Psychological disturbance

II. Assessment

A. Soft-tissue injury (see Sprains/Strains, Chap. 90)

B. Fracture/dislocation (see Fractures/Dislocations, Chap. 168)

C. Acute transient synovitis of the hip
1. Subjective data: pain in anteromedial aspect of thigh and/or knee
2. Objective data
   a. Antalgic limp
   b. Possible low grade fever, usually not over 100°F (37.75°C)
   c. Local tenderness on palpation of anterior aspect of hip joint
   d. Limitation of joint motion
      (1) Internal rotation
      (2) Abduction
      (3) Extension
   e. No bony abnormalities seen on x-ray

D. Osgood-Schlatter disease (tendonitis of distal portion of patellar tendon)
1. Subjective data
   a. Local pain in anterior aspect of knee
   b. Aggravation of pain on running, climbing stairs, jumping, or kneeling
   c. Increase of pain by
      (1) Forced knee extension against resistance
      (2) Squatting with knee in full flexion

d. Decrease or disappearance of pain with rest

2. Objective data
   a. Enlargement of tibial tuberosity
   b. Maximal tenderness at insertion of patellar tendon to bone
   c. No effusion in knee joint
   d. Increase of pain by
      (1) Forced knee extension against resistance
      (2) Squatting with knee in full flexion
   e. No significant bony abnormality seen on x-ray

E. Nocturnal pains ("growing pains")

1. Subjective data
   a. Pain that varies in frequency and intensity
   b. Pain that may wake child at night
   c. Pain that is *not* present during day
2. Objective data
   a. More common sites in calves and feet
   b. No point tenderness
   c. No signs of systemic infection
   d. No significant abnormality found in objective data

F. Psychological disturbance

1. Subjective data
   a. Indication of mild emotional problems in client and/or family
   b. Inconsistency in complaints of pain
2. Objective data: no findings in data collection of swelling or true abnormality

III. Management

A. Acute transient synovitis

1. Treatments/medications
   a. Bedrest
      (1) With skin traction if pain is significant
      (2) With traction forces in line with flexion deformity of hip
   b. Possible need for aspiration if
      (1) Definite widening of joint space on x-ray
      (2) Marked limitation of hip motion
   c. Continued non-weight-bearing for 7 to 10 days after normal hip motion is restored
      (1) Bedrest until normal hip motion
      (2) Crutches for 7 to 10 days thereafter
   d. Aspirin, every 4 to 6 h for pain relief, if necessary
2. Counselling/prevention
   a. Stressing importance and reason for non-weight-bearing
      (1) To decrease pain
      (2) To prevent possible complications
   b. Devising method of traction at home
   c. Using crutches
   d. Stressing importance of follow-up
   e. Explaining value of maintaining contact with school and peers during absence
3. Follow-up
   a. In 2 to 3 days to examine range of motion of hip and to observe progress
   b. In 7 to 10 days to ensure no recurrence before resuming full weight bearing and normal activity
   c. In 2 to 3 months for repeat x-rays to rule out avascular necrosis of femoral head
4. Consultations/referrals

   Note to school nurse and/or teacher anticipating absence from school, use of crutches, and gradual return to normal activity

B. Osgood-Schlatter disease

1. Treatments/medications
   a. In cases of mild pain, simple restriction of excessive physical activity until joint is pain-free
      (1) Active sports
      (2) Running and jumping
   b. If significant pain on stance-phase activities, splinting in full extension until symptoms abate
   c. When pain-free, isometric exercises to restore strength of quadriceps
2. Counselling/prevention
   a. Consideration of problems caused by limitation of activity
   b. Stressing importance of follow-up
   c. Advising of possibility of enlarged tibial tubercle and possible need for later excision
3. Follow-up
   a. In 10 days
      (1) To reaffirm diagnosis
      (2) To evaluate effect of limited activity
      (3) To plan exercise program
   b. Sooner if pain increases
   c. Further follow-up as symptoms warrant
4. Consultations/referrals

   Note to school nurse and/or teacher explaining limitation of activity

C. Nocturnal pains

1. Treatments/medications
   a. Massage or application of low heat to relieve symptoms
   b. Mild analgesics
      (1) Aspirin
      (2) Acetaminophen
2. Counselling/prevention

a. Determining type and temperature of heat application
b. Being cautious concerning use of analgesics (If required often, follow-up visit is necessary.)
c. Explaining cause
   (1) Exact cause is unknown
   (2) Possibly the difference in growth rate between muscle and bone
d. Avoiding overexertion
e. Reassuring that no serious abnormality exists

3. Follow-up
   a. In 3 to 4 weeks if symptoms persist
   b. Sooner, depending on level of parental anxiety
4. Consultations/referrals: none

D. Psychological disturbance

1. Treatments/medications: none
2. Counselling/prevention
   a. Reassurance that no specific abnormality was found
   b. Consideration of causes and possible need for family counselling
3. Follow-up
   a. In 2 to 3 weeks if symptoms persist
   b. Sooner if pain increases, swelling occurs, or other abnormalities arise
4. Consultations/referrals
   a. Family counselling service if appropriate
   b. Psychologist or psychiatrist if significant disturbance exists

Table 88-1 Medical Referral/Consultation

Diagnosis	Clinical Manifestations	Management
CONGENITAL DISEASES		
Sickle cell anemia (hereditary disorder characterized by abnormal hemoglobin in the red blood cells)	Possible presenting symptoms in infants: swelling of hands and feet Chronic anemia Acute crises with possibility of Severe abdominal pain with vomiting Warm, swollen, and painful joints Involvement of liver, central nervous system, lungs, heart, or kidney Possible growth retardation	Referral to physician See Anemia, Chap. 39
TRAUMA		
Foreign body	Unilateral History of trauma and often evidence of scar Possible point tenderness Chronic pain and swelling Possibly not visible on x-ray	Referral to physician Probable need for excision
INFECTION		
Acute suppurative arthritis (inflammation of the joint caused by pus-forming organisms)	In most cases, history of recent injury or infection Joint pain with acute onset Antalgic limp or inability to walk if lower limb involved	Immediate referral to physician/orthopedist

Table 88-1 Medical Referral/Consultation *(continued)*

Diagnosis	Clinical Manifestations	Management
	Signs of systemic infection Elevated temperature, possibly as high as 104°F (40°C) Irritability Anorexia Warm and swollen infected joint Extreme pain during active and passive motions of joint	
Tuberculous arthritis (tuberculosis of the joint usually due to hematogenous spread from a primary focus)	Common sites: vertebral column, hip, knee, and ankle Chronic pain and swelling Probable limitation of motion and muscle atrophy Possible slight limp Positive tubercular skin test Visualized on x-ray	Referral to physician/orthopedist Counselling Stressing importance of medical attention and continued follow-up Helping client anticipate prolonged treatment Notifying Department of Health
Rheumatic fever (an inflammatory disease which follows an infection with Group A streptococci)	Possible association with any combination of the following Carditis Polyarthritis Chorea Erythema marginatum Subcutaneous nodules Probable elevated temperature Laboratory findings of Increased ESR Leukocytosis Evidence of preceding streptococcal infection	Referral to physician/pediatrician See Acute Rheumatic Fever, Chap. 145
ACQUIRED DISEASES		
Slipped femoral capital epiphysis (adolescent coxa vara—mechanical derangement of epiphyseal plate)	Possible acute or chronic pain in hip or knee Antalgic limp Restriction of motion in internal rotation, abduction, and flexion Visualized on x-ray	Referral to physician/orthopedist Counselling Stressing importance of immediate medical attention and follow-up to prevent permanent damage
Osteochondritis dissecans	Most common in knee joint Intermittent pain and swelling Severe pain if fragment detached Possible clicking or locking of joint Probable atrophy of controlling muscles and limited motion of joint	Referral to physican/orthopedist

Table 88-1 Medical Referral/Consultation *(continued)*

Diagnosis	Clinical Manifestations	Management
Popliteal cyst (Baker's cyst)	Usually unilateral Swelling, commonly On medial side of posterior aspect of knee Distal to knee crease No knee joint dysfunction	Referral to physician/orthopedist Possible need for surgical excision if cyst is large and causing symptoms
Juvenile rheumatoid arthritis (Still's disease—a generalized systemic autoimmune disease)	Polyarthritis in most cases Effected joints that are warm, painful on motion, and swollen Possible Elevated temperature Skin rash Splenomegaly Lymphadenopathy Anemia Onset usually before age 5	Referral to physician/pediatrician Rest, alternating with controlled activity Correction of anemia Aspirin Steroids if necessary Prevention and correction of deformity Possible surgery if conservative treatment not adequate Synovectomy Procedures to correct deformities
TUMORS		
Malignant bone tumor	Possible pain Possible palpable mass Possible elevated temperature and leukocytosis Diagnosis by x-ray and biopsy	Immediate referral to physican/orthopedist See Neoplastic Disease, Chap. 148

bibliography

Alexander, Mary M., and Brown, Marie Scott. Performing the neurologic examination. *Nursing 76* **6**: (1976).

———, and ———. Performing the neurologic examination, part 2. *Nursing 76* **6**: (1976).

———, and ———. Physical examination, The musculoskeletal system. *Nursing 76* **6**: (1976).

Barnett, Henry L., and Einhorn, Arnold H. *Pediatrics* (16th ed.). New York: Appleton Century Crofts, 1977.

DeAngelis, Catherine. *Pediatric primary care* (2d ed.). Boston: Little, Brown, 1979.

Ferguson, Albert Barnett, Jr. *Orthopedic surgery in infancy and childhood* (4th ed.). Baltimore: Williams & Wilkins, 1975.

Green, Morris, and Haggerty, Robert J. *Ambulatory pediatrics II*. Philadelphia: Saunders, 1977.

Hughes, James G. *Synopsis of pediatrics* (4th ed.). St. Louis: Mosby, 1975.

Kempe, C. Henry, et al. *Current pediatric diagnosis and treatment* (4th ed.). Los Altos, Calif.: Lange, 1976.

Mital, Mohinder A., and Matza, Richard A. Osgood-Schlatter disease: The painful puzzler. *The Physician and Sports-medicine*, **5**:60–67 (1977).

Tachdjian, Mihran O. *Pediatric orthopedics*, Philadelphia: Saunders, 1972.

89 Leg Length Inequality

CAROLYN B. COLWELL

ALERT

1. Any discrepancy greater than $\frac{1}{2}$ in or 1 cm
2. Obvious limp, creating physical or psychological problems for the child

I. Etiology

A. Congenital diseases

1. Congenital dislocation of hip
2. Hypoplasia of long bones of lower extremity
3. Myelodysplasia

B. Trauma

1. Epiphyseal fractures
2. Fractures of shaft of long bones

C. Infection

1. Bone—osteomyelitis
2. Joint—suppurative arthritis
3. Neurogenic—poliomyelitis

D. Acquired diseases

1. Legg-Calvé-Perthes disease
2. Slipped femoral capital epiphysis
3. Fibrous dysplasia
4. Cerebral palsy

E. Tumors

1. Benign unicameral bone cyst
2. Malignant neoplasm

II. Assessment: Leg length discrepancy of less than 1/2 in or 1 cm

A. Subjective data

No serious problems created by limp

B. Objective data

1. Apparent limp, but of minor degree and not disabling
2. Absence of infection

III. Management: Leg length discrepancy of less than 1/2 in or 1 cm

A. Treatments/medications: none

B. Counselling/prevention

1. Reassurance to parent(s) and children that no evidence of significant problem exists
2. Consideration of importance of cosmetic appearance and suggestions to achieve the optimum
   a. Utilization of long pants and skirts
   b. Type of shoes
   c. Inside lift to shoe if appropriate
3. If emotional overreaction by child or parent(s), consider cause and need for further counselling

C. Follow-up

1. In 3 to 6 months to recheck findings
2. Sooner if limp develops or progresses

D. Consultations/referrals: none

Table 89-1 Medical Referral/Consultation: Leg length discrepancy *greater* than 1/2 in or 1 cm

Diagnosis	Clinical Manifestations	Management
Congenital Disease		
Congenital dislocated hip	If infant Limited passive abduction of hip in 90° flexed position Asymmetry of skin folds of thigh and/or gluteal and popliteal creases Apparent shortening of femur—Galeazzi's sign and/or Allis' sign Presence of Ortolani click Positive Trendelenburg's test if over age 3 Abnormal gait, with instability and gluteus medius lurch Visualized on x-ray	Referral immediately to physician/orthopedist Counselling/prevention Vital importance of immediate medical attention and continued follow-up and treatment Reassurance concerning nonpreventability Positive outlook if detected early Anticipation of cast care if appropriate Possibility of hospitalization if over age 2
Trauma		
Epiphyseal fracture	History of trauma Significant measured discrepancy Abnormal gait Visualized on x-ray	Referral to physician/orthopedist Counselling Need for complete medical workup to determine type of treatment Availability of surgical procedure to correct discrepancy Shortening procedures Lengthening procedures
Infection		
Osteomyelitis	History of acute infection with Localized acute pain Systemic signs of infection Significant discrepancy of more than ½ in or 1 cm Abnormal gait Visualized on x-ray	Referral to physician/orthopedist Counselling: see under Trauma, above
Acquired Disease		
Fibrous dysplasia	There may be café au lait spots on the skin. Pain, if present, may indicate pathological fracture. Females may have associated endocrine disturbances. It can be visualized on x-ray.	Referral to physician/orthopedist
Cerebral palsy (impaired neurological function caused by deficient structure, growth, or development of the central nervous system)	Delayed developmental milestones Abnormality of muscle tone Faulty motor movement of limb and trunk muscles, with varying distribution of muscle groups Presence of joint contracture common Possible associated problems Mental retardation Visual and sensory defects Speech defects	Referral to physician/orthopedist See Cerebral Palsy, Chap. 151 Counselling Necessity for complete medical evaluation Importance of comprehensive therapeutic program

Table 89-1 Medical Referral/Consultation: Leg length discrepancy *greater* than 1/2 in or 1 cm *(continued)*

Diagnosis	Clinical Manifestations	Management
Tumors	Pain Deformity sometimes evident Possible pathological fracture Diagnosed with x-ray and biopsy	Referral to physician/orthopedist Counselling Necessity of further medical evaluation to determine exact diagnosis and treatment

bibliography

Alexander, Mary M., and Brown, Marie Scott. Physical examination, the musculoskeletal system. *Nursing 76*, **6**(4) (1976).

———, and ———. Performing the neurologic examination. *Nursing 76*, **6**(6) (1976).

———, and ———. Performing the neurologic examination, Part 2. *Nursing 76*, **6**(7) (1976).

Ferguson, Albert Barnett, Jr. *Orthopedic surgery in infancy and childhood* (4th ed.). Baltimore: Williams & Wilkins, 1975.

Lloyd-Roberts, G. C. *Orthopaedics in infancy and childhood.* London: Butterworth, 1971.

Tachdjian, Mihran O. *Pediatric orthopedics.* Philadelphia: Saunders, 1972.

90 Sprains/Strains

CAROLYN B. COLWELL

ALERT

1. Joint instability or laxity
2. Severe pain and swelling
3. Open wound
4. Inadequate circulation to extremity

I. Etiology—Low-Velocity Trauma

A. Sports injury

B. Bicycle injury

C. Miscellaneous accidental injury

II. Assessment

A. Partial ligamentous or muscle tear

1. Subjective data
   a. In less severe injuries, pain may appear 4 to 12 h following accident.
   b. Pain may occur immediately and persist.
   c. Pain may increase if the ligament is stressed.
   d. The affected part will be painful on palpation.
2. Objective data
   a. Swelling
   b. May be palpable defect in muscle mass
   c. May be change in surface contour of muscle
   d. Limited range of motion
   e. Possible slight instability
   f. No obvious deformity or displacement
   g. If weight-bearing extremity, may have antalgic limp

B. Back strain

1. Subjective data
   Mild muscle spasm and pain
2. Objective data
   a. Normal function of extremities
   b. Normal neurological exam

III. Management

A. Partial ligamentous or muscle tear

1. Treatments/medications
   a. Apply ice packs to the injured area.
      (1) Apply immediately for 30 to 45 min.
      (2) Repeat 2 times per day until acute symptoms subside.
   b. Elevate the affected extremity.
   c. Compression strap the involved extremity with ace bandages.
      (1) In position of comfort and function
      (2) Inclusion of joint proximal and joint distal to injured area
   d. If the wrist or finger is affected, splint in a position of comfort and function until symptoms subside.
   e. If it is an upper extremity, apply a sling for comfort and rest.
   f. For a lower extremity, use crutches to avoid immediate weight bearing.
   g. When acute pain and swelling subside, apply warm soaks for 15 min several times a day.
   h. Give for pain relief, if necessary,
      (1) Acetaminophen
      (2) Aspirin
   i. The client can gradually return to active exercise and weight bearing after the pain and swelling have subsided.
2. Counselling/prevention
   a. Necessity for immediate follow-up if circulatory impairment suspected at any time
   b. Signs and symptoms indicating inadequate circulation to the extremity
      (1) Pain, persistent and increasing
      (2) Pale to blue color
      (3) Cool to cold temperature
      (4) Decreased or tingling sensation

(5) Increased swelling
(6) Inability to move extremity

c. Importance of rest and elevation in decreasing pain and swelling
d. Instruction on rewrapping ace bandages twice a day or if the pain increases or the wrapping loosens
e. Use of crutches and safety aspects concerning this
f. Importance of use of voluntary, active exercises after acute pain and swelling have subsided
g. Emphasis on gradual return to full activity when full range of motion restored
h. Accident prevention if appropriate

3. Follow-up
   a. In 48 h to observe improvement and reaffirm diagnosis
   b. Sooner if pain and swelling persist or increase despite treatment
   c. In 1 week to evaluate exercise program and for possible repeat x-ray
4. Consultations/referrals
   Note to school nurse and/or teacher explaining activity limitations

B. Back strain

1. Treatments/medications
   a. Bed rest in semi-Fowler's position with firm mattress
   b. Application of heat to affected area of back
   c. Analgesics if necessary
   d. Low-back exercise program to begin when pain-free
   e. Gradual return to full activity
2. Counselling/prevention
   a. Use of heating pad and safety precautions involved
   b. Importance of follow-up
   c. Reassurance that symptoms should resolve with treatment
   d. Importance of gradual return to full activity (include parent and child)
3. Follow-up
   a. In 1 week to check progress and reaffirm diagnosis
   b. Sooner if pain persists or increases despite treatment
4. Consultations/referrals: note to school nurse and/or teacher explaining activity limitations

Table 90-1 Medical Referral/Consultation

Diagnosis	Clinical Manifestations	Management
Complete rupture, or moderate to severe sprain or strain	Significant pain and swelling Change in surface contour of extremity Palpable defect Unstable joint Deformity perhaps evident Visualized on stress films	Referral to physician Temporary treatment Assure the absence of associated serious injury, to the head, or from shock. Apply ice to the injured area. Splint in a position of optimum comfort. Counselling/prevention Importance of immediate medical treatment Keeping extremity elevated Care in transporting client
Fracture/dislocation	See Fractures/Dislocations, Chap. 168	

bibliography

Alexander, Mary M., and Brown, Marie Scott. Physical examination, the musculoskeletal system. *Nursing 76*, **6**:4 (1976).

________, and ________. Performing the neurologic examination. *Nursing 76*, **6**:6 (1976).

________, and ________. Performing the neurologic examination, Part 2. *Nursing 76*, **6**:7 (1976).

Cox, J. S., and Brand, Robert L. Evaluation and treatment of lateral ankle sprains. *The Physician and Sportsmedicine*, **6**:5 (1977).

Gellis, Sydney S., and Kagen, Benjamin M. *Current pediatric therapy 8*. Philadelphia: Saunders, 1978.

Green, Morris, and Haggerty, Robert J. *Ambulatory pediatrics II*. Philadelphia: Saunders, 1978.

Hughes, James G. *Synopsis of pediatrics* (4th ed.). St. Louis: Mosby, 1975.

Kalenak, A., et al. Athletic injuries: Heat vs. cold. *American Family Physician*, 1975.

Kempe, C. Henry, et al. *Current pediatric diagnosis and treatment* (4th ed.). Los Altos, Calif.: Lange, 1976.

Tachdjian, Mihran O. *Pediatric orthopedics*. Philadelphia: Saunders, 1972.

91 Knee Injury

CAROLYN B. COLWELL

ALERT

1. Significant pain and limitation of function
2. Significant swelling
3. Draining wound
4. Impaired circulation of limb distal to injury

I. Etiology

A. Low-velocity injury
1. Sports
2. Bicycle
3. Fall from moderate height (under 8 ft)

B. High-velocity injury
1. Automobile
2. Motorcycle
3. Fall from significant height (over 8 ft)

II. Assessment

A. Mild sprain/strain—(see Sprains/Strains, Chap. 90)

B. Mild traumatic synovitis
1. Subjective data
   a. Pain usually mild
   b. Low-velocity injury
2. Objective data
   a. Effusion, usually developing gradually over 5 or 6 h
   b. Tender to palpation
   c. Limitation of motion due to pain and/or fluid
   d. Swelling of mild to moderate degree

III. Management—Mild Traumatic Synovitis

A. Treatments/medications
1. Ice packs if within first 48 h
2. Compression with ace bandage until swelling and pain subside
3. Elevation of knee
4. Joint protection—if moderate injury
   a. Splint—in 5° lacking full extension
   b. Crutches
5. Warm, moist heat, 15 to 20 min, 3 to 4 times a day, starting 48 h after injury
6. Active assisted exercises several times a day within tolerance, after initial symptoms subside

B. Counselling/prevention
1. Importance of elevation of extremity
2. Use of crutches
3. Warm bath or warm towels with plastic covering, probably best means of securing moist heat
4. Demonstration of active and isometric exercises with emphasis on active aspect
5. Importance of follow-up if pain or swelling increase despite treatment
6. Gradual resumption of normal activity
7. Accident prevention

C. Follow-up
1. In 2 to 3 days to observe knee and possibly begin exercises
2. Sooner if pain and swelling persist or increase despite treatment
3. Again in 1 to 2 weeks to ensure complete recovery

D. Consultations/referrals: note to school nurse and/or teacher explaining temporary limitation of activity

Table 91-1 Medical Referral/Consultation

Diagnosis	Clinical Manifestations	Management
Fracture/dislocation	See Fractures/Dislocations, Chap. 168, Table 168-3.	
Foreign body	History of trauma often associated with glass, wood, or cinders Chronic pain and swelling, if long-standing injury May be point tenderness May not be visible on x-ray	Referral to physician/orthopedist for probable excision
Traumatic dislocation of patella	Usually lateral dislocation Often reduces spontaneously History of direct blow to knee—usually on inner side of patella Swelling Tenderness, especially on medial aspect of patella Active extension of leg impossible X-ray showing position of patella and presence or absence of chip fracture	Consultation with physician Treatment If still dislocated, reduce by extending knee with hip flexed while gently pushing patella medially into normal position. Immobilize with cast or splint in 5° lacking full extension. Repeat x-ray after reduction to assure proper position and absence of fracture. Counselling/prevention Elevation of knee if significant swelling Skin care with splint or cast Importance of follow-up Possibility of surgery if recurrence more than 3 times Accident prevention Return visit in 10 days to reexamine knee and possibly begin isometric and active exercise program Sooner if pain and swelling persist Note to school nurse or teacher explaining temporary limitation of activity
Traumatic hemarthrosis	Swelling, immediately after injury Pain Limitation of motion Presence of blood from joint aspiration	Consultation with physician/orthopedist and referral if needed to aspirate knee Treatment Joint aspiration—may need to be repeated Ice packs first 24–48 h after injury Compression with ace bandage or knee immobilizer until swelling and pain subside Elevation of knee Crutches, if appropriate (should not bear weight) Active or active assisted exercises several times a day within tolerance after initial symptoms have subsided

Table 91-1 Medical Referral/Consultation *(continued)*

Diagnosis	Clinical Manifestations	Management
		Counselling/prevention Importance of elevation Use of crutches if indicated Explanation of appropriate exercises Importance of follow-up to ensure absence of joint damage Gradual resumption of normal activity Accident prevention Return visit in 2–3 days to observe knee and possibly begin exercises; sooner if pain and swelling persist or increase despite treatment; again in 1–2 wk to ensure progress toward complete recovery Consultations/referrals To physician if recurrent, for consideration of possible bleeding disorder Note to school explaining activity limitation

bibliography

Ferguson, Albert Barnett, Jr. *Orthopedic surgery in infancy and childhood* (4th ed.). Baltimore: Williams & Wilkins, 1975.

Green, Morris, and Haggerty, Robert J. *Ambulatory pediatrics II*. Philadelphia: Saunders, 1978.

Kempe, C. Henry, et al. *Current pediatric diagnosis and treatment* (4th ed.). Los Altos, Calif.: Lange., 1976.

Sharrand, W. J. W. *Pediatric orthopaedics and fractures*. Oxford, Engl.: Blackwell, 1971.

Tachdjian, Mihran O. *Pediatric orthopedics*. Philadelphia: Saunders, 1972.

92 Toe-walking

CAROLYN B. COLWELL

ALERT
1. Unilateral with leg length discrepancy
2. Associated neuromuscular abnormality
3. Associated with severe pain

I. Etiology

A. Congenital abnormalities
1. Short tendo calcaneus
2. Charcot-Marie-Tooth disease
3. Club foot (talipes equinovarus)

B. Trauma: Achilles tendonitis

C. Infectious diseases: poliomyelitis

D. Acquired diseases
1. Muscular dystrophy
2. Sever's disease
3. Cerebral palsy

II. Assessment

A. Normal developmental toe-walking
1. Subjective data
   a. Common in second year of life
   b. May be familial history of toe-walking
2. Objective data
   a. Usually bilateral toe-walking gait
   b. Equinus position of feet
      (1) Assumed when walking
      (2) More pronounced when hurrying
   c. Feet showing passive dorsiflexion to right angle without force
   d. Normal neurological exam

B. Painful heels ("pump bumps")
1. Subjective data
   a. Common in females ages 6 to 12
   b. May be heel pain
2. Objective data
   a. Presence of callus and underlying bursa on heel from shoe with tight heel fit
   b. Normal range of motion of foot
   c. Normal neurological exam
   d. No signs of systemic illness

C. Achilles tendonitis
1. Subjective data
   Usually occurs after strenuous activity
2. Objective data
   a. Swollen and tender Achilles tendon near insertion
   b. May be crepitus over tendon on palpation
   c. Normal range of motion of foot and ankle
   d. Absence of instability or muscle abnormality

D. Sever's disease (epiphysitis of the calcaneus)
1. Subjective data
   a. Heel pain, unilateral or bilateral
   b. Most common at age 10 or 11
   c. Aggravated by activity; improves with rest
2. Objective data
   Tenderness over insertion of tendo calcaneus

III. Management

A. Normal developmental toe-walking
1. Treatments/medications
   a. If muscle tightening, passive stretching exercises
   b. High-top, hard-soled shoes
2. Counselling/prevention
   a. Reassurance of absence of abnormality
   b. Normal developmental pattern when first walking
   c. Probability of heel-toe gait developing in 3 to 6 months
   d. Demonstration of exercises if indicated
3. Follow-up

a. In 1 month to reaffirm diagnosis and observe for normal development
b. Sooner if progressive, or if anxiety of parent indicates need

4. Consultations/referrals: none

B. Painful heels

1. Treatments/medications
   Change shoe style to decrease stress on posterior heel
2. Counselling/prevention
   a. Explanation of how callus formed
   b. Importance of working with the client
      (1) To achieve relief of pain and a normal gait
      (2) To find footwear that is esthetically pleasing to client
   c. Remote possibility of surgery if bursa persists
3. Follow-up
   a. In 2 to 3 months to note progress
   b. Sooner if pain persists
4. Consultations/referrals: none

C. Achilles tendonitis

1. Treatments/medications
   a. Small lift added to heel
   b. Curtailment of sports, running, jumping, and prolonged walking until symptoms subside
2. Counselling/prevention
   a. How to obtain lift for shoe
   b. Importance of limiting activity to allow healing
   c. Reassurance that normal activity will be resumed eventually
3. Follow-up
   a. In 3 to 4 weeks to observe progress and confirm diagnosis
   b. Sooner if pain persists despite treatment
4. Consultations/referrals: note to school nurse and/or teacher to excuse from physical education

D. Sever's disease

1. Treatments/medications
   a. Limitation of activity until pain subsides
   b. Plastic heel cup—foam rubber heel pad for shoe
2. Counselling/prevention
   a. Guidance in obtaining heel cup and pad
   b. Importance of temporary limitation of activity—discussion with child and parent
3. Follow-up
   a. In 3 to 4 weeks to observe improvement
   b. Sooner if pain increases despite treatment
4. Consultations/referrals: none, unless severe

Table 92-1 Medical Referral/Consultation

Diagnosis	Clinical Manifestations	Management
Congenital short tendo calcaneus (or contracture of triceps surae muscle)	Abnormal gait Toe-toe pattern Awkward, with hyperextended knee when heel-toe gait is attempted Limited range of dorsiflexion Variable degree of equinus deformity Normal neurological exam	Consultation with physician/orthopedist Probable need for Passive stretching exercises of triceps surae muscle by parent(s) 15–20 times Several times daily Splint or bivalved cast at night If permanent contracture Walking cast Gait training on removal of cast Counselling/prevention Importance of regularity of exercises and splint Prevention of skin breakdown with splint or cast Possible need for surgery if conservative treatment fails
Charcot-Marie-Tooth disease (peroneal muscular atrophy)	Onset of symptoms, usually between 5 and 15 yr Difficulty in walking or wearing shoes	Referral to physician Probable need for Passive stretching exercises

Table 92-1 Medical Referral/Consultation *(continued)*

Diagnosis	Clinical Manifestations	Management
	May be muscle cramps and paresthesia in legs Symmetrical muscle atrophy, first of intrinsic muscles of feet Gradual progression of involvement to calf muscles and possibly upper limbs	Night splints to prevent fixed deformity Active exercises to maintain strength of muscles Regular muscle testing Counselling/prevention Importance of regular exercises Prevention of skin breakdown with night splints Necessity for medical follow-up Possible need for surgery Support and guidance in view of chronic and progressive nature of disease Referral for genetic counselling
Club foot	See Foot Deformities, Chap. 86	

bibliography

Alexander, Mary M., and Brown, Marie Scott. Physical examination, The musculoskeletal system. *Nursing 76,* **6**:4 (1976).

________, and ________. Performing the neurologic examination. *Nursing 76,* **6**:6 (1976).

________, and ________. Performing the neurologic examination, Part 2. *Nursing 76,* **6**:7 (1976).

Blockey, N. J. *Children's orthopaedics—Practical problems.* London: Butterworth, 1976.

Ferguson, Albert Barnett, Jr. *Orthopedic surgery in infancy and childhood* (4th ed.). Baltimore: Williams & Wilkins, 1975.

Sharrard, W. J. W. *Pediatric orthopaedics and fractures.* Oxford: Blackwell Scientific Publications, 1971.

Tachdjian, Mihran O. *Pediatric orthopedics.* Philadelphia: Saunders, 1972.

93 Abnormal Gait

CAROLYN B. COLWELL

ALERT
1. Localized pain, swelling, and fever
2. Progressive or disabling
3. Generalized neuromuscular involvement and/or signs of increased intracranial pressure
4. Vertigo

I. Etiology

A. Congenital diseases
   1. Bone malformations, giantism
   2. Joint dislocations
   3. Myelodysplasia
   4. Arthrogryposis multiplex congenita
   5. Achondroplasia

B. Trauma
   1. Fractures
   2. Dislocations
   3. Foreign body
   4. Soft-tissue injuries
      a. Sprains and strains
      b. Skin and subcutaneous tissue

C. Infection
   1. Osteomyelitis
      a. Bacterial *(Staphylococcus aureus)*
      b. Acid-fast bacilli (tubercle bacillus)
   2. Suppurative arthritis
   3. Poliomyelitis
   4. Rheumatic fever

D. Acquired diseases
   1. Aseptic necrosis
      a. Legg-Calvé-Perthes disease—of hip
      b. Köhler's disease—of tarsal navicular
   2. Neuromuscular disorders
      a. Cerebral palsy
      b. Muscular dystrophy
      c. Friedreich's ataxia
      d. Vertigo
   3. Juvenile rheumatoid arthritis
   4. Acute transient synovitis
   5. Slipped capital femoral epiphysis
   6. Rickets
   7. Blount's disease

E. Tumors
   1. Benign
   2. Malignant

F. Psychological problems
   Hysteria

II. Assessment

A. Trauma
   1. Soft-tissue injuries (see Sprains/Strains, Chap. 90)
   2. Fractures/dislocations (see Fractures/Dislocations, Chap. 168)

B. Positional alterations
   1. Bow legs (see Leg Deformities, Chap. 87)
   2. Knock-knees (see Leg Deformities, Chap. 87)
   3. In-toeing
      a. Hip—femoral anteversion (see Leg Deformities, Chap. 87)
      b. Knee—internal tibial torsion (see Leg Deformities, Chap. 87)
      c. Foot (see Foot Deformities, Chap. 86)
   4. Out-toeing (see Foot Deformities, Chap. 86)
   5. Toe-walking (see Toe-Walking, Chap. 92)

C. Mimicry
   1. Subjective data
      a. No symptoms or indication of disease or abnormality
      b. Similarity of gait to individual in child's environment or association

2. Objective data
   Abnormal gait which may be similar to that of family member or associate

III. Management—Mimicry

A. Treatments/medications: none

B. Counselling/prevention: reassurance to parent that no abnormality is present

C. Follow-up: return in 2 to 3 months if gait abnormality persists

D. Consultations/referrals: none

Table 93-1 Medical Referral/Consultation

Diagnosis	Clinical Manifestations	Management
Congenital diseases		
Myelodysplasia (neurologic deficit resulting from a myelomeningocele)	History of myelomeningocele at birth Varying levels of neurologic deficit T12 or L1—probable scoliosis L3 or L4—probable hip dislocation Possible deformity and decreased function of lower extremities Incontinence—bowel and bladder	Referral to physician Comprehensive rehabilitation program, depending on degree of neurologic impairment
Arthrogryposis multiplex congenita (incomplete fibrous ankylosis of many or all of the joints)	Contractures in either flexion or extension Enlarged and cylindrical joints Poor muscle power Probability of other congenital anomalies	Referral to physician Possibility of bracing or surgery Usually long-term comprehensive therapeutic program required
Trauma		
Fractures (see Fractures/Dislocations, Chap. 168)	History of trauma Visualization on x-ray Possible displaced alignment Pain and swelling	Referral to physician Immediate treatment Splint as it lies. Move child with great care. Possible hospitalization
Infection		
Acute hematogenous osteomyelitis (pyogenic infection of metaphysis of bone)	Local symptoms Acute, severe pain Swelling, warmth, and erythema Limited function of involved area due to pain Systemic symptoms Fever Malaise Decreased appetite May be history of previous skin infection Elevated white blood count (WBC) and sedimentation rate	Immediate referral to physician Probable hospitalization and anticipation of Intravenous antibiotics Immobilization of involved extremity Antipyretics and analgesics Possibly surgery Incision and drainage Closed irrigation system
Poliomyelitis (acute viral infection causing destruction of anterior horn cells)	History of acute infection Atrophic muscles Varying degree Varying distribution May be leg length discrepancy May be scoliosis or kyphosis	Referral to physician Oral trivalent attenuated vaccine Comprehensive rehabilitation program Possibility of reconstructive orthopedic procedures Tendon transfer Arthrodesis

Table 93-1 Medical Referral/Consultation *(continued)*

Diagnosis	Clinical Manifestations	Management
Acquired diseases		
Aseptic necrosis Legg-Calvé-Perthes disease	Persistent pain in hip or *knee* Limp—often of slow onset Limitation of motion Abduction Internal rotation Normal lab findings X-ray findings Joint effusion Varying degrees of necrosis of bone	Referral to physician Possible hospitalization Protection by avoidance of weight bearing Braces Cast Possible surgery if deformity of epiphysis results
Neuromuscular disorders Duchenne's muscular dystrophy (hereditary, pseudohypertrophic, progressive disease)	Delayed walking and running Difficulty climbing stairs and rising from floor Waddling gait Pseudohypertrophy of calf muscles Lumbar lordosis	Referral to physician No specific treatment Maintenance of independent ambulation as long as possible Utilization of various disciplines in achieving maximum potential
Friedreich's ataxia (hereditary, progressive spinocerebellar degeneration)	Ataxic gait Incoordination Clumsiness Delayed walking Speech defects (later) Pes cavus Horizontal nystagmus Loss of deep tendon reflexes	Referral to physician No specific treatment available
Tumors		
Bone tumors	Pain Deformity sometimes evident Possible pathologic fracture Diagnosed with x-ray and biopsy	Immediate referral to physician Anticipation of hospitalization
Psychological problems		
Hysteria	Gait abnormality: usually bizarre—no consistent abnormal pattern Evidence of emotional disturbance in child and/or family	Referral to physician Probable need for psychotherapy

bibliography

Alexander, Mary M., and Brown, Marie Scott. Physical examination, The musculoskeletal system. *Nursing 76*, **6**:4 (1976).

———, and ———. Performing the neurologic examination. *Nursing 76*, **6**:6 (1976).

———, and ———. Performing the neurologic examination, Part 2. *Nursing 76*, **6**:7 (1976).

DeAngelis, Catherine. *Pediatric primary care* (2d ed.). Boston: Little, Brown, 1979.

Ducroquet, Robert, et al. *Walking and limping, A*

study of normal and pathological walking. Philadelphia: Lippincott, 1965.

Ferguson, Albert Barnett, Jr. *Orthopedic surgery in infancy and childhood* (4th ed.). Baltimore: Williams & Wilkins, 1975.

Green, Morris, and Haggerty; Robert, Jr. *Ambulatory pediatrics II*. Philadelphia: Saunders, 1977.

Hughes, James G. *Synopsis of pediatrics* (4th ed.). St. Louis, Mosby, 1975.

Lloyd-Roberts, G. C. *Orthopaedics in infancy and childhood.* London: Butterworth, 1971.

Tachdjian, Mihran O. *Pediatric orthopedics.* Philadelphia: Saunders, 1972.

94 Back Pain

HARRIETT S. CHANEY

ALERT

1. Paresthesias and/or paralysis
2. Excruciating flank pain radiating to genitalia
3. Inability to raise legs
4. Urinary frequency, hesitancy, dysuria, hematuria, anuria
5. Lateral deviation of the spine
6. Back stiffness
7. Uterine malposition

I. Etiology

A. Pain produced by stretching or incomplete tearing of the muscles, tendons, ligaments of the back, in the absence of gross structural change

B. Sources

1. Trauma as a result of a mild blunt blow to the back
2. Lifting of heavy objects
3. Maintenance of an abnormal posture
4. Movement with the spine in a position of improper mechanical balance, as when lifting and turning simultaneously
5. Strenuous participation in sporting events

II. Assessment: Back Strain

A. Subjective data

Mild to moderately severe pain located across lumbosacral area, precipitated or exaggerated by activity or improper body posture

B. Objective data

1. Localized pain and/or muscle spasm upon palpation of lumbosacral area
2. Minimal or no pain when raising leg straight
3. Normal laboratory data

III. Managment: Back Strain

A. Treatments/medications

1. Activity
   a. For moderately severe pain, bed rest
   b. For minimal pain, restrict activity, specifically lifting
2. Sleeping surface
   a. Firm mattress, or
   b. Move mattress to the floor, or
   c. Place $\frac{1}{2}$- to $\frac{3}{4}$-in plywood between mattress and boxspring
3. Local applications
   a. Ice bag or cold-water bottle to reduce swelling during acute phase (1 to 3 days)
   b. After 3 days application of heat to increase circulation and relax muscle spasms
   c. Back-support device such as a belt, girdle, brace
4. Medications
   a. Analgesics: aspirin, acetaminophen, Darvon, and codeine (prescribed only by physician)
   b. Muscle relaxants: meprobamate, Valium, Soma, Robaxin (not used for children)
   c. Mild tranquilizers: meprobamate, Valium, Librium (not for children—consult physician)

B. Counselling/prevention

1. Medications
   a. Importance of taking analgesics before pain is very severe
   b. Importance of taking prescribed medications properly
2. Instruction in body positions
   a. Sit in a straight chair with a firm back for a short period of time; keep knees higher than hips by using a foot stool.

b. Drive automobile with seat forward so knees are higher than hips; wear lap and shoulder safety belts.
c. Stand for short periods of time, shifting from one foot to the other; wear low shoes.
d. Lie on one side with knees and hips flexed or on back with knees slightly elevated—do *not* lie on stomach.
e. Do not make beds or vacuum carpets, participate in sporting events, or attend physical education classes during episodes of acute pain.

3. Instruction in weight reduction if indicated
4. Demonstration of correct body mechanics for lifting
5. Demonstration of exercises to be initiated following periods of acute pain (see Fig. 94-1)

C. Follow-up: return visit in 3 weeks

D. Consultations/referrals

1. Refer to a physician after 4 weeks if the condition is not markedly improved.
2. Inform the school health nurse or employer of limitations.
3. Refer to a physicial therapist for local treatment applications or exercise training.

Fig. 94-1 Exercises for alleviating back pain. Exercises should be done as the client is able to tolerate them. Progress will become apparent as the abdominal muscles are strengthened *(c, f)* and back muscles are stretched and strengthened *(a, b, c, d, e, g)*.

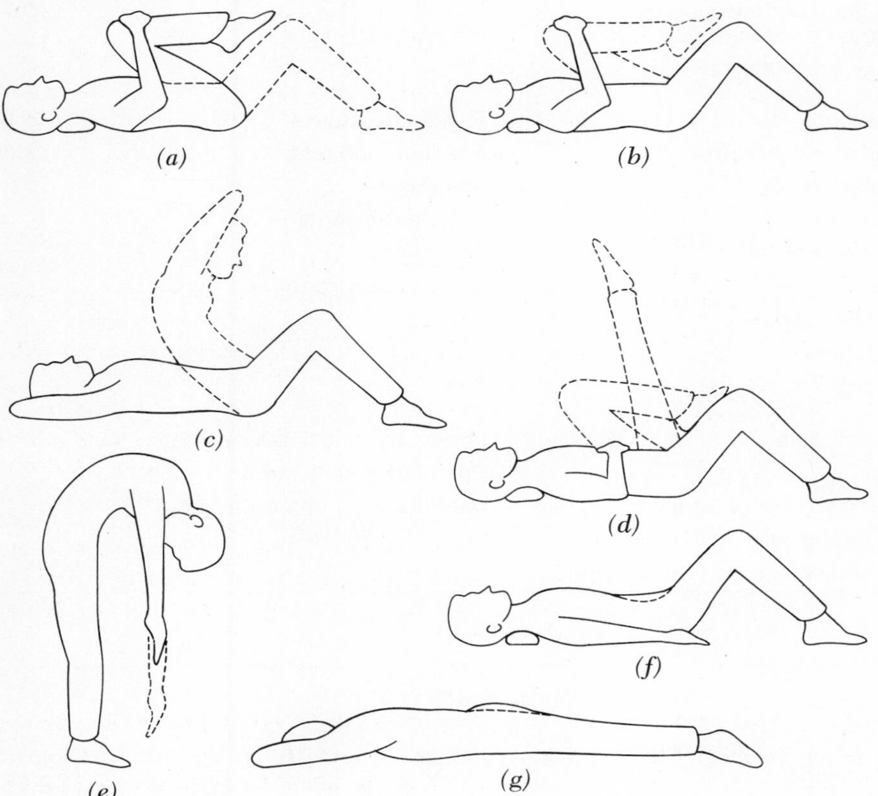

Table 94-1 Medical Referral/Consultation

Diagnosis	Clinical Manifestations	Management
Acute pyelonephritis	Fever with shaking chills Nausea, vomiting, diarrhea Dysuria, frequency Tenderness upon bimanual palpation of the kidney region Bacteriuria, pyuria, hematuria Leukocytosis	Physician referral Antibiotics Force fluids Follow-up urinalysis with cultures
Arthritis of spine	Pain centered in spine Limitation of motion and stiffness X-ray revealing spur formation, lipping Negative rheumatoid factor	Consultation with physician Acetylsalicylic acid Moderate exercise Local heat Physical therapy
Gynecological	Uterine malposition: retroversion, descensus, prolapse Uterosacral ligament invasion by endometrioses or carcinoma Late weeks of pregnancy	Physician referral
Ruptured intervertebral disk	Abnormal posture Limitation of spine motion Radicular back pain Paresthesias Course twitching or fasciculations Muscle spasms Impaired tendon reflexes Muscle weakness Muscle atrophy	Physician referral Absolute bed rest Analgesics Muscle relaxants Myelogram Corrective surgery
Infectious Pott's Disease or osteomyelitis	Nocturnal back pain Spinal ache Fever, night sweats Percussion tenderness Intervertebral disk and vertebral lesions	Immediate physician referral Spinal immobilization Multiple drug chemotherapy

bibliography

Bergerson, Berry S. *Pharmacology in nursing.* St. Louis: Mosby, 1976.

Caldwell, A. B., and Chase, C. Diagnosis and treatments of personality factors in chronic lowback pain. *Clinical Orthopedics* and *Related Research,* **129**:144–149 (1977).

Fowkes, William C., and Hunn, Virginia K. *Clinical assessment for the nurse practitioner.* St. Louis, Mosby, 1973.

Harvey, A. M., Johns, R. J., Owens, A. H. and Ross, R. S. (eds.). *The principles and practices of medicine.* New York: Appleton-Century-Crofts, 1976.

Hoole, A. J., Greenberg, R. A., and Pickard, C. G. *Patient care guidelines for family nurse practitioners.* Boston: Little, Brown, 1976.

Hudak, C. M., Redstone, P. M., Hokanson, N. L., and Suzuki, I. E. *Clinical protocols: A guide for nurses and physicians.* Philadelphia: Lippincott, 1976.

Nealon, Thomas F. (ed.). *Management of the patient with cancer.* Philadelphia: Saunders, 1976.

Newman, R. I., et al. Multidisciplinary treatment of chronic pain: long-term follow-up of low back pain patients. *Pain,* **4**(3):283–292 (1978).

Thorn, G. W. et al. *Harrison's principles of internal medicine.* New York: McGraw-Hill, 1977.

Tucker, S. M., Breeding, M. A., Canobbio, G. D., Paquette, E. H., Wells, M. E., and Willmann, M. E. *Patient care standards.* St. Louis: Mosby, 1975.

Wallach, Jacques. *Interpretation of diagnostic tests.* Boston: Little, Brown, 1974.

95 Crooked Back (Scoliosis)

M. CONSTANCE SALERNO

I. Etiology

A. Nonstructural
1. Poor posture
2. Pain
3. Muscle spasm
4. Short leg

B. Structural
1. Idiopathic (most common)
2. Congenital
3. Neuromuscular

II. Assessment: Idiopathic Scoliosis

A. Subjective data
1. Family history of crooked back
2. Client and/or parent(s) may complain of
   a. Poor posture
   b. Slouching
   c. High shoulder
   d. Crooked neck
   e. Lump on back
   f. One leg longer
   g. Hemline crooked
   h. Waist not the same on either side
   i. One breast larger
   j. Hip prominent

B. Objective data (see Fig. 95-1)
1. Client in upright position
   a. Head not centered over pelvis
   b. Shoulder elevated
   c. Scapula prominent
   d. Hip prominent (pelvic asymmetry)
   e. Asymmetric waist crease
   f. Exaggerated flank crease
   g. Asymmetrical arm-bone distance (one arm apparently longer than other)
   h. Curves less than 25° perhaps not visible in this position
2. Client in forward-bend position
   a. Small curves of 5 to 10° detected
   b. Observe anteriorly asymmetry of thorax
   c. Observe posteriorly asymmetry of trunk
3. Standing anterior/posterior spinal x-ray confirming extent of curve

III. Management: Idiopathic Scoliosis

A. Treatments/medications (see Table 95-1)

B. Counselling/prevention
1. The only sure way of preventing the severe curvatures of idiopathic scoliosis is by *early recognition* and treatment.
2. Screening before age 10 years should include boys as well as girls (see Fig. 95-1).
3. Clients with curves less than 15° should be alerted to the possibility of progression.
4. All siblings should be periodically evaluated for curvatures.

C. Follow-up

An orthopedist should determine the need for correction and examine the child at regular intervals to detect any progression of the curve.

D. Consultations/referrals
1. Consult a physician.
2. Refer to an orthopedic surgeon if lateral curvature is detected.

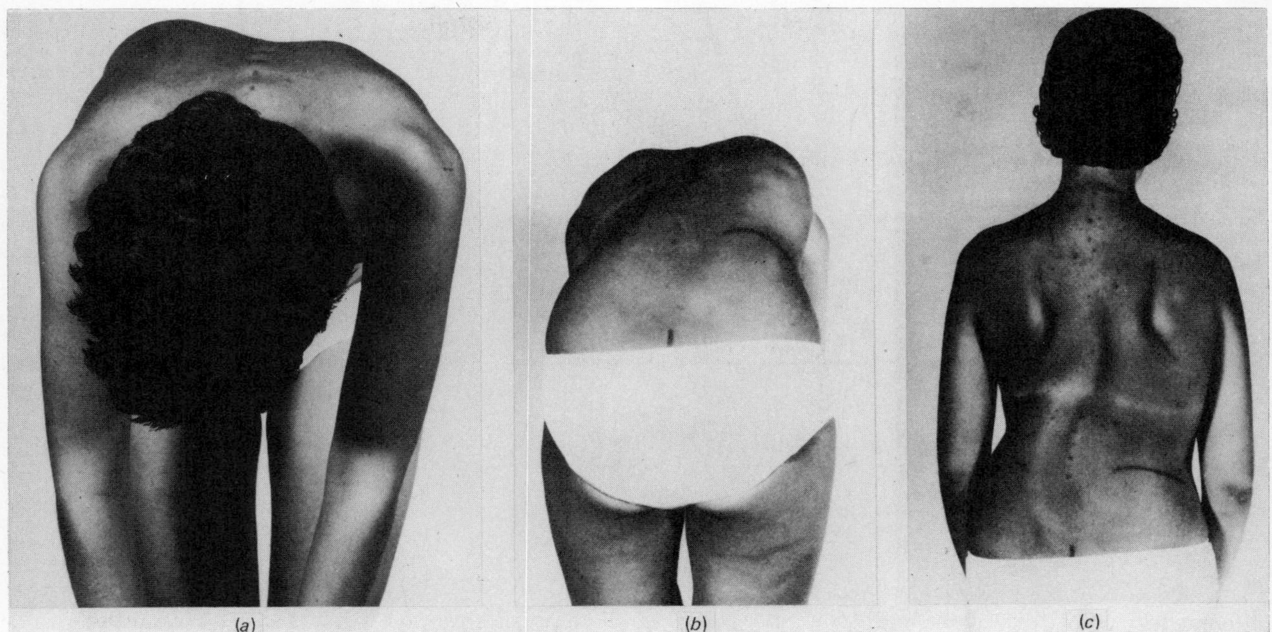

Figure 95-1 (a to c) Idiopathic scoliosis in a 14-year-old girl. First visit to orthopedist. Screening positions: standing and forward bend. Observe for: (1) general posture and alignment of the spine: (a) lateral angulation and (b) balance of head, neck, and shoulders over pelvis; and (2) asymmetry: (a) exaggerated flank crease—more prominent on opposite side, (b) high shoulder, (c) position of scapulae, (d) convexity on side of major curve (caused by protruding ribs), (e) prominent hip, and (f) one arm longer than other when hanging free in a forward bend position. *(From Ingalls, A. J., and Salerno, M. C. Maternal and child health nursing (4th ed.). St. Louis: Mosby, 1979, p. 567. Photos courtesy of the Naval Regional Medical Center, San Diego.)*

Table 95-1 Medical Referral/Consultation: Structural Scoliosis

Diagnosis	Clinical Manifestations	Management
Congenital—one side of vertebral column grows faster than the other	Misalignment of spine and asymmetry	Hospitalization Surgical correction at 1 or 2 yr of age perhaps indicated to prevent greater asymmetrical growth
Neuromuscular—result of disorders such as poliomyelitis, cerebral palsy, muscular dystrophy, etc.	Misalignment of spine and asymmetry	In order to prevent respiratory complications, some type of stabilization of spine must be considered using an external support or surgery.
Idiopathic	See II, A and B, above	An orthopedist should determine the need for correction and examine the child at regular intervals to detect any progression of the curve.

Table 95-1 Medical Referral/Consultation: Structural Scoliosis *(continued)*

Diagnosis	Clinical Manifestations	Management
Curve less than 20°	Misalignment of spine and asymmetry	Continued observation by orthopedic surgeon
Curve greater than 20° but less than 45°		Milwaukee brace and exercise program (see Fig. 95-2)
Curve greater than 50° (see Fig. 95-3)	Misalignment of spine and asymmetry; high shoulder; prominent hip; uneven legs (see Fig. 95-1)	Surgical correction; procedure consisting of a posterior fusion of the involved vertebrae with internal stabilization by distraction rods (see Fig. 95-4 and Fig. 95-5)

Figure 95-2 *(a)* A 13-year-old girl wearing a Milwaukee brace with right thoracic pad, left axillary sling, and left lumbar pad. Overall alignment is good. *(b)* Same girl, front view. Brace is contoured close to the body. *(c)* Brace can be worn under clothing without being noticed. *(From Ingalls and Salerno, p. 569.)*

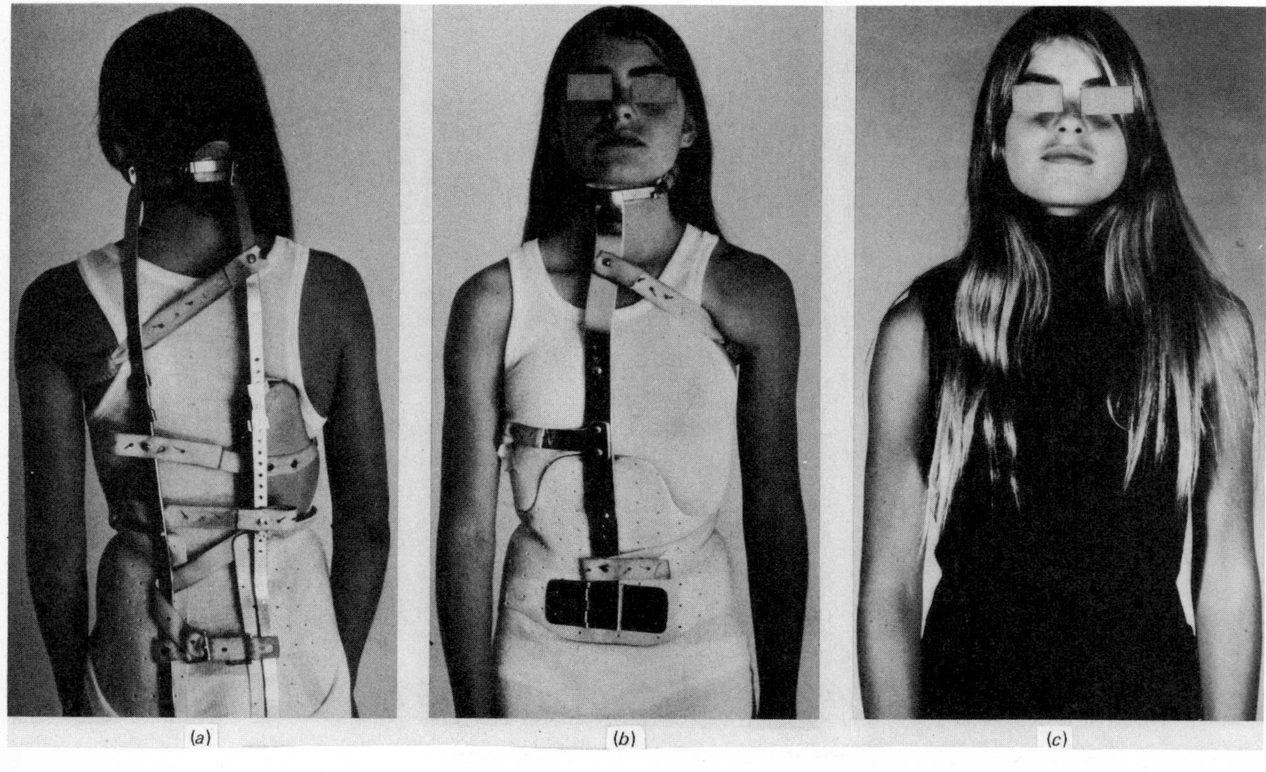

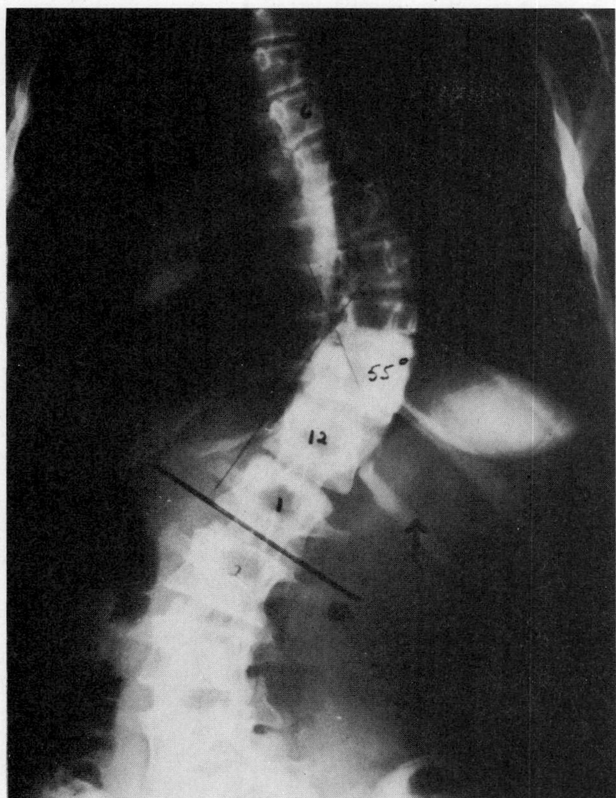

Figure 95-3 Roentgenogram of a 14-year-old girl (same as in Fig. 95-1) shows a 55° right thoracic curve of the spine. *(From Ingalls and Salerno, p. 568.)*

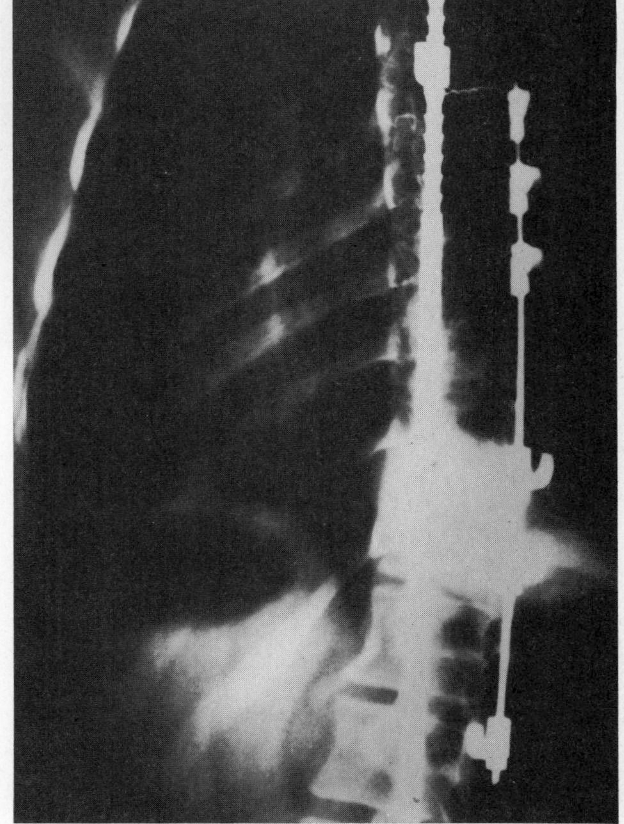

Figure 95-4 Roentgenogram of the back of the same client as in Fig. 95-3 6 months after spinal fusion and Harrington instrumentation. *(From Ingalls and Salerno, p. 570.)*

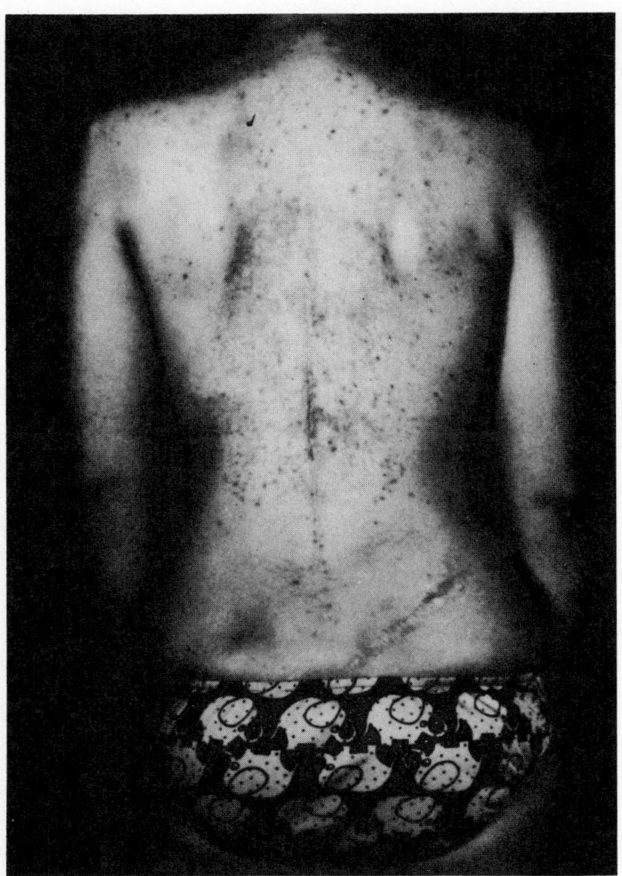

Figure 95-5 Postoperative standing position shows girl's spine reasonably well compensated. *(From Ingalls and Salerno, p. 570.)*

bibliography

Asher, M. A. Orthopedic screening. *Pediatric Clinics of North America,* **24**:713–721 (1977).

Dunn, B. H., Hakala, M. W., and McGee, M. E. Scoliosis screening. *Pediatrics,* **61**:794–797 (1978).

Holt de Toledo, C., et. al. The patient with scoliosis. *American Journal of Nursing,* **79**:1587–1612 (1979).

Keim, H. A. Scoliosis. *Clinical Symposia,* **30**:1. Summit, NJ: Ciba Pharmaceutical Co., 1978.

Love-Minogna, S. Scoliosis. *Nursing 77,* **7**:50–55 (1977).

Sigil, C. Current concepts in the management of scoliosis. *Nursing Clinics of North America,* **11**:691–698 (1976).

section 10

the integumentary system

INTRODUCTION JANE A. FOX

I. Subjective Data

A. Age
B. Description of problem; rash
C. Onset—progression, location
D. Characteristics at onset
E. Associated symptoms
1. Pruritis
2. Fever
3. Swollen glands
4. Nausea/vomiting
5. Headache
6. Stiff neck
7. Weakness
8. Abdominal pain
9. Bleeding

F. Urine and stool patterns
G. Sleeping patterns
H. Present medications, creams or oils, and medications used in the past which were helpful
I. Past/present history
1. Rashes
2. Allergies (eczema, asthma)
3. Anemia
4. Cutaneous tumors
5. Chronic problems

J. Nutritional history
K. Recent contagious disease or contact with contagious plant or infected person
L. History of trauma
M. Immunization history
N. Family history of skin rashes, chronic problems, allergies, acne, cancer, neurofibromatosis
O. Social history—housing and living conditions, economics, school, employment, recent trips

II. Objective Data

A. Physical examination
1. In newborn or infant, conduct a complete physical examination: Carefully inspect mouth for thrush and inspect diaper area, noting type of diapers worn.
2. In older children, conduct a problem-oriented physical examination: head, skin, lymph nodes, mouth, throat, nose, chest, heart, abdomen; neurological exam (in specific cases); muscular-skeletal exam if extremities involved.
3. Carefully inspect and palpate skin for turgor, texture, temperature, color, discolorations. Note and describe rashes and lesions. Palpate for tenderness and pain. Inspect condition of nails.
4. Inspect mouth for ulcers, and note condition of mucous membranes.
5. Palpate lymph nodes.

6. Palpate abdomen for tenderness and percuss and palpate for organomegaly.

B. Laboratory data—the following may be indicated

1. Culture of lesion
2. Gram stain of lesion
3. Scraping of lesion for fungus
4. Wood's lamp examination
5. Patch testing in severe cases of poison ivy/poison oak; deferral until eruption is cleared—may aggravate symptoms
6. Skin testing to rule out allergy (by physician)
7. X-ray

96 Vascular and Pigmented Nevi (Birthmarks)

JACALYN PECK DOUGHERTY

ALERT

1. Vascular nevi
   a. Port-wine stain in distribution of trigeminal nerve
   b. Cavernous hemangioma interfering with bodily function or near body orifice
   c. Rapid growth, change in status
   d. Repeated subjection to trauma, irritation

2. Pigmented nevi
   a. Recent change in size, color, status
   b. Repeated subjection to trauma, irritation
   c. Congenital giant, or bathing-trunk, nevus
   d. More than six café au lait spots on skin
   e. Appearance of pigmented nevi with halo

I. Etiology

A. Vascular nevi: overgrowth of blood vessels
1. Flat hemangiomas
   a. Salmon patch
   b. Port-wine stain
2. Raised hemangioma: strawberry
3. Other: cavernous

B. Pigmented nevi: overgrowth of pigment cells
1. Freckles (ephelis)
2. Mongolian spot
3. Café au lait spot
4. Junctional nevi
5. Compound nevi
6. Intradermal nevi
7. Blue nevi
8. Benign juvenile melanoma
9. Malignant melanoma
10. Halo nevi
11. Giant pigmented nevi

II. Assessment

A. Salmon patch
1. Subjective data
   a. Present at birth
   b. Transient
   c. Lesions fading and disappearing, or perhaps persisting faintly into adult life
   d. May reappear during crying episodes
2. Objective data
   a. Present at birth
   b. Salmon color to bright red
   c. Located on nape of neck, upper eyelids, glabella
   d. Flat
   e. Blotchy, irregular shape
   f. Blanch on pressure
   g. Size variable
   h. Transient

B. Port-wine stain
1. Subjective data
   a. Present at birth
   b. Usually persists
   c. Does not enlarge
2. Objective data
   a. Present at birth
   b. Red to dark reddish purple
   c. Sharply demarcated
   d. Flat
   e. Usually located on face, occipital area of scalp, or neck
   f. Occasionally located on extremities or other areas of body
   g. Usually unilateral
   h. Size variable
   i. May disappear but usually persists
   j. Does not enlarge

C. Strawberry hemangioma
1. Subjective data

a. Present at birth or appearing in newborn period
b. May enlarge rapidly in infancy
c. In newborn, may appear first as blanched area
d. Spontaneous involution usual

2. Objective data
a. Present at birth or appearing in newborn period
b. In newborn, may appear first as blanched area
c. Bright-red to bluish red "strawberry" appearance
d. Sharply demarcated
e. Slightly raised
f. Located primarily on shoulders, but any area of body may be involved
g. Size variable
h. Involutes spontaneously
i. Involution heralded by pale purple or gray spot
j. Involution proceeding centrally outward

D. Cavernous hemangioma

1. Subjective data
a. Present at birth
b. Lesions sometimes growing rapidly in infancy
c. Spontaneous involution usual
d. Involution first appearing as gray center

2. Objective data
a. Present at birth
b. Soft, rounded, compressible tumor
c. Normal overlying skin with blue to purplish coloration
d. Blanches with pressure
e. Raised
f. Poorly circumscribed
g. Located primarily on head but may occur anywhere on body
h. May occur in sites other than skin
i. Size variable
j. Disappears spontaneously

E. Freckles (ephelis)

1. Subjective data
a. First apparent in early childhood
b. Accentuated by exposure to sun
c. Familial tendency

2. Objective data
a. First apparent in early childhood
b. Color tan to dark brown
c. Irregularly shaped or rounded
d. Flat
e. More prevalent in sun-exposed areas of skin
f. Size variable
g. Most common in individuals with red hair

F. Mongolian spot

1. Subjective data
a. Present at birth
b. Does not enlarge
c. Generally fades by age 4 years

2. Objective data
a. Present at birth
b. Color pale blue to dark brown to black
c. Poorly demarcated, irregular
d. Flat
e. No blanching with pressure
f. Usually located over sacrum and buttocks, but may be located over extremity
g. Size variable
h. Usually solitary
i. Common in dark-skinned races

G. Café au lait spots

1. Subjective data
a. Present at birth or developing in early childhood
b. Lesions persisting
c. Numbers increasing with age
d. May be familial history for neurofibromatosis
e. May complain of skin tumors in childhood or at puberty

2. Objective data
a. Present at birth or developing in early childhood
b. Tan to brown areas of increased pigmentation
c. Irregularly shaped or oval
d. Sharply demarcated
e. Flat
f. Size and number variable
g. Possibly associated with flaccid tumors on palpation with unaffected overlying skin
h. Located anywhere on body

H. Junctional nevi

1. Subjective data
a. Few at birth—usually appearing during childhood
b. Numbers increasing with age
c. Size and appearance perhaps changing with age
d. Characteristics perhaps altered by recurrent trauma or repeated exposure to carcinogenic agents or sun

2. Objective data
a. Usually appears during childhood
b. Color light brown to dark brown or black
c. Flat or slightly elevated

d. Usually hairless
e. Located on all parts of skin, including genitalia, mucous membranes
f. Size, shape, and number variable

I. Compound nevi
1. Subjective data
a. Usually appears during childhood
b. Numbers increasing with age
c. Size and appearance perhaps changing with age
d. Appearance and characteristics perhaps altered by recurrent trauma or repeated exposure to carcinogenic agents or sun
2. Objective data
a. Usually appearing during childhood
b. Color pale brown to dark brown or reddish brown
c. Usually raised
d. Located on all parts of skin
e. Size, shape, and number variable

J. Intradermal nevi
1. Subjective data
a. Usually appearing during childhood
b. Numbers increasing with age
c. Size and appearance perhaps changing with age
d. Characteristics perhaps altered by recurrent trauma or repeated exposure to carcinogenic agents
2. Objective data
a. Usually appearing during childhood
b. Color flesh to brown or blue
c. Usually raised and dome-shaped
d. Surface smooth and uniform
e. Usually hair bearing
f. Located on all parts of skin
g. Size, shape, and number variable

K. Blue nevi
1. Subjective data
a. Usually present since birth
b. Usually solitary
2. Objective data
a. Usually present at birth
b. Color light blue to dark blue to blue-black
c. Flat, raised, or nodular
d. Surface smooth
e. Solitary
f. Usually located on dorsal hands, on face, or on buttocks
g. Size and shape variable

L. Benign juvenile melanoma
1. Subjective data
a. Appearing in childhood, before puberty
b. Size/appearance may change with age
c. Characteristics perhaps altered by recurrent trauma or repeated exposure to carcinogenic agents or sun
2. Objective data
a. Appearing during childhood
b. Color flesh to reddish brown to brown-black
c. Nodular or raised
d. Surface smooth
e. Usually hairless
f. Usually located on face or extremities

III. Management

A. Salmon patch
1. Treatments/medications: none
2. Counselling/prevention
a. Advise parent(s) lesion benign, transient
b. Advise parent(s) lesion may disappear or fade with persistence into adulthood
3. Follow-up: none
4. Consultations/referrals: none

B. Port-wine stain
1. Treatments/medications: none except cosmetic coverings
2. Counselling/prevention
a. If present at birth, support parent(s) for normal grieving process
b. Advise use of Covermark or other cosmetic covering
c. Counsel for psychological trauma if needed
d. If lesion in distribution of trigeminal nerve, advise parent(s) that lesion may be associated with Sturge-Weber disease (see Table 96-1)
e. If lesion located over large extremity, advise parent(s) that lesion may be associated with Klippel-Trénaunay-Weber syndrome (see Table 96-1)
3. Follow-up
a. If lesion on face, careful observation for development of signs of Sturge-Weber disease (seizures, hemiplegia, glaucoma, retardation)
b. If lesion located over extremity, careful observation for development of hypertrophy of limb
4. Consultations/referrals: referral to physician for evaluation of possible Sturge-Weber disease or Klippel-Trénaunay-Weber syndrome

C. Strawberry hemangioma
1. Treatments/medications: none
2. Counselling/prevention

a. Lesion may present at birth as blanched area of skin.
b. Advise parent(s) best treatment is observation.
c. Lesion may grow rapidly before resolution.
d. Resolution usually occurs by age 5 to 9 years.
e. Suggest counselling if needed for psychological trauma.
f. Offer emotional support for period of rapid growth or while awaiting resolution.

3. Follow-up: careful periodic observation to monitor growth or resolution
4. Consultations/referrals: referral to physician for evaluation if located near body orifice or of large size, or if there is superficial ulceration or secondary bacterial infection

D. Cavernous hemangioma

1. Treatments/medications: none unless marked growth when located near body orifice, which significantly compromises function
2. Counselling/prevention
   a. If it is present at birth, support the parent(s) in the normal grieving process.
   b. Advise parent(s) that the best treatment is observation, unless it is located near a body orifice whose function may be compromised.
   c. Lesion may grow rapidly before resolution.
   d. Resolution usually occurs by age 5 to 9 years.
   e. Suggest counselling for psychological trauma, if needed.
   f. Offer emotional support for the period of rapid growth and while awaiting resolution.
3. Follow-up
   a. Careful periodic observation to monitor growth or resolution, especially if located near body orifice
   b. If very large, careful periodic evaluation for thrombocytopenia (see Table 96-1, Kasabach-Merritt syndrome)
4. Consultations/referrals: referral to physician for evaluation if located near body orifice or if very large

E. Freckles (ephelis)

1. Treatments/medications: none
2. Counselling/prevention
   a. Freckles are found most frequently in children with red hair.
   b. Individuals with freckling should avoid exposure to sunlight.
   c. Protective sunscreening ointments should be used when prolonged sun exposure is anticipated.
3. Follow-up: none
4. Consultations/referrals: none

F. Mongolian spot

1. Treatments/medications: none
2. Counselling/prevention
   a. Most American Indian, black, and Oriental infants have mongolian spots.
   b. Lesions are benign.
   c. Lesions fade with time but may persist into adulthood.
   d. Lesions are not bruises.
3. Follow-up: none
4. Consultations/referrals: none

G. Café au lait spots

1. Treatments/medications: none
2. Counselling/prevention
   a. If a positive family history exists, more than six lesions may indicate Recklinghausen's neurofibromatosis (see Table 96-1).
   b. Less than six lesions generally indicate a benign extraneous finding.
3. Follow-up: careful periodic observation for development of tumors in skin or neurological involvement
4. Consultations/referrals: referral to physician if child has more than six lesions and/or presence of cutaneous tumors or neurological involvement

H. Junctional and compound nevi

1. Treatments/medications: none, unless subject to recurrent irritation or trauma, for cosmetic reasons, or if changing in size, color, or status; then total excision required
2. Counselling/prevention
   a. Numbers may increase with age.
   b. Monitor periodically for change in size, color, status.
   c. Avoid repeated exposure to sun, irritation, carcinogenic agents.
   d. Removal may be indicated if there is repeated trauma or irritation, or if nevi are located on mucous membrane.
   e. If removal is indicated, excision should be total.
3. Follow-up: none, other than periodic monitoring
4. Consultations/referrals: to dermatologist if history of recent change in size, color, or status, or for consideration of cosmetic removal

I. Blue nevi

1. Treatments/medications: none unless subject to recurrent irritation or trauma, for cosmetic reasons, or if changing in size, color,

or status; then total excision required

2. Counselling/prevention
   a. Usually solitary
   b. Monitoring periodically for change in size, color, status
   c. Avoidance of repeated exposure to sun, irritation, carcinogenic agents
   d. Removal perhaps indicated for nevi repeatedly subjected to trauma or irritation
   e. If removal indicated, total excision desirable
   f. Generally benign
   g. Often present at birth
3. Follow-up: none, other than periodic monitoring
4. Consultation/referrals: to dermatologist if history of recent change in size, color, or status, or for consideration of cosmetic removal

Table 96-1 Medical Referral/Consultation

Diagnosis	Clinical Manifestations	Management
Sturge-Weber disease	Port-wine stain covering at least upper eyelid or supraorbital region of face and scalp (trigeminal nerve distribution) Associated signs of hemiparesis, glaucoma, seizures, retardation, neurologic deficits	Referral to physician Medications as needed for management of glaucoma and seizures; physical therapy for hemiparesis Emotional support of client/parent(s) Follow-up: by physician as needed for management of signs and symptoms
Klippel-Trénaunay-Weber syndrome	Port-wine stain covering an extremity or part of an extremity Hypertrophy of involved limb	Referral to physician Surgery sometimes required Emotional support of client/parent(s) Follow-up: by physician as needed for management of signs and symptoms
Kasabach-Merritt syndrome	Large cavernous hemangioma Anemia, thrombocytopenia secondary to platelet trapping within hemangioma	Referral to physician Prednisone and/or surgery perhaps required Emotional support of client/parent(s) Follow-up: by physician as needed for signs and symptoms
Cavernous hemangioma	Location near body orifice Rapid growth with potential or actual interference with bodily function	Referral to physician Prednisone and/or surgery perhaps required Emotional support of client/parent(s) Follow-up: by physician as needed for signs and symptoms of bodily function compromise
Recklinghausen's disease (neurofibromatosis)	Familial history of neurofibromatosis Presence of more than six café au lait spots May have tumors arising in skin or elsewhere prior to or with onset of puberty Associated signs and symptoms may include retardation, skeletal deformities, seizures, hearing and vision impairment	Referral to physician, geneticist Emotional support of client/parent(s); genetic counselling Follow-up: by physician as needed for management of signs and symptoms

Table 96-1 Medical Referral/Consultation *(continued)*

Diagnosis	Clinical Manifestations	Management
Malignant melanoma	Found primarily in adults New lesion or recent change upon existing pigmented lesion Recent change in size, color, status Bleeding, crusting, ulceration, inflammation, pain, or itching Flesh to red-brown-black Color diffuse at periphery Irregular or variegated pigment Irregular or smooth surface Usually hairless	Consultation with physician Immediate referral to dermatologist Total excision Reassurance of client/parent(s) Routine and careful observation of remaining nevi by client/parent(s) essential Periodic observation of remaining nevi by health care practitioner
Halo nevi	Circular area of depigmentation surrounding pigmented nevus	Consultation with physician Immediate referral to dermatologist Total excision Reassurance of client/parent(s) Routine and careful observation of remaining nevi by client/parent(s) essential Periodic observation of remaining nevi by health care practitioner
Giant pigmented nevi (bathing-trunk nevus)	Pigmented lesion extending over large percentage of body surface Color dark brown to black Irregularly shaped Hair bearing after first few years of life May show malignant change Congenital	Consultation with physician Immediate referral to dermatologist Partial or total excision Support of parent(s) for normal grieving process Emotional support of client/parent(s) Some congenital giant pigmented nevi showing malignant changes and requiring excision Follow-up: by physician as needed to monitor status

bibliography

Behrman, T., Labow, T. A., and Rozen, J. H. *Common skin diseases—Diagnosis and treatment* (2d ed.). New York: Grune & Stratton, 1971.

Kempe, C. H., Silver, H. K., and O'Brien, D. *Current pediatric diagnosis and treatment* (5th ed.). California: Lange, 1978.

Stewart, W. D., Danto, J. L., and Maddin, S. *Dermatology: Diagnosis and treatment of cutaneous disorders* (2d ed.). St. Louis: Mosby, 1970.

———, ———, and ———. *Synopsis of dermatology.* St. Louis: Mosby, 1970.

Weinberg, S., Leider, M., and Shapiro, L. *Color atlas of pediatric dermatology.* New York: McGraw-Hill, 1975.

97 Scaly Scalp

MARILYN GREBIN

I. Etiology (unknown)

II. Assessment

A. Cradle cap
1. Subjective data
   a. Occurs in infants
   b. Worsened by the use of creams and oils
2. Objective data
   a. Mildly erythematous base
   b. Greasy, scaling of the scalp

B. Dandruff
1. Subjective data
   a. May occur anytime after infancy
   b. Active in the spring and fall
   c. Positive family history
   d. Mild pruritis
   e. Vague discomfort
2. Objective data
   a. Erythematous, scaling plaques
   b. Found on scalp, forehead, eyebrows, face, and axillae

C. Atopic dermatitis (eczema)
1. Subjective data
   a. History of family allergies and/or asthma
   b. Most common in infants and young children
   c. Intense pruritis
2. Objective data
   a. Infants and young children
      (1) Erythematous, scaling, crusty lesions
      (2) Found on face, ears, neck, scalp, popliteal spaces, antecubital fossa
      (3) Regional adenopathy
   b. Older children
      (1) Erythematous, scaling, crusty lesions
      (2) Found on the nape of the neck and behind the ears, and on the arms and legs

D. Psoriasis
1. Subjective data
   a. Older than 10 years of age
   b. Rare in younger children
2. Objective data
   a. Lesions small, erythematous, and circumscribed
   b. Dry, silvery scales
   c. Found on extremities, trunk, and scalp
   d. Fingernails pitted

E. Fungal infection of the scalp (tinea capitus)
1. Subjective data
   a. Occurrence at any age
   b. Recent contagion contact
2. Objective data
   a. Lesions are small, circumscribed, erythematous, grey, scaly patches
   b. Patches of alopecia where lesion presents
   c. Fluorescence under Wood's lamp

F. Pediculosis capitus (see Lice, Chap. 108)
1. Subjective data
   a. Intense pruritis
   b. Recent contagion contact
2. Objective data
   a. Ova (nits) attached to hair shaft, giving the appearance of dandruff
   b. Occipital or cervical adenopathy

III. Management

A. Cradle cap
1. Treatments/medications: shampoo daily with mild soap and water, using a soft brush.
2. Counselling/prevention
   a. Avoid the use of creams, lotions, or oils.
   b. Keep the head dry.
3. Follow-up: revisit in 2 weeks

4. Consultations/referrals: none

B. Dandruff

1. Treatments/medications: shampoo twice weekly with Selsun Blue.
2. Counselling/prevention: avoid hairdryers, which increase flaking.
3. Follow-up: return visit in 2 months if dandruff not controlled with shampoos
4. Consultations/referrals: none

C. Atopic dermatitis (Eczema)

1. Treatments/medications
   a. Alpha-Keri oil baths twice per week
   b. Use of soap substitute (Lowila Cake)
   c. Alpha-Keri lotion application 3 times per day
   d. Antibiotics for secondary skin infection
2. Counselling/prevention
   a. Fingernails kept clean and short
   b. Use of cotton clothing
   c. Diet free from acid foods, milk
   d. Removal of possible environmental allergens
      (1) Animals
      (2) Wool
      (3) Dust
      (4) Feathers
3. Follow-up
   a. Return visit in 2 weeks for check
   b. Follow monthly until controlled
4. Consultations/referrals
   a. Allergy skin testing by allergist
   b. In uncontrollable cases, referral to dermatologist

D. Psoriasis of the scalp

1. Treatments/medications
   a. Daily mineral oil applications to remove scales
   b. Followed by hot towels (turban fashion) for 10 min each time, $\frac{1}{2}$ h before shampooing
   c. Polytar shampoo
   d. Synalar solution rubbed into scalp
2. Counselling/prevention
   a. Avoid scratching.
   b. Encourage compliance with treatment regimen.
   c. Explain psoriasis and its control with persistent treatment.
3. Follow-up
   a. Weekly visits
   b. Communication with parent(s) by telephone about progress
4. Consultations/referrals: Dermatology consultation if not controlled in 1 month

E. Fungal infection of the scalp (tinea capitus)

1. Treatments/medications
   a. Whitfield's ointment (12% benzoic acid and 6% salicylic acid)
   b. Tinactin or Micatin ointment applied twice daily for 14 days
   c. Griseofulvin, in severe cases by the physician only
2. Counselling/prevention
   a. Avoid scratching.
   b. Encourage compliance with medication regimen.
   c. Use hot water; soap, and ammonia to clean clothing, especially hats.
   d. Dry-clean clothing.
3. Follow-up: return visit after 14 days
4. Consultation/referral: severe cases should be referred to the physician.

F. Pediculosis capitus

1. Treatments/medications
   a. Kwell shampoo once (may be repeated)
   b. Bacitracin ointment for secondary skin infection for 7 days
2. Counselling/prevention
   a. Examination of all family members
   b. Special laundering of clothing and linens
      (1) Separate from those of other family members.
      (2) Add ammonia solution to the wash water.
      (3) Use hot water.
      (4) Clothing may be boiled.
      (5) Steam press clothing.
      (6) Dry clean
3. Follow-up
   a. Revisit in 2 days
   b. For excessive secondary skin lesion infection, another visit in 1 week
4. Consultations/referrals
   a. School nurse
   b. Public health nurse for families continually reinfected

bibliography

DeAngelis, Catherine. *Pediatric primary care* (2d ed.). Boston: Little, Brown, 1979.

Gellis, Sydney S., and Kagan, Benjamin M. *Current pediatric therapy 8* (2d ed.). Philadelphia: Saunders, 1978.

Hurwitz, Sidney, Grebin, Burton, and Grebin, Marilyn. Newer developments in pediatric dermatology. *Pediatric Nursing* **4**(6):36–40 (1978).

98 Diaper Rash

CAROL ANN BROWN

ALERT

1. Newborn with more than erythematous papulovesicular lesions in diaper area, i.e., bullous or pustular lesions
2. Persistent diaper rash, inspite of therapy, beyond 1 week
3. Diaper rash accompanied by adverse systemic symptoms

I. Etiology

A. Infection
1. Viral
2. Bacterial
3. Fungal

B. Contact
1. Soaps, detergents, creams, powders
2. Feces, ammonia and other breakdown products from urine

C. Mechanical
1. Disposable diapers—occlusive
2. Rubber pants—occlusive
3. Obesity—increased intertriginous areas

D. Improper hygiene

E. Underlying skin problem
1. Atopic dermatitis
2. Seborrheic dermatitis

II. Assessment

A. Infection
1. Viral
   a. Subjective data
      (1) Fever
      (2) Upper respiratory infection (URI)
      (3) Sudden onset
      (4) Other children at home with upper respiratory infections and/or similar rash
   b. Objective data
      (1) Erythematous maculopapular, papulovesicular, even pustular lesions over diaper area, usually extending to other parts of body
      (2) Fever, symptoms of upper respiratory infection, and regional lymphadenopathy
      (3) Moderately ill-looking child because of the above
2. Fungal—*Candida albicans*
   a. Subjective data
      (1) Moderate to sudden onset
      (2) May report crying with wet and/or soiled diaper
      (3) Mother may have history of vaginal infection during pregnancy or current infection
      (4) Parent(s) may report "milk" stuck to oral mucosa
   b. Objective data
      (1) Erythematous papulovesicular lesions over perineum with extension of lesions to abdomen and redness in groin folds
      (2) Diaper area perhaps red and parchmentlike, with scalloped edges
      (3) Occasionally seen with oral candidiasis—white patches on oral mucosa or tongue

B. Contact—soaps, detergents, creams, powders, feces, urine-breakdown products
1. Subjective data
   a. Sudden prolonged onset
   b. Frequent loose stools, strong odor to urine
   c. Low fluid intake
   d. Strong detergent used in washing; poor

rinse of diapers, infrequent changing of diapers, poor cleansing of diaper area after urine and stool

e. Perfumed soaps, creams, and powders used during diaper changes

2. Objective data
   a. Erythematous, shinning, peeling exfoliation to bullae and papules over diaper area sparing folds without satellite lesions to abdomen
   b. Male with reddened ulcers on head of penis, with slight dryness
   c. Can be associated with an ID bracelet reaction—defined as disseminated eczematous lesions developing over all parts of body in response to the primary problem
   d. Fecal irritation—mainly involves perianal area and buttocks
   e. Ammonia diaper dermatitis—may begin with burnlike, bullous lesions with resultant red, glazed, sunburnlike rash and postinflammatory hypopigmentation
   f. Aside from above, physical exam usually normal and child appearing well
   g. Strong smell to diaper

C. Mechanical
1. Subjective data
   a. Usually prolonged onset
   b. Disposable diapers or cloth with plastic pants used
   c. Infrequent changes of diapers
   d. Report of long naps and sleeping through night with drying of diaper between wetting
2. Objective data
   a. Erythematous, excoriated, dry, and at times just hyperpigmented areas where plastic pants or disposable diaper rub against skin
   b. Maceration of skin from sweat retention caused by above
   c. Tide-mark diaper rash—scaly areas of upper thighs and at diaper margins from frequent wetting and subsequent drying of diaper
   d. Child appearing well otherwise

D. Improper hygiene
1. Subjective data
   a. Faulty washing of cloth diapers, poor cleansing of diaper area at changes
   b. Other children with rashes and poor hygiene
2. Objective data
   a. Can be any of the above presentations
   b. General hygiene poor

E. Underlying skin problems
1. Atopic dermatitis
   a. Subjective data
      (1) Positive family history of allergies
      (2) History of food allergies
      (3) Report of child being uncomfortable, itching skin
      (4) Introduction of too many new foods too fast
   b. Objective data
      (1) Erythematous, papulosquamous, dry lesions in patches over diaper area or confluent
      (2) Other areas of involvement—cheeks, antecubital and popliteal fossae, extensor surfaces of extremities, back
      (3) May have areas of excoriation from scratching
2. Seborrheic dermatitis
   a Subjective data—any of above
   b. Objective data
   (1) Erythematous, papulosquamous lesions developing a yellow, oily, easily removed crust that generally forms in intertriginous areas and usually begins in genitocrural folds
   (2) Lesions perhaps annular and erythematous, resembling ringworm
   (3) Other areas of involvement—scalp, eyebrows, retroauricular area

III. Management

A. Prevention
1. Frequent diaper changes
2. Good cleansing at changes
   a. Milk soaps and water with hand or washcloth
   b. Cotton balls with mineral oil (baby oil) or baby lotion
3. Protecting cream/ointment at first sign of redness, i.e., Desitin, A&D ointment, petroleum jelly
4. Proper care of cloth diapers
   a. Borate solution soaking
   b. Washing with milk soap with borate powder added to wash
   c. Double rinsing good at times
   d. Drying in the sun if possible

B. General management of diaper rash
1. Treatments/medications
   a. Creams applied to protect and dry skin: Desitin, A&D ointment, Zinc oxide paste
   b. For weeping and sunburnlike lesions, use of Burow's 1:20 aluminum acetate solution on clean cloths or gauze 4 times a day

2. Counselling/prevention
   a. To dry the lesions
      (1) Increase exposure to air or sunlight; at nap and bedtime, place the child on an absorbent pad without a diaper, and change the child's position frequently.
      (2) Apply cornstarch to the diaper area at changes.
      (3) Use one layer of cloth diapers, loosely attached.
      (4) Use two layers of cloth diapers at night, if the child sleeps long periods.
      (5) Discontinue rubber pants and disposable diapers.
   b. Change to mild soaps and discontinue the use of perfumed creams, powders, and fabric softeners.
   c. Advise the mother regarding proper soaking, rinsing, and washing of cloth diapers (see Prevention, III, A above).
   d. Wash the diaper area with mild soap and water, especially after stool, and pat dry with a clean towel or cloth; use nonalkaline soaps such as Basis Soap, Lowila Cake, Aveeno soap.
   e. Do not mix creams and powders.
   f. For severe rashes, change diapers at night while sleeping.
   g. Increase fluids in diet to decrease concentration of urine, making urine less irritating.
   h. The person diapering the child should wash hands well with soap and water before handling the child, before and after diaper changes.
3. Follow-up:
   Maintain phone contact, scheduling a visit if the rash does not improve within 2 weeks.
4. Consultations/referrals
   a. Visiting nurse service—if need evaluation of home or assistance of teaching diaper care in home
   b. Physician—if not resolving with above treatments, or severe dermatitis

C. Infection

1. Viral
   a. Treatments/medications: see General management of diaper rash, III, B, 1 above.
   b. Counselling/prevention: see General management of diaper rash, III, B, 2 above.
   c. Follow-up: Schedule a visit in 48 h, with good phone contact in between visits.
   d. Consultations/referrals: see General management of diaper rash, III, B, 4 above.
2. *Candida albicans*
   a. Treatments/medications
      (1) Nystatin cream to affected area 3 times a day or Mycolog Cream (nystatin, steroid, and antibiotic) sparingly to affected area 2 to 3 times a day
      (2) If oral candidiasis present —nystatin (Mycostatin) oral suspension (100,000 units/mL) 1 mL orally 4 times a day for 1 week or more; best applied with cotton ball and rubbed on affected areas
   b. Counselling/prevention: see General management, III, B. 2 above.
   c. Follow-up: 1 week
   d. Consultations/referrals: see General management, III, B, 4 above.

D. Mechanical contact and improper hygiene

1. Treatments/medications
   a. Refer to General management, III, B, 1 above.
   b. Acute, resistant, and/or chronic dermatitis may need application of steroid cream (hydrocortisone 1%, Valisone 0.1%, Kenalog 0.1%) sparingly 3 times a day.
2. Counselling/prevention: see General management, III, B, 2 above.
3. Follow-up
   a. Revisit should be scheduled in 1 week to check for improvement or resolution of dermatitis.
   b. Maintain good phone contact.
4. Consultations/referrals: see General management, III, B, 4 above.

E. Atopic dermatitis—seborrheic dermatitis

1, Treatments/medications
   a. See General management, III, B, 1 above.
   b. Apply a steroid cream (Hydrocortisone 1%, Valisone 0.1%, Kenalog 0.1%) sparingly 3 times a day to affected area.
2. Counselling/prevention
   a. See General management, III, B, 2 above.
   b. See Allergies, Chap. 137.
3. Follow-up: return visit in 1 week with good phone contact
4. Consultations/referrals: see General management, III, B, 4 above.

Table 98-1 Medical Referral/Consultation

Diagnosis	Clinical Manifestations	Management
Herpes simplex type II—primary	Vescular lesions with yellow membrane which after rupturing leaves an ulcer May have systemic symptoms: fever, irritability, pain Usually occurs when another member of the household (who has close contact with child) has a herpes recurrent infection, i.e., cold sore	Referral to physician No medication See General Management
Staphylococcal diaper dermatitis	Usually secondarily infected chemical, mechanical, or contact dermatitis Erythematous pustular lesions with easily sloughed surfaces Large bullous lesions with easily sloughed surfaces that appear flaccid and wrinkled Can be associated with fever, irritability, and poor feeding Laboratory: Gram's stain positive—culture showing staphylococcal infection	Referral to physician—may need hospitalization depending on systemic symptoms Cloxacillin oral suspension 125 mg/5 mL, 500–200 mg/kg per day orally in divided doses every 6 h See General Management
Streptococcal diaper dermatitis	Papulovesicular lesions with honey-colored crust formation May be an older child in home with similar lesions around mouth or nose (most common) Laboratory: Gram's stain positive—culture showing streptococci and some staphylococci	Consultation with physician Medications Less than 60 lb, 600,000 units LA Bicillin IM Oral Pen Vee K 25 mg/kg per day in four divided doses for 10 days See General Management Follow-up: return visit in 2 days to check progress and again at 1 wk

bibliography

Burgoon, Carroll F., et al. Diaper dermatitis. *Pediatric Clinics of North America,* **8**:835–856 (1961).

Chard, Marilyn A., and Dudding, Georgia Scoggins. Common skin problems in the newborn and infant. *Issues in Comprehensive Pediatric Nursing,* **1**:27–38 (July/August, 1977).

DeAngelis, Catherine. *Pediatric primary care* (2d ed.). Boston: Little, Brown, 1979.

Hoole, Axalla J., and Greenberg, Robert A. *Patient care guidelines for family nurse practitioners.* Boston: Little, Brown, 1976, pp. 93–96.

Jacobs, Alvin H. Eruptions in the diaper area. *Pediatric Clinics of North America,* **25**:209–224 (1978).

Koblenzer, Peter J. Diaper dermatitis—An overview, *Clinical Pediatrics,* **12**:386–390 (1973).

Lack, Edward B., and Esterly, Nancy B. Some common dermatologic problems of the first year of life. *Pediatric Digest,* June:11–19 (1974).

Nelson, Waldo E., et al. *Textbook of pediatrics* (10th ed.). Philadelphia: Saunders, 1975, pp. 1550, 1558.

Perlman, Henry Harris. A guide to some common dermatologic problems in childhood. *Hospital Medicine,* April:84–98 (1969).

———. The formulary of dermatologicals for children. *Drug Therapy,* January:85–96 (1975).

99 Prickly Heat (Miliaria)

M. CONSTANCE SALERNO

I. Etiology

A. Sweat retention in crystalline form associated with overheating and tight clothing

B. Keratin plugs at various levels of the sweat duct

II. Assessment

A. Subjective data

1. Itching and/or stinging
2. Rash appearing in area of maceration

B. Objective data

1. A minute transparent vesicle appears if the plug is superficial.
2. A discrete (2 to 5 mm) erythematous papulovesicular rash appears when deeper plugging occurs.
3. The most frequently involved areas are the face, neck, trunk, and diaper area, and any areas where perspiration is common or friction is frequent.
4. Rash may include pustular lesions.

III. Management

A. Treatments/medications

1. Reduction of environmental temperature by avoiding overdressing
2. Reduction of body temperature by use of antipyretics
3. Skin lotion containing hydrocortisone (triamcinolone acetonide lotion: 0.025% Kenalog)
4. Calamine lotion may be used as a drying agent

B. Counselling/prevention

1. Prevention is easier than treatment—avoid overdressing.
2. Lightweight, absorbent clothing is preferred.
3. In a very humid climate, a cool starch bath (1 cup cornstarch to a tub of tepid water) will help.
4. Avoid oily skin ointments and creams.

C. Follow-up

1. None unless secondary infection presents
2. For secondary monilial or bacterial infection, addition of Mycolog cream or other specific antibiotic to treatment regimen

D. Consultations/referrals: none

bibliography

McGuire, J. Other diseases of the skin. In A. M. Rudolph (ed.), *Pediatrics* (16th ed.). New York: Appleton-Century-Crofts, 1977, pp. 901–902.

Noojin, R. O. Pediatric dermatology. In H. C. Shirkey (ed.), *Pediatric therapy* (5th ed.). St. Louis: Mosby, 1975, p. 882.

Vaughan, V. C., McKay, R. J., and Nelson, W. E. *Textbook of pediatrics.* Philadelphia: Saunders, 1975, p. 1519.

100 Poison Ivy/Poison Oak

COLLEEN CAULFIELD

ALERT

1. Evidence of severe hypersensitivity response
2. Involvement of face, eyes, mucous membranes, genitalia
3. Widespread involvement and/or severe discomfort
4. Secondary infection

I. Etiology

A. Delayed or cell-mediated contact dermatitis caused by contact with oleoresins ("urushiols") in the *sap* of roots, stems, leaves, seeds, flowers, and fruits of the *Rhus* plant family (poison ivy, oak, and sumac)

Prior sensitization required for response; initial contact with allergen followed by a 7- to 21-day sensitization period; initial contact may not result in a response but subsequent exposures will

B. Eruption

1. May develop within hours to days after contact
2. New lesions usually continuing for 1 to 5 days, giving the appearance of a spreading rash

C. Severity of response influenced by

1. Quantity of antigen
2. Sensitivity to the antigen
3. Skin thickness; response more intense in areas of lesser thickness

D. Mode of transfer

1. Direct contact with oleoresin
   a. Oleoresin on skin surface may actively persist for 3 days.
   b. Oleoresin on clothes, pet fur, etc., may persist for more than a week.
2. Indirect contact by passive transfer of oleoresin via hands, clothes, etc., to other body areas; groin and eyelids frequently affected
3. Eruption not spread by vesicular fluid

II. Assessment

A. Subjective data

1. Sequential vesicular rash
2. Pruritus, burning
3. History of exposure or previous *Rhus* sensitivity

B. Objective data

1. Linear distributed vesicles at point of contact with *Rhus,* usually on an extremity that has brushed past the plant.
2. Secondary contact points that appear as haphazard, asymmetrical vesicles on different parts of the body, of varying severity, and on skin of varying thickness
3. Blotchy erythema
4. Reactive edema

III. Management

A. Treatments/medications

1. Acute vesicular stage
   a. Mainstay—Burow's solution (1:20—1:40) on intermittent compresses; frequency and intervals determined by severity
      (1) Mild to moderate—at 1-h intervals, 3 times a day
      (2) Severe—15 min every 1 to 2 h; continuous if very severe or widespread involvement
   b. Topical fluorinated corticosteroid creams 0.5% sparingly after each compress
2. After vesicular stage, discontinuance of com-

presses and application of calamine lotion and/or steroid cream (if needed), 3 times a day

3. Relief of pruritus; sedation
   a. Baths
      (1) Starch—add $\frac{1}{2}$ box cornstarch to a tub of tepid water; soak 20 to 30 min
      (2) Oatmeal—add 1 cup colloidal oatmeal to a tub of tepid water; soak 20 to 30 min
   b. Lotions
      Calamine lotion with 0.25% phenol applied 3 times a day, more frequently if needed
   c. Antihistamines
      (1) Diphenhydramine
      (2) Trimeprazine
      (3) Cyproheptadine
4. Severe widespread involvement: systemic corticosteroids after physician consultation
5. Secondary infection
   a. Appropriate antibiotics, usually for *Staphylococcus aureus* or *Streptococcus*
   b. Benzyl penicillin
   c. Erythromycin
6. Hyposensitization
   a. Not recommended except in severely sensitized individuals who cannot avoid exposure
   b. Results in only a milder response and is associated with significant adverse reactions
   c. Defer until acute dermatitis resolved

B. Counselling/prevention

1. Acute episode
   a. Eliminate antigen source.
   b. Instruct regarding treatment regimen, especially application of compresses.
   c. Avoid getting soap and water on those areas, except with compresses.
   d. Keep the areas clean, dry, and well aired.
   e. Wear soft, light, nonirritating clothing.
   f. Avoid the itch-scratch-itch cycle
   g. Cut fingernails short to prevent trauma; young children may need to wear mittens while sleeping
   h. Wash hands frequently to prevent secondary infection.
2. Instruction on identification of plant
3. Destruction of plants in the area
4. Teach how to avoid e.g., wearing protective clothing
5. If exposure occurs in the future
   a. Wash contact areas immediately with soap and water, being sure to rinse thoroughly.
   b. Wash all clothing, being careful not to spread antigen while removing clothing.

C. Follow-up

1. Telephone in 3 days to report progress.
2. Return in 3 days if there is no improvement.
3. Return immediately if there is evidence of secondary infection.

D. Consultations/referrals

1. Refer to a physician if the conditions in the Alert occur.
2. Send a note to the school nurse regarding treatment.
3. Notify the public health nurse if there is the suspicion of noncompliance of if there is difficulty with the treatment regimen.

bibliography

Dahl, M. V. The poisons of summer: updating your clinical checklist. *Modern Medicine.* July-August: 94–100 (1978).

Graef, J. W., and Core, T. E. *Manual of pediatric therapy.* Boston: Little, Brown, 1976.

Hoole, A. J., et al. *Patient care guidelines for family nurse practitioners.* Boston: Little, Brown, 1976, pp. 112–114.

Koblenzer, P. J. Contact dermatitis; Poison ivy dermatitis. In S. S. Gellis and B. M. Kagan (eds.), *Current pediatric therapy 6.* Philadelphia: Saunders, 1973, pp. 473–474.

Moschella, S. L., et al. *Dermatology.* Philadelphia: Saunders, 1975, pp. 250–255.

Noojiin, R. O. Pediatric dermatology. In H. C. Shirkey (ed.), *Pediatric Therapy* (5th ed.). St. Louis: Mosby, 1975, pp. 863–864.

101 Scabies

LESLIE LIETH

I. Etiology

A. *Sarcoptes scabiei*

B. Mode of transmission

1. Direct personal contact
2. Indirect contact
   a. Bed clothes
   b. Towel

C. Secondary infection common

1. Staphylococci
2. Streptococci

II. Assessment

A. Subjective data

1. Itchy rash
2. Fever
3. History of recent trip outside the United States by client/family
4. May have family members or friends with similar lesions

B. Objective data

1. Skin examination may reveal three types of lesions.
   a. 1 to 2 cm, curving or S-shaped or subcorneal burrows which may terminate in a small vesicle, usually located on sides of fingers
   b. Firm, indurated, erythematous, ½-cm excoriated nodules, occurring on interdigital webs, volar surfaces of wrists, penis, and scrotum
   c. 0.2- to 0.5-cm urticarial papules, which may be capped by a pinpoint-crusted excoriation, occurring on lower abdomen, buttocks, and thighs
2. To confirm diagnosis, it is necessary to identify the female mite, her eggs, or her feces.

III. Management

A. Treatments/medications

1. Kwell lotion or cream (1% Gamma benzene hexachloride)
   a. Apply over entire skin surface for 24 h.
   b. Then wash off.
   c. A second or third application may be made at 1-week intervals.
2. Shower or hot bath with soap and water
3. Secondarily infected lesions: topical antibiotic ointments

B. Counselling/prevention

1. Instruct regarding medications and treatments.
2. Explain transmission of parasite.
3. Explain importance of screening all family members.
4. Treat all infected family members.
5. Contacts and family members can be treated prophylactically.
6. Prevent spread of parasite.
   a. After treatment begins, use only fresh-laundered linen and bed clothes.
   b. Clean previously used clothing and linen.
      (1) Boiling
      (2) Ironing with hot iron
   c. Client should sleep alone.
7. Prevent scratching, if possible.
   a. Use mittens.
   b. Trim fingernails, toenails; keep clean.
   c. Hold child frequently.
8. Instruct to telephone if
   a. Increase in itching/discomfort
   b. Lesions become red, appear infected
   c. High fever

C. Follow-up

1. Return visit every week until resolved
2. Then 4 to 6 weeks later

D. Consultations/referrals

1. Public health nurse
2. School nurse

bibliography

Hazeirgg, D. E., et al. Diagnosis of scabies. *Southern Medical Journal*, **68**(5):549–551 (1975).

Orkin, Milton, and Maibach, Howard I. Scabies in children. *Pediatric Clinics of North America*, **25**:371–386 (1978).

Shirkey, Harry C. *Pediatric therapy*. St. Louis: Mosby, 1975.

102 Abscesses

ASHER H. WEINSTEIN

I. Etiology

A. Abscesses—bacterial infection
1. From penetrating wounds
2. Furuncles, carbuncles (boils)
3. Infected cysts
4. Infected blisters

B. Carbuncles, furuncles
1. Ingrown hair (folliculitis)
2. Usually *Staphylococcus*
3. Single-draining site (carbuncle)
4. Multiple-draining site (furuncle)

C. Cysts—sebaceous gland obstructed
1. Poor hygiene
2. Chemical obstruction (such as from makeup)
3. Oily skin

D. Blisters
1. Mechanical, as irritation from tools
2. From burns

II. Assessment

A. Subjective data
1. Pain
2. Possible history of trauma

B. Objective data
1. Abscess
   a. Fluctuant area
   b. Erythema around region
   c. Edematous
   d. Raised
   e. Pain on palpation
   f. Exudate
2. Carbuncle/furuncle
   a. Induration
   b. Erythema around region
   c. Superficial or deep
   d. Single-drain site (carbuncle)
   e. Multiple-drain site (furuncle)
   f. Exudate seeping from region
3. Cysts
   a. Fixed, raised lump
   b. Central core area on surface (follicle opening)
   c. Single or multiple sites
   d. Foul-smelling, nonpurulent sebum at core opening
   e. Infected, draining, purulent discharge
4. Blisters
   a. Thin membranous covering
   b. May be painful on palpation
   c. Contains a clear watery liquid
   d. May or may not be infected

III. Management

A. Abscesses
1. Treatments/medications
   a. Incision and drainage under local anesthesia (lidocaine)
   b. Pack with suitable material (iodoform gauze)
   c. Culture and sensitivity of drainage
   d. Dry, sterile dressing and absorbent gauze
   e. Appropriate antibiotic therapy if large abscess
   f. Laboratory screen for diabetes
2. Counselling/prevention
   a. Body hygiene
   b. Avoidance of local irritation
   c. Dressing kept dry and clean
3. Follow-up: revisit in 3 days for removal of packing and dressing change, then as needed
4. Consultations/referrals: as needed according to severity

B. Carbuncle/furuncle

1. Treatments/medications
   a. Warm compress or evaporating soaks using 1 oz white vinegar to 1 pt water; soak a piece of gauze; apply and allow to evaporate dry twice a day; dry, sterile dressings with antiseptic ointment in between soaks
   b. Incision and drainage of any formed abscesses that are fluctuant
   c. Culture and sensitivity of drainage
   d. Appropriate antibiotic therapy
   e. Laboratory screening for diabetes
2. Counselling/prevention
   a. Hygiene
   b. Avoidance of tight-fitting clothing
3. Follow-up: revisits at 2- to 3-day intervals for evaluation of site
4. Consultations/referrals: referral to physician if abscess forms for incision and drainage

C. Cysts

1. Treatments/medications
   a. If no infection, none
   b. If infection, follow III, A, 1 above
2. Counselling/prevention: hygiene
3. Follow-up: as needed
4. Consultations/referrals: asymptomatic and clients recovered from infections should be referred to a surgeon for elective excision of the cyst to prevent possibility of infection

D. Blisters

1. Treatments/medications
   a. Intact, unbroken blisters may be left alone and protected by plain gauze.
   b. Broken or infected blisters should be debrided and then dressed with gauze and antiseptic ointment.
2. Counselling/prevention
   a. Safety
   b. Avoidance of tight-fitting shoes
3. Follow-up: revisit in 3 days if needed and for any additional debridement
4. Consultations/referrals: none

bibliography

Anndt, Kenneth A. *Manual of dermatologic therapeutics*. Boston: Little, Brown, 1974.

Krupp, Marcus A, and Chatton, Milton J. *Current medical diagnosis and treatment* (2d ed.). Los Altos, Calif.: Lange, 1979.

Sauer, Gordon C. *Manual of skin diseases* (3d ed.). Philadelphia: Lippincott, 1973.

Schwartz, Seymour I. *Principles of surgery*. (3d ed.) New York: McGraw-Hill, 1979.

103 Nail Injury/Infection

ASHER H. WEINSTEIN

I. Etiology

A. Nail injury
1. Traumatic avulsion, partial or complete
2. Crush injury

B. Nail infection
1. Bacterial, usually *Staphlococcus*
2. Fungal
3. Ingrown toenails
4. Infection of a hangnail (paronychia)

II. Assessment

A. Fungal infection
1. Subjective data
   a. Long-standing, chronic, progressive involvement
   b. Usually no history of pain
   c. No history of trauma
   d. One or more nails involved
2. Objective data
   a. Nail thickened, raised, discolored, undermined
   b. Nail not tender on palpation

B. Bacterial infection
1. Subjective data
   a. Drainage from margin of nail
   b. Obvious abscess
   c. Pain, short duration, rapid onset 2 to 5 days
   d. History of injury to the cuticle
   e. Tendency for toenails to ingrow
2. Objective data
   a. Tender on palpation
   b. Obvious area where nail is ingrown into the tissue
   c. Exudate from the area

C. Nail injury
1. Subjective data
   a. Painful nail or pain in surrounding area
   b. History of trauma: crush/avulsion
2. Objective data
   a. Nail perhaps avulsed or crushed
   b. Possible concurrent injury to underlying bone
   c. If infection, exudate visible
   d. Obvious subungual abscess

III. Management

A. Fungal infections
1. Treatments/medications
   a. The nail should be filed lightly with an abrasive stick to remove the glaze.
   b. Then an antifungal agent, such as Lotrimin 1% cream or lotion, should be applied to all parts of the nail twice a day.
2. Counselling/prevention
   The "cure," if effective, may take as long as 1 year. Client compliance is essential.
3. Follow-up: revisit at 6-week to 2-month intervals to trim nails and record progress and compliance.
4. Consultations/referrals:
   a. Consult a physician.
   b. If the fungal infection is severe or widespread, then the client should be referred to a physician for oral agents.

B. Bacterial infections
1. Treatments/medications
   a. Mild, early paronychia infections which are minimally painful to palpation may be treated with alcohol soaks for 24 to 48 h. The nail should be soaked in alcohol 70% for 2 h and then dry for 4 h, repeated throughout the day.
   b. Severe cases, or nails that don't improve with the above treatment, should be re-

sected back to the matrix of the nail. The amount of nail to be removed should be in proportion to the area of infection and should be done with digital block anesthesia lidocaine 2% and then dressed as in Nail Injury, III, C below.

2. Counselling/prevention
   a. Care not to injure cuticles of the nail
   b. Care and instruction about the cutting of toenails
3. Follow-up
   a. Schedule a revisit for redressing and reevaluation in 3 days.
   b. For ingrown toenails, follow-up at home should include 3-min, twice-a-day scrubs with an antiseptic soap, followed by a dry, sterile dressing with antiseptic ointment.
4. Consultations/referrals
   a. Consult a physician.
   b. Severe infections may progress to an osteomyelitis, and these cases should be referred to an orthopedist surgeon.

C. Nail injury

1. Treatments/medications
   a. X-ray for underlying bone damage, crush, or fracture.
   b. Thoroughly clean and irrigate the region with an appropriate antiseptic solution.
   c. If the nail is still for the most part attached, then apply antiseptic ointment and nonadherent gauze with a dry sterile dressing.
   d. If the nail is avulsed and attached at only a small region, the nail should be removed under local anesthesia lidocaine 2% digital block and the wound dressed as above.
   e. Tetanus prophylaxis may be needed.
2. Counselling/prevention
   Safety regarding shoes, etc.
3. Follow-up
   a. Schedule a revisit in 2 to 3 days for dressing change and reevaluation of the wound.
   b. If there is any complication of infection at the recheck, then a culture should be done and appropiate antibiotic therapy begun.
4. Consultations/referrals:
   a. Consult/refer to a physician for nail removal.
   b. Refer to a physician/orthopedist if the bone is involved by infection or fracture.

bibliography

Anndt, Kenneth A. *Manual of dermatologic therapeutics*. Boston: Little, Brown, 1974.

Eckert, Charles D. *Emergency room care* (2d ed.). Boston: Little, Brown, 1971.

Krupp, Marcus A., and Chatton, Milton J. *Current medical diagnosis and treatment* (2d ed.). Los Altos, Calif.: Lange, 1979.

104 Minor Trauma

ASHER H. WEINSTEIN

ALERT
1. Deep lacerations
2. Lacerations involving damage to tendons or motor and sensory nerves
3. Lacerations involving major vessels

I. Etiology

A. Abrasion: rubbing or scraping of outer layers of skin
1. From falling, slipping, etc.
2. From scuff burns from carpet, etc.

B. Laceration
1. Incised wounds, caused by sharp instrument, knife, razor, glass
2. Tear wounds
   a. Produced by blunt trauma
   b. Blunt instrument under force
   c. Falling against blunt object

C. Puncture
1. Caused by sharp instrument such as a needle, knife, or nail
2. Usually a deep wound with a small entry point

D. Contusion
1. Caused by blunt trauma without a break in the skin
2. Vessels in tissue damaged causing interstitial hemorrhage

II. Assessment—Abrasion, Laceration, Puncture, Contusion (see Etiology, above)

A. Subjective data: symptoms vary and depend upon
1. Cause
2. Elapsed time
3. Pain
4. Loss of movement of injured part
5. Contamination
6. Tetanus prophylaxis

B. Objective data: findings vary and depend upon
1. Type of wound and cause
2. Site and size of wound
3. Depth of injury
4. Foreign body
5. Hemorrhage
6. Infection or exudate from wound
7. Loss of movement of part
8. Sensory loss

III. Management

A. Abrasion
1. Treatments/medications
   a. Clean wound with antiseptic soap (Betadine, pHīsoHex) and lukewarm water to remove all foreign substances, such as dirt.
   b. Air dry or dry with a sterile gauze.
   c. Apply an ointment such as Betadine or Bacitracin to the area, and cover with a nonadherent mesh such as vaseline gauze or Xeroform and a gauze pad, and secure with roller gauze.
   d. Be sure client has tetanus immunization.
2. Counselling/prevention
   a. Dressing should be kept clean and dry.
   b. Dressing should be kept in place for 5 days.
   c. Client should be instructed about safety.
3. Follow-up
   a. Return visit in 5 days for reevaluation and dressing change
   b. Return sooner if malodorous dressing, increased pain, or purulent drainage, fever, or erythema
4. Consultation/referral: none

B. Laceration

1. Treatments/medications
   a. Clean thoroughly with antiseptic soap and water.
   b. Inspect the wound for any foreign body.
   c. If the wound is clean and superficial and there is no tension on the skin, then it may be closed with Steri-Strips or a butterfly bandage, painted with Betadine, and covered with a dry sterile bandage.
2. Counselling/prevention
   a. Keep the bandage dry and clean.
   b. Steri-Strips should be kept in place for 5 to 7 days.
   c. Advise on appropriate safety precautions.
3. Follow-up
   a. Return visit in 24 to 48 h for dressing change and reevaluation; bandage perhaps changed but Steri-Strips should remain in place
   b. Return sooner if malodorous dressing, discharge from wound, fever, or erythema
4. Consultation/referral
   a. If the wound is grossly contaminated or deep, a physician should be consulted regarding surgical debridement and/or suture closure and appropriate antibiotic therapy.
   b. Referral should also be made if there is loss of movement of the part or significant sensory loss because of possible tendon or nerve damage.

C. Puncture

1. Treatments/medications
   a. The wound should be cleaned with antiseptic soap and water and painted with Betadine, and no attempt should be made to close the wound by suture or other means.
   b. A sterile dressing should be applied.
   c. Tetanus prophylaxis should be assured.
   d. Appropriate antibiotic therapy is called for if the wound is deep or grossly contaminated.
2. Counselling/prevention
   a. Keep the wound clean and dry until healed.
   b. Advise on appropriate safety precautions.
3. Follow-up
   a. Schedule a return visit in 24 to 48 h for reevaluation and redressing.
   b. The wound should be inspected for signs of infection, and the client should be advised to return if there is any drainage, erythema, fever, or increased pain.
4. Consultations/referrals

   Deep or grossly contaminated or infected puncture wounds should be referred to a physician to examine for possible underlying structure damage or for surgical debridement.

D. Contusion

1. Treatments/medications
   a. The area of contusion should be treated with an ice pack applied intermittently for the first 24 to 48 h, followed with applications of heat.
   b. No dressing is required.
2. Counselling/prevention: Appropriate safety precautions
3. Follow-up: Unless there are specific complications such as an expanding hematoma or infection, no follow-up is indicated.
4. Consultation/referral: none, except as outlined in Follow-up above

bibliography

Eckert, Charles D. *Emergency room care* (2d ed.). Boston: Little, Brown, 1971.

Schwartz, Seymour I. et al. *Principles of surgery* (3d ed.) New York: McGraw-Hill, 1979.

Wilson, John L. *Handbook of surgery* (5th ed.). Los Altos, Calif.:Lange, 1973.

105 Weeping Lesions

MARILYN GREBIN

ALERT
1. High fever
2. Vesicles over eczematous lesions
3. Toxic appearance
4. Petechiae

I. Etiology
A. Infection
   1. Bacterial
   2. Viral
B. Allergy
C. Miscellaneous

II. Assessment
A. Infection
   1. Impetigo contagiosa (staphylococci and streptococci)
      a. Subjective data
         (1) Recent contact with infected individual
         (2) Scratching of infected area
         (3) Recent history of infection
      b. Objective data
         (1) Uncleanliness of skin and nails
         (2) Mucopurulent rhinorrhea
         (3) Vesicular, straw-colored lesions and crusts on face, ears, around nares, posterior neck, scalp
         (4) Scratch marks
   2. Bullous impetigo (staphylococci, streptococci)
      a. Subjective data
         (1) Infants
         (2) Recent infection of skin or upper respiratory tract
         (3) Recent contagious contact
      b. Objective data
         (1) Uncleanliness of skin and nails
         (2) Erythematous papules on moist surfaces or creases
         (3) Forming of bullae filled with clear or cloudy straw-colored fluid
         (4) When bullae rupturing, the skin appearing scalded with straw-colored or brown crusts
   3. Herpes simplex
      a. Subjective data
         (1) Recent contact
         (2) Irritability
         (3) Anorexia
         (4) Mouth pain and odor
         (5) History of fever
         (6) History of eruption 3 to 5 days prior to crusts
      b. Objective data
         (1) Fever
         (2) Clusters of small vesicles on an erythematous base
         (3) Lesions appearing anywhere on the skin and mucous membranes
         (4) Yellow crusts forming upon vesicular rupture
         (5) May have gingivostomatitis
   4. Varicella (chickenpox)
      a. Subjective data
         (1) Cough
         (2) Coryza
         (3) Fever
         (4) Malaise
         (5) Anorexia
      b. Objective data
         (1) Papular eruption beginning on the chest
         (2) Vesicles on an erythematous base
         (3) Centripetal spread (teardrop on a rose petal)
         (4) Vesicles rupturing and crusting

(5) Fever

5. Herpes zoster (shingles)
   a. Subjective data
      (1) Chills
      (2) Fever
      (3) Malaise
   b. Objective data
      (1) Clustered vesicular eruption in a dermatome of innervation
      (2) Appears on fourth or fifth day
      (3) Neuralgia along rash site
      (4) Vesicles rupturing and crusting

B. Allergic

1. Atopic dermatitis (eczema)*
   a. Subjective data
      (1) Allergies to foods or medication
      (2) Chronic upper respiratory infections
      (3) Positive family history of eczema, allergies
      (4) Presence of pruritis
   b. Objective data
      (1) Erythematous patches of papules on face, trunk, neck and popliteal and anticubital areas
      (2) Serous weeping areas
      (3) Crusting found in younger children
      (4) Clear nasal drainage
      (5) Scratch marks with bleeding
      (6) Skin texture dry
      (7) Child sometimes having episodes of wheezing
2. Allergic contact dermatitis (see Poison Ivy/Poison Oak, Chap. 100)
   a. Subjective data
      (1) Contact with poison ivy or poison oak plants
      (2) Any age group
      (3) Intense pruritis
   b. Objective data
      (1) Vesicles of various sizes on erythematous base
      (2) Vesicles rupturing and crusting
      (3) Intense pruritis with scratch marks that spread lesions to unaffected areas of the body

III. Management

A. Infection

1. Impetigo contagiosa
   a. Treatments/medications: Bacitracin ointment 500 units/g
   b. Counselling/prevention
      (1) Isolation of toilet articles from other family members
      (2) Nails kept clean and cut short
      (3) Instruction to parent(s) in the proper cleansing technique
   c. Follow-up: revisit 5 to 7 days
   d. Consultations/referrals: none
2. Bullous impetigo
   a. Treatments/medications
      (1) Oxacillin for 7 to 10 days, or
      (2) Long-acting Bicillin, or
      (3) Penicillin for 10 to 14 days, divided into three doses per day, or
      (4) For children allergic to penicillin, erythromycin for 10 to 14 days
   b. Counselling/prevention
      (1) Instruct parent(s) in the importance of compliance with the treatment regime.
      (2) Isolate the child's toilet articles from those of other family members.
   c. Follow-up
      (1) Revisit in 7 days to check progress.
      (2) Revisit in 14 days upon completion of medication.
   d. Consultations/referrals: If there is no response to medication at either of the follow-up visits, consult with the physician.
3. Herpes simplex
   a. Treatments/medications
      (1) No treatment for skin lesions; healing effected within 10 days
         (a) For gingivostomatitis lesions, hydrogen perioxide diluted 1:1 for oral rinse; Cēpacol mouthwashes for oral hygiene
         (b) Acetaminophen for fever
   b. Counselling/prevention
      (1) Prevention of dehydration by drinking cold, nonacid liquids
      (2) Diet including soft, bland foods
      (3) Reassurance to the parent(s) because the child may be very irritable
      (4) Lesions may last 4 to 10 days
   c. Follow-up: revisit in 7 days.
   d. Consultations/referrals: Physician should examine the child with gingivostomatitis.
4. Varicella (chickenpox)
   a. Treatments/medications
      (1) Aspirin or acetaminophen for fever
      (2) Caladryl lotion
   b. Counselling/prevention
      (1) Keep fingernails clean and cut short.
      (2) Cotton mittens may be necessary for a small child.

*See Allergies, Chap. 137.

(3) Bathe carefully with soap and water—after vesicles crust.

(4) Isolate from high-risk clients or persons who have not had varicella.

(5) Reassure the parent(s) that the vesicles will be completely erupted in 3 to 5 days and will begin to dry and crust by 7 to 10 days.

(6) When all lesions are crusted, the child may return to school.

c. Follow-up: by telephone in 6 days

d. Consultations/referrals

(1) None in uncomplicated cases

(2) Physician intervention if the child is at risk

(3) School nurse

5. Herpes zoster (shingles)

a. Treatments/medications

(1) Aspirin for pain

(2) If the pain is severe, physician may prescribe codeine

b. Counselling/prevention

(1) The child should be encouraged to rest.

(2) Isolate toilet articles from those of other family members.

(3) Isolate from high-risk individuals.

(4) Reassure the parent(s).

c. Follow-up: revisit within 7 to 10 days

d. Consultations/referrals: Physician should be aware of the child and the condition.

B. Allergic

1. Atopic dermatitis (eczema)

a. Treatments/medications

(1) Take Alpha-Keri oil baths twice per week (avoid excessive bathing).

(2) Use soap substitutes such as Lowila Cake.

(3) Apply Alpha-Keri lotion 3 times per day.

(4) Antibiotics are indicated for secondary skin infections.

(5) For weeping lesions, use wet compresses with Burow's solution 15 min each hour; rinse and reapply.

(6) Topical corticosteroids may be prescribed by the physician.

(7) Immunizations should be determined by the allergist after testing.

b. Counselling/prevention

(1) Instruct parent(s) in bathing and skin care techniques.

(2) Reassure parent(s) that this disorder can be controlled if the regimen is followed.

(3) Keep child's fingernails short.

(4) Use cotton clothing.

(5) Diet should be free from acid foods and milk.

(6) Remove possible environmental allergens such as dust, wool, animals, etc.

(7) Mittens may be necessary for small children.

c. Follow-up

(1) Revisits should be frequent until there is some control of the dermatitis.

(2) A home visit can assist the parent(s) in preparing the environment.

d. Consultations/referrals

The child should be seen by an allergist for testing and case review.

2. Allergic contact dermatitis

a. Treatments/medications

(1) Wash skin lesions with soap and water.

(2) Apply Caladryl lotion.

(3) In severe cases, the physician may prescribe Prednisone 2 mg/kg per day for 5 days; decreasing the dosage after 5 days.

b. Counselling/prevention

(1) Instruct parent(s) in proper cleansing technique.

(2) Isolate toilet articles from those of other family members.

(3) Have the parent(s) investigate the source of the contact irritant if it is in the child's near environment.

c. Follow-up: revisit in 5 days

d. Consultations/referrals: severe cases with bullous lesions must be seen by the physician.

bibliography

DeAngelis, Catherine. *Pediatric primary care* (2d ed.). Boston: Little, Brown, 1979.

Gellis, Sydney, S., and Kagan, Benjamin M., *Current pediatric therapy 8*. Philadelphia: Saunders, 1978.

Hurwitz, Sidney, Grebin, Burton, and Grebin, Marilyn. Newer developments in pediatric dermatology. *Pediatric Nursing*, **4**(6):36–40 (1978).

Weinberg, Samuel, Leider, Morris, and Shapiro, Lewis. *Color atlas of pediatric dermatology*. New York: McGraw-Hill, 1975.

Table 105-1 Medical Referral/Consultation

Diagnosis	Clinical Manifestations	Management
Ecthyma (streptococcus, staphylococcus)	Encompasses entire epidermis to the upper dermis Appears as a firm crust on an ulcer surrounded by erythema	Referral to the physician
Erysipelas (Group A beta hemolytic streptococcus)	Toxic appearance Fever Chills Malaise Lesions circumscribed and erythematous Vesicles and bullae rupturing and crusting	Referral to the physician
Eczema herpeticum or dermatitis herpetiformis	Herpetic vesicles covering all the areas of eczema Weeping—crusting of the lesions High fever Severe toxicity Fatal if complicated by bacterial infection	Referral to the physician
Stevens-Johnson syndrome	Wheals, bullae, and urticarial lesions of the mouth, eyes, genitalia High fever Severe toxicity Petechiae Hemorrhagic crusting	Referral to the physician
Pemphigus	Rare in children Vesicles appearing on uninflamed skin Weeping and crusting	Referral to the physician

106 Hives (Urticaria)

M. CONSTANCE SALERNO

ALERT
1. Acute respiratory distress
2. Anaphylaxis

I. Etiology

A. Hives (urticaria)
1. Skin manifestation associated with erythema, pruritus, and wheal formation
2. Usually caused by the release of a chemical mediator, histamine, following an antigen-antibody interaction

II. Assessment

A. Subjective data
1. Known possible causes
2. Rapid onset of pruritic skin lesions
3. Past history of similar symptoms

B. Objective data
1. Skin lesions are characteristically erythematous and raised (wheals or welts), often annular, and sometimes coalescent.
2. Distribution may be localized or generalized with lesions appearing in successive crops.
3. Hives may be associated with edema of eyelids, lips, tongue, genitalia, hands, and/or feet.

III. Management

A. Treatments/medications
1. Search for cause and elimination of offending allergens, including foods, drugs, insect bites, parasitic infestations, plants, and other environmental agents
2. Antihistamines (see Table 137-2) may be given every 4 to 6 h on a regular schedule and continued for several days after the lesions disappear
   a. Chlorpheniramine maleate (Chlor-Trimeton)
   b. Diphenhydramine hydrochloride (Benadryl)
   c. Tripelennamine hydrochloride (Pyribenzamine)
3. Aqueous epinephrine 1:1000 subcutaneously (s.c.) for rapid relief of widespread intense pruritis, followed by prescribed antihistamine regimen
4. Tepid starch bath

B. Counselling/prevention
1. Determine allergen and avoid.
2. Avoid heat or cold exposure.
3. Stress compliance with medication.
4. Instruct for starch bath (1 cup cornstarch in a tubful of water, blotting skin dry after bathing).
5. Lesions should disappear in 48 h.

C. Follow-up: Return visit if condition worsens or does not resolve in 48 h.

D. Consultations/referrals: Refer to physician if condition does not resolve in 48 h.

Table 106-1 Medical Referral/Consultation

Diagnosis	Clinical Manifestations	Management
Erythema multiforme	Sudden appearance of macular, erythematous, urticarial rash on skin and sometimes mucous membranes	Referral to physician/allergist Search for cause, especially bacteria or viral infections or drugs

Table 106-1 Medical Referral/Consultation *(continued)*

Diagnosis	Clinical Manifestations	Management
		Supportive and symptomatic treatment Antihistamines
Severe form of Stevens-Johnson syndrome	Typical iris or target skin lesions Mucous membranes, especially mouth conjuctiva and urethra, perhaps involved	Immediate referral to physician Hospitalization
Anaphylaxis (severe allergic reaction occurring minutes after exposure to etiological agent, particularly bee sting)	Diffuse flushed skin Intense pruritis Hoarseness Dyspnea—may be fatal!	Early recognition sometimes life saving Epinephrine (aqueous 1:1000) twice at 20-min intervals Maintenance of airway Supportive Follow-up by pediatric allergist

bibliography

Bailit, I. W., and Mueller, H. L. Allergic disorders. In H. C. Shirkey (ed.), *Pediatric therapy* (5th ed.). St. Louis: Mosby, 1975, pp. 897–901.

Ferrara, A. Rashes (urticaria). In S. K. Dube and S. H. Pierog (eds.), *Immediate care of the sick and injured child.* St. Louis: Mosby, 1978, pp. 55–56.

Mueller, H. L. Stinging-insect allergy. *Pediatric Annals,* 3:43–53 (1974).

Vaughan, V. C., McKay, R. J., and Nelson, W. E. *Textbook of pediatrics* (10th ed.). Philadelphia: Saunders, 1975, pp. 512–518.

107 Bites

ASHER H. WEINSTEIN

ALERT

1. Bites involving the face and the hands
2. Infection of a bite involving the hands
3. Bite from wild or unknown animal

I. Etiology

A. Wild animals
B. Domestic animals
C. Human bites

II. Assessment: Signs and symptoms vary, pertinent information is:

A. Subjective data

1. Type of bite, animal/human
2. Time since the injury
3. Immunization status of animal if known
4. Immunization status of client
5. Contamination of wound
6. Previous treatment

B. Objective data

1. Size and depth of wound
2. Contamination
3. Hemorrhage
4. Function of the part injured

III. Management

A. Human bites

1. Treatments/medications
   a. Bite wounds should never be sutured because of the high index of infection in almost all bites, except when serious cosmetic defect is present.
   b. Irrigate and clean the wound with normal saline and/or suitable antiseptic solution.
   c. Debridement is indicated according to the depth of the wound
   d. Apply antiseptic ointment and petroleum jelly packing.
   e. Apply a sterile dressing.
   f. Tetanus prophylaxis is indicated.
   g. Appropriate antibiotic therapy is indicated for all but the slightest human bite wounds.
   h. Immobilize as needed.
2. Counselling/prevention
   a. Instruct on observing for signs of inflammation and infection.
   b. Stress that the dressing is to be kept clean and dry.
3. Follow-up
   Revisit in 48 h for reevaluation and redressing, and also to check for signs of infection
4. Consultations/referrals
   All hand and face wounds should be referred to a surgeon for adequate debridement and/or cosmetic repair, or for possible loss-of-function and infection complications.

B. Animal bites (see Table 107-1)

1. Treatments/medications
   a. Bite wounds should never be sutured except when a serious cosmetic defect is present.
   b. Irrigate and clean the wound with normal saline and/or suitable antiseptic solution.
   c. Debridement is indicated according to the depth of the wound.
   d. Apply antiseptic ointment and petrolatum packing.
   f. Apply a dry sterile dressing.
   g. Tetanus prophylaxis is indicated.
   h. If rabies prophylaxis is indicated, the animal should be confined for observation, if possible.

2. Counselling/prevention
   a. Safety in dealing with animals, domestic and wild
   b. Dressing to be kept clean and dry
3. Follow-up
   Revisit in 48 h for dressing change and re-evaluation of the wound
4. Consultations/referrals
   a. Refer to physician any client bitten by an unknown, wild, or rabid animal.
   b. Face and hand wounds, with or without infection, should be referred to a surgeon for definitive care for cosmetic and functional reasons.
   c. Report to the health department.

Table 107-1 Medical Referral/Consultation

Diagnosis	Clinical Manifestations	Management
Rabies or suspicion of rabies	Bite by bat, raccoon, skunk, fox, or other wild animal Unprovoked attack from unimmunized or unknown dog or cat Headache Apprehension Fever Paresis/paralysis Pharyngeal spasm on thought or sight of water	*Immediately* refer to physician. Notify health department. Confine animal for observation for 10 days. If animal was killed, save carcass, for evaluation by local health laboratory. Immediately cleanse and flush wound with soap and water.

bibliography

Benenson, Abram S. (ed.). *Control of communicable diseases in man* (12th ed.). Washington, DC.: American Public Health Association, 1975, pp. 250–257.

Eckert, Charles D. *Emergency room care* (2d ed.). Boston: Little, Brown, 1971.

Wilson, John L. *Handbook of surgery* (5th ed.). Los Altos, Calif.: Lange, 1973.

108 Lice

MARILYN GREBIN

I. Etiology

A. *Pediculus humanus*
1. Var. *capitis*
2. Var. *corporis*

B. *Phthirius pubis* (crab louse)

II. Assessment

A. Pediculosis capitis
1. Subjective data
   a. Recent contact
      (1) Home
      (2) School
   b. Pruritis
2. Objective data
   a. Presence of ova attached to hair shaft
   b. Skin lesions
      (1) Flat erythematous base
      (2) Areas of excoriation on the scalp
      (3) Bloody crusts on the scalp
   c. Occipital lymphadenopathy

B. Pediculosis corporis
1. Subjective data
   a. Recent contact
      (1) Home
      (2) School
   b. Pruritis
2. Objective data
   a. Presence of ova along seams of clothing or attached to pubic hair
   b. Skin lesions
      (1) Flat erythematous base
      (2) Areas of excoriation on the body
      (3) Bloody crusts on the skin
   c. Axillary, inguinal lymphadenopathy

III. Management

A. Pediculosis capitis
1. Treatments/medications
   a. Kwell shampoo once (may be repeated)
   b. Bacitracin ointment for secondary skin infection for 7 days
2. Counselling/Prevention
   a. Examination of all family members
   b. Special care for clothing and linens
      (1) Separate from the clothing of other family members.
      (2) Add ammonia solution to the wash water.
      (3) Use all hot water.
      (4) Clothing may be boiled.
      (5) Steam-press clothing, paying strict attention to seams.
      (6) Dry cleaning is recommended.
3. Follow-up
   a. Revisit in 2 days
   b. For excessive secondary skin lesion infection, another visit in 1 week
4. Consultations/referrals
   a. School nurse
   b. Public health nurse for families continually reinfected

B. Pediculosis corporis
1. Treatments/medications
   a. Kwell lotion applied to affected area once, may be repeated again in 24 h
   b. Topicide (benzyl-benzoate-DDT-benzocain emulsion) applied to affected areas
   c. Bacitracin ointment for secondary skin infection
2. Counselling/prevention (see Pediculosis capitus above). Counsel parent(s) to prevent the child's putting the affected, medicated body part into his or her mouth.
3. Follow-up (see Pediculosis capitus above)
4. Consultations/referrals (see Pediculosis capitus above)

bibliography

Barnett, Henry L. *Pediatrics* (16th ed.). New York: Appleton-Century-Crofts, 1976.

Billstein, S. Diagnosis and treatment of lice. *Journal of School Health,* **47**(6):356–357 (1977).

Harlin, V. K. Pediculosis: its transmission and treatment in schools. *Journal of School Health,* **47**(6):348 (1977).

Harlin, V. K. Role of other school health team members. *Journal of School Health,* **47**(6):360–362 (1977).

Slack, P. Head infestation. *Nursing Times,* **72**(6):225–227 (1976).

109 Corns/Calluses/Warts

ASHER H. WEINSTEIN

I. Etiology

A. Corns and calluses—mechanical in origin

1. Ill-fitting footwear
2. Friction
3. Unequal weight distribution
4. Excessive body weight
5. Abnormality in bone structure of feet

B. Plantar warts—viral in origin

II. Assessment

A. Corns

1. Subjective data
   a. Pain on weight bearing
   b. New footwear
2. Objective data
   a. Pain and point tenderness on palpation
   b. Hard, dry skin in small area
   c. Small diameter, glassy core, translucent

B. Calluses

1. Subjective data
   a. Burning sensation of feet while walking
   b. Long hours standing at work
2. Objective data
   a. Possible diabetes
   b. General thickening of skin over large area
   c. Dry skin

C. Plantar warts

1. Subjective data
   a. History of other household members with warts
   b. Pain and tenderness around the lesion rather than point tenderness
   c. One or multiple sites
2. Objective data
   a. Soft, grainy appearance
   b. Raised or flat lesion
   c. Capillary bleeding on paring of the lesion
   d. Fissures
   e. Pain not on palpation but rather from "pinching"

III. Management

A. Corns

1. Treatments/medications
   a. Paring with a surgical blade after soaking to soften the skin
   b. A thin, soft, felt pad with a hole at the site of the corn
   c. Correction of mechanical abnormalities with a shoe insert
   d. Relief of friction point in footwear
2. Counselling/prevention
   a. Correctly fitting footwear
   b. Home care including use of a pumice stone for paring
3. Follow-up: return visit in 4 to 6 weeks for re-evaluation
4. Consultations/referrals: referral to podiatrist for evaluation and possible fitting of shoe inserts for correction of abnormalities

B. Calluses

1. Treatments/medications
   a. Paring of thickened tissue with a surgical blade after soaking
   b. Use of a keratolytic agent, such as a compound of salicylic acid, acetone, and collodion, applied at night as a paste and covered with a piece of adhesive and then removed in the morning; done on a daily basis
2. Counselling/prevention
   a. Properly fitting footwear and daily change
   b. Home care with a pumice stone
   c. Liberal use of skin cream to keep skin soft

3. Follow-up: return visit in 4 to 6 weeks for re-evaluation
4. Consultations/referrals: none

C. Plantar warts
1. Treatments/medications
   a. Surgical excision
   b. Application of liquid nitrogen to the wart at 1 week intervals, until blanching occurs
   c. Keratolytic agents as for calluses, above
2. Counselling/prevention
   a. Warts may clear up spontaneously.
   b. Warts may not respond to treatment.
   c. Care should be taken in not touching or picking at warts.
3. Follow-up: visits at 1-week intervals for treatment and evaluation
4. Consultations/referrals: referral to podiatrist for surgical excision

bibliography

Chatton, Milton J. *Handbook of medical treatment* (13th ed.). Los Altos, Calif.: Lange, 1972.

Degowin, Elmer L., and Degowin, Richard L. *Bedside diagnostic examination* (3d ed.). London: Macmillan, 1976.

Krupp, Marcus A., and Chatton, Milton J. *Current medical diagnosis and treatment* (2d ed.). Los Altos, Calif.: Lange, 1979.

Prior, John A., and Silberstein, Jack S. *Physical diagnosis* (4th ed.). St. Louis: Mosby, 1973.

110 Acne/Blackheads/Pimples

JANE A. FOX/ANN M. NEWMAN

ALERT
1. Neonate
2. Those receiving steroids, anticonvulsants, or oral contraceptives
3. Secondary bacterial infection
4. Severe nodulocystic acne
5. Draining sinuses and cysts
6. Those unresponsive to therapy

I. Etiology

A. Onset of puberty causes increased androgen levels, which cause the pilosebaceous glands to enlarge and produce sebum. Acne may develop when
1. Excess sebum is produced.
2. Follicular openings are too small to accommodate the flow of sebum.
3. Excessive sebum reduces the size of the follicular openings.

B. Precipitating factors may include
1. Familial predisposition
2. Stress
3. Lack of sleep
4. Menses
5. Hot, humid weather
6. Occlusive cosmetics and creams

II. Assessment

A. Acne neonatorum
1. Subjective data
   a. Family history may reveal one or both parents had severe acne.
   b. It usually occurs in an infant less than 3 months of age, but it may occur in a child up to 2 years of age.
   c. Parent(s) may report "pimples" on face of infant/child.
2. Objective data
   a. Incidence higher in males during first 3 months of life
   b. Lesions appearing as erythematous papules, papulopustules, and comedones (whiteheads and blackheads); a nodulocystic lesion, which causes a pitted scar, rarely produced
   c. Cheeks most common site, but forehead and chin may be involved

B. Prepubescent acne
1. Subjective data
   a. Usually appearing between the ages of 6 and 8 years
   b. Family history of acne in one or both parents or siblings
   c. Parent(s) stating that child has "pimples, blackheads, or whiteheads"
2. Objective data
   a. Comedones, erythematous papules, papulopustules, even nodulocystic lesion noted
   b. Most common on forehead and chin, but may appear anywhere on face
   c. Culture of pustule or nodule revealing higher incidence of *Corynebacterium* acne

C. Acne vulgaris
1. Subjective data
   a. Chief complaint usually pimples, blackheads, whiteheads, bumps, or "zits"
   b. Usual onset between 9 and 20 years of age; most severe in females 14 to 17 years and males 16 to 19 years
   c. May have family history of acne
   d. History may reveal increased stress, poor sleeping habits, use of occlusive cosmet-

ics, participation in sports which require protective headgear

e. Sometimes condition worsens prior to menses

2. Objective data

a. Comedones (small, closed papules = whiteheads; open papules with dark plugs = blackheads), inflammatory papules, pustules, nodules, cysts, and scars may be noted on the skin.

b. The most common sites are the face, back, shoulders, upper chest, and neck.

c. The skin is shiny and oily in the area of the lesions.

III. Management

A. Acne neonatorum

1. Treatments/medications

a. Usually no treatment indicated

b. Mild topical agents (see Table 110-1) after physician consultation

2. Counselling/prevention

a. Reassure parent(s) that condition is usually mild and of short duration.

b. Describe condition and progression of symptoms.

c. Reassure about parenting capability.

d. Instruct on any medications.

3. Follow-up

a. Telephone call in 72 h to report condition, and again in 10 days

b. Return visit if condition worsens or as needed for parental reassurance and well-child visits

4. Consultations/referrals

a. Refer to a dermatologist all severe cases and those of long duration.

b. Consult a physician if medication is needed.

B. Prepubescent acne

1. Treatments/medications

a. Topical drying agents (see Tables 110-1 and 110-2)

b. Frequent washing of face

c. Acne soaps (Table 110-3)

d. See also Acne vulgaris, III, C below

2. Counselling/prevention

a. Instruct on treatment regimen.

b. Parent(s) should be instructed to observe when the face gets greasier, and facial washings should be done at that time.

c. Assist parent(s) in identifying/predicting stressful situations for the child so that they may be avoided or lessened when possible.

d. See also Acne vulgaris, III, C below.

3. Follow-up

a. As determined by dermatologist

b. Telephone calls to report progress

c. Return visits as needed for reassurance, health teaching, and well-child care

4. Consultations/referrals

a. Refer to a dermatologist for appropriate medications.

b. Notify the school nurse.

C. Acne vulgaris

1. Treatments/medications

a. Topical peeling and drying agents (see Table 110-1) or benzoyl peroxide preparations (see Table 110-2)

b. Soaps and scrubs (see Table 110-3)

c. Ultraviolet light therapy

d. Comedo extraction

e. Systemic therapy after consultation with physician

f. By physician

(1) Acne surgery

(2) Cryotherapy

(3) Dermabrasion

2. Counselling/prevention

a. Carefully explain the cause and prolonged course of the disease, that it is not curable but it is controllable.

b. Reassure the client that the condition is *not* related to masturbation, sexual activity or lack of it, sexual fantasies, venereal disease, or dirt.

c. Explain the treatment regimen and the importance of the client's active and willing participation. Include a written, detailed description of the home treatment schedule, i.e., the times the medication is to be given and the topical agents applied, and the frequency, dosages, amounts, and time restrictions.

d. Instruct and observe proper skin cleansing. Wash the face and/or other affected areas with warm, soapy water 3 to 4 times daily for 1 min. Rinse well with warm water. Use a clean washcloth with each washing.

e. Inform of any possible side effects of the prescribed treatment.

f. Discuss with the client the rationale for keeping hands away from the face, i.e., residual scarring could occur.

g. Hair should be styled away from the face and shampooed regularly.

h. Greasy and occlusive cosmetics and creams should be avoided.

i. Females should be instructed in the application of water-based makeup, which may help to improve appearance.

j. If a sun lamp (ultraviolet light therapy) is prescribed, instruct in the proper, safe usage.
   (1) Exposure should be limited.
   (2) Eyes should be properly shielded.
   (3) The distance from the lamp should always be constant.
   (4) An automatic timer or another person should be used to limit exposure with each use.
   (5) Initial exposure should be 30 s, gradually increasing until the desired results are obtained. Then continue with one to two treatments per week.

k. Instruct client/parent in extraction of comedones.
   (1) Purchase a comedo extractor at a local pharmacy.
   (2) Place the hole at the end of the extractor over comedo and gently press against skin with a mild sliding motion.
   (3) The face should be thoroughly washed with warm, soapy water before and after removal.
   (4) Hot towels may be placed on the skin prior to extraction.
   (5) The extractor should be carefully washed with soap and water before and after use and kept in alcohol between usage.

l. Individual and/or group counselling may be beneficial for peer acceptance, approval, and support.

3. Follow-up
   a. Arrange for a telephone call in 72 h to determine the effectiveness of and compliance with the treatment.
   b. Schedule a return visit in 1 week if on systemic therapy and 2 weeks if on topical therapy, to assess effectiveness and compliance. Have the client demonstrate face cleansing and comedo extraction; review health teaching and continue appropriate counselling.
   c. Schedule return visits monthly, or sooner if indicated.
4. Consultations/referrals
   a. Refer to dermatologist those with
      (1) Severe acne
      (2) Nodulocystic lesions
      (3) Acne unresponsive to prescribed therapy
      (4) Draining cysts and sinuses
      (5) Scars
      (6) Chronic diseases, i.e., diabetes
      (7) Secondary bacterial infections
      (8) Current history of corticosteroid therapy
   b. Professional counselling as needed

Table 110-1 Peeling and Drying Agents

Product	Description	Use
Acnederm Lotion (flesh tinted)	Contains zinc oxide and sulfur	Apply several times daily.
Acne-Dome Creme and Lotion	Contains sulfur and resorcinol monoacetate	Apply sparingly to affected areas 2 times daily.
Acnomel Cream and Cake (flesh tinted)	Contains sulfur and resorcinol	Apply cream 1 to 2 times daily; cake 2 to 3 times daily.
Bensulfoid Lotion	Contains sulfur and resorcinol	Apply once a day to affected areas.
Exzit Medicated Creme and Lotion	Contains sulfur and resorcinol monoacetate	Apply 2 times daily.
Fostril Drying Lotion (flesh tinted)	Contains sulfur	Apply thin film 1 to 2 times a day.
Klaron Lotion	Contains salicylic acid and sulfur	Apply 1 to 2 times a day to affected areas.
Komed Acne Lotion	Contains sodium thiosulfate, salicylic acid, and resorcinol	Apply 1 to 2 times a day to affected areas.
Neutrogena Acne Drying Gel pH 6	Contains witch hazel and isopropyl alcohol	Apply 1 to 2 times a day.
Pernox	Contains sulfur and salicylic acid	Apply 1 to 2 times a day.

Table 110-1 Peeling and Drying Agents *(continued)*

Product	Description	Use
Postacne Lotion (flesh tinted)	Contains sulfur	Apply 1 to 2 times a day.
Rezamid Lotion (flesh tinted)	Contains resorcinol and sulfur	Apply 1 to 2 times a day.
Sulfacet-R Lotion (flesh tinted)	Contains sulfonamides and sulfur	Apply 1 to 3 times daily.
Transact Medicated Acne Gel	Contains laureth-4, sulfur, and alcohol	For sensitive skin, use once every other day; apply once daily after 2 to 3 days; increase use as tolerance develops.

Note: These agents may cause excessive drying, reddening, or scaling of the skin. For best results thoroughly cleanse skin before use.

Table 110-2 Benzoyl Peroxide Preparations

Product and Concentration	Use	Remarks
Benzagel 5 or 10%	Apply once or more daily.	Benzoyl peroxide preparations are antibacterial.
Desquam Gel 5 or 10%	Apply 1 to 2 times daily.	Benzoic acid is a breakdown product which acts as an irritant to cause a drying and peeling effect on the skin.
Epi Clear Squibb Antiseptic Lotion for Acne 5 or 10%	Apply 1 to 2 times daily.	Allergic contact dermatitis and severe erythema have been reported with use of topical benzoyl peroxide.
Loroxide Lotion (flesh tinted) 5.5%	Apply 1 to 2 times daily.	Concentration and/or frequency of use must be modified according to client's response.
Pan Oxyl Gel 5 or 10%	Apply 1 to 2 times daily.	Harsh abrasive cleaners should not be used simultaneously, and ultraviolet and cold quartz light therapy should be used in lesser amounts. These preparations should not be used by anyone with a sensitivity to benzoyl peroxide.
Persadox Acne Cream and Lotion 5 to 10%	Apply once daily. If dryness, redness, or peeling does not occur in 3 to 4 days, increase use to 2 times daily.	It may also bleach colored fabrics.
Persa-Gel 5 to 10%	Apply once daily. Increase to 2 times daily as tolerance develops.	
Sulfoxyl Lotion Regular and Strong 5 to 10%	Apply 1 to 2 times daily.	
Vanoxide Lotion 5%	Apply 1 to 2 times daily.	
Xerac BP 5 to 10%	Apply 1 to 2 times daily.	

Table 110-3 Soaps and Scrubs

Product	Description	Use
Acne-Dome Medicated Cleanser	Contains colloidal sulfur and salicylic acid	2 times daily
Epi Clear Acne Soap	Contains sulfur	2 times daily
Epi Clear Scrub Cleanser	Contains aluminum oxide particles	2 times daily.
Exzit Medicated Cleanser	Contains colloidal sulfur and salicylic acid	2 times daily

Table 110-3 Soaps and Scrubs *(continued)*

Product	Description	Use
Fostex Cake Acne Skin Cleanser	Contains sulfur and salicylic acid	2 times daily
Komex Scrub	Contains sodium tetraborate decahydrate in a base	1 to 2 times daily
Neutrogena Acne Cleansing Soap with Lipid Solvents	Ethanol amine based soap	1 to 3 times daily
Seba-Nil acne and oily skin cleanser	Contains alcohol	Daily as needed

bibliography

Caro, Ivor. Acne vulgaris: Recent advances in pathogenesis and treatment. *The Journal of Family Practice*, **5**:747–750 (1977).

Evans, Jane Cooper, and Singleton, Carolynn Elaine. Acne: The scourge of adolescence. *Issues in Comprehensive Pediatric Nursing*. New York: McGraw-Hill, 1976.

Farber, Eugene. Acne vulgaris. *Scientific American medicine*. New York: Scientific American, 1978, pp.2–7.

Farber, George A., et al. Football acne—An acniform eruption. *Cutis*, **20**:356–360 (1977).

Fulton, James E., and Bradley, Sara. The choice of vitamin A acid, erythromycin or benzoyl peroxide for the topical treatment of acne. *Cutis*, **17**:560–564 (1976).

Goldman, Leon. Acne prevention in the family. *American Family Physician*, **16**:68–72 (1977).

Hurwitz, Sidney. Acne vulgaris—Concepts of pathogenesis and treatment. . .A practical approach. *Pediatric Basics*, No. 20 (February 1978).

Kligman, Albert, and Plewig, Gerd. Classification of acne. *Cutis*, **17**:520–522 (1976).

MacKenzie, Albert. Use of Buf-Puf and mild cleansing bar in acne. *Cutis*, **19**:370–371 (1977).

Mysliborski, Judith Ann, and Lumpkin, Lee R. Treating acne vulgaris. *American Family Physician*, **15**:86–91 (1977).

Rasmussen, James E. A new look at old acne. *Pediatric Clinics of North America*, **25**:285–303 (1978).

Reisner, Ronald M. The rational therapy of acne. *Cutis*, **17**:527–530 (1976).

Strauss, John S., et al. The role of skin lipids in acne. *Cutis*, **17**:485–487 (1976).

Vaughan, Victor C., and McKay, R. James (eds.). *Nelson textbook of pediatrics* (10th ed.). Philadelphia: Saunders, 1975, pp. 1518, 1562–1563.

section 11

developmental concerns

INTRODUCTION KAREN A. BALLARD

I. Subjective data

A. Identification of problem
1. Behavior—normal, abnormal
2. Developmental task

B. Description of problem
1. Age at onset
2. Precipitating events
   a. Pain
   b. Anger
   c. Frustration
   d. Jealousy
   e. New situations
   f. Strange people
   g. Frightening experiences
   h. Limit setting
   i. Discipline
   j. Noncompliance
   k. Separation
   l. Sibling rivalry
   m. Departure, loss of friend
   n. Illness, operation, hospitalization
   o. Death in family
3. Frequency of episodes
   a. Time of day or night
   b. Daily, weekly, monthly
4. Duration
5. Description of behavior
   a. What is said or done
   b. Individual's reaction to own behavior
   c. Parental response to behavior

C. Prenatal history
1. Planned or unexpected pregnancy
2. Mother's general health
   a. Toxemia
   b. Eclampsia
   c. Hypertension

D. Birth history
1. Birth weight
2. Respiratory status
3. Apgar score(s)

E. Developmental history
1. Identification of present developmental stage and its inherent tasks
2. Previous handling of developmental tasks
3. Previous and present response to limit setting

F. Past medical history
1. Date of last physical examination
2. Hospitalizations
3. Acute or chronic illnesses
4. Need for invasive procedures
5. Child's and parent(s)' reaction
6. Date and result of last hearing and vision test
7. Past or present history of

In problems which affect the school-age child and adolescent, it is often important to interview the parent(s) and child separately. The child may not be as expressive in the company of the parent(s).

a. Rituals before being able to perform an activity
b. Nail biting
c. Tics
d. Vocal disturbances
(1) Stuttering
(2) Stammering
e. Other repetitive acts
f. Rapid performance of tasks and play activities

G. Diet history

H. Sleep pattern
1. Number of hours sleep night/day
2. Rituals
a. Favorite toys
b. Bedtime stories
c. Songs
d. Night light
3. Sleep disturbances
a. Refusal
b. Dream and nightmare activity

I. Elimination patterns
a. Bowel and bladder control
b. Toilet-training methods

J. Discipline
1. Description of child-rearing philosophy
2. Methods
3. Parental reaction
4. Child's reaction
5. Effectiveness

K. School history (see also Social history, I., L. below)
1. School attended
2. Number of students in class
3. School performance
4. Parental expectations of child for performance
5. Performance as compared to other siblings
6. Amount of homework
7. Assistance with school work: home, tutoring
8. Description of school behavior
9. Parental knowledge of child's IQ
10. Anxiety about child's performance
11. Parent/teacher conference
12. Child's like or dislike of classroom, teacher, and/or classmates
13. Child's understanding of school work
14. Place in the classroom
15. Favorite subject
16. Least-liked subject

L. Social history
1. Changes in family constellation
a. Death of family member
b. Separation or divorce
c. Marriage
d. Birth of a sibling
2. Stresses in home environment
a. Maternal anxiety
b. Marital disharmony
c. Parental quarreling
d. Parental inconsistency
e. Emotional absence of a parent
f. Change in main care giver
g. Change in baby-sitter(s)
h. Parental illness
i. Sibling illness
j. Change in bed or room assignment
k. Increase/decrease in assigned responsibilities
l. Relocation of family
m. Economic difficulties
n. Alcoholism, drug abuse
3. Stresses in peer/school/work environment
a. "Special" friendships
b. Change in peer group
c. Peer illness
d. Loss of friendship
e. Formation, joining, or exclusion from a "gang"
f. Introduction to school (play group, nursery school, new grade/school)
g. Teacher-pupil relationship
h. New curriculum
i. School performance
j. New job
k. Work performance
l. Work evaluations
m. Promotion

II. Objective Data

A. Physical examination
1. The thoroughness of the physical examination will depend upon the existing data base, the severity of the presenting concern, and the practitioner's familiarity with the family.
2. In some instances, a physical examination is not necessary, unless the practitioner wishes to utilize it as a means of interacting with the child (all infants should be thoroughly examined).
3. Vision and hearing screens should be done yearly.

B. Laboratory data—the following tests may be indicated
1. Complete blood count (CBC) and differential
2. Urinalysis

e. EEG
4. Stool for ova and parasites

C. Other

1. Bender-Gestalt
2. Draw-A-Person (Goodenough-Harris)
3. Denver Developmental Screening Test
4. Wechsler Intelligence Scale for Children (WISC)
5. School performance report

D. Assessment of parent-child relationship

1. Interview the parent(s) separately from the child.
2. Interview the child.
3. Assess parent-child interactions.

111 Thumb-sucking/Pacifiers/Comforters

CAROL ANN BROWN

ALERT

1. Excessive use of comforter, interfering with normal activities
2. Poor parent-child relationship
3. Escape from reality
4. Regression—severe

I. Etiology

A. Infant

1. Not enough sucking from feeding
2. Increased sucking need

B. Toddler/preschooler

1. Developmental struggle between independence and dependence
2. Attempt to recapture the security of infancy—regression

II. Assessment

A. Infant

1. Not enough sucking from feeding
   a. Subjective data
      (1) Usually less than 3 months of age
      (2) Too little time spent on breast because of enforced time limit on each breast: less than 15 min
      (3) Too little sucking from bottle because of large hole in nipple
      (4) Mother reporting rapid elimination of 10 P.M. and 2 A.M. feedings
      (5) Early discontinuance of breast-feeding (parent not likely to stop bottle-feeding early to opt for cup feeding)
      (6) Infant rooting and sucking hands excessively after feedings
      (7) Infant may be irritable and crying frequently throughout day between feedings
   b. Objective data
      (1) Physical examination usually normal
      (2) Large hole in nipple on bottle
      (3) Mother unsure how to breast-feed infant—periods at breast too short
      (4) Crying infant with active rooting and sucking reflexes
      (5) Child calms when sucking
2. Increased nonnutritive sucking need
   a. Subjective data
      (1) Usually less than 3 months of age
      (2) Parent(s) reporting sucking and rooting even after
         (a) Proper breast- and bottle-feeding
         (b) Long periods at breast or bottle
         (c) Frequent feedings during day—every 2 to 4 h
      (3) Fretful infant
   b. Objective data
      (1) The physical examination is usually normal, with very active sucking and rooting reflexes.
      (2) After feeding, the child appears to want more sucking.
      (3) The parent(s) exhibits good feeding techniques.

B. Toddler/preschooler

1. Developmental struggle between independence and dependence
   a. Subjective data
      (1) The parent(s) may report the child began using a comforter (suckable, strokable) in infancy.
      (2) The child may have discontinued using the comforter and then begun again with some family upset, such as a new sibling, parental discord, separation.
      (3) The child needs the comforter when in

stress: tired, unhappy, hungry.

(4) There are too many limits set on the child, including harsh discipline/punishment.

(5) The parent(s) is beginning to feel uncomfortable about the child's use of a comforter.

(a) Punishes (or ridicules) child for using comforter

(b) Responds to child positively when using comforter which reinforces use of comforter by child

b. Objective data

(1) Usually normal physical examination

(a) May have upper lip and slight upper teeth protrusion secondary to use of pacifier and thumb

(b) May have callus on thumb (or finger) from sucking

(2) Child usually using comforter during exam because of stressful situation

(3) May observe harsh limits or ridicule from parent(s)

(4) May observe detached parent-child relationship

2. Attempt to recapture the security of infancy—regression (see II, B, 1 above)

III. Management

A. Suckable comforters

1. Treatments/medications: none

2. Counselling/prevention

a. If there is not enough sucking from feeding, increase the sucking time on breast or bottle.

(1) Feed at one breast for feeding and let infant suck as long as wants, or

(2) Feed at both breasts, allowing sucking to continue until the need is fulfilled at the last breast.

(3) For bottle-fed infants

(a) Check nipples—they should have small holes.

(b) Advise parent(s) that the child should take at least 20 min to empty the bottle.

(c) Tighten the cap to decrease the air flow into the bottle and decrease the milk flow out per suck.

(d) Go slower in eliminating the 10 P.M. and 2 A.M. feedings.

(e) Encourage the use of a pacifier to fulfill sucking needs if unable to change feeding.

(4) Reassure the parent(s) that it is not abnormal for a child to need more sucking.

(5) Place a pacifier in the mouth when the child is well fed and looking around for something to suck on.

b. Pacifiers are often used to prevent thumb-sucking.

(1) Less chance of malocclusion

(2) Usually given up by 1 to 2 years of age

c. Counsel parent(s) on safety measures for pacifiers.

(1) One-piece rubber pacifiers

(2) Nuk exerciser-pacifier designed for fewer orthodontal problems

(3) Pacifier *not* to be worn around neck on string

(4) Frequent inspection of pacifier important to make sure it is not worn

d. Instruct parent(s) to

(1) Decrease the use of the pacifier gradually by limiting its use and taking it away during times least needed (advantage over thumb-sucking).

(2) Avoid misuse of pacifier: to keep child placid or quiet, and in place of parental attention.

(3) Attach the pacifier to a favorite animal so that when the child wants to discontinue its use, there is still the animal for security.

(4) Remove the pacifier from the mouth when the child is sleepy or drowsy.

e. Be sure parent(s) is aware of child's developmental needs for independence beginning at 6 months of age.

(1) The child can get pleasure and security from a comforter without giving up independence.

(2) The comforter is something which the child can control.

(3) Advise the parent(s) not to make a struggle of their child's striving for independence.

(4) Review with the parent(s) the limits set on the child, to determine if they are fair and not overburdening.

f. Reassure parent(s) this is a normal need of children during times of stress, sleep, hunger, and boredom.

g. Advise parent(s) to have the child on a regular schedule so the child can predict what will come next and feel secure.

h. Encourage strokable comforters if the child needs security at nap or nighttime.

i. The parent(s) may need to be more attentive to the child during difficult times.
   (1) Hold the child quietly.
   (2) Have special reading storytimes.
   (3) Rock the child in a rocking chair.
   (4) Rub the child's back at bedtime.
   (5) Establish a bedtime ritual.
j. Reassure the parent(s) that displacement of teeth is not a problem until after 6 years of age, unless the child sucks excessively or with intense pressure on the upper teeth.
k. Normally sucking should not interfere with regular activity.

3. Follow-up: good phone contact with return visits as needed for counselling or referrals.
4. Consultations/referrals
   a. Dentist—if malocclusion or child over 6 years of age
   b. Physician—if excessive thumb-sucking

B. Strokable comforter, i.e., blanket, animals

1. Treatments/medications: none
2. Counselling/prevention
   a. Set limits for the use of the comforter.
      (1) Only in home
      (2) Only at bedtime—easier for an older child
   b. Arrange to wash it tactfully.
      (1) Split in half or have a duplicate
      (2) Take it away after the child is asleep to launder it.
   c. If the child displays any allergic reaction,
      (1) Avoid wool blankets.
      (2) Restuff kapok-stuffed animals with hypoallergenic materials.
   d. Reassure the parent(s) that dependency usually stops at 5 or 6 years of age.
   e. Advise stressing positives in the child's development.
      (1) How grown-up child has become, with examples of grown-up behavior
      (2) Mentioning going to school and how child will not need comforter there
   f. Stress to parent(s) the importance of stimulating planned and consistent activity for the child not involving the comforter.
      (1) Trips to parks
      (2) Art work
      (3) Games, imaginary play
   g. Make parent(s) aware of how they reinforce the use of the comforter as an attention-getting mechanism, and advise positive reinforcement when the child is not using the comforter.
   h. If there is a new sibling in home, advise parent(s) to accept increased or new use of comforter patiently until the child works out feelings of jealousy and place in the family.
   i. Explore the causes of unrest at home with the parent(s), and offer appropriate referrals.
   j. Urge the parent(s) to avoid punishment or ridicule, which may increase the dependency.
3. Follow-up
   a. Good phone contact
   b. Regular, periodic, well-child visits
4. Consultations/referrals: for family problems —social worker, family counselling services

bibliography

Brazelton, T. Berry. *Infants and mothers: differences in development.* New York: Delacorte Press, 1969.

Cruzon, M. E. J. Dental implications of thumbsucking. *Pediatrics,* **54**(2), 1974.

Illingworth, Ronald S. *The normal child.* New York: Churchill Livingstone, 1975.

Jenson, George D. *The well child's problems.* Chicago: Year Book, 1962.

Spock, Benjamin. Avoiding behavior problems. *Journal of Pediatrics,* **27**:363–382 (1945).

———. *Baby and child care.* New York: Pocket Books, 1976.

112 Stranger Anxiety

KAREN A. BALLARD

ALERT
Child over 2 years of age

I. Assessment

A. Subjective data

1. Parent(s) reports that infant reacts to strangers with
   a. Crying
   b. Restlessness
   c. Tense extremities
   d. Clinging to mother/care giver
2. Stranger anxiety
   a. Peaks between 6 and 8 months
   b. May last several months to a year
   c. May hurt the feelings of relatives/friends, who feel rejected
3. "Looming effect" occurs when infant reacts with fear to the approaching person as a large, fast-moving object with the potential to hurt/harm

B. Objective data: Physical examination is normal.

II. Management

A. Treatments/medications: none, see II, B, below

B. Counselling/prevention

1. At 6 months, infant normally
   a. Is aware of a person as a whole object
   b. Establishes patterns of familiarity with person(s)
   c. Imitates familiar person(s)
   d. Shows beginning signs of anxiety when a person is unfamiliar
2. The infant should be allowed to establish his or her own pace at becoming comfortable with strangers.
   a. Strangers should approach the infant slowly.
   b. If holding the infant, the parent should speak quietly to the infant and the stranger and should stop advancing toward the stranger either a few feet away or at signs of infant anxiety.
   c. The infant must *not* be thrust into the arms of strangers.
   d. The infant should be securely held and comforted.
3. The introduction of the infant before 6 months to potential strangers may help reduce anxiety. (Parent(s) should be present.)
   a. Close relatives who are frequently in home
   b. Baby-sitters
   c. This method is less effective if the infant is introduced to too many individuals.
4. Encourage parent(s) to realize that this fear is normal and related to the process of individualization.
   a. Reflects threats to infant's basic sense of security
   b. Indicates awareness that parent(s) and infant are separate individuals

C. Follow-up

1. This depends on the severity of the stranger anxiety.
2. The focus should be on helping the parent(s) to identify behaviors which facilitate the child's interactions with strangers.

D. Consultations/referrals: none

Table 112-1 Medical Referral/Consultation

Diagnosis	Clinical Manifestations	Management
Excessive stranger anxiety, either In frequency and quality under 2 yr, or Persisting past 2 yr	Inability to tolerate presence of strangers or being in strange places Excessive crying, restlessness, tenseness, and clinging to parent(s)	Refer for professional counselling.

bibliography

Bowlby, John. *Deprivation of maternal care—A reassessment of its effects.* New York: Schocken Books, 1966.

Church, Joseph. *Understanding your child from birth to three.* New York: Pocket Books, 1976.

Dunn, Judy. *Distress and comfort (the developing child).* Cambridge: Harvard, 1977.

Lewis, Melvin. *Clinical aspects of child development.* Philadelphia: Lea & Febiger, 1971.

Mahler, Margaret. *On human symbiosis and the vicissitudes of individualization.* New York: International Universities Press, 1968.

Sharin, K. Cognitive and contextual determinants of stranger fear in six and eleven-month-old infants. *Child Development,* **48**:537–544 (1977).

113 Teething/Tooth Eruption

CAROL ANN GRUNFELD

ALERT

1. Significant fever: greater than 38.5°C (101.3°F) orally or 39°C (102.2°F) rectally
2. Severe pain
3. Evidence of stomatological lesions
4. Symptoms of systemic illness (teething sometimes concurrent with, but cannot be deemed responsible for, systemic illness)

I. Etiology

Tooth eruption is a normal developmental process influenced by stages of root formation and hormones

II. Assessment

A. Normal eruption of primary or permanent teeth (teething without complication)

1. Subjective data
   a. Infant or young child *may* be restless or fretful.
   b. Infant *may* exhibit a decreased appetite or reluctance to nurse.
   c. Older child or young adult *may* complain of gum soreness.
   d. Infant seems to put everything within reach into the mouth.
   e. Increased salivation occurs (may be developmentally coincidental with the eruption of primary teeth).
2. Objective data
   a. Inflammation of gingival tissue
   b. Mild edema of gingival tissue
   c. Excoriation of gingival tissue secondary to emergence of the crown of a tooth

B. Eruption hematoma

1. Subjective data: see normal eruption, II, A above
2. Objective data: bluish purple, elevated area of gingival tissue above erupting tooth

C. Eruption sequestra

1. Subjective data: see normal eruption, II, A, above
2. Objective data: minute splinter of bone overlying the crown of an erupting tooth (usually a molar)

III. Management

A. Normal eruption

1. Treatments/medications
   a. Provide infant with firm, blunt, and perhaps cold objects to chew, such as zwieback toast, a rubber teething ring or toy, a large piece of raw carrot, or an ice cube tied in a cloth napkin or diaper.
   b. Cup feeding may be less irritating than bottle-feeding for infants.
   c. A soft diet is preferable for children and adults.
   d. For relief of pain associated with teething, when necessary, suggest
      (1) Topical preparations applied 3 to 4 times daily to affected tissues for temporary relief (see Table 113-1)
      (2) Systemic analgesics, such as aspirin or acetaminophen
2. Counselling
   a. Teething causes no symptoms other than pain and possibly increased salivation; systemic disturbances may be coincidental with, but are not caused by, teething. Teething is a normal developmental occurrence.
   b. Keep small, sharp, or brittle toys and objects out of an infant's reach.
   c. Older painted furniture and toys, in addi-

tion to walls and fixtures, may be sources of lead-based paint—which is potentially toxic when ingested. Today virtually all infant furniture and painted toys have been painted with leadless paint.

d. Infants may exhibit nighttime wakefulness secondary to teething pain. It is preferable to reinforce this as little as possible, for an occasional child may develop a persistent habit of waking.

e. Medication should be reserved for the most severe pain or eruption.
   (1) Teach how to apply local preparations.
   (2) Teach how to measure and administer oral medications to infants and children.

f. Teething is a convenient condition to blame for diarrhea, coryza-rhinorrhea, excessive crying, wakefulness at night, and a grab bag of other ill-defined symptoms. There is a risk of ignoring signs and symptoms of serious disease as well as a risk of missing the opportunity to discuss normal developmental issues.

3. Follow-up
   a. If symptoms persist for more than 1 week without eruption of a tooth, telephone for assistance.
   b. If systemic symptoms (e.g., fever, diarrhea, or exanthem) develop, telephone for assistance.
4. Consultations/referrals
   a. Note to "day-care mother" explaining infant's behavior change
   b. Note to school nurse and/or teacher if administration of medication is required during school session

B. Eruption hematoma—no clinical significance; treat as normal eruption

C. Eruption sequestra—no clinical significance; treat as normal eruption

Table 113-1 Topical Preparations for Relief of Teething Pain

Product (manufacturer)	*Ingredients* (analgesic/anesthetic)
Baby Oragel (Commerce)*	Benzocaine—viscous, water-soluble base
Dr. Hands Teething Lotion (Roberts)*	Tincture of pellitory; menthol; clove oil; hamamelis water; alcohol, 10%
Numzit (Pure Pac)*	Glycerin; alcohol, 10%; gel vehicle
Orabase (Hoyt)*	Benzocaine
Ora-Jel-d (Commerce)*	Benzocaine, clove oil, benzyl alcohol, adhesive base
Teething lotion (DeWitt)*	Propylene glycol, 44%; glycerin, 29%; benzocaine, 5.6%; benzyl alcohol, 2.5%; tincture of myrrh, 4.5%; alcohol
Whiskey or comparable alcholic beverage	40%–100% alcohol
Herbal tea†	From roots of goldthread, *Coptis groenlandica;* for use as mouthwash for babies suffering from teething soreness

**American Pharmaceutical Association. Handbook of nonprescription drugs* (5th ed.). Washington, D.C.: Author, 1977, p. 261.
†Fielder, Mildred. *Plant medicine and folklore.* New York: Winchester Press, 1977, p. 172.

Table 113-2 Medical Referral/Consultation

Diagnosis	Clinical Manifestations	Management
Supernumerary teeth	Variation in eruption sequence	Consultation with physician/referral to dentist Extraction—at the discretion of the dentist after radiologic exam
Missing teeth	Variation in eruption sequence	Consultation with physician/referral to dentist

Table 113-2 Medical Referral/Consultation *(continued)*

Diagnosis	Clinical Manifestations	Management
		Radiologic exam—probably dental Requires construction of space maintainer to prevent shifting of adjacent teeth
Impaction	Failure of tooth to erupt (third molars and maxillary cuspids most commonly involved)	Referral to dentist Surgery and orthodontics required
Natal teeth	Teeth present at birth or erupting shortly after birth, either supernumerary or part of the deciduous dentition	Consultation with physician/referral to dentist Probably remove, to facilitate nursing and avoid the risk of aspiration
Ectopic eruption	A permanent tooth that is out of alignment erupting into the position of a neighboring tooth—cessation of eruption or premature loss of a primary tooth	Consultation with physician/referral to dentist The dentist may be able to correct the path of eruption of the permanent tooth. A space maintainer is required if the primary tooth is lost prematurely.
Infection associated with eruption (usually related to eruption of third molars)	Client appearing toxic Fever Pain Edema and inflammation of surrounding tissue Possibly purulent discharge	Consultation with physician/referral to dentist Systemic antibiotic Systemic and/or topical analgesic May require excision and draining
Stomatological lesions	See Mouth Sores, Chap. 44.	

bibliography

Honig, Paul J. Teething—Are today's pediatricians using yesterday's notions? *Journal of Pediatrics,* **87**(3):415–417 (1975).

Illingworth, R. S. *Common symptoms of disease in children* (4th ed.). London:William Clowes and Sons, 1973, pp. 137, 241, 311.

Kempe, C. Henry, et al. *Current pediatric diagnosis and treatment* (4th ed.). Los Altos, Calif.: Lange, 1978.

McDonald, Ralph E. *Dentistry for the child and adolescent* (2d ed.). St. Louis: Mosby, 1974, p. 74.

Neaderland, Ralph. Teething—A review. *Journal of Dentistry for Children,* **19**:127 (1952).

Radbill, S. X. Teething as a medical problem, Changing viewpoints through the centuries. *Clinical Pediatrics,* **4**:556 (1956).

Schaad, T. D., et al. Extreme ectopic eruption of lower permanent lateral incisors. *American Journal of Orthodontics,* **66**(3):280–286 (1974).

Tanner, H. A., and Kitchen, K. N. An effective treatment for pain in the eruption of primary and permanent teeth. *Journal of Dentistry for Children,* **31**:289–292 (1964).

Van Der Horst, Ronald L., et al. On teething in infancy. *Clinical Pediatrics,* **12**:607–610 (1973).

114 Rhythmic Movements/ Rocking

KAREN A. BALLARD

ALERT
1. Prolonged rocking
2. Immature behavior
3. Self-destructive behavior

I. Assessment

A. Subjective data

1. Most habitual rhythmic movements are a means of self-stimulation
   a. Age at onset
      (1) Body rocking—5 to 12 months
      (2) Head rolling—6 to 36 months
      (3) Head banging—6 to 36 months
   b. Usually lasting a few months
   c. Stopping spontaneously between 2 and 3 years
   d. May persist into toddler stage, sometimes into preadolescence
2. Parent(s) describes behavior as
   a. Usually occurring in bed
   b. Prior to falling asleep
   c. Apparently pleasurable
   d. Difficult activity to stop

B. Objective data

1. Physical examination is essentially normal; however,
   a. Occipital hair loss may be present because of head rolling.
   b. Facial and head bruises may be present as a result of head banging.
2. Laboratory data is normal.
3. Parent(s) appears comfortable and relaxed with the child.

II. Management

A. Treatments/medications: recommend that parent(s)

1. Hold child more often and for longer periods.
2. Rock the child to sleep.
3. Stroke the child when rocking starts.
4. Pad and anchor the crib/bed.

B. Counselling/prevention: counsel parent(s) that

1. 15 to 20 percent of normal children engage in some form of rhythmic movement (body rocking, head rolling, head banging).
2. The rhythmic movement serves to relieve tension and provides libidinal gratification, similar to masturbatory activities.
3. It almost always resolves spontaneously.

C. Follow-up

1. Follow-up depends on the severity of the behavior and parental anxiety.
2. Support should focus on encouraging the parent(s) to follow the treatment plan closely.

D. Consultations/referrals: nursery school teacher

Table 114-1 Medical Referral/Consultation

Diagnosis	Clinical Manifestations	Management
Child neglect	Child shows signs of failure to thrive (see Chap. 134). Parent(s) is uncomfortable when holding the child.	Professional counselling Referral to child protection agency See Battered/Abused Child, Chap. 159
Mentally deficient and/or brain damaged	Poor performance ratio on the Denver Developmental Screening Test Developmental lag	Pediatric neurologist Professional counselling
Otitis media	Frequent pulling/rubbing at ear Tympanic membrane red, bulging	See Ear Pain/Discharge, Chap. 23 Antibiotics Counselling regarding medications and importance of thorough treatment, prevention, follow-up
Cataracts	Decreased visual acuity Prolonged rocking	Referral to pediatric ophthamologist

bibliography

Barnett, Henry. *Pediatrics* (16th ed.). New York: Appleton-Century-Crofts, 1977.

Caetano, Anthony, and Kaufman, James. Reduction of rocking mannerisms in two blind children. *Education of the Visually Handicapped,* 7:101–105, (1975).

DeAngelis, Catherine. *Pediatric primary care* (2d ed.). Boston: Little, Brown, 1979.

Friedman, Stanford. *The pediatric clinics of North America—Symposium on behavioral pediatrics* (vol. 22, no. 3). Philadelphia: Saunders, 1975.

Illingworth, Ronald. *The normal child* (6th ed.). New York: Churchill Livingstone, 1975.

Kanner, Leo. *Child psychiatry* (4th ed.). Springfield, Ill.: Charles C Thomas, 1972.

115 Separation Anxiety

KAREN A. BALLARD

ALERT

1. Excessive, incapacitating separation anxiety
2. Decreased hearing

I. Assessment

A. Subjective data

1. Parent(s) reports child reacts to separation with
   a. Crying, screaming
   b. Temper tantrums
   c. Attempts to follow parent(s)
   d. Period of protest followed by acceptance
   e. Breath holding
2. Separation anxiety
   a. Occurs between 12 and 24 months
   b. May last into third year
   c. Occurs independently or concurrently with stranger anxiety
   d. Is very prominent in hospitalized children, especially under 5 years
3. Variables which influence separation tolerance/anxiety are
   a. Degree of parent/child symbiosis
   b. Number and quality of previous successful separations
   c. Other concurrent stresses on child
      (1) Developmental
      (2) Familial
      (3) Social
      (4) Environmental

B. Objective data: Physical examination and developmental assessment are normal.

II. Management

A. Treatments/medications: none

B. Counselling/prevention

1. Advise parent(s) that separation anxiety is
   a. *Normal* and expected
   b. Indicates child has successfully established a basic trust relationship with another person
   c. Involved with child's self-image
   d. A fear of loss of main love object and a fear of loss of part of self
2. Counsel parent(s) to
   a. Avoid prolonged, voluntary breaks in mother-child relationship during the first 3 years.
   b. Introduce the child by 6 months to a few alternative care givers.
      (1) Baby-sitters
      (2) Close relatives
   c. Play separation-mastery games with the child.
      (1) Peek-a-boo
      (2) Hide and seek
   d. Plan for separations by
      (1) Providing child with transitional objects which symbolically represent mother (keys, scarf, stuffed animals, blanket)
      (2) Introducing child to care giver
      (3) Never attempting to sneak away; stating day and time of return.

C. Follow-up

1. Follow-up depends on the severity of the separation anxiety.
2. Focus should be on helping parent(s) understand and appropriately support the child through this period.

D. Consultations/referrals: none

Table 115-1 Medical Referral/Consultation

Diagnosis	Clinical Manifestations	Management
Excessive, incapacitating separation anxiety, either In frequency and quality under 3 yr, or Persisting past 3 yr	Inability to tolerate absence of mother Excessive crying, restlessness, and clinging to mother, sometimes progressing to head banging and self-biting	Refer for professional counselling.
Childhood psychosis—symbiotic type	Child usually shows developmental lag Delayed speech Extreme panic when separated from mother Many autistic features	Refer for professional counselling.
Deafness	Inattentiveness Developmental lags Poor speech development Fearfulness	See Deafness/Defective Hearing/Hearing Changes, Chap. 26.

bibliography

Bowlby, John. *Deprivation of maternal care—A reassessment of its effects.* New York: Schocken Books, 1966.

Church, Joseph. *Understanding your child from birth to three.* New York: Pocket Books, 1976.

Fraiberg, Selma. *The magic years.* New York: Scribner, 1959.

Klaus, Marshall, and Kennell, John. *Maternal-infant bonding.* St. Louis: Mosby, 1976.

Schmeltz, K. An early latency child's use of obsessional ritual to master separation anxiety. *Maternal Child Nursing Journal,* **6**:117–134 (1977).

Scipien, Gladys, et al. *Comprehensive pediatric nursing* (2d ed.). New York: McGraw-Hill, 1979.

Smith, L. Effects of brief separation from parent on young children. *Journal of Child Psychology and Psychiatry and Allied Disciplines,* **16**:245–254 (1975).

116 Sibling Rivalry

KAREN A. BALLARD

ALERT

1. Destructive acts toward sibling or self
2. Regression without expected improvement

I. Assessment

A. Subjective data

1. Precipitating events
   a. Birth of sibling
   b. Adoption
   c. Foster child
   d. Marriage
   e. Divorce, separation
   f. Stepchildren
2. Characteristics which may be noted by parent(s)
   a. Rivalry keener in children of same sex
   b. More common in boys than girls
   c. More intense when sibling is 2 to 4 years old when next child is born
   d. Decreases as children grow older
   e. Older children sometimes demonstrating "envy" of baby role in family
   f. Envy of older siblings sometimes forcing younger child to attempt tasks beyond capacity
3. Parent(s) may demonstrate confusion about setting consistent limits with various children.

B. Objective data

Physical examination is normal—school report will provide a guide for social adjustment outside the family unit.

II. Management

A. Treatments/medications: Goals of treatment are to teach parent(s)

1. The meaning of "equivalent" love, not "equal" love, which is unrealistic
2. Reasonable limitations
3. The freedoms appropriate to a child's age

B. Counselling/prevention

1. Sibling rivalry is the child's normal initiation into competitive living and can be constructive and strengthening.
2. Parent(s) should be advised to
   a. Relax
   b. Identify and meet the parent(s)' own needs
   c. Be positive in self-evaluation
   d. Be calm in interactions with the sibling(s)
3. Counsel parent(s) that sibling rivalry is normal and
   a. Allows child to test values and behaviors as learned from parent(s)
   b. Helps the child explore his or her limits and potential
   c. Helps child learn to share satisfactions and frustrations
   d. Allows expression of aggression within a framework
   e. Provides companionship, separate and distinct from peer group and friends
4. Since sibling rivalry can be exacerbated with the birth of a new sibling, advise parent(s) to
   a. Make any room changes before the baby comes
   b. Put the crib away prior to birth
   c. Introduce nursery school before birth, if possible
   d. Tell the child the baby will be helpless and need care: deemphasize "playmate" aspect
   e. Call sibling(s) from the hospital
   f. Bring a gift home
   g. Deemphasize any signs of regression in sibling(s)
      (1) Demanding behaviors

(2) Abandonment of toilet training
(3) Use of baby bottle

C. Follow-up

1. Follow-up depends on severity of behavior.
2. The focus should be on helping parent(s) and child explore adaptive behaviors.

D. Consultations/referrals: none

Table 116-1 Medical Referral/Consultation

Diagnosis	Clinical Manifestations	Management
Excessive, maladaptive behavior	Regression without expected improvement Destructive acts toward siblings Self-destructive acts Mutism Fecal smearing	Professional counselling

bibliography

Barnett, Henry. *Pediatrics* (16th ed.). New York: Appleton-Century-Crofts, 1977.

DeAngelis, Catherine. *Pediatric Primary Care* (2d ed.). Boston: Little, Brown, 1979.

Erickson, Marcene. *Assessment and management of developmental changes in children.* St. Louis: Mosby, 1976.

Gochros, J. S. Notes from a family counselor . . . On helping the older child survive the new baby. *American Baby,* **38**:28 (1976).

Lidz, Theodore. *The person* (2nd ed.). New York: Basic Books, 1976.

Roth, P. G. Sibling rivalry. *American Baby,* **39**:36–38 (1977).

Spock, Benjamin. *Baby and child care.* New York: Pocket Books, 1972.

117 Discipline

KAREN A. BALLARD

ALERT
1. Evidence of physical abuse/neglect
2. Abuse present in maternal/paternal childhoods
3. Utilization of harsh disciplinary methods

I. Assessment: Acceptable Discipline

A. Subjective data

1. Each parent
   a. Shares similar philosophy of child discipline
   b. Accepts responsibility to discipline
   c. Understands discipline is only appropriate when utilized correctly
   d. Understands the potential for abuse
2. Acceptable disciplinary episodes are
   a. Related to an appropriate precipitating event
      (1) Disobedience
      (2) Noncompliance
      (3) Excessive fighting
   b. *Not* related to developmental tasks
      (1) Toilet training
      (2) Self-feeding
      (3) Self-dressing
   c. Consistent with parent(s) general child-rearing philosophy
   d. Age appropriate
      (1) Young, preschool child—brief scolding
      (2) School-age child—brief scolding/spanking, deprivation of favorite activities
      (3) Adolescent—scolding; deprivation of favorite activities; assignment of extra chores
   e. Similarly applied to all children.
3. Acceptable disciplinary methods are
   a. Scolding—2 to 3 min
   b. Assignment of extra work or chores
   c. Deprivation of favorite activities
   d. Brief spanking using a hand and *only* on the child's buttocks
4. Child responds to discipline with
   a. Increase/decrease in undesirable behavior
   b. Increase in general acting-out behavior
   c. Child's mood may be
      (1) Compliant and obedient
      (2) Withdrawn and sullen
      (3) Angry and belligerent

B. Objective data

1. Physical examination within normal limits
2. No evidence of physical abuse

II. Assessment: Unacceptable Discipline

A. Subjective data

1. Important to evaluate whether disciplinary methods are actually child abuse (see Battered/Abused Child, Chap. 159); occasional use of unacceptable discipline is human and understandable and should not be harshly or precipitously judged
2. Each parent may
   a. Disagree regarding philosophy of child discipline
   b. Have difficulty accepting individual responsibility to discipline
   c. Have difficulty recognizing the potential for abuse
   d. Indicate that discipline is a parenting problem
3. Unacceptable disciplinary episodes are
   a. Often not related to an appropriate precipitating event
   b. Related to developmental tasks of child

c. Related to parental frustrations and feelings
d. Reflections of inappropriate parenting and child-rearing practices
e. Frequent, inconsistent, and not age appropriate

4. Unacceptable disciplinary methods are
   a. Threats of
      (1) Abandonment
      (2) Loss of parental love
      (3) Physical mutilation
   b. Depreciation of child's self-image
   c. Prolonged spanking, hitting, and any physical force
5. Abuse present in maternal/paternal childhoods

B. Objective data

1. Physical examination may show
   a. Child to be pale and poorly nourished
   b. Bruises, welts
   c. Chronic/acute otitis media
   d. Hearing loss
   e. Present/past skeletal injuries
2. Assessment of parent-child relationship may indicate
   a. Poor eye contact between parent(s) and child
   b. Little or no physical contact
   c. Child withdrawn
   d. Parent(s) uncomfortable handling child

III. Management

A. Treatments/medications: none

B. Counselling/prevention

1. Discipline is a necessary part of every child's development; children raised without discipline can become fearful, insecure, and unsure of parental love.
2. Some goals of discipline are to teach children
   a. Behavior which is acceptable to society
   b. Respect for the rights and property of others
   c. The ability to distinguish between safe and unsafe
3. Advise parent(s) that acceptable discipline is
   a. Immediate and not delayed
   b. Not done in anger
   c. Age and event appropirate
   d. Consistent
   e. Identified by a reasonable time limit
4. Encourage parent(s) to
   a. Reinforce good behavior
   b. *Not* discipline for acts beyond the child's control
      (1) Thumb-sucking
      (2) Stress-related enuresis
5. Help parent(s) identify behaviors which usually will require discipline.
   a. Unreasonable fighting with siblings/peers
   b. Dangerous activities
   c. Open defiance of family rules
   d. Rebellion against family/societal morals and standards
6. Support parent(s) in dealing with fears regarding spoiling and overregulating the child.
7. Counsel parent(s) to
   a. Mutually accept responsibility for discipline.
   b. Be reasonably consistent.
   c. Administer discipline in private.
   d. Identify and discuss misbehavior with the child before initiating discipline.
   e. Avoid comparing sibling/peer behaviors.
   f. Keep all discipline simple and brief.
8. Encourage parent(s) to discuss their feelings regarding
   a. Their own childhood and disciplinary experiences
   b. What discipline means to them
   c. How it feels to discipline

C. Follow-up: dependent upon parental ability to establish satisfactory disciplinary methods

D. Consultations/referrals: professional counselling if parental problems continue

bibliography

Brown, Marie Scott, and Murphy, Mary Alexander. *Ambulatory pediatrics for nurses.* New York: McGraw-Hill, 1975.

Church, Joseph. *Understanding your child from birth to three.* New York: Pocket Books, 1976.

Clemmens, Raymond, and Kenny, Thomas. Prevention of emotional problems in childhood: A philosophy for child rearing. *Clinical Pediatrics*, **16**:122–123 (1977).

DeAngelis, Catherine. *Pediatric Primary Care* (2d ed.). Boston: Little, Brown, 1979.

Drabman, Ronald, and Jarvie, Greg. Counselling parents of children with behavior problems: The use of extinction and time-out techniques. *Pediatrics*, **59**:78–85 (1977).

Flinders, N. J. How to teach children right from wrong. *Parents' Magazine*, **50**:31–32 (1975).

Foster, Randall. Parenting the child with a behavior disorder: A family approach. *Pediatric Annals*, **6**:29–43 (1977).

Friedman, David, and Sevinger, Hershel. Discipline and alternatives to punishment. *Pediatric Annals*, **6**:25 (1977).

Hyman, I. A. Paddling, punishing and force: Where do we go from here? *Children Today*, **6**:17–25 (1977).

Illingworth, Ronald. *The normal child* (6th ed.). New York: Churchill Livingstone, 1975.

Murphy, Mary Alexander. Discipline. *Pediatric Nursing*, **2**:28–32 (1976).

Rouslin, Sheila. Developmental aggression and it's consequence.*Perspectives in Psychiatric Care*, **13**:170–175 (1975).

Spock, Benjamin. *Raising children in a difficult time*. New York: Pocket Books, 1974.

118 Breath-holding

KAREN A. BALLARD

ALERT

1. Loss of consciousness
2. Breath-holding episodes in children over 6 years of age

I. Assessment

A. Subjective data

1. Most common between 1 and 5 years with onset usually before 18 months; may be present in 50 percent of younger children
2. Episodes possibly occurring several times a day or only once every few months
3. Possibly history of previous aggressive behavior
   a. Biting
   b. Hitting
   c. Kicking
4. Precipitating events can be
   a. Pain
   b. Anger
   c. Frustration
   d. Limit setting
   e. Conflict
   f. Discipline
   g. Separation from mother or home

B. Objective data

1. Appears to be more common in males and white children
2. Typical breath-holding episodes identified by the following sequence
   a. Precipitating event
   b. Child crying out 2 to 3 times
   c. Child holding breath on expiration
   d. Period of apnea for 5 to 10 s
   e. May be cyanotic, and slight twitching may or may not be observed
   f. Child recovering in 2 to 3 min
   g. If precipitating event is pain, child sometimes becoming pallid instead of cyanotic and losing consciousness without crying out
   h. Heart rate slowing
   i. Blood pressure dropping acutely
3. Hematocrit and hemoglobin sometimes revealing concurrent iron deficiency anemia

II. Management

A. Treatments/medications: none, unless iron deficiency anemia present

B. Counselling/prevention

1. The family should be counselled to view a breath-holding episode as a form of temper tantrum.
2. During an episode, advise and support parent(s) to
   a. Make every effort to ensure child's safety.
   b. Maintain a calm manner.
   c. React with a minimum of fuss and interest.
   d. DO *NOT* throw cold water on the child or slap the child's face.
3. Keep a record of episodes and attempt to identify precipitating events.
4. Discuss methods of distracting the child at time of exposure to a known precipitator.

C. Follow-up

1. Follow-up depends on frequency and severity of breath-holding episodes.
2. Focus of visits should be on counselling and supporting the parent(s).

D. Consultations/referrals

1. Pediatrician
2. Pediatric neurologist
3. Teacher and/or school nurse if child is in nursery school or play groups

Table 118-1 Medical Referral/Consultation

Diagnosis	Clinical Maniifestations	Management
Seizure disorder	Does not follow orderly sequence of breath-holding episode Usually no precipitating event Clonic-tonic movements Cyanosis usually following episode and loss of consciousness Loss of sphincter control	Immediate referral to pediatric neurologist See Blackout Spells/Seizures, Chap. 79 Support, reassurance, and education of parent(s)
Breath-holding episode after 6 yr of age	Infantile aggressive pattern indicative of a more severe emotional problem	Referral to pediatric neurologist Professional counselling Consultation with school nurse

bibliography

Bakwin, Harry, and Bakwin, Ruth. *Behavior disorders in children.* Philadelphia: Saunders, 1972.

DeCastro, F., Rolfe, U., and Drew, J. K. *The pediatric nurse practitioner* (2d ed.). St. Louis: Mosby, 1976.

Illingworth, Ronald. *The normal child* (6th ed.). New York: Churchill Livingstone, 1975.

Mitchell, Ross (ed.). *Disease in infancy and childhood* (7th ed.). Baltimore: Williams & Wilkins, 1973.

Reece, Robert, and Chamberlain, John. *Manual of emergency pediatrics.* Philadelphia: Saunders, 1974.

119 Anger

KAREN A. BALLARD

ALERT
1. Delinquent and antisocial behaviors
2. Child harms self or others

I. Assessment

A. Subjective data

1. Normal anger is belligerent, defiant behavior which does not develop into either delinquent or antisocial acts.
2. There are two main types.
   a. Internal/passive—characterized by
      (1) Depression
      (2) Inability to express anger and aggressive feelings
      (3) Endless attempts to please others; fear of loss of love and social isolation
      (4) Avoidance of conflict and controversy
      (5) Uncomfortableness when anger is expressed by others
      (6) Child usually made to feel guilty or inadequate by parent(s); parental affection dependent on child's obedience
   b. External/aggressive—characterized by
      (1) Quarreling
      (2) Fighting
      (3) Open defiance
      (4) Physical/verbal abuse of peers and siblings
      (5) Parent(s) usually negligent in setting firm, loving limitations on child's behavior
3. Anger can also be a stage in the normal grief and mourning process of the child.
4. The age at the onset of the anger makes a difference in its expression.
   a. Toddler—anger often undifferentiated
   b. Adolescent—generally an increase in angry outbursts
5. The precipitating event might be any of the following.
   a. Death and/or loss of love object
   b. Frustration of wishes by parents, siblings, or peers
   c. Periods of separation
6. Behavior might be any of the following.
   a. Verbal outbursts
   b. Physical fights
   c. Quarreling
   d. Open defiance
   e. Protest
   f. Complaining
   g. Withdrawal
   h. Sullenness

B. Objective data: physical examination is within normal limits.

II. Management

A. Treatments/medications: none

B. Counselling/prevention

1. Parent(s) can be reassured that the emotional health of all children requires that they learn appropriate, socially acceptable expressions of anger.
   a. Protest
   b. Complaining
   c. Safe physical outlets
2. Parent(s) must ensure that allowing expressions of anger does not permit the child to harm him- or herself or others.
3. Parent(s) should be advised that sometimes children need to be reassured that they have not alienated parental love by their expression of anger.

C. Follow-up

1. Follow-up depends on the severity of the behavior.
2. Angry behavior patterns in children usually respond well to short-term counselling of parent(s) and child by a sympathetic counsellor.

D. Consultations/referrals: professional counselling

Table 119-1 Medical Referral/Consultation

Diagnosis/Problem	Manifestations	Management
Prolonged, excessive anger	Behavior continues to persist over a 3-mo period of time after onset of counselling by practitioner. Child physicially harms self or others	Immediate referral for professional counselling
Delinquent and antisocial behaviors	Angry behaviors escalate (running away, truancy, setting fires, stealing, etc.)	Immediate referral for professional counselling

bibliography

Anderson, L. S. The aggressive child. *Children Today,* **7**:11–14 (1978).

Gochros, J. S. Only spank when you're angry. *American Baby,* **39**:34–35 (1977).

Harrison, Saul, and McDermott, John. *Childhood psychopathology.* New York: International Universities Press, 1972.

Joint Commission on Mental Health of Children (Task Forces I, II, and III and the Committees on Education and Religion). *Mental health: From infancy through adolescence.* New York: Harper & Row, 1973.

LeShan, Eda. Getting mad is quite OK. *Woman's Day,* **41**:56–58 (1978).

Lewis, Melvin. *Clinical aspects of child development.* Philadelphia: Lea & Febiger, 1971.

Schwartz, Jane Lenker, and Schwartz, Lawrence. *The psycho-dynamics of patient care.* Englewood Cliffs: Prentice-Hall, 1972.

120 Negativism

KAREN A. BALLARD

I. Assessment

A. Subjective data

1. Most frequently occurs in
   a. Toddlers
   b. Adolescents
2. Can be exacerbated by concurrent
   a. Hunger
   b. Fatigue
   c. Insecurity
   d. Jealousy
3. Precipitating events can be
   a. Frustration
   b. Jealousy
   c. Noncompliance
   d. Limit setting
   e. Sibling rivalry
4. Parent(s) describes that
   a. "No" is a frequent verbal response.
   b. Oppositional behaviors are frequent.
   c. Reluctance is noted in compliance with requests.
   d. Crying, shouting behaviors are present.
   e. There is voluntary isolation from family activities.

B. Objective data

1. Physical examination normal
2. Intelligence screening
   a. Expected to be normal
   b. Negativism possibly a reflection of underlying learning problems

II. Management

A. Treatments/medications: none

B. Counselling/prevention

1. Advise parent(s) that negativism is a normal developmental problem and reflects the need to learn control of self and others.
   a. Toddlers—negativism a response to parental demands that behavior(s) reflect appropriate family, cultural, and social norms
   b. Adolescents/young adults—negativism a result of the struggle to achieve final independence and individuation
2. Counsel parent(s) to understand the use of the word "no."
   a. Means not just "no" but also indicates "I won't"
   b. Can mean "yes" and reflects the ambivalence of the dependent/independent conflict
   c. Becomes a powerful tool if its use receives reinforcement from the parent(s)
3. Parent(s) can be counselled to
   a. Help child with activities
   b. Reinforce positive behaviors
   c. Avoid the use of
      (1) Opposition as a control of the negativism
      (2) Frequent orders/commands
      (3) Interrupting activities

C. Follow-up

1. Follow-up depends on the severity of the negativistic behaviors.
2. The focus should be on counselling and supporting parental participation in positive, shared activities.

D. Consultations/referrals: none

bibliography

Brown, Marie Scott, and Murphy, Mary Alexander. *Ambulatory pediatrics for nurses.* New York: McGraw-Hill, 1975.

Fraiberg, Selma. *The magic years.* New York: Scribner, 1959.

Illingworth, Ronald. *The normal child* (6th ed.). New York: Churchill Livingston, 1975.

121 Temper Tantrums

KAREN A. BALLARD

Definitive elimination of all organic causes is *imperative.* A complete history and physical examination should precede investigation of psychological causes.

I. Assessment

A. Subjective data

1. Usually between 1 and 3 years of age
2. Children with determined, aggressive personalities more prone
3. Precipitating events may be
   a. Failure to get own way
   b. Resistance to complying with parental wishes or demands
   c. Deprivation
   d. Jealousy
4. Behavior during tantrum
   a. Kicking
   b. Screaming
   c. Throwing objects
   d. Breath-holding
5. Predisposing factors
   a. Child's own personality
   b. Child's desire to practice new skills
   c. Imitativeness—family member, friend, or sibling with temper pattern which has been observed by child.
   d. Presence of insecurity in child
   e. Child's level of intelligence
   f. Previous parental patterns of overindulgence, overprotection, and domination
   g. Parental inconsistency in limit setting
   h. Parental fatigue, impatience, or unhappiness

B. Objective data: Physical examination is within normal limits.

II. Management

A. Treatments/medications: none

B. Counselling/prevention

1. The clue to managing temper tantrums is in prevention and in recognition of them as a normal development problem.
2. Parent(s) of toddlers and preschoolers should be counselled to
   a. Keep the child occupied
   b. Provide opportunities for appropriate peer play
      (1) Community play programs
      (2) Nursery school
      (3) Visiting friends
   c. Provide assistance to the child in acquiring and practicing new skills
3. Intervention is formulated on what is effective for the child and comfortable for the parent(s).
   a. Hold and comfort the child; do *not* attempt to bribe or give rewards.
   b. Remove the child physically from the situation, and place him or her in a safe area until the tantrum ceases.
      (1) Own room
      (2) Play yard
   c. Ignore the child until the tantrum ceases.
   d. Distract the child from the tantrum.
      (1) Suggest play activity.
      (2) Play music.
      (3) Play with water or give a bath.
4. Encourage parent(s) to attempt to identify

precipitating events and manipulate them to avoid the tantrum.

a. Assist the child in performing frustrating tasks.
b. Interrupt sibling and/or peer arguments.
c. Provide imaginative play equipment.

C. Follow-up: as needed to offer support and reassurance to parent(s)

D. Consultations/referrals: professional counselling if no improvement within 3 to 6 months

Table 121-1 Medical Referral/Consultation

Diagnosis	Clinical Manifestations	Management
Chronic infection	Low-grade fever Malaise Elevated or decreased white blood cells	Consult a physician.
Deafness	Inattentive Poor response to noise Poor speech development Conductive hearing loss	Consult a physician, refer to an ear, nose, and throat specialist. See Deafness/Defective Hearing/Hearing Changes, Chap. 26.
Mental retardation	Below appropriate growth and development level Poor speech development Lag in social skills	Consult a physician. Refer to a child development clinic.
Cerebral tumor	Abnormal neurological exam Change in level of consciousness Ataxia	Consult a physician/refer to a pediatric neurologist.
Degenerative diseases of nervous system	Abnormal neurological exam Failure to thrive Abnormal developmental milestones	Consult a physician/refer to a pediatric neurologist.

bibliography

Barnett, Henry. *Pediatrics* (16th ed.), New York: Appleton-Century-Crofts, 1977.

Brown, Marie Scott, and Murphy, Mary Alexander. *Ambulatory pediatrics for nurses.* New York: McGraw-Hill, 1975.

Church, Joseph. *Understanding your child from birth to three.* New York: Pocket Books, 1976.

DeAngelis, Catherine. *Pediatric Primary Care* (2d ed.) Boston: Little, Brown, 1979.

Illingworth, Ronald. *The normal child* (6th ed.). New York: Churchill Livingstone, 1975.

Radl, S. L. Children are not for breaking. *American Baby,* **39**:56–57 (1977).

Raley, W. Toddlers and their temper tantrums. *American Baby,* **38**:20 (1976).

Shaw, Charles. *When your child needs help.* New York: Morrow, 1972.

Steward, Martin. Temper, temper . . . How to deal with tantrums. *Parents' Magazine,* **54**:75–76 (1979).

122 Toilet Training

KAREN A. BALLARD

ALERT

1. Bed-wetting (enuresis) after age 5
2. Stool incontinence (encopresis) after age 4

I. Assessment: Readiness and Appropriateness for Toilet Training

A. Subjective data

1. Before initiation of toilet training, the child must
   a. Be physiologically mature
      (1) Between 1 and $2\frac{1}{2}$ years
         (a) Bladder sensation develops.
         (b) The child can sense and indicate the urge to void.
         (c) The child is physically capable of initiating voiding when bladder capacity reaches 90 mL.
         (d) Once started, the child cannot interrupt the stream.
      (2) Between $2\frac{1}{2}$ and $4\frac{1}{2}$ years
         (a) Gains control over reflexes
         (b) Becomes involved in being able to inhibit voiding
         (c) When bladder can accommodate between 300 and 350 mL, is able to stay dry throughout night
   b. Have regular bowel movements
   c. Have awareness of desired behavior
      (1) Has eliminated
      (2) Is eliminating
      (3) Is about to eliminate
   d. Understand what training chair and/or toilet is and be willing to sit on it
   e. Be psychologically ready
      (1) Secure and gratifying parent-child relationship
      (2) Have desire to please parent(s)
      (3) Child's wish to control impulses
2. The stress of toilet training can contribute to concurrent problem(s) which are alleviated when toilet-training practices are moderated.
   a. Temper tantrums
   b. Eating disturbances
   c. Sleeping disturbances

B. Objective data

1. The physical examination is normal.
2. The laboratory data is normal.
3. Developmental assessment shows evidence of sufficient motor and emotional maturation.
4. The parent-child relationship is adequate.

II. Management

A. Treatments/medications: none

B. Counselling

1. Discuss toilet-training plan *before* child reaches 15 months by
   a. Helping parent(s) withstand pressures for early toilet training
   b. Exploring appropriate and inappropriate methods
   c. Helping parent(s) understand importance of relaxed, unpressured approach
   d. Preparing parent(s) for child's mistakes and relapses
2. Suggest the following toilet-training program (modification of method described by Brazelton, 1962) (copyright American Academy of Pediatrics, 1962).
   a. Use a potty chair, as it is more comfortable than a potty seat on a toilet.
   b. Introduce the child to his or her potty seat as just another chair; allow for a period of familiarity.

c. Initially, allow the child to sit on the chair, fully clothed, while a brief story is read.
d. After 1 week, the child can be placed on the chair without diapers but with no attempt at collection.
e. Change the child's soiled diapers in front of the chair and drop the diapers into the pot.
f. Finally, put the child on the chair for collection.
g. Collection time should be limited to 15 min unless the child is successful or too distracted to remain on the chair.

3. Three processes of the child to be explored with parent(s) are
   a. Bowel control
   b. Waking control of the bladder
   c. Sleeping control of the bladder
4. Support the parent(s) in their efforts and suggest that
   a. One or two willing, significant adults devote time and effort to the toilet-training process and share the responsibility.
   b. Significant adult and child develop mutual communication.
      (1) Word(s) for urine
      (2) Word(s) for feces
   c. Positive reinforcement should follow all successes.
   d. There should be no harsh punishment for failure and/or disinterest.
   e. There should be no coercion or use of suppositories
5. Assist parent(s) in identifying and anticipating events which can cause relapse in control.
   a. Excitement
   b. Play situation(s)
   c. Stress
   d. Illness/hospitalization
   e. Absence of significant adult(s)
6. Counsel parent(s) that fecal smearing and increased touching of genitalia during toilet training are normal behaviors; they should be treated in a matter-of-fact way and will diminish as control increases.

C. Follow-up

1. Follow-up depends on how the parent(s) and the child adapt to the toilet-training program.
2. The focus should be on direction and support of the parent(s).

D. Consultations/referrals: none

Table 122-1 Medical Referral/Consultation

Diagnosis	Clinical Manifestations	Management
Enuresis	Involuntary loss of urine Presence after 3 yr, persisting past 5 yr Two types In children who have never developed bladder control In children who had bladder control but lost it	See Bed-wetting, Chap. 77 Urological evaluation Consultation with physician
Encopresis	Involuntary passage of feces Occurs in children 7–9 yr 3 times more prevalent in boys than girls Approximately 50% had originally controlled bowel movements	Referral to physician See Stool Incontinence (Encopresis), Chap. 50 Evaluation for organic cause

bibliography

Berg, I., Fielding, D. and Meadow, R. Psychiatric disturbance, urgency, and bacteriuria in children with day and night wetting. *Archives of Disease in Childhood,* **52**:651–657 (1977).

Brazelton, T. Berry. A child-oriented approach to toilet training. *Pediatrics,* **29**:121–128 (1962).

Brown, Marie Scott, and Murphy, Mary Alexander. *Ambulatory pediatrics for nurses.* New York: McGraw-Hill, 1975.

Church, Joseph. *Understanding your child from birth to three.* New York: Pocket Books, 1976.

DeAngelis, Catherine. *Pediatric Primary Care* (2d ed.). Boston: Little, Brown, 1979.

DeVrais, Marten, and DeVries, Rachel. Cultural relativity of toilet training readiness: A perspective from East Africa. *Pediatrics,* **60**:170–177 (1977).

Erickson, Marcene L. *Assessment and management of developmental changes in children.* St. Louis: Mosby, 1976, pp. 217–227.

Fraiberg, Selma. *The magic years.* New York: Scribner, 1959.

Tsai, Sherry Woodruff. Enuresis: The management challenge. *Pediatric Nursing,* **2**:33–37 (1976).

123 Tooth Grinding

KAREN A. BALLARD

ALERT

1. Acute and sudden onset of tooth grinding
2. Changes in level of consciousness

I. Assessment

A. Subjective data

1. Usually considered normal when occurring in sleep; can be normal in awake state
2. May accompany dream activity or occur as a reaction to daytime stress
3. Can persist into adulthood

B. Objective data

Persistent tooth grinding results in flattened tooth cusps and/or worn incisors.

II. Management

A. Treatments/medications: none

B. Counselling/prevention

1. Parent(s) should be assisted in understanding that tooth grinding can have underlying emotional cause.
2. The individual's everyday life must be evaluated in order to identify specific stresses.
   a. Peer group
   b. Learning tasks
   c. Family relationships
3. Particular attention should be paid to modifying any life stress which has a high aggression-stimulating potential.

C. Follow-up

1. Follow-up depends on the frequency and severity of the behavior.
2. Focus should be on support and encouraging verbalization of feelings.

D. Consultations/referrals

1. Professional counselling
2. School teacher and nurse
3. Dentist

Table 123-1 Medical Referral/Consultation

Diagnosis	Clinical Manifestations	Management
Meningitis or other consciousness-altering infection	Acute onset of tooth grinding Stiff neck Alteration in level of consciousness Positive Kernig's and/or Brudzinski's sign	Immediate physician referral
Dental abnormalities	Loss of dental enamel Change in structure of teeth	Referral to dentist See "Dental Health" in Chap. 9
Mental retardation	Abnormal developmental milestones Poor speech development Lag in social skills	Consult a physician. Refer to a child development clinic.

bibliography

Barnett, Henry. *Pediatrics* (16th ed.). New York: Appleton-Century-Crofts, 1977.

Chapman, A. H. *Management of emotional problems of children and adolescents* (2d ed.). Philadelphia: Lippincott, 1974.

DeAngelis, Catherine. *Pediatric Primary Care* (2d ed.). Boston: Little, Brown, 1979.

Illingworth, Ronald. *The normal child.* New York: Churchill Livingstone, 1975.

Mikami, D. B. A review of psychogenic aspects and treatment of bruxism. *Journal of Prosthetic Dentistry,* **37**:411–419 (1977).

Mitchell, Ross (ed.). *Disease in infancy and childhood* (7th ed.). Baltimore: Williams & Wilkins, 1973.

Reece, Robert, and Chamberlain, John. *Manual of emergency pediatrics.* Philadelphia: Saunders, 1974.

124 Biting

KAREN A. BALLARD

ALERT
Biting behavior after 5 years of age

I. Assessment

A. Subjective data

1. Most common in the preverbal child who is unable to express frustration
2. Early form of aggressive behavior and, developmentally, is followed by hitting and kicking
3. Usually becomes a problem in the last half of the first year of life when the child begins to acquire teeth; may have later, sudden onset between 2 and 3 years
4. Precipitating events may be
   a. Discipline
   b. Frustration in a task, developmental and/or manual
   c. Peer/sibling conflict
   d. Poor communication skills
5. Parent(s) sometimes state that child bites self and others

B. Objective data

The physical examination is within normal limits.

II. Management

A. Treatments/medications: none

B. Counselling/prevention

1. Biting should be identified to the parent(s) as both an aggressive behavior and a maladaptive method of communication.
2. If the biter is an infant who is being breast-fed, counsel the parent(s) to provide a biting substitute with zwieback, teething ring, spoon, or hard rubber toy.
3. If the biter is a preschool child (under 5 years), the behavior is probably related to a frustrating social situation. Suggest to parent(s) to
   a. Simplify the play situation.
      (1) Small peer-group play
      (2) Short, specific playtimes
   b. Attempt to reduce any high-level competitiveness in the child's play.
   c. Provide more adult supervision in all situations which seem to provoke biting.
      (1) Adult intervention should be aimed at preventing behavior rather than punishment.
      (2) Do *not* bite child back or wash child's mouth out with soap as an intervention.
      (3) Child may be isolated by the adult from the group each time a biting episode occurs.
   d. Encourage child to verbalize frustrations and difficulties.

C. Follow-up

1. Follow-up depends on the severity of the behavior.
2. The focus of visits is on counselling and support of the parent(s).

D. Consultations/referrals: teacher of nursery school or play group

Table 124-1 Medical Referral/Consultation

Diagnosis	Clinical Manifestations	Management
Dental abnormalities	Retarded dental growth	Refer to a dentist.
	Presence of infection and/or caries	See Dental Health in Chap. 9.
	Any malformation or abnormality in mouth	See Mouth Sores, Chap. 44.
Biting behavior after 5 yr of age	May be manifestation of more serious emotional problems	Consultation with physician Professional counselling

bibliography

Brown, Marie Scott, and Murphy, Mary Alexander. *Pediatric history taking and physical diagnosis for nurses*. New York: McGraw-Hill, 1979.

Church, Joseph. *Understanding your child from birth to three*. New York: Pocket Books, 1976.

Dodson, Fitzhugh. *How to parent*. New York: New American Library, 1970.

Fraiberg, Selma. *The magic years*. New York: Scribner, 1959.

Ilg, Frances, and Ames, Louise Bates. *Child behavior*. New York: Harper & Row, 1966. (Originally published, 1955.)

McGuire, P. F. Debbie won't stop biting her playmates: Behavior modification in family medicine. *Journal of the Maine Medical Association*, **68**:267–268 (1977).

Spock, Benjamin. *Raising children in a difficult time*. New York: Pocket Books, 1974.

125 Fighting

KAREN A. BALLARD

ALERT
Increased fatigue

I. Assessment

A. Subjective data

1. Fighting usually occurs mostly in childhood and is developmentally progressive in its expression/description.
   a. 2 to 3 years—biting, hitting
   b. 3 to 7 years—rough, tumble games with pretend killing and shooting
   c. 7 to 12 years—cowboys and Indians, war games, hitting
   d. 12 to 18 years—rough contact sports, fist-fighting, group/gang fighting
2. Aggressive, fighting behaviors can usually be identified in child's home environment.
3. Boys fight more outside the home than girls.
4. Fighting in childhood is normal, and concern should develop with excessive or abusive fighting.
5. Precipitating events may be
   a. Failure to get own way
   b. Jealousy
   c. Anger
   d. Frustration
   e. Limit setting
6. Fighting behavior(s) may be described as
   a. Spontaneous/planned
   b. Controlled/uncontrolled
   c. Kicking
   d. Hitting
   e. Inside/outside home
   f. Self or others injured
7. Predisposing factors may be
   a. Child's own personality
   b. Child's desire to practice new skills
   c. Imitativeness—family member, friend, or sibling with aggressive, fighting behaviors
   d. Presence of insecurity in child
   e. Child's level of intelligence
   f. Fatigue

B. Objective data

1. Physical examination should be within normal limits.
2. Laboratory data are normal, and intelligence screening indicates normal functioning.

II. Management

A. Treatments/medications: none

B. Counselling/prevention

1. The difficulty in managing fighting behaviors is the decision of when to intervene; the clue is *prevention* of the behavior.
2. A parent can encounter difficulty with fighting because of that parent's own difficulty in handling aggression, especially when it is directed toward another person with the intention of hurting.
3. Advise parent(s) that determined attempts to curtail fighting in children often result in its continuation as an attention-seeking device. Some fighting is normal.
4. Counsel parent(s) to
   a. Help children learn to settle their own disputes.
   b. Anticipate when limits are reached.
   c. Separate children as necessary.
   d. Learn to provide appropriate, diversionary, aggressive outlets.
      (1) 2 to 3 years—pound-a-peg toys, clay
      (2) 3 to 7 years—punching toys, jungle gyms
      (3) 7 to 12 years—organized team sports

(soccer, baseball), supervised boxing, target games

(4) 12 to 18 years—organized team sports (baseball, basketball, football, soccer), athletic leagues (boxing, bowling, archery)

5. Advise parent(s) that siblings often quarrel, tease, bicker, and fight; parent(s) should be assisted in differentiating normal from excessive sibling behavior.
6. Assist parent(s) in identifying the child's underlying problem.
   a. Difficulty with feelings
      (1) Jealousy
      (2) Anger
      (3) Frustration
      (4) Insecurity
   b. Learning difficulties
      (1) Mild retardation
      (2) Perceptual problems
      (3) Teacher-student relationship
      (4) Inappropriate educational goals
   c. Interpersonal difficulties
      (1) Isolation by peer group
      (2) Insecurity in peer group
   d. Family difficulties
      (1) Parental fighting
      (2) Harsh, punitive discipline
      (3) Sibling bullying/tyranny

C. Follow-up

1. Follow-up depends on the frequency and severity of fighting behaviors.
2. The focus of visits should be on identifying underlying problems and counselling the parent(s).

D. Consultations/referrals

1. Teacher and/or school nurse if fighting is present in and/or associated with school
2. Professional counselling if
   a. Underlying problem severe
   b. Behavior not modified by counselling within 3 months

bibliography

Brown, Marie Scott, and Murphy, Mary Alexander. *Pediatric history taking and physical diagnosis for nurses.* New York: McGraw-Hill, 1979.

Parker, D. The aggressive child . . .Should you worry. *American Baby,* **37**:20 (1975).

Redl, Fritz. *When we deal with children.* New York: Free Press, 1966.

Shaw, Charles. *When your child needs help.* New York: Morrow, 1972.

Spock, Benjamin. *Raising children in a difficult time.* New York: Pocket Books, 1974.

126 Jealousy

KAREN A. BALLARD

I. Assessment

A. Subjective data

1. Most often associated with
   a. Perceptions of favoritism
   b. Difficulty with a new sibling
   c. Normal oedipal feelings
2. Child fears losing something previously possessed
   a. Love
   b. Feeling of importance
   c. Feeling of being wanted
3. Behavior
   a. Overt signs
      (1) Verbalization of feeling
      (2) Aggression toward perceived favorite
      (3) Selfishness
      (4) Inferiority complex
   b. Occult signs
      (1) Regression to infantile behaviors
         (a) Thumb-sucking
         (b) Enuresis
         (c) Infantile speech pattern
      (2) Quarrelsomeness
      (3) Negativism
      (4) Aggression
4. Jealousy most common in firstborn and if not resolved, can lead to permanent personality traits of aggressiveness, selfishness, and inferiority
5. Jealousy can be exaggerated by feelings of insecurity related to
   a. Overprotection
   b. Parental impatience
   c. Parental domination
   d. Discord in family
   e. Poor limit setting
   f. Threats of and/or actual abandonment by a parent
6. Intensity of jealousy usually decreases as family size increases
7. The smaller the age difference between two siblings, the greater the chance of jealousy

B. Objective data

Physical examination is normal.

II. Management

A. Treatments/medications: none

B. Counselling/prevention

1 Advise parent(s) that jealousy responds best to
   a. Love
   b. Understanding
   c. Limit setting in a secure environment
2. Prevention is the key to handling jealousy; help parent(s) anticipate high-risk areas.
   a. School performance favoritism—avoidance of comparisons between siblings
   b. Birth or adoption of a new sibling should be accompanied by
      (1) Sibling involvement in planning
      (2) Supervised playtime for siblings with the child
      (3) Sibling participation in care
3. Distract a jealous sibling into an activity; this could be "special" and define this child's more advanced status in the family.

C. Follow-up

1. Follow-up depends on the intensity of the problem.
2. Focus on counselling the parent(s), and support the child in verbalizing or playing-out feelings.

D. Consultations/referrals: professional counselling if no improvement in 6 months

bibliography

Bernstein, Anne C. Jealousy in the family. *Parents' Magazine,* **54**:47–51 (1979).

DeAngelis, Catherine. *Pediatric Primary Care* (2d ed.). Boston: Little, Brown, 1979.

Illingworth, Ronald. *The normal child* (6th ed.). New York: Churchill Livingstone, 1975.

Lidz, Theodore. *The person* (2d ed.). New York: Basic Books, 1976.

Shaw, Charles. *When your child needs help.* New York: Morrow, 1972.

Spock, Benjamin. *Raising children in a difficult time.* New York: Pocket Books, 1974.

127 Fears

KAREN A. BALLARD

ALERT
Excessive incapacitating fears

I. Etiology

Fears are usually learned by

A. Observation
B. Suggestion
C. Threats

II. Assessment

A. Subjective data

1. Fears are one of the most common emotional symptoms in childhood and can persist into adulthood.
2. Fears fall into three main categories.
   a. Normal fears, which serve to protect and prevent accidents
      (1) Hot versus cold
      (2) Fire
      (3) Perils of traffic
   b. Mild fears, usually learned from others or resulting from one's misinterpretation of the environment; most *normal* childhood fears in this category
      (1) Strange people
      (2) New situations
      (3) Animals
      (4) Dark and night
      (5) Thunder and loud noises
      (6) Getting hurt
      (7) Doctors and hospitals
      (8) Injections
      (9) Ghosts
      (10) Death
      (11) Hell
      (12) Abandonment
   c. Excessive fears, which are distorted ideas causing problems in daily life
      (1) Being flushed down toilet into drain
      (2) Death occurring in sleep
      (3) A "bad" thought becoming reality
3. Different kinds of fears occur most commonly at different ages.
   a. 6 months—fear of strangers
   b. 18 months—fear of separation
   c. 2 to 3 years—fear of dogs, cats, toilets, darkness
   d. 8 years—fear of death
   e. 12 to 18 years—fear of loss of autonomy, illness and death
   f. Adults—fear of animals, heights, travel, intimacy and commitment, illness and death
4. Precipitating events may be
   a. New situations
   b. Strange people
   c. Thunder and loud noises
   d. Animals
   e. Hospitals, doctors, and nurses
   f. Fires
5. Behavior may be described as
   a. Crying, screaming
   b. Hiding
   c. Running away

B. Objective data

1. Physical examination is within normal limits.
2. Those with high IQs have potential for more fears.

III. Management

A. Treatments/medications: none

B. Counselling/prevention

1. All normal individuals have fears which are

generally related to their developmental level and life experiences.
2. Parent(s) can be reassured that, since fears are related to the child's developmental level, many fears are outgrown.
3. All adults involved should realize the fear is real and should be respected.
4. It is not beneficial or effective to tease, ridicule, or ignore the fear.
5. Most fearful children respond well when the adult is patient, sympathetic, and supportive of child's functioning.
6. The parent(s) can desensitize children to fearful objects by allowing manipulation and play until the child feels safe.
7. Counselling for the adolescent and young adult should be directed toward a mature lifestyle which supports independent functioning. This can be accomplished by appropriate educational, vocational, and professional counselling.

C. Follow-up
1. Follow-up depends on the severity of the fears.
2. Focus should be on counselling and supporting parent(s) and the child and encouraging verbalization and/or playing-out of feelings.

D. Consultations/referrals
1. Professional counselling
2. Teacher and school nurse

Table 127-1 Medical Referral/Consultation

Diagnosis	Clinical Manifestations	Management
Excessive, incapacitating fears	Inability to leave home or separate from parent(s) Panic episodes when placed in fearful situation Activities of daily living impeded	Refer immediately for professional counselling

bibliography

Astin, E. W. Self-reported fears of hospitalized and nonhospitalized children aged ten to twelve. *Maternal-Child Nursing Journal,* **6**:17–24 (1977).

Barnett, Henry. *Pediatrics* (16th ed.). New York: Appleton-Century-Crofts, 1977.

Brown, Marie Scott, and Murphy, Mary Alexander. *Pediatric history taking and physical diagnosis for nurses.* New York: McGraw-Hill, 1979.

Fraiberg, Selma. *The magic years.* New York: Scribner, 1959.

Illingworth, Ronald. *The normal child* (6th ed.). New York: Churchill Livingstone, 1975.

Johnson, J. E., et al. Easing children's fright during health care procedures. *Maternal Child Nursing,* **1**:206–210 (1976).

Parness, E. Effects of experiences with loss and death among preschool children. *Children Today,* **4**:2–7 (1975).

Shaw, Charles. *When your child needs help.* New York: Morrow, 1972.

128 Sleep Disturbances

KAREN A. BALLARD

ALERT
1. Seizure disorder
2. Ear pain or decreased hearing
3. Rectal itch (pinworms)
4. Separation anxiety

I. Assessment

A. Subjective data

1. Sleep disturbances are characterized by
   a. Occurrence during "active period" of sleep when the individual can be observed as having body and rapid eye movements (REM)
   b. Presence of daytime stresses
   c. Fears
   d. Concurrent developmental stresses
2. Sleep disturbances can be identified as
   a. Sleep refusal seen in children below 3 years; can persist into later years
   b. Nightmares seen in children below 3 years and in others at times of stress
   c. Night terrors seen most commonly in preschoolers
3. Possible to identify specific differences in sleep disturbances
   a. Sleep refusal is particularly related to fear of losing parent when asleep and is associated with separation anxiety.
   b. Nightmares occur in individuals who confuse fantasy with reality and have dreams about monsters, ghosts, animals, and frightening experiences.
   c. Night terrors occur during sudden arousal from non-REM sleep and present as
      (1) Distressed, inconsolable agitation
      (2) A sudden sitting up in bed, accompanied by screaming
      (3) Limited in time (10 to 15 min)
      (4) Not remembered in morning
4. Parent(s) may have incorrect attitudes
   a. Wrong ideas concerning the amount of sleep required
   b. Overanxiety
   c. Rigid child-rearing and disciplinary methods
   d. Frequent checking on child during sleep
5. Precipitating events may be
   a. Absence of parent(s)
   b. Introduction to school
   c. Change in home or school
   d. Sibling rivalry
   e. Illness or hospitalization
   f. Frightening experience

B. Objective data

1. The physical examination is normal, but the child may present as anxious and fearful.
2. Laboratory tests are normal.

II. Management

A. Treatments/medications

1. An aberrant sleep treatment program should include
   a. Allowance for expression of parental feelings
   b. Keeping a record of sleep and naps
   c. Separate sleeping area for child
   d. Well-ventilated room
   e. Warm bath prior to sleep
   f. Safe, comforting toys
   g. Establishment of a bedtime hour
   h. Night-light
   i. Quiet play/rituals
   j. Presence in home of trusted adult(s)—parent(s), baby-sitters

k. Removal of environmental and external stresses
l. Assistance of parent(s) in identifying and modifying precipitating events
(1) Separation anxiety
(2) School difficulties
(3) Sibling rivalry
(4) Fear of dark
(5) Fear of objects in room
(6) Fear of falling asleep
(7) Frightening experiences/memories
(8) Illness and hospitalization
2. In severe cases, medication (e.g. chloral hydrate, diphenhydramine, phenobarbital) may be administered at bedtime for 7 to 10 days in an attempt to alter pattern; however, this intervention is only moderately effective.

B. Counselling/prevention
1. Anticipatory guidance should include informing the parent(s) that
a. Normal sleep habits are associated with the dark and night and develop with individual maturity.
(1) 3-month-old—some daytime wakefulness and nocturnal sleep
(2) 8- to 9-month-old—sustained periods of daytime wakefulness; one to two daytime naps and nocturnal sleep
(3) Toddlers—sustained daytime wakefulness; could benefit from a nap
(a) 2 years—numerous rituals
(b) 3 years—fewer rituals, more compliant, increased nightmare activity
(4) Older children and adolescents—pattern of daytime wakefulness and nocturnal sleep can be adjusted to complement daily activities
b. Most individuals establish a sleep pattern which suits them.
2. Counsel parent(s) that
a. The child should *not* be allowed to sleep in the parental bed.
b. Bed should never be used as punishment.
c. Presleep rituals help to allay fears, but they can become negative reinforcers if the child uses them to postpone sleep.
d. Certain requests after bedtime can be fulfilled, and the parent(s) should set firm and consistent limits.
3. The practitioner must remember to
a. Support all positive parental efforts to establish a sleep program and modify the child's behavior.
b. Acknowledge the inherent frustrations.
c. Encourage the parent(s) to get sufficient sleep.

C. Follow-up
1. Schedule biweekly visits.
2. The child should respond well to short-term counselling; parent(s) needs support until necessary maturation occurs.

D. Consultations/referrals: professional counselling

bibliography

Beardslee, E. W. The sleep of infants and young children: A review of the literature. *Maternal Child Nursing*, **5**:5–14 (1976).

DeAngelis, Catherine. *Pediatric Primary Care* (2d ed.). Boston: Little, Brown, 1979.

Erickson, Marcene. *Assessment and management of developmental changes in children*. St. Louis: Mosby, 1976.

Fraiberg, Selma. *The magic years*. New York: Scribner, 1959.

Friedman, Stanford. *The pediatric clinics of North America—Symposium on behavioral pediatrics*, (vol. 22, no. 3). Philadelphia: Saunders, 1975.

Illingworth, Ronald. *The normal child* (6th ed.). New York: Churchill Livingstone, 1975.

Inglis, S. The nocturnal frustration of sleep disturbance. *Maternal Child Nursing*, **1**:280–287 (1976).

Mitchell, Ross (ed.). *Disease in infancy and childhood* (7th ed.). Baltimore: Williams & Wilkins, 1973.

Redl, Fritz. *When we deal with children*. New York: Free Press, 1966.

Shepherd, M., Oppenheim, B., and Mitchell, S. *Childhood behavior and mental health*. New York: Grune & Stratton, 1971.

Winter, Ruth. Good night, sleep tight . . . please! *Parents' Magazine*, **53**:56 (1978).

Table 128-1 Medical Referral/Consultation

Diagnosis	Clinical Manifestations	Management
Seizure disorder	Usually no precipitating event	Immediate referral to pediatric neurologist
	Tonic-clonic movements	See Blackout Spells/Seizures, Chap. 79.
	Cyanosis usually following episode and loss of consciousness	Support, reassurance, and education of parent(s) and client
	Loss of sphincter control	

129 School Phobia

KAREN A. BALLARD

ALERT
1. Bizarre, panic reactions
2. Isolation and withdrawal
3. Minimal peer interactions

I. Etiology

A. Anxiety about separating from parent(s)
B. Frightening experience at school
C. Fear of traveling
D. Social withdrawal

II. Assessment

A. Subjective data
1. School phobia is
   a. Not a true phobia but a fear of being away from parent(s), especially mother
   b. Most common in passive, immature, dependent children
   c. Acute in younger children; more insidious in older
   d. When present in adolescence, almost always a sign of more severe psychiatric problems
2. School phobia is strongly influenced by
   a. Marital disharmony
   b. Parental doubt that child will be able to stay in school
   c. Child's perception that integrity of home depends upon his or her physical presence
   d. Family has an illness orientation
   e. Reality factors influencing attendance
3. Age at onset
   a. At entry into school—5 to 7 years
   b. Change in school level—10 to 12 years
   c. Late in school experience—14+ years
4. Precipitating events may be
   a. Minor accident
   b. Illness, operation
   c. Change of school, class
   d. Departure, loss of school friend
   e. Death, illness in family
5. Child may complain of
   a. Nausea and vomiting
   b. Shortness of breath
   c. General aches and pains
   d. Generalized anxiety
   e. Acute panic
6. Developmental history may reveal
   a. Stranger anxiety
   b. Separation anxiety
   c. Other fears
7. School information will show
   a. Actual number of days missed
   b. Record of illnesses
   c. Child's actual and performance ability
   d. Indication of whether there are real external hindrances
   e. Evaluation of child's behavior with
      (1) Family
      (2) Peers
      (3) Teachers

B. Objective data
1. Physical examination is normal.
2. Laboratory data is normal and the school report should indicate absences; actual and performance ability; behavior with teachers.
3. Parent-child interactions may show
   a. Acute anxiety in child
   b. Increased anxiety in parent
   c. Overwhelming demands by child or parent
   d. Maternal insecurity

III. Management

A. Treatments/medications

1. All must agree that the child is to return to school.
2. Frequency of counselling is dependent on family's success in achieving short-term and long-term goals.
3. All adolescents should be involved in psychotherapy.

B. Counselling/prevention

1. Reassure child and parent(s) that
   a. Physical complaints are real and not deliberate lies.
   b. Something can be done.
   c. Tears and distress on starting school are neither unusual nor abnormal.
2. Identify the quality of the child's behavior when not under the stress of school attendance (weekends, holidays).
3. Counsel parent(s) that successful attendance at school is indicator of the child's mental health.
   a. Separation/individuation
   b. Challenge of new experiences and learning
   c. New social experiences
   d. Spirit of competitiveness
4. Emphasize positive behavior modification, not negative punishment.
   a. School accomplishments should receive positive parental reaction.
   b. Nonattendance should receive neutral reaction from parent(s).
5. Parent(s) and teacher should form a therapeutic alliance.
   a. Meet frequently
   b. Compare results
   c. Avoid criticism

C. Follow-up

1. Schedule visits weekly for 3 months.
2. Encourage parent(s) to enter family therapy if symptoms exacerbate or are not alleviated within 3 months.
3. The focus should be on supporting more adaptive behaviors in child and parent(s).

D. Consultations/referrals

1. Professional counselling
2. School teacher(s)
3. School nurse

bibliography

Andersen, L. S. When a child begins school. *Children Today,* **5**:16–19 (1975).

Boder, Elena. School failure—Evaluation and treatment. *Pediatrics,* **58**:394–403 (1976).

Carey, W., Fox, M., and McDevitt, S. Temperament as a factor in early school adjustment. *Pediatrics,* **60**:621–624 (1977).

Flaugher, C. School refusal: A therapeutic approach. *Journal of Psychiatric Nursing,* **15**:23–26 (1977).

Friedman, Stanford. *The pediatric clinics of North America—symposium on behavioral pediatrics* (vol. 22, no. 3). Philadelphia: Saunders, 1975.

Harrison, Saul, and McDermott, John. *Childhood psychopathology.* New York: International Universities Press, 1972.

Menkes, John H. On failing in school. *Pediatrics,* **58**:392–393 (1976).

Mitchell, Ross (ed.). *Disease in infancy and childhood* (7th ed.). Baltimore: Williams & Wilkins, 1973.

Rutter, Michael. *Helping troubled children.* New York: Free Press, 1966.

———, and Hersov, Lionel (eds.). *Child psychiatry—Modern approaches.* Oxford: Blackwell Scientific Publications, 1977.

Shaw, Charles. *When your child needs help.* New York: Morrow, 1972.

Wader, P. R., et al. School phobia. *Pediatric Clinics of North America,* **22**:605–617 (1975).

Table 129-1 Medical Referral/Consultation

Diagnosis	Clinical Manifestations	Management
Severe emotional problem, psychosis	Presence of school phobia in adolescence Severe behavior in child, indicating Loss of contact with reality Marked withdrawal Destructive behavior	Professional counselling
Severe, excessive fears	Child's behavior includes other fears Water Dogs/cats Cars/buses Dark Death	Professional counselling See Fears, Chap 127
Truancy—willful avoidance of school	Child shows no evidence of fear. Child admits to deliberate avoidance.	Professional counselling See Truancy, Chap. 132

130 Lying/Stealing/ Cheating

KAREN A. BALLARD

I. Assessment

A. Subjective data

1. Lying, stealing, and cheating are common problems of almost 25 percent of the normal school-age population; they are usually protest reactions to increased emotional stress and indicate unmet needs. Precipitating events may include:
   a. Increase in chores and family responsibilities
   b. Too many activities
   c. Lack of personal time
   d. Poor school performance
2. There are differences in these behaviors depending upon age.
   a. 3 to 7 years—frequent experimentation with lying and stealing
   b. 7 to 12 years—frequent episodes of cheating in school environment
   c. 12+ years—persistent lying, stealing, and cheating perhaps developing into a pervasive delinquent pattern
3. Cheating, most prevalent in the school environment, can be understood as
   a. Learned by child from parental cheating behaviors (e.g., cheating on IRS forms or in business transactions)
   b. A need to break acknowledged "rules" in an attempt to reach desired goal (e.g., cheating on examination for a specific grade)
4. Cheaters who are not caught will often act up in other areas in order to receive punishment as satisfaction for their "guilty" consciences; this allows them to continue cheating.
5. Lying is an intentional misstatement of fact with a specific end goal; in the preschool child, lying can be fantasy translated into storytelling. Reasons for lying are to
   a. Win praise
   b. Gain prestige/recognition
   c. Boost the ego
   d. Gain friends
   e. Escape parental punishment or displeasure
6. Major lying episodes usually represent
   a. Rebellion against morals and parental standards
   b. Repressed hostility
   c. An inadequate identification with acceptable morals and standards of behavior
7. Stealing can have a developmental origin, as in the preschool child who lacks the ability to discriminate between "mine" and "others"; these children usually take
   a. Small toys from friends
   b. Objects from neighborhood stores, frequently while with parent
8. In the older individual, stealing can be understood as
   a. An expression of the need to be loved
   b. A bribe for friendship
   c. An expression of hostility and rebellion against parent(s) and parental morals and standards
   d. A counterphobic behavior in which one flirts with the feared danger
   e. An act performed as a "gang"; a peer group ritual
9. Characteristics of stealing
   a. It may occur inside/outside the home.
   b. Objects stolen may be things denied the child.

c. Objects may have a symbolic significance (e.g., stealing food = parental love; stealing money = parental power).

10. Some stealing can be classified as dissocial when it occurs in a society which tolerates minor thievery as long as one is not caught.
11. Kleptomania is repetitive stealing which gives the individual strong sensual excitement and occurs mainly in late adolescence and adulthood.

B. Objective data

The physical examination should be normal, unless the stress of poor school performance is due to a previously unrecognized visual or hearing defect.

II. Management

A. Treatments/medications: none

B. Counselling/prevention

1. General advice to parent(s)
   a. First offenses and isolated occurrences of lying, stealing, and cheating, if handled wisely and with tact, will usually subside.
   b. Examine the offense, the environment in which it occurred, and the individual(s) involved before intervening.
2. Lying behaviors
   a. Counsel parent(s) to evaluate the aim of the lie and its meaning to the child.
   b. Parent(s) should communicate displeasure to the child by brief scolding and simply stating the social and moral unacceptability of the behavior.
3. Stealing and cheating behaviors
   a. Parent(s) should explain objects which belong to others may not be taken.
   b. Parent(s) should state the social and moral unacceptability of the behaviors.
4. If cheating, lying, and stealing continue, parent(s) can employ other appropriate disciplinary actions (see Discipline, Chap. 117).

C. Follow-up

1. Follow-up depends on the severity of the behavior.
2. The focus should be on counselling and supporting the family and encouraging verbalization of feelings.

D. Consultations/referrals

1. Professional counselling
2. Teacher and school nurse

---

bibliography

Barnett, Henry (ed.). *Pediatrics* (16th ed.). New York: Appleton-Century-Crofts, 1977.

Brown, Marie Scott, and Murphy, Mary Alexander. *Ambulatory pediatrics for nurses.* New York: McGraw-Hill, 1975.

Elkind, David. *A sympathetic understanding of the child—birth to sixteen.* Boston: Allyn and Bacon, 1974.

Harrison, Saul, and McDermott, John. *Childhood psychopathology.* New York: International Universities Press, 1972.

Illingworth, Ronald. *The normal child* (6th ed.). New York: Churchill Livingstone, 1975.

Lewis, Melvin. *Clinical aspects of child development.* Philadelphia: Lea & Febiger, 1971.

Metz, J. R., Allen, C. M., and Shinefield, G. B. H. A pediatric screening examination for psychosocial problems. *Pediatrics,* **58**:595–606 (1976).

Mitchell, Ross (ed.) *Disease in infancy and childhood* (7th ed.). Baltimore: Williams & Wilkins, 1973.

Stumphauzer, Jerome. Elimination of stealing by self-reinforcement of alternative behavior and family contracting. *Journal of Behavior Therapy and Experimental Psychiatry,* **6**:265–268 (1976).

131 Juvenile Delinquency

KAREN A. BALLARD

I. Etiology

A. The line between delinquent and nondelinquent behavior is very fine.

B. Causes are always multifaceted.

1. Serious family problems
2. Lack of parental love or concern
3. Chronic insecurity
4. Presence of cruelty in home
5. Financial insecurity
6. Peer pressure
7. Environmental stress

II. Assessment

A. Subjective data

1. Youthful antisocial behavior which violated the law
2. More prevalent in boys than girls and in individuals of normal intelligence
3. Precipitating events
   a. New situations
   b. Parental discipline
   c. New peer group
   d. Formation of a gang
4. The delinquent expresses feelings of
   a. Rejection
   b. Inadequacy
   c. Guilt
   d. Jealousy
5. Separate interviews may indicate troubled areas in the parent-child relationship.
   a. Discipline
   b. Unrealistic expectations
   c. Unmet needs
   d. Poor communication
6. An interview with the teacher can
   a. Identify school behaviors
   b. Illuminate peer relationships
   c. Indicate performance level
   d. Identify academic potential
7. Delinquent behavior may be identified as
   a. Neurotic—recent, uncharacteristic misbehavior which represents an attempt to communicate unmet needs
   b. Sociological or social—occurring in subcultures whose members share antisocial standards of conduct and sanction illegal activities by individuals who are usually well-adjusted members of their peer groups
   c. Characterological—marked by aggressive and impulsive behavior coupled with a lack of attachment to or consideration of others and reflecting a serious personality disorder

B. Objective data

Physical examination is normal.

III. Management

A. Treatments/medications: Parent(s) and child will need to be involved in psychotherapy and/or counselling.

1. The neurotic type responds to short-term counselling which focuses on the unrecognized needs and supports alternative behaviors.
2. The characterological type requires extensive, in-depth psychotherapy and, sometimes, residential treatment.
3. The sociological or social type responds to involvement in social action programs.
   a. Job corps
   b. Youth action groups

B. Counselling/prevention

1. The practitioner must recognize that man-

agement will require intensive, multifaceted input.

a. Any combination of individual, family, and group psychotherapy
b. Vocational guidance and job training
c. Social action programs
d. Behavior modification

2. Counsel parent(s) to avoid harsh and punitive responses.
   a. See Discipline, Chap. 117.
   b. Firm limit setting should be identified and encouraged.

C. Follow-up

1. Weekly visits utilizing appropriate modalities
2. Focus on behavior modification and satisfaction of needs

D. Consultations/referrals

1. Professional counselling
2. Teacher(s) and school nurse
3. Vocational counsellor

bibliography

Andrew, J. M. Delinquency, sex and family variables. *Social Biology,* **23**:168–171 (1976).

Austrin, H. R., et al. Interpersonal trust and severity of delinquent behavior. *Psychological Reports,* **40**:1075 (1977).

Fagin, Claire (ed.). *Readings in child and adolescent psychiatric nursing.* St. Louis: Mosby, 1974.

Friedman, Standford (ed.). *The pediatric clinics of North America—Symposium on behavioral pediatrics* (vol. 22, no. 3). Philadelphia: Saunders, 1975.

Joint Commission on Mental Health of Children (Task Forces I, II, and III and the Committees on Education and Religion). *Mental health: From infancy through adolescence.* New York: Harper & Row, 1973.

Weiner, I. B. Symposium on behavioral pediatrics: Juvenile delinquency. *Pediatric Clinics of North America,* **22**:673–684 (1975).

132 Truancy

MARILYN GREBIN

I. Etiology

A. Dislike of school
1. Low intelligence—underachiever
2. Superior intelligence—boredom
3. Language deficiency

B. Fear of punishment
1. Parent(s)
2. School

C. Parental attitudes
1. Parental dislike of school system
2. Keeping the child truant for personal reasons
3. Praise of one sibling over another

D. Psychological conflicts
1. Home and family
2. Fantasy world
3. Peer group rejection

E. Physical illness

II. Assessment

A. Parental reasons
1. Parental dislike of school system
2. Keeping child truant for selfish reasons
3. Performance expectations greater than the child can achieve
4. Parent(s) not assisting the child with schoolwork
5. Chronic fighting, separation, or divorce situation within the home

B. Child's reasons
1. Inconsistency within the home
   a. Parental disputes
   b. Illnesses
2. Poor rapport with the teacher
3. Physically the child perhaps not fitting in with peers (obesity, uncoordination)
4. Vision or hearing difficulty in the classroom
5. Decreased comprehension of the classwork

III. Management

A. Treatments/medications: none

B. Counselling/prevention
1. Child
   a. Spend one or two visits with the child to establish rapport.
   b. Most children will identify the reason for the behavior.
   c. Allow the child to express any fears or concerns about the environment at home and school.
   d. Assist the child in making decisions about particular problems.
   e. Have the child keep a diary of experiences that were uncomfortable, including how difficulties were resolved.
2. Parent(s)
   a. Have the parent(s) spend more time with the child (working on homework and activities).
   b. Advise the parent(s) about communicating with the teacher.
   c. Parent(s) and teacher(s) should encourage the child's efforts to achieve.
   d. Parent(s) and teacher(s) should be less punitive.
   e. Encourage peer relationships.

C. Follow-up
1. Schedule weekly or biweekly visits.
2. Communicate frequently with parent(s) and teacher to assure continuity in dealing with the child's problems.

D. Consultations/referrals

1. If a child is exhibiting aggressive behavior and communication is hampered
   a. Professional counselling
   b. Neurologist
   c. Audiologist
2. Psychologist for psychometric testing
3. School guidance counsellor

bibliography

Tyrrell, Rosalie. Psychological crisis of childhood and adolescence. *Issues in Comprehensive Pediatric Nursing,* **1**(6):18–29 (1977).

section 12

nonspecific complaints and problems

133 Paleness/Pallor

JENNIFER L. PIERSMA

Paleness or pallor is a common symptom of illness in the child or young adult. It is most frequently associated with the hematological system. It is anticipated that pallor, when accompanied by other more specific signs/symptoms, may direct the primary health care provider to the involved body system.

ALERT

1. Newborn
2. Altered level of consciousness
3. Signs/symptoms of circulatory disturbance
4. Signs/symptoms of respiratory distress
5. Signs/symptoms of blood loss
6. History of blood dyscrasia
7. Iron deficiency anemia unresponsive to iron therapy after 2 to 4 weeks

I. Etiology

A. Skin tone
B. Infection
C. Blood loss

II. Subjective Data

A. Age
B. Onset
C. Associated symptoms
D. Recent illnesses
E. Recent hospitalizations (blood transfusions)
F. Accidents
G. Medications
H. Allergies
I. Birth history
J. Medical/family history: bleeding disorders, sickle cell, malignancy, alcoholism; Mediterranean ancestry, black ancestry
K. Environmental history: lead, dirt, paint eating (pica)
L. Developmental history: delays in milestones—language, psychosocial, fine motor, gross motor
M. Nutritional history
N. Complete review of systems (client)

III. Objective Data

A. Physical examination

1. Complete physical examination
2. Skin and lymph: petechiae, ecchymoses, extent of pallor; nailbeds, enlarged lymph nodes
3. Mouth: color and moistness of oral mucosa, tongue
4. Eyes: sclera, conjunctivae
5. Cardiorespiratory: blood pressure, pulse(s), respiration; murmurs, cyanosis
6. Abdomen: bowel sounds, tenderness, distention, masses; enlarged liver and/or spleen
7. Rectal: masses, stool for occult blood
8. Extremities: palmar creases for pallor
9. Neurological: state of consciousness, total response of the child

B. Laboratory data

1. Hematocrit
2. Hemoglobin
3. Smear of peripheral blood
4. Reticulocyte, if indicated
5. Urinalysis
6. Stool for occult blood

IV. Assessment

A. Pale complexion

1. Subjective data
   a. Familial and/or genetic characteristic
   b. Indoors a great deal
2. Objective data
   a. Normal physical examination
   b. Normal hemoglobin/hematocrit
   c. Other laboratory screening tests within normal limits

B. Simple fatigue

1. Subjective data
   a. Overwork and/or overactivity; life crisis
   b. Deviation from normal sleep patterns: illness, hospitalization, fears, night terrors (dreams)
2. Objective data
   a. Normal physical examination
   b. Normal hemoglobin/hematocrit
   c. Other laboratory screening tests within normal limits

C. Infection

1. Subjective data
   a. Associated symptoms
      (1) Fever
      (2) Irritability
      (3) Others, dependent on involved body system
   b. Recent illness in family/client
2. Objective data
   a. Increased or decreased white blood cell count (serum)
   b. Positive cultures(s) related to specific body system
   c. Other abnormal screening tests

D. Iron deficiency anemia

1. Subjective data
   a. Age: 6 months to 2 years (most common)
   b. No overt clinical signs and symptoms if mild anemia
   c. Poor dietary intake of iron
   d. Associated symptoms may include
      (1) Fatigue
      (2) Irritability
      (3) Anorexia
      (4) Fat and flabbiness
      (5) Feeding problems (secondary to anorexia and irritability)
      (6) Delayed motor development
      (7) Beeturia
2. Objective data
   a. General appearance: irritability, fat and flabbiness, delayed development
   b. Pallor
   c. Tachycardia
   d. Splenomegaly
   e. Extremities: pallor, poor muscle tone; good weight gain
   f. Delayed motor development for age may be observed
   g. Lowered hemoglobin for age
   h. Decreased hematocrit
   i. Decreased hemoglobin to hematocrit ratio (1:3)
   j. Characteristics of red blood cells: microcytic, hypochromic (may also be poikilocytic and anisocytic)
   k. Decreased number of red blood cells (serum), decreased mean corpuscular volume (MCV)
   l. Decreased mean corpuscular hemoglobin concentration (MCHC)
   m. Reticulocyte count perhaps elevated early in illness or low in moderate to severe anemia
   n. Decreased serum iron, increased iron-binding capacity (if done) later in the illness

V. Management

A. Pale complexion

1. Treatments/medications: none
2. Counselling/prevention
   a. Reassure parent(s) and client that this paleness is within the range of normal.
   b. Explain the role of melanin in producing differences in skin tones(s).
   c. Discuss paleness in relation to body image.
   e. Increase time spent outdoors (if desired).
3. Follow-up: none
4. Consultations/referrals: none

B. Simple fatigue

1. Treatments/medications: none
2. Counselling/prevention
   a. Reassure parent(s)/client that this state is not pathologic.
   b. Discuss rest/sleep principles.
   c. Discuss measures to promote relaxation.
   d. Discuss measures to lessen pain, anxiety, fear, and/or stress.
3. Follow-up
   a. Return visit if fatigue becomes a chronic problem
   b. Return visit if other signs/symptoms occur
4. Consultations/referrals: none indicated unless simple fatigue becomes a chronic problem due to psychosocial stressors or physiological imbalance

C. Infection
1. Treatments/medications: as indicated for identified organism and involved body system
2. Counselling/prevention: as indicated by involved system, disease agent, antibiotics, and other medications prescribed
3. Follow-up: as indicated by culture(s) and/or resolution of signs/symptoms
4. Consultations/referrals: as indicated

D. Iron deficiency anemia
1. Treatments/medications
   a. Oral iron: 1.5 to 2 mg/kg elemental iron (ferrous sulfate) 3 times daily
   b. Diet: Increase in intake of iron-rich foods; decrease in milk intake, if indicated
2. Counselling/prevention
   a. Iron-fortified formula during the first year of life
   b. Discussion of the importance of a well-balanced diet with adequate iron
   c. Parental education regarding medication
      (1) Importance of giving prescribed amounts at the times indicated
      (2) How to give medications based on the developmental age of the client
      (3) Oral iron given with ascorbic acid (vitamin C)
      (4) Avoidance of giving with meals due to unpleasant taste and decreased absorption
      (5) Medication kept in original container, out of reach of children
      (6) See Oral Medications, Appendix 2
   d. Oral iron preparations sometimes staining teeth; encouragement of brushing of teeth
   e. Instruction that oral iron may turn stools black
3. Follow-up
   a. Return visit in 7 to 14 days
   b. Check of reticulocyte, hemoglobin, or hematocrit
   c. Seen monthly until anemia has cleared
   d. Review Counselling/prevention, V, D, 2 above
4. Consultations/referrals
   a. Refer to physician if anemia unresponsive to therapy after 2 to 4 weeks.
   b. Notify the community health nurse for a home visit if the client or family is noncompliant.

Table 133-1 Medical Referral/Consultation

Diagnosis	Clinical Manifestations	Management
Leukemia	Petechiae Ecchymoses Bone pain Lymph nodes enlarged Hepatosplenomegaly Blasts predominating on peripheral blood smear Thrombocytopenia	Immediate referral to physician/hematology specialist Diagnostic workup: see Preparation for Hospitalization, Part 7, and Neoplastic Disease, Chap. 148 Counselling Explanation of diagnosis, treatment plan, prognosis to family (to client if agreed upon) Requires close supervision Ongoing family counselling, professional consultation if indicated Follow-up: intense
Hypothyroidism	Large tongue Hoarse cry (voice) Hypothermia Pale, cool, or mottled skin Poor muscle tone Bradycardia Delayed intellectual development Delayed closure of fontanels	Referral to physician Treatments/medications Thyroid function tests Levothyroxine or desiccated thyroid per physician plan Counselling Explanation of diagnosis, treatment plan, prognosis to family Requires close supervision

Table 133-1 Medical Referral/Consultation *(continued)*

Diagnosis	Clinical Manifestations	Management
Addison's disease	Weakness Episodes of nausea, vomiting, diarrhea Increased desire for salt Hypotension Dehydration Increased areas of pigmentation	Referral to physician Treatments/medications may include hydrocortisone, cortisone, increased salt intake, or supplemental desoxycorticosterone Counselling Explain diagnosis, treatment plan, prognosis to the family. Teach signs/symptoms. Salt retention Overdose Dehydration Readjust medications during stressful periods.
Shock	Agitation Confusion Decrease in responsiveness Pale, cold, or mottled skin Nailbeds cyanotic Poor capillary refill Tachycardia Tachypnea In a newborn: lethargic, pale, slightly gray, with decreased skin temperature	Immediately refer to a physician. Lie flat, and elevate the legs if there is no respiratory distress. Ensure that airway is clear, and client is getting adequate oxygen. Maintain circulation.

bibliography

Barness, Lewis A. *Manual of pediatric physical diagnosis* (4th ed.). Chicago: Year Book, 1973.

DeAngelis, Catharine. *Pediatric Primary Care* (2d ed.) Boston: Little, Brown, 1979.

Illingsworth, R. S. *Common symptoms of disease in children* (5th ed). Oxford: Blackwell Scientific Publications, 1975.

Kempe, C. H., Silver, H. K., and O'Brien, D. *Current pediatric diagnosis and treatment* (5th ed.). Los Altos, Calif.: Lange, 1978.

Rudolph, Abraham M. (ed.). *Pediatrics* (16th ed.). New York: Appleton-Century-Crofts, 1977.

Wasson, J., Walsh, T., Thompkins, R., and Sox, H. *The common symptom guide*. New York: McGraw-Hill, 1975.

134 Failure to Thrive

LESLIE LIETH

"Failure to thrive, besides being the inability to maintain adequate weight gain in relation to birth weight, can be defined as a growth failure syndrome in infancy and early childhood lacking clear evidence of primary systemic disease" (Barbero and Shaheen, 1967). Table 134–1 will alert the practitioner to some of the organic causes that should have been ruled out when failure to thrive syndrome is diagnosed.

I. Etiology: Unknown

II. Subjective Data: Complete, Detailed History

III. Objective Data

A. Complete physical examination

1. Accurate plotting of measurements—including height, weight, and head circumference
2. Observation of parent-child interaction closely during visit, with more than one observer if possible

B. Laboratory

1. Usually indicated
   a. Complete blood count
   b. Urinalysis with microscopic examination, and culture
   c. Chest x-ray; wrist x-ray for bone age
   d. Stool examination for fat particles, pH
   e. Thyroid function studies
2. Sometimes indicated
   a. Electrolytes, blood urea nitrogen (BUN), calcium, phosphorus, creatinine
   b. Sweat chloride test
   c. Electrocardiogram
   d. Liver enzymes
   e. Venous lead level

IV. Assessment

A. Subjective data

1. Usually normal birth weight
2. Poor appetite or refusal to take food
3. Chronic vomiting
4. Chronic diarrhea or constipation
5. Sickly child (according to parent(s))
6. Irritability or excessive crying
7. Listlessness or lethargy
8. Sleep disturbances
9. Breath-holding episodes
10. Caloric intake usually inadequate
11. Parental history may reveal
    a. Poor historian
    b. Lack of support from or absence of spouse, family, friends
    c. Emotional disturbance or maladaption—such as drug abuse, mental retardation, alcoholism, immaturity, psychiatric illness
    d. Marital discord
    e. Physical illness
    f. Many pregnancies and children at short intervals
    g. Unwanted pregnancy
    h. Difficult delivery in which complications seemed to threaten life of mother or baby
    i. Family illness
    j. Financial insecurity

B. Objective data

1. Avoids eye contact, stares into space, disinterested
2. Unable to respond normally to love and attention
3. Makes few sounds
4. Appears not well cared for physically
5. Can appear malnourished
6. Signs of dehydration

7. Muscle wasting
8. Anemia
9. Developmental milestones perhaps delayed
10. Height and weight below 3rd percentile
11. Parental height normal
12. Bone age x-rays normal
13. Infant held stiffly away from parent

V. Management

A. Treatments/medications

1. If workup to rule out organic disease not complete, must be done, see Laboratory, III, B above.
2. Removal of child from current environment sometimes necessary—hospitalization if suffering from acute illness or not responding to outpatient therapy
3. Actively involving parent(s) in therapy and setting mutually agreed upon goals
4. Diet appropriate for age
5. Infant/child stimulation program
   a. See Well-Child Care, Chap. 9 for stimulation appropriate for age.
   b. Encourage play at mealtimes.
   c. The child should not be left in the crib for long periods—change the child's position frequently.
   d. Vocalize with the child.
   e. Encourage eye and physical contact.

B. Counselling/prevention

1. Identify those women at risk during pregnancy.
2. Offer more prenatal parenting classes in preparation for parenthood.
3. Rooming-in and parent-care pavillions in hospitals can be expanded.
4. Explain failure to thrive syndrome to parent(s) once organic disease is ruled out, anticipating such parental reactions as feelings of inadequacy, extreme frustration, guilt, anxiety, and anger.
5. Support, not criticism, is essential.
6. Explain the baby's needs to the parent(s), reinforcing positive aspects of parental behavior.
7. Encourage the parent to take an afternoon off each week and get out of the house alone.
8. Encourage participation by other family members in the baby's care and stimulation.

C. Follow-up

1. Schedule visits every 2 to 4 weeks.
2. Get a detailed history at each visit of activity, nutritional assessment, psychosocial changes.
3. Closely monitor growth and development.

D. Consultations/referrals

1. Coordination of health team members is essential in multidisciplinary approach to treatment.
2. Consult with the pediatrician.
3. Refer to a nutritionist for counselling.
4. Refer to the visiting nurse service.
5. The family may need homemaker services.
6. Refer to a part-time day-care center.
7. Refer to community mothers' groups.
8. Refer to a social worker for assessment and help with pressing social problems.
9. Refer to or consult with a psychologist regarding an infant stimulation program.
10. Refer to a local community infant stimulation program, if one exists.
11. Refer parent(s) to a professional counsellor for individual or family therapy when indicated.

Table 134-1 Medical Referral/Consultation

Diagnosis	Clinical Manifestations	Management
Renal disease	Chronic urinary tract infection Any urinary tract symptom, i.e., dysuria, polyuria, frequency Family history of renal disease Adequate appetite and food intake Abnormal urinalysis and can have positive urine culture Growth below normal for age Altered electrolytes Hypertension	Refer to the physician.

Table 134-1 Medical Referral/Consultation *(continued)*

Diagnosis	Clinical Manifestations	Management
Cardiac disease	Tires easily Poor feeder Fatigue or distress seen when observing child feeding Color cyanotic or pale on exertion Murmur Hypertension Growth below normal Hemoglobin sometimes higher than normal	Refer to the physician.
Gastrointestinal disease	Chronic or acute vomiting Alterations in stools Poor feeder or can have good appetite Growth below normal Jaundice Hepatomegaly Abnormal liver enzymes Explosive stools	Refer to the physician.
Endocrine disorders	Poor feeder Subnormal temperature Recent loss of weight Delayed height or weight or both Developmental delay Hyper or hypotonia Low thyroid function studies Truncal obesity with delayed height X-ray of long bones revealing delay in osseous development Abnormal facies	Refer to the physician.
Chronic lead intoxication	Decreased appetite Apathy Irritability Vomiting Constipation Delayed growth Slowdown of development Presence of lead in environment Pica Hyperactivity Abdominal pain and tenderness, masses Clumsiness Convulsions Anemia High blood-lead level	Refer to the physician. See Lead Poisoning, Chap. 155.

Table 134-1 Medical Referral/Consultation *(continued)*

Diagnosis	Clinical Manifestations	Management
	Ataxia	
	Lead line on gum margins	
	Pale color	
	Hepatosplenomegaly	
CNS disorders	Poor feeding history	Refer to the physician.
	Delayed growth	
	Delayed development	
	Prenatal history of toxemia, bleeding, infection, placental insufficiency	
	Natal history of prolonged labor, meconium staining, other evidence of fetal distress or complications	
	Neonatal history of cyanosis, jaundice, infection, seizures	
	Abnormal neurological examination	

bibliography

Barbero, A., and Shaheen, E. Environmental failure to thrive: a clinical view. *Journal of Pediatrics,* **71**:639–644(1967).

Bowlby, John. *Attachment and loss* (Vol. 1). New York: Basic Books, 1969.

Corcoran, Marya McClay. Nursing role and management of failure-to-thrive clients. *Issues in Comprehensive Pediatric Nursing,* **3**:29–40 (October 1978).

Graef, John, and Cone, Thomas E. *Manual of pediatric therapeutics.* Boston: Little, Brown, 1974.

Green, Morris, and Haggerty, Robert J. *Ambulatory pediatrics II.* Philadelphia: Saunders, 1977.

Roper, Karen E., et al. Failure to thrive: An opportunity for innovative nursing. *Pediatric Nursing,* **2**:43–45 (1976).

Rubin, Reva. Basic maternal behavior. *Nursing Outlook,* **9**:683+ (1961).

Smith, C. A., and Berenberg, W. The concept of failure to thrive, *Pediatrics,* November:661–663 (1970).

Suran, Bernard, and Hatcher, Roger P. The psychological treatment of hospitalized children with failure-to-thrive. *Pediatric Nursing,* **1**:10–17 (1975).

135 Itching[1]

MARY ALEXANDER MURPHY

Generalized Itching

ALERT
1. No improvement within 24 h
2. Any suspected systemic disease

I. Etiology
- **A.** Environmental factors
  1. Bathing with strong alkaline soaps
  2. Winter weather
  3. Low humidity
- **B.** Disease conditions
  1. Diabetes mellitus
  2. Drug reactions
  3. Lymphomas
  4. Renal failure
  5. Liver malfunctions

II. Subjective data
- **A.** Age
- **B.** Onset
- **C.** Description of problem
- **D.** Associated symptoms
  1. Bites
  2. Pain
  3. Rash
  4. Weight loss
  5. Bloody urine
  6. Overeating
  7. Excessive drinking
  8. Fever
  9. Vaginal discharge
  10. Rectal itch
- **E.** Diet history
  1. Foods which effect itch
  2. New foods in diet
- **F.** Elimination pattern
  1. Any changes from normal pattern
  2. Cleansing technique, i.e., toilet paper
  3. Exposure to pinworms
- **G.** Sleeping habits: itching disturbs sleep
- **H.** Clothing
  1. Exposure to new clothing
  2. Type of clothing worn
     - a. Tight or loose fitting
     - b. Woolen
  3. Type of detergents and other products added to wash
- **I.** Bathing
  1. Frequency
  2. Type of soap used
  3. Use of bubble bath
- **J.** Exposures
  1. Insects
  2. Plants
  3. Animals
- **K.** Present/past history of
  1. Diabetes
  2. Cancer
  3. Renal failure
  4. Hepatic malfunctions
- **L.** Current medications, i.e., antibiotic therapy
- **M.** History of itching
  1. Frequency
  2. Sequence of lesions
  3. Previous treatments and results
- **N.** Allergies
- **O.** Family history for chronic problems, genetic diseases, allergies, and skin disorders
- **P.** Social history

[1]Itching (pruritis) is frequently broken into two large categories: *generalized* and *localized.*

III. Objective Data

A. Physical examination (complete)

1. Careful inspection and palpation of skin
   a. Total number and location of lesions
   b. Primary and secondary lesions
      (1) Redness, dryness, roughness—diffuse or definite
      (2) Linear scratch marks
      (3) Excoriations, thickening of skin, scarring, oozing
2. Fingernails worn from scratching
3. Palpation of lymph nodes for enlargement

B. Laboratory data

1. Culture any drainage
2. Microscopic inspection—insect bite, scaling

IV. Assessment

A. Environmental factors

1. Subjective data
   a. Itch generally over total body
   b. Itch several specific areas
   c. Itch disrupting daily life or sleep, or only at specific times
2. Objective data
   a. Normal skin
   b. Dry, rough skin
   c. Red, excoriated patches
   d. Scratch marks

B. Drug reactions

1. Subjective data
   a. Sudden onset
   b. Severe itching
   c. Drug ingestion
2. Objective data
   a. Lesions may be tiny, erythematous, macular, papular, vesicular, or wheallike.
   b. They may be symmetrically distributed.
   c. Lesions cover large body areas.

V. Management

A. Environmentally caused itching

1. Treatments/medications
   a. Aspirin or acetaminophen—dose appropriate for age
   b. Antihistamines
   c. Corticosteroids—oral and local
   d. Tranquilizers and sedatives
   e. Bathing
      (1) Avoid excessive bathing; 1 to 2 times per week is suggested.
      (2) Use bland, mild soap, such as Ivory.
      (3) Add oils to the bath water, such as Alpha-Keri, Lubath.
      (4) Pat (rather than rub) dry after the bath.
      (5) Promptly apply soothing emollient lotion.
   f. Avoidance of hot, overheated rooms
   g. Avoidance of scratchy woolen clothing
   h. Sleeping between cotton sheets, not under woolen blankets
2. Counselling/prevention
   a. Instructions on bathing
   b. Proper clothing and sleeping covers
   c. Proper drug usage
3. Follow-up
   a. Telephone call after 48 h to report progress
   b. If no improvement—return visit within 1 week
4. Consultations/referrals
   a. Consultations on medications
   b. Referrals to pediatrician or dermatologist if itching not improved within week

B. Disease condition causing itching (Table 135–1)

Table 135-1 Medical Referral/Consultation

Diagnosis	Clinical Manifestations	Management
Diabetes mellitus	Polyuria Polydipsia Leg and abdominal cramping Enuresis Emotional upset Lethargy Weight loss Mild itching	Immediate referral to pediatrician Insulin Diet Urine testing Follow-up—need for team approach
Lymphomas	Depressed appetite Lethargy	Immediate referral to pediatrician

Table 135-1 Medical Referral/Consultation *(continued)*

Diagnosis	Clinical Manifestations	Management
	Weight loss Fever Muscular weakness Enlarged lymph nodes Mild itching	See Neoplastic Disease, Chap. 148 Follow-up—need for team approach
Renal failure	Nausea Vomiting Inactivity Sleepiness Paleness Muscular twitching Mild itching	Immediate referral to pediatrician See Preparation for Hospitalization, Part 7 Follow-up—need for team approach
Liver malfunctions	Excessive fatigue Anorexia Enlarged abdomen Enlarged liver Weight loss Paleness Possible jaundice Mild to moderate itching	Immediate referral to pediatrician See Preparation for Hospitalization, Part 7 Follow-up—need for team approach.

Localized Itching

I. Etiology

A. Circumscribed neurodermatitis
1. Habit—cycle of itch, scratch, itch, scratch, etc.
2. Bites
   a. Scabies
   b. Bedbugs
   c. Mosquitoes
3. Nervousness and tiredness

B. Scalp and neck
1. Seborrheic dermatitis
2. Contact dermatitis

C. Extremities
1. Seborrheic dermatitis
2. Contact dermatitis
3. Atopic dermatitis
4. Hives

D. Anal region
1. Atopic dermatitis
2. Contact dermatitis (chemical contacts)
3. Moisture
4. Tight clothing—panties, diapers, rubber pants
5. Harsh, alkaline soaps
6. Home remedies
7. Pinworms
8. Oral antibiotics
9. Friction and rubbing
10. Psoriasis

E. Vulva
1. *Monilia*
2. *Trichomonas*
3. Diabetes
4. Antibiotic treatment
5. Harsh chemicals—bubble bath, douches
6. Contraceptive jellies or creams

F. Scrotum
1. Tinea infection
2. Tight clothing
3. Harsh soaps
4. Contact chemicals

II. Subjective Data: See generalized itching, II, above

III. Objective Data: See generalized Itching, II, above

IV. Assessment

A. Circumscribed neurodermatitis
1. Subjective data
   a. Nervousness, agitation
   b. Irritability
2. Objective data
   a. Bites
      (1) Scabies
      (2) Lice
      (3) Bedbugs
      (4) Fleas
   b. Primary lesions—small, localized, and like a bite
   c. Secondary lesions—excoriated, skin thickening, scarring
   d. Common locations
      (1) Posterior hairline
      (2) Wrists
      (3) Ankles
      (4) Ears
      (5) Anal region

B. Scalp and neck
1. Seborrheic dermatitis
   a. Subjective data
      (1) Upset mother
      (2) Calm infant—mild scratching
   b. Objective data
      (1) Oily scalp and skin
      (2) Scaliness
      (3) Greasy flakes
      (4) Reddened areas—especially on forehead and cheeks
      (5) Some crusting
2. Contact dermatitis
   a. Subjective data
      (1) Severe itching
      (2) Upset child
   b. Objective data
      (1) Erythema—well circumscribed
      (2) Oozing
      (3) Vesicles
      (4) Edema
      (5) Common locations
         (a) Posterior neck
         (b) Legs
         (c) Face
         (d) Genitalia
         (e) Posterior hands
         (f) Scalp

C. Extremities
1. Seborrheic dermatitis—as above
2. Contact dermatitis—as above
3. Atopic dermatitis
   a. Subjective data
      (1) Mild to severe itching
      (2) May disrupt daily activities
   b. Objective data
      (1) Dry skin
      (2) Erythema
      (3) Papules
      (4) Excoriations and scratch marks
      (5) Oozing and crusting
      (6) Common locations
         (a) Infants
            1. Scalp
            2. Face
         (b) Toddlers and older
            1. Face
            2. Neck
            3. Ears (especially behind)
            4. Hands and wrists
            5. Antecubital areas of arms
            6. Popliteal leg sections
4. Hives (urticaria)
   a. Subjective data
      (1) Sudden, severe itching
      (2) Itching perhaps appearing before wheal
   b. Objective data
      (1) Reddened, macular areas
      (2) Wheals
      (3) Vesicles and/or bullae perhaps following

D. Anal region
1. Atopic dermatitis—as above
2. Contact dermatitis—as above
3. Moisture
   a. Subjective data
      (1) Child may not complain of discomfort.
      (2) Child may show irritation only at specific times of day.
   b. Objective data
      (1) Damp skin
      (2) Erythematous area
      (3) May have macular, papular, or vesicular lesions

4. Tight clothing
   a. Subjective data
      (1) Child may not be complaining.
      (2) Mother may be upset.
   b. Objective data
      (1) Marks left from tight elastic
      (2) Type of clothing—rubber soakers, nylon panties, nylon crotch reinforcements
      (3) Erythematous area
5. Harsh, alkaline soaps
   a. Subjective data
      (1) Child may not be complaining.
      (2) Itch may be after bathing.
   b. Objective data
      (1) Erythema
      (2) Scratch marks
6. Home remedies
   a. Subjective data
      (1) Mother treating child with household remedy.
      (2) Itching began with treatment or soon after.
   b. Objective data
      (1) Erythema of area where remedy was applied
      (2) Scratch marks
7. Pinworms
   a. Subjective data
      (1) Presence of worms in bed clothing in morning
      (2) Siblings with pinworms
      (3) Mild to severe anal itching at night
   b. Objective data
      (1) Erythema
      (2) Scratch marks
      (3) Signs of vaginitis—some girls may develop vaginitis with pinworms
8. Oral antibiotics
   a. Subjective data
      (1) History of recent antibiotic ingestion
      (2) Recent illness
   b. Objective data
      (1) Highly variable
      (2) Macular, papular rash
      (3) Vesicles or wheals sometimes developing
      (4) Large, symmetrical distribution
      (5) Vaginal *Monilia* infection—in girls
9. Friction and rubbing
   a. Subjective data
      (1) Mild itching
      (2) Certain clothing or bathing may aggravate
   b. Objective data
      (1) Restricted erythematous area
      (2) Scratch marks
10. Psoriasis
   a. Subjective data
      (1) Upset mother
      (2) Child calm—mild itching
   b. Objective data
      (1) Early droplike, isolated lesions
      (2) Bright-red patches
      (3) Silvery, dried, scaly patches, which can be removed
      (4) Common locations
         (a) Scalp
         (b) Elbows
         (c) Knees
         (d) Base of spine
         (e) Feet
         (f) Nails

E. Vulva

1. *Monilia*
   a. Subjective data
      (1) Mild itching
      (2) Voiding sometimes causing burning or increased itching
   b. Objective data
      (1) Early lesions—isolated, tiny, red areas
      (2) Definite borders
      (3) Oozing
      (4) Thick, cheesy vaginal discharge
2. *Trichomonas*
   a. Subjective data
      (1) Rare before puberty
      (2) Mild to severe itching
   b. Objective data
      (1) Redness
      (2) Edema
      (3) Pale, white, frothy discharge
3. Diabetes—as above
4. Antibiotic treatment—as above
5. Harsh chemicals
   a. Subjective data
      (1) Exposure to chemicals
      (2) Mild to severe itching
   b. Objective data
      (1) Variable
      (2) Erythema
      (3) Macular, papular lesions to vesicular, bullae-type lesions
6. Contraceptive jellies or creams
   a. Subjective data
      (1) Exposure to jellies or creams
      (2) Mild to severe itching
   b. Objective data

(1) Variable
(2) Erythema
(3) Macular, papular lesions to vesicular, bullae-type lesions

F. Scrotum

1. Tinea infection
   a. Subjective data
      (1) Exposure
      (2) Severe itching
   b. Objective data
      (1) Symmetrical, rounded lesions
      (2) Margins containing scaly, erythematous areas, with some vesicles
      (3) Lesion sometimes showing clearing in center
2. Tight clothing—as above
3. Harsh soaps—as above
4. Contact chemicals—as above

V. Management

A. Circumscribed neurodermatitis

1. Treatments/medications
   a. Aspirin or acetaminophen
   b. Antihistamines
   c. Sedation—chloral hydrate
   d. Corticosteroid creams
   e. Application of bland, mild lotions
      (1) Calamine
      (2) Use of soap substitutes
   g. Avoidance of harsh toilet tissue
   h. Application of cold, wet dressings for 30 min 3 times per day; choice of following
      (1) Plain tap water
      (2) Saline (2 tsp salt to 1 qt water)
      (3) Boric acid solution (1 Tbsp to 1 qt water)
      (4) Diluted milk
      (5) Starch (1 box to a tub of cool to lukewarm water)
      (6) Oatmeal (1 cup to a tub of water)
2. Counselling/prevention
   a. Explanation of condition to parent and child and need to avoid all scratching
   b. Instructions on soaks
   c. Instructions on nail care—short, clean, smooth
   d. Instructions on daily hygiene
   e. Instructions on medications
3. Follow-up
   a. Telephone call after 48 h for progress
   b. If no improvement, reappointment
4. Consultations/referrals
   a. Consultation on medications
   b. Referrals to pediatrician or dermatologist if itching not improved within week

B. Scalp and neck

1. Seborrheic dermatitis
   a. Treatments/medications
      (1) Medication for mild seborrheic dermatitis: nothing
      (2) Medication for severe seborrheic dermatitis
         (a) Sedatives
         (b) Oral or local steroids
         (c) Antibiotics for secondary infections
      (3) Shampoo
         (a) Infants
            1. Daily with mild soap
            2. Thorough rinsing
            3. Firm pressure—even over fontanels
         (b) Older children
            1. 1 to 3 times weekly with special shampoo (Sebulex, Selsun, etc.)
            2. Thorough rinsing
      (4) Reduction in number of baths
      (5) Use of mild soap and copious rinsings
   b. Counselling/prevention
      (1) Instructions on bathing and/or soaks
      (2) Instructions on general hygiene to prevent repeat
      (3) Demonstration of firmness needed in shampooing hair
      (4) Instruction on nail care—short, smooth, clean
   c. Follow-up
      (1) Telephone call after 1 week for progress
      (2) If no improvement, reappointment
   d. Consultations/referrals
      (1) Consultation on any prescription drugs
      (2) Referral to dermatologist if itching does not improve
2. Contact dermatitis
   a. Treatments/medications
      (1) Antihistamines
      (2) Mild sedatives
      (3) Oral or topical corticosteroids
      (4) Removal of causative agent
      (5) Cold, frequent soaks or compresses
   b. Counselling/prevention
      (1) Instructions on bathing and/or soaks
      (2) Instructions on general hygiene and avoidance of causative agent
      (3) Instructions on nail care—short, smooth, clean
   c. Follow-up
      (1) Telephone call after 48 h for progress
      (2) If no improvement, reappointment

d. Consultations/referrals
   (1) Consultation on prescription medications
   (2) Referrals to pediatrician if itching not improved

C. Extremities

1. Seborrheic dermatitis—as above
2. Contact dermatitis—as above
3. Atopic dermatitis
   a. Treatments/medications
      (1) Antihistamines
      (2) Antibiotics for secondary infections
      (3) Topical steroids
      (4) Bathing
         (a) Take bland, mild baths with milk, oatmeal, or starch.
         (b) Avoid strong soaps.
      (5) Stay out of overheated rooms.
      (6) Keep humidity low—perspiration increases discomfort.
      (7) Avoid woolen clothing next to the skin.
      (8) Monitor diet for any cause-and-effect foods.
   b. Counselling/prevention
      (1) Bathing and soaking instructions
      (2) Nail and hygiene care
      (3) Environmental control to avoid causative agents
   c. Follow-up
      (1) Telephone call after 48 h for progress
      (2) If no improvement, reappointment
   d. Consultations/referrals
      (1) Consultations on prescription medications
      (2) Referral to dermatologist if no improvement
4. Hives (urticaria)
   a. Treatments/medications
      (1) Antihistamines
      (2) Sedatives
      (3) Epinephrine
      (4) Antibiotics for secondary infection
      (5) Oral or topical steroids
      (6) Removal of causative agent if possible
      (7) Soothing baths several times daily
         (a) Plain water
         (b) Starch
         (c) Oatmeal
         (d) Oil
   b. Counselling/prevention
      (1) Bathing and soaks instructions
      (2) Nail and hygiene care
      (3) Environmental control to avoid causative agents
   c. Follow-up
      (1) Telephone call after 48 h for progress
      (2) If no improvement, reappointment
   d. Consultations/referrals
      (1) Consultation on prescription medications
      (2) Referral to dermatologist if itching remains

D. Anal region

1. Atopic dermatitis—as above
2. Contact dermatitis—as above
3. Moisture, tight clothing, harsh soaps, home remedies, and friction and rubbing
   a. Treatments/medications
      (1) Removal of causative agent
      (2) Loose, cotton underclothing
      (3) Careful washing and rinsing of area
      (4) Medications: none
   b. Counselling/prevention
      (1) Instructions on bathing
      (2) Instructions on general hygiene
      (3) Instructions on clothing
   c. Follow-up
      (1) Parent to call for new appointment if condition does not improve.
      (2) Check condition at next regular appointment.
   d. Consultations/referrals
      (1) Consultation if condition does not improve
      (2) Referral to pediatrician
4. Pinworms
   a. Treatments/medications
      (1) Povan
      (2) Monopar
      (3) Gentian violet
      (4) Daily clean underclothing to be worn all the time—even to bed
      (5) Frequent, careful washing of all bed linens—for entire family
      (6) Short, clean nails
      (7) Frequent bathing and separate towels and washcloths.
   b. Counselling/prevention
      (1) Instruction on medications
         (a) When to take and for how long
         (b) Alert to parent that Povan turns stools red
      (2) Instructions on individual bathing and sleeping—if possible
      (3) Instructions on general hygiene
         (a) Washing hands
         (b) Short nails
   c. Follow-up

(1) Retest for eggs following completion of medication.
(2) Retreat for additional infestations.
d. Consultations/referrals
(1) Consultation on prescription medications
(2) Referral to public health nurse to help family with hygiene
5. Oral antibiotics—as above
6. Psoriasis
a. Treatments/medications
(1) Mild tranquilizers
(2) Topical steroids
(3) Petroleum-based ointment to areas
(4) Daily bathing
(a) Remove scales.
(b) Soak in tub and use a soft brush to remove further scales.
(c) Apply ointment.
(5) Encouragement of exposure to the sun
b. Counselling/prevention
(1) Give instruction on bathing and scrubbing.
(2) There is no prevention.
c. Follow-up
(1) Continual support and encouragement until remission
(2) Reappointment to change medication or soaking instructions
d. Consultations/referrals
(1) Chronic problem—may need psychological support
(2) Referral to dermatologist for additional treatments

E. Vulva

1. *Monilia*
a. Treatments/medications
(1) Nystatin or Mycolog cream topically
(2) Gentian violet swabbed on area
(3) Dry, clean genital area
(a) For infant—diaper care
(b) For older child—clean panties and maybe extra padding to avoid staining clothing
(4) General hygiene
b. Counselling/prevention
(1) Instructions on general hygiene
(2) Instructions on applying medication and avoiding clothing damage
c. Follow-up
(1) Telephone call from parent if no improvement within 1 week
(2) Reappointment
d. Consultations/referrals
(1) Consultation on medications
(2) Referral to pediatrician if infection persists
2. *Trichomonas*
a. Treatments/medications
(1) Flagyl for 10 days
(2) Acidic vaginal douches—1 Tbsp white vinegar to 1 qt water
(3) General hygiene to area
(a) Careful cleansing after bowel movements
(b) Careful washing and copious rinsing
(c) Clean, cotton panties
(4) Avoidance of intercourse during therapy
b. Counselling/prevention
(1) Instructions on genital hygiene
(2) Instructions on medications
c. Follow-up
(1) Treat sexual partner, if infected
(2) Make a return appointment for reoccurrence.
d. Consultations/referrals
(1) Consultation on medications
(2) Referral to specialist for continued infection
3. Diabetes—as above
4. Antibiotic treatment—as above
5. Harsh chemicals—as above
6. Contraceptive jellies or creams
a. Treatments/medications
(1) Avoidance or change of current jelly or cream
(2) General hygiene to area
(a) Careful bathing and rinsing
(b) Dry, cotton panties
(3) Medications: none
b. Counselling/prevention
(1) Instructions to avoid intercourse until irritation clears
(2) Instructions on general hygiene
c. Follow-up
(1) Return appointment if no improvement
(2) Recheck of area at next regular appointment
d. Consultations/referrals
(1) None
(2) Referral for gynecologist if persistent

F. Scrotum

1. Tinea
a. Treatments/medications
(1) Griseofulvin
(2) Tinactin topically: caution against over treatment which causes relapse

(3) Frequent bathing with mild soap and copious rinsing.
(4) Dry, clean cotton undergarments
(5) Avoidance of high humidity, which may aggravate condition

b. Counselling/prevention
(1) Instructions on medications
(2) Instructions on hygiene
(3) Instructions on avoiding high humidity

c. Follow-up
(1) Return appointment following medication if no improvement seen
(2) Recheck at next regular appointment

d. Consultations/referrals
(1) Consultation for prescription medication
(2) Referral to pediatrician if infection persists

2. Tight clothing—as above
3. Harsh soaps—as above
4. Contact chemicals—as above

bibliography

Behrman, Howard T., Labor, Theordore, and Rozen, Jack. *Common skin diseases: diagnosis and treatment* (3rd ed). New York: Grune & Stratton, 1978.

Collar, Maureen, and Brown, Marie. Over-the-counter-drugs for skin disorders. *The Nurse Practitioner,* **2**(5):14–17, 35–38 (1977).

Derbes, Vincent. Rashes: recognition and management. *Nursing '78,* **8**(3):54–59(1978).

Kempe, C. Henry, Silver, Henry K., and O'Brien, Donough. *Current pediatric diagnosis and treatment.* Los Altos, Calif.: Lange, 1978.

Jacobs, Alvin. Atopic dermatitis: clinical expression and management. *Pediatric Annals,* **5**(12):763–771 (1976).

Weinberg, Samuel, and Hoekelman, Robert. *Pediatric dermatology for the primary care practitioner.* New York: McGraw-Hill, 1978.

Weston, William, and Huff, J. Atopic dermatitis: etiology and pathogenesis. *Pediatric Annals,* **5**(12):759–762 (1976).

136 Drowsiness/Tiredness/Fatigue

HARRIETT S. CHANEY

ALERT

1. Abnormal neurological assessment
2. Recent head trauma: days or 1 to 2 weeks
3. Fever, nausea, vomiting, photophobia, nuchal rigidity
4. Poison ingestion
5. Unexplained fatigue sometimes the first symptom of an infectious process such as hepatitis, tuberculosis, infectious mononucleosis, flu, or other systemic viruses
6. Hypokalemia
7. Slow pulse
8. Anemia
9. Weight loss
10. Diabetes mellitus
12. Allergies
13. Hoarseness, intolerance to cold, decreased sweating, skin dry and rough, eyelids puffy, anorexia, increased weight

I. Etiology

A. Drowsiness—pathological objective state in which the client cannot remain in a wakeful state despite stimulation

1. Trauma resulting in localized or generalized brain edema, subdural hematoma, acute epidural hemorrhage
2. Cerebral hemorrhage due to trauma, aneurysm, hypertensive vascular disease
3. Infectious process such as meningitis, encephalitis

B. Tiredness, fatigue—a subjective complaint reflective of weariness and loss of a sense of well being

1. Nonpathophysiological processes
   a. Prolonged physical exertion
   b. Physical or mental overworking
   c. Decreased motivation regarding school and interests
   d. Drugs: depressants, recreational drugs, diuretics
   e. Malnutrition
   f. Depression
   g. Anxiety
   h. Lack of physical exercise
   i. Insufficient sleep
   j. Physical and psychosocial adjustments of adolescents
   k. Improper infant feeding
   l. Familial turmoil
2. Pathological processes
   a. Infectious process such as meningitis, hepatitis, tuberculosis, infectious mononucleosis, flu
   b. Hematopoietic disorders such as anemia
   c. Endocrine disorders such as diabetes mellitus, primary aldosteronism, Addison's disease, hypothyroidism, hyperparathyroidism, Cushing's disease
   d. Cardiovascular disease such as derangements of the heart beat

II. Subjective Data: A complete history including

A. Problem-oriented history

1. Onset
2. Duration
3. Associated with headache, weight loss, shortness of breath, leg cramps, fever, sore throat, hoarseness, intolerance to cold, decreased sweating, anorexia, weight gain, skin changes, syncope, stiff neck, photo-

phobia, bleeding, tarry stools, polydipsia, polyuria, polyphagia

4. Recent exposure to hepatitis, flu, tuberculosis, infectious mononucleosis, meningitis
5. Drugs: prescription, nonprescription, recreational
6. Dietary patterns
7. Normal daily activities
8. Sleep patterns
9. Description of school and activities of interest to determine presence of dissatisfaction
10. Recent unpleasant events: death, absence of achievement, relocation, medical illness, emotional crisis, physical trauma
11. Past history of diabetes, cardiovascular disease

B. Immunization history

C. Allergies

D. Family history of tuberculosis, hepatitis, cardiovascular disease, endocrine disorders

E. Social history to determine economic capabilities, recreational interests, socializing potentials

III. Objective Data

A. Physical examination—because of the nature of drowsiness, tiredness, and fatigue, the existence of pathology assumed until ruled out; therefore, a complete physical examination required, including a neurological assessment

B. Laboratory data—complete blood count (CBC)

C. Psychosocial assessment

IV. Assessment: Tiredness or Fatigue Due to Nonpathophysiological Processes

A. Subjective data—history may reveal presence of one or more of the following factors

1. Feelings or observation of "no ambition," "no pep," "no activities," "turned off," "fed up"
2. Great physical exertion or prolonged mental or physical labor
3. Limited number of daily activities which are not challenging mentally or physically
4. Abnormal sleeping pattern: terminal insomnia, difficulty falling asleep, or fitful, light, or intermittent sleep
5. Recent unpleasant event
6. School and/or activity dissatisfaction
7. Inadequate nutrition due to ignorance, lack of resources, life-style
8. Very limited or inadequate self-image

B. Objective data

1. Normal physical examination and laboratory data
2. Personal judgments based upon observation of client: flat affect, listless, sad, tense, anxious

V. Management: Tiredness or Fatigue Due to Nonpathophysiological Processes

A. Treatments/medications: none

B. Counselling/prevention

1. Report the occurrence of any new symptoms, such as fever, nausea, vomiting, diarrhea, body aches, headache, sore throat, cough.
2. Explore alternatives for instances of school and/or activity dissatisfaction.
3. Recommend a program of *regular* physical exercise, in instances where the client fails to challenge his or her body physically, such as walking, bicycling, jogging, swimming, bowling, tennis, squash, golf. Provide or recommend current literature in this area available through the U.S. Government Printing Office or local bookstores.
4. Discourage the use of any over-the-counter sleeping aids and daytime naps. Suggest as sleeping aids regular daily physical exercise, warm baths, reading and/or relaxation techniques.
5. Review components of adequate nutrition and provide take-home literature on this matter (available through the Government Printing Office, local extension offices).
6. Explore socialization opportunities with the client.
7. Discuss elements relevant to adolescent adjustments and/or family turmoil.

C. Follow-up

1. Advise the client to phone immediately with the onset of additional symptoms.
2. Schedule a return visit in 2 weeks.

D. Consultations/referrals

1. If a depressed client does not respond to the aforementioned interventions, refer for professional counselling.
2. Refer to governmental social programs instances of malnutrition and social deprivation.

Table 136-1 Medical Referral/Consultation

Diagnosis	Clinical Manifestations	Management
Drowsiness	Inability to remain in wakeful state despite stimulation *Always* pathological in etiology	Immediate physician or emergency room referral Emergency vehicle transportation perhaps necessary
Brain edema, subdural hematoma, acute epidural hemorrhage	Fatigue progressing to drowsiness and coma following recent or recent past trauma Nausea, vomiting, headache, confusion Abnormal neurological findings, such as Babinski's sign (after 2 years of age), muscle weakness, abnormal pupil response	Immediate physician or emergency room referral Emergency vehicle transportation perhaps necessary
Meningitis	Fatigue progressing to drowsiness and coma Fever, headache, stiff neck and back Petechial or purpuric skin eruption Positive Kernig's and Brudzinski's sign Tense or bulging anterior fontanel in infant	Immediate physician referral
Encephalitis	Fatigue progressing to stupor or coma Fever, confusion, convulsions Aphasia, hemiparesis, asymmetry of tendon reflexes, Babinski's sign Ataxia, myoclonic jerks, nystagmus, facial weakness	Immediate physician referral
Hepatitis	Fatigue perhaps earliest symptom Headache, anorexia, fever Nausea, vomiting, diarrhea, dark urine Jaundice Leading clue: exposure to hepatitis	Physician referral
Tuberculosis	Fatigue perhaps early symptom Night sweats, fever Anorexia, weight loss Cough—hemoptysis, purulent sputum Leading clue: exposure to TB	Physician referral
Infectious mononucleosis	Fatigue perhaps an early symptom Headache, sore throat, fever Cervical lymphadenopathy, palatine petechiae Splenomegaly occurring in 50% of clients Lymphocytosis with atypical forms Heterophil agglutination—positive Leading clue: exposure to mononucleosis	Physician consultation Symptomatic therapy Salicylates, acetamenophen Gargle Rest, fluids
Flu	Fatigue perhaps early symptom General body aching	Symptomatic therapy Salicylates, acetamenophen

Table 136-1 Medical Referral/Consultation *(continued)*

Diagnosis	Clinical Manifestations	Management
	Fever, headache, cough, nausea, vomiting, diarrhea Leading clue: exposure to flu	Antinausea, antidiarrhea Rest, fluids
Anemia	Fatigue perhaps early symptom Pallor of skin and mucous membrane Anorexia, heartburn, headache, vertigo, irritability Palpitations, shortness of breath Decreased to absent reflexes Frank or occult bleeding Decreased hematocrit and hemoglobin	Physician referral See Anemia, Chap. 39
Derangement of heart beat, dysrhythmias	Slow apical pulse—bradycardia Irregular apical pulse reflective of sinoarterial arrest or block; sinus arrhythmia; premature atrial, junctional, or ventricular contraction; blocks; atrial fibrillation Near fainting, syncope, vertigo Rapid apical pulse reflective of tachycardia, PAT, atrial flutter, junctional tachycardia, ventricular tachycardia Nausea, vomiting	Physician referral See Heart Beat/Rate Changes/Murmurs, Chap. 35 See Congenital Heart Defects, Chap. 146
Hypokalemia	Tiredness and fatigue early symptoms Polyuria; emotional lability Leg weakness and muscle cramps ECG showing prominent U wave Cardiac dysrhythmias; abdominal distention Hypokalemia found in digitalis intoxication, diuretic usage, adrenal virilism, aldosteronism, diabetic acidosis, dehydration	Immediate physician referral
Diabetes mellitus	Fatigue early symptom Polydipsia, polyuria, polyphagia Weight loss, nocturia, vulvar pruritis, blurred vision Glucosuria	Physician referral
Addison's disease	Insidious to progressive fatigability Anorexia, nausea, vomiting, weight loss Cutaneous and mucosal pigmentation of unexposed areas Hypotension, hyperkalemia Voice failure	Physician referral
Cushing's syndrome	Easy fatigability Truncal obesity, hypertension, amenorrhea, hirsutism Abdominal striae, edema Glucosuria May be due to adrenal hyperplasia, neoplasms, exogenous, iatrogenic use of steroids	Physician referral

Table 136-1 Medical Referral/Consultation *(continued)*

Diagnosis	Clinical Manifestations	Management
Hypothyroidism	Unexplained fatigue Intolerance to cold; "doughy" skin Eyelids puffy; hoarseness; decreased sweating Sluggishness and/or weight gain in older clients; growth failure in newborn; feeding problem in infant Constipation Pseudomyotonia	Physician referral
Hyperparathyroidism	Fatigue and muscle weakness Hyporeflexia, cardiac dysrhythmias Bone pain upon weight bearing, shortened stature Dehydration Symptoms and findings associated with kidney stones and duodenal uclers	Physician referral

bibliography

Harvey, A. M., Johns, R. J., Owens, A. H., and Ross, R. S. (eds.). *The principles and practice of medicine.* New York: Appleton-Century-Crofts, 1976.

Thorn, G. W., Adams, R. D., Braunwald, E., Isselbacker, K. J., and Petersdorf, R. G. (eds.). *Harrison's principles of internal medicine.* New York: McGraw-Hill, 1977.

Tucker, S. M., Breeding, M. A., Canobbio, G. D., Paquette, E. H., Wells, M. E., and Willmann, M. E. *Patient care standards.* St. Louis: Mosby, 1975.

Wallach, Jacques. *Interpretation of diagnostic tests.* Boston: Little, Brown, 1974.

137 Allergies

RITA M. CARTY

ALERT[1]

1. Difficulty breathing
2. Sudden onset of wheezing, abdominal cramps, vomiting, diarrhea

I. Etiology

A. Antigen-antibody union

1. The reaction occurs when the level of resistance (threshold) is exceeded.
2. It is caused by higher-than-usual concentrations of allergens and by lowered resistance due to infection.
3. After the first attack, the threshold is permanently lowered.
4. Once the antigen-antibody reaction is established, the client is affected by allergens, infection, psychological stress.

B. Inhalants (pollens, spores, molds, etc.)

C. Contactants (metals, cosmetics, drugs, plants, etc.)

D. Ingestants (food and drugs)

E. Injectables (drugs, vaccines, animal serum, and saliva)

II. Subjective Data

A. Age

B. Presenting problem(s)

1. Onset
   a. Time of day, season, year
   b. Location
2. Frequency of occurrence
3. Treatments—relief
   a. Home remedies
   b. Prescribed medications
4. Hospitalizations related to problem
5. Past evaluations
   a. Allergy skin tests
   b. Desensitization therapy
   c. Elimination diet
6. Restriction of activities
7. Number of days absent from school last year due to illness

C. Present or past history of

1. Itchy ears, nose, eyes, throat
2. Red, watery eyes
3. Frequent sneezing
4. Clear, watery nasal discharge
5. Wheezing
6. Cough
7. Rash/hives
8. Recurrent eyes and/or ear infections
9. Increased ear wax
10. Postnasal drip
11. Frequent "colds"
12. Sores on lips, tongue, gums
13. Shortness of breath
14. Dyspnea on exertion
15. History of croup/pneumonia
16. Colic
17. Diarrhea
18. Vomiting
19. Constipation
20. Fatigue
21. Irritability
22. Frequent outbursts of inappropriate laughter, speech, or crying
23. Disruptive behavior in school
24. Difficulty with urination
25. Enuresis
26. Headaches
27. Convulsions

[1]For any client in whom allergies are suspected, a complete history and physical examination is indicated.

D. Relationship between each of the following and the onset of symptoms
1. Seasons
   a. House dust and respiratory infections (winter)
   b. Trees (spring)
   c. Weeds (summer to fall)
   d. Grasses (spring or summer)
2. Molds
   a. Outdoor seasonal molds (wet, warm periods)
   b. Mildew
   c. Old storage areas (attics, damp basements)
   d. Moldy foods
3. Animals
   a. House pets
   b. Clothing made of animal hair or hide
      (1) Belts
      (2) Wool
4. Cosmetics and perfumes
5. Paints/sprays
6. Medicines
   a. Penicillin
   b. Aspirin
   c. Sulfur
   d. Others
7. Emotional and/or social factors
   a. Change in family constellation
      (1) Mother working
      (2) Separation
      (3) Divorce
   b. Moves
   c. Change in school

E. Environmental history
1. Number and relationship of people residing in home
2. Apartment or private house
3. Description of home
   a. Length of time in present house
   b. Age of house
   c. Type of heating and cooling and its location (attic or basement)
   d. Pets and/or animals in house
   e. Location of house—near vacant lots, wineries, open fields, factories
4. Description of child's room
   a. Location
   b. Shared with siblings
   c. Type of pillows, blankets, bedspread, mattress, and drapes
   d. Stuffed toys or dolls
   e. Floor coverings (rugs, pads)
   f. Covering on windows (venetian blinds, shades, curtains)
   g. Storage in room

F. Family history—should include, at least, both parents; all siblings and grandparents
1. Asthma
2. Eczema
3. Hay fever
4. Hives
5. Sinusitis
6. Headaches
7. Known allergies to foods or drugs
8. Serious infections
9. Chronic and/or genetic disorders
10. Cancer

G. Prenatal history
1. Medications
2. Illnesses

H. Infancy
1. Problems/illnesses
   a. Milk intolerance
   b. Colic
   c. Rashes, eczema
   d. Diarrhea
   e. Choking
   f. Frequent/recurrent illness
2. Feeding
   a. Bottle or breast
   b. Type of formula used

I. Dietary history (should be detailed)
1. Food likes/dislikes
2. Number of meals per day
3. Sample menu or 24 h diet recall
4. Description of mealtimes
   a. Tensions
   b. Family members present
   c. Same or varied time of day
5. Normal activity before and after meals

III. Objective Data

A. Physical examination
1. A complete physical examination is usually indicated, with emphasis on eyes, ears, nose, mouth, throat, heart, lungs, abdomen, and skin.
2. The following physical findings may suggest allergy.
   a. Eyes
      (1) Allergic shiners (black eyes)
      (2) Muddy, injected conjunctiva
      (3) Cobblestone appearance of upper and lower torsal conjunctiva
      (4) Long, silky eyelashes
      (5) Sties
      (6) Excessive lacrimation

(7) Rubbing or excessive blinking

b. Ears
  (1) Drainage
  (2) Decreased hearing
  (3) Absent or distorted cone of light
  (4) Immobile tympanic membrane on pneumoscopy

c. Nose
  (1) Allergic salute (transverse nasal crease)
  (2) Enlarged adenoids
  (3) Pale, boggy mucous membranes
  (4) Watery, mucoid nasal discharge
  (5) Nasal polyps
  (6) Tender frontal and maxillary sinuses

d. Mouth/throat
  (1) Gaping, open-mouthed expression
  (2) Red throat
  (3) Swollen lips or tongue
  (4) Gingival hyperplasia
  (5) Dental deformities (malocclusion)
  (6) Geographic tongue

e. Lungs
  (1) Barrel chest
  (2) Pigeon chest
  (3) Prominent lump in upper back
  (4) Harsh breath sounds
  (5) Wheezes

f. Skin
  (1) Rashes
  (2) Dryness
  (3) Scaliness
  (4) Scratch marks
  (5) Inflammations
  (6) Pallor
  (7) Hives

B. Laboratory data

1. CBC including eosinophils
2. Nasal and bronchial smears for eosinophils
3. Tuberculin test
4. Throat culture
5. After consultation with a physician and if respiratory symptoms present, pulmonary function tests
6. Skin testing by allergist
7. Chest x-ray done on all clients presenting with first attack of wheezing

IV. Assessment (see Table 137-1)

V. Management:General

A. Treatments/medications

1. Elimination of known allergen(s)
2. If unable to control or eliminate allergen(s) from environment—immunotherapy to decrease sensitivity to allergens
3. Antihistamines (see Table 137-2), expectorants, bronchodilators sometimes necessary for symptomatic relief
4. Environmental control—need to "desensitize" room (see Fig. 137-1)

B. Counselling/prevention

1. If immunotherapy is necessary, explain to parent(s) and child what to expect, how it will feel, and the goal of therapy.
2. Describe what it means to have an allergy(s) and different ways of manifestation.
3. Instruct client/parent to keep a diary of what symptoms appear when and the circumstances surrounding the onset.
4. Stress the child as a person, do not stress the allergy. The allergy should not be a frequent topic of conversation, nor should the child be allowed to use it as an excuse.
5. Help parent(s)/child to recognize and avoid known allergens.
6. Teach how to control the environment, desensitize a room, remove known allergens.
7. When known allergies exist, medications should be used with care. Acetaminophen may be less apt to cause sensitivity than aspirin.
8. If there is a known drug allergy, parent(s)/client should know and have in writing the names of the drug, both generic and trade, so they may notify future health professionals. A tag may be worn around the neck.
9. Encourage the parent(s) to allow the child as much freedom as is safe for normal development, both physically and psychologically.
10. Encourage the child to become involved in own care, and give appropriate education.
11. Normal health maintenance is very important in prevention and early detection of associated problems in allergic children.
12. Discuss financial ability with parent(s). Many expenses are tax deductible and receipts should be saved.

C. Follow-up

1. Dependent upon severity of symptoms and parental understanding and ability to cope; initially, may be necessary for bimonthly visits for support and reeducation
2. Regular well-child visits

D. Consultations/referrals

1. Allergist
2. School nurse/teachers

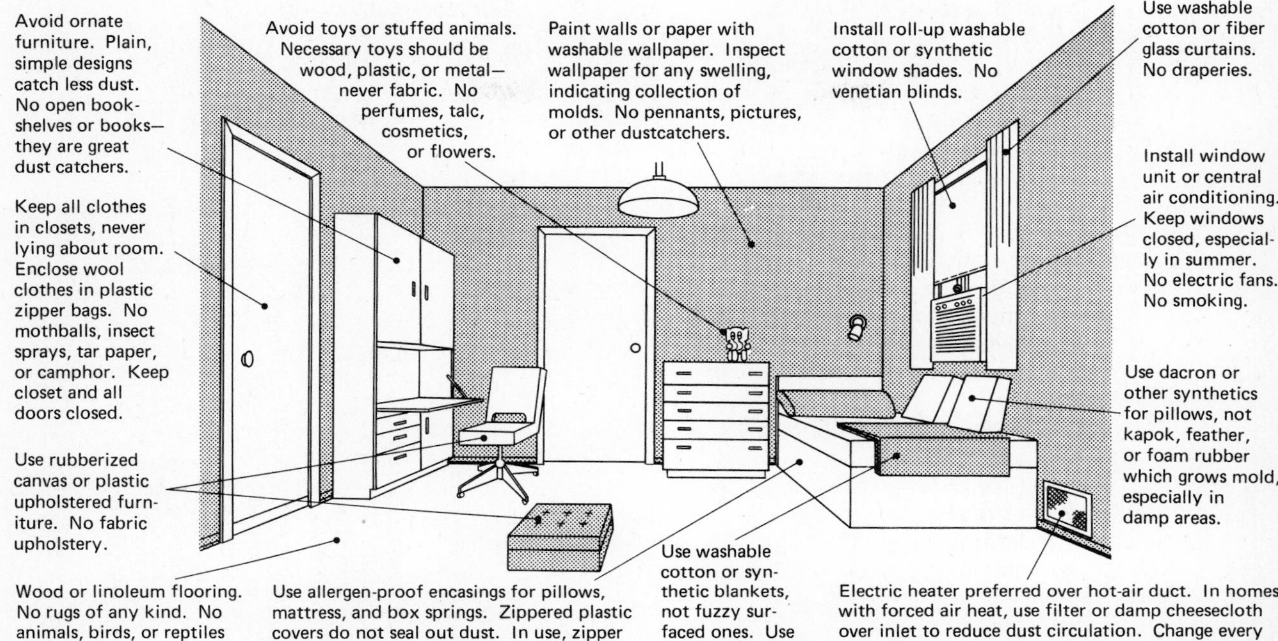

Figure 137-1 Guide to "desensitizing" a room. Cleaning tips: Wet-dust twice a day. Damp-mop floor with a solution of disinfectant. Oil-mop baseboards. Vacuum only if room is aired afterward. Use tank-type cleaner. Attach a second hose to outlet, placing end outside window or in hall to prevent redistributing allergens. *(From Guide to "desensitizing a room. Richmond, VA: A. H. Robins Co.)*

bibliography

Bridgewater, Sharon C., and Voignier, Ruth R. Allergies in children: teaching. *American Journal of Nursing,* **78**(4):620–623 (1978).

———, ———, and Smith, C. Steven. Allergies in children: recognition. *American Journal of Nursing,* **78**(4):614–616 (1978).

Buckley, Rebecca H. Advances in asthma/allergy. *Pediatric Nursing,* **5**(2):B–D (1979).

Carty, Rita M. Some facts about allergies. *Pediatric Nursing,* **3**(2):7–9 (1977).

Gellis, Sydney S., and Kagan, Benjamin M. *Current pediatric therapy* 8. Philadelphia: Saunders, 1978, pp. 675–706.

LaBella, Ginger. The nurse practitioner and the allergic child. *Pediatric Nursing,* **5**(2): E–F (1979).

McGeady, Stephen J., and Sherman, Brock V. Management of the child with recurrent asthma. *Pediatric Annals,* **6**(8):11–23 (1977).

The Philadelphia Regional Pediatric Pulmonary Disease Program. Emergency room treatment of acute asthma. *Pediatric Annals,* **6**(8):7–10 (1977).

Table 137-1 Assessment and Management of Allergic Disorders

Assessment	Allergic Rhinitis	Atopic Dermatitis (Eczema)	Asthma	Urticaria	Gastrointestinal Allergy	Tension Fatigue Syndrome
Subjective data	Itchy, runny (clear mucus) nose Frequent sneezing Nasal obstruction Itchy eyes, palate, ears Recurrent epistaxis Family history positive for allergies	Intensely itchy rash Parent(s) sometimes reporting child scratches vigorously at night Family history positive for allergies	Coughing Difficulty breathing Chest pain Severe cases sometimes having vomiting and abdominal pain Family history positive for allergies	Itching and stinging welts	Nausea Vomiting Headache Anorexia Diarrhea Mother sometimes noting baby not gaining weight Anal itching Rectal bleeding May have history of other allergic diseases Positive family history for allergies	Parent(s) or client describing alternating periods of tension and fatigue; may have any of the following symptoms Hyperactivity Clumsiness Inability to relax Sleep problems Muscle pains Fatigue Nasal stuffiness, itching Sneezing Cough Abdominal pain Headache Bedwetting (enuresis) School problems
Objective data	Bilateral nasal congestion Nasal mucosa bluish and edematous Mouth breathing Allergic shiners Nasal smear—increased eosinophils	Erythematous, papulovesicular weeping lesions—crusting sometimes noted Increased skin markings Hyper/hypopigmentation of skin Common sites Infant: scalp, neck, cheeks, hands, extensor	Coarse and/or fine rales Prolonged expiration with expiratory and, occasionally, inspiratory wheeze May have rales, rhonchi Diaphoresis Nasal flaring	Edematous, red plaques or welts with sharp borders May be generalized or limited to the palms, soles of the feet, or pressure points Usually fade in less than 12 h	Pallor Poor weight gain May have any of the following signs Cracked, inflamed lips Circumoral or chin eczema Swelling of tongue Canker sores (aphthous stomatitis)	Allergic shiners Edema around eyes Wheezing Pallor—especially of face Diaphoresis Signs of allergic rhinitis

Table 137-1 Assessment and Management of Allergic Disorders *(continued)*

Assessment	Allergic Rhinitis	Atopic Dermatitis (Eczema)	Asthma	Urticaria	Gastrointestinal Allergy	Tension Fatigue Syndrome
		surfaces of extremities Child (more than 2 yr): face, scalp, flexor surfaces Morgan's fold—definite wrinkle below lower eyelid	Intercostal retractions		Uvular edema Hives (urticaria) Wheezing Nasal smear—increased eosinophils	
Treatments/medications	Avoidance of suspected allergens Antihistamines (diphenhydramine or Chlor-Trimeton) Temporary use of topical nasal corticosteroids (Turbinaire, 2 puffs each nostril tid) Immunotherapy perhaps indicated	Keep temperature constant; use humidifier, vaporizer, air conditioner. Bathe only twice a week in tepid water with mild soap (Neutrogena or Lowila); do not take bubble baths. Avoid harsh clothing and bedding; use cotton. Keep nails short, filed, and clean. Avoid changes in family routine. For weeping lesions, apply cool tap-water compresses qid for 20 min; pat skin dry. Apply topical corticosteroids (Synalar,	Severe attack Aqueous epinephrine 1:1000 subcutaneous injection 0.01 mL/kg May repeat 2 times at 10–15 min intervals If client clears, give Sus-Phrine 0.005 mL/kg 20 min after last dose of epinephrine Environmental control Immunotherapy Infrequent attack (1–2/yr) bronchodilators when needed Systemic corticosteroids prescribed by the physician	Mild cases: diphenhydramine or chlorpheniramine maleate Antipruritic relief Cool-water baths Addition of Aveeno to bath water Severe cases Adrenalin in oil 1:500 IM Laryngeal edema—adrenalin 1:1000 IM or IV Long-lasting, subacute urticaria: oral steroids	Identification and elimination of causative food from diet Daily food diary Infant: substitution of nonmilk formula—note which type of carbohydrate in formula Older infant and child: trial diet milk substitute, 1 grain, 1 vegetable, 1 fruit, 1 meat Avoidance of prepared baby foods and all additives Addition of new food every 2 wk Vitamins and iron perhaps needed Skin testing perhaps indicated	Food elimination diet—no milk, dairy products, and chocolate Reintroduce milk products in 1 mo to see if symptoms reoccur. If no improvement with above elimination, eliminate wheat and eggs. If symptoms improve, eliminate causative agents from the diet. Skin testing may be indicated if there is no improvement with the above.

Table 137-1 Assessment and Management of Allergic Disorders *(continued)*

Assessment	Allergic Rhinitis	Atopic Dermatitis (Eczema)	Asthma	Urticaria	Gastrointestinal Allergy	Tension Fatigue Syndrome
		Aristocort, Kenalog, Valisone) 3–4 times per day Ointment—dry plaques Cream—weeping lesions Only for limited time—danger of absorption in young children After improvement, hydrocortisone 1% Antihistamine (diphenhydramine) for antipruritic and sedative effect				
Counselling/ Prevention	See Management, V above. Discuss the condition and the different ways the child may respond to the allergen(s) i.e., reacting 1 day but not another. Allergic reaction lowers resistance, making the person more susceptible to infection.	See Management, V above. Discuss chronicity of condition, causes, and medication. Discuss the importance of keeping the skin lubricated. Advise that the client avoid stress.	See Management, V above. Provide parent(s) with information about cause of "attack" and condition. Support parent(s) and reassure about child's condition. Parent(s) needs to understand that "toughening up" the child will not prevent symptoms. Explain how infection, stress,	Keep diary to attempt to determine the offending agent. Instruct regarding medications. Avoid scratching.	In families where there is a high incidence of allergy, suggest that mothers breast-feed their newborns. Instruct regarding daily food diary—mother to record ingested food, time eaten, and any symptoms experienced. Instruct on diet and reassure parent(s) that child is getting enough food.	Instruct client and parent(s) on above treatment and importance of following diet exactly Write out all diet instructions Parent(s) need support in dealing with child's behavior

Table 137-1 Assessment and Management of Allergic Disorders *(continued)*

Assessment	Allergic Rhinitis	Atopic Dermatitis (Eczema)	Asthma	Urticaria	Gastrointestinal Allergy	Tension Fatigue Syndrome
			and allergens combine to cause the symptoms.			
Follow-up	Return visit if symptoms not improved or cleared in 3–5 days, or if symptoms recur	Exacerbation—telephone call every other day, return visit 1 wk	Telephone call in 4 h after return home from acute attack to report progress Return visit in 10 days or sooner if symptoms reappear or as needed for counselling and reassurance	Return visit in 3 days if symptoms persist	Return visit in 3–5 days if symptoms persist Return visit if symptoms reoccur Phone contact as needed for questions and reassurance	Phone call in 48 h for report on symptoms Return visit in 5 days
Consultations/ referrals	Allergist School nurse Camp counsellor	Referral to physician/allergist /dermatologist Severe cases Those with secondary bacterial infections Those who fail to respond to treatment in 2 wk School nurse	Referral to physician/allergist Children less than 2 yr of age Those with first attack of wheezing Those who fail to respond to treatment Those with repeat attacks School nurse/teacher	Immediate referral to physician if suspected laryngeal edema Consultation with allergist if chronic, recurrent episodes lasting more than 1 wk	Consultation with the allergist School nurse/teacher Referral to physician—severe cases Dietitian	Consultation with physician Referral to an allergist if skin testing indicated Dietitian School nurse

Table 137-2 Classification of Antihistamines

Drug (Generic and Trade Name)	Manufacturer	Preparations Available	Dosage
ETHANOLAMINES			
Diphenhydramine			
(Benadryl)	Parke-Davis	Capsules: 25 and 50 mg	5 mg/kg per day in 3 or 4 divided doses
(Bax)	McKesson	Elixir: 10 mg/4 mL	Children over 10 kg:
(SK)	SKF	Injection: 10 and 50 mg/mL	12.5 to 25 mg 3 or 4 times a day
(Fenyhist)	Mallard		
Carbinoxamine			
(Clistin)	McNeil	Tablets: 4 mg Repeat action: 8 and 12 mg Elixir: 4 mg/5 mL	0.4 mg/kg per day in 3 or 4 divided doses Children 1–3 yr: 2 mg 3 or 4 times a day Children 3–6 yr: 2–4 mg 3 or 4 times a day Children over 6 yr: 4 mg 3 or 4 times a day
ETHYLENEDIAMINES			
Tripelennamine			
(Pyribenzamine)	CIBA	Tablets: 25 and 50 mg Delayed action: 50 and 100 mg Elixir: 37.5 mg/5 mL	5 mg/kg per day in 3 or 4 divided doses Children: not to exceed 300 mg/24 h
Methapyrilene hydrochloride			
(Histadyl)	Lilly	Pulvules: 25 and 50 mg Syrup:20 mg/5 mL Injection: 20 mg/mL	5 mg/kg per day in 3 or 4 divided doses Children over 6 yr: 25 mg 3 or 4 times a day
ALKYLAMINES			
Chlorpheniramine maleate			
(Chlor-Trimeton)	Schering	Tablets: 4 mg Repeat action: 8 and 12 mg Syrup: 2 mg/5 mL Injection: 100 mg/mL	0.4 mg/kg per day in 3 or 4 divided doses Children over 6 yr: 2 mg 3 or 4 times a day Infants: 1 mg 3 or 4 times a day
(Teldrin)	SKF	Spansules: 8 and 12 mg	Long-acting preparations
(Histaspan)	USV	Spansules: 8 and 12 mg	Children 6–12 yr: 8 mg A.M. or P.M.
(Cosea)	Alcon	Spansules: 8 and 12 mg	Children over 12 yr: 8 mg 2 times a day
(Histex)	Mallard	Sustained release capsules: 12 mg	
(Drize M)	Ascher	Sustained release capsules: 8 mg	
(Allerbid Tymcaps)	Amfre-Grant	Sustained release capsules: 8 mg	
Brompheniramine maleate			
(Dimetane)	Robins	Tablets: 4 mg Repeat action: 8 and 12 mg Elixir: 2 mg/5 mL Injection: 10 and 100 mg/mL	0.4 mg/kg per day in 3 or 4 divided doses Children over 6 yr: 2 mg 3 or 4 times a day

Table 137-2 Classification of Antihistamines *(continued)*

Drug (Generic and Trade Name)	Manufacturer	Preparations Available	Dosage
PIPERAZINES			
Cyclizine hydrochloride (Marezine)	Burroughs Wellcome	Tablets: 50 mg	3 mg/kg per day in 3 divided doses Children over 6 yr: 25 mg 3 or 4 times a day
PHENOTHIAZINES			
Promethiazine (Phenergan)	Wyeth	Tablets: 12.5 and 25 mg Syrup: 6.25 mg/5 mL Fortes syrup: 25 mg/5 mL Suppositories: 25 and 50 mg Injection: 25 and 50 mg/mL	2 mg/kg per day in 3 or 4 divided doses Children over 6 yr: 6.25 to 12.5 mg 3 times a day
(Lemprometh) (Remsed)	Lemmon Endo	Tablets: 25 and 50 mg	
MISCELLANEOUS			
Cyproheptadine hydrochloride (Periactin)	Merck, Sharp & Dohme	Tablets: 4 mg Syrup: 2 mg/5 mL	0.25 mg/kg per day in 3 or 4 divided doses Children over 6 yr: 4 mg 2 or 3 times a day not to exceed 16 mg/day; Periactin not used in newborn or premature infants
Hydroxyzine (Atarax)	Roerig	Tablets: 10, 25, 50, and 100 mg Syrup: 10 mg/5 mL	2 mg/kg per day in 3 or 4 divided doses Children over 6 yr: 50 to 100 mg in divided doses Children under 6 yr: 50 mg/day in divided doses
(Vistaril)	Pfizer	Capsules: 25, 50, and 100 mg Suspension: 25 mg/5 mL Injection: 25 and 50 mg/mL	

From Siegel, Sheldon C. Allergic rhinitis. In Gellis, S. S., and Kagan, B. M., *Current pediatric therapy 8.* Philadelphia, Saunders, 1978, pp. 677–678.

Table 137-3 Medical Referral/Consultation

Diagnosis	Clinical Manifestations	Management
Anaphylaxis	Mild local or generalized itching and/or burning of the skin Diaphoresis Apprehension Hives Flushing Mild cough Pallor Elevated blood pressure Nausea/vomiting Diarrhea Abdominal pain Chest tightness or pain Wheezing Rapid, weak pulse	Immediate referral to physician Initiation of treatment Epinephrine hydrochloride (adrenalin) 1:1000, 0.2–0.5 mL IM or SC into arm (opposite limb of where allergy shot given) Massage area Application of tourniquet above antigen injection site Injection of epinephrine hydrochloride 1:1000, 0.2 mL locally into the antigen injection site Lay client flat with feet elevated; keep client warm Injection of diphenhydramine hydrochloride 20–30 mg IM Blood pressure checked frequently Give oxygen, if needed

PART 4

communicable diseases

INTRODUCTION JANE A. FOX

I. Subjective Data

A. Age and sex
B. Reason for visit and description of problem
C. Onset
D. Known exposure
E. Associated symptoms
1. Rash
2. Pruritis
3. Fever
4. Conjunctivitis
5. Photophobia
6. Visual changes
7. Ear pain
8. Runny nose
9. Sore throat and/or difficulty swallowing
10. Slurred speech
11. Swollen glands
12. Stiff neck
13. Cough
14. Nausea, vomiting, and/or diarrhea
15. Abdominal pain
16. Testicular pain and/or swelling
17. Painful joints
18. Headache
19. Anorexia
20. Lethargy and/or malaise
21. Irritability
22. Weakness

F. Immunization history
G. Diet history: food and fluid intake in past 24 h
H. Current medications
I. Allergies
J. Chronic conditions
K. Family history
1. Recent illness
2. Immunization status
3. Chronic conditions

L. Social history, including school attendance

II. Objective Data

A. Physical examination
1. Temperature
2. Height and weight
3. General appearance
4. Inspection of skin
5. Palpation of lymph nodes for enlargement and tenderness
6. Fundoscopic examination
7. Inspection of mouth and pharynx
8. Otoscopic examination
9. Auscultation of heart for murmurs
10. Auscultation and percussion of lungs
11. Inspection, auscultation, percussion, and palpation of abdomen for masses and tenderness
12. Palpation of testes in postpubertal male for pain and swelling (when mumps suspected)
13. Neurological examination

B. Laboratory data
1. Usually none indicated
2. Serum antibody samples sometimes indicated to confirm diagnosis—collected as early as possible and repeated in 2 weeks

138 Roseola Infantum (Exanthem Subitum)

MARTHA FRISBY

ALERT

1. Convulsions
2. Lack of improvement within 3 days from initial temperature spike

I. Etiology: Thought To Be Viral; No Organism Isolated

II. Assessment

A. Subjective data

1. Age: 6 months to 3 years most common
2. Child's activity decreased
3. High temperature—103 to 105° F (39.4 to 40.5° C) in the afternoon
4. Rash, appearing as temperature returns to normal

B. Objective data

1. Generally very little hard data
2. Mild pharyngitis—one-third cases
3. Mild otitis media—one-fourth cases—generally not associated with significant pain
4. Lymphadenopathy
   a. Moderately firm, nontender, freely movable
   b. Not more than 0.5 to 1.5 cm
   c. Suboccipital, postcervical, postauricular
5. WBC
   a. First 24 to 36 h: leukocytosis (12,000 to 15,000), slight increase in neutrophils
   b. Second to third day: leukopenia with absolute neutropenia and relative lymphocytosis
   c. Within a week: normal, lymphocytosis possibly lasting longer
6. Rash
   a. Rose-pink
   b. Predominantly on the neck and trunk
   c. Discrete, small, often irregular in shape; small macules or maculopapules
   d. Fades on pressure
   e. Begins to fade shortly after appearance
   f. May persist 1 to 2 days

III. Management

A. Treatments/medications

1. Symptomatically prescribed
2. For lowering temperature
   a. Aspirin
   b. Acetaminophen
   c. Tepid sponge bath as needed until the temperature is below 102° F (38.9° C)

B. Counselling/prevention

1. Instruct parent(s) on medications and temperature control
2. Instruct parent(s) on progression of illness

C. Follow-up: none

D. Consultations/referrals: physician if convulsions (see Table 138-1)

Table 138-1 Convulsions in Roseola Infantum

Convulsions	Treatment
Tonic-clonic Short-duration Temperature-related	*Immediate* referral to physician Medications Aspirin Acetaminophen Phenobarbital Tepid sponge bath See Blackout Spells/Seizures, Chap. 79

bibliography

Berenberg, William, and Wright, Stanley. Roseola infantum (exanthem subitum). *New England Journal of Medicine*, **241**:253 (1949).

Berliner, Benjamin C. A physical sign useful in diagnosis of roseola infantum before the rash. *Pediatrics*, **25**:1034 (1960).

Clemmens, Harry H. Exanthem subitum (roseola infantum): Report of 80 cases. *Journal of Pediatrics*, **26**:66 (1945).

Juretic, M. Exanthema subitum: A review of 243 cases. *Helvetica Paediatrica Acta*, **18**:80–95 (1963).

Krupp, Marcus A., and Chatton, Milton. *Current medical diagnosis and treatment*. Los Altos, Calif.: Lange, 1979.

Yow, M. D. (chairman). *Report of the Committee on Infectious Diseases*. Evanston, Ill.: American Academy of Pediatrics, 1977.

139 Rubella (German Measles)

M. CONSTANCE SALERNO

I. Etiology: Rubella Virus

II. Assessment

A. Subjective data

1. History of exposure
2. Headache
3. Malaise
4. Tender, swollen suboccipital, postauricular, and cervical nodes
5. No rubella immunization

B. Objective data

1. Fever
2. Rash
   a. Maculopapular eruption beginning on face, progressing rapidly downward to trunk and extremities
   b. Rash subsiding within 3 days

III. Management

A. Treatments/medications

1. Supportive
2. Aspirin or acetaminophen for headache, malaise, or lymph node pain

B. Counselling/prevention

1. Live rubella virus vaccine recommended for boys and girls between age 15 months and puberty; affords long-term protection
2. Transmission by direct contact with nasopharyngeal secretions of infected person
3. Incubation period from 14 to 21 days
4. Communicable for from 7 days before to 5 days after appearance of rash
5. Highly contagious
6. Should be reported to local public health authority
7. Isolate only to protect susceptible pregnant women (see "Immunizations" in Chap. 9).

C. Follow-up: none

D. Consultations/referrals

1. Notify schoolteacher and/or school nurse
2. Physician referral for exposed pregnant woman

bibliography

Benenson, A. (ed.). *Control of communicable diseases in man* (12th ed.). Washington, D.C.: American Public Health Association, 1975, pp. 272–276.

Krugman, S., Ward, R., and Katz, S. L. *Infectious diseases in children* (6th ed.). St. Louis: Mosby, 1977, pp. 274–292.

Steigman, A. J. (ed.). *Report of the Committee on Infectious Diseases* (18th ed.). Evanston, Ill.: American Academy of Pediatrics, 1977, pp. 242–249.

140 Measles (Rubeola)

M. CONSTANCE SALERNO

1. Etiology: Measles Virus

II. Assessment

A. Subjective data

1. Exposure to measles
2. No measles immunization or inadequate immunization
3. Runny nose
4. Cough
5. Fever
6. Malaise
7. Rash
8. Anorexia

B. Objective data

1. Koplik spots appear 2 days before the rash and are pathognomonic (tiny white spots surrounded by a bright red halo on buccal membrane).
2. High fever.
3. Coryza, conjunctivitis, and cough.
4. Erythematous, maculopapular, discrete rash erupts on face and neck, over the trunk and extremities.
5. Rash appears 4 days after initial illness and begins to fade on the third day after appearance.
6. Generalized lymphadenopathy.

III. Management

A. Treatments/medications

1. Supportive
2. Cool environment
3. Acetaminophen or aspirin for fever
4. Fluids should be encouraged
5. Bed rest during acute phase
6. Subdued light if photophobia present
7. Isolation from onset of catarrhal stage through third day of rash

B. Counselling/prevention

1. Incubation period is from 10 to 12 days.
2. Period of communicability is from fifth day of incubation period through third day of rash.
3. Highly contagious until after the third day of the rash.
4. May return to school after fifth day of rash.
5. Confers life-long immunity.
6. All exposed susceptibles (i.e., those who have not had measles and who have not received live attenuated vaccine) should be protected with immune serum globulin.
7. Measles can be prevented by immunization.
8. Complications of measles are common and serious. Instruct parent(s) carefully regarding symptomatic management and recognition of the complications listed below.

C. Follow-up: if condition worsens, return visit

D. Consultations/referrals

1. Referral to physician
   a. Otitis media
   b. Pneumonia
   c. Encephalitis
2. Notification of school nurse and/or school teacher

bibliography

Grossman, M. Contagious diseases of childhood. In H. C. Shirkey (ed.), *Pediatric therapy* (5th ed.). St. Louis: Mosby, 1975, pp. 528–533.

Krugman, S., Ward, R., and Katz, S. L. *Infectious diseases in children* (6th ed.). St. Louis: Mosby, 1977, pp. 132–148.

Steigman, A. J. (ed.): *Report of the Committee on Infectious Diseases* (18th ed.). Evanston, Ill.: American Academy of Pediatrics, 1977, pp. 132–137.

141 Chickenpox (Varicella)

M. CONSTANCE SALERNO

ALERT
Immunologically compromised children

I. Etiology: Varicella-Zoster (V-Z) Virus

A. Primary infection: varicella
B. Reactivation of latent infection: herpes zoster

II. Assessment

A. Subjective data
1. History of exposure
2. Low-grade fever which increases proportionately to the severity of the eruption
3. Headache, malaise, and anorexia accompanying fever
4. Pruritis

B. Objective data
1. Simultaneous appearance of skin lesions in various stages of development; macule progresses rapidly to a papule, vesicle (teardrop on a rose petal), and finally to a crust or scab.
2. Lesions usually appear in crops on any area of body, with greatest concentration on the trunk.
3. Vesicles may appear on mucous membrane of mouth.
4. New lesions continue to appear for 5 to 6 days.

III. Management

A. Treatments/medications
1. Symptomatic
2. Acetaminophen or aspirin for pain
3. Calamine lotion to reduce pruritis

B. Counselling/prevention
1. Incubation period is 10 to 20 days.
2. Period of communicability is from 1 day before rash to 5 to 6 days after the last crop of vesicles.
3. Highly contagious until all lesions have crusted.
4. Exclude from school for 1 week after initial eruption and avoid exposure to infants and high-risk children.
5. Fingernails should be kept short and clean to minimize secondary bacterial infection caused by scratching.
6. Condition is spread chiefly by direct contact.
7. Confers life-long immunity, but reactivation of latent virus may cause herpes zoster.
8. Chickenpox may be prevented in exposed susceptible children by zoster immune globulin (ZIG) if given within 72 h of exposure. (ZIG is available in limited amounts from the Sidney Farber Cancer Institute, Division of Microbiology, 44 Benney St., Boston, Mass., telephone: 617–732–3121).

C. Follow-up
1. None
2. Return visit for systemic antibiotic therapy if secondary pyogenic infection occurs

D. Consultations/referrals
1. Immediate medical referral for exposed children who are at risk, such as children receiving immunosuppressive therapy, children with antibody-deficiency disease, and infants under 6 months
2. Notification of schoolteacher and/or school nurse

bibliography

Benenson, A. (ed.). *Control of communicable diseases in man* (12th ed.). American Public Health Association, Washington, D.C., 1975, pp. 69–71.

Hoole, A. J., Greenberg, R. A., and Pickard, C. G. (eds.). *Patient care guidelines for family nurse practitioners.* Boston: Little, Brown, 1976, pp. 324–327.

Grossman, M. Contagious diseases of childhood. In H. C. Shirkey (ed.), *Pediatric therapy* (5th ed.). St. Louis: Mosby, 1975, pp. 536–539.

Krugman, S., Ward, R., and Katz, S. L. *Infectious diseases in children* (6th ed.). St. Louis: Mosby, 1977, pp. 451–471.

Steigman, A. J. (ed.). *Report of the Committee on Infectious Diseases* (18th ed.). Evanston, Ill.: American Academy of Pediatrics, 1977, pp. 304–310.

142 Mumps (Epidemic Parotitis)

MARTHA FRISBY

ALERT
1. Nuchal rigidity
2. Change in level of consciousness
3. Ataxia of trunk or extremities
4. Lethargy and/or irritability
5. Abnormal eye movements
6. Slurred speech
7. Vomiting
8. Severe testicular pain and swelling
9. Signs of cerebellar ataxia

I. Etiology: Mumps Virus

II. Assessment

A. Parotid or salivary gland form (parotitis)

1. Subjective data
   - a. Exposure to mumps 14 to 21 days previously
   - b. Bilateral or unilateral painful swelling in front of the ears
   - c. Mild abdominal pain
   - d. Possibly mild respiratory symptoms
2. Objective data
   - a. Fever
   - b. Tender enlargement of the salivary glands affected
     - (1) Swelling aligned with the long axis of the ear and the ramus of the mandible, tapering on each side
     - (2) Submaxillary or sublingual gland swelling—glands possibly seem fused
   - c. Lymphedema of face possibly present (makes margins of swelling indistinct)
   - d. Obliteration of angle of mandible
   - e. Orifice of Stensen's duct possibly reddened and swollen
   - f. Relative lymphocytosis possibly present
   - g. Serum amylase possibly elevated
   - h. Fourfold rise in complement-fixing antibodies in paired serums—diagnostic
   - i. Isolated mumps virus from saliva, pharynx, or urine

B. Orchitis or oophoritis

1. Subjective data
   - a. Fever
   - b. Chills
   - c. Testicular pain and swelling (male)
   - d. Lower abdominal pain (female)
2. Objective data
   - a. Fever
   - b. Testicular pain and swelling on palpation
   - c. Lower abdominal pain on palpation

III. Management

A. Parotid or salivary gland form (parotitis)

1. Treatments/medications
   - a. Bed rest during the febrile period
   - b. Aspirin or acetaminophen for temperature or pain
   - c. Soft diet
   - d. Isolation until swelling subsides
2. Counselling/prevention
   - a. Observation for and prevention of further spread of mumps
     - (1) Spread by respiratory droplet
     - (2) Infectious 1 day prior to swelling until swelling subsides
     - (3) Incubation period 14 to 21 days
   - b. Vaccine for others in the family
     - (1) Cannot prevent infection in persons already exposed—takes 28 days to develop antibodies
     - (2) Particularly good for pubescent males

to avoid orchitis

c. Prevention through immunization of all children 15 months of age and older with live attenuated mumps virus vaccine

3. Follow-up: none
4. Consultations/referrals: school nurse

B. Orchitis

1. Treatments/medications
   a. Strict bed rest
   b. Scrotal support
   c. Ice to area
   d. Analgesic—aspirin or acetaminophen
2. Counselling/prevention
   a. Rarely results in sterility
   b. Unilateral in 75 percent of cases
   c. Subsides within 2 weeks
3. Follow-up: return visit within 1 week
4. Consultations/referrals
   a. Immediate referral to physician for severe swelling
   b. May require surgical intervention

C. Oophoritis

1. Treatments/medications
   a. Symptomatic only
   b. Aspirin (ASA) or acetaminophen for pain
2. Counselling/prevention
   a. Medication
   b. Progression of disease
3. Follow-up: return if symptoms worsen
4. Consultations/referrals: none necessary unless condition worsens—then to physician

Table 142-1 Medical Referral/Consultation

Diagnosis	Clinical Manifestations	Management
Meningoencephalitis	Lethargy Fever Nuchal rigidity, headache Nausea and vomiting Decreased level of consciousness Cerebrospinal fluid (CSF) Lymphocytic pleocytosis Elevated protein Normal glucose Signs of increased intracranial pressure	Immediate referral to physician Hospitalization possibly necessary See Preparation for Hospitalization, Part 7 Aseptic meningitis Bed rest Maintainance of fluid balance ASA or acetaminophen as necessary for pain or temperature Encephalitis Adequate ventilation Intracranial pressure to be decreased Symptomatic support
Pancreatitis	Epigastric pain Pain radiating to back Position of comfort upright and forward Nausea and persistent vomiting High fever Chills Prostration Increased serum amylase Leukocytosis	Immediate referral to physician Hospitalization possibly necessary See Preparation for Hospitalization, Part 7 Rest Gastric suction Electrolyte and fluid replacement Control of pain
Orchitis—severe	Severe pain Severe swelling of the testes Both pain and swelling uncontrolled by supportive treatment	Immediate referral to physician May require hospitalization See Preparation for Hospitalization, Part 7 May require referral to surgeon 1% procaine solution injected into spermatic cord at external inguinal ring (20–30 mL)—by physician *only*

Table 142-1 Medical Referral/Consultation *(continued)*

Diagnosis	Clinical Manifestations	Management
		Codeine 30 mg po q4h for pain—ordered by physician Hydrocortisone sodium succinate 100 mg IV followed by 20 mg po q6h for 2–3 days Incision of tunica
Cerebellar ataxia	Ataxia of trunk and extremities—possibly quite severe or mild Hypotonia and tremor of extremities possibly present Possible nystagmus or other abnormal eye movements Speech possibly affected Irritable Vomiting Sensory and reflex testing usually normal No signs of increased intracranial pressure CSF showing few lymphocytes	Immediate referral to physician May require hospitalization See Preparation for Hospitalization, Part 7 Supportive therapy Chlorpromazine if client is irritable or vomiting

bibliography

Gray, J. A. Mumps. *British Medical Journal*, **1**:338–340 (1973).

Kempe, Henry C., Silver, Henry K., and O'Brien, Donough. *Current pediatric diagnosis and treatment.* Los Altos, Calif.: Lange, 1978.

Krupp, Marcus A., and Chatton, Milton. *Current medical diagnosis and treatment.* Los Altos, Calif.: Lange, 1979.

Modlin, John F., Orenstien, Walter A., and Brandling-Bennett, A. David. Current status of mumps in the United States. *Journal of Infectious Diseases*, **132**:106–108 (1975).

Yow, M. D. (chairman). *Report of the Committee on Infectious Diseases* (18th ed.). Evanston, Ill.: American Academy of Pediatrics, 1977.

PART 5

conditions requiring long-term management

section 1

diseases

143 Hemophilia[1]

RACHEL FELDMAN FRANK

ALERT
1. Prolonged or inexplicable bleeding
2. A known hemophiliac with a history of major trauma

I. Etiology

A. Genetically transmitted absence or inactivity of 1 of the 12 clotting factors (see Genetic Evaluation, Chap. 3)

B. Different factors have different modes of inheritance:
1. Factors VIII and IX—sex-linked—most common
2. Von Willebrand's disease—autosomal dominant
3. Factors I, II, V, VII, X, XI, XII, and XIII—autosomal recessive

II. Subjective Data

A. Client with undiagnosed bleeding disorder
1. Bleeding history
   a. Circumcision
   b. Dental procedures
   c. Surgery
   d. Nosebleeds
   e. Abnormal sequelae following minor trauma
2. Family history
   a. Known hemophiliac relatives
   b. Family bleeding history
3. Social history
   a. Family's ability to cope with a chronic genetic illness
   b. Ability to cope with financial burden

[1]*Note:* This disease should be managed by a hematologist. The practitioner can be instrumental in early detection and long-term management.

B. Known hemophiliac
1. History of bleeding
   a. Onset
   b. Duration
   c. Pain
   d. Swelling
   e. Limitation of motion
2. Social impact of episode on client
   a. Absence from school or work
   b. Missed social events
   c. Financial implications
3. Impact of episode on family
   a. Financial burden
   b. Necessity for rearranging plans and commitments
   c. Attention of parent(s) diverted from other siblings and from each other

III. Objective Data

A. Physical examination
1. Complete physical examination for undiagnosed client
   a. Joint and muscle function
   b. Skin color
   c. Inspect, auscultate, palpate, and percuss abdomen for organomegaly and tenderness.
2. For a known hemophiliac
   a. Brief generalized examination
   b. Thorough investigation of site of bleeding for
      (1) Range of motion
      (2) Visible swelling
      (3) Localized tenderness
      (4) Compromised bodily functions related to site of bleeding, for example
         (a) Neurological impairment

(b) Gastrointestinal or genitourinary dysfunction

B. Laboratory data

1. Screening tests
   a. Complete blood count (CBC) with platelets, differential, and reticulocyte count
   b. Prothrombin time (PT) and partial thromboplastin time (PTT)
   c. Liver function studies—baseline
   d. Australian Antigen (AA)
   e. Blood type
2. Specific tests ordered after consultation with a hematologist
   a. Specific factor assays
   b. Bleeding time
   c. Ristocetin and aspirin studies
   d. X-rays of major joints

IV. Assessment

A. Subjective data

1. Positive bleeding history
2. Positive family history
3. Client's perception of pain or limitation related to bleeding site
   a. Tingling
   b. Weakness

B. Objective data

1. Findings while no bleeding is occurring
   a. Often no positive findings
   b. Joint deformities
   c. Loss of muscle mass or strength
   d. Laboratory findings
      (1) Normal CBC
      (2) Normal PT
      (3) Prolonged PTT in severe hemophilia; PTT possibly normal in mild cases
      (4) Liver function studies and AA possibly altered following exposure to repeated transfusions
      (5) Joint x-rays may show soft tissue and/or bony abnormalities at sites of repeated hemarthroses.
2. Findings during an episode related to the bleeding site
   a. Joints and muscles
      (1) Swelling
      (2) Limitation of motion
      (3) Splinting
   b. Head
      (1) Local swelling or bruise
      (2) Abnormal neurologic function
   c. Visible bleeding
      (1) Cuts and abrasions
      (2) Hematuria
      (3) Epistaxis
      (4) GI bleeding
      (5) Drop in hemoglobin or hematocrit indicating blood loss

V. Management

A. Treatments/medications

1. Prescribed only by physician
2. Almost always requires replacement therapy with appropriate factor concentrates
3. Joint and muscle bleeding
   a. Replacement therapy
   b. Immobilization followed by passive then active exercises
4. Head injuries
   a. Immediate physician contact
   b. Immediate replacement therapy to achieve 100 percent factor activity
5. Visible bleeding
   a. Cuts and abrasions often treatable by local measures alone
   b. Replacement therapy for all other types of visible bleeding
6. Lowered hemoglobin and hematocrit
   a. Arrest of bleeding
   b. Iron therapy for mild deficiency
   c. Blood transfusion for severe deficiency
7. Possible to use Amicar in place of or in conjunction with factor replacement therapy in certain instances such as dental procedures
   a. Used to prevent the breakdown of the clot once it is formed
   b. Not used when fast clot reabsorption is desired

B. Counselling/prevention

1. Education of client and family
   a. Nature of disease
   b. Treatment protocols
   c. Activities to be avoided and encouraged
   d. Home care (self-infusion) teaching when appropriate
2. Counselling of client and family
   a. Acceptance by family of a child with a genetic disease
      (1) Guilt versus blame
      (2) Altered marital, parent-child, and sibling relationships
   b. Recognition of common deviant behavior problems
      (1) Denial
      (2) Passive dependency
      (3) Overtly daredevil behavior
   c. Reinforcement of positive family interactions

3. Education of community
   a. Teachers and employers
   b. Physicians and nurses within the community

C. Follow-up

1. Encouragement of adherence to treatment protocols
2. Continuous availability to client and family in times of stress

D. Consultations/referrals

1. Immediate consultation with hematologist for
   a. Major trauma
   b. Head injuries
2. Orthopedic problems
   a. Physical therapy
   b. Orthopedist
3. Dental
   a. Routine care every 6 months
   b. Coordinated dental/hematology coverage for surgical procedures
4. Mental health personnel
   a. Social service
   b. Psychology/psychiatry
   c. Genetic counselling
5. Community agencies
   a. Hemophilia Foundation
   b. Vocational rehabilitation

bibliography

Jones, Peter. *Living with hemophilia.* Philadelphia: Davis, 1974.

Levine, Peter. Comprehensive health care clinic for hemophiliacs, *Archives of Internal Medicine* (July 1976).

Mouche, Jan. Comprehensive care of the hemophiliac 1978. *Infusion* (September–October 1978).

National Heart and Lung Institutes Blood Resource Studies. *Pilot study of hemophilia treatment in the United States.* Bethesda, MD: National Blood Resource Program, National Institute of Health, Department of Health, Education, and Welfare, 1972.

144 Cystic Fibrosis

LINDA MEYER DITE

This condition should be managed in collaboration with a physician. The treatment regimen should be initiated and periodically evaluated at a cystic fibrosis treatment center.

ALERT
1. Chronic cough
2. Recurrent pneumonia
3. Heat intolerance
4. Failure to thrive
5. Bulky, shiny, foamy, smelly stools
6. Voracious appetite
7. Rectal prolapse
8. Hemorrhagic disease of the newborn

I. Etiology

A. Genetic: Mendelian recessive

B. Abnormal function of exocrine glands

II. Subjective Data—Complete History with Special Attention to

A. Birth history

B. Past health history
1. Review of symptoms
2. Developmental history
3. Allergies
4. Immunizations
5. Frequency of previous digestive or respiratory illnesses

C. Family history
1. Family members known to have cystic fibrosis
2. Children or young adults with chronic obstructive lung disease, severe asthma, etc., in family
3. Infant deaths due to pneumonia, dehydration, unknown causes, etc., in family

D. Social history
1. Educational
2. Economic
   a. Eligibility for county, state, or federal aid
   b. Insurance
   c. Income
   d. Other resources or debts

E. Family's knowledge and understanding of disease: interview of child and family individually, then together (see Family Assessment, Chap. 1)
1. Previously acquired information
2. Previous experiences (undiagnosed or misdiagnosed)
3. Support systems
4. Expectations
   a. Effect cystic fibrosis will have on daily life
   b. Prognosis
   c. Health care system
5. Personal feelings and values of child and family members

III. Objective Data

A. Physical examination
1. Complete physical examination
2. Height and weight plotted on growth chart

B. Laboratory data
1. Ordered by practitioner
   a. Sweat test(s)
   b. Chest x-ray
   c. TB testing
   d. Sputum culture and sensitivity
   e. Complete blood count (CBC) with differential and immunodiffusion
   f. Routine urinalysis

2. Ordered after consultation with a physician
   a. Pulmonary function tests
   b. Stools for trypsin
   c. Duodenal aspiration for trypsin levels

C. Family assessment
1. Level of, and ability in understanding of disease process
2. Child and family's developmental and emotional status
3. Present stage in long-term grieving process

IV. Assessment

A. Subjective data
1. Recurrent colds or respiratory infections
2. Chronic cough, dyspnea, hemoptysis
3. Recurrent pneumonia or pneumonia in first year of life (right upper lobe or right middle lobe atelectasis)
4. Unusually frequent, foul-smelling flatus or bulky, foamy, oily, foul-smelling stools
5. Meconium ileus or intestinal obstruction
6. Poor weight gain despite voracious appetite
7. Salty taste to skin, heat intolerance, dehydration
8. Prolonged neonatal jaundice
9. Nasal polyps, sinusitis
10. Hemorrhagic disease of the newborn
11. Rectal prolapse
12. Abdominal distention
13. Decreased exercise tolerance

B. Objective data
1. Physical examination
   a. Poorly nourished appearance
   b. Digital clubbing
   c. Barrel chest
   d. Cyanosis, jaundice, edema, visible salt crystals on skin
   e. Productive and/or spasmotic cough; cough causing cyanosis or vomiting
   f. Abdominal distention
   g. Hepatosplenomegaly
   h. Inguinal hernia
   i. Poorly developed secondary sex characteristics, undescended testicles
   j. Respiratory infection, hemoptysis
   k. Salty taste to skin
   l. Nasal polyps, sinusitis
   m. Hemorrhagic disease of the newborn
   n. Rectal prolapse
2. Laboratory data
   a. Borderline or positive sweat test (iontophoresis)
      (1) Borderline: 40 to 60 meq/L sodium, potassium, chloride. Repeat test several times (if normal, but history strongly suggestive, also repeat several times.)
      (2) Positive sweat test is greater than 60 meq/L.
      (3) Test is unreliable if insufficient amount of sweat is collected, client is acutely ill, and with certain endocrine disorders.
      (4) Sweat test is positive in 99 percent of all cystic fibrosis clients.
   b. Increased markings, atelectasis, collapse, or pneumothorax, on chest X-ray
   c. Normal immunodiffusion
   d. Decreased pulmonary function
   e. Stools with golden yellow droplets or decreased trypsin levels
   f. Decreased trypsin levels on duodenal aspiration

V. Management

A. Treatments/medications
1. Postural drainage (see Figs. 144–1 to 144–10) and breathing exercises to maintain pulmonary hygiene (mist tent therapy and inhalations almost entirely abandoned)
2. Normal carbohydrate, high-protein, low-fat diet with liberal use of salt (except when cor pulmonale exists)
3. Environmental considerations should include air temperature of 68°F, air conditioning, light to moderate clothing, and reduced stresses, e.g., heat, pollution, etc.
4. Surgical intervention for repeated lung collapse or intestinal obstruction
5. Bronchoscopy for hemoptysis
6. Vitamins A, D, E, K
7. Pancreatic extracts, e.g., Viokase, Cotazym, or pancreatin
8. Antibiotics (see Table 144–1).
9. Other medications, e.g., mucolytics, anabolic steroids, flu vaccine
10. Routine immunizations especially measles and diphtheria-pertussis-tetanus
11. Antihistamines and cough suppressants contraindicated because coughing serves to remove mucus

B. Counselling/prevention
1. Practitioner should examine personal values and feelings about genetic diseases, chronic illness, and death. Plan how to avoid placing personal values on family.
2. Amount of information presented should be individually planned after family assessment and physical assessment of client's present condition.

3. Genetic counselling: Cystic fibrosis is the most common lethal genetic disease in the Caucasian population, affecting approximately 1:1500 live births. It is 5 times more common in the overall United States population than the next most common genetic disease, sickle cell anemia. Of the Caucasian population 3 to 5 percent carry the gene for cystic fibrosis. It is presently impossible to determine the carrier state or if a fetus is affected. There is a 25 percent chance of producing a child with cystic fibrosis *with each pregnancy.* Both sexes are affected equally. Approximately 2 percent of all diagnosed cystic fibrosis clients are black. The incidence in the Mongolian race is approximately 1:90,000.
4. Prognosis
   a. Cystic fibrosis can be difficult to diagnose. The onset of recognizable symptoms can occur at any time between birth and adolescence. All accurately diagnosed cases of meconium ileus have cystic fibrosis, with few exceptions. Approximately 10 percent of all cystic fibrosis clients have meconium ileus at birth and may have a more serious disease process. The disease is manifested in a variety of ways (pulmonary, GI, or both), and in varying degrees of severity. Cystic fibrosis is a progressive disease, the median survival age being 17.2 years. Death is usually due to blockage of the bronchial tree with infected mucus causing eventual respiratory failure and/or cor pulmonale secondary to chronic hypoxia.
   b. Early diagnosis brings earlier treatment to slow the progression of the disease process; however, it may also mean the symptoms are more severe, making them more recognizable, and indicating the disease process is more severe.
5. Additional concerns
   a. In 85 percent of all cystic fibrosis clients there are little or no pancreatic enzymes. In spite of a good or voracious appetite, these people have impaired digestion and malabsorption and lose fat-soluble vitamins.
   b. Sugar intolerance or blockage of intrahepatic bile ducts yielding biliary cirrhosis can be an additional complication. The gallbladder and submaxillary glands can also be involved. The disease process may become more complicated in females at or during puberty and in pregnancy.
   c. Most males are sterile due to arrested development of the vas deferens, epididymis, and seminal vesicle. Although females have no specific abnormality, they do have an increased difficulty with conception due to scant viscous mucus in the cervix.
6. Practitioner responsibilities
   a. Support—ongoing, especially at the prediagnostic stage, the diagnostic phase, during hospitalizations, at the terminal stage, at death, and after death as well as at normal stress periods, e.g., entering school
   b. Education of client and family, significant others, e.g., grandparents, baby-sitters, etc., the community, school personnel, employers, neighbors, and community health agencies
   c. Counsellor
   d. Providing anticipatory guidance, e.g., regarding peer relationships, expectations for self, and educational and career goals
   e. Client and family advocate
   f. Coordinator of the health care team
   g. Education of the public
7. Issues of particular concern to families
   a. Parents—guilt and blame, fear of unknown, fear of inability to care for child, fear of loss and death, and social isolation
   b. Client—interference with daily activities, parental overprotectiveness, lack of independence, and body image
   c. Role of practitioner—encouraging normal activity to the extent physical condition permits, providing hope and encouragement to keep up with demands of treatment regimen, dealing with fear of death, and helping families to keep cystic fibrosis as a part of their lives but not the center of it
8. Additional supports
   a. Introduction of new families to other families with cystic fibrosis child
   b. Additional psychological counselling for families, particularly when death seems imminent and then does not occur on repeated hospital admissions
   c. Group counselling for clients and parents

C. Follow-up

1. Close telephone contact
2. Return visits as determined by physician and as needed for counselling
3. Home visit after initial diagnosis to determine if environment suitable to carry out treatment

regimen; additional home visits possibly indicated after hospitalizations and to teach various procedures to family members or other care givers

4. If client should die, contact maintained with family to help them readjust their life-style and regain independence

D. Consultations/referrals

1. Cystic Fibrosis Foundation
   National Headquarters
   6000 Executive Boulevard, Suite 309
   Rockville, Maryland 20852
   a. Information for clients, families, teachers, and professionals
   b. List of cystic fibrosis treatment centers
   c. Fund raising—research, program development
   d. Financial resources available to cystic fibrosis clients for education, etc.
2. Various medical and surgical specialists as indicated by client's presenting problem
3. Public health nurse
4. Vocational and educational guidance
5. Ongoing communication with health team at nearest cystic fibrosis treatment center.
6. Notification of school nurse and classroom teacher
7. Genetic counselling
8. Employer, if client desires

Table 144-1 Antibiotics

Usual Organisms	Antibiotics
Staphylococcus aureus	Semisynthetic penicillins, cephalosporins—PO Methicillin, cephalosporins—IV
Hemophilus influenzae	Gantrisin, cephalosporins—PO
Escherichia coli *Bacillus proteus* *Klebsiella*	Cephalosporins, aminoglycosides, carbenicillin, ticarcillin—IV
Pseudomonas (most troublesome organism; usually in later disease stages, but can occur at any age)	Aminoglycosides—IV: gentamicin, tobramycin, amikacin Coly-Mycin or colistin Carbenicillin Ticarcillin

POSTURAL DRAINAGE

A person should be carefully trained in the technique before performing postural drainage.

Postural drainage, or segmental bronchial drainage, involves the utilization of gravity and physical maneuvers (vibrating and clapping) to stimulate the movement of accumulated mucus. Movement of secretions and coughing assist in relieving airway obstruction (Figs. 144–1 to 144–10).

Postural drainage should be performed with regard to the needs or constraints of the child's physical condition. A schedule of 2 or 3 times a day, with 2 min of clapping per position, can be a general guideline.

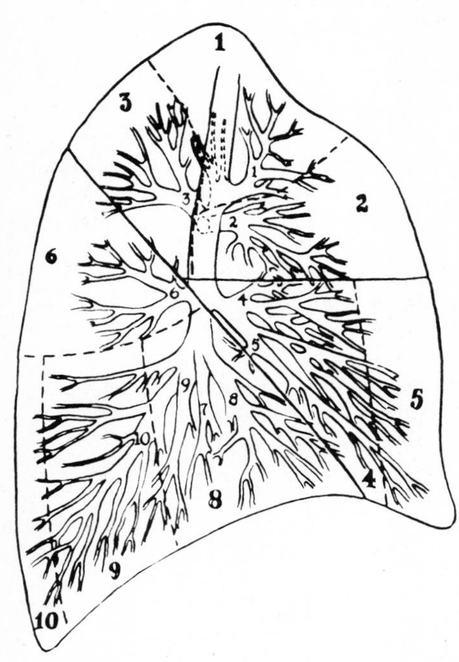

Name/Locations	Number/Key
RIGHT UPPER LOBE	
Apical	1
Anterior	2
Posterior	3
RIGHT MIDDLE LOBE	
Lateral	4
Medial	5
RIGHT LOWER LOBE	
Superior	6
Medial	7
Anterior Basal	8
Lateral Basal	9
Posterior Basal	10
LEFT UPPER LOBE	
Apical-Posterior	1-3
Anterior	2
Lingula	
Superior	4
Inferior	5
LEFT LOWER LOBE	
Superior	6
Anteriomedial Basal	7-8
Lateral Basal	9
Posterior Basal	10

Figure 144-1 Bronchopulmonary segments. For each position the segment and the airway leading to it are identified by the same number. The numbers show which area of the chest surface should be clapped to assist gravity in the drainage of secretions. Figures 144-2 through 144-10 show the various positions to use for drainage of particular segments. *(Figures taken from Cystic Fibrosis Foundation. Segmental bronchial drainage for CF patients. Used with permission.)*

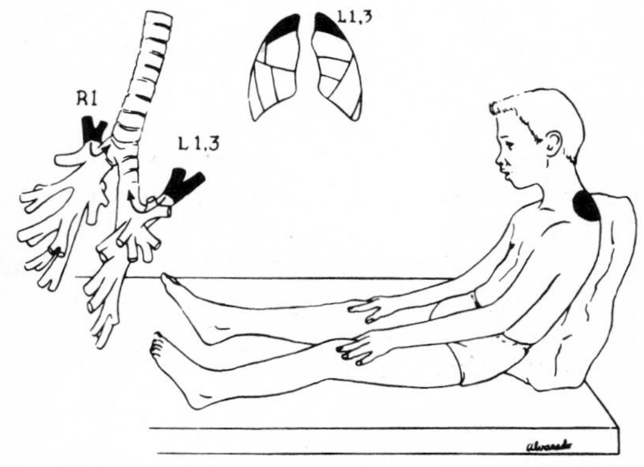

Figure 144-2 Upper lobes: apical segment. Client sits on the bed or drainage table, which is in a flat position, and is leaned back on a pillow at a 30° angle against the care giver. The care giver claps with a cupped hand over the area between the clavicle (collarbone) and scapula (shoulder blade) on each side. The area for clapping shown is the apical-posterior segment of the left upper lobe, L-1-3. The apical segment of the right upper lobe, R-1, is drained by the same position, with clapping on the right side.

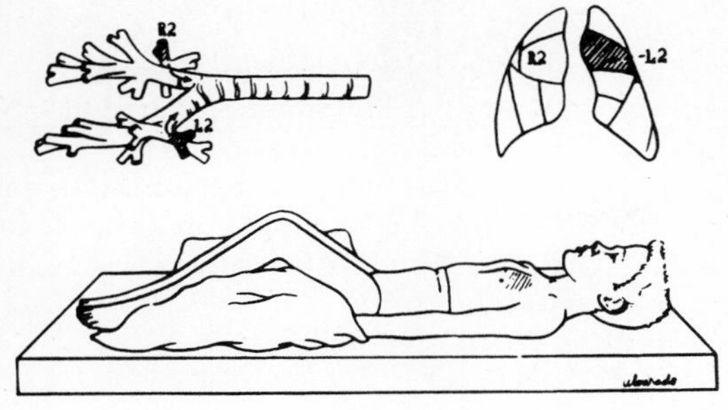

Figure 144-3 Upper lobes: anterior segments. The client lies on his or her back on the bed or drainage table, which is in a flat position. The care giver claps between the clavicle and nipple on each side. The area for clapping shown is the anterior segment of the left upper lobe, L-2.

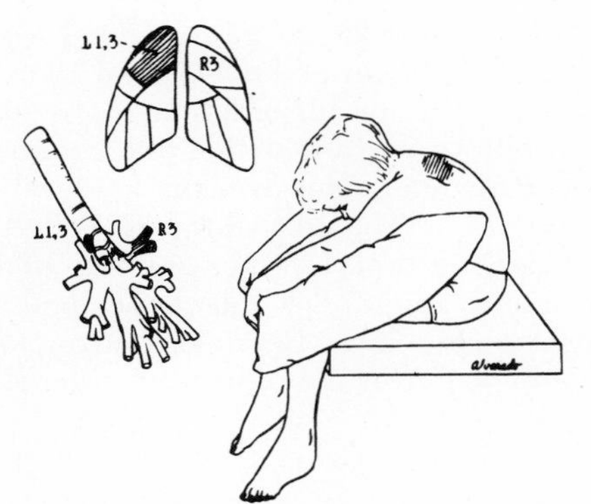

Figure 144-4 Upper lobes: posterior segment, right; apical-posterior segments, left. The client sits on the bed or drainage table, which is in a flat position, and leans forward over a folded pillow at a 30° angle. The care giver stands behind and claps over the upper back on both sides. The area for clapping shown is for the apical-posterior segment of the left upper lobe, L-1-3. The posterior segment of the right upper lobe, R-3, is drained in the same position with clapping on the right side of the chest.

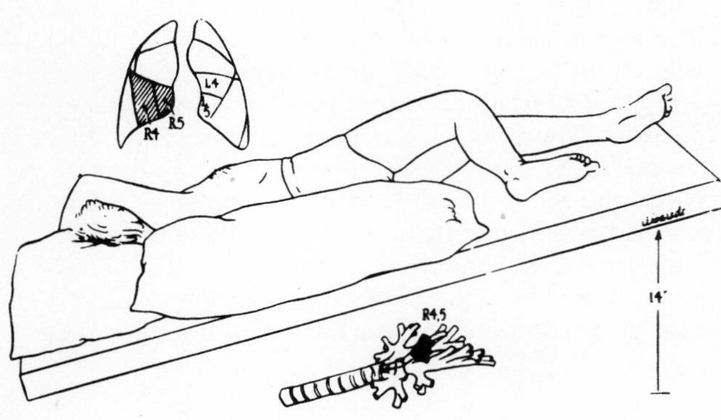

Figure 144-5 Right middle lobe: lateral segment, medial segment. The foot of the table or bed is elevated 14 in (about 15°). The client lies head down on the left side and rotates one quarter turn backward. A pillow may be placed behind the client (from shoulder to hip). Knees should be flexed. The care giver claps over the right nipple. In female clients with breast development or tenderness, a cupped hand should be used with heel of hand under the axilla (armpit) and fingers extending forward beneath breast. Area shown is the right middle lobe, R-4-5.

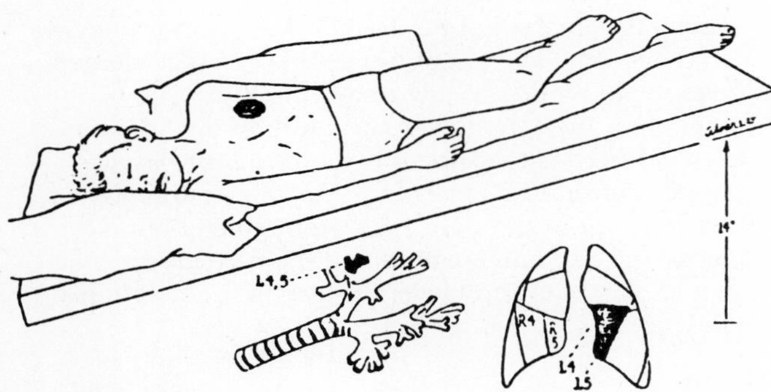

Figure 144-6 Left upper lobe: lingular segment—superior segment, inferior segment. The lingular segment of the left upper lobe, L-4-5, is drained by placing the client in the same head-down position except that he or she lies on the right side and rotates one quarter turn backward. The care giver claps over the left nipple.

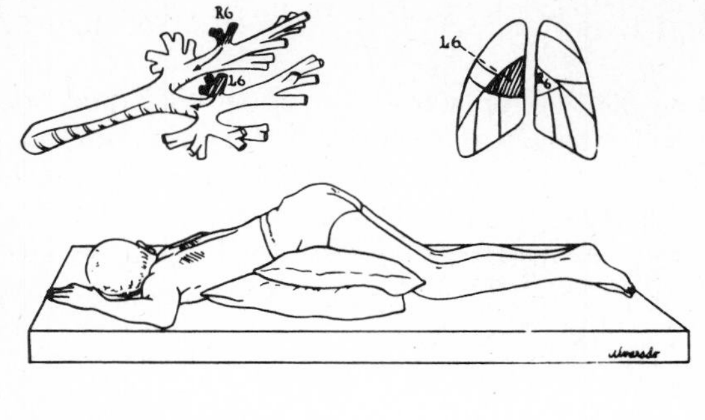

Figure 144-7 Lower lobes: superior segments. Client lies on his or her abdomen on a bed or table, which is in a flat position, with two pillows under the hips. The care giver claps over the middle part of the back at the tip of the scapula on either side of the spine. The area shown is the superior segment of the left lower lobe, L-6.

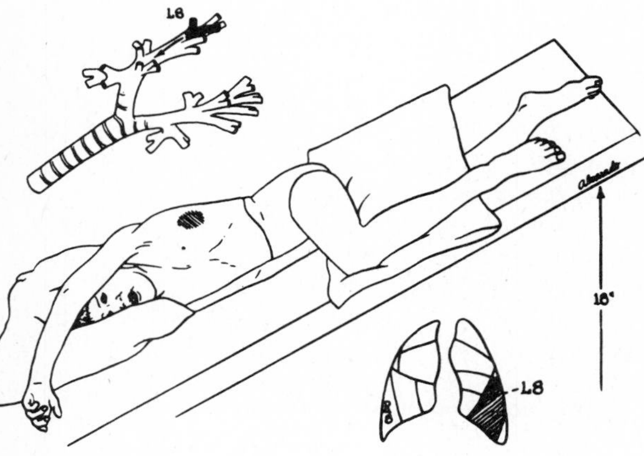

Figure 144-8 Lower lobes: anterior basal segments. The foot of the table or bed is elevated 18 in (about 30°). The client lies on his or her side at a 90° angle in the head-down position with a pillow under one knee. The care giver claps over the lower ribs just beneath the axilla. The area shown is the left anterior basal segment, L-8. For drainage of the right anterior basal segment, R-8, the client should lie on his or her left side in the same position and the care giver should clap over the right side of the chest.

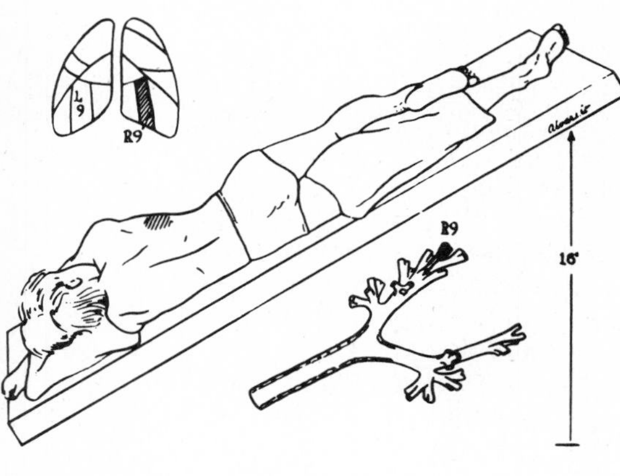

Figure 144-9 Lower lobes: lateral basal segments. The foot of the table is elevated 18 in (about 30°). The client lies on his or her abdomen, head down, and rotates one quarter turn upward from a prone position. The upper leg is flexed over a pillow for support. The care giver claps over the uppermost portion of the lower ribs. The area shown is the right lateral basal segment, R-9. For drainage of the left lateral basal segment, L-9, the client should lie on his or her right side in the same position and the care giver should clap over the left side of the chest.

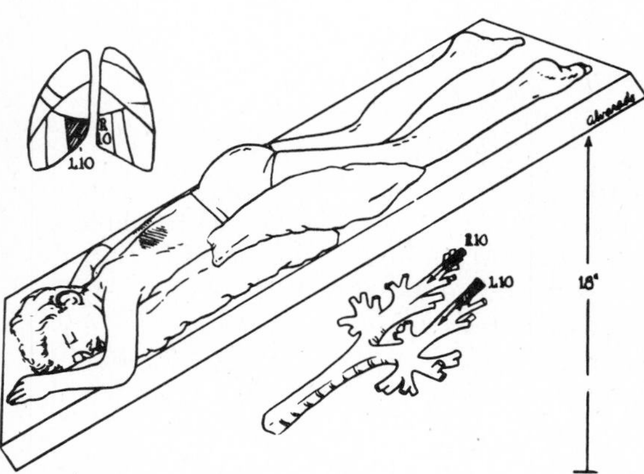

Figure 144-10 Lower lobes: posterior basal segments. The foot of the bed or table is elevated 18 in (about 30°). The client lies on his or her abdomen, head down, with a pillow under the hips. The care giver claps over the lower ribs close to the spine on each side. The area shown is the posterior basal segment of the left lower lobe, L-10. For drainage of this segment of the right lower lobe, the client is placed in the same position and the care giver should clap over the lower ribs on the right side of the chest.

Clapping Cup hand on chest wall over segment to be drained. Hand should conform to chest wall and trap a cushion of air to soften the blow of clapping.

Vibration Press flattened hand firmly on chest wall over segment to be drained. Tense upper arm and shoulder as in isometric contractions. Perform only during exhalation. Client should exhale as slowly and completely as possible saying "fff" or "sss."

Deep breathing Deep inhalation with forced, but not strained, exhalation.

Assisted coughing Support sides of lower chest to decrease strain and increase effectiveness of coughing.

bibliography

Burton, Lindy. *Family life of sick children: A study of families coping with chronic childhood disease.* Boston: Routledge, 1975.

Crozier, D. N. Cystic fibrosis: A not-so-fatal disease, *Pediatric Clinics of North America,* **21**(4):935–950 (1974).

Ingram, Carol. Of service to families with children having cystic fibrosis. In Hall and Weaver (eds.), *Nursing of families in crisis.* Philadelphia: Lippincott, 1974, pp. 205–215

McCollum, Audrey, and Gibson, Lewis E. Family adaptation to the child with cystic fibrosis. *The Journal of Pediatrics,* **77**(4):571–578 (1970).

National Cystic Fibrosis Research Foundation. *Guide to drug therapy in patients with cystic fibrosis.* Atlanta, National Cystic Fibrosis Research Foundation, 1974.

Patterson, Paul K., Denning, Carolyn R., and Kutscher, Austin (eds.). *Psychosocial aspects of cystic fibrosis: A model for chronic lung disease.* New York: Foundation of Thanatology, 1973.

Selekman, Janice. Cystic fibrosis: What is involved in the home treatment program for these children, adolescents, and young adults? *Pediatric Nursing,* March/April: 32–35 (1977).

Steele, Shirley (ed.). *Nursing care of the child with long-term illness.* New York: Appleton-Century-Crofts, 1971.

Tropault, A., Franz, M. and Dilgard, V. Psychological aspects of the care of children with cystic fibrosis. *American Journal of Diseases of Children,* **119**:424–432 (1970).

145 Acute Rheumatic Fever

ILENE BURSON GOTTESFELD

ALERT
1. Child under 6 years old
2. Past history of acute rheumatic fever (ARF)
3. Recent past history of untreated or inadequately treated streptococcal infection

I. Etiology: Group A Beta-Hemolytic Streptococci

II. Subjective Data
A. Onset/age
B. Associated symptoms
   1. Chest pain
   2. Anorexia
   3. Joint pain
   4. Fever
   5. Chorea
C. Recent history
   1. Upper respiratory infection
   2. Sore throat
   3. Otitis media
   4. Exposure to strep infection
   5. Sinusitis with or without epistaxis
D. Medications
E. Allergies
F. Immunization history
G. Family history of rheumatic fever and/or rheumatic heart disease, recent illnesses, and allergies
H. Social history—to determine living conditions and ability of family to comply with treatment regimen

Note: Any client in whom acute rheumatic fever (ARF) is suspected should be referred immediately to a physician.

III. Objective Data
A. Physical examination
   1. Perform complete physical examination.
   2. Take temperature.
   3. Carefully palpate cervical nodes for tenderness or swelling.
   4. Carefully inspect nails in infant for excoriation.
   5. Auscultation of lungs and heart sounds should be given special attention.
   6. Inspect skin for rashes.
   7. Palpate wrists, knees, elbows, and spinous processes of thoracic and lumbar vertebrae for nodules.
   8. Observe movements of extremities.
B. Laboratory data
   1. ECG
   2. Antistreptolysin-O titer (ASLO)
   3. Complete blood count (CBC) with white blood cell differential
   4. ESR (erythrocyte sedimentation rate)
   5. C-reactive protein (CRP)
   6. Chest x-ray posterior-anterior (PA) and lateral
   7. Echocardiogram by physician
   8. Throat culture

IV. Assessment
The clinical diagnosis of ARF is based on the Jones criteria. There must be two major or one major and two minor manifestations plus an antecedent streptococcal infection in order to make the diagnosis more definitive.

A. Jones criteria
   1. Major manifestations
      a. Carditis

b. Polyarthritis
c. Chorea
d. Erythema marginatum
e. Subcutaneous nodules

2. Minor manifestations
   a. Clinical
      (1) History of previous rheumatic fever
      (2) Evidence of preexisting rheumatic heart disease
      (3) Arthralgia
      (4) Fever
   b. Laboratory
      (1) Electrocardiogram—prolonged P-R interval
      (2) Increased ASLO greater than 333; rises 1 to 2 weeks after infection
      (3) Increased erythocyte sedimentation rate (ESR)
   c. Other tests not in Jones criteria
      (1) Throat culture positive for group A beta-hemolytic streptococci
      (2) Elevated ESR—higher with anemia, lower with conjestive heart failure
      (3) CRP positive

V. Management

A. Treatments/medications

1. Alternatives in universal treatment for eradication of streptococcal infection (choose one)
   a. Benzathine penicillin G: single dose of 600,000 U IM for child under 10 years; 900,000 U for child older than 10 years
   b. Aqueous procaine penicillin: 600,000 U IM daily for 10 days
   c. Procaine penicillin with aluminum monostearate in vial: 300,000 U IM every 3 days repeated 3 times in child under 10 years and 600,000 U in older child
   d. Oral penicillin G: 250,000 U 3 times daily for 10 days
   e. AP Bicillin: 900,000 to 1.2 million U IM in single dose
   f. If penicillin allergy exists
      (1) Erythromycin: 50 mg/kg per day for 10 days
      (2) Lincomycin: 25 to 50 mg/kg per day for 10 days
      (3) Cephalothin: 50 mg/kg per day IM
   g. Antistreptococcal prophylaxis
      (1) Initiated immediately after diagnosis
      (2) Medication alternatives
         (a) Benzathine penicillin G: 1.2 million U monthly IM
         (b) Oral penicillin: 400,000 U 2 times a day
         (c) Gantrisin or sulfadiazine: 0.5 g 2 times a day
         (d) Erythromycin: 100 mg orally 2 times daily if allergic to penicillin

B. Counselling/prevention

1. Contact with individuals known to have intercurrent strep infection to be avoided
2. Parent(s) and child instructed in medication administration and antistreptococcal prophylaxis
3. Compliance with treatment protocol assessed and emphasized

C. Follow-up

1. Repeat throat culture 1 week after treatment initiated; monthly for 2 to 4 months
2. Return visit in 1 week, sooner if other symptoms develop

D. Consultations/referrals

1. School nurse to be informed
2. Public health nurse visit to evaluate compliance with treatment regimen
3. Physician, if other symptoms are present
4. Dentist to be informed of subacute bacterial endocarditis prophylaxis prior to extractions or deep cavity drilling

Table 145-1 Medical Referral/Consultation

Diagnosis	Clinical Manifestations	Management
Carditis	Usually developing 2 weeks after onset of disease Pallor Anorexia Easy fatigue Shortness of breath Chest pains	Referral to physician and/or cardiologist Treatment dependent upon severity Bed rest Modified activity Acetylsalicylic acid and prednisone Fluid restriction Counselling Involvement of client and parent(s) in therapy

Table 145-1 Medical Referral/Consultation *(continued)*

Diagnosis	Clinical Manifestations	Management
	Associated symptoms Cough Diaphoresis Abdominal pain/discomfort Low-grade fever Rapid, sweeping pulse Signs of congestive heart failure Puffiness of face—periorbital edema Sacral edema (infant) Hepatomegaly Absence of prior organic heart disease	Topics of education Rheumatic fever and heart disease Medications and side effects Need to prevent respiratory infection Importance of prophylaxis penicillin during dental procedure or minor surgery Penicillin prophylaxis; parental benzathine penicillin G 1–2 million U/month for minimum of 5 years Advising in assessment of appropriateness of future plans and lifestyle with respect to prognosis Regular weekly follow-up Informing of school nurse and referral to public health nurse for home evaluation, compliance, support
Polyarthritis	Severe joint pain—usually two or more large joints (ankles, knees, elbows, wrists) Limitation of movement Joint pain migratory Hot, red, swollen joint or joints identified Duration of joint involvement 1–5 days per joint Surrounding muscles in spasm Total joint involvement for 2–4 weeks Aspiration of joint yielding clear, serous, sterile, high-protein fluid	Referral to physician and/or cardiologist Treatment Bed rest Modified activity Acetylsalicylic acid Wet compresses to affected joint Provision of adequate joint support to affected limb Counselling/prevention Rheumatic fever prophylaxis Instruction of client and parent(s) Observation for any bruising Necessity of seeking treatment quickly for suspected tonsillitis Throat cultures for all family members All positive cultures to be treated Weekly visits and lab tests until asymptomatic Notification of school nurse and referral to public health nurse
Chorea (Sydenham's, St. Vitus' dance)	Emotional instability Confusion Irritability Insomnia Nervousness Frequent dropping of things Common in girls 7–14 years old Incoordinant movements of face, trunk, extremities Poor hand-eye coordination—finger to nose test	Referral to physician and/or cardiologist Treatments/medications Antistreptococcal prophylaxis Usually self-limited—not significant enough to treat Bed rest Drugs for sedation: phenobarbital, chlorpromazine, or valium Counselling/prevention Assuring family that this is transient Encouragement of rest and independent functioning when possible Follow-up as needed for rheumatic fever

Table 145-1 Medical Referral/Consultation *(continued)*

Diagnosis	Clinical Manifestations	Management
	Gait and/or speech possibly impaired Muscle strength diminished Diffuse ECG change Diagnosis possible by having client count fast	Informing school nurse and teacher in the event of possible communication problems Referral to public health nurse
Subcutaneous nodules	Found most commonly in severe carditis Duration several weeks to months Symmetrical, clustered, or singular nodules—attached loosely to joint capsules and tendon sheaths on periosteum Freely moveable under skin Painless Commonly found over scalp, joints, and vertebrae Size varies from that of a pea to an almond Palpable and visible in indirect light	Referral to physician and/or cardiologist See V., Management, in this chapter
Erythema marginatum	Transient rash over trunk, inner aspects of arms, thighs, not face; no itching Accentuated by heat Pink, raised macules with sharp margin and normal center Typical pattern of wavy, thin red line surrounding an area of intact skin about 1–2 cm in size	Referral to physician and/or cardiologist See V., Management, in this chapter

bibliography

Jones criteria (rev.). New York: American Heart Association, 1967.

Markowitz, M., and Kuttner, A. G. *Rheumatic fever: Major problems in clinical pediatrics.* Philadelphia: Saunders, 1967.

Markowitz, M. Eradication of rheumatic fever: an unfulfilled hope. *Circulation,* **41:**1077 (1970).

Markowitz, M., and Gordis, L. *Rheumatic fever.* Philadelphia: Saunders, 1972.

Nadas, Alexander, and Filer, Donald C. *Pediatric cardiology* (3rd ed.). Philadelphia: Saunders, 1972.

146 Congenital Heart Defects[1]

ELEANOR RUDICK

ALERT (See Table 146-1)

A. Infant

1. Paroxysmal tachypnea (hypoxic spells)
2. Syncope
3. Hemiplegia, convulsions
4. Cardiac failure
   a. Tachycardia
   b. Enlargement of the liver
   c. Rapid respiration
   d. Prominent third heart sound
   e. Rales (usually late symptom)
   f. Pitting edema (late manifestation)

B. Older Child Requiring Immediate Evaluation

1. Shortness of breath
2. Decreased exercise tolerance
3. Cyanosis
4. Abnormalities of heart rate or rhythm
5. Cardiac enlargement
6. Long systolic murmur
7. Any diastolic murmur
8. Changing cardiac murmurs or heart sounds
9. Cardiac failure
10. Hypertension
11. Retardation of growth/development
12. Progression of any signs or symptoms

I. Etiology

A. Unknown in most instances

B. Multifactorial inheritance hypothesis

C. Environmental influences during pregnancy—infection, drugs, radiation; more likely in mothers 40 to 44 years of age; incidence apparently higher in clients living in high altitudes

II. Subjective Data (A complete history is needed if not previously recorded.)

A. Prenatal history

B. Birth history

C. Neonatal problems

D. Infancy

1. Tachypnea—at feeding times
2. Fatigability
3. Failure to gain weight
4. Increased sweating
5. Developmental milestones (delayed)

E. Older child

1. Developmental history
2. Exercise tolerance
   a. Need for frequent rest
   b. Kind of play
3. Dyspnea on exertion
4. History of rheumatic fever

F. Family history

1. History of congenital cardiac disease
2. History of rheumatic fever

G. Social history

1. Family constellation
2. Living conditions
3. Economic status and supportive others—to determine ability to cope with long-term problem, possibly life-threatening condition

III. Objective Data

A. Complete physical examination

B. Laboratory data

1. Complete blood count (CBC)
2. Urinalysis

[1]Any child suspected of having a congenital heart defect should be referred to a pediatrician or cardiologist *immediately*.

3. Hemoglobin
4. Hematocrit
5. Chest x-rays—anterior-posterior (AP) and lateral
6. Electrocardiogram (ECG)

IV. Assessment of Cardiac Status (see Table 146-1)

V. Management

A. Treatments/medications

1. Depending on nature and severity of lesion, and the age of the child, a program is prescribed by the physician.
2. For operable lesions, surgery may be postponed until infant is older.
3. Hospitalization may be necessary for treatment and diagnostic procedures (phonocardiography, cardiac catheterization).

B. Counselling/prevention

1. Counsel parent(s) about the following:
   a. The lesion—hemodynamics
   b. Medication
   c. Need for careful supervision
   d. Nutritional needs and special aids for feeding
2. Instruct parent(s) to observe infant for signs of impending failure.
   a. Easy fatigability
   b. Poor weight gain
   c. Development of or increase in cyanosis
   d. Tachypnea
   e. Increased sweating and hypoxic spells (due to decreased pulmonary blood flow)
   f. Knee-chest position
3. When time for surgery is determined, prepare for hospitalization and surgery.
4. Encourage parent(s) to allow the child as normal a life as possible. Discourage overprotection.
5. Child should attend school.
6. If murmur is benign, parent(s) need to know that heart is normal and child needs no restrictions.
7. Infants need not be restricted—crawling, walking, crying, and resting comfortably at will should be allowed.
8. For older children, an appropriate plan of activity can be prescribed after cardiac status and functional capacity have been determined.
9. Prevention of bacterial endocarditis. Children with congenital heart defects are at risk for bacterial endocarditis. Prophylactic antibiotics should be given before dental work and for 2 days following, and before GU tract and GI tract surgery or instrumentation. Prophylaxis should continue after cardiac surgery.

C. Follow-up

1. Well-child supervision should be continued with attention to immunizations, dental care, and developmental assessment.
2. Provide telephone availability and visits as needed to reassure parent(s).

D. Consultations/referrals

1. Refer to public health nurse.
2. Refer to social service agency depending on family's ability to cope.

Table 146-1 Assessment of Cardiac Status

Observation	Infant	Older Child
Color	Cyanosis May appear at birth, shortly after, or months later Polycythemia usually developing with persistent cyanosis Pallor—suggests anemia and should be treated to reduce heart work	Cyanosis Persistent, progressive; subsequent polycythemia Clubbing associated with long-standing cyanosis and polycythemia Pallor—possibly due to anemia, which itself may underlie murmurs or heart enlargement
Growth and development	Failure to gain weight indicative of serious heart problem—in cyanotic infant, alert! Weight increase due to edema—late indication of severe failure	Growth retardation possible with large left-to-right shunts in severe cyanosis Sudden weight gain possibly indicative of edema accompanying failure
Fatigue/exercise tolerance	Young infant Very lengthy feeding periods interrupted by shortness of breath	Majority able to lead normal active lives May seek less active play, rest more frequently

Table 146-1 Assessment of Cardiac Status *(continued)*

Observation	Infant	Older Child
	Labored breathing possibly occurring with defecation Older infant—shortened duration of effort in creeping, walking	Activity of most cyanotic children self-limited; squat or require carrying Failure to improve exercise tolerance during childhood: need for reevaluation
Respiration	Change in rate/character often early indicators of distress Tachypnea suggestive of onset of failure Paroxysmal tachypnea and cyanosis occurring with cyanotic lesions—due to hypoxia not failure	Dyspnea on exertion: need for reevaluation Severe dyspnea in cyanotic child: need for rest, squatting Paroxysmal tachycardia—indicative of severe hypoxia
Pulse and blood pressure	Paroxysmal tachycardia determined by rate at rest (> 200); may result in failure if persistent (more than 1 h); specific treatment required Easily palpable radial pulse and faint or absent femoral pulse indicative of coarctation of aorta	Pulse possibly revealing of abnormal cardiac rates or rhythms; confirmation by ECG Upper and lower extremity pulses and blood pressure to be carefully noted Pulse below 70 possible suggestion of heart block; confirmed by ECG
Cardiac size and configuration	Size and configuration of heart and vascularity of lungs determined by serial x-rays. Caution: danger of excessive radiation	Serial x-rays helpful in assessment of progressive increase in size of heart and/or changes in vascular markings. Caution: danger of excessive radiation
Cardiac sounds and murmurs	Murmur in newborn possibly disappears later Murmur resulting from malformation possibly not apparent until later in infancy or early childhood Continuous murmur over upper left chest commonly due to patent ductus arteriosus—usually audible by 2 months of age	Change in quality of sounds or rhythms: need for reevaluation "Innocent" murmurs Extremely common Never accompanied by cardiac symptoms/laboratory evidence of heart disease Organic murmurs Systolic with thrill usually organic Harsh systolic and thrill close to sternum or over base of heart: congenital rather than acquired heart disease Diastolic murmurs (other than venous hum): organic. Must differentiate between short diastolic murmur and normal third heart sound Apical (basal diastolic) murmurs with cardiac enlargement present in some congenital malformations and also in acute rheumatic fever (ARF) and rheumatic heart disease (RHD) (see Acute Rheumatic Fever, Chap. 145).

bibliography

Coats, Kathryn. Non-invasive cardiac diagnostic procedures. *American Journal of Nursing,* **75:**1980–1985 (1975).

Eugle, Mary Alen. Congenital heart disease and rheumatic fever. In Helen Wallace et al. (eds.), *Maternal and child practices.* Springfield, Ill.: Charles C Thomas, 1973, pp. 1074–1085.

Gottesfeld, Ilene Burson. The family of the child with congenital heart disease. *Maternal Child Nursing,* **4**:101–104 (1979).

Jackson, Patricia Ludder. Digoxin therapy at home: keeping the child safe. *Maternal Child Nursing,* **4**:105–109 (1979).

Klaus, Marshall H., and Fanaroff, Avroy A. *Care of the high-risk neonate.* Philadelphia: Saunders, 1973, pp. 228–253.

Kupst, Mary Jo, et al. Helping parents cope with the diagnosis of congenital heart defect: An experimental study. *Pediatrics,* **59**:266–271 (1977).

Nadas, Alexander S., and Fyler, Donald C. *Pediatric cardiology* (3d ed.). Philadelphia: Saunders, 1972, pp. 3–20; 293–661.

Smith, Kathleen Moreau. Recognizing cardiac failure in neonates. *Maternal Child Nursing,* **4**:98–100 (1979).

147 Juvenile Diabetes

M. CONSTANCE SALERNO/DIANA W. GUTHRIE

I. Etiology

A. Unknown
B. Genetic—may be inherited; exact pattern of inheritance unknown
C. Viral
D. Hormonal
E. Tumors
F. Steroid-induced
G. Other

II. Subjective Data

A. Complete history on initial visit
B. Interval history at each visit (see Fig. 147-1)

Figure 147-1: Diabetes Interval History

Name ____
Date ____

Date/age of onset:

Interval since last exam:

Interval history (change in diet, insulin, activity):

Problems or questions:

Diet
Calories: Distribution:
Food: weighed/measured/estimated
Breakfast time: Snack time:
Lunch time: Snack time:
Supper time: Snack time:

Insulin

Time	Dose (mL/U)	Type of Insulin
A.M.:____	A.M.:____	NPH:____ Reg:____ Other:____
Noon:____	Noon:____	Reg:____
P.M.:____	P.M.:____	NPH:____ Reg:____ Other:____

Total 24-h dose:____ Strength:____
Injection site:
Arms____ Abdomen____ Thigh____
Buttocks____ Other____
Who gives the injection and when?
Hypoglycemia:
Date
Description:

Infections:
Date:
Description:

(continued)

Variations in calorie intake:
- Are snacks always eaten?
- Is food plan satisfactory?
- Is food adjusted with activity?
- Is food adjusted with illness?
- If yes, how?

Usual activity pattern (describe):

Weekend variation: more/less/same
Emotional status
Participation in class: all/some/none
Reliability of record:
Understanding of care:
Participation in diabetic management:

Urine Tests
Test used for sugar:
- Frequency of test for sugar:
- % negative:___ % positive:___

Test used for acetone:
- When do you test for acetone?
- Number of positive tests:
- Who tests specimens?

Control rating:
Understanding of care: good/fair/poor

Physical Exam Temp: Pulse: Resp: BP:

Head:	Teeth:	Lungs:	Back:
Eyes:	Throat:	Abdomen:	Deep reflexes:
Ears:	Neck:	Genitalia:	Superficial reflexes:
Nose:	Chest:	Extremities:	Nuchal rigidity:
Mouth:	Heart:	Skin:	Posture:

General development and other comments:

Impression:

Treatment (prn):

Nurse/dietician comments:

Lab results: Clinitest:
Acetest:
Protein:

Dextrostix:
Insulin (time):
Food (time): pH:

Recommendations:
Date of return: ____________________

Examiner's signature: ____________________

III. Objective Data

A. Physical examination, complete

B. Laboratory data

1. Urinalysis
2. Blood sugar
3. Glucose tolerance test with insulin
4. Composite blood analysis test, e.g., SMAC 20
5. Other (e.g., A, C Hgb, urine function studies, etc.)

IV. Assessment

A. Subjective data

1. Family history of diabetes
2. Symptoms appearing abruptly
3. Polyuria
4. Polydipsia
5. Polyphagia
6. Weight loss
7. Fatigue and weakness

8. Bed-wetting
9. Dry, itchy skin
10. Visual disturbances
11. Headache
12. Malaise
13. Abdominal pain

B. Objective data

1. Flushed face
2. Poor skin turgor
3. Soft, sunken eyes
4. Dry mucous membrane
5. Fruity-smelling breath
6. Deep, rapid respirations
7. Weak, rapid pulse
8. Dullness
9. Stupor
10. Loss of consciousness
11. Laboratory data
    a. Glucose in urine
    b. Ketones in urine
    c. Elevated blood sugar
    d. Elevated ketone concentration in blood
    e. Low plasma bicarbonate
    f. Low blood pH
    g. Low CO_2
    h. Elevated or decreased serum potassium
    i. Decreased total-body potassium
    j. Increased amino acid concentration

V. Management

A. Acute (see medical referral/consultation, Table 147-1)

B. Long-term (beginning after initial hospitalization and control of ketoacidosis)

C. Goals

1. To maintain a high level of metabolic control
2. To teach the child and parent(s) the skills of self-care
3. To foster the development of a happy, useful, and productive citizen

D. Objectives: To assist the child and/or parent(s)

1. To acquire an accurate understanding of the disease and its consequences
2. To eliminate overt symptoms of diabetes
3. To prevent ketoacidosis
4. To prevent hypoglycemia
5. To accept increasing responsibility for his or her own management

E. Treatments/medications

1. Insulin (see Table 147-2)
2. Meal plan
    a. Exchange system
    b. Point system (1 point = 75 cal)
    c. Total available glucose (TAG)
3. Urine test
    a. Clinitest (copper reduction) for control
    b. Tes-Tape, Diastic, and Clinistix (glucose oxidase) for travel and school
4. Exercise
    a. Planned (i.e., aerobics, etc.)
    b. Unplanned
5. Keeping records

F. Counselling/prevention

1. Instruction and demonstration
    a. Dynamics of insulin (short-acting and intermediate insulins) (see Table 147-2)
        (1) Onset
        (2) Peak
        (3) Duration of action
        (4) Adverse reactions
    b. Administration of insulin
        (1) Withdrawing
        (2) Injection
        (3) Rotation of sites
        (4) Mixing
        (5) Care of supplies and insulin
    c. Glucagon
        (1) Action
        (2) Use
        (3) Adverse reaction
    d. Following a meal plan *(suggested guide)*
        (1) 30 cal/lb for prepubescent and pubescent
        (2) 30 cal/kg for postpubescent varied according to level of exercise
        (3) Diet should supply sufficient calories to meet the needs of exercise, growth, and appetite:

Protein	15 to 20 percent of calories
Fat	30 to 40 percent of calories
CHO	40–55 percent + of calories

        (4) Caloric intake should be divided into three meals and two or three snacks based upon the individual's lifestyle and upon the dynamics of insulin absorption.
    e. Collecting and testing urine specimens
        (1) Time
            (a) Fractional specimen
            (b) 24-h specimen
            (c) Single-voided
            (d) Double-voided
        (2) Method
            (a) Two-drop Clinitest (Ames)
            (b) Acetest or Ketostix

f. Balancing exercise
   (1) Anticipate and vary food intake.
   (2) Increase food with increased physical activity.
   (3) Give less food with less than usual exercise.
   (4) Decrease insulin only when increased level of food intake is not tolerated or if individual is overweight.

g. Infection/illness
   (1) Alter insulin dosage as needed.
   (2) Supplement with doses of regular insulin when needed.
   (3) Provide special diet with fewer calories.

h. Hygiene
   (1) Care of teeth
   (2) Care of skin
   (3) Care of feet

i. Record keeping
   (1) Purpose: assessment of changing needs
   (2) To be recorded accurately:
      (a) Daily urine tests
      (b) Insulin dosage; site and time of injections
      (c) Adverse reactions and treatment (see Table 147-3)
      (d) Diet variations
      (e) Exercise
      (f) Illness
      (g) Stressful situations

2. Evaluation
   a. Initial assessment and reassessments of the child's physical, social, and emotional needs
   b. Reassessment of the child's and/or parent(s)'s knowledge and understanding of diabetes and application of skills in the home
   c. Methods of assessment
      (1) Questionnaire (written or verbal)
      (2) Demonstration (home visit if possible)
      (3) interview (regular ongoing visits)
   d. Purpose
      (1) to assist the child and parents in the home
      (2) to monitor the child's progress
      (3) to motivate the child toward increased self-care

G. Follow-up
1. Periodic evaluation of child's clinical course
2. Periodic assessment of the child's growth and development
3. Continued reeducation and reinforcement necessary on a regular schedule

H. Consultations/referrals: Management of the child with diabetes is accomplished through a team approach. Referral or consultation should be made with the appropriate member whenever necessary. A collaborative relationship with each member—the physician, the nurse (hospital, clinic and/or nurse educator), school nurse whenever applicable, the nutritionist, social worker, and the family members and especially the child with diabetes is essential.

Table 147-1 Medical Referral Consultation

Diagnosis	Clinical Manifestation	Management
Diabetic ketoacidosis (severe hyperglycemia)	Dehydration Abdominal pain Acetone breath Kussmaul's respirations Cardiac arrhythmia Coma	Hospitalization—intensive care Perfused doses of insulin IV or $\frac{1}{2}$ SC (or IM)/$\frac{1}{2}$ IV Fluid and electrolyte replacement Careful monitoring of: Blood glucose Electrolytes Urine glucose and acetone levels Vital signs—impending circulatory collapse Cardiac stability (ECG): Hyperkalemia—abnormal T wave Hypokalemia—addition of U wave Level of consciousness
Insulin shock (severe hypoglycemia)	Convulsions Loss of consciousness	Patent airway IV glucose (treatment of choice) or glucagon ($\frac{1}{2}$ mg below 3 yr, 1 mg 3 yr and over)

Table 147-2 Action Time and Appearance of Most Commonly Used Insulins

			Previously reported action* h			Revised action† h		
Type of insulin	Appearance	Action	Onset	Peak	Duration	Onset	Peak	Duration
Regular	Clear	Rapid	½	2–4	5–7	½–1	2–4	6–8
Semilente	Cloudy	Rapid	½	4–8	12–16	½–1	2–4	8–10
Globin	Clear	Intermediate	1–2	8–10	18–24	1–2	6–8	12–14
NPH	Cloudy	Intermediate	2–4	12–18	24–28	1–2	6–8	12–14
Lente	Cloudy	Intermediate	2–4	12–18	24–28	1–2	6–8	14–16
PZI	Cloudy	Long	4–6	18–26	36–72	4–6	18±	36–72
Ultralente	Cloudy	Long	4–6	18–26	36–72	4–6	8–12	24–36

*These are the standard values for onset, peak action, and duration of action of insulins found in standard medical texts. They have been widely accepted for many years.

†These are revised values for insulin action based on careful and accurate diurnal blood glucose measurements in large numbers of diabetic children under carefully controlled conditions of dietary intake and standardized activity patterns. These studies were performed at the University of Missouri and reported in 1975.

Source: From Elizabeth L. Burke, *Insulin,* in Diana W. Guthrie, and Richard A. Guthrie, (eds.), *Nursing management of diabetes mellitus,* St. Louis, Mosby, 1977, p. 87.

Table 147-3 A Comparison of Hypoglycemia and Hyperglycemia

	Hypoglycemia	Hyperglycemia
Causes	Too much insulin	Too little insulin
	Increased exercise without increased food intake	Eating improperly
	Decreased food intake	Decreased exercise without decreased food intake
	Drugs (oral hypoglycemic agents)	Emotional stress
		Infection
		Drugs
Symptoms	Nervous	Weak
	Shaky	Increased thirst
	Weak	Frequent urination
	Sweaty	Dry mouth and soft eyes
	Headache	Decreased appetite or polyphagia
	Impaired vision	Nausea and vomiting
	Hunger	Abdominal pain
	Irritability	Coma
	Lability of mood	Acetone breath
	Convulsions	
Laboratory findings		
Urine	Glucose—negative	Glucose—positive
	Acetone—negative but may be positive	Acetone—positive
	Diacetic acid—negative	Diacetic acid—positive

Table 147-3 A Comparison of Hypoglycemia and Hyperglycemia *(continued)*

	Hypoglycemia	Hyperglycemia
Blood	Glucose—60 mg/dL or lower Acetone—negative CO_2—usually normal	Glucose— ± 250 mg/L Acetone—usually positive CO_2—< 20 meq/L Leukocytosis—present, may be very high
Treatment	Sugar: ingestion of sweetened fluids, such as soda pop or juice, or 2 tsp sugar Glucagon: ½ to 1 mg given subcutaneously or intramuscularly Glucose: 10 to 20 mL 50% dextrose given intravenously	Administration of regular insulin Fluid replacement Intravenous Oral Frequent monitoring of urine glucose and acetone levels Observation for circulatory collapse

Source: From Judy Jordan, Acute care of diabetes, in Diana W. Guthrie, and Richard A. Guthrie (eds.), *Nursing management of diabetes mellitus,* St. Louis, Mosby, 1977, p. 74.

bibliography

Guthrie, Diana, W., and Guthrie, Richard, A. (eds.). *Nursing management of diabetes mellitus.* St. Louis: Mosby, 1977.

Kohler, Elaine. Diabetic day: Setting goals for a child-directed ambulatory program. *Clinical Pediatrics* **17**:24–28 (1978).

Vaughan, V.C., McKay, R.J., and Nelson, W.E. (eds.). Diabetes mellitus. In *Textbook of pediatrics* (10th ed.). Philadelphia: Saunders, 1975, pp. 1259–1271.

Weil, W.B. Diabetes mellitus. In M. Green and R. J. Haggerty (eds.). *Ambulatory pediatris II,* Philadelphia: Saunders, 1977, pp. 339–347.

148 Neoplastic Disease

ELEANOR RUDICK

ALERT
1. Enlarged abdomen
2. Petechiae
3. Increased intracranial pressure (headache, vomiting, papilledema)
4. Bone pain

I. Etiology

Cancer in children displays a distinctly different pattern from that found in the adult population. It is therefore highly probable that different causes underlie the development of many malignant processes in children. For example, cancer is found in the neonatal period, indicating that prolonged exposure to environmental factors can be excluded from consideration for at least some cases of the disease (Evans, 1976).

A. Viruses
B. Immune defects
C. Genetics
D. Environment

II. Subjective Data

A. Problem-oriented history (A complete history is needed if not previously recorded.)
   1. Onset of symptoms
   2. Recent infection
      a. Upper respiratory infection (URI)
      b. Fever
      c. Swollen glands
   3. Fatigue
   4. Shortness of breath
   5. Pallor
   6. Masses
   7. Bone pain
   8. Headache
   9. Bleeding
   10. Vomiting

B. Developmental history
   1. Milestones
   2. Illnesses

C. Past health history
   1. Immunizations
   2. Frequency of health care visits
   3. Chronic/genetic disorders

D. Family history for chronic and/or genetic disorders

E. Social history
   1. Family constellation and financial capability
   2. Living conditions—as basis for assessing family's ability to cope
   3. Significant and supportive others

III. Objective Data

A. Physical examination: complete physical examination (see Chap. 7)

B. Laboratory data
   1. Complete blood count (CBC) with differential
   2. Hemoglobin
   3. Erythrocyte sedimentation rate (ESR)
   4. Urinalysis
   5. Chest x-ray

Note: When neoplastic disease is suspected, an immediate referral should be made to the physician. The practitioner will be instrumental in successful management.

Table 148-1 Medical Referral/Consultation

Diagnosis	Clinical Manifestations	Management
Acute lymphocytic leukemia (ALL)	Pallor Petechiae Fatigue Infection Joint pain Enlarged nodes Immature WBCs (peripherally) Blasts in marrow Hepatomegaly Splenomegaly	Referral to physician Treatments/medications, possibly including Chemotherapy Radiotherapy Hospitalization Surgery Immunotherapy Counselling—discussion with parent(s) Remission, consolidation; maintenance Multimodel therapy—effects of staging Individualized therapy based on Location of primary tumor Type of malignancy Grade of malignancy Size of tumor or number of cells (ALL) Age of client Presence or absence of gross metastases Likelihood of long-term disease-free survival Goals of therapy Directed to eradication of localized disease as well as eradication of distant metastases (visible or microscopically presumed to be present) Every effort made to minimize significant long-term toxicity when considering type and intensity of each treatment modality Supports to decrease associated problems Infection control Strict attention to toxic effects of drugs Nutrition Blood/blood fractions Psychological aspects Sharing diagnosis and protocols with children and families Initial period of adjustment before remission Periods of adjustment during course of remissions and relapses Life planning Follow-up Well-child supervision Attention to maintenance regime Referral pattern from the pediatrician to a tumor or hematology center for positive diagnosis and treatment regimen; then back to the pediatrician and primary health care practitioner for follow-
Brain tumor	Signs of increased intracranial pressure Infant Child Visual and fundoscopic changes Gait disturbance Vomiting Morning headache Pain with position change Peak age 5–9 yrs	
Hodgkin's disease	Enlarged (painless) nodes Present symptoms determined by location of nodes Night sweats Fever Weight loss	
Neuroblastoma	Mass: adrenal glands; cervical, thoracic, abdominal, sympathetic ganglia Fever Pain Pallor Irritability Majority metastatic at diagnosis	
Wilms's tumor	Abdominal mass Pain Hematuria Anemia Hypertension	
Soft-tissue sarcoma; rhabdomyosarcoma	Head and neck region Genitourinary tract Extremities Trunk—chest wall and retroperitoneal area	

Table 148-1 Medical Referral/Consultation *(continued)*

Diagnosis	Clinical Manifestations	Management
	High incidence of metastases at diagnosis (lymph node, lung, bone marrow, bone, and liver)	through with prescribed regimen; with return to tumor center for periodic reevaluation of status and rehabilitation
Malignant bone tumor Osteogenic sarcoma	Predominantly in adolescent age group In long bones—distal femur, proximal tibia, proximal humerus Pain Swelling and soft-tissue mass Usually history of trauma (not thought to be causal)	
Ewing's sarcoma	Primarily age 10–20 yrs Pain and swelling at site Commonly long bones of extremities Flat bones of trunk Simulates osteomyelitis	

references

Evans, Audrey E., et al. Childhood cancer: Basic considerations in diagnosis and treatment. *Pediatric Clinics of North America,* **23** (1976).

bibliography

Bruya, Margaret, Auld, T., and Madeira, Nancy Powell. Stomatitis after Chemotherapy. *American Journal of Nursing,* **75**(8):1349–1352 (1975).

Creene, Patricia. The Child with leukemia in the classroom. *American Journal of Nursing,* January:86–87 (1975).

Evans, Audrey E., et al. (eds.). "Pediatric oncology. *Pediatric Clinics of North America,* February (1976).

Foley, Genevieve, and McCarthy, Ann Marie. The Child with leukemia. *American Journal of Nursing,* July:1108–1122 (1976).

Hersh, Stephen P. *NIMH to Physicians #2, Psychosocial management of leukemias in children and youth.* Washington, D.C.: National Institute of Mental Health, 1974.

Hofmann, Adele D., et al. *The hospitalized adolescent.* New York: The Free Press, 1976.

Leventhal, Brigid D., and Hersh, Stephen. Modern treatment of childhood leukemia: The patient and his family. *Nursing Digest,* July/August (1975).

Martinson, Ida M., et al. Home care for children dying of cancer. *Pediatrics,* **62**:106–113 (1978).

section 2

developmental disabilities

149 Learning Disabilities[1]

KAREN A. BALLARD

I. Etiology

- **A.** Toxemia
- **B.** Eclampsia
- **C.** Major illness during pregnancy
- **D.** Birth trauma
- **E.** Low birth weight
- **F.** Perinatal anoxia
- **G.** Seizures
- **H.** Neonatal jaundice
- **I.** Failure to thrive
- **J.** Infection
- **K.** Head trauma

II. Subjective Data: A complete history with special emphasis on

- **A.** Description of problem
- **B.** Age at onset
  1. Present prior to formal schooling
  2. Present since beginning of education
  3. Initially good school performance with disintegration noted in later years
  4. Relation of onset to any stressful situation
- **C.** Response to problem
  1. Client
  2. Parent(s)
- **D.** School
  1. Description of school and typical school day
  2. Number of students in class
  3. Seating position in classroom
  4. Subjects liked/disliked
  5. Complaints or concerns of teacher(s)
  6. Grades
- **E.** Child-rearing philosophy and methods
- **F.** Family history
  1. Similar disabilities in siblings
  2. Parental history of learning disabilities
  3. Behavior disorders
  4. Chronic problems
  5. Psychiatric disorders
- **G.** Social history
  1. Description of living situation
  2. Changes in family constellation
     - a. Divorce or marriage
     - b. Death of a family member
     - c. Birth of a sibling
  3. Stresses in home environment
     - a. Relocation
     - b. Parental quarrelling
  4. Stresses in peer/school/work environment
  5. Relationships with family members, friends, significant others
- **H.** Patterns and habits
  1. Changes in sleep pattern
  2. Changes in personal hygiene
  3. Eating disturbances
- **I.** Past/present history
  1. Speech defect
  2. Hearing problem and/or frequent ear infections
  3. Vision problem
  4. Behavior problem
  5. Prolonged and/or serious illness
  6. Allergies
  7. Frequent upper respiratory infections
- **J.** Hospitalizations
- **K.** Prenatal history
- **L.** Birth history
- **M.** Developmental history
- **N.** Careful, thorough review of systems

[1]*Note:* A child with a learning disability should be managed by the practitioner in consultation with a physician.

III. Objective Data: (see Introduction to Section 8)

A. Physical examination: complete physical examination including

1. Vision testing
2. Hearing testing; audiometric studies
3. Complete neurological examination

B. Laboratory data

1. Complete blood count (CBC)
2. Urinalysis
3. Other tests as indicated

C. Psychological screening

1. Draw-A-Person
2. Denver Developmental Screening Test—up to 6 years of age
3. Wechsler Intelligence Scale for Children-Revised (WISC-R)—6 to 16 years of age

IV. Assessment (see Table 149-1)

A. Subjective data

1. One out of every twenty school children may have some form of learning disability; of these there are 4 times as many boys as girls.
2. Parent(s) may identify the difficulty as
   a. Physical illness
   b. Speech problem
   c. Hearing problem
   d. Behavior problem
   e. School performance problem
3. The child is usually described as
   a. Distractible
   b. Having a short attention span
   c. Hyperactive
   d. Impulsive
   e. Emotionally labile
   f. Socially immature
   g. Explosive, bad-tempered
   h. Inadequate in school adjustment
      (1) Reading difficulties
      (2) Abstracting difficulties
      (3) Arithmetic problems
      (4) Handwriting problems
      (5) Poor peer relationships
4. Similar disabilities may be identified in parent(s) and/or siblings.
5. Developmental history often reveals
   a. Unevenness in the developmental sequence
   b. Weaning and feeding difficulties
   c. Clumsiness
   d. Poor motor coordination
   e. Delayed, atypical language development
   f. Difficulty with toilet training
6. Previous history may reveal the following problems, which may either be indicative of hyperactive systems or have contributed to developmental problems by the interruption of normal functioning.
   a. Allergies
   b. Chronic ear-nose-throat (ENT) infections
   c. Colic
   d. Celiac disease
   e. Headache
   f. Vomiting
   g. Hospitalization(s)
   h. Seizures
   i. Strabismus
7. There are statistically higher incidences of learning disabilities in children when their mothers' pregnancies and their birth histories had complications of the following nature.
   a. Toxemia
   b. Bleeding during pregnancy
   c. Hypertension
   d. Blood incompatibility (Rh, ABO)
   e. Viral illnesses
   f. Birth trauma
   g. Premature birth
   h. Birth and neonatal anoxia

B. Objective data

1. Physical examination should be normal unless there is a previously unrecognized physical problem which is contributing to learning difficulty.
   a. Visual deficit
   b. Hearing loss
   c. Chronic infection
   d. Pinworms
   e. Hyperthyroidism
2. Positive "soft" neurological signs may vary greatly in learning disabled children and may change with age; difficulty may be observed in the following.
   a. Running, skipping movements
   b. Writing coordination
   c. Harmonious movement of body parts
   d. Willingness to move a body part
   e. Performing directional movements
   f. Awareness of the relationship of one object to another
3. Poor performance levels may occur in the following tests.
   a. Draw-A-Person, which serves as a gross guide to general intellect, body image, and emotional integrity
   b. Bender gestalt test

c. WISC-R
d. Denver Developmental Screening Test
e. Standardized scholastic achievement tests
4. There has been observed a high correlation of concurrent allergic manifestations.

V. Management

A. Treatments/medications

1. The main areas of disability which are considered in treatment are
   a. Visual
   b. Motor
   c. Auditory and language
   d. Comprehension (dyslexia)
2. Treatment modalities
   a. Educational
      (1) Regular classroom—appropriate modification of curriculum; can include special tutoring
      (2) Special classroom—a specially trained teacher providing appropriately geared curriculum to children with similar disabilities
      (3) Private tutoring—either to substitute for lack of special programs or in conjunction with formal education
   b. Medical
      (1) Frequent exchange of information and collaboration with involved professionals
      (2) Medication as determined by physician (Benadryl, Dexedrine, Cylert, and Ritalin; see Table 149-2)
      (3) Indications for medication
         (a) Absence of severe emotional problems
         (b) Near-normal intelligence potential
         (c) Behavior consistently below expected performance level
         (d) Symptoms of minimal brain dysfunction
      (4) Carefully monitored medication regimen
         (a) Start with minimal dose.
         (b) Titrate until relief of symptoms and/or side effects is observed.
         (c) Maintain a balance between minimum side effects and maximum effectiveness.
   c. Psychological
      (1) Individual therapy
      (2) Parental therapy
      (3) Child/parent therapy
      (4) Family therapy
3. Treatment should aim to
   a. Correct interpretation of sensory stimuli (visual)
   b. Encourage development of gross motor training (hopping, skipping, jumping, moving)
   c. Encourage use of auditory capacities (awareness of sound; development of appropriate responses; sound discrimination)
   d. Encourage articulation (ability to remember and reproduce sounds; word sequencing; sentence development)
   e. Develop reading skills and promote correct comprehension (dyslexia)

B. Counselling/prevention

1. Counsel parents *not* to depend on diagnostic labels or to expect only limited responses from their child.
2. Counsel parents to do the following.
   a. Communicate their love and acceptance.
   b. Demonstrate acceptance.
   c. Understand the normalcy of their own ambivalent feelings, conflicting expectations, and feelings of guilt.
   d Avoid seeking blame.
   e. Avoid overprotection and indulgent behavior.
   f. Set firm, consistent limits.
   g. Use appropriate discipline.
   h. Provide an organized environment.
   i. Allow and support child in simple decision making.
   j. Establish predictable family routines around the activities of daily living.
   k. Allow child to assume responsibilities for simple chores.
   l. Assist other family members in understanding the child.
   m. Understand and appreciate their child's unique worth, abilities, and contributions.
   n. Remain parent(s) and not assume the "professsional" role.
   o. Recognize and identify side effects of medications (see Table 149-2).

C. Follow-up

1. There should be periodic complete physical examinations with CBC, urinalysis, and liver function tests.
2. If medications are prescribed, evaluation should be maintained on a weekly basis until medication level is established, then biweekly or monthly.

3. Regular counselling visits can be scheduled as needed, depending on needs of child and family.

D. Consultations/referrals; any of the following may be appropriate.

1. Pediatric neurologist
2. Psychologist/psychiatrist
3. Ophthalmologist
4. Social worker
5. Teacher
6. Speech and hearing therapist
7. American Foundation for Learning Disabilities, 30 Rockefeller Plaza, New York, NY 10020
8. Association for Children with Learning Disabilities, 5225 Grace Street, Pittsburgh, PA 15236
9. Closer Look, Box 1492, Washington, DC 20013
10. The Orton Society, Suite 115, 84115 Bellona Lane, Towson, MD 21204

bibliography

Bax, Martin C. O. The assessment of the child at school entry. *Pediatrics,* **58**:403–407 (1976).

Binder, Florence Z., and Butler, Joan E. Children with learning disabilities. *Issues in Comprehensive Pediatric Nursing.* **3**:1–14 (September 1978).

Cline, F. W. (ed.). The Nurse Practitioner and Learning Disorders. *Nurse Practitioner,* **2**:31–32 (1977).

Denhoff, Eric. Learning disabilities: An office approach. *Pediatrics,* **58**:409–411 (1976).

Hogan, Gwendolyn, and Ryan, Nell J. Evaluation of the child with a learning disorder. *Pediatrics,* **58**:407–409 (1976).

Huessy, Hans Rosenstock, and Cohan, Alan Howard. Hyperkinetic behaviors and learning disabilities followed over seven years. *Pediatrics,* **57**:4–10 (1976).

Koppitz, E. M. *The Bender-gestalt test for young children.* New York: Grune & Stratton, 1963.

McCormick, David P. Pediatric evaluation of children with school problems. *American Journal of Diseases of Children,* **131**:318–322 (1977).

Smith, M. D., et al. Intellectual characteristics of school labelled learning disabled children. *Exceptional Children,* **43**:352–357 (1977).

Williams, J. F. Learning disabilities: A multi-faceted health treatment. *Journal of School Health,* **46**:515–516 (1976).

Table 149-1 Differential Diagnosis of Disturbed Educational Development*

Cause	History of High-Risk Factors	Developmental Milestones	Physical Examination	Neurologic Examination	EEG
Specific learning disability	Possible relation to complications of pregnancy and delivery	May exhibit isolated developmental delays (e.g., speech or motor coordination)	Usually normal	Usually normal; may detect "soft" or "subtle" neurologic signs	Usually normal
Mental retardation	Possible relation to complications of labor and delivery; genetic faults	Delays may be noted in all areas of development	Usually normal findings as related to specific syndromes (e.g., Down's syndrome)	Varies with extent of central nervous system damage	Varies from normal to abnormal
Organic handicap (e.g., hearing loss)	May have history of infections or trauma (e.g., chronic otitis media)	Usually normal; developmental delay may be isolated (e.g., delayed speech)	Abnormality may be apparent on examination (e.g., scarred tympanic membrane)	Abnormality of affected organ	Usually normal
Somatic illness	Usually none	Usually normal; occasionally development is irregular	Depends on specific type of somatic disorder (e.g., cardiac, renal, etc.)	Usually normal unless a problem of nervous system	Usually normal; question of some abnormalities
Psychosis	Usually none	Usually normal	Usually normal	Usually normal or minor abnormalities	Usually normal
Behavioral disorders	Usually none	Usually normal	Usually normal	Usually normal	Usually normal
Socioeconomic (cultural) deprivation	Usually none; possible history of poor prenatal care	Usually normal	Usually normal	Usually normal	Usually normal

*In part adapted from Schulman, J. L. *Management of emotional disorders in pediatric practice,* Chicago: Year Book, 1967.

Source: Gottlieb, Marvin I. Educational health and development. In Hughes, James G. *Synopsis of pediatrics* (4th ed.). St. Louis: Mosby, 1975.

Table 149-1 Differential Diagnosis of Disturbed Educational Development* *(continued)*

Teachers' Observations	School Achievement	Psychologic Evaluation (WISC)	Parents' Observations	General Remarks
Puzzling, child may perform well in some areas academically and socially	Depressed in affected areas and gradually spreads	Some normal performances and some areas are depressed	Usually no problems except for school difficulty; does well with friends	May have no problems until starting school; preschool identification encouraged; may have superimposed behavioral disorder
Child unable to compete at grade level or with children of same age	Depressed for age; functions better in Special Education Program	Usually depressed in all areas	Usually no family disruption; plays with younger children	Suspicions may be aroused in preschool period because of developmental delays or dull affect
Academically, functions well in uninvolved areas; peer rapport good	Depressed in areas that require use of affected sensory skill	Depressed in area requiring use of affected modality	Functions well in uninvolved areas	Occasionally exhibits associated behavioral difficulties; deficits a medical challenge
Change in performance related to onset of illness	Poor performances during periods of illness, otherwise normal achievement	May be depressed as result of illness	No difficulty except for illness	Family aware of acute or chronic nature of illness
Bizarre responses; may be withdrawn and unresponsive	Erratic but usually very poor	Bizarre responses, possibly with islands of normal function	Disturbed parent-child relationships; siblings, peer, and social relationships are poor	Preschool behavior may be obviously that of a disturbed child
Attention-seeking behaviors; may annoy classmates; acting out behavior; islands of good behavior	Varies; can and frequently does do well	Good results if child cooperates	Better on a 1 to 1 basis; occasional parent-child disturbances	Behavioral disorder may have onset with start of school or exaggerated when school begins
May be characterized as "poorly motivated"	Generally performance is poor when in competitive academic atmosphere	Generally depressed; can reflect cultural bias of test items	Functions well in our cultural environment; friends with similar circumstance	Evidences of socioeconomic depression; functions well at home and with neighborhood peers; slow in school

Table 149-2 Medications

Drug	Dosage	Side Effects	Remarks
Diphenhydramine hydrochloride (Benadryl)	5 mg/kg per 24 h divided into 4 doses; not to exceed 300 mg per day	Drowsiness Dryness of mouth, nose, and throat Confusion Nervousness and restlessness Nausea and vomiting Diarrhea or constipation Tightness of chest Thickening of bronchial secretions	Basically a potent antihistamine with anticholinergic, antitussive, antiemetic, and sedative effects Can be used in very young children except in premature or newborn infants Can be taken with food One of the safest psychoactive drugs
Dextroamphetamine sulfate (Dexedrine)	In children 3 to 5 yrs: 2.5 mg/day po with weekly increments of 2.5 mg In children 6 yrs and older: 5 mg/day po, with weekly increments of 5 mg Total dosage should not exceed 40 mg/day	Insomnia Anorexia Irritability Headache Dryness of mouth Gastrointestinal distress Paradoxical reactions High potential for abuse	Contraindicated in Children under 3 yrs Hypertensive clients Used with caution in presence of diabetes Should be taken 1 h before meals If administered twice a day, should be given before breakfast and lunch Blood pressure and pulse to be checked Weight taken twice weekly Instruction of parent(s) on signs of overdose Restlessness Tremor Rapid respiration Confusion Assaultiveness Panic states Nausea, vomiting Abdominal cramps Convulsions Coma Psychological dependency possible
Pemoline (Cylert)	Over 6 yrs: 37.5 mg per day po, with weekly increments of 18.75 mg to average dose of 56.25–75 mg per day; not to exceed 112.5 mg per day	Insomnia Anorexia Weight loss Irritability Headache Drowsiness Mild depression Skin rashes Temporary suppression of growth rate	Should be administered in single morning dose Not recommended for children under 6 yrs Clinical improvement gradual, possibly taking 3–4 wks Advisable to interrupt drug once or twice a year in order to test continued need

Table 149-2 Medications *(continued)*

Drug	Dosage	Side Effects	Remarks
Methylphenidate hydrochloride (Ritalin)	Over 6 yrs: 5 mg per day po, with weekly increments of 5–10 mg to average dose of 20–30 mg per day; not to exceed 60 mg per day	Growth retardation Anorexia Weight loss Lowered seizure threshold Irritability Insomnia Dizziness Headache Skin rashes Blood dyscrasias (anemia, leukopenia, thrombocytopenia)	Administered before breakfast and lunch Contraindicated in Children under 6 yrs Hypertension Convulsive disorders Agitation Psychological dependency possible Blood pressure and pulse to be checked Weighing twice weekly Instruction of parent(s) on signs of overdose High blood pressure Cardiac arrythmias Tachycardia Agitation Nausea and vomiting Personality changes

150 Down's Syndrome[1]

MARILYN GREBIN

I. Etiology: Genetic

A. Trisomy 21—91 percent
B. Trisomy 21/normal mosaicism—4 percent
C. Translocation—1 percent

II. Subjective Data

Complete history with special emphasis upon:

A. Prenatal history
B. Birth history
C. Neonatal history
D. Growth and development history
E. Past medical history
F. Family history for genetic disorders
G. Social history

III. Objective Data

A. Physical examination (complete)
B. Laboratory data (done by physician)

1. Chromosome analysis
   a. Child (to confirm diagnosis)
   b. Parent(s) (useful for genetic counselling)
2. Thyroid studies
3. Pelvic x-rays

IV. Assessment

A. Down's syndrome

1. Subjective data; the parent(s) may bring the child to the primary health care provider for any one of the following problems.
   a. Respiratory infection
   b. Conjunctivitis
   c. Seizures
   d. Dry or mottled skin
   e. Slow growth
   f. Tongue protrusion
   g. Chronic rhinitis
2. Objective data
   a. Head
      (1) Third to twentieth percentile
      (2) Brachycephalia
      (3) Sagittal fontanel—2 cm anterior to posterior fontanel
      (4) Possible late closure of fontanels (may have third fontanel)
      (5) Thin cranium
   b. Eyes
      (1) Upturned palpebral fissures
      (2) Bilateral epicanthal folds
      (3) Small bony orbits
      (4) Brushfield's spots
      (5) Strabismus (30 percent)
      (6) Cataracts (1.3 percent)
      (7) Nystagmus (15 percent)
   c. Ears
      (1) Small—with decreased length
      (2) Cartilaginous anomalies: overfolding of angulated upper helix
      (3) Low placement
   d. Nose
      (1) Small
      (2) Low nasal bridge
   e. Neck
      (1) Short
      (2) Possibly webbed
   f. Hair
      (1) Possibly a midline parietal hair whorl
      (2) Fine, soft, sparse
      (3) Pubic hair straight at adolescence
   g. Skin
      (1) Excessive on back of neck

[1]*Note:* The client with this syndrome must be evaluated by a physician. The practitioner may be called upon to manage a stable child.

(2) Dry
(3) Mottled appearance

h. Mouth
(1) Small oral cavity
(2) Hypoplasia of the mandible
(3) Tongue protrusion; scrotal tongue
(4) Small, irregular teeth

i. Hands and feet
(1) Brachydactylia
(2) Hypoplasia of midphalanx of fifth finger (60 percent) with clinodactylism (50 percent)
(3) Simian crease of palm (45 percent)
(a) Unilaterally
(b) Bilaterally
(4) Ulnar loop dermal ridge all digits
(5) Wide gap between first and second toes
(6) Syndactyly of second and third toes

j. Musculoskeletal
(1) Hypotonia—very prominent
(2) Hyperflexibility of joints
(3) Diastasis recti
(4) Umbilical hernia
(5) Pelvic abnormalities (x-ray findings)
(a) Broad ilia
(b) Small acetabular angles
(c) Elongated ischia
(6) Funnel or pigeon chest

k. Growth and development
(1) Slow
(2) Height attained by age 15 years

l. Genitalia
(1) Infantile genital development
(2) Cryptorchidism

m. Mental status
(1) IQ range 25 to 50 (Studies now indicate that Down's syndrome children reared at home achieve a higher IQ.)
(2) Happy
(3) Friendly
(4) Perhaps mischievous and obstinate
(5) Rowdy voice

n. Associated problems
(1) Congenital heart disease
(a) Atrioventricular canal
(b) Ventricular septal defect
(2) Lower respiratory infections
(3) Chronic rhinitis
(4) Chronic conjunctivitis
(5) Periodontal disease
(6) Leukemia—1 percent of population
(7) Polycythemia—15 percent
(8) Seizures—5 percent
(9) Duodenal stenosis (in a small percentage)
(10) Lens opacities

B. Cretinism (athyreotic hypothyroidism or goitrus cretinism)

1. Subjective data
a. Recognized after 2 months of age
b. History of constipation
c. Possibly lethargic
d. History of feeding difficulties

2. Objective data
a. Head normal size, possible third fontanel, with immature facial bone structure
b. Eyes normal size and slanted with puffy eyelids
c. Low nasal bridge
d. Tongue thick, large, protruding
e. Hoarse cry
f. Respiratory distress
g. Linear growth retarded, weight increased
h. Enlarged abdomen
i. May have umbilical hernia
j. Hands and feet short and square
k. Skin dry and coarse
l. Hair dry and coarse
m. Thyroid function tests: low serum T^4 concentration and high serum TSH concentration
n. Chromosomal pattern normal

V. Management

A. Down's syndrome

1. Treatments/medications: none

2. Counselling/prevention
a. Provide genetic counselling for the parent(s) to determine the likelihood of producing another child with Down's syndrome.
b. Encourage and support the parent(s) to manage the child within the home setting.
c. Assist parent(s) to express feelings of rejection.
d. Encourage parent(s) to join parent groups of others with Down's syndrome children.
e. Give parent(s) published information about Down's syndrome.
f. Encourage parent(s) to participate in infant stimulation programs
g. Inform about educational availabilities.
h. Amniocentesis should be done on mothers at risk.

3. Follow-up
a. By the interdisciplinary team as often as the parent(s) requires support
b. By the team for evaluation of the child's status and progress

4. Consultations/referrals
   a. Support for practitioner in following the Down's syndrome child and family from
      (1) Pediatrician
      (2) Genetic counsellor
      (3) Cardiologist
      (4) Psychologist
      (5) Speech pathologist
   b. For genetic counselling and treatment referrals:
      National Genetics Foundation
      250 West 57th Street
      New York, NY 10019

B. Cretinism

1. Treatments/medications: levothyroxine (prescribed by the physician)
   a. Infant and young child: 25 μg daily and increased by increments of 25 μg at 1-week intervals to reach a daily dose of 100 μg after 3 to 4 weeks. Then, the dose is increased slowly to maintain serum T_4 concentrations between 9 and 12 μg/100 mL.
   b. Older children and adult: Initial daily dose should not exceed 50 μg with increments every 2 to 3 weeks until normal metabolic state is obtained and serum T_4 concentration is around 9 to 12 μg/100 mL.
2. Counselling/prevention
   a. Encourage compliance with the medical regimen.
   b. Provide explanation of the disorder and recovery.
3. Follow-up: by the pediatrician and endocrinologist
4. Consultations/referrals
   a. Pediatrician
   b. Endocrinologist

---

bibliography

Coleman, Mary. Down's syndrome. *Pediatric Annals,* **7**(2):36–39 (1978).

Gellis, Sydney S. *Down's syndrome; informing the parents: A study of parental preferences.* In William F. Gayton and Linda Walker (eds.), *The year book of pediatrics.* University of Rochester, 1975, pp. 429–430.

Golden, William, Pashayan, Hermine M. The effect of parental education on the eventual mental development of non-institutionalized children with Down's syndrome. *Journal of Pediatrics,* **89**:603–605 (1976).

Greenwood, Ronald D., and Nadas, Alexander S. The clinical course of cardiac disease in Down's syndrome. *Pediatrics,* **58**:893–897 (1976).

Smith, David W. *Recognizable patterns of human malformation.* Philadelphia: Saunders, 1976, pp. 6–9.

Vaughan, Victor C., III, and McKay, R. James. *Nelson textbook of pediatrics* (10th ed.). Philadelphia: Saunders, 1975.

William, Robert H. (ed.). *Textbook of endocrinology.* Philadelphia: Saunders, 1974.

151 Cerebral Palsy[1]

HELEN M. LERNER

ALERT
1. Infants under 1 year undiagnosed
2. Children not under comprehensive care
3. Parent(s) who deny existence of handicap
4. Overly protective parent(s)
5. Developmental lags in two or more areas

I. Etiology
- **A.** Events occurring during pregnancy
  1. Genetic
  2. Malnutrition and infection
  3. Anoxia
  4. Toxemia
- **B.** Events during labor and delivery
  1. Excessive drugs or anesthesia
  2. Malposition and cephalopelvic disproportion
  3. Anoxia due to bleeding or pressure on cord
- **C.** Events during perinatal period
  1. Premature birth
  2. Anoxia
  3. Hyperbilirubinemia
- **D.** Events during early childhood
  1. Trauma
  2. Infections of central nervous system
  3. Poisoning

II. Subjective Data
- **A.** Age
- **B.** Prenatal history
- **C.** Labor and delivery
- **D.** Birth history
- **E.** Developmental history
  1. Social—responsiveness, feeding
  2. Gross motor—locomotion, body control
  3. Language—imitating sounds, use of language
  4. Fine motor—toys
- **F.** Nutrition
  1. Sample menu
  2. Difficulty in sucking, swallowing, or chewing
- **G.** Previous health problems and hospitalization
- **H.** Sources of health care
- **I.** Social history
  1. Living conditions
  2. Knowledge of child's condition
  3. Ability to care for handicapped child
     - a. Physical and emotional
     - b. Financial
- **J.** Child's ability to carry out activities of daily living
- **K.** Family history
  1. Genetic diseases
  2. Previous neurological handicaps

III. Objective Data
- **A.** Physical examination (complete)
  1. Measurement of head—charted on graph
  2. Musculoskeletal examination
  3. Careful neurological exam with special attention to
     - a. Inspection of head
     - b. Gross motor abilities
     - c. Fine motor abilities
     - d. Muscle tone
     - e. Infants under 1 year
       - (1) Presence or absence of appropriate infantile reflexes
       - (2) Persistence of infantile reflexes
     - f. Eye exam and vision test

[1]*Note:* This condition should be managed in consultation with a physician.

g. Hearing test

B. Laboratory data: none

C. Denver Developmental Screening Test

IV. Assessment

A. Spastic cerebral palsy

1. Subjective data
   a. History of premature birth, anoxia
   b. Report of developmental lag in one or more areas
2. Objective data
   a. Resistance to passive movement
   b. Increased stretch and deep tendon reflexes
   c. Strabismus
   d. Scissor gait
   e. Dysarthria

B. Athetoid cerebral palsy

1. Subjective data
   a. Perinatal brain injury, anoxia, kernicterus
   b. Developmental lag in one or more areas
2. Objective data
   a. Involuntary movements involving major joints
   b. Lurching gait
   c. Strabismus
   d. Low-tone hearing loss
   e. Hands severely affected
   f. Persistent infantile reflexes

C. Ataxic cerebral palsy

1. Subjective data
   a. Birth injury
   b. Infectious disease of central nervous system
   c. Drug toxicity
   d. Head injury
   e. Slow motor development, especially walking
   f. Nausea
2. Objective data
   a. Broad-based, staggering gait
   b. Falls easily
   c. Nystagmus
   d. Intention tremor
   e. Hypotonia
   f. Slow, monotonous speech

V. Management

A. Treatments/medications

1. No general treatment; adapted to child's special abilities and disabilities
2. Medications as needed for seizure disorders and muscle relaxation

B. Counselling

1. Family needs
   a. Encourage family members to verbalize feelings regarding child's condition and prognosis.
   b. Help with realistic planning for periods of stress, present needs, and future.
2. Nutrition
   a. Infants under 1 year
      (1) Provide special nipples when sucking reflex is weak.
      (2) Stimulate lips to encourage sucking.
      (3) Retrusion tongue reflex may persist for many months.
   b. Older children
      (1) Spoon with special handle may be needed.
      (2) Encourage water play with spoon to gain fine motor control.
      (3) May need thickened liquids if problem with swallowing.
      (4) ENCOURAGE SELF-FEEDING: Parent(s) may continue process long past need.
3. Toilet training—see Toilet Training, Chap. 122
   a. From 9 to 18 months: choose appropriate potty chair.
      (1) Special support to keep child's trunk in sitting position possibly necessary
      (2) Foot support—so abdominal muscles can be assisted with bowel evacuation
      (3) Raised sides for balance support
      (4) Foam strips to prevent slipping
   b. From 19 months to 4 years:
      (1) Make bathroom available—no slippery floors or obstacles.
      (2) Prevent constipation.
         (a) Provide adequate fluid and roughage: abdominal muscles have decreased tone.
         (b) Put child in squatting position for short periods of time.
4. Hygiene
   a. Position forward to prevent Moro reflex from interfering with bath.
   b. Wash child in symmetrical position.
   c. Have rubber mat or rings in tub.
   d. Children with athetoid cerebral palsy should sit with legs straight out—sling useful.
   e. For children with spastic cerebral palsy:
      (1) Seat in tub aids balance.
      (2) With severe spasticity the child should lie in tub with little water.
      (3) Head rests are useful.

(4) Muscle spasms are relaxed in tub of warm water.

f. Aids for self-bathing
   (1) Mitt-type washcloth
   (2) Nailbrush with dented sides for grip
   (3) Long-handled back brush
   (4) Tray with suction cups for brush and soap

5. Dressing
   a. Child lies or sits up, back to dresser.
   b. Severely handicapped child can lie down with pillow.
   c. Sitting balance is essential for independent dressing.
   d. Hemiplegic can balance on unaffected side and dress affected arm and leg first.
   e. Stretchy clothes with large openings are best.
6. Play
   a. Infants under 1 year
      (1) Position changed frequently—can't do for self
      (2) Position to see activity and other parts of room
   b. Older children
      (1) Large heavy balls for athetoid and ataxic children
      (2) Small balls for spastic children to grasp
   c. All children—play as appropriate to developmental skills
7. Well-child care
   a. Preventive health care
      (1) Regular health care
      (2) Immunizations
         (a) Need for divided doses of routine immunizations
         (b) Pertussis vaccine immunizations perhaps not given
   b. Prevention of complications due to acute illness resulting from handicapping condition
      (1) Pneumonia
      (2) Dehydration
      (3) Seizures with high fever

C. Follow-up: visits for well-child care and as needed for parental support

D. Consultations/referrals

1. Pediatric neurologist—for evaluations and general assessment, protocols for seizure medication
2. Social worker-family needs, financial problems, programs available
3. Occupational therapist—assistance in developing skills for activities of daily living (ADL) and play
4. Speech therapist—speech and language problems
5. Psychiatrist—mental health problems interfering with coping ability and maximizing potential for development
6. Psychologist—testing and evaluation
7. Educator—appropriateness of available programs—joint planning for child's learning
8. Physical therapist—for evaluation of child's potential for developing musculoskeletal system in terms of ADL and ambulation

bibliography

Barnard, Kathryn E., and Powell, Marcene L. *Teaching the mentally retarded child—a family care approach*. St. Louis: Mosby, 1972.

Finnie, Nancy R. *Handling the young cerebral palsied child at home*. New York: Dutton, 1970.

Haslam, Robert H. (ed.). Symposium on habilitation of the handicapped child. *Pediatric Clinics of North America*, **20**:27–44 (1973).

152 Autism

PAULENE S. JOHNSON

I. Etiology

A. Psychogenic

1. Extreme negative interpersonal environment during the critical periods of development
   a. 0 to 6 months—object relationships
   b. 6 to 9 months—language and locomotion
   c. 18 to 24 months—child begins to shape relationships with the environment
2. Maternal deprivation

B. Organic

1. Inborn disturbances of affective contact
2. Gross perceptual hyposensitivity
3. Sequela of encephalitis

II. Subjective Data

A. Reasons of parent(s) for seeking help

B. Child's response to parent(s)

C. Child's method of communication

D. Method used by parent(s) in communicating with child

E. Description by parent(s) of child's behavior and personality from infancy to the present time, i.e., was the child easily comforted as an infant? How does the child relate to siblings and peers?

F. Associated problems

1. Head banging
2. Remaining motionless for long periods of time during periods of wakefulness
3. Constant body rocking
4. Continuous screaming
5. Self-inflicted injuries
6. Extreme inattentiveness

Note: This condition should be managed in consultation with a physician. A multidisciplinary approach is most effective.

G. Mode of parent(s) in controlling child's behavior

H. Prenatal history

I. Birth history—Apgar score, oxygen needed

J. Neonatal history—milestones, age achieved

K. History of head trauma

L. Exposure to encephalitis

M. Family history for hearing problems, emotional disorders, and mental retardation

N. Social history to determine history of stresses in the home, primary child care giver, siblings, living conditions, and family's ability to comply with treatment regimen

III. Objective Data

A. Physical examination

1. Complete physical examination
2. Eye examination (difficult with autistic child due to profound withdrawal); findings which indicate light perception and some visual acuity:
   a. Direct and consensual pupillary constriction
   b. Blink reflex
   c. Optokinetic nystagmus
   d. Hand-eye coordination
3. Hearing (difficult to test due to profound withdrawal)
   a. Acoustic blink
   b. Evoked-response audiometric examination
4. Thorough neurological examination
5. Observation of parent-child relationship for
   a. Eye contact
   b. Parent looking at child when child's name is mentioned

c. Touching and stroking between parent and child
d. Closeness and/or distancing in seating arrangements
e. Consistency in mode of communication

B. Laboratory data—Denver Developmental Screening Test or Preschool Attainment Record

IV. Assessment

A. Subjective data

1. Mutism or language that doesn't seem intended for interpersonal communication
2. Ritualistic behavior
3. Lack of response to normal sounds
4. Nondistractibility
5. Profound social withdrawal
6. Parent(s) reporting:
   a. Failure of child to assume anticipatory posture as an infant
   b. As infant, was not easily comforted
   c. Demonstrates extreme resistance to any changes in daily routine
   d. Constant head banging
   e. Continuous body rocking
7. History of birth trauma
8. History of emotional discord in the home
9. Distancing behavior between mother and child

B. Objective data

1. Physical findings including vision, hearing, and neurological examinations determined to be within normal limits
2. Lack of eye contact
3. Normal growth pattern
4. Normal gross- and fine-motor adaptive development
5. Delayed language development
6. Delayed personal-social development

V. Management

A. Treatments/medications

1. *Parentectomy.* The child is removed from parental influence and placed in a residential home for treatment. This was an early mode of treatment, and some psychotherapists still believe a parentectomy is essential to successful treatment.
2. Psychotherapy with parent(s) as cotherapists. In this type of treatment, the parent(s) are reeducated and learn how to create highly impactful affective stimulation and offer a wide variety of sensory experiences through tactile, kinesthetic, and proprioceptive experiences.
3. Family training programs
   a. Parent(s) gain insight into the existing pattern of interaction within the family unit.
   b. They learn to modify their patterns of initiating and reciprocating exchanges with the child.
   c. Utilizing the above knowledge, the parent(s) are taught to modify the child's verbal behavior and bizarre behavior.
4. Behavior modification. This is the most common treatment, and is usually carried out in conjunction with family training programs.
   a. Reward (food, praise, encouragement) must be given immediately and consistently after the approved behavior is completed.
   b. Behavior not to be reinforced is not rewarded.
5. Medications—none

B. Counselling/prevention; supportive therapy is required regardless of mode of treatment.

1. Reinforce prescribed treatment.
2. Allay feelings of guilt which are common, and are often exacerbated by the harsh appearance of behavior modification techniques.
3. Stress need for consistency in parent-child interaction.
4. Food is most frequently used as a reward to reinforce positive behavior. To avoid problems of obesity and dental caries, it is necessary to consider the sugar and calorie content of the food being offered.
5. Autistic children often enjoy playing with audiovisual devices. If the child has a special interest in this area, permitting the use of a television, radio, or tape recorder may prove to be a more satisfactory reward than food. More importantly, these devices, especially a tape recorder, may prove to be an invaluable aid in language training. The child's fascination with any communication device should be communicated to the therapist or school personnel.
6. Children who are autistic continue to explore their world through their senses of taste and smell long after the toddler stage has passed. For this reason, it is recommended that substances which are harmful when ingested be kept well out of reach of the older autistic child as well as the toddler.

7. "Time out areas" are used to socially isolate for a short period of time (1 to 20 min) the child who is behaving in a socially unacceptable manner. If this is included in the child's training program, it is important to reinforce with the parent(s) the following.
   a. The child must know the exact amount of time he or she is to spend in the isolation area (bedroom, hallway, etc.). Giving the child a timer set for 1, 2, 3, or more minutes is helpful in conveying this information.
   b. Each time the child repeats the unacceptable behavior, the amount of time spent socially isolated is increased.
   c. It seems most effective if only one behavior is treated in this manner at any given time.
8. Management of temper tantrums is best accomplished by ignoring the child while he or she is screaming and giving lots of attention, praise, and reward once the tantrum stops.
9. Many autistic children are particularly fearful of new social situations. When planning a family outing, it is best to prepare the child in advance through words and phrases which may lend familiarity to the situation and prevent complete bewilderment by new surroundings. Taking the child's favorite toys and clothes will also prove helpful. Increase the scope of social interaction gradually.
10. The autistic child is especially prone to be upset by failure. Therefore, it is important when teaching new tasks to do so in simple steps, making links with skills which are already familiar and which give pleasure.

C. Follow-up: well-child-care visits initially. Frequent visits (preferably in the home) to assess family's acceptance of, and ability to follow, therapeutic regimen. Maintaining ongoing dialogue between parent(s) and school staff is essential. Frequently, parent(s) will develop ways of assisting at home that can be included at school, and the carry-over of the school program into the home setting is necessary for the child's optimum treatment.

D. Consultations/referrals: all presumptive autistic syndromes should be referred to physician, psychiatrist, or psychologist.

bibliography

Bachrach, Ann W. *Developmental therapy for young children with autistic characteristics.* Baltimore: University Park Press, 1978.

Bettleheim, B. *The empty fortress: infantile autism and the birth of self.* New York: The Free Press, 1967.

Hargrave, Elizabeth, and Swisher, Linda. Modifying the verbal expression of a child with autistic behaviors. *Journal of Autism and Childhood Schizophrenia,* **5**(2):147–153 (1975).

Kanner, L. Early infantile autism. *Pediatric Clinics of North America,* no. **5** (1958).

Rimland, B. The differentiation of childhood psychosis: An analysis of checklists. *Journal of Autism and Childhood Schizophrenia,* **1**:175–189 (1971).

———, *Infantile autism.* New York: Appleton Century Crofts, 1967.

153 Duchenne's Muscular Dystrophy[1]

MARILYN GREBIN

I. Etiology: Genetically Determined Myopathy

II. Subjective Data: a complete history including

A. Age and sex

B. History of the present problem

1. Description of child climbing stairs
2. Presence of muscle cramps
3. Difficulty running with excessive falling
4. Awkward posture
5. Difficulty rising from chair, bed, floor
6. Weakness of shoulders or hips
7. Facial expression, difficulty smiling or frowning
8. Floppy baby
9. Difficult feeding, with choking or dysphagia
10. Inability to fully close eyes
11. Poor grasp

C. Complete developmental history

D. Family history—genetic disorders or mental retardation

E. Past hospitalizations, reasons

F. Past treatments or diagnoses

III. Objective Data

A. Complete physical examination

1. Facial ptosis or weakness
2. Ocular movements
3. Musculoskeletal examination
   a. Gait
   b. Posture
   c. Stair climbing
   d. Rising from floor
   e. Scapular size and position
   f. Balance
   g. Muscular weakness, grip
   h. Presence of contractures, bony deformities
4. Neurodevelopmental
   a. Developmental milestones
   b. Deep tendon reflexes
   c. Hand opposition
   d. Finger to nose
   e. Outstretched arms
   f. Extension of tongue
   g. Smile
   h. Pursing of lips
   i. Grip
   j. Fasciculations, especially of tongue or thumb
5. Cardiovascular
   a. Presence of murmurs
   b. Abnormal rhythms

B. Laboratory data—the following tests should be ordered after consultation with or by a physician.

1. Creatine phosphokinase (CPK)
2. Glutamic-oxaloacetic transaminase (GOT)
3. Electromyogram (EMG)
4. Electrocardiogram (ECG)
5. Muscle biopsy
6. Genetic typing

IV. Assessment: Duchenne's Muscular Dystrophy

A. Subjective data—the parent(s) may present with any or all of the following problems in a male child older than 3 years

1. Delayed motor milestones
2. Inability to climb stairs
3. Muscle cramps

[1]*Note:* All children in whom the diagnosis of Duchenne's muscular dystrophy is suspect must be examined and diagnosed by the physician.

4. Difficulty running, with excessive falling
5. Awkward, slow posturing
6. Difficulty rising from chair, bed, floor

B. Objective data

1. Male
2. Pseudohypertrophy of gastrocnemius muscle (80 percent)
3. Proximal weakness
4. Lumbar lordosis
5. Protuberant abdomen
6. Waddling gait, talipes equinovarus
7. Positive Gowers' sign—use of hands climbing up the legs when rising from the floor
8. Deep tendon reflexes normal in early disease
9. Knee jerks, disappearing with disease progression
10. Ankle jerks remaining intact
11. Mild mental retardation (IQ 70 to 75)
12. Obesity
13. Inability to walk by age 12 years
14. Decreased fine-motor movements
15. Muscles of face and neck affected in the terminal stages
16. Cardiac arrythmias
17. Weakness of the shoulder girdle
18. CPK elevated during early disease
19. EMG confirming myopathic changes
20. Muscle biopsy abnormal
21. Genetics—X-linked

V. Management: Duchenne's Muscular Dystrophy

A. Treatments/medications

1. Medications—none
2. Treatments
   a. Physical therapy to prevent contractures
   b. Brace when ambulation begins to decrease
   c. Wheelchair with a firm seat and vertebral support

B. Counselling/prevention

1. Explain the course of the disorder.
   a. Progressive weakness
   b. Confinement to wheelchair by age 12 yr
2. Provide genetic counselling for the parent(s) and family members.
3. Educate parent(s) for care at home.
   a. Encourage school, social, and interpersonal activities as long as possible.
   b. Encourage self-care skills even though the child may do them slowly.
   c. Discourage immobility, bed rest, or prolonged sitting activities.
   d. Encourage consistent health care follow-up.
   e. Maintain active exercises, walking at least 4 h/day.
   f. Prevent obesity by a balanced caloric diet.
   g. Maintain upright sitting posture during feeding to avoid choking.
   h. Learn postural drainage techniques (see Cystic Fibrosis, Chap. 144) or IPPB use to prevent pneumonia as weakness increases.
4. Counsel parent(s) to understand the psychology of chronic disease.
   a. Low frustration level of the child who cannot do tasks
   b. Preoccupation with self or withdrawal
   c. Manipulation of environment
   d. Emotional immaturity
   e. The need to foster independence
   f. Problem of the premature death for the child and family members
   g. Decreasing parental overprotection
   h. Dealing with sibling reactions to the handicapped child
   i. Disciplining the child; setting limits
5. Support of parental problems can be handled in parent group sessions or health care provider–parent conferences.
6. Give the parent(s) the opportunity to express fears and concerns about care.
7. Discourage "shopping around" for cures by keeping parent(s) informed.
8. Suggest the use of home health aids—over-the-bed bars, hand rails, grab bars, raised toilet seats, bed cradles, foot boards.

C. Follow-up: multidisciplinary team approach (These team members should supply input as often as parental support warrents.)

1. Physicians—pediatrician, neurologist, psychiatrist, geneticist, physiatrist
2. Primary health care practitioner
3. Physical therapist
4. Public health nurse
5. Social worker
6. Professional counsellor—psychologist
7. Genetic counsellor

D. Consultations/referrals

1. All people in the multidisciplinary team plus
2. School nurse
3. Special educator
4. Muscular Dystrophy Association in the area

Table 153-1 Medical Referral/Consultation: Common Muscular Dystrophies

Diagnosis	Clinical Manifestations	Management
Becker's muscular dystrophy (late-onset, X-linked)	Over 20 years of age Maternal uncles or male siblings affected Ability to walk until age 15 Physical characteristics (see Duchenne's) Muscle enzymes rarely elevated Subtle changes revealed by muscle biopsy CPK elevated in most women carriers	Referral to physician See Management, V
Limb girdle muscular dystrophy (autosomal recessive)	Male or female 10–20 years of age Weakness of shoulder girdle Difficulty combing hair Weakness of pelvic girdle—difficulty running or climbing stairs or rising from chair Findings similar to Duchenne's muscular dystrophy Weakness progresses slowly Positive Gowers' sign with severe onset Scapular winging Contractures of Achilles tendon with talipes equinovarus CPK levels elevated early (values do not equal one-half of Duchenne's) EMG and muscle biopsy show nonspecific myopathy	Referral to physician See Management, V
Congenital muscular dystrophy (autosomal recessive)	Weakness since birth—"floppy baby" Poor feeding Limited movement Delayed milestones Weakness of face and extraocular muscles Deep tendon reflexes decreased or absent Weak respirations Floppy appearance Limited active mobility Joint contractures Mild to severe mental retardation CPK mildly increased EMG mildly myopathic Abnormal muscle biopsy	Referral to physician See Management, V
Facioscapulohumeral dystrophy (Landouzy-Déjerine) (autosomal dominant)	More than 20 years of age Weakness of face and scapular muscle Difficulty closing eyes Unable to close eyes against force Unable to smile or whistle or pucker lips Unable to raise arms over head	Referral to physician See Management, V

Table 153-1 Medical Referral/Consultation *(continued)*

Diagnosis	Clinical Manifestations	Management
	Impassive facial expression—face unlined Unable to hold air in oral cavity Winged scapula Weak lower extremities—foot drop, contractures Kyphoscoliosis and lumbar lordosis Serum enzymes are normal EMG—similar changes as Duchenne's muscular dystrophy	
Myotonic dystrophy childhood form (autosomal dominant)	Age 5–15 years Delayed motor development Awkward gait Facial weakness Delayed motor milestones, mental retardation Ptosis, facial diplegia, bitemporal muscle atrophy Myotonia Spasm of superior recti muscle after forced closure of eyes Fasciculation of tongue; depression furrow remains after percussion Abductor spasm of the thumb after percussion Inability to quickly release grip of objects Distal weakness in older child Adolescent development of frontal baldness, gonadal atrophy, cataracts Cervical kyphosis Dysarthric or nasal speech, mouth drooping open Foot drop Deep tendon reflexes diminish with disease progress EMG—classic myotona with increase and decrease of discharge over seconds Enzymes rarely elevated ECG abnormal	Referral to physician See Management, V
Ocular muscular dystrophy (oculopharyngeal muscular dystrophy) (autosomal dominant)	Possible occurrence of symptoms in the adolescent Weakness of facial muscles Dysphagia Ptosis, strabismus Weakness of facial muscles; distal and neck weakness Limited eye movement CPK normal EMG—myopathy	Referral to physician See Management, V

bibliography

Downey, John, and Low, Neils. *The Child with disabling illness*. Philadelphia; Saunders, 1974, pp. 217–228.

Furukawa, Tetsuo, and Peter, James. Muscular dystrophies and related disorders, I. The muscular dystrophies, *Journal of the American Medical Association,* **239**(15): 1537–1542 (1978).

———, and ———. The Muscular dystrophies and related disorders, II. Diseases simulating muscular dystrophies. *Journal of the American Medical Association,* **239**(16):1654-1659 (1978).

Hymovich, Debra. Parents of sick children. *Pediatric Nursing,* **2**(5):9-13 (1976).

Slater, Gerald, and Swaiman, Kenneth. Muscular dystrophies of childhood. *Pediatric Annals,* **6**(3):51–93 (1977).

154 Cleft Lip/Cleft Palate

MARILYN GREBIN

I. Etiology

A. Unknown

B. Failure of fusion of maxillary and premaxillary process between fifth and eighth week of intrauterine life

II. Subjective data

A. Age (usually infants)

B. Sex

C. Prenatal history

D. Birth history

E. Any other congenital anomalies

F. Feeding problems

1. Method used
2. Presence of choking

G. Respiratory distress

H. Oral bleeding

I. Family history for congenital anomalies and/or others with genetic disorders

J. Social history

1. Child's care givers
2. Economic status
3. Sleeping arrangements

K. Psychological status of family members

1. Reaction of parent(s) to this child
2. Reaction of siblings to this child
3. Ability of parent(s) to care for child

III. Objective Data

A. Physical examination (complete)

1. Emotional status (observe)
   a. Child
   b. Mother
2. Description of cleft lip and/or cleft palate
3. Condition of tongue and gums; and number and conditon of teeth (if any)
4. Inspection of posterior pharynx for depth and length of cleft palate
5. Observe sucking ability
6. Observe feeding technique of parent(s)
7. In the older child, an articulation and phonation screen

B. Laboratory data: x-ray by physician prior to surgical procedures

IV. Assessment

A Subjective data

1. Infant
   a. Feeding problems
      (1) Inability to suck properly on the nipple
      (2) Regurgitation of food into the nasopharynx
      (3) Aspiration of food or fluids causing increased respiratory distress
   b. Parent(s) demonstrate excessive anxiety in handling the child
2. Older child
   a. Articulation and phonation problems possibly the presenting symptom if the child has progressed in age with either cleft lip or cleft palate
   b. Poor dentition
   c. Oral bleeding

B. Objective data

1. Cleft lip and/or hard or soft cleft palate
2. Poor nutritional status
3. Anxious mother
4. Irritable child
5. Otitis media
6. Upper respiratory infection
7. Mild ocular hypertelorism
8. Poor sucking reflex
9. Increased nasal drainage

10. Irregular dentition
11. Poor articulation in the older child

V. Management

A. Treatments/medications

1. Feeding (to prevent aspiration)
   a. Liquids should be given in a paper or soft cup with the child in a sitting position.
   b. Solids should be diluted with the liquids or fed in very small amounts, very slowly, by a spoon placed on the child's tongue to avoid nasal regurgitation.
2. For the infant with only cleft palate, a duck-billed nipple may be obtained for feeding or a duck-billed pacifier for comfort.
3. Surgical correction will be determined by the physician.

B. Counselling/prevention

1. Since the child may be hospitalized for long periods, the parental attachment process may become altered, and it is necessary to help parent(s) overcome fantasies about the perfect child and form new expectations that take into account the child's limitations.
2. Parent(s) should be taught
   a. About the anomaly and the basis for treatment, in order to decrease their guilt and anxiety.
   b. To decrease anxieties when handling the child, the parent(s) should hold the infant upright, talk to the baby, smile, and relax before feeding.
   c. Appropriate feeding techniques.
3. The practitioner should be available to the parent(s) for guidance and support.
4. Explanation of the child's anomaly and the treatment should be provided several times during the regimen to ensure understanding.
5. Help parent(s) overcome feelings of guilt.
   a. Allow and encourage expression of positive and negative feelings.
   b. Have parent(s) share home care experiences in parent groups or counselling sessions.
6. Developmental growth should be shared with the parent(s) at each level to demonstrate that normal growth and development is in progress.
7. Give parent(s) written materials to assist in the education process.

C. Follow-up

1. The practitioner should follow the child's progress
   a. Telephone communication
   b. Home visits
   c. Outpatient visits
   d. During hospitalization to ensure continuity of counselling with other staff
2. To ensure teaching of progressive handling and feeding techniques

D. Consultations/referrals

1. Plastic surgeon
2. Orthodontist
3. Speech pathologist
4. Psychological evaluation
   a. Older child
   b. Parent(s) who continues to have anxieties

bibliography

Gellis, Sydney S., and Kagen, Benjamin M. *Current Pediatric Therapy 8*. Philadelphia: Saunders, 1978.

Gracely, Katherine, A. Parental attachment to a child with congenital defect. *Pediatric Nursing*, **3**(5):15–17 (1977).

Hymovich, Debra. Parents of sick children. *Pediatric Nursing*, **2**(5):9–13 (1976).

section 3

social disorders

155 Lead Poisoning[1]

LESLIE LIETH

ALERT
1. Elevated lead level over 50 μg/dL whole blood
2. Free erythrocyte protoporphyrin (FEP) over 120 μg/dL
3. Irritability
4. Lethargy
5. Ataxia
6. Hepatosplenomegaly
7. Abdominal tenderness

I. Subjective Data

A. Same data base needed for suspected case and known case

B. Complete history, including:

1. History of present illness
   a. Decrease in appetite
   b. Anorexia
   c. Apathy
   d. Irritability
   e. Vomiting
   f. Constipation
   g. Slowdown of development
   h. Behavior or personality changes
   i. Hyperactivity
   j. Episodic lethargy or stupor
   k. Convulsions
   l. Coma
2. Developmental history
   a. History of pica
   b. Developmental milestones
   c. Denver Developmental Screening Test (DDST)
3. Family history
   Any other children or adults in family with history of lead poisoning or pica
4. Social history
   a. Does client live in old (before 1940) or new building?
   b. Does client live near any factories? smelters?
   c. Does client visit or stay with persons who live in old buildings or near factories or smelters?
   d. Name the following sources of lead, and ask informant if this source is present in the environment.
      (1) Peeling plaster or paint
      (2) Painted furniture
      (3) Inadequately glazed pottery
      (4) Painted toys—particularly old, tin toys
      (5) Newspaper print, especially colored ads and comics
      (6) House and outdoor dust and dirt
      (7) Airborne lead from restoration of old houses, heavily trafficked areas, burning batteries for heat, shooting galleries
      (8) Bootleg whiskey
      (9) Lead toys
      (10) Plastic jewelry coated with lead to simulate pearls
      (11) Paint pigments used by artists
      (12) Swallowed lead weights (curtain weights, fishing sinkers)
5. Past medical history
   a. History of previously documented lead poisoning or treatment for same?
   b. Previous testing for lead poisoning? Results?

[1]Any client with a blood lead level over 50 μg/dL should be referred to a physician.

II. Objective Data

A. Suspected case

1. Problem-oriented physical examination, including skin, lymph, head, eyes, ears, mouth, teeth, nose, throat, neck, chest, lungs, heart, abdomen, musculoskeletal, neurological
2. Developmental screening
3. Height, weight, and temperature
4. Laboratory
   a. FEP (free erythrocyte protoporphyrin) test
   b. Hemoglobin, reticulocyte count, white blood cell count with differential
   c. Venous lead level
   d. Urinalysis
   e. Also possibly
      (1) Flat plate of abdomen
      (2) X-ray, posterior-anterior views of wrists, knees
      (3) Urine sample for lead (if available)
      (4) Hair sample for lead (if available)

B. Known case

1. Physical examination—same as for suspected case
2. Developmental screening
3. Height, weight, and temperature
4. Laboratory
   a. Venous lead level
   b. FEP
   c. Hemoglobin, reticulocyte count, white blood cell count with differential
   d. Urinalysis
   e. Flat plate of abdomen
   f. X-ray, posterior-anterior views of wrists, knees
   g. Urine sample for lead (if available)
   h. Hair sample for lead (if available)

III. Assessment

A. Normal child, but at risk

1. Subjective data
   Presence of one or more risk factors, i.e., pica, presence of lead in environment, poor housing, city dweller, family history of lead poisoning (see also Social history section, I, B, 4)
2. Objective data
   a. Normal values for FEP, venous lead, hemoglobin, etc.
   b. Normal physical examination

B. Lead intoxication—minimally elevated

1. Subjective data
   a. Asymptomatic
   b. Usually presence of one or more high risk factors as discussed above (III, A, 1)
2. Objective data
   a. FEP between 60 and 119 μg/dL whole blood
   b. Lead level between 30 and 49 μg/dL whole blood
   c. Physical examination: can have pale color, otherwise negative

C. Lead intoxication—moderately elevated

1. Subjective data
   a. Usually presence of one or more high-risk factors (see III, A, 1)
   b. Symptoms can include
      (1) Constipation
      (2) Slow growth
      (3) Slow development
      (4) Clumsiness
      (5) Lethargy
      (6) Abdominal pain
      (7) Hyperactivity
      (8) Poor appetite
2. Objective data
   a. Venous lead level between 50 and 79 μg/dL whole blood
   b. FEP elevated, 120 to 189 μg/dL whole blood
   c. Lead deposits in long bones revealed by x-ray
   d. Hemoglobin usually low for age
   e. Physical examination can reveal
      (1) Developmental delay
      (2) "Lead line" along gum margins
      (3) Irritability
      (4) Lethargy
      (5) Abdominal tenderness
      (6) Fever
      (7) Hepatosplenomegaly
      (8) Lymphadenopathy
      (9) Clumsiness
      (10) Hyperactivity
      (11) Ataxia
      (12) Pale skin, pale conjunctivas

D. Lead intoxication—extremely elevated

1. Subjective data: see III, C, 1
2. Objective data
   a. Elevated venous lead level greater than 80 μg/dL whole blood
   b. Elevated FEP greater than 190 μg/dL
   c. Lower than normal hemoglobin
   d. Lead deposits in long bones shown on x-ray
   e. Physical examination
      (1) See III, C, 2, e.
      (2) Can also have convulsions.

IV. Management

A. At-risk child with normal FEP and lead level

1. Treatments/medications: none
2. Counselling/prevention: Provide family with information about lead poisoning, recognizing potential sources, etc.
3. Follow-up
   a. Visits every 4 to 6 months
   b. FEP periodically, especially during peak season (May to October)
4. Consultations/referrals: none

B. Lead intoxication—minimally elevated levels

1. Treatments/Medications
   a. Complete blood count (CBC) with reticulocytes if not done recently
   b. Serum iron level
   c. Oral iron if anemic (see Anemia, Chap. 39)
2. Counselling/prevention
   a. Identify sources of lead in environment.
   b. Familiarize family with sources of lead; provide information concerning prevention of lead poisoning, possible signs and symptoms of intoxication.
3. Follow-up
   a. Make appointment for 2 to 3 months.
   b. Retest lead levels every 2 to 3 months until stabilized, then every 6 months until not at risk.
4. Consultations/referrals
   a. Refer to medical protocol or consult with physician.
   b. Refer to public health nurse to help identify source of lead and to reinforce counselling.

C. Lead intoxication—moderately to extremely elevated levels

1. Treatments/medications
   a. Remove child from environment until source of lead is eliminated.
   b. Test all other persons in household for lead intoxication.
   c. Use of chelating agents by physician. Commonly used agents are calcium disodium edetate (EDTA); dimercaprol (BAL); and d-penicillamine.
   d. If client is also iron deficient at the same time, chelation therapy should not begin until iron therapy is stopped.
2. Counselling/prevention
   a. Prepare family for hospitalization (see Part 7, Preparation for Hospitalization)
   b. See V, B, 2
3. Follow-up
   a. Follow lead levels periodically, even after history of elimination of lead sources.
   b. Follow client periodically, at least school-age children, checking for developmental problems and/or neurological sequelae.
4. Consultations/referrals
   a. Refer to physician for therapy and hospital admission.
   b. Involve department of health to find source of lead and have a joint effort with them to have source eliminated.

bibliography

Chisolm, J. J., et al. Poisoning: Lead toxicity from suspicion to therapy. *Patient Care,* **10**:80–94 (1976).

Croft, H., et al. Children and lead poisoning. *American Journal of Nursing,* **75**:102–104 (1975).

———, and ———. Exposure to lead: sources and effects. *New England Journal of Medicine,* **297**:943–945 (1977).

Graef, John, and Cone, Thomas. *Manual of pediatric therapeutics.* Boston: Little, Brown, 1974.

Jonides, Linda, and Heindl, Mary C. Difficulties in treating lead poisoning. *Pediatric Nursing,* **1**:24–28 (1975).

Rice, C., et al. Unsuspected sources of lead poisoning. *New England Journal of Medicine,* **296**:1416 (1977).

156 Obesity/Overweight

PENELOPE S. PECKOS

ALERT
Manifestation of excessive adiposity (fatness)
1. Upper arms, neck, face
2. Panniculus (abdominal fat padding)
3. Thighs

I. Etiology

A. Overeating
B. Underexercising
C. Genetic potential
D. Chronic illness (immobility due to accident, polio, etc.)
E. Hyperplastic obesity (early-onset obesity with increased number of fat cells)
F. Psychological factors—trauma, severe illness, death of one parent, fragmented family—separation or divorce, alcoholism
G. Social factors
1. Ethnic and cultural milieu
2. Money available from earnings/liberal allowance

II. Subjective Data: Interview Parent(s) and Client Separately

A. Age at onset and present age
1. Infant weight record valuable
2. School height-weight record valuable

B. Chronological position of the client to other siblings
C. Nutritional history
1. 24-h recall at time of examination (client)
2. 7-day dietary intake record preferred later
3. Previous dieting experience of client
4. Eating patterns of family:
   a. Dietary history—parent(s)
   b. Ethnicity—cultural foods

D. Family history
1. Ethnic background of each parent—current age
2. History of weight of parent(s) and siblings (with ages)

E. Menstrual history
1. Age at onset
2. Erratic or regular

F. Past or present history
1. Acne
2. Bed-wetting
3. Nail biting
4. Eye problems (glasses or other)
5. Orthodontics (dental problems)

G. Mild and/or severe physical or psychological disabilities
1. Dyslexia
2. Diabetes
3. Mental retardation (degree, if any)
4. Bone or skeletal malformations; growth problems

H. Social history
1. Physical activity—at school: frequency, type
2. Physical activity—during nonschool time: frequency, type
3. Preferred entertainment (sports, movies, television, etc.); participatory or spectator
4. Family activities
   a. Vacation plans (together or separate)
   b. Camp experience of client, if any (or sleep-away experience)
5. Academic achievement
6. Social behavior of client
   a. Available money to spend (source and how spent)
   b. Ability to separate from parent(s)
   c. School socials—friends involved (one,

few, many)
  d. Peer relationship (loner, shy, gregarious)
7. Mealtimes—family together or separate; sociability of family unit
8. Alcohol consumption—client, parent(s)

III. Ojective Data

A. Physical examination

1. Complete physical examination
2. General appearance and dress
3. Height and weight—plotted on graph
4. Skinfold measurement of adiposity
   a. Lange skinfold caliper
   b. Midtriceps and subscapular areas
   c. Distribution of adiposity (hips, thighs, chest, arms)
5. Level of physical development
   a. Hirsuteness of males—primary and secondary sex characteristics
   b. Females—primary and secondary sex characteristics
6. Thorough inspection of skin for acne—face, back
7. Nail-biting: inspection of nails for evidence
8. Evaluation of psychological status
9. Evaluation of parent-child relationship

B. Laboratory data

1. Complete blood count (CBC)
2. Urinalysis
3. Endocrine and/or hormonal assays if indicated
4. Other bioassays as indicated; blood lipid levels
   a. At initial visit
   b. Repeated at mid adolescence
5. X-ray of the wrist to determine bone age

IV. Assessment

A. Subjective data

1. Increased food intake recently
2. Lessened physical activity
3. History of physical illness and/or disability
   a. Chronic problems
   b. Nonspecific problems
   c. Gastrointestinal problems
4. Family crisis (death, severe illness, etc.)
5. Academic problems (learning disability)
6. Social problems (peer and authority figures)
7. Behavior aberrations (school, home, peers)
8. History of acne, bed-wetting, nail-biting, eye problems, orthodontics
9. Early onset of menarche (10 years old)
10. Possible history of overweight in family

B. Objective data

1. Increased developmental changes
   a. Musculature—normal for age
   b. Skeletal development—normal for age
   c. Fat padding
      (1) Normal for female; menarche; previous increases in fat padding
      (2) Increased adiposity—chest, back, waist, abdomen, thighs
   d. Weight chart—depicting large gains in weight over short periods of time (months to a year)
   e. Lange skinfold measurements over 20 mm (midtriceps reading)
2. Endocrine pathology possibly revealed by laboratory tests
3. Body language indicates
   a. Shyness or aggressiveness
   b. Eye contact—or its absence
   c. Relaxed or fidgety
4. Parent-child interaction—physical and/or nonphysical; passive dependency of client

V. Management

A. Treatments/medications

1. Anorexigenic drugs contraindicated for children and adolescents due to undesirable side effects in most instances
2. Available fad diets are contraindicated for children and adolescents because they
   a. Lack in general essential nutrients
   b. Produce ketosis (absence of carbohydrates and high-fat)
   c. Are monotonous
3. Use of hormones contraindicated unless obesity a result of endocrine pathology
4. Behavior modifications (if indicated)—limited success; relatively new approach, more research needed
5. Dietary modification most successful approach to date (see Table 156-1); nutritionally adequate—high protein, moderate fat, low carbohydrate
   a. Meets nutrient requirements for growth and development
   b. Varied and satisfying—no restrictions of any food (except quantity)
   c. Satisfies social and cultural environment of client—snacks, eating out, parties, etc.
   d. Weight loss not to exceed 2 lb per week
   e. Caloric intake for girls—recommended 1200 kcal/day or more, depending on age

f. Dietetic foods not recommended; not always available for teenager
g. Artificial sweetener allowed in beverages only
h. Occasional low-calorie soft drink allowed; one or two per day

B. Counselling/prevention

1. Client
   a. Dietary modification
      (1) Nutrition education needed
         (a) Function of food and nutrients in the body
         (b) Understanding of energy balance, calories
         (c) Relation of frequency and quantity of all foods eaten to weight gain
      (2) Normalcy of diet—greater success in weight loss
   b. Increased physical activity
      (1) School sports activities
      (2) Walking or jogging
      (3) Dancing, calisthenics, ice skating
      (4) Bowling, tennis, swimming
      (5) Encouragement of whatever adolescent enjoys
      (6) Consistency of activity important—once a week, twice a week, or whatever schedule is comfortable and achievable
2. Parent(s)
   a. Parent(s) involvement essential to success
      (1) Understand client's needs and wants.
      (2) Provide dietary assistance (proper and variety of foods).
      (3) Cease nagging, bribing, and ridicule.
      (4) Allow client to assume responsibility for food intake.
      (5) Show love for the client as he or she is—not what parent(s) want the child to be.
      (6) Praise for success achieved is important.
      (7) Offer only limited criticism.
   b. "4 L's" for parent(s)
      (1) Listen to your child.
      (2) Love your child (equated with respect).
      (3) Let your child grow up (mature).
      (4) Limit your child.
3. Prevention of obesity
   a. Should begin prenatally (weight gain) and at birth
      (1) Avoidance of overfeeding
      (2) Early training in exercise and activity
   b. Nutrition education for parent(s) and child

C. Follow-up: by nutritionist if available—others as needed

1. Weekly for first month
2. Biweekly if progress is satisfactory
3. Monthly for rest of year
4. Telephone calls between visits permitted ad lib

D. Consultations/referrals

1. Physician for treatment of medical problems
2. Nutritionist
3. Social worker, psychologist, school nurse, as indicated
4. Professional counselling
   a. Determined by family history and problems
   b. Assessment by physician, nurse, social worker
   c. Psychological and nutritional counselling concurrently, depending upon the complexity of the problem

bibliography

Buskirk, E. R. Obesity: A brief overview with emphasis on exercise. *Federation Proceedings,* **33**:1948–1951 (1974).

Golden, Michael P. An approach to the management of obesity in childhood. *Pediatric Clinics of North America,* **26**(1):187–197 (1979).

Mayer, J. Genes and obesity. In *Overweight: Causes, cost, and control.* Englewood Cliffs, N.J.: Prentice-Hall, 1968.

Peckos, P. S., Spargo, M. A., and Heald, F. P. Program and results of a camp for obese adolescent girls. *Postgraduate Medicine* **27**:527 (1960).

Rome, H. P. The dimensions of obesity. In F. J. Ingelfinger, A. S. Relman, and M. Finland (eds.), *Controversy in internal medicine.* Philadelphia: Saunders, 1966, pp. 464–473.

Stern, J. S., and Greenwood, M. R. C. A review of development of adipose cellularity in man and animals. *Federation Proceedings* **33**:1952–1955 (1974).

Van Itallie, R. B., and Campbell, R. C. Multidisciplinary approach to the problem of obesity. *Journal of the American Dietetic Association,* **61**:385 (1972).

Table 156-1 Sample Menus

Breakfast
4 oz orange juice
⅔ cup any cold cereal
6 oz low-fat (1%) milk or skimmed milk

or

½ grapefruit
1 toasted English muffin
1 tablespoon butter or margarine
8 oz low-fat (1%) milk or skimmed milk

Lunch
Lean meat or fish or chicken sandwich: 2 pieces thin-sliced bread—white or whole wheat; 2 oz lean meat, fish, or chicken
Lettuce and sliced tomato or celery and carrots
1 fresh fruit, any kind
8 oz low-fat or skimmed milk

Midafternoon or before bed (not both)
1 cup bouillon
2 saltines
1 slice American cheese (1 oz)

or

1 fresh fruit
8 oz low-cal soft drink
(1 12-oz can permitted per day)

Dinner
6 oz lean meat, fish, or fowl
1 cup any cooked vegetable
1 bowl salad
1 tablespoon regular salad dressing
½ cup jello or 1 fresh or canned fruit
8 oz skim milk

or

2 2-oz hamburgers
1 1-oz slice cheese
10 French fries
Lettuce and tomato—ad lib
½ cup cole slaw
8 oz skim milk
2 chocolate chip cookies

Snacks
3 times a week
- Small package M & M's or 1 small package peanuts
- 1 small Hershey bar
- 1 small box raisins

Desserts
1–3 times a week
- 2-in square of angel food cake or sponge cake
- 2 cookies
- $\frac{1}{10}$ of an 8-in apple pie
- ½ cup sherbet or ice cream
- 2-in square of gingerbread
- 2-in^2 brownie

157 Drug Abuse

ANTHONY S. MANOGUERRA, JR.

ALERT
1. Lethargy, coma
2. Hypotension
3. Irregular cardiac rhythm or severe tachycardia or bradycardia
4. Seizures
5. Hallucinations and/or delirium
6. Evidence of aspiration
7. Hypothermia or hyperthermia
8. Problems associated with IV drug use, i.e., venous thrombosis, infection, etc.

I. Etiology: Unknown

II. Subjective Data

A. History of drug intake
1. What was taken?
2. How much?
3. Route of administration?
4. Time of administration: If chronic, when did client begin using drug or chemical? Has tolerance developed (increased dose needed to produce effect)?
5. Symptoms experienced?
6. Time of onset of symptoms?
7. If not an acute overdose, what has caused the client to seek medical care at this time?

B. Immunization history: date of last tetanus vaccination

C. Family history: other members of family with drug or chemical abuse problems

D. Social history
1. Helps determine reasons for using drugs; possible then to estimate likelihood of treatment success
2. Living conditions
3. School/job
4. Recent stresses

III. Objective Data

A. Physical examination
1. Perform complete physical examination.
2. Inspect for evidence of infection or other associated problems, such as hepatitis, phlebitis, liver or kidney damage, bone marrow suppression.

B. Laboratory data
1. Urine and blood tests can be used to confirm what drugs or chemicals are being abused.
2. Histories given by drug abuse clients are notoriously unreliable, and often the diagnosis can be made only after finding substances in the client's blood or urine.

IV. Assessment

A. See Table 157-1 for signs and symptoms of commonly abused drugs.
1. Initial presentation of client will vary considerably from person to person and depending on time since exposure.
2. Multiple drug abuse is the rule rather than the exception, so the clinical picture may not implicate a particular drug.

B. Table 157-2 shows the symptoms of drug withdrawal.

C. Table 157-3 lists the signs and symptoms of commonly abused chemicals. Chemical abuse (paint, glue, solvents) is particularly prevalent in adolescents.

D. Table 157-4 lists some common plants or plant extracts that may be abused for their hallucinogenic effects.

V. Management

A. Treatments/medications
1. Acute overdose
   a. Support respiratory and cardiovascular

function.

b. Arrange for transport of client to hospital emergency facility.

c. If there was oral ingestion, and client does not have a contraindication, induce vomiting with syrup of ipecac. Contraindications: coma, seizures, severe lethargy, ingestion of corrosive substances, or petroleum distillates.

d. Treat any infectious complications with appropriate antibiotics.

2. Chronic exposure

a. Make sure no immediate threat to life exists, and provide supportive care if necessary.

b. Treat any infectious complications with appropriate antibiotics.

B. Counselling/prevention

1. Provide supportive and nonjudgmental atmosphere.
2. Attempt to identify for the client aspects of lifestyle that may contribute to drug use so that positive change may be effected.
3. Provide support to family, in particular spouse, children, or parent(s).
4. Each community's resources for dealing with drug abuse problems will vary. The practitioner should be familiar with the local counselling services so that accurate referrals can be made.
5. No effective method of prevention has been developed to date. With adolescents who may be using drugs because of peer pressure or boredom, it may be necessary to divert energies into activities such as sports, music, etc., which will decrease idle time.

C. Follow-up: Ascertain by telephone or visit whether client has entered a treatment program, and continue to provide positive psychological support as needed.

D. Consultations/referrals

1. All drug abuse clients should receive a psychiatric evaluation.
2. Clients should be referred to detoxification programs or counselling programs as needed.
3. All physicians who have prescribed medications for the client should be informed of the identified abuse problem.
4. Family of the client should be referred for counselling.

Table 157-1 Signs and Symptoms of Drug Overdose

Drug	Signs and Symptoms	Laboratory
OPIATES AND SYNTHETIC DERIVATIVES (Heroin, morphine, codeine, propoxyphene, methadone, meperidine, etc.)	CNS depression; respiratory depression; hypotension; pin-point pupils; pale, cool, damp skin; cyanosis. Needle marks ("tracks") may be visible. If hypoxia has resulted in cerebral damage, pupils may be dilated instead of pin-point. Also, combinations of drugs may alter this finding.	Rarely useful. Opiates may be detected in the urine.
BARBITURATES (Secobarbital, pentobarbital, phenobarbital, amobarbital, etc.)	CNS depression, respiratory depression hypotension, absent bowel sounds, cutaneous bullae.	Barbiturate blood levels may not accurately reflect the degree of intoxication. Useful for verifying diagnosis.
GLUTETHIMIDE (Doriden)	CNS depression, hypertension followed by hypotension, respiratory depression, decreased or absent bowel sounds, dilated pupils, dry mouth, irritability and seizures, urinary retention. Coma may be cyclical in nature.	Blood levels do not correlate with degree of toxicity.
AMPHETAMINES AND SYNTHETIC DERIVATIVES	Restlessness, irritability, insomnia, hyperactivity, seizures, tachycardia, fever, dilated pupils, diaphoresis, nausea, vomiting, anorexia. Chronic use: malnutrition, weight loss, suicidal tendencies, paranoia.	Detectable in urine (qualitative).

Table 157-1 Signs and Symptoms of Drug Overdose *(continued)*

Drug	Signs and Symptoms	Laboratory
ANTICHOLINERGIC DRUGS (Antihistamines, phenothiazines, over-the-counter sleep aids, plants such as Jimson weed, antidepressants)	Anxiety, delirium, disorientation, hallucinations, seizures, tachycardia, fever, dilated pupils, vasodilation, urinary retention, decreased bowel activity, drying of secretions Severe poisoning leads to coma, respiratory depression, cardiac arrhythmias.	Difficult to detect in both urine and blood due to low concentrations
BENZODIAZEPINES (Diazepam, chlordiazepoxide, flurazepam, clonazepam, lorazepam, nitrazepam, oxazepam)	Excitement followed by drowsiness	Not useful
ETHCHLORVYNOL (Placidyl)	CNS depression, respiratory depression, hypotension, hypothermia, cardiac arrest Coma possibly prolonged (250–300 h)	Blood levels available; however, do not correlate well with level of consciousness
LSD	Visual and auditory hallucinations. When these symptoms unpleasant or intolerable, referred to as "a bad trip"	Not useful
MEPROBAMATE (Equanil)	Drowsiness or light coma, nystagmus, muscle weakness, arrhythmias, convulsions Severe cases: coma and respiratory depression, hypothermia	Blood levels Therapeutic 4–5 mg% Toxic > 5 mg%
METHAQUALONE (Quāālude, Sopor, Parest, Somnafac)	Mild to severe coma preceded by hyperexcitability and hyperreflexia; myoclonic jerking, convulsions, tachycardia	Poor correlations between blood levels and clinical effects. Most clients intoxicated if blood level > 2.5 mg/100 mL
METHYPRYLON (Noludar)	CNS depression, hypotension, respiratory depression, tachycardia, hypo or hyperthermia	Blood levels Toxic > 3–6 mg/100 mL Therapeutic < 1 mg/100 mL
PHENCYCLIDINE (PCP)	Excitation, paranoid behavior, horizontal and vertical nystagmus, tachycardia, hypertension, hypotension (late), seizures, hyperreflexia Severe poisoning: respiratory depression and coma	Qualitative urine test readily available
PEYOTE-MESCALINE	CNS stimulation (similar to amphetamines) Nausea, vomiting, perspiration may precede hallucinations Hypertension, tachycardia, nystagmus, ataxia, mydriasis, hyperreflexia	May be detected in urine
COCAINE	CNS stimulation, euphoria, restlessness, headache, nausea, vomiting, fasciculations, bradycardia, hypertension, tachypnea Severe overdose: seizures, arrhythmias, coma, respiratory failure	Qualitative urine test readily available

Table 157-2 Drug Withdrawal

Drug	Potential for Physical Addiction*	Symptoms of Withdrawal
OPIATES AND SYNTHETIC NARCOTICS	+++	Anxiety, sweating, dilated pupils, piloerection, occasionally vomiting and abdominal pain, insomnia
BARBITURATES	+++	Anxiety, sleep disturbances, nausea, vomiting, irritability, restlessness, tremulousness, postural hypertension, seizures, fever, psychosis
BENZODIAZEPINES	++	Similar to barbiturates
AMPHETAMINES	+	Apathy, somnolence, depression
COCAINE	0	None
ALCOHOL	++	Tremulousness, hallucinations, seizures, delirium

* +++ = high potential; 0 = low potential.

Table 157-3 Signs and Symptoms of Chemical Abuse

Chemical	Signs and Symptoms	Method of Exposure
TOLUENE, XYLENE (Commonly found in glues, metallic patents, and as solvent for other chemicals)	Acute: bronchial and laryngeal irritation, transient euphoria, headache, giddiness, vertigo, ataxia. High dose: coma, renal tubular acidosis, proteinuria. Chronic: Liver and renal damage.	Inhalation
GASOLINE (Contains mixtures of petroleum distillates including toluene and xylene)	Same as for toluene.	Inhalation
BUTYL NITRITE (Locker room odorizer commonly sold as Locker Room, Jock Aroma, and other names)	Euphoria, headache, sensation of slowing of time. High doses may produce syncope due to hypotension. Chronic use multiple times a day may theoretically lead to methemoglobinemia.	Inhalation
TRICHLOROETHANE (Found in dry-cleaning agents and spot removers)	CNS depression, hypotension, arrhythmias.	Inhalation

Table 157-4 Selected Plant Substances of Abuse

Name of Plant or Plant Extract	Active Ingredient	Signs and Symptoms
JIMSON WEED (Jamestown weed, stinkweed)	Atropine and scopolamine	Hallucinations, delirium, fever, dry mouth, tachycardia, dilated pupils, decreased GI motility. Large doses: coma, seizures.

Table 157-4 Selected Plant Substances of Abuse *(continued)*

Name of Plant or Plant Extract	Active Ingredient	Signs and Symptoms
NUTMEG AND MACE (Seed of *Myristica fragrans*)	Myristicin	Hallucinations, lightheadedness, abdominal pain, flushed skin, drowsiness, stupor, mydriasis, blurred vision, tachycardia, (similar to atropine poisoning).
AMANITA MUSCARIA (Mushroom)	Ibotenic acid Muscimol	Onset 30–90 min after ingestion: drowsiness, confusion, dizziness, ataxia, euphoria, muscle cramps, delirium, hallucinations. Severe drowsiness and coma lasting 4–8 h usually terminates the episode.
PSILOCYBE MEXICANA (Mushrooms)	Psilocybin Psilocin	Hallucinations, dysphoria, mydriasis, vertigo, ataxia, muscle weakness, drowsiness progressing to sleep lasting 4–6 h. In children hyperpyrexia and seizures may occur.

bibliography

Bourne, P. G. *A treatment manual for acute drug abuse emergencies.* Washington, DC: United States Government Printing Office, NCDAI publication no. 16, 1974.

Kramer, J., Manoguerra, A., and Schnoll, S. H. When drug abuse enters the differential. *Patient Care,* **10:**110–131 (1976).

———, ———, and ———. Treating the acute overdose victim. *Patient Care,* **11:**76–103 (1977).

Rumack, B. H. *Poisindex.* Denver: Micromedex, 1979.

Smith, D. E., and Wesson, D. R. *Diagnosis and treatment of adverse reactions to sedative-hypnotics.* Washington DC: United States Government Printing Office, DHEW publication no. 75–144, 1975.

158 Alcohol Abuse

CAROL R. NOTARO

ALERT
1. Marked behavioral changes
2. Hallucinations
3. Memory impairment
4. Episodes of "blackouts"

I. Etiology

A. Unknown

B. Proposed theories of causation

1. Disturbance in developmental pattern
   a. Fixation at oral stage of development
   b. Sugerego/ego dystonia
2. Family system disturbances
   a. Presence of alcohol abuse/alcoholism in family members
   b. Dysfunctional family unit
3. Biological/chemical components
   a. Intolerance to alcohol
   b. Presence of alcoholism in family members
4. Psychobiosocial changes of adolescence

II. Subjective Data

A. History of problem

1. Onset
2. Alcohol consumption pattern
   a. Amount of intake
   b. Frequency of intake
   c. Location where intake occurs
   d. Social context of intake
3. Behavior pattern
   a. Onset of changes
   b. Change in school attendance
   c. Change in scholastic achievement
   d. Change in peer group associations
   e. Attitudinal change
   f. Changes in family relationships

B. Family history

1. Alcohol abuse/alcoholism in family members
2. Emotional problems in family members
3. Discord in family unit

C. Social History

D. Legal history

1. Arrests for intoxication
2. Juvenile authority involvement

III. Objective Data

A. Physical examination

1. Perform problem-oriented physical examination—ears, nose, throat, heart, lungs, abdomen, neurological.
2. Note odor of alcohol on breath.
3. Note if slurring of speech is present.
4. Check for impaired motor coordination.

B. Laboratory: blood alcohol level

IV. Assessment

A. Alcohol abuse

1. Subjective data
   a. Excessive alcohol intake
   b. Consumption of alcoholic beverages before, during, and/or after school or work hours
   c. Behavior pattern changes
      (1) Decrease in scholastic achievement
      (2) Disrupted family relationships
      (3) Change in peer associations
      (4) Changes in attitudes
2. Objective data: indications of intoxication
   a. Odor of alcohol on breath
   b. Impaired motor coordination
   c. Slurring of speech
   d. Blood alcohol level over 100 mg/100 mL

B. Alcoholism
1. Subjective data
   a. Excessive alcohol intake
   b. Consumption of alcoholic beverages before, during, and/or after school or work hours
   c. Changes in behavior patterns
      (1) Change in scholastic achievement
      (2) Disrupted family relationships
      (3) Change in peer associations
      (4) Changes in attitudes
      (5) Inability to stop drinking despite the wish to stop
   d. History of arrests for intoxication/driving while intoxicated
2. Objective data
   a. Evidence of frequent intoxication
      (1) Odor of alcohol on breath
      (2) Impaired motor coordination
      (3) Slurring of speech
   b. Juvenile authority record
   c. Blood alcohol level over 100 mg/100 mL

V. Management

A. Alcohol abuse
1. Treatment
   a. Group discussion alternatives
      (1) Values-clarification group
      (2) Young People's Alcoholics Anonymous
      (3) Rap group
   b. Support of family members—nonjudgmental attitude
   c. Support of nurse practitioner
2. Counselling/prevention
   a. Reinforcement of therapeutic intervention
   b. Education regarding the following:
      (1) Place of alcohol use in society
      (2) Need for establishing and maintaining open lines of communication between parent(s) and child
      (3) Recognition of early signs of emotional distress in the child
3. Follow-up
   a. Maintain contact with client for supportive purposes.
   b. Maintain contact with therapist regarding course of therapy.
   c. Maintain contact with parent(s) for support.
4. Consultations/referrals
   a. Physician/child psychiatrist referral if behavioral problems antedate onset of alcohol abuse
   b. Group discussion alternatives
      (1) Psychotherapist offering values-clarification group
      (2) Rap group
      (3) Young People's Alcoholics Anonymous (AA), located through Alcoholics Anonymous in area

B. Alcoholism
1. Treatment
   a. Detoxification
   b. Group therapy/family therapy
   c. Young People's AA group
2. Counselling/prevention
   a. Reinforcement of therapeutic intervention through supportive measures and encouragement
   b. Education regarding the following
      (1) Place of alcohol use in society
      (2) Need for establishing and maintaining open lines of communication between parent(s) and child
      (3) Recognition of early signs of emotional distress in the child
3. Follow-up
   a. Maintain contact during detoxification period.
   b. Maintain contact with client during course of treatment.
   c. Maintain contact with parent(s) for purpose of support and reinforcement of treatment.
4. Consultations/referrals
   a. Physician/child psychiatrist referral for evaluation for detoxification/hospitalization
   b. Physician/child psychiatrist referral if behavioral problems antedate alcohol usage
   c. Psychotherapist offering group therapy and family therapy
   d. Young People's AA group, located through Alcoholics Anonymous in area

Table 158-1 Medical Referral/Consultation

Diagnosis	Clinical Manifestations	Management
Behavior disorder	Antisocial behavior Delinquency Explosive behavior Paranoid behavior Truancy Withdrawn behavior	Consult physician; refer to child psychiatrist/community mental health center for psychodiagnostic testing. Support therapeutic intervention by maintaining contact throughout course of treatment. Behavior modification. If problem severe and family support system lacking, residential treatment may be indicated.
Mixed substance abuse	Alcohol use combined with use of another substance; barbiturates, amphetamines, marijuana, cocaine, chemicals, inhalants Hallucinations Antisocial behavior Paranoid behavior	Consult physician; refer to child psychiatrist. Refer to drug treatment center. Maintain contact with client and family for purpose of support and encouragement. See Drug Abuse, Chap. 157.

bibliography

Chafetz, Morris E., Hertzman, Marc, and Berenson, David. Alcoholism: a positive view. In Silvano Arieti (ed.), *The american handbook of psychiatry* (2d ed.). New York: Basic Books, 1974, vol. 3, pp. 367–392.

Chafetz, Morris E., Blane, Howard T., and Hill, Marjorie J. *Frontiers of alcoholism.* New York: Science House, 1970.

Gale, Leonard, and Frances, Allen. Super-ego factors in alcoholics. *American Journal of Psychotherapy,* **29**:235–242 (1975).

Josselyn, Irene M. Adolescence. In Silvano Arieti (ed.), *The American handbook of psychiatry* (2d ed.). New York: Basic Books, 1974, vol. 1, pp. 382–398.

National Council on Alcoholism. Criteria for the diagnosis of alcoholism. *American Journal of Psychiatry,* **129**: 127–135 (1972).

Steinglas, Peter, and Weiner, Sheldon. Familial interactions and determinants of drinking behavior. In Nancy K. Mello and Jack H. Mendelson (eds.), *Recent advances in studies of alcoholism: An interdisciplinary symposium.* Washington, D.C.: United States Government Printing Office, 1971, pp. 687–705.

Young people and alcohol. *Alcohol Health and Research World,* Summer 1975, pp. 2–10.

159 Battered/Abused Child

LESLIE LIETH

I. Etiology

Trauma caused by burns or other forms of abuse

II. Subjective Data: Complete history including

- **A.** Age
- **B.** Reason for visit
- **C.** Nutritional history
- **D.** Developmental history, including DDST, behavior, school performance
- **E.** Clinic or physician providing primary care
- **F.** Social history
- **G.** Family history
- **H.** Immunization history
- **I.** Past medical history, including prenatal, natal, postnatal, accidents, burns, hospitalizations

III. Objective Data

- **A.** Physical examination: complete physical examination including thorough skin exam, neurological, behavioral and developmental assessment, parent-child interaction
- **B.** Laboratory data
  1. Complete body x-rays
  2. CBC and urinalysis
  3. DDST

IV. Assessment

- **A.** Subjective data
  1. Bizarre accidents.
  2. Multiple accidents or accidental poisonings.
  3. Unexplained injury.
  4. Child is given inappropriate food, drink, or drugs.
  5. Child is seen as "different" or "bad" by parent(s).
  6. Parent(s) presents contradictory history.
  7. Parent(s) delays in bringing child for care.
  8. Parent(s) projects cause of injury onto a sibling or third party.
  9. Parent(s) is misusing drugs or alcohol.
  10. Parent(s) overreacts or underreacts to seriousness of situation.
  11. Parent(s) is reluctant to give information.
  12. Parent(s) refuses consent for further diagnostic studies or admission to hospital.
  13. Parent(s) has unrealistic expectations of child.
  14. Parent(s) "shops" for hospital care.
  15. Past history of abuse in upbringing of parent(s).
  16. Parent(s) may admit to using severe punishment or abusive behavior.
  17. Parent(s) complains that child gets him or her uptight and frustrated.
  18. Parent(s) has little support from family, friends, and may lead isolated life.
  19. Child is expected to support, comfort, and reassure parent(s).
  20. History of abuse with another child.
  21. Unwanted pregnancy, difficult delivery, or complications at time of birth.
  22. History of interruption of maternal-infant bonding.
- **B.** Objective data
  1. Bruises, welts, or scars on body
  2. Burns (round, uniform, often multiple burns are from cigarettes)
  3. Buttock and foot burns with clear line of de-

Note: Suspicion of battered or abused child must be referred to physician.

marcation
4. Old and new scars occurring simultaneously
5. Fractures in different stages of healing
6. Skull and long bone fractures in infants
7. Intra-abdominal injuries presenting with vomiting, distention, and localized tenderness
8. Limitation of motion of an extremity
9. Poor hygiene
10. Marked passivity and watchfulness, fearful expression in child
11. Malnourished-looking child
12. Developmental retardation
13. Subdural hematomas
14. Signs of sexual abuse
15. Parental loss of control during interview
16. Parental detachment
17. Injury present that is not mentioned in history

V. Management

A. Treatments/medications (see Counselling/prevention, B.)

B. Counselling/prevention

1. Immediate care for injury.
2. Suspected child abuse must be reported immediately to local protective services agency.
3. Immediate care is protection of child—the decision to hospitalize child is made by physician or physician with protective services worker.
4. Inform parent(s) that case is being reported.
5. Assure parent(s) that hospital staff is going to help him or her and the child.
6. Be truthful and honest with parent(s).
7. Attempt to help parent(s) establish trust and confidence in hospital personnel.
8. Involve law enforcement officers only in instances of parental uncooperation.
9. During initial encounter, attempts by hospital staff to identify the agent of an injury or to determine if neglect or abuse was "intentional" may be ill advised.
10. Do a skeletal survey for fractures.
11. If and when child is returned to the home, an ongoing treatment program is essential. This may include
    a. Family therapy or individual therapy
    b. Parent support groups
    c. Parenting classes or a parent-teaching program hospital- or community-based
    d. Coordination of child-abuse team workers for mutual plan and goals
    e. Infant stimulation program
    f. Individual psychotherapy for child
    g. Therapeutic play groups
    h. Child companion; Big Brother or Big Sister program
    i. Job training for mother
    j. Homemaker services/baby-sitter
    k. Crisis intervention—hotline phone, etc.
12. Measures to prevent child abuse would include
    a. Identify those parent(s) at risk and intervene with educational and training experiences.
    b. Provide day care which involves parent(s).
    c. Parenting classes in schools (high school, college, adult education).
    d. Accessible family planning services; reducing the number of unwanted pregnancies.
    e. Expanded prenatal education programs to involve the entire family and to extend beyond birth of baby.
    f. Assigning lay person as mother-baby helper to each newborn and mother to help establish positive bonding in hospital.
    g. Visiting nurses or trained lay persons should visit all discharged mothers and newborns for support and guidance during early postpartum period in the home.

C. Follow-up

1. Periodic reports to protective services by hospital team usually required
2. Careful screening for subsequent abuse
3. Visits scheduled every 1 to 4 weeks during initial period of treatment

D. Consultations/referrals

1. Suspected child abuse warrants immediate referral to physician and protective services agency.
2. Hospital social worker for further assessment, support of parents, and treatment.
3. Visiting nurse for reinforcement of parenting teaching and support.
4. Psychologist or psychiatrist for evaluation and/or further treatment.
5. Refer to abusive parents program, if available in community, as well as parent support groups.

bibliography

Green, Morris, and Haggerty, Robert J. *Ambulatory pediatrics II*. Philadelphia: Saunders, 1977.

Helfer, Ray E., and Kempe, C. Henry (eds.). *Child abuse and neglect: The family and community*. Cambridge, Mass.: Ballinger, 1976.

Kempe, C. Henry, and Helfer, Ray E. *Helping the battered child and his family*. Philadelphia: Lippincott, 1972.

Koocher, G. P. (ed.). *Children's rights and the mental health professions*. New York: Wiley, 1976.

Reinhart, John B. Syndromes of deficits in parenting: Abuse, neglect and accidents. *Pediatric Annals*, **6**:7–24 (1977).

160 Sexual Abuse

CHRISTINA M. GRAF

Because of the complexities inherent in the problem of sexual abuse, a single approach to this problem cannot be defined. Appropriate management, follow-up, and referral must take into consideration the nature and extent of the abuse, the legal implications, the resources available within the community, and the strengths and weaknesses of the family and individual family members. The specific approach must be determined by the professionals involved, and individualized for the particular family. Therefore, the practitioner must become familiar with the laws dealing with sexual abuse of children and the resources available within the community and then incorporate these into any approach to the sexually abused child.

I. Subjective Data

A. Problem-oriented history
1. Description of incidents which occurred
   a. Type and sites of abuse
   b. Frequency and times
   c. Places
   d. Person or persons involved
   e. Use of threats or force
2. Associated physical symptoms
3. Anxiety symptoms

B. Behavioral problems, including school problems

C. Family/social history

D. Response of child

E. Response of parent(s)

II. Objective Data

A. Complete physical examination
1. Particular attention to sites of abuse identified on history
2. Pelvic examination usually not necessary in preadolescent girls unless rape has occurred

B. Laboratory data
1. Endocervical smear for gonorrhea if indicated by history
2. Appropriate laboratory exams for conditions identified on history and physical (vaginitis, urinary tract infections, etc.)

III. Assessment

A. Subjective data
1. History of incidents
   a. May range from exhibitionism or fondling to rape
   b. Aggressor
      (1) Stranger or person to whom the family has no commitment—usually easier for the family to deal with
      (2) Member of the family constellation—presents a conflict for family with loyalty divided between victim and aggressor
         (a) Brother-sister—most frequently occurring, but usually transient; fewer long-term consequences unless it occurs persistently
         (b) Father-daughter—potentially most damaging; indicates disordered family functioning
         (c) Mother-son—occurs infrequently; indication of severe pathology
         (d) Father-son—occurs rarely
2. Associated physical symptoms possibly present
   a. Symptoms of urinary tract infection
   b. Symptoms of vaginitis, pelvic inflammatory

disease, or venereal disease

3. Anxiety symptoms may include insomnia, irritability, depression
4. Behavioral problems possibly present
   a. Inability to form peer relationships
   b. Delinquency
   c. Declining grades and truancy
   d. Attempts to run away from home
5. Family/social history
   a. Sexual abuse occurring within the family constellation is indicative of a disordered family.
   b. If the father is the aggressor, family characteristics usually include
      (1) Sexual problems between the parents
      (2) Sanction of mother, who suspected or knew of the abuse, but avoided direct confrontation
      (3) Fear of family disintegration among family members
   c. Other children in the family may have been sexually abused.
   d. Family may have a history of sexual abuse over several generations.
6. Response of child
   a. Younger children respond primarily to approach of aggressor rather than to the actual abuse.
      (1) If aggressor is kind and gentle, child perceives events only as a demonstration of caring.
      (2) If aggressor is threatening, child will exhibit fear.
      (3) Reactions following disclosure of incidents will be influenced by behavior of parent(s) and others.
   b. Preadolescents and adolescents react to the actual abuse.
      (1) If the abuse is not discovered, may experience fear and shame, low self-esteem.
      (2) If the abuse is discovered, with subsequent separation from family, some may see this as punishment which reinforces low self-esteem; others may feel responsible for family disintegration.
7. Response of parent(s)
   a. If aggressor is outside of family constellation, parent(s) may demonstrate anger and feelings of guilt.
   b. If aggressor is part of the family, responses may include shock, denial, disbelief, anger toward victim, shame, fear of incident's becoming known, attempts to conceal.

B. Objective data

1. May demonstrate redness, swelling, or bruising of genitalia.
2. Bruises, lacerations, etc., indicative of physical abuse may be present.
3. Concurrent genitourinary conditions may be present (refer to discussion of specific conditions elsewhere in this book).

IV. Management

A. Goals of management

1. Protect child from further abuse.
2. Assist parent(s) and child to deal with stress of situation.
3. Provide immediate counselling and practical assistance.
4. Prepare parent(s) and child for subsequent steps in process.
5. Determine treatment services required and coordinate available resources to provide these.
6. Promote resolution of crisis to return family to normal functioning, or to strengthen family functioning.

B. General principles

1. Interview parents and child separately.
2. Approach child in a relaxed, tactful, and supportive manner.
3. Approach parents in an honest and supportive manner.
4. Remain with child through all procedures, explain procedures, and answer questions.

C. If aggressor is outside of family constellation

1. Provide opportunity for parent(s) and child to explore feelings and reactions.
2. Inform parent(s) of all procedures and results of procedures.
3. Assure parent(s) that, if the event is handled calmly and reasonably, the child will not experience long-term, negative effects.
4. Assist the parent(s) to utilize appropriate resources in dealing with the crisis.

D. If the aggressor is within the family constellation, management will require extensive counselling, including the following:

1. Counselling of individual family members
2. Counselling of parent(s)
3. Counselling of individual parent(s) with child
4. Family counselling

bibliography

Gianetti, Henry. The treatment of father-daughter incest: A psycho-social approach. *Children Today,* **5**(4):2–5, 34 (1976).

Gorline, Lynne Lesak, and Ray, Mary Moore. Examining and caring for the child who has been sexually assaulted. *Maternal Child Nursing,* **4**:110–114 (1979).

Leaman, Karen. The sexually abused child. *Nursing 77,* **7**(5):68–72(1977).

Leone, Dolores M. Sexual abuse of children. *AORN,* **27**(4):642–644 (1978).

Nakashima, Ida I., and Zakus, Gloria E. Incest: Review and clinical experience. *Pediatrics,* **60**(5):696–701 (1977).

Sarles, Richard M. Incest. *Pediatric Clinics of North America,* **22**(3):633–642 (1975).

161 Rape[1]

CHRISTINA M. GRAF

I. Elements of the Legal Definition of Rape

A. Penetration of the penis into the female genitalia (not necessarily coitus)

B. Nonconsent on the part of the female, including nonvalid consent if the victim is any of the following.

1. Younger than the statutory age of consent
2. Mentally incompetent
3. Intoxicated or drugged

C. Compulsion by means of fear, verbal threats, physical assault, etc.

II. Subjective Data

A. Problem-oriented history

1. Description of events in the order of occurrence—identification of times wherever possible
   a. Where victim was contacted
   b. Identity of assailant, if known
   c. Threats or violence used
   d. Circumstances of the rape itself
      (1) Extent of penetration
      (2) Whether anal or oral intercourse occurred
2. Events following rape, i.e., did victim do any of the following.
   a. Bathe or douche
   b. Change clothing
   c. Talk with family, friends, etc.
   d. Delay in reporting assault

B. Medical and social history

1. Last normal menstrual cycle
2. History of illness, including venereal disease
3. Use of contraceptives
4. Date of most recent intercourse prior to assault
5. Possibility of pregnancy prior to assault

III. Objective Data

A. Complete physical examination

1. Complete perineal and pelvic examination (in young girls, this may need to be done under anesthesia)
2. Inspection of rectum and perianal area
3. Particular attention to signs of physical violence
4. Notation of breast development in young girls
5. Evaluation of emotional status

B. Laboratory data

1. Vaginal, anal, oral smears and aspirates
2. Specimen of pubic hair
3. CBC, ESR, serology, urinalysis, pregnancy test
4. Suspected hair, blood, or seminal stains transferred from assailant
5. Stained or damaged clothing

IV. Assessment

A. Subjective data

1. History of penetration of the penis into the female genitalia without consent of the female
2. Possible history of physical abuse

B. Objective data

1. Scratches, lacerations, bruises, petechiae, or erythema of genitalia possibly present
2. Hymen may be absent/present
3. Mucoid exudate possibly observed in vagina

[1]*Note:* Because of the physical, emotional, and legal implications of rape, treatment of the rape victim requires a multidisciplinary approach, with the initial examination and treatment managed by the physician.

4. Possibly erythema, lacerations, or scratches of anus and surrounding area
5. Other signs of physical abuse may be observed

V. Management

A. General principles

1. Approach victim in a supportive and nonjudgmental manner.
2. Obtain appropriate consents prior to physical examination.
3. Remain with victim throughout procedures and explain all aspects of procedures and treatments.
4. Observe physical and emotional status throughout procedures.
5. Ensure that all specimens are accurately labelled and appropriately handled (usually they will be transferred personally by the physician and receipts obtained).

B. Treatments/medications

1. Treatment appropriate for physical injuries (lacerations, fractures, bruises, etc.)
2. Prevention of venereal disease
   a. Probenecid 1 g po, followed by procaine penicillin 4.8 million U IM, or ampicillin 3.5 g po
   b. If allergic—spectinomycin 4 g IM
3. Prevention of pregnancy for victim at risk
   a. Diethylstilbestrol 25 mg twice a day for 5 days (must be initiated within 72 h of exposure) (prescribed by physician)
   b. Antiemetics possibly required since nausea and vomiting are common side effects
4. Relief of pain from contusions, lacerations, etc.
   a. Warm sitz baths
   b. Hydrocortisone cream
   c. Analgesics

C. Counselling

1. Remain supportive and nonjudgmental.
2. Explain all procedures and explain what may be expected through the various stages of the process.
3. Provide opportunity to express feelings and concerns.
4. Provide support to husband and/or family.

D. Follow-up

1. Contact physician if menses fails to occur within 1 week following completion of estrogen therapy.
2. Return for repeat cultures for test of cure 7 to 14 days after treatment for venereal disease.
3. Make phone call or visit to victim within 1 week following initial contact for further support; then continue as needed (coordinate with other disciplines involved).

E. Consultations/referrals

1. Rape Crisis Center or other appropriate community agencies and professionals
2. Psychiatric referral for severe or prolonged emotional disturbance
3. Inclusion of husband/family in referrals

bibliography

Breen, James L., Greenwald, Earl, and Gregori, Caterina A. The molested young female: evaluation and therapy of alleged rape. *Pediatric Clinics of North America*, **19**(3):717–726 (1972).

Clark, Terri Patricia. Counseling victims of rape. *American Journal of Nursing*, **76**(12):1964–1966 (1976).

Hunt, Glenn R. Rape: An organized approach to evaluation and treatment. *Annals of Family Practice*, **15**(1):154–158 (1977).

Massey, J. B., Garcia, Celso-Ramon, and Emech, J. P. Management of sexually assaulted women. *Obstetrical and Gynecological Survey*, **27**(3):190–192 (1972).

Shaw, Bernice L. "When the problem is rape. *RN*, **35**(4):25–28 (1972).

Woodling, Bruce A., Evans, Jerome R., and Bradbury, Michael D. Sexual assault: Rape and molestation. *Clinical Obstetrics and Gynecology*, **20**(3):509–530 (1977).

PART 6

emergencies

162 Respiratory Arrest

ILENE BURSON GOTTESFELD

I. Assessment and Management: Unwitnessed or Witnessed Cardiac Arrest (One Rescuer)

A. Establish unresponsiveness.
1. Shake the child.
2. Ask, Are you okay?

B. Open airway.
1. Infant or small child
   a. Gently tilt head back while child is lying flat on back.
   b. Do not hyperextend neck too much.
2. Late-school-age child and adolescent
   a. Place right hand under neck, left hand on forehead.
   b. Gently lift up on neck and push on forehead to hyperextend neck.

C. Establish breathlessness.
1. Place ear close to child's mouth or stoma.
2. Simultaneously observe for rise and fall of chest.

D. Ventilate—four quick breaths.
1. Infant or small child
   a. Inhale and place mouth over mouth and nose or stoma of child to form seal (make certain seal is formed and mouth and nose closed).
   b. Exhale quickly and with enough force to see chest rise, but not too forcefully.
   c. It may be helpful to the rescuer to release seal of mouth slightly or puff cheeks during exhalation.
2. School-age child and adolescent
   a. Inhale and place mouth over child's mouth, and pinch nostrils, or place mouth to child's mouth and nose or stoma.
   b. Exhale quickly and forcefully enough to see chest rise.

E. Establish pulselessness.
1. Place two fingers lightly on carotid closest to rescuer—5 to 10 s.
2. Place hand gently over precordium—5 to 10 s.

F. Create artificial circulation.
1. Infant under 15 lb
   a. Encircle chest, having fingers on back and two thumbs over midsternum.
   b. Provide back support.
   c. Tips of index and middle fingers should be placed midsternum.
   d. Compress $\frac{1}{2}$ to $\frac{3}{4}$ in.
   e. Compress chest 80 to 100 times per minute—five compressions to one breath (alternate).
2. Small child
   a. Place heel of one hand midsternally.
   b. Compress $\frac{3}{4}$ to $1\frac{1}{2}$ in.
   c. Keep ratio of five compressions to one ventilation.
3. Large child or adolescent
   a. Landmark with right hand, kneeling so that left knee is opposite shoulder.
   b. Place right index and two middle fingers of hand on base of sternum (xyphoid process).
   c. Immediately to left of these fingers, place heel of left hand.
   d. Place right hand on top of left hand, fingers interlocking.
   e. Rocking forward with elbows locked, compress 1½ to 2 in.
   f. Compress 60 to 80 times per minute.

G. Continue cycle until spontaneous breathing and circulation have been restored or
1. Another responsible person takes over.

2. A physician assumes responsibility.
3. Client has been transferred to a health care institution.
4. Rescuer is exhausted.

H. After 1 min and every few minutes thereafter, check carotid pulse and pupils.

I. Accident victim—same as above, except do not move child. Open airway by placing hands on either side of head to maintain neutral position.

II. Assessment and Management: Obstructed Airway

A. Establish unresponsiveness—as in cardiac arrest.

B. Open airway.

C. Establish breathlessness.

D. Ventilate—if this fails, precede to E below.

E. Reposition and attempt ventilation.

F. Roll child toward you, or turn head to side.

G. Open mouth; cross index and middle fingers on right hand and sweep fingers down cheek toward pharynx.

H. Reposition and attempt ventilation if still obstructed.

I. Roll over or turn upside down—two sharp blows between shoulder blades with heel of hand.

J. Look for foreign body; turn head to side; sweep out mouth.

K. Reventilate.

L. Triple airway maneuver

1. Place right knee opposite forehead.
2. Grasp lower jaw near angles with both hands.
3. Open mouth and lift jaw upward.
4. Tilt head back.
5. Open lips with thumbs.

M. Ventilate by mouth-to-mouth breathing, sealing nose with cheek if still obstructed.

N. Repeat blows, and attempt to ventilate.

III. Counselling/Prevention

A. Increase community awareness

1. Give lecture series on accidents and other common causes of death in which cardiopulmonary resuscitation (CPR) would be necessary
2. Offer certification course in CPR.
3. Devise list of available community emergency services and their phone numbers.

B. Increase family awareness

1. Alert family to community resources.
2. Provide instruction in resuscitation techniques if the situation warrants (e.g., child has illness which involves cardiopulmonary system or which may precipitate future respiratory or circulatory arrests).
3. Offer education on accident prevention and safety hazards in the house.
4. Alert family to signs and symptoms of a forthcoming collapse should the child's health indicate close observation.

C. Provide death and dying counselling should resuscitation efforts fail.

bibliography

American Heart Association, *Cardiopulmonary resuscitation and emergency cardiac care,* 1975.

Ungvarski, Peter J., Argondizzo, Nina T., and Boos, Patricia K. CPR current practice revised. *American Journal of Nursing,* February 1975.

163 Burns ASHER H. WEINSTEIN

I. Assessment and Management

A. Scene of accident

1. If victim is in flames, log-roll to extinguish.
2. Immerse injured body part in cool water; avoid ice water and ice packs.
3. Immediately transport victim to hospital for burns involving large body area. Do not immerse in water, as that may cause hypothermia and cardiac arrhythmias.
4. Chemical burns—continuously irrigate area with large amounts of water for minimum of 10 min if eyes or skin are involved.
5. While immersing or irrigating injured part, remove burned clothing.
6. Do not use sprays, ointments, home remedies.
7. Give nothing by mouth.
8. Notify physician and/or transport to emergency room.

B. Immediately after accident or upon arrival at health care facility

1. Victim is usually awake and conscious, so all procedures and treatments should be carefully explained.
2. Determine airway patency.
   a. Singed nasal hairs
   b. Darkened sputum
   c. "Smoky" odor to breath
   d. Inspect for burns of oral and nasal mucosa or obvious soot or carbon
   e. Inspiratory wheeze
   f. Increased hoarseness
   g. Difficulty breathing
3. Begin intravenous solution of lactated Ringer's solution (usually not necessary for minor burns).
4. Treat shock and bleeding if present.
5. Description of accident: time, place, surrounding circumstances, heat source. Danger to respiratory tract exists if accident occurred in an enclosed space.
6. Brief medical history: allergies to food and medications (especially penicillin), illnesses, chronic diseases, current medications, last tetanus shot. A complete history and physical examination should be done once emergency treatment is initiated.
7. Assess burn.
   a. Causative agent
   b. Depth (see Table 163-1)
   c. Body surface area involved (see Fig. 163-1)
   d. Body parts involved
   e. Age of client
   f. Other injuries
8. Monitor vital signs (temperature, pulse, respiration, blood pressure), and obtain body weight and height.
9. All victims with large burns should have blood gas and pH determinations to monitor respiratory status.
10. Institute appropriate emergency care (see Table 163-2).
11. The following burns usually require hospitalization.
    a. Full-thickness burns (third-degree) of more than 5 percent of body surface area
    b. In a child 4 years of age and under
    c. Partial-thickness burns (second-degree) of more than 15 percent of body surface area
    d. Burns involving face, eyes, ears, nose, hands, perineum, feet
    e. Chemical burns
    f. Electrical burns
12. Minor burns can be managed at home.

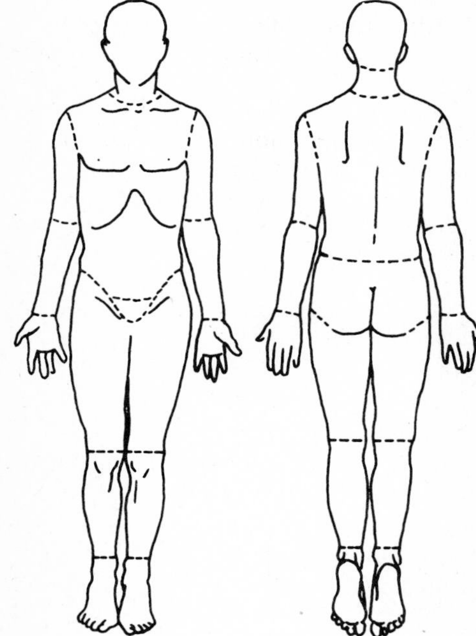

AREA	1 Yr.	1-4 Yrs.	5-9 Yrs.	10-14 Yrs.	15 Yrs.	Adult	2°	3°
Head	19	17	13	11	9	7		
Neck	2	2	2	2	2	2		
Ant. Trunk	13	13	13	13	13	13		
Post. Trunk	13	13	13	13	13	13		
R. Buttock	2½	2½	2½	2½	2½	2½		
L. Buttock	2½	2½	2½	2½	2½	2½		
Genitalia	1	1	1	1	1	1		
R.U. Arm	4	4	4	4	4	4		
L.U. Arm	4	4	4	4	4	4		
R.L. Arm	3	3	3	3	3	3		
L.L. Arm	3	3	3	3	3	3		
R. Hand	2½	2½	2½	2½	2½	2½		
L. Hand	2½	2½	2½	2½	2½	2½		
R. Thigh	5½	6½	8	8½	9	9½		
L. Thigh	5½	6½	8	8½	9	9½		
R. Leg	5	5	5½	6	6½	7		
L. Leg	5	5	5½	6	6½	7		
R. Foot	3½	3½	3½	3½	3½	3½		
L. Foot	3½	3½	3½	3½	3½	3½		
TOTAL								

Figure 163-1 Lund and Browder chart. The Burn Extent Estimator is a convenient method of estimating the client's total body surface area in square feet, the percent of body surface burned, and the approximate surface area of the burn in square feet. The figures can be shaded to show the burn area(s) on the client's body, and the chart can be used to estimate the percentage of the burn. *(From Artz, C. P., and Moncrief, J. A. The treatment of burns (2d ed.). Philadelphia: Saunders, 1969, p. 91.)*

a. First-degree burn (superficial)
   (1) Cold, wet compresses to relieve pain
   (2) Bactericidal cream, if needed

b. Second-degree burn (partial-thickness)
   (1) Immediately immerse newly received burn in cold water for 30 min to prevent tissue damage and relieve pain.
   (2) Keep wound clean—gently pat with mild soap and tap water, do not rub.
   (3) Air-dry.
   (4) Apply antimicrobial cream, i.e., sulfadiazine ointment (Silvadene), and cover with a porous, nonadherent dressing with a thick layer of sterile roller gauze, and secure with tape.
   (5) Pain medication: aspirin or acetaminophen as needed.
   (6) Encourage good fluid intake.
   (7) Return visit in 24 h for dressing change and then at appropriate intervals not to exceed 3 or 4 days.

13. In infant and young child if history does not fit the injury, consider the possibility of child abuse (see Battered/Abused Child, Chap. 159).

II. Counselling/Prevention

A. Explain all procedures and treatments to client and family.

B. Encourage and answer all questions.

C. Reassure client and family and describe what to expect if hospitalization is needed.

D. If hospitalization is indicated, maintain close contact with client and family. The recovery period is long, painful, and stressful. The continual support of many health professionals is needed.

E. Instruct on home management of minor burns.

1. Provide pain relief.
2. Keep wound clean—when instructed, wash

daily with mild soap and tap water.

3. How to perform dressing changes (when instructed).
   a. Remove dressing after thoroughly soaking in soapy tap water.
   b. Change daily.
   c. Observe during dressing change for signs of infection; telephone immediately if signs are present.

F. Prevention

1. See "Accident Prevention" in Chap. 9.
2. Avoid prolonged exposure to sun and sun lamps.
3. Explain safety regarding chemicals.
4. Provide fire prevention education in all schools and to parent groups to inform and encourage fire prevention practices.

bibliography

Artz, C. P., and Moncrief, J. A. *The treatment of burns,* (2nd ed.). Philadelphia: Saunders, 1969.

Feller, Irving, and Jones, Claudella Archambeault. *Nursing the burned patient.* Ann Arbor, Mich.: Institute for Burn Medicine, 1973.

Finley, Robert K. Assessing and treating burns. *Nursing '76,* **6**(9):54–55 (1976).

Frye, Susan, and Sander, Julie. The initial management of the acutely burned child. *Issues in Comprehensive Pediatric Nursing,* March-April:39–59 (1976).

Henderson, John. *Emergency medical guide* (4th ed.). New York: McGraw-Hill, 1978, pp. 240–251.

Miur, I. F. K., and Barclay, T. L. *Burns and their treatment* (2d ed.). Chicago: Year Book, Medical Publishers. 1974.

Penoff, James. In Barry, Jeanie (ed.), *Emergency nursing.* New York: McGraw-Hill, 1978, pp. 347–354.

Wagner, Mary M. Emergency care of the burned patient. *American Journal of Nursing,* **77**(11): 1788–1791 (1977).

Table163-1 Categories of Burn Depth

Degree	Cause	Surface Appearance	Color	Pain Level	Histologic Depth	Healing Time
First All are considered minor unless under 18 months, over 65, or with severe loss of fluids.	Flash, flame, ultraviolet (sunburn)	Dry, no blisters, edema	Erythematous	Painful	Epidermal layers only	2 to 5 days with peeling, no scarring, may have discoloration
Second (partial-thickness) Minor—less than 15% in adults, less than 10% in children. Moderate—15–30% in adults, or less than 15% with involvement of face, hands, feet, or perineum; minor chemical or electrical; in children, 10–30% Severe—more than 30%	Contact with hot liquids or solids, flash flame to clothing, direct flame, chemical	Moist blebs, blisters	Mottled white to pink, cherry red	Very painful	Epidermis, papillary, and reticular layers of dermis; may include fat domes of subcutaneous layer	Superficial—5 to 21 days with no grafting; deep with no infection—21 to 35 days; if infected, converts to full thickness
Third (full-thickness) Minor—less than 2% Moderate—2–10% any involvement of face, hands, feet, or perineum. Severe—more than 10% and major chemical or electrical.	Contact with hot liquids or solids, flame, chemical, electricity	Dry with leathery eschar until debridement, charred blood vessels visible under eschar	Mixed white (waxy-pearly), dark (khaki-mahogany), charred	Little or no pain, hair pulls out easily	Down to and includes subcutaneous tissue; may include fascia, muscle, and bone	Large areas require grafting that may take many months; small areas may heal from edges after weeks

Source: Wagner, Mary M. Emergency care of the burned patient. *American Journal of Nursing,* **77**(11):1790 (1977).

Table 163-2 Summary Chart for the Emergency Care of Burns

Classification of burns
- Agent: Thermal, electrical, chemical
- Depth: First-degree: red skin
  - Second-degree: red skin plus blisters
  - Third-degree: red skin plus blisters plus crust or pure white skin or loss of all skin
- Surface area: rule of nines

ED treatment
- First-degree: Cold towels
- Second-degree: Remove blebs and dress with Xeroform and Kerlix
- Third-degree: Hospitalize

Treatment of hospitalized burns
- Tetanus immunization
- Tracheostomy evaluation
- Evaluation of burning agent
  - If chemical, flush well
  - If electrical, get ECG
- IVs: Normal saline solution and indwelling catheter; run IV at rate to get urinary output of 30 to 50 mL/h
- Local treatment: Cleanse the burn with saline and dress with appropriate dressing (probably Silvadene for all large burns)
- Systemic antibiotics: None or penicillin for 5 days
- Special treatment (ears, hands): Close attention to problems of ears, and hands in position of function
- Oral intake: All large burns nothing by mouth (NPO); consider nasogastric tube

Source: Penoff, James. The emergency treatment of burns. In Jeanie Barry (ed.), *Emergency nursing.* New York: McGraw-Hill, 1978, pp. 353.

164 Heat Stroke/Exhaustion

ASHER H. WEINSTEIN

I. Assessment and Management

A. Heat stroke[1]

1. Signs
   a. Dry, flushed, hot skin
   b. Elevated body temperature
   c. Victim possibly collapsed or unconscious
2. Treatment
   a. Reduce body temperature quickly.
      1. Move to cool, shady area.
      2. Remove clothing.
      3. If possible, immerse in tub of cold water.
      4. Wrap victim in wet, cold towels and turn on electrical fans or hand fan.
   b. Low, semireclining position is preferred.
3. Transport to hospital as soon as possible.

B. Heat exhaustion

1. Signs
   a. Skin is cool, clammy, and pale (appears "white")
   b. Normal body temperature
   c. Fatigue, faintness
   d. Weak and thready pulse
   e. Shallow respirations
2. Treatment
   a. Move to cool area.
   b. Loosen or remove clothing.
   c. Place in supine position.
   d. Cool body: put cool cloths to face and wrists.
   e. May need to raise legs—Trendelenburg position.
   f. If conscious may give cool drink by mouth to replace salt and electrolytes, i.e., salt water, salt tablets, Gatorade, iced coffee.
   g. Maintain reclining position until fully recovered.
   h. Consult physician.
   i. If unconscious, transport to hospital.

C. Heat exhaustion and/or heat stroke usually occurs on very hot, humid days.

[1]Heat stroke is a medical emergency and requires *immediate* treatment.

II. Counselling/Prevention

A. Explain all procedures to client and family.

B. Instruct on avoidance of reexposure to hot environment because of increased sensitivity to heat stroke after exposure which may persist for a long period of time.

C. Instruct on appropriate apparel for warm temperature: light-colored, loose-fitting, absorbent.

D. The importance of maintaining adequate fluid and salt intake, especially during periods of high humidity and hot temperatures, should be explained to the client and family.

E. Teach clients, especially athletes, on prevention of heat stroke/exhaustion:

1. Limit activity on hot days and during hottest part of day (11 A.M. to 2 P.M.).
2. Gradually increase exercise tolerance over a long time period.
3. When exercising, take frequent rests and increase fluid and salt intake.
4. Wear light-weight, light-colored clothing.
5. Avoid exercise during illness.

bibliography

Henderson, John. *Emergency medical guide* (4th ed.). New York: McGraw-Hill, 1978, pp. 255–258.

Pascoe, Delmer J., and Grossman, Moses (ed.). *Quick reference to pediatric emergencies*. Philadelphia: Lippincott, 1973, pp. 281—282.

165 Frostbite

ASHER H. WEINSTEIN

I. Assessment and Management

A. Deep frostbite[1]

1. Signs
   a. Involved tissue white and waxy in appearance
   b. Skin "hard" to the touch
   c. Blisters
   d. Loss of sensation
   e. Signs of necrosis or gangrene
2. Treatment
   a. Must begin immediately.
   b. If possibility of refreezing, do *not* begin rewarming.
   c. Remove all wet clothing.
   d. Rapidly rewarm injured part in water 40 to 44°C (approximately 104 to 112°F.) for 20 to 40 min. Keep water temperature constant, and injured part surrounded by water. Procedure may be painful.
   e. Keep client warm (not hot) with blanket.
   f. Avoid movement or weight bearing on injured part.
   g. Keep involved area clean; cover with sterile dressing.
   h. Keep blisters intact.
   i. If client is conscious, may be given hot liquids, i.e., tea, coffee. *Avoid* alcohol and tobacco.
   j. Once involved part is completely thawed, begin rhythmically raising and lowering it to stimulate circulation.
   k. Tetanus prophylaxis.
   l. Analgesics for pain if needed.
3. Transport to hospital as soon as possible.
4. When frostbite is present, *never* do the following.
   a. Rub injured area
   b. Rub with snow or ice
   c. Attempt to thaw involved area slowly
   d. Attempt rewarming with hot water or over an open flame
   e. Try to rewarm by movement or exercise

B. Superficial frostbite

1. Signs
   a. Involved area feels extremely cold and appears white.
   b. Skin feels hard on the surface but doughy underneath.
   c. Loss of normal sensation.
2. Treatment
   a. Gently warm involved area.
   b. Cover with sterile dressing.

C. Impending frostbite

1. Most commonly involved: ears, nose, hands, feet, chin, cheeks
2. Extent of injury dependent upon
   a. Duration of exposure
   b. Temperature
   c. Humidity
   d. Windchill factor
3. Children, alcoholics, nervous or easily excitable people more prone to frostbite
4. Warning signs of frostbite
   a. Tingling sensation or numbness
   b. Involved area perhaps red, cold, and painful
5. Treatment
   a. Return indoors.
   b. Hold fingers in armpits.
   c. Blow warm air on involved part.

[1]Deep frostbite is a medical emergency and requires *immediate* treatment.

II. Counselling/Prevention

- **A.** Dress appropriately for weather conditions.
- **B.** Avoid prolonged exposure in cold weather.
- **C.** Know area in which traveling.
- **D.** Keep alert to signs of impending frostbite and take appropriate action.
- **E.** In minor frostbite pain may persist for 2 to 4 days.
- **F.** Protect injured part from reexposure to cold—recurrence is common after injury.
- **G.** Explain all procedures and offer reassurance as needed.
- **H.** If treated at home, keep injured part elevated and return visit in 24 h and as needed thereafter.

bibliography

Henderson, John. *Emergency Medical Guide* (4th ed.). New York: McGraw-Hill, 1978, pp. 251–254.

Pascoe, Delmer J., and Grossman, Moses (eds.). *Quick Reference to Pediatric Emergencies.* Philadelphia: Lippincott, 1973, pp. 283–285.

166 Head Injury

M. CONSTANCE SALERNO

I. Assessment and Management

A. If client is unconscious, notify and refer to physician/neurologist.[1]

B. Assess immediately
1. General state
2. Level of consciousness
3. Pupil response
4. Motor function
5. Vital signs

C. Changes in the client's degree of alertness or vital signs indicate need for prompt medical attention.

D. If client is conscious and alert, obtain history of the injury.
1. Time
2. Place
3. Type (accidental/nonaccidental) and description
4. Related signs and symptoms (any loss of consciousness)

E. A complete physical examination with careful neurological assessment should be done on any client with a head trauma.

F. If any questions as to the severity of the head injury, client should be admitted to hospital for observation.

G. Clean and assess abrasions or lacerations.

H. Large lacerations should be sutured.

I. No medications should be given to small children.

[1]Have an emergency resuscitation cart available.

J. Aspirin or acetaminophen may be given for headache in older children.

K. Client may be discharged to competent parent(s) or adult if physical examination and neurological assessment are negative including normal vital signs.

II. Counselling/Prevention

A. Observe for 24 h after injury.

B. Check every hour including at night.

C. Signs and symptoms that indicate need for reevaluation and/or hospitalization:
1. Changes in degree of alertness, e.g., slurred speech, drowsiness, confusion, inability to answer simple questions
2. Persistent vomiting, particularly of a projectile type
3. Asymmetry of pupils, constriction of pupil, double vision
4. Weakness of arms or legs especially on one side of body
5. Twitching or convulsions
6. Spinal fluid otorrhea or rhinorrhea
7. Slowed pulse
8. Irregular respirations
9. Elevated temperature
10. Elevated blood pressure

D. Have name and telephone number of emergency room and/or physician to call if any of the above findings are present or if concerned during immediate post-injury period.

bibliography

Kunkel, Joyce, and Wiley, John K. Acute head injury. *Nursing '79,* **9**:23–33 (1979).

Meyed, C. J. Acute brain trauma. *American Journal of Nursing,* **78**:40–43 (1978).

Reuben, R.N. Central nervous system emergencies. In S. K. Dube, and S. H. Pierog (eds.), *Immediate care of the sick and injured child.* St. Louis: Mosby, 1978, pp. 106–109.

Singer, H. S., and J. M. Freeman, Head trauma for the pediatrician. *Pediatrics,* **62**:819–825 (1978).

Shillito, J., Jr. Head injuries. In M. Green and R. J. Haggerty, *Ambulatory pediatrics II.* Philadelphia: Saunders, 1977, pp. 247–252.

167 Drowning

ELIZABETH HAWKINS-WALSH

It is not well known that there are *two* types of drowning: inhalation of water *(wet drowning)* and laryngospasm *(dry drowning)*. All victims of submersion should be seen by a physician in a hospital facility. Initially, all victims should be assumed to have aspirated.

I. Assessment and Management

A. Scene of retrieval

1. Position victim so that emergency resuscitative measures can be performed. Place salt-water victims in slight Trendelenburg position. *Note:* No attempt should be made to drain water from lungs other than by positioning described for salt-water victims. Fresh water is rapidly absorbed. *Rescue efforts must not be interrupted for even a few seconds.*
2. Establish and maintain clear airway.
   a. In absence of mechanical suction, swab mouth and hypopharynx with fingers wrapped in absorbent material.
   b. Place head in maximum extension and lift jaw.
3. Evaluate respiratory effort (if necessary, initiate *mouth-to-mouth breathing* immediately).
   a. Apnea
   b. Rate and depth of respirations
   c. Cyanosis
   d. Flaring, retractions
4. Assess circulation.[1]
   a. Pulses—carotid, femoral, or radial. If pulse rate feeble or unable to be determined, *external cardiac massage*
   b. Heart sounds—auscultation
   c. Blood pressure—when equipment available
5. Summon emergency vehicle.
6. 100% F_1O_2 if possible, when necessary cardiopulmonary resuscitation (CPR)

B. Upon stabilization and arrival at hospital facility

1. Physical examination should then include
   a. Adequacy of respiratory effort
      (1) Inspection—symmetrical movement of chest wall; hyperpnea; cyanosis; retractions; nasal flaring
      (2) Palpation—depth of excursion; crepitation
      (3) Percussion—dullness, hyperresonance
      (4) Auscultation—adventitious sounds: quality of breath sounds bilaterally
   b. Circulation
   c. Patency of airway—repeated vomiting frequently seen subsequent to
      (1) Ingestion of large quantities of fluid
      (2) Distention of abdomen during resuscitative efforts
   d. Vital signs
   e. Neurological examination—level of consciousness; orientation; responsiveness; reflexes–pupillary response
   f. Areas of trauma
   g. Skin—mottling, color, temperature, clammy
2. Laboratory data
   a. Arterial blood gases (pH, pCO_2, pO_2 and bicarbonate)
   b. Chest x-ray
   c. Whole blood hemoglobin, hematocrit, plasma hemoglobin

[1]Fixed and dilated pupils can not be used as absolute criteria for circulatory arrest.

d. Serum electrolytes
e. Alveolar-arterial O_2 gradient
f. Electrocardiogram

3. Objective findings in victims of near drowning are directly related to
   a. Duration of submersion
   b. Quantity of water aspirated
   c. Type of water aspirated
   d. Immediacy of effective resuscitation

C. Hospital therapy

1. Complete physical examination with neurological check
2. 100% F_1O_2 by inhalation (until arterial blood gases (ABGs) prove it unnecessary)
3. Ventilatory assistance—if required
4. $NaHCO_3$ (0.3 to 0.4 meq/L) IV—give in emergency room until ABGs drawn; then, as needed
5. Arterial blood gases
6. IV's—lactated Ringer's solution until electrolyte changes known
7. Antibiotics—broad-spectrum if aspiration
8. Stomach decompression if distended
9. Serial chest x-rays
10. Monitor respiratory rate, temperature, heart rate, arterial blood pressure/central venous-pressure; urinary output
11. Nonaspiration—observation overnight; cough and deep-breathe F_1O_2
12. Therapeutic hypothermia occasionally indicated with severe, persistent hypoxemia

D. Follow-up: At least an overnight hospital stay with careful monitoring is usually indicated. All victims should be seen at least once following discharge from the hospital to rule out possibility of residual or late-appearing problems.

II. Counselling/Prevention

A. Primary prevention/counselling

1. Parental
   a. Impress parent(s)/guardian(s) with high incidence of drowning.
      (1) Highest incidence occurs between 10 and 19 years of age.
      (2) 85 percent drowning victims are male.
      (3) Potential exists for drowning of unattended infants in bath water.
      (4) Swimming pools are most frequent site of infant drownings.
         (a) Lack of adequate enclosures
         (b) Improper supervision
         (c) Undrained pools in winter, wells, ponds
      (5) Peak season and time—summer, holiday weekend, 12 to 3 P.M.
   b. Promote awareness of child's need for adequate supervision despite presence of lifeguards.
   c. Swimming ability is primary deterrent to drowning.
      (1) Early swimming lessons
      (2) Danger of false assurance
      (3) 35% of drowning victims able to swim
      (4) Voluntary hyperventilation prior to submersion, possibly fatal
      (5) Danger of repeated diving at brief intervals
   d. "Buddy system" is crucial for children with seizure disorders or transient ischemic attacks and those on medication.
   e. Life preservers are to be worn by all small children in vicinity of water, docks, boats.
2. Public education
   a. Promote education programs in schools, camps, places of employment.
   b. Incidence of drowning expected to increase with increasing popularity of water sports.
   c. "Drown-proofing" technique—promote awareness by all, especially swimmers and boaters.
      (1) Take a breath.
      (2) Passively allow oneself to sink below water surface to one's "natural" level (usually eyebrow level).
      (3) Resurface in 8 to 10 s.
      (4) Exhale, then inhale.
      (5) Repeat sinking process.
      (6) This can be continued for longer than 6 h without fatigue or circulatory or respiratory difficulties.
   d. Alcohol use implicated in large number of drownings—alcohol and drugs are absolute contraindications around water sports.
   e. Danger of swimming alone.
   f. Boating and fishing accidents.
   g. Skin/scuba diving.
      (1) Lack of proper equipment or knowledge
      (2) Nitrogen narcosis (common at 150 ft)
   h. Black victims of drowning 3 times the number of white victims
   i. Swimming lessons
      (1) School system—mandatory?
      (2) Youth organizations
      (3) Red Cross

B. Secondary prevention

1. Broad public awareness
   a. Lifesaving technique
      (1) Danger of panic and appropriate response
      (2) Modes of victim retrieval
   b. Cardiopulmonary resuscitation (CPR)
      (1) Immediate resuscitation
      (2) Uninterrupted resuscitation
      (3) Transport of every suspected victim to hospital
2. Adequate equipment and personnel trained in its use at all public beaches
3. Insurance of monitoring closely all victims within a hospital
4. Improved hospital support and health professionals informed of current techniques in treating the drowning victim

bibliography

Battaglia, Jane Donahue, and Lockhart, Charles H. Drowning and near-drowning. *Pediatric Annals,* **6**:95–106 (1977).

Craig, A. B., Jr. Summary of 58 cases of loss of consciousness during underwater swimming and diving. *Medicine and Science in Sports,* **8**:171–175 (1976).

Dietz, D. E., and Baker, S. P. Drowning, epidemiology and prevention. *American Journal of Public Health,* **64**:303–312 (1974).

Modell, J. H. *Pathophysiology and treatment of drowning and near-drowning.* Springfield, Ill.: Charles C Thomas, 1971.

Modell, J. H. Graves, S. A., and Ketover, A. Clinical course of 91 consecutive near-drowning victims. *Chest,* **70**(2):231–238 (1976).

Near-drowning: Strategy for survival. *Emergency Medicine,* **2**:16–21(1970).

Redding, J. Saving victims of near drowning. *Medical Opinion,* **5**:32–38 (1976).

Ryna, Allan J. Drowning's deadly toll: Can more be saved? *Sports Medicine,* **5**:28–41 (1977).

168 Fractures/Dislocations

CAROLYN B. COLWELL

I. Assessment and Management

A. Obtain history from client/parent(s).
1. Age
2. Specifics of accident or injury
   a. Time of occurrence
   b. Velocity of impact
   c. Major sites of impact
   d. Bone snap heard?
3. Previous treatment
4. Previous injury
5. Present complaints of pain
   a. Exact location
   b. Onset
   c. Severity
6. Date of last tetanus shot

B. General physical examination for possible shock[1] and/or associated injury; if traumatic incident occurred, carefully examine head, trunk, back, abdomen.

C. Examine injured part for
1. Drainage
2. Swelling
3. Deformity or displacement
4. Point of maximum tenderness
5. Instability, compared with opposite side
6. Voluntary function
7. Range of motion, active or active-assistive

D. Observe for limp, if lower extremity involved.

E. Perform neurological examination of involved extremity.
1. Muscle exam
2. Sensory exam
3. Reflexes

F. The following require, *immediate* referral to orthopedist.
1. Open (compound) fracture
2. Displacement or deformity

G. The following are signs of fracture (referral to orthopedist is usually indicated).
1. Pain and/or local tenderness
2. Swelling
3. Deformity
4. Discoloration
5. Inability to move injured part
6. Shock

H. For fracture management see Table 168-1.

I. Immobilize injured part with splint before movement is attempted (see Table 168-2).

J X-ray possibly both sides for comparison.

K. For diagnosis and management of common fractures and dislocations (see Table 168-3).

II. Counselling/Prevention

A. Importance of maintaining bandage, splint, or cast in place

B. Instruction on skin care with cast or splint and exercises associated with it

C. Discussion of activity restrictions with client and family

D. Instruction on the importance of follow-up

E. Accident prevention (see Chap. 9)

F. Counselling for specific fractures/dislocations (see Table 168-3)

G. Write note to school nurse to explain activity limitation.

[1]If shock or obvious fracture is present, immobilize and institute appropriate management immediately; refer to orthopedist.

Table 168-1 Fracture Management: General Principles of Care

Avoid unnecessary handling.

Immobilize (see Table 168-2).

Apply clean dressings to wounds.

Control hemorrhage with direct pressure (tourniquets are a last resort in hemorrhage control and may lead to loss of the involved limb).

Check for the "5 P's" of vascular occlusion distal to injury:
- Pain
- Pulselessness
- Paresthesia
- Pallor
- Paralysis

Source: Barry, Jeanie (ed.). *Emergency nursing.* New York: McGraw-Hill, 1978, p. 321.

Table 168-2 General Considerations in Splint Application*

Immobilize before moving the client or applying traction—"splint" 'em where they lie."

Do *not* straighten dislocations.

If an open fracture, stop bleeding and dress wound before splinting; do *not* push protruding bone back inside.

Immobilize broken bone or dislocated joint one joint above and one joint below point of injury.

Apply slight traction (steady downward pull) while splinting and maintain until splint is in place.

Splint tightly; but do not interfere with circulation.

Check pulse, color, pain, and sensation distal to injury before and after splinting.

Suspect injury to neck or spine in any accident which could cause fracture or dislocation.

Pad the splint carefully to prevent pressure points and discomfort to the area.

*These guidelines represent basic principles of management for any type of orthopedic injury.

Source: From Barry, Jeanie (ed.). *Emergency nursing.* New York: McGraw-Hill, 1978, p. 323.

Table 168-3 Common Fractures and Dislocations*†

Diagnosis	Clinical Manifestations	Management
Undisplaced fractured clavicle	History of injury to area Possible pain on change of position of upper limb Local swelling, tenderness, and crepitation over fracture sites Absence of displacement Fracture visualized on x-ray	Immobilization via figure-of-eight, nonelasticized bandage Restriction of activity from strenuous sports for 3 to 4 weeks Aspirin or acetaminophen for pain if necessary *Counselling:* Importance of maintaining bandage in place and tightening daily Caution regarding excessive pressure on axillary vessels and possible circulatory impairment

Table 168-3 Common Fractures and Dislocations*† *(continued)*

Diagnosis	Clinical Manifestations	Management
		Need to check for skin irritation and pressure sores Reassurance, if visible callus is present, that it will disappear in 6 to 9 months Return visit in 3 days to ensure maintenance of strapping; sooner if pain increases In 4 to 6 weeks x-ray repeated; probable removal of strapping and gradual return to full activity
Radial head dislocation or pulled elbow	History of trauma causing traction on elbow Acute pain with point tenderness over radial head Unwillingness to extend elbow Supination of forearm causes severe pain Most common ages 1 to 3 years Click possibly heard or felt in child's elbow by person who pulled it X-ray to assure absence of fracture	*Dislocation reduced:* forearm gently manipulated into full supination and elbow into full extension A click usually heard and/or felt as reduction occurs Often immediate relief of pain Sling can be used for 1 week If recurrent dislocation, splint protection for 3 to 4 weeks Gentle, graduated active exercises following removal of splint If any question that reduction occurred, child sent home with sling to return on following day *Counselling:* Reassurance of likelihood of immediate recovery Explanation of how dislocation occurs, and thus how it might be prevented Support and reassurance if necessary because of guilt feelings of parent(s) Return visit: On following day to ensure child is pain-free and fully using arm In 2 weeks to evaluate return to normal activity; sooner if continued pain or recurrence
Undisplaced fracture or dislocation of phalanges in the hand	History of trauma to finger Pain Significant difficulty moving adjacent joint Swelling X-ray revealing either dislocation without fracture, or fracture without displacement	*Dislocation:* Reduced with gentle traction on finger Immobilized with splint continuously for 10 days *Undisplaced fracture:* Splint in position of function, including adjacent joints or adjacent fingers, for 10 to 14 days Splint to be used in sports activities for additional 10 days If dominant hand, discussion of possible problems with schooling

Table 168-3 Common Fractures and Dislocations*† *(continued)*

Diagnosis	Clinical Manifestations	Management
		Return visit: In 10 days to assure proper position, sooner if increased pain and swelling Consultation with orthopedist if difficulty with reduction
Fracture of toe	History of trauma Pain Swelling Undisplaced fracture revealed on x-ray	Fractured toe strapped to adjacent toe with tape Gauze pad placed between two toes Foot elevated if significant pain and swelling Weight-bearing as tolerated; crutches if necessary *Counselling:* Reassurance of nondisplacement Importance of immobilization until x-ray shows healing Return visit in 10 days for possible removal of splint; sooner if pain and swelling increase
Torus fracture of distal radius and ulna	History of fall on outstretched hand Mild pain and swelling Minimal deformity or displacement X-ray revealing crumbled dorsal cortex and intact volar cortex	Consultation with physician/orthopedist Treatment below elbow cast or volar splint for 3 weeks Reassurance of nondisplacement, but emphasis on importance of temporary immobilization Return visit: In 3 weeks to repeat x-ray, assure healing and remove splint, sooner if problems arise
Stress fracture (caused by continued excessive stress, increased bony resorption, and, thus, weakened bony cortex)	No history of acute trauma, although possible recent participation in vigorous activity that was unusual for client Antalgic limp, usually of gradual onset, if lower limb Local pain Aggravated by activity Relieved by rest Variable swelling and tenderness on palpation Adjacent joints retaining full range of joint motion with exception of hip fracture Able to visualize callus or fracture on x-ray	Consultation with physician/orthopedist Resting the affected part If tibia, may need above-knee walking cast for 3–4 weeks If fibula, adhesive elastic strapping applied *Counselling:* Clarification of activity limitation Cast care, if one is indicated Explanation of cause; need for rest of afflicted part Return visit: In 3 weeks for repeat x-ray and evaluation of activity

Table 168-3 Common Fractures and Dislocations*† *(continued)*

Diagnosis	Clinical Manifestations	Management
Traumatic fracture dislocation (with exception of those discussed previously)	History of trauma involving significant stress to bone or joint Pain with localized tenderness Swelling Loss of function of adjacent joint Possible deformity or displacement Fracture or dislocation visualized on x-ray	Immediate referral to physician/orthopedist *Temporary treatment:* Absence of serious associated injury ensured Bleeding stopped with direct pressure if open wound Extremity splinted "as it lies" if feasible If necessary, realignment attempted with gentle traction only Pain relief as needed *Counselling:* Necessity for immediate medical treatment Reassurance and calming measures to client and parent(s) Care in transporting Importance of elevating involved extremity Possible need for hospitalization Send adequate records with client to health facility
Congenital dislocated hip	*Newborn or infant* Ortolani sign (click is heard when hip is abducted with hips and knees in flexed position) Asymmetry of skin folds of thigh and/or of gluteal and popliteal creases Limited passive abduction of hips, with hips and knees flexed Apparent shortening of femur (Galeazzi's sign)—difference in knee levels with knees and hips flexed at right angles, and infant lying on firm surface *Beyond age 3* Abnormal gait Contralateral tilt of pelvis with each step Lateral deviation of spine towards affected side If bilateral, a ducklike waddle Positive Trendelenburg test (dropping of pelvis on normal side as child stands on dislocated hip) Visualized on x-ray	Refer immediately to physician/orthopedist *Counselling:* Vital importance of continued follow-up and treatment Reassurance concerning nonpreventability Positive outlook if detected early Anticipation of cast care, if appropriate Possibility of hospitalization, if beyond age 2 months
Recurrent dislocation of patella	Common in girls, age 6 through adolescence	Referral to physician/orthopedist If still dislocated, reduced by extending

Table 168-3 Common Fractures and Dislocations*† *(continued)*

Diagnosis	Clinical Manifestations	Management
	Recurrent pain and/or swelling of knee Common complaint that "knee gives out" Acute apprehension when patella is passively pushed over lateral condyle with knee 30° flexed May be palpable and/or audible click if client sits with knees flexed and is told to extend them If within 48 h of dislocation, swelling possibly present X-ray revealing any bony abnormalities	knee with manual pressure on patella in medial direction Splinted in full extension Anticipation of immobilization in cast, followed by exercises
Pathologic fractures of diverse etiology	Pain Gait abnormality if lower extremity involved Absence of history of traumatic episode, or history of trivial injury May be deformity May be associated symptoms Café au lait spots and endocrine disturbances with fibrous dysplasia History of multiple fractures, blue sclerae, and short stature with osteogenesis imperfecta Visualization of fracture on x-ray	Refer immediately to physician/orthopedist Splinted "as it lies" for transfer
Battered child syndrome (nonaccidental injury)	Unexplained injury Discrepancies in history Repeated accidents Delay in seeking medical attention Multiple old and new signs of trauma Signs of fear or emotional disturbance in parent(s) Signs of emotional deprivation in child Often multiple fractures, old and new, visualized on x-ray	Referral to physician See Battered/Abused Child, Chap. 159

*For general management and counselling/prevention see I and II in this chapter.

†Physician and/or orthopedist consultation or referral is usually indicated.

bibliography

Alexander, Mary M., and Brown, Marie Scott, Performing the neurologic examination, part 1. *Nursing '76,* **6**:6 (1976).

———, and ———. Performing the neurologic examination, part 2. *Nursing '76,* **6**:7 (1976).

———, and ———. Physical examination, the musculoskeletal system. *Nursing '76,* **6**:4 (1976).

Barnett, Henry L., and Einhorn, Arnold H. *Pediatrics* (16th ed.). New York: Appleton Century Crofts, 1977.

DeAngelis, Catherine. *Pediatric primary care.* Boston: Little, Brown, 1979.

Dods, Virginia R. Emergency care of orthopedic injuries. In Jeanie Barry (ed.), *Emergency nursing.* New York: McGraw-Hill, 1978, pp. 317–345.

Ferguson, Albert Barnett, Jr. *Orthopedic surgery in infancy and childhood* (4th ed.). Baltimore: Williams & Wilkins, 1975.

Green, Morris, and Haggerty, Robert J. *Ambulatory pediatrics II.* Philadelphia: Saunders, 1977.

Kempe, C. Henry, et al. *Current pediatric diagnosis and treatment* (5th ed.). Los Altos, Calif.: Lange, 1978.

Lloyd-Roberts, G. C. *Orthopaedics in infancy and childhood.* London: Butterworth, 1971.

Sharrard, W. J. W. *Pediatric orthopaedics and fractures.* Oxford: Blackwell, 1971.

Tachdjian, Mihran O. *Pediatric orthopedics.* Philadelphia: Saunders, 1972.

169 Choking

JANE A. FOX

I. Assessment and Management

A. If the victim is breathing and coughing, he or she is not truly choking.

B. The truly choking client[1] will

1. Be *unable* to speak or cry.
2. Turn blue.
3. Collapse.

C. If a person is choking, do the following.

1. Open victim's mouth and reach in with your fingers to attempt to dislodge the obstruction.
2. If no results, give one forceful blow between the shoulder blades (lay child over your knees).
3. If the object is not dislodged from the windpipe, begin the Heimlich maneuver (same for child and adult)—a quick, inward, upward pressing of the abdomen.
   a. Stand behind the victim.
   b. Place one of your fists, thumb-side in, against the victim's abdomen. Your hand should be placed below the rib cage and slightly above the navel. Grasp your fist with your other hand.
   c. Press firmly into the victim's abdomen with a quick upward thrust.
   d. Repeat, if object not dislodged.
   e. If victim is an infant or a child in the supine position
      (1) Face victim.
      (2) Place the heel of your bottom hand over the abdomen below the rib cage, above the navel.
      (3) Give a quick upward and inward thrust.

D. If the above methods are unsuccessful, transport victim immediately to a hospital.

E. Once breathing is restored, the victim should be evaluated for complications.

II. Counselling/Prevention

A. The primary treatment of choking is prevention. This is especially important in children.

B. The parent(s) should be taught at different well-child visits—at 6 months, 9 months, 12 months, and again, if necessary—how to handle a choking emergency.

C. Mass public education should be instituted in preparing people to effectively respond in a choking emergency.

D. Parent(s) should be educated in *preventing* choking incidents.

1. Introduce solid foods only after the child has teeth for chewing. Solid foods should be strained, and progression should be to finger food (i.e., soft, cooked carrots).
2. Remove small objects which can easily be placed in mouth.
3. Carefully check toys, dolls, games for loose pieces and other objects easily swallowed.
4. No child under 3 years of age should be allowed hard candy, cough drops, gum, peanuts, popcorn, or kernel corn.
5. Never allow child to eat while overly active or lying down.
6. Children learn by example from parent(s)—adults should not put or hold small objects to mouth.

[1]If the client is truly choking, the object must be dislodged within 4 min!

bibliography

Block, Charles R., and Block, Constance E. Help, my child is choking. *Pediatric Nursing,* **2**:48–49 (1976).

Henderson, John. *Emergency medical guide* (4th ed.). New York: McGraw-Hill, 1978. pp. 109–116.

Hoekelman, Robert A. *Principles of pediatrics: health care of the young.* New York: McGraw-Hill, 1978, p. 1936.

Snyder, Donald R., et al. *Handbook for emergency medical personnel.* New York: McGraw-Hill, 1978. pp. 22–27.

170 Poisoning[1]

JANE A. FOX

I. Assessment and Management

A. By telephone

1. Obtain name, address, telephone number.
2. Determine client's condition and age.
3. Identify poison, if known, and also
   a. Amount ingested
   b. Time of ingestion
4. Determine toxicity.
   a. If nontoxic substance (see Table 170-1), reassure caller.
   b. For substance to be qualified as nontoxic, it must meet certain criteria (Mofenson and Greensher, 1977).
      (1) Positive identification of the substance
      (2) Assurance that *only one* substance was ingested
      (3) The words *Danger, Poison, Warning,* or *Caution not* shown on container
      (4) An adequate determination of the amount ingested
      (5) Client without symptoms
      (6) Possible for practitioner to call back to determine client's condition
      (7) Client under 5 years of age
5. Follow-up appointment should be made in the near future to review accident prevention with parent(s)/care giver(s).
6. If toxicity unknown, call local Poison Control Center and begin treatment.
7. If toxic substance, begin treatment listed below, unless contraindicated, and arrange immediate transportation to nearest hospital. Notify hospital of client's expected arrival, type of substance ingested, time, amount, and present physical condition. Instruct parent(s)/care giver(s) to bring bottle containing ingested substance and any vomitus to hospital.
8. Plant ingestion—to determine toxicity see Table 170-2.

B. Treatment

1. Remove ingested substance.
   a. *DO NOT* induce vomiting if the following apply to the client.
      (1) Unconscious
      (2) Having seizures
      (3) Ingested substance caustic, i.e., toilet-bowl cleaner, drain cleaner
      (4) Ingested substance hydrocarbon, i.e., paint thinner or remover, gasoline, lighter fluid
      (5) Ingested agent an antiemetic
   b. To induce vomiting
      (1) Give syrup of ipecac
         (a) 15 mL
         (b) Follow with one to two glasses of noncarbonated liquid, i.e., water.
         (c) If no vomiting within 20 to 30 min, repeat dose.
         (d) Wait another 20 min; if still no vomiting—gastric lavage is necessary.
      (2) If syrup of ipecac not available, give one to two glasses of water and stroke back of throat with blunt object.
      (3) Instruct parent(s)/care giver(s) to save all vomitus and bring to hospital.
   c. Gastric lavage is performed by physician at hospital facility.
2. Inactivate poison.
   a. Activated charcoal (effective absorbent of many poisons)
      (1) Given after emesis or gastric lavage.

[1]*Note:* This is the most frequent medical emergency in the pediatric age group. Over 2 million children in the United States ingest a poisonous substance each year (Mofenson and Greensher, 1977).

(2) *Do not* give simultaneously with syrup of ipecac.
(3) Give 5 to 6 tsp of activated charcoal in glass of water.
(4) Should be given within 30 min after poison ingestion.

b. Give specific antidote, if known (see Table 170-3).

3. Perform careful physical examination and initiate life-supporting measures.
   a. Establish patent airway.
   b. Determine respiratory status.
   c. Treat shock.
   d. Determine circulatory status.
   e. Maintain fluid and electrolyte balance.
   f. Monitor vital signs.
   g. Determine neurological status—control seizures.
4. Be aware of inaccurate emergency instructions (Mofenson and Greensher, 1977).
   a. DO NOT give vinegar or fruit juice (acid) to neutralize ingestion of an alkali corrosive.
   b. DO NOT give sodium bicarbonate if acids have been ingested.
   c. DO NOT use milk as a diluent; use *only* water.
5. Suspect poisoning in the following situations.
   In any ill client
   (1) With abrupt onset of illness
   (2) Age 1 to 4 years
   (3) With past history of poison ingestion
   (4) Signs of a multiple-system involvement that does not suggest a single disease process (McMillan, Nieburg, and Oski, 1977).
6. Possible that specific symptoms may suggest the poison or drug involved (see Table 170-4)

II. Counselling/Prevention

A. See "Accident Prevention" in Chap. 9.

B. Poison prevention should be a part of every well-child visit. It is an ongoing educational process and parent(s)/care giver(s) need to be aware of potential dangers for their developing child.

C. Assist parent(s)/care giver(s) in identifying potential dangers and offer suggestions to correct the dangers.

D. Reassure parent(s) and encourage verbalization during and after a poisoning accident.

E. Prevention—see Table 9-5 in "Accident Prevention" in Chap. 9.

F. Provide additional counselling and close follow-up for children at risk for accidental poisoning, i.e., those with previous poisoning incident, overactive or impulsive children, families under stress.

bibliography

Arena, Jay M. *Poisoning: Toxicology-symptoms-treatment* (3d ed.). Springfield, Ill.: Charles C Thomas, 1975.

———. *The treatment of poisoning.* Summit, N.J.: CIBA Pharmaceutical Company, 1977.

———. The clinical diagnosis of poisoning. *Pediatric Clinics of North America,* **17**:477–494 (1970).

Lovejoy, Frederick H., and Alpert, Joel J. In Sydney S. Gellis and Benjamin M. Kagan (eds.), *Current pediatric therapy 8.* Philadelphia: Saunders, 1978, pp. 709–710, 713–723.

Lybarger, Patricia M. Accidental poisoning in childhood: An ongoing problem. *Issues in Comprehensive Pediatric Nursing,* **1**(6):30–39 (1977).

McMillan, Julia A., Nieburg, Philip I., and Oski, Frank A. *The whole pediatrician catalog.* Philadelphia: Saunders, 1977, p. 424.

Minnear, John H. The poisoning emergency. *American Journal of Nursing,* **77**(5):842–844 (1977)

Mofenson, Howard C., and Greensher, Joseph. Controversies in the prevention and treatment of poisoning. *Pediatric Annals,* **16**(11):60–74 (1977).

Mofenson, Howard C., and Greensher, Joseph. Poisonings—an update. *Clinical Pediatrics,* **18**(3):144–146 (1979).

———, and ———. The unknown poison. *Pediatrics,* **54**:336–342 (1974).

Neadlam, Nerman K., et al. Demographic characteristics of adolescents with self-poisoning. *Clinical Pediatrics,* **18**(3):147–154 (1979).

Pascoe, Delmer J., and Grossman, Moses. *Quick reference to pediatric emergencies.* Philadelphia: Lippincot, 1973, pp. 299–337.

Table 170-1 Frequently Ingested Products That Are Usually Nontoxic

Abrasives
Adhesives
Antacids*
Antibiotics
Baby-product cosmetics*
Ballpoint pen inks
Bathtub floating toys
Battery (dry cell) (1/5 MLD of mercuric chloride)
Bath oil (Castor oil and perfume)*
Bleach (less than 5% sodium hypochlorite)*
Body conditioners*
Bubble-bath soaps (detergents)
Calamine lotion*
Candles (beeswax or paraffin)
Caps (toy pistols) (potassium chlorate)
Chalk (calcium carbonate)
Cigarettes or cigars (nicotine)
Clay (modeling)
Colognes
Contraceptive pills
Corticosteroids*
Cosmetics*
Crayons (marked AP, CP)
Dehumidifying packets (silica or charcoal)
Detergents (phosphate)
Deodorants
Deodorizers (spray and refrigerator)
Elmer's glue*
Etch-A-Sketch*
Eye makeup*
Fabric softeners
Fertilizer (if no insecticides or herbicides added)*
Fish-bowl additives
Glues and pastes*
Golf ball (core may cause mechanical injury)
Grease*
Hair products (dyes, sprays, tonics)*
Hand lotions and creams*
Hydrogen peroxide (medicinal 3%)*
Incense*
Indelible markers
Ink (black, blue)
Iodophil disinfectant*
Laxatives*
Lipstick*
Lubricant*
Lubricating oils*
Lysol brand disinfectant (not toilet-bowl cleaner)*
Magic markers
Makeup (eye, liquid facial)*
Matches
Mineral oil*
Newspaper*
Paint (indoor, latex)
Pencil (lead-graphite, coloring)
Perfumes
Petroleum jelly (Vaseline)
Phenolphthalein laxatives (Ex-Lax)*
Play-Doh
Polaroid picture coating fluid
Porous-tip ink marking pens
Prussian blue (fericyanide)*
Putty (less than 2 oz)
Rouge*
Rubber cement*
Sachets (essential oils, powder)
Shampoos (liquid)
Shaving creams and lotions
Soap and soap products
Spackles*
Suntan preparation*
Sweetening agents (saccharin, cyclamates)
Teething rings (water sterility)
Thermometers (mercury)
Thyroid tablet*
Toilet water*
Toothpaste (with or without fluoride)
Vaseline*
Vitamins (with or without fluoride)
Warfarin*
Watercolors*
Zinc oxide*
Zirconium oxide*

*Indicates new additions to the list of nontoxic ingestions.
Source: Mofenson, Howard C., and Greensher, Joseph. Controversies in the prevention and treatment of poisonings. *Pediatric Annals,* **16**(11):72 (1977).

Table 170-2 Poisonous Plants

Plant	Toxic Part and Substance	Symptoms	Treatment
	House plants		
Arnica *(Arnica montana, sororia, cordifolia)*	Flowers and roots	GI symptoms, drowsiness, coma	Gastric lavage or emesis; symptomatic
Arum family: calla lily *(Caladium),* dumbcane *(Dieffenbachia),* elephant's ear *(Colocasia), Alocasia, Philodendron, Dracunculus, Amorphophallis*	All parts (calcium oxalate, unidentified principles)	Severe burning of mucous membranes with swelling of tongue and throat; nausea; vomiting; diarrhea; salivation; rarely, direct systemic effects	Gastric lavage or emesis; symptomatic

Table 170-2 Poisonous Plants *(continued)*

Plant	Toxic Part and Substance	Symptoms	Treatment
	House plants (continued)		
Castor bean *(Ricinus communis)*	Seed (ricin, if chewed; if swallowed whole, the hard seed coat prevents absorption and poisoning).	Severe GI symptoms, convulsions, uremia	Immediate gastric lavage or emesis; supportive; 5 to 15 g sodium bicarbonate daily to alkalinize urine
Mistletoe *(Phoradendron flavescens)*	Berries (β-phenylethylamine and tyramine)	GI symptoms, and bradycardia similar to digitalis	Gastric lavage or emesis; supportive; potassium, procainamide, quinidine sulfate, or disodium salt of EDTA
Rosary pea, jequirity bean, precatory bean, prayer bean, love bean, or lucky bean *(Abrus precatorius)*	Poisoning unlikely unless bean (abrin) is chewed; if chewed, causes agglutination and hemolysis even in weak dilution.	(Symptoms may be delayed 1 to 3 days); severe GI symptoms, drowsiness, coma, circulatory collapse, hemolytic anemia, oliguria, fatal uremia	Gastric lavage or emesis; maintenance of circulation; blood transfusions to correct hemolytic anemia; sodium bicarbonate to alkalinize urine
	Flower Garden Plants		
Bleeding heart or Dutchman's breeches *(Dicentra pucilla, cucullaria)*	All parts (isoquinoline-type alkaloids such as apomorphine, protoberberine, and protopine)	Trembling, ataxia, respiratory distress, convulsions	Symptomatic
Daphne *(Daphne mezereum)*	All parts (daphnin)	Abdominal pain, vomiting, bloody diarrhea, weakness, convulsions	Gastric lavage or emesis; symptomatic
Foxglove *(Digitalis purpurea)*	Leaves (digitalis glycosides)	Nausea, diarrhea, stomach pain, severe headache, irregular heartbeat and pulse, tremors, convulsions	Gastric lavage or emesis; supportive; atropine, potassium, procainamide, quinidine sulfate, or disodium salt of EDTA
Hyacinth *(Hyacinthus orientalis)*	Bulb	Severe GI symptoms	Gastric lavage or emesis; symptomatic
Indian tobacco *(Lobelia inflata)*	All parts (α-lobeline)	Progressive vomiting, weakness, stupor, tremors, contraction of pupils, coma	Gastric lavage or emesis; artificial respiration; atropine, 2 mg IM as necessary
Jessamine or yellow jessamine *(Gelsemium sempervirens)*	All parts (gelsemine and gelseminine)	Profuse sweating, muscular weakness, convulsions, respiratory depression	Gastric lavage or emesis; atropine, 2 mg IM as necessary; artificial respiration

Table 170-2 Poisonous Plants *(continued)*

Plant	Toxic Part and Substance	Symptoms	Treatment
	Flower Garden Plants (continued)		
Lantana, red sage, wild sage *(Lantana camara)*	All parts (lantanin), especially the green berries	Photosensitization with increase in severity from sunlight; acute symptoms resemble belladonna alkaloid (atropine) poisoning.	Gastric lavage or emesis; symptomatic and supportive
Lily-of-the-valley *(Convallaria majalis)*	Leaves and flowers (convallatoxin and other glycosides)	Irregular heartbeat, stomach upset	Gastric lavage or emesis; supportive; potassium, procainamide, quinidine sulfate, or disodium salt of EDTA
Narcissus family: daffodil, jonquil *(Narcissus pseudonarcissus, jonquilla)*	Bulb	GI symptoms	Gastric lavage or emesis; symptomatic
Nutmeg *(Myristica fragrans)*	Seeds (myristicin)	Hallucinations and elation, stomach pain, red skin, dry mouth, drowsiness, stupor, double vision, delirium (Two nutmegs can be fatal.)	2 to 4 oz mineral or castor oil, followed by gastric lavage and demulcents
Oleander *(Nerium oleander)*	Leaves (oleandrin and nerioside)	Nausea, severe vomiting, stomach pain, dizziness, slowed pulse, irregular heartbeat, marked dilation of pupils, bloody diarrhea, drowsiness, unconsciousness, paralysis of lungs (One leaf can kill an adult.)	Gastric lavage or emesis; symptomatic and supportive; potassium, procainamide, quinidine sulfate, or disodium salt of EDTA
Sweet pea *(Lathyrus odoratus)*	All parts, but especially seeds (β-amino-propionitrile, α-γ-aminobutyric acid)	Paralysis; slow, weak pulse; respiratory depression; convulsions	Gastric lavage or emesis; symptomatic
	Vegetable Garden Plants		
Rhubarb *(Rheum rhaponticum)*	Leaves only (oxalic acid)	Nausea, vomiting, abdominal pain, anuria, hemorrhages	Gastric lavage or emesis with limewater, chalk, or calcium salts; calcium gluconate; forced IV fluids; supportive
	Ornamental Plants and Trees		
Black locust *(Robinia pseudocacia)*	Bark, foliage, and seed (phytotoxin)	Nausea, vomiting, weakness, depression	Symptomatic

Table 170-2 Poisonous Plants *(continued)*

Plant	Toxic Part and Substance	Symptoms	Treatment
	Ornamental Plants and Trees (continued)		
Elderberry, black and scarlet elder *(Sambucus canadensis, pubens)*	Leaves, shoots, and bark (sambunigrin, a cyanogenic glycoside)	Nausea, vomiting, diarrhea	Gastric lavage or emesis; commercially available cyanide kit
Heath family: azaleas, *Rhododendron,* laurels *(Kalmia)*	All parts (andromedotoxin)	Salivation, lacrimation, rhinorrhea, vomiting, convulsions, slowing of pulse, hypotension, paralysis	Gastric lavage or emesis; activated charcoal, atropine, hypotensive drugs
Wisteria *(Wisteria sinensis)*	Pods (resin and glycoside, wisterin)	Severe GI symptoms, collapse	Gastric lavage or emesis; symptomatic
Yew *(Taxus baccata)*	All parts (alkaloid taxine)	GI symptoms, dilation of pupils, muscular weakness, coma, convulsions, cardiac and respiratory depression	Gastric lavage or emesis; meperidine to control pain; otherwise, symptomatic
Cherries, wild and cultivated *(Prunus)*	Twigs, foliage, and seeds (cyanide-releasing compound)	Stupor, vocal cord paralysis, tremors, convulsions, coma	Gastric lavage or emesis; use cyanide kit if indicated
	Plants that Grow in the Wild		
Buttercup family: crowfoot or buttercup *(Rananculus),* cowslip or marsh marigold *(Caltha palustris),* larkspur *(Delphinium),* monkshood *(Acontium)*	All parts; for monkshood, especially roots and seeds	Paresthesia, burning sensation of mouth and skin, nausea, vomiting, hypotension, weak pulse, convulsions	Atropine, 2 mg IM and repeat as necessary; maintenance of blood pressure; artificial respiration
Deadly nightshade *(Atropa belladonna)*	Berries, leaves, and roots (atropine and related alkaloids)	Fever; rapid heartbeat; dilation of pupils; skin hot, flushed, dry	Gastric lavage (4% tannic acid solution) or emesis; pilocarpine for dry mouth and visual disturbances
Laurel: mountain, black, sheep, American. See Heath family, above			
Mushrooms *(Amanita muscaria and phalloides).*	All parts	Stomach cramps, thirst, difficulty breathing	Gastric lavage, saline catharsis, activated charcoal, atropine IM
Pokeweed, pokeberry, scoke, or inkberry *(Phytalocca americana)*	All parts, especially root (saponin and glycoprotein); glycoproteins in African species produce	Burning bitter taste in mouth, persistent vomiting, amblyopia, slowed respiration, dyspnea, weakness,	Gastric lavage or emesis; symptomatic

Table 170-2 Poisonous Plants *(continued)*

Plant	Toxic Part and Substance	Symptoms	Treatment
Plants that Grow in the Wild (continued)			
	lymphocytes that resemble those in Burkitt's lymphoma.	tremors and convulsions, peripheral blood plasmacytosis (May be fatal)	
Poison hemlock *(Conium maculatum)*	All parts (alkaloid coniine)	GI symptoms, necrosis, muscular weakness, respiratory paralysis, convulsions	Gastric lavage or emesis; saline cathartic; maintenance of clear airway; oxygen and artificial respiration; anticonvulsive therapy
Thornapple, jimsonweed, or stinkweed *(Datura stramonium)*	All parts (atropine and related alkaloids)	Thirst, dilation of pupils, dry mouth, red skin, headache, hallucinations, rapid pulse, high blood pressure, delirium, convulsions, coma	Gastric lavage or emesis; pilocarpine for dry mouth and visual distrubances; barbiturates for convulsions
Water hemlock or cowbane, beaver poison *(Cicuta maculata, virosa)*	Roots (resin cicutoxin)	GI symptoms, convulsions, respiratory depression	Gastric lavage or emesis; symptomatic; parenteral short-acting barbiturates to control convulsions

Source: Arena, Jay M. Poisonous plants. *Clinical Symposia,* **30**(2):30–32, CIBA Pharmaceutical Company, Division of CIBA-GEIGY Corporation, 1977.

Table 170-3 Treatment of Specific Poisons

Drug	Toxicity and Excretion	Symptoms	Treatment
Acetaminophen (Tylenol, Tempra, Liquiprin)	Potential hepatotoxicity with ingestions of > 15 g in adolescent and > 5 g in child. Hepatotoxicity with serum level > 300 μg/mL 4 h following ingestion Major route of excretion—hepatic metabolism	Nausea, vomiting, diaphoresis; 36 to 48 h following ingestion—jaundice, elevated hepatic enzymes and bilirubin, prolonged prothrombin time; fully reversible or progresses to hepatic failure; renal and myocardial toxicity	Removal with emesis or lavage, activated charcoal, support for hepatic failure, treatment of hepatic failure, (cysteamine, methionine, acetylcysteine)
Acids (Lysol)	Toxicity related to concentration and duration of exposure	Corrosive burns of mucous membranes, mouth, esophagus, and stomach; pain in area of burns; circulatory collapse and shock; complications—esophageal and gastric perforation, glottic edema, pulmonary edema, pneumonia, stricture formation of esophagus and pylorus	Emetics and lavage are contraindicated; immediate removal from esophagus with water or milk: neutralization with an alkali not advised; opiates for pain; intravenous therapy for shock
Alkali (Lye, Drano, Saniflush, Clinitest)	Toxicity to esophagus related to concentration and duration of exposure	Corrosive burns of mucous membranes of mouth and esophagus; pain in area of burns; circulatory collapse and shock; complications—esophageal and gastric perforation, glottic edema, pulmonary edema, pneumonia, stricture formation of esophagus	Emetics and lavage are contraindicated; immediate removal from esophagus with water or milk; neutralization with an acid not advised; opiates for pain; intravenous therapy for shock; with evidence of esophageal or gastric burn (clinically, by esophagoscopy or by esophagram), prednisone, 2 to 3 mg/kg per 24 h for 3 weeks and then tapered over 1 week; broad-spectrum antibiotic coverage while on steroids; following therapy, upper gastrointestinal series for evidence of stricture; dilation of stricture if present
Ammonium hydroxide (Ammonia)	Toxicity to esophagus related to concentration and duration of exposure	Corrosive burns of mucous membranes of mouth and esophagus; circulatory collapse and shock; complications include esophageal and gastric perforation, glottic edema, pulmonary edema, pneumonia	Emetics and lavage are contraindicated; immediate removal from esophagus with water or milk; neutralization with acid not advised

Table 170-3 Treatment of Specific Poisons *(continued)*

Drug	Toxicity and Excretion	Symptoms	Treatment
Amphetamines (Benzedrine, Dexedrine, Dexamyl)	Symptoms when therapeutic dose exceeded. Lethal dose in man estimated at 20 to 25 mg/kg Major route of excretion—hepatic metabolism; minor route—renal	Nervousness, hyperactivity, mania, psychotic-like state; tachycardia, hypertension, cardiac arrhythmias, hyperpyrexia; convulsions and shock	Emesis or lavage; activated charcoal; control of seizures with barbiturates or diazepam; support for cardiovascular and respiratory failure; acidification of urine with ammonium chloride to increase excretion of drug; chlorpromazine; phenoxybenzamine or phentolamine for hypertensive emergencies
Aniline	Induces methemoglobinemia. Cyanosis with methemoglobin levels of greater than 15%; lethargy with levels greater than 40%, potential lethal levels at greater than 70% Major route of excretion—hepatic metabolism	Apathy and headache, cyanosis with dyspnea, hypotension and convulsions, circulatory and respiratory failure, intravascular hemolysis	Emesis or lavage; removal from source of exposure; oxygen; methylene blue; transfusion therapy for intravascular hemolysis
Antihistamines and cold medications (Dimetapp, Congesprin, Actifed, Contac, Sudafed, Allerest, Triaminic)	Symptoms when therapeutic dose exceeded Major route of excretion—hepatic metabolism	Excitation, disorientation, drowsiness, coma; anticholinergic syndrome—dry mouth, dilated pupils, fever, flushed skin, tachycardia, absent bowel sounds, urinary retention; hypertension, hypotension; convulsions; arrhythmias; cardiovascular collapse and respiratory depression	Emesis or lavage; activated charcoal; vigorous gastrointestinal catharsis; treatment of fever; maintenance fluid therapy; support for circulatory and respiratory failure; treatment of seizures with barbiturates or Valium; treatment with physostigmine
Arsenic	Major toxicity—gastrointestinal, hepatic, renal and central nervous system Major route of excretion—renal	Sweetish metallic taste in mouth; burning sensation in throat; diarrhea, vomiting, dehydration; delirium, convulsions, coma, hyperreflexia, seizures; pulmonary edema; hemolysis; arsenic in gastrointestinal tract—radiopaque on x-ray; toxic effects on liver, kidney and marrow	Emesis or lavage; intravenous hydration; treatment of liver and renal decompensation; transfusion therapy for hemolytic anemia; dimercaprol (BAL) therapy indicated when unknown amount ingested, with symptoms or when toxic levels exist
Atropine (Atropine- and scopolamine-containing agents)	Symptoms when therapeutic dose exceeded Major route of excretion—hepatic metabolism	Excitation, disorientation, drowsiness, coma; anticholinergic syndrome—dry mouth, dilated pupils, fever, flushed skin, tachycardia, absent bowel sounds, urinary retention; hypertension, hypotension;	Emesis or lavage; activated charcoal; vigorous gastrointestinal catharsis; treatment of fever; maintenance fluid therapy; support for circulatory and respiratory failure; treatment of seizures with barbiturates or

Table 170-3 Treatment of Specific Poisons *(continued)*

Drug	Toxicity and Excretion	Symptoms	Treatment
		convulsions; arrhythmias; cardiovascular collapse, and respiratory depression	diazepam; treatment with physostigmine
Barbiturates (Amobarbital, secobarbital, pentobarbital, phenobarbital)	Potentially fatal dose 40 to 50 mg/kg for short-acting barbiturates, and 65 to 75 mg/kg for long-acting barbiturates. Blood levels of 3 to 4 mg/100 mL for short-acting barbiturates and 10 to 15 mg/100 mL for long-acting barbiturates found with severe overdose (grades III–IV). Excretion of short-acting barbiturates—hepatic metabolism Excretion of long-acting barbiturates—renal and hepatic metabolsim	Mental confusion, drowsiness, coma; ataxia, vertigo, slurred speech; decreased deep tendon reflexes, decreased response to pain; hypotension, hypothermia; pulmonary edema with short-acting barbiturates; respiratory failure	Emesis or lavage; activated charcoal; forced fluid diuresis for long-acting barbiturates; alkalinization of urine for long-acting barbiturates; osmotic agents and diuretics for long-acting barbiturates; maintenance fluids for short-acting barbiturates; support for respiratory and cardiovascular failure; dialysis for long-acting barbiturates
Bleach (Clorox, Purex, Sani-Chlor)	Major toxicities to intestinal mucosa and central nervous system Major route of excretion—renal	Irritation and pain to mouth and esophagus; stricture and perforation extremely unlikely; nausea and vomiting; delirium, obtundation, and coma; hypotension	Removal with lavage if vomiting has not occurred; removal from skin by flooding with water; support for central nervous system and circulatory failure; treatment as caustic (acid-alkali) not necessary
Boric acid	Fatal dose is estimated at 0.1 to 0.5g/kg Major route of excretion—renal	Bloody diarrhea and dehydration; erythroderma and exfoliation; lethargy, convulsions; jaundice; hypotension; anuria; coma	Removal from skin, with ingestion emesis or lavage, intravenous fluids, treatment of seizures with barbiturates and diazepam
Bromides	Bromides produce toxicity by displacing chlorides from plasma and cells. Bromide toxicity occurs at > 50 mg/100 mL Major route of excretion—renal	Acute ingestion causes nausea, vomiting, paralysis and coma; chronic poisoning causes confusion, ataxia, slurred speech, irritability, delusions, psychotic behavior, stupor	Emesis or lavage; sodium chloride, 5 g/day in divided doses for 1 to 4 weeks (in adolescent) to hasten excretion; hemodialysis
Camphor (Campho-Phenique, camphor liniment)	Fatal dose for a 1-year-old child is approximately 1 g Major route of excretion—hepatic	Headache; burning in mouth and throat; camphor odor on breath; nausea and vomiting; feeling of warmth, excitement, irrational behavior, muscle spasms, convulsions, coma; circulatory and respiratory collapse	Emesis or lavage; activated charcoal; treatment of seizures with barbiturates or diazepam; support for respiratory and circulatory failure

Table 170-3 Treatment of Specific Poisons *(continued)*

Drug	Toxicity and Excretion	Symptoms	Treatment
Carbon monoxide	Cellular hypoxia as a result of high affinity of carbon monoxide for hemoglobin Major route of excretion—respiratory	At 20% carboxyhemoglobin—headache, vertigo, shortness of breath; at 40 to 50% carboxyhemoglobin—coma, cherry-red color to lips and skin, cardiac arrhythmias and ischemia, respiratory failure, irreversible brain damage	Removal of client from site of exposure to uncontaminated air; 100 % oxygen by mask for 30 min to 2 h; with respiratory depression, artificial respiration with 100 % oxygen; maintain temperature and blood pressure; recognition and treatment of cerebral edema
Carbon tetrachloride	Toxic dose by ingestion is as low as 3 to 5 ml. Causes injury to liver, kidneys, myocardium, central nervous system. Major exposure—oral or by inhalation Major route of excretion—hepatic metabolism	Abdominal pain, nausea and vomiting; headache and confusion; obtundation, coma, respiratory depression; circulatory collapse; renal, hepatic and myocardial damage	Emesis or lavage; maintenance hydration; avoid epinephrine and related compounds; respiratory support; management of renal and hepatic damage
Cathartics (Mineral oil, Ex-Lax, phenolphthalein, Metamucil)	Generally of low toxicity	Irritation of gastrointestinal tract causing tenesmus, vomiting, diarrhea; rarely hypotension, collapse, coma	With large ingestion, emesis or lavage; milk to decrease gastrointestinal irritation; if severe symptoms, hydration, medication for pain, treatment of shock
Chloral hydrate	Dose greater than 50 mg/kg causes hypnotic effects Major route of excretion—hepatic metabolism	Drowsiness, mental confusion, coma, shock, respiratory depression	Emesis or lavage, maintenance fluids, respiratory support
Cyanide	Cyanide exerts toxicity on cellular cytochrome oxidase systems causing cytotoxic anoxia. Severe and rapid onset of toxicity. Routes of exposure include ingestion and inhalation. Survival for 4 h often associated with recovery	Death in 10 to 15 min; bitter almond smell; tachycardia, bradycardia; absence of cyanosis; coma; hypotension; convulsions	Respiratory support with 100% oxygen; removal to uncontaminated atmosphere and removal of contaminated clothing; lavage after antidotes have been given; immediate use of amyl nitrite by inhalation followed by sodium nitrite; sodium thiosulfate
Detergents, soaps, and cleaners	Variable toxicity	Anionic detergents (Tide, Cheer, Ajax, Top Job, Comet, Windex, Mr. Clean, Lestoil, Joy, Spic'n Span, bar soap, bubble bath, household detergents) cause mild vomiting and diarrhea; cationic detergents (pHisoHex,	For anionic detergents-supportive therapy; no removal necessary. For cationic detergents: emesis or lavage, support for coma and respiratory failure, and treatment of seizures with barbiturates or diazepam. For

Table 170-3 Treatment of Specific Poisons *(continued)*

Drug	Toxicity and Excretion	Symptoms	Treatment
		Zephiran, Diaparene) cause nausea, vomiting, convulsions, coma; electric dishwasher and laundry granules cause caustic burns	treatment of dishwater and laundry granule burns, see under Alkali
Digitalis	Toxic symptoms when therapeutic dose exceeded Major route of excretion—hepatic metabolism with biliary and renal excretion of metabolites	Nausea, vomiting, altered color vision, slow and irregular pulse, hypotension, arrhythmias due to increased myocardial irritability	Emesis or lavage; activated charcoal; maintenance fluids; potassium, quinidine, Pronestyl, Xylocaine as determined by type of arrhythmias
Ergot derivatives (Sansert, ergotamine)	Toxic symptoms when therapeutic dose exceeded. Low toxicity Major route of excretion—hepatic metabolism	Diarrhea, vomiting; convulsions; hypotension; coma; constriction of blood vessels with numbness, coldness and gangrene of extremities with chronic ingestion	Emesis or lavage; control of seizures with barbiturates and diazepam; respiratory and cardiovascular support; vasodilators may be required with chronic ingestion
Ethyl alcohol (Ethanol, isopropyl alcohol, cologne, perfume)	Blood level: 0.05 to 0.15 %, mild; 0.15 to 0.3%, moderate; 0.3–0.5%, severe; above 0.5%, coma Major route of excretion—hepatic metabolism	Initial excitation, delirium and inebriation; later depression, stupor, coma; alcohol odor on breath; hypoglycemia; slurred speech and muscle incoordination; respiratory failure	Emesis or lavage, glucose for hypoglycemia, maintenance fluids, support for respiratory and circulatory failure, hemodialysis
Fluoride	Of low toxicity with 50 to 200 mg/kg as the estimated fatal dose. Fluorides act as cellular poisons interfering with calcium metabolism and enzyme mechanisms. Major route of excretion—renal	Nausea, vomiting, and diarrhea; salivation and irritation of mucous membranes; tremors and convulsions; respiratory failure; complications include jaundice, oliguria, anemia, leukopenia	Emesis or lavage, intravenous fluids, oxygen, support for cardiovascular and respiratory failure, calcium gluconate by mouth as local antidote to bind ingested fluoride
Hormones (Enovid, Ortho-Novum, Oracon, Norlestrin, Premarin)	Low toxicity	Nausea and vomiting, fluid retention, vaginal bleeding in girls	Emesis or lavage if more than 15 to 20 tablets have been ingested
Hydrocarbons (Kerosene, gasoline, mineral spirits, paint thinner, lighter fluid, barbecue fluid, dry cleaning fluid)	Toxicity to lungs and central nervous system Major route of excretion—hepatic metabolism	Hydrocarbon smell in mouth and on breath; burning in the mouth and esophagus; vomiting; pulmonary symptoms—cough, fever, bloody sputum, cyanosis, rales, pulmonary infiltrates; central nervous system drowsiness, mild coma, seizures	Removal is not indicated with petroleum distillate hydrocarbon ingestions in children. If very large amounts (> 100 mL) are taken (as in a suicide attempt), in alert client emesis with ipecac syrup is a safer method of removal than lavage. For

Table 170-3 Treatment of Specific Poisons *(continued)*

Drug	Toxicity and Excretion	Symptoms	Treatment
			pneumonia use of oxygen and antibiotics with signs of superinfection; use of steroids not indicated. Supportive therapy for central nervous system depression and seizures; avoid epinephrine; appropriate support for hepatic, renal, cardiac and bone marrow toxicity
Chlorinated hydrocarbon insecticides (DDT, dieldrin, lindane)	Variability of toxicity among compounds. Routes of absorption include gastrointestinal and cutaneous. Variability of absorption from cutaneous route	Vomiting, excitation, numbness, weakness, incoordination, tremors, seizures, circulatory and respiratory failure	Decontamination of skin, removal with emesis or lavage, gastrointestinal catharsis, support for respiratory or circulatory failure, control of seizures with barbiturates and diazepam
Organophosphate insecticides (Parathion, chlorthion, Bidrin, Dimetilan, Sevin)	Major route of excretion—hepatic metabolism with metabolites often pharmacologically active	Blurred vision, sweating, miosis, tearing, salivation, papilledema, cyanosis, seizures, pulmonary edema	Decontamination of skin, removal with emesis or lavage, gastrointestinal catharsis, support for respiratory or circulatory failure, control of seizures with barbiturates and diazepam, atropine sulfate, pralidoxime chloride
Carbamate insecticides		Same as for organophosphate insecticides	Decontamination of skin, removal with emesis or lavage, gastrointestinal catharsis, support for respiratory or circulatory failure, control of seizures with barbiturates and diazepam, atropine sulfate
Ipecac syrup	Amounts greater than 30 mL are potentially toxic	Nausea and vomiting; tachycardia, arrhythmias, hypotension; dyspnea; cardiac, hepatic and marrow toxicity; coma	Removal by emesis or lavage, activated charcoal, observation for arrhythmias or heart failure, treatment of hepatic or marrow toxicity
Iron (Ferrous sulfate, ferrous gluconate, ferrous fumarate, vitamins with iron)	Serum level of $> 400\ \mu g/100$ mL associated with systemic toxicity. Major toxicities—gastrointestinal, central nervous system, liver and vasculature Major route of excretion—renal	Symptoms occur $\frac{1}{2}$ to 4 h post ingestion; vomiting, diarrhea, melena; drowsiness, lethargy, pallor; metabolic acidosis; hepatic damage and coagulation defects; coma and shock; stricture of gastrointestinal tract; iron tablets, radiopaque on x-ray	Emesis or lavage; bicarbonate or phosphates to precipitate iron and prevent absorption; fluid therapy and expanders for shock. If (a) shock and coma, (b) serum iron level of greater than 400 $\mu g/100$ mL, (c) overdose in lethal range, (d) positive provocative chelation, treat with deferoxamine.

Table 170-3 Treatment of Specific Poisons *(continued)*

Drug	Toxicity and Excretion	Symptoms	Treatment
			Hemodialysis or exchange transfusion for renal failure
Lead	Toxicity by ingestion and inhalation. Symptoms with blood level > 40 μg/100 mL. Danger of encephalopathy with levels greater than 80 μg/100 mL	Ingestion causes chronic toxicity, inhalation, acute toxicity; abdominal pain, nausea, vomiting; opaque lead particles on x-ray; lethargy, ataxia; encephalopathy and coma	Emesis or lavage; gastrointestinal catharsis; treatment for renal failure and encephalopathy; calcium EDTA and/or BAL or d-penicillamine therapy
Lomotil (Atropine and diphenoxylate hydrochloride)	Toxicity when therapeutic dose exceeded (combined toxicity of atropine and diphenoxylate hydrochloride) Major route of excretion for both drugs—hepatic metabolism	Atropine signs 1 to 2 h following ingestion occur infrequently; diphenoxylate signs 2 to 5 h after ingestion; pinpoint pupils; lethargy, coma; respiratory depression; hypotension; convulsions	Emesis or lavage; activated charcoal; gastrointestinal catharsis; naloxone hydrochloride; ventilatory support for respiratory failure
Mercury Inorganic	Exposure from inorganic mercury found in rodenticides, mercury amalgam, diuretics	Major toxicity to gastrointestinal tract, kidneys, and liver; bloody diarrhea, metallic taste in mouth; abdominal pain; renal tubular damage and anuria; hepatic damage	Emesis or lavage; fluid therapy and transfusion therapy; treatment of liver and renal failure; dimercaprol (BAL)
Organic	Exposure from manufacturing plants and agricultural usage Major route of excretion—renal and gastrointestinal tract	Major toxicity to central nervous system; paresthesias, hypesthesia; weakness, apathy, inability to concentrate, loss of memory; ataxia, tremors, chorea; hearing difficulty; coma, seizures	N-acetyl penicillamine
Methyl alcohol (Wood alcohol)	2 tsp is toxic. Toxic blood level greater than 10 to 20 mg/100 mL. Major toxicities at > 50 mg/100 mL. Toxicity caused by methanol and metabolic breakdown products formaldehyde and formic acid Major route of excretion—hepatic metabolism	Headache and dizziness, nausea and vomiting, visual impairment, metabolic acidosis, coma, cyanosis, hypotension, respiratory failure	Emesis or lavage, monitoring for acidosis and correction with sodium bicarbonate, ethanol therapy, hemodialysis in association with ethanol therapy
Naphthalene (Mothballs, repellent cakes, deodorizer cakes)	Greater than 1 tsp is toxic Major route of excretion—hepatic metabolism	Nausea, vomiting, abdominal cramps; convulsions; coma; intravascular hemolysis with G6PD deficiency; oliguria and anuria	Emesis or lavage; control of seizures with barbiturates and diazepam. For intravascular hemolysis, intravenous fluids and alkalinization of the urine with bicarbonate to prevent

Table 170-3 Treatment of Specific Poisons *(continued)*

Drug	Toxicity and Excretion	Symptoms	Treatment
			precipitation of hemoglobin in tubules. Support for respiratory and circulatory failure; transfusion for anemia
Narcotic analgesics (Morphine, codeine, Demerol, methadone, propoxyphene, pentazocine)	Symptoms when therapeutic dose exceeded Major route of excretion—hepatic metabolism	Lethargy, coma; pinpoint pupils; respiratory depression; hypotension; convulsions	Emesis or lavage, activated charcoal, gastrointestinal catharsis, naloxone hydrochloride, ventilatory support for respiratory failure
Nicotine	Fatal dose of nicotine is about 40 to 60 mg. Swallowed as tobacco, nicotine is less toxic because of poor absorption from the stomach Major route of excretion—hepatic metabolism and renal excretion of metabolites	Nausea and vomiting, tachycardia, hypertension, headache, sweating, convulsions, coma, respiratory failure	Emesis or lavage, activated charcoal, control of seizures with barbiturates and diazepam, support for respiratory failure, atropine for parasympathetic overstimulation
Nitrates and nitrites	Individual susceptibility varies considerably. Ability to cause methemoglobinemia Major route of excretion—renal	Nausea and vomiting, headache, flushed skin, dizziness, hypotension, respiratory failure, coma	Emesis or lavage, oxygen, blood transfusion, methylene blue therapy, support for respiratory and circulatory failure
Phencyclidine (PCP, "Angel Dust," Peace Pill)	Widespread use. Passed. Alleged to be THC, LSD, psilocybin and mescaline Major route of excretion—hepatic metabolism with renal excretion of metabolites	*Low dose*—excitation, paranoid behavior, miotic pupils, nystagmus, increased blood pressure, pulse and respiration, slurred speech, drowsiness *High dose*—decreased reflexes, coma, seizures, opisthotonus, hypotension, respiratory depression	Emesis or lavage; reduction of sensory stimuli; diazepam, 0.5 mg/kg per 24 h for control of agitation, opisthotonus; acidification of urine with ammonium chloride to enhance renal excretion; support for respiratory and circulatory failure
Polishes and waxes (Pride, Old English, O'Cedar, Jubilee, Kleer Floor Wax, Bruce Cleaning Wax, Aerowax, Armstrong 1-step, Pledge Furniture polish, Stanley Furniture Cream)	Main toxicity is pulmonary, caused by aspiration. Central nervous system signs less severe, secondary to absorption from lungs	Burning of the mouth and esophagus; vomiting and diarrhea; pulmonary involvement—cough, fever, dyspnea, rales, cyanosis, pulmonary infiltrates; infiltrates clear over 1 to 4 weeks	Do not induce emesis for pulmonary involvement: oxygen, moisture, antibiotics when clinical course or sputum examination indicate superinfection; supportive therapy for central nervous system depression and seizures

Table 170-3 Treatment of Specific Poisons *(continued)*

Drug	Toxicity and Excretion	Symptoms	Treatment
Psychedelic drugs (LSD, mescaline, psilocybin, STP, DMT)	Duration and intensity of effect varies from drug to drug and from individual to individual Major route of excretion—hepatic metabolism	Dilation of pupils, tachycardia, mild hypertension, incoordination, visual hallucinations, distortion of sensory perception, exaggerated sense of comprehension	"Talking down" in quiet nonthreatening atmosphere; diazepam, 0.5 mg/kg per 24 h for sedative effect; avoidance of chlorpromazine with STP or DMT
Salicylates (St. Joseph's, Bayer, Bufferin, Rexall, Empirin, Anacin, Excedrin, Congesprin, Ben Gay)	Symptoms at 150 mg/kg or greater or at serum levels greater than 30 mg/100 mL; 50 to 80 mg/100 mL, mild symptoms; 80 to 100 mL severe symptoms; greater than 100 mg/100 mL, potentially fatal Major route of excretion—renal; minor route—hepatic	Vomiting, hyperventilation, fever, thirst, sweating, hypoglycemia or hyperglycemia, prolonged prothrombin time, confusion, delirium, coma, convulsions. In small children, metabolic acidosis; in older children, respiratory alkalosis	Emesis or lavage; activated charcoal; forced fluid diuresis (1 to 2 times maintenance); colloid for volume expansion; glucose for hypoglycemia; sponging for fever; vitamin K_1 for hypoprothrombinemia; alkalinization of urine with bicarbonate; hemodialysis, peritoneal dialysis or exchange transfusion with (a) levels greater than 100 to 150 mg/100 mL (b) anuria, (c) heart disease preventing forced fluid diuresis
Strychnine (Rodenticides)	Fatal dose for an adolescent is 15 to 30 mg. Toxicity due to increased reflex excitability	Increased deep tendon reflexes with muscle stiffening and opisthotonus; respiratory failure	Emesis or lavage, control of seizures with barbiturates and diazepam, prevention of peripheral stimuli and enforcement of quiet, support for respiratory and circulatory failure
Sympathomimetics (Ephedrine, epinephrine, Isuprel, Neo-Synephrine)	Toxic symptoms when therapeutic dose exceeded Major route of excretion—hepatic metabolism	Nervousness; tachycardia, arrhythmias; dilated pupils; blurred vision; convulsions, respiratory failure; coma	Emesis or lavage, treatment of seizures with barbiturates or diazepam, support for respiratory and circulatory failure
Thallium	Single doses of 8 to 10 mg/kg have been fatal in children Major route of excretion—renal	Abdominal pain, vomiting, diarrhea; diaphoresis, hyperpyrexia, salivation; hypotension, hypertension; ataxia, tremors, choreiform movements, paresthesias, coma; peripheral neuropathies; alopecia	Emesis or lavage; vigorous gastrointestinal catharsis; potassium chloride, 5 to 25 g/day orally to augment rate of excretion; prussian blue (potassium ferric hexacyanoferrate) and Dithiocarb under investigation and of unclear value at this time
Theophylline (Caffeine, aminophylline,	Toxicity when serum levels exceed 25/μg/mL. Nausea and vomiting seen between 15 and 25 μg/mL	Agitation, restlessness; vomiting, hematemesis; fever; tachycardia and cardiac arrhythmias; convulsions;	Emesis or lavage; enemas for rectally administered overdose; avoidance of sympathomimetics; supportive

Table 170-3 Treatment of Specific Poisons *(continued)*

Drug	Toxicity and Excretion	Symptoms	Treatment
slophylline)	Major route of excretion—hepatic metabolism	vasomotor collapse; respiratory failure	therapy for dehydration, seizures, arrhythmias and hypotension
Thyroid (Cytomel, Synthroid, desiccated thyroid, Choloxin)	Toxicity when therapeutic dosage exceeded. Thyroxine is about 200 times and triiodothyronine 800 to 1000 times as potent as desiccated thyroid. Long half-life of 6 to 7 days Major route of excretion—hepatic metabolism	Palpitation, rapid pulse; headache; tremors, nervousness, delirium; diaphoresis, hyperpyrexia; vomiting; symptoms may occur up to 1 week post ingestion	Emesis or lavage, supportive care for hyperpyrexia and central nervous system excitation
Tranquilizers (Mellaril, Equanil, Miltown, Placidyl, Doriden, Noludar, Dalmane, Librium, Valium)	Toxicity when therapeutic dosage exceeded Major route of excretion—hepatic metabolism	Sleepiness, weakness, unsteadiness, incoordination, hypotension, cyanosis, respiratory failure, coma	Emesis or lavage, activated charcoal and gastrointestinal catharsis, maintenance of an adequate airway and oxygen, support for respiratory and circulatory failure, supportive therapy during coma
Turpentine and other volatile oils (xylene, benzene, toluene)	Predominant central nervous system toxicity Major route of excretion—hepatic metabolism	Nausea, vomiting, central nervous system excitation, lethargy, coma; pneumonia and pulmonary edema; renal, hepatic and bone marrow toxicity	Emesis or lavage, treatment of seizures with barbiturates and diazepam, ventilatory support for respiratory failure, treatment of renal, hepatic or bone marrow failure
Tricyclic antidepressants (Imipramine, amitriptyline)	Symptoms when therapeutic dose exceeded Major route of excretion—hepatic metabolism	Excitation, disorientation, drowsiness, coma; anticholinergic syndrome—dry mouth, dilated pupils, fever, flushed skin, tachycardia, absent bowel sounds, urinary retention; hypertension, hypotension; convulsions; arrhythmias; cardiovascular collapse and respiratory depression	Emesis or lavage, activated charcoal, vigorous gastrointestinal catharsis, treatment of fever, maintenance fluid therapy, support for circulatory and respiratory failure, treatment of seizures with barbiturates or diazepam

Table 170-3 Treatment of Specific Poisons *(continued)*

Drug	Toxicity and Excretion	Symptoms	Treatment
Vitamin A	Of low toxicity with symptoms from ingestion of 200,000 to 300,000 units	Fatigue, anorexia, vomiting, bulging fontanelle, increased intracranial pressure	Emesis or lavage with large ingestions
Vitamin D	Of low toxicity with symptoms from ingestions of 100,000 to 150,000 units Major route of excretion—hepatic metabolism and biliary excretion	Elevation of serum calcium, metastatic calcifications, renal damage	Emesis or lavage with large ingestions; support for renal failure
Warfarin (Dicumarol)	Repeated doses needed to cause symptoms. Only single ingestions that are massive in amount will cause symptoms.	Prolonged prothrombin time and clinical bleeding occurring a few days to a few weeks following ingestion	Emesis or lavage following a very large single ingestion, monitoring of prothrombin time, vitamin K_1 transfusion therapy

Source: Lovejoy, Frederick H., Jr., and Alpert, Joel J. Treatment of specific poisons. In Gellis, Sydney S., and Kagan, Benjamin M. (eds.). *Pediatric therapy 8.* Philadelphia: Saunders, 1978, pp. 713–723.

Table 170-4 Guidelines for Unknown Poison

Symptoms and Signs	Possible Poison
Agitation, hallucinations, dilated pupils, bright red color to the skin, dry skin, and fever	Atropinelike agents LSD
Marked activity, tremors, headache, diarrhea, dry mouth with foul odor, sweating, tachycardia, arrhythmia, dilated pupils	Amphetamines
Slow respirations, pinpoint pupils, euphoria, or coma	Opiates
Salivation, lacrimation, urination, defecation, miosis, and pulmonary congestion	Organic phosphates or poison mushrooms
Sleepiness, slurred speech, nystagmus, ataxia	Barbiturates or tranquilizers
Hypernea, fever, and vomiting	Salicylates
Oculogyric crisis, ataxia, and unusual posturing of head and neck	Phenothiazines
Nausea, vomiting, sweatiness, and pallor are early manifestations; late manifestations include stupor and signs of liver failure	Acetaminophen

Source: McMillan, Julia A., et al. *The whole pediatrician catalogue.* Philadelphia: Saunders, 1977, p. 423.

PART 7

preparation for hospitalization

NANCY ANN CALLAND HART

I. Importance of Preparing the Child and Family for Hospitalization and/or Surgery

General considerations

1. Anxiety-producing situation
   a. Child is faced with threats and fears.
   b. Having had a previous experience with hospitalization and/or surgery does not necessarily reduce fears.
2. Individualized family preparation can reduce the stress and anxiety of hospitalization and surgery.
   a. Anxiety interferes with the learning process.
   b. Acquisition of knowledge will give the family more control over the situation.
   c. Parent(s) will be able to support the child better if anxiety level is kept low.
   d. Child will be more likely to gain mastery of the experience and understand it.
   e. Child will be less likely to have adverse reactions upon discharge.
3. Goals
   a. Child/parent(s) can effectively deal with the anxiety-producing situations of hospitalization and/or surgery.
   b. Family can utilize adequate defense to cope; will provide a sound base for future times of crisis.

II. Role of the Practitioner in Providing Anticipatory Guidance

A. Establish warm, trusting relationship with family.

B. Initial assessment should include

1. Psychological factors
2. Family, social factors
3. Physical factors
4. Developmental factors
5. Extent of knowledge
   a. Of child
      (1) Ask directly, "What do you know about your illness? Hospitalization? Surgery?"
      (2) Observe child at play.
         (a) Engage child in dramatic play regarding events of hospitalization.
         (b) In play, child often reveals concerns, fears.
         (c) When talking to child, be on child's eye level and maintain eye contact.
   b. Of family
      (1) Ask directly what they have been told.
      (2) Question carefully to determine level of understanding.
6. Determine how much and what type of information parent(s) want child to have.
   a. Must respect wishes of parent(s).
   b. Explain benefits to child of a thorough preparation.
7. Determine sequelae of previous experiences with hospitalization/surgery.
   a. Physical
   b. Emotional/psychological
   c. Developmental
8. Obtain special information needed to facilitate adjustment to hospitalization.
   a. Peer relationships
   b. Play patterns—favorite games, stories, music
   c. Eating patterns
      (1) Special likes and dislikes
      (2) Usual manner of eating
   d. Sleeping patterns
      (1) Any nighttime fears
      (2) Usual type of bed
      (3) Nap—length and frequency

(4) Special routines
e. Self-care activities
(1) Dresses self? Brushes own teeth?
(2) Tell mother child may regress in hospital.
f. Pertinent school history
g. Normal activity level
h. Unusual fears or habits, e.g., thumb-sucking
i. Language development
(1) Level of understanding
(2) Special words child uses for bowel movement, urination
j. Child's usual reaction to pain
(1) Does child have a high or low threshold?
(2) Does child seem to be comforted by presence of parent(s)?
(3) Has parent(s) instructed child that "big boys (girls) don't cry?"
(a) If child is not allowed to express emotions freely, a greater burden is placed on child.
(b) Tell parent(s) the benefits of allowing child to cry if in pain.
k. Any special routines
l. Any special needs of the child
9. Explore possible parental concerns.
a. Financial
b. Effect of hospitalization on other children
(1) How to explain situation
(2) How to deal with their reactions
(a) May feel more vulnerable: they could be next
(b) May feel jealous of attention "sick" child is getting
(3) Specific techniques to deal with whatever problem exists for parent(s)
c. Care of other children
(1) Does parent(s) have reliable care givers?
(2) Parents can rotate remaining at hospital so children at home won't feel deserted.
d. Effect hospitalization will have on other family members, e.g., spouse, grandparents
e. Maintenance of home
f. Job disturbances
g. Outcome of surgery, hospitalization
(1) Physical
(2) Emotional
(3) Developmental
h. Distorted perceptions of parent(s) relating to prior or present hospitalization

C. Identify major problem areas.
D. Plan nursing interventions appropriate to the problem.
E. Evaluate interventions, making alterations when appropriate.
F. Educate the family.
1. Consider the following factors.
a. Age
b. Developmental level
c. Cognitive level, language development
d. Prior experiences with health care system
e. Nature of operation, procedures
f. Readiness to learn
g. Level of anxiety
h. Cultural background
i. Ability of parent(s) to teach child
2. Determine existing misconceptions.
a. Ask parent(s)/child what they know.
b. Ask parent(s) what the child has been told.
c. Listen to child at play.
3. Give family new knowledge.
a. Whenever possible assist parent(s) with teaching child. Instruct parent(s) *how* to teach if necessary. This depends on assessment of the teaching abilities of the parent(s). Teach whatever is pertinent for the child to know (e.g., blood tests, x-rays to be done, etc.). This depends on the individual situation.
(1) Maintains role of parent(s).
(2) Gives child a sense of security.
(3) Primary health care practitioner should act as resource to parent(s), e.g., provide appropriate teaching materials as needed.
b. Use principles of teaching.
(1) Assess readiness to learn.
(2) Begin with basic concepts and proceed to complex ones.
(3) Use words the family can understand and use in verbal communication.
(4) Utilize short teaching periods.
(a) 15 to 30 min is usually adequate.
(b) Length depends on individual attention span.
(5) Be sensitive to verbal and nonverbal cues of family and respond according to their needs.
c. Surgery
(1) Establish what knowledge physician has given; clarify and build on this.
(2) Avoid giving specific details of surgery.
(3) Avoid use of threatening words, e.g., *cut, taking out*

d. Evaluate teaching frequently.
   (1) Check for understanding.
   (2) Repetitions may be necessary.
e. Answer questions as they are raised.
   (1) Do not assume that child/family has no questions because none are asked.
   (2) Answers should be honest, clearly stated, and as short as possible.
f. Familiarize parent(s) with hospital prior to child's admission.
   (1) Location
   (2) Type of institution—teaching, research, private
   (3) Tour of typical hospital unit
   (4) Type of nursing care available
   (5) Admission procedures
   (6) Visiting hours
   (7) Provisions for staying overnight
   (8) Mealtimes
   (9) Eating facilities available
   (10) Parking facilities
   (11) Public transportation
   (12) Smoking regulations
   (13) Health team members who will care for child
   (14) Personal belongings child may bring
   (15) Phone number of unit
g. Specific information for child
   (1) Typical room
   (2) Playroom, if available
   (3) Admission procedure—taught close to the time when events will occur
   (4) Introduction to health team members

4. Help parent(s) cope with child's hospitalization by making them aware of *possible* reactions.
   a. Aggression, anger
   b. Feelings of guilt, of being punished
   c. Specific fears, e.g., needles, hospital noises
   d. Regression to previous stage of development, e.g., toilet-trained child possibly needing diapers again
      (1) Emphasize that it is best to allow the regression to occur.
      (2) Inform parent(s) that child will shortly resume previous level of functioning.
      (3) Inform parent(s) that hospitalization is not the time to teach new skills or to insist child use newly developed skills.
   e. Separation anxiety
      (1) Stress that this is normal.
      (2) Emphasize to be honest with child and not to "sneak" out.
      (3) If available and appropriate, encourage rooming in.
   f. Following discharge parent(s) may see
      (1) Sleep disturbances
      (2) Regression
      (3) Demanding behavior
      (4) Irritability
      (5) Clinging to parent(s)
      (6) Fears

      (Important to stress that these reactions are not abnormal unless they persist)

5. Apprise parent(s) of child's special needs during hospitalization.
   a. Warm, supporting parent(s)
   b. Expressive play
   c. Honest explanations, simply stated
   d. Physiologic and security needs (determinants of behavior of child)

6. Teaching methods
   a. Booklets, pamphlets
   b. Body diagrams
   c. Hospital tours
   d. Preadmission "parties"
   e. Play techniques
      (1) Invite but *never* force a child to play.
      (2) Use self to play for child unable to participate personally.
   f. Films
   g. If appropriate allow family to talk with children who have experienced similar surgery.
   h. Hold group discussions if several families are facing similar experiences.
   i. Make appropriate books regarding hospitalization available to child/family (see bibliography).[1]

7. Timing of preparation
   a. Toddler
      (1) Younger toddler will not absorb much factual information—present facts immediately preceding event.
      (2) Older toddler may grasp basic facts—tell just prior to admission.
   b. 4 to 6 years old
      (1) Tell no more than 1 week in advance.
      (2) If told sooner, child may forget.
   c. 7 years old and older
      (1) Can receive information as soon as it's known hospitalization will be necessary.

[1]Institutions can order a "Children's Hospital" toy from Sales Department, Fisher-Price Toys, 70 Church Street, East Aurora, N.Y. 14052.

(2) Use child's questions and responses as a guideline.
(3) If child asks no questions, begin approximately 10 days to 2 weeks in advance.

III. Provide Support to Child/Family Before, During, and After Hospitalization.

IV. Act as Liaison Between Family and Hospital Personnel.

A. Provide hospital health care workers with pertinent information regarding the child/family.
1. Ideally this is done just prior to admission.
2. Information can be used by hospital personnel as part of an ongoing nursing process; will provide continuity of care and eliminate unnecessary questioning of family.

B. Remain alert to changing needs.

C. Assist in planning, implementation, and evaluation of prehospitalization teaching programs.

V. Assess Postoperative Status in Conjunction with Other Health Team Members.

A. In hospital (if have hospital privileges)
1. Encourage verbalizations of feelings.
2. Initiate any teaching necessary.
3. Keep communication lines open with rest of health team.

B. Post discharge
1. Evaluate adaptation
   a. Physical
   b. Psychological
   c. Developmental
2. Notify physician in case of
   a. Prolonged emotional reactions
   b. Prolonged developmental delays
   c. Physical complications

VI. Community Education

A. Plan, implement, and evaluate programs designed to inform the well child about hospitalization.

B. Utilize existing groups, e.g., Association for the Care of Children in Hospitals (ACCH).

VII. Groups in Need of Special Attention

A. General principles for special-needs group
1. Be active in identifying special-needs groups.
   a. Work closely with physicians, courts, community health nurses.
   b. Let other health team members know that special cases should be referred to practitioner.
2. Thorough assessment of each particular situation is essential.
3. Be aware of available resources in community; refer when necessary.
4. Provide supportive relationship for child/family.
5. Practitioner can be very useful in providing continuity of care.
6. Be aware of available educational materials to use in training of professionals regarding special needs.

B. Child from children's home
1. Anxiety level may be higher due to lack of sense of security.
2. Establish supportive one-to-one relationship.

C. Delinquent child
1. Hospitalization may seem a retribution.
2. Child may become depressed or belligerent in hospital.
3. Set clear limits.
4. Use firm, supportive, positive approach.
5. Be honest and nonjudgmental.

D. Single-parent families
1. Needs depend on specific situation.
   a. If divorce, separation, or death was recent, family still in state of crisis and in need of crisis techniques.
   b. If family unit has stabilized, crisis intervention not necessary.
2. Assess family needs.
   a. Financial
   b. Support systems available
   c. Emotional
   d. Physiologic
3. Child especially vulnerable to effects of hospitalization may view himself or herself as the causative agent of separation or death of other parent.
4. Provide support, close relationship.
5. Refer to appropriate sources for additional help.

E. Retarded child
1. Make careful assessment.
   a. Special attention to child's ability to comprehend and verbalize spoken language
   b. Convey to other health team members any pertinent information
2. Dispel myths.
   a. Staff may think retarded child does not need explanations.

b. Staff may not be aware that a retarded child is often very sensitive to what others say and do.

3. Support family as needed.

F. Handicapped child

1. Do careful assessment of self-care activities.
2. Family interaction needs careful assessment.
   a. Feelings of hostility, guilt may exist.
   b. Feelings are often ambivalent.
3. Dispel myths—staff may treat all handicapped children as if they were retarded.

G. Child with chronic illness

1. Needs careful assessment.
   a. Family resources may be exhausted.
   b. Needs vary according to length, severity of illness.
   c. Situation may have caused distorted perceptions.
2. Repeated hospitalizations
   a. Hospitalization may still be anxiety-producing.
   b. Need for preparation still exists.

H. Poverty-level families

1. Poor living conditions
2. Widespread disorganization of family life
3. Often have emotional, intellectual, and various behavioral problems as well as various health problems
4. Typical personality constellation
   a. Fatalistic
   b. Present-oriented
   c. Authoritarian
   d. Distrust of outsiders
   e. Low self-esteem
   f. Little belief in own coping capacities
   g. Limited verbal communication
   h. Become anxious and defensive when confronted with new situations
5. Effects of illness, hospitalization on child
   a. The child may feel defenseless (e.g., child who was a "tough street kid" and depends on physical strength for identity).
   b. Hospital may provide sense of security and comfort.
      (1) May have been deprived of nutrition, medical attention, love, and belonging and/or esteem.
      (2) Sense of regularity provides structure.
      (3) May be a growth-promoting experience.
      (4) Child may simulate illness in order to be able to stay in hospital.
6. Interventions
   a. Make careful assessment.
   b. Help child to recognize individual importance by valuing what he or she communicates.
   c. Moderate authoritarian approach is least likely to alienate family.
   d. Do not engage family in lengthy discussion or great deal of talk about the future.
   e. Frequently check on child's adjustment to home situation.

I. Suspected child abuse

1. Assessment of family interactions essential
   a. Parental feelings often vary.
      (1) Guilt over incident
      (2) Fear of being punished
      (3) Hostility toward child
   b. Observe and record interactions of family members.
2. Observe reactions of child to hospitalization.
   a. May feel relief
   b. May be very fearful
   c. May not want to return home
3. Report suspected cases to proper authorities.
4. See Poverty-level families, VII, H if applicable

J. Attempters of suicide (see Suicide, Chap. 85)

1. Assess present suicidal potential.
2. Very important to be seen by suicidal person as a trusting friend.
   a. Treat with respect, honesty.
   b. Be accessible for support, to listen.
3. Educate staff about special needs.
   a. Unsuccessful attempter may be treated with scorn by hospital staff.
   b. An attempter needs firm, clear limits.

K. Addicted/alcoholic child

1. Often feels alienated.
2. Provide one-to-one relationship.
3. Be cognizant of current laws.

VIII. Emergency Admissions

A. Effect on child

1. Very stressful situation
   a. Unfamiliar surroundings
   b. Subjected to many painful and frightening procedures
   c. Comes in contact with many strangers in short period of time
2. Many fears possibly aroused
3. Fears intensified if child lacks knowledge, e.g., may fear injection will leave a hole and blood will all flow out
4. Fears possibly intensified by seeing (or hearing) other persons undergoing procedures

B. Possible parental reactions
1. May direct efforts towards helping child
2. Anger at child, themselves
3. Guilt over incident, feel responsible
4. Fearful of outcome
5. Time to teach child a lesson
6. Feels threatened

C. Interventions
1. Establish rapport.
   a. State what child is probably feeling, e.g., "You must feel scared not knowing what these tubes are for," or, "You must feel angry that all this is happening so quickly to you."
      (1) This will give child feeling of security; knowing someone guesses how he or she feels.
      (2) It enables child to express feelings.
   b. Begin immediately to explain to child what is happening.
2. Provide emotional support to decrease anxiety.
   a. Spend time with family.
   b. Answer questions in language they can understand.
   c. Give short, honest explanations of events.
      (1) Having to wait for explanations will cause a family to become anxious.
      (2) You may need to repeat.
      (3) Use calm, soothing voice.
      (4) Child needs *frequent reassurance* other parts of the body are not damaged.
   d. Correct misconceptions.
   e. Provide for ventilation of feelings.
   f. Show parent(s) the child is the main focus.
   g. Nonverbal support is very important.
   h. Be aware of family's nonverbal cues.
3. Involve parent(s) in care whenever possible.
   a. Allows parent(s) to gain some control over situation.
   b. Decreases feelings of role conflict.
   c. Depends on situation; in some cases more traumatic for parent(s) to participate.
   d. If parent(s) cannot stay, have them leave personal article with child to reassure child parent(s) will return.
4. Act as liaison between emergency room experience and transition to ward if child is admitted.
5. Provide training of emergency room personnel in child development and the needs of children in a stressful situation.

IX. Ambulatory Surgery

A. Considerably shortens hospital stay

B. Interventions
1. Encourage child/parent(s) to attend preadmission orientation program.
2. Have visual materials available for the family in advance of the surgery.
3. Keep in frequent contact with family in the role of liaison person.

Preparing the Family for Hospitalization of a Child

Developmental Needs	Primary Causes of Stress	Interventions	Behaviors Indicating Stress
		Infant	
Establishing mother-infant bond Establishing sense of trust Continuity of care giver, routines Needs met quickly Provision of comfort measures	Separation from mother Separation from familiar surroundings	If hospitalization is needed immediately following birth: *If at all possible,* arrange for infant to go home with mother. Home environment more conducive to establishment of mother-infant bond. Parent-child relationship needs a relaxed, private atmosphere.	Feeding difficulties Sleep disturbances Retarded development

Preparing the Family for Hospitalization of a Child *(continued)*

Developmental Needs	Primary Causes of Stress	Interventions	Behaviors Indicating Stress
		Infant (continued)	
		Instruct mother in importance of establishing relationship with baby. Provide opportunities for mother and infant to be alone. Provide reassurance, support. Encourage mother to hold, cuddle, stroke infant, establish eye-to-eye contact. Hospitalization for older infant If possible, arrange for mother to stay with child. Explain that child may regress. Give thorough explanation of what will happen, any special equipment.	
		Toddler	
Development of sense of autonomy Supervised freedom to explore Sense of security determined primarily by presence and love of mother. Regression as a result of separation most evident in this age group Beginning to learn control of body functions Learning to communicate and to think Increasingly able to understand others and express self Able to think about problems; may solve simple problems	Unable to be autonomous; behaviors restricted Painful, unpredictable experiences	Encourage parent(s) to stay with hospitalized child as much as possible. Explain child may violently protest when mother leaves. Stress this is normal whereas feelings of despair and denial upon separation are more harmful. Stress that parent(s) be honest at all times; do not sneak out on child. Instructions to toddler should be: Brief Honest Immediately prior to event Allow toddler to explore as far as safety allows.	Crying and protesting Resisting

Preparing the Family for Hospitalization of a Child *(continued)*

Developmental Needs	Primary Causes of Stress	Interventions	Behaviors Indicating Stress
		Toddler (continued)	
Thinking is egocentric and magical, i.e., things happen because they are wished		Encourage staff to follow toddler's usual routines as much as possible. Encourage parent(s) to bring familiar objects from home. Favorite toy, book, blanket Picture of family Support mother to increase continuity and quality of mothering.	
		Preschooler	
Developing a sense of initiative Main fear—abandonment by parents Pain and illness viewed as a punishment Has concerns about body injury Understanding of anatomy and physiology often distorted May think having their blood drawn will cause them to lose all blood Has more precise control of language than toddler, but has a limited ability to understand complex sentences and words Need for information; understanding of environment Active fantasy life	Separation from family Intrusive procedures Pain	Encourage parent(s) to stay with child as much as possible. Give honest, simple explanations. Use play as method of teaching. Dolls, puppets Free-form activities such as paints, clay Parent(s) encouraged to play with child Dramatic play Important to give *whys* of painful procedures to reduce guilt feelings. Carefully explain what body parts will be operated on. Very important to uncover child's misconceptions in this area Use of body diagrams helpful to pinpoint exact area Encourage participation of preschool child in self-care.	Many fears Sleep disturbances, especially nightmares
		School-Age Child	
Developing a sense of industry Success in school Recently has won control of body; may be	Unrealistic fears, especially regarding surgery, anesthesia Inadequate preparation	Needs thorough explanations. If child is to have surgery, explain: Will not wake up during surgery	Regression, withdrawal Increased dependency Depression

Preparing the Family for Hospitalization of a Child *(continued)*

Developmental Needs	Primary Causes of Stress	Interventions	Behaviors Indicating Stress
		School-Age Child (continued)	
preoccupied with bodily functions Fear of death and bodily injury often exaggerated Needs exact information Can solve problems and manipulate symbols More reality-based than preschooler		*Will* wake up after surgery Able to understand past, present, and future; give child timing of events. Fears may not be expressed. May seem so terrible, afraid to verbalize them. May feel embarrassed to admit fear. Tell child it is normal to have fears and it helps to talk about them. Allow child to handle equipment. Can teach how things work, e.g., child will enjoy taking the nurse's blood pressure. Child enjoys technical explanations.	
		Adolescent	
Developing a sense of identity and sense of intimacy Involved in struggle of independence and dependence; emancipation from parents Satisfactory relationship with opposite sex Acceptance of new body image Peer group very important Making decisions about future vocation Achieving integrated personality	Has fragile self-esteem and body image Fears unacceptance from peers	Explanations can be detailed and technical; on adult level. Will demonstrate practitioner's respect for adolescent. Assess to determine if teenager is understanding correctly. Allow as much participation in decision-making process as possible. If possible, organize group of adolescents with the same health problem. Allow time for adolescent to express feelings and thoughts in creative ways. Poetry Music Art	Continually challenges authority figures Increased rebelliousness

Preparing the Family for Hospitalization of a Child *(continued)*

Developmental Needs	Primary Causes of Stress	Interventions	Behaviors Indicating Stress
		Adolescent (continued)	
		Reassure adolescent that need for privacy from others will be respected.	

ADDITIONAL INFLUENCING FACTORS WHICH AFFECT ALL AGE GROUPS:

1. Individual differences in personality
2. Family dynamics, parent(s)-child relationship
3. Cultural and ethnic differences
4. Religion
5. Previous hospital experience
6. Attitudes of family
7. Quality of preparation

bibliography

Books

Bergman, Thesi. *Children in the hospital.* New York: International Universities Press, 1965.

Petrillo, Madeline, and Sanger, Sirgay. *Emotional care of hospitalized children.* Philadelphia: Lippincott, 1972.

Plank, Emma N. *Working with children in hospitals* (2d ed.). Cleveland: Case Western Reserve University, 1971.

Oremland, Evelyn K., and Oremland, Jerome D. *The effects of hospitalization on children.* Springfield, Ill.: Charles C Thomas, 1973.

Articles

Canright, Patricia, and Campbell, Mary Jo. Nursing care of the child and his family in the emergency room. *Pediatric Nursing,* **3:**43–45 (1977).

Kunzman, Lucy. Some factors influencing a young child's mastery of hospitalization. *Nursing Clinics of North America,* **7:**13–26 (1972).

Petrillo, Madeline. Preventing hospital trauma in pediatric patients. *American Journal of Nursing,* **68:**1468–1473 (1968).

Resnick, Rene, and Hergenroeder, Elizabeth. Children and the emergency room. *Children Today,* September-October: 5–8 (1975).

Visintainer, Madelon A., and Walter, John A. Psychological preparation for surgical pediatric patients: The effect on children's and parents' stress responses and adjustment. *Pediatrics,* **56:**187–202 (1975).

Audiovisual media

These can be utilized by practitioner for teaching professionals and parents.

I. The American Journal of Nursing Company
Educational Services Division
10 Columbus Circle
New York, NY 10019

A. *The hospitalized child*
   1. 44 min, 16-mm film, sound, black andwhite
   2. Discusses difficulties, fears, and fantasies of children in accepting hospitalization.

B. *Play therapy and the hospitalized child*
   1. 26 min, black and white
   2. Describes how to assist children in adjusting to hospitalization through play therapy.

C. *Psychiatric-Mental Health Nursing: The crisis of loss*
   1. 30 min. videotape, sound, color
   2. Problems of loss and mourning are discussed using crisis theory as a framework.

II. Children's Hospital National Medical Center
111 Michigan Avenue, NW
Washington, DC 20010

To prepare a child
   1. 32 min, 16-mm, sound, color with study guide and bibliography
   2. The child-care staff demonstrates the qual-

ity of care needed to prepare children for hospitalization.

III. Trainex Corporation
Subsidiary Medcom Inc.
PO Box 116
Garden Grove, CA 92642

A. *Admission and orientation of the child*
   1. 35-mm filmstrips, audio-tape-cassettes, 33⅓ LP, color
   2. Discusses fears and anxieties of child and parents. Techniques are indicated for reducing the stress of hospitalization. Includes emotional needs of the child and the value of parental participation.

B. *Parents and their ill child*
   1. 35-mm filmstrip, audio-tape-cassette, 33⅓ LP, color
   2. Parents are given suggestions to help prepare themselves and their child for hospitalization

C. *Preparing the child for procedures*
   1. 35-mm filmstrip, audio-tape-cassettes, 33⅓ LP, color
   2. Designed to help health care personnel minimize the emotional trauma of hospitalization of a child.

IV. Films designed for child viewing

A. Trainex Corporation: *Stephen goes to the hospital*
   1. 35-mm filmstrip, audio-tape-cassettes, 33⅓ LP, color
   2. Told by Stephen's doctor; begins in doctor's office and shows Stephen's various experiences during hospitalization, ending with discharge from the hospital.

B. Children's hospital national medical center: *A hospital visit with clipper*
   1. 16-mm filmstrip, color, 25 min
   2. Using puppets, the child is introduced to the hospital environment.

Books which prepare children for hospitalization

Bemelmans, Ludwig. *Madeline.* New York: Viking Press, 1939. For all ages 3–9 years.

My tour with clipper book. Washington D.C.: Children's Hospital National Medical Center. For ages 2–12 years.

Michael's heart test. Philadelphia: Children's Hospital of Philadelphia, 1967. For ages 3–12 years.

Margaret's heart operation. Philadelphia: Children's Hospital of Philadelphia, 1969. For ages 3–12 years.

Clark, Bettina, and Coleman, Lester L. *Pop-up going to the hospital.*New York: Random House, 1971. Grades Kindergarden to 3.

Deegan, Paul J. *A hospital: Life in a medical center.* Mankato, Minn.: Amecus Street, 1971. Grades 4–7.

Falk, Ann Mari. *The ambulance.* Toronto: Burke Publishing Co., 1966. For ages 3–9 years.

Froman, Robert. *Let's find out about the clinic.* New York: Franklin Watts, Inc., 1968. Grades Kindergarden to 3.

Haas, Barbara Schuyler. *The hospital book.* Baltimore, Md.: John Street Press, 1970. For ages 4–10 years.

Hallqvist, Britt G. *Bettina's secret.* New York: Harcourt, Brace, & World, 1967. Grades 3–7.

Kay, Eleanor. *The clinic.* New York: Franklin Watts, 1971. Grades 4–6.

The emergency room. New York: Franklin Watts, 1970. Grades 5–7.

Welzenbach, John F., and Cline,Nancy. *Wendy Well and Billy Better say "hello hospital"; Wendy Well and Billy Better visit the hospital see-through machine; Wendy Well and Billy Better meet the hospital sandman; Wendy Well and Billy Better ask a "mill-yun" hospital questions.* Chicago: Med-Educator, 1970. For ages 3–12 years.

Wolde, Gunilla. *Tommy goes to the doctor.* Boston: Houghton Mifflin, 1972. For ages 2–5 years.

appendixes

1 Intramuscular Injections

COLLEEN CAULFIELD

Administering intramuscular (IM) injections to children of all ages can be very stressful for both the child and the nurse. The procedure is also painful, and it is difficult for a nurse to inflict pain on a child. Many uncertainties and questions exist in the mind of the concerned nurse—why? how? can the pain, psychological and physical, be relieved? The purpose of this appendix is to review the basic principles of safe intramuscular injection to a child. A developmental approach will be used. Discussion will include

1. A review of the indications for intramuscular injection.
2. A review of the hazards of intramuscular injection with implications for prevention.
3. A review of four sites used in intramuscular injection.
4. Means of reducing the physical pain associated with an intramuscular injection.
5. Developmental considerations in administering intramuscular injections to children.

INDICATIONS FOR INTRAMUSCULAR INJECTIONS

The efficacy and safety of some medications are strongly influenced by the route of administration. Choice of route is based on an accurate knowledge of the pharmacokinetic properties of the drug and an assessment of the child. The major indications for giving a drug intramuscularly include

1. The child is unable to or unwilling to take the medication orally.
2. Parent compliance with administering the drug is questionable. An injection will ensure that the child receives the needed medication.
3. A local effect is desired.
4. A prolonged effect is desired (i.e., long-acting penicillin).
5. The therapeutic margin of drug safety is limited, and a precise dose is required.
6. Drug effect from other routes may be unpredictable.
7. A rapid effect is desired.
8. The medication cannot be administered orally with predictable effects or without irritation to the gastrointestional tract.

HAZARDS OF INTRAMUSCULAR INJECTIONS

An intramuscular injection is not an innocuous procedure. The intact skin is the body's first line of defense, and any intrusion into this barrier provides a porthole for serious complications. Bones, muscles, nerves, tissues, and blood vessels may be injured. The following conditions have been reported following improper intramuscular injection technique: abscesses, anesthesia, arteriolar spasm, cysts, foot drops, edema, hematomas, hypesthesia, muscular dystrophy, fibrosis, numbness in the extremities, necrosis with sloughing, paralysis, pedal growth arrest, peripheral neuritis, transverse myelitis, periostitis, vasospastic disease, and wrist drop.

Table A1-1 outlines the major complications of intramuscular injections with implications for prevention.

SITES FOR INTRAMUSCULAR INJECTIONS

Selection of an injection site should not be haphazard and based on the convenience of the nurse or the child. Many of the complications of intramuscular injections can be prevented by careful selection of a site. Site selection should be based upon

1. Knowledge of the locations of major nerves and vessels in relation to the site selected.
2. Assessment of the muscle mass to be injected into. Muscle mass size changes during childhood, reflecting the necessity of approaching site selection from a developmental point of view.
3. Assessment of the surrounding tissues with the aim of permitting retention and consistent absorption of the drug.

Figures A1-1, A1-3, A1-4, and A1-5 illustrate four injection sites suitable for use in children.[1] Information regarding preparation of the child and injection technique follows.

The Vastus Lateralis (Fig. A1-1)

The vastus lateralis is the major muscle of the quadriceps femoris group. The muscle is well developed at birth and is recommended by many as the preferred site for intramuscular injections in infants and children. When correctly identified, the site is far removed from major vessels and nerves and is of sufficient size to permit repeated injections. However, this area is not without complications. The vastus lateralis and the anterolateral upper thigh are not synonymous with the thigh; indiscriminate injection into the medial thigh is dangerously close to the sciatic nerve and the femoral arteries and veins. Needle length should be limited to 1 in when this site is used.

[1]The author would like to thank Laurie Kallsen for her illustrations of the injection sites.

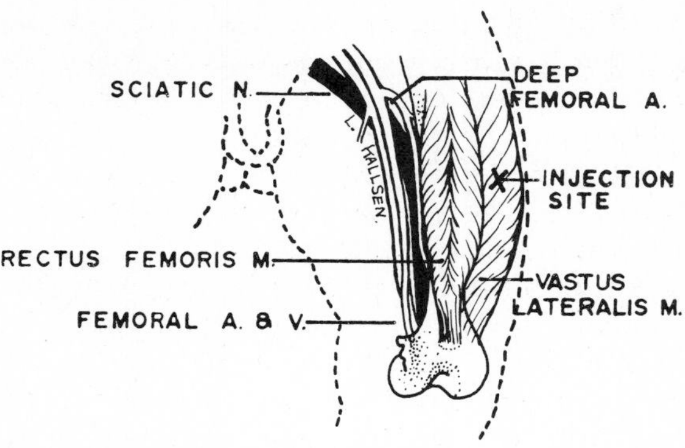

Figure A1-1 The vastus lateralis.

Preparation and Positioning The site is accessible with the child supine, prone, sitting, or in the lateral recumbent position. Figure A1-2 illustrates a position which permits adequate visualization and restraint in young children.

Technique The area between the greater trochanter and the patella is divided into thirds. The injection is given in the middle third, lateral to

Figure A1-2 A position of restraint for intramuscular injection in the vastus lateralis. The mother holds the child on her lap; the nurse stabilizes the leg to be injected between her knees. Mother's lap is a familiar position and gives the child emotional as well as physical security. Continuous comforting is possible, and immobility is limited to a minimun. *(Photo courtesy of Richard Trottier.)*

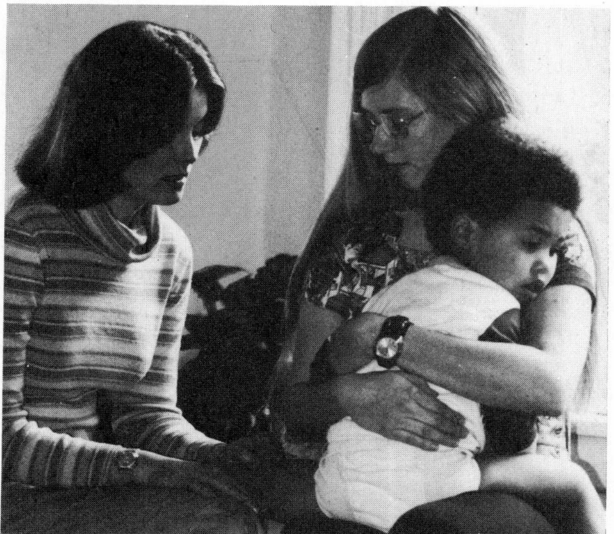

the midline of the anterior thigh, in a straight, front-to-back course. Compressing the tissue between the fingers will increase the penetrable muscle mass and help to stabilize the extremity in infants, small children, and very thin adolescents or adults. The tissue should be held taut in well-developed adolescents and adults.

Anterolateral upper thigh The injection site is the lateral thigh, upper outer quadrant, at the juncture of the mid and distal thirds. The needle should be directed distally and inserted at a 45° angle to the horizontal long axis of the leg, pointing toward the knee. Penetration should never be deeper than 1 in.

The Ventral Gluteal Area (Fig. A1-3)

The ventral gluteal area, also called von Hochstetter's site, has gained increasing recognition and is recommended by some as the preferred intramuscular site in children. The gluteus medius and gluteus minimus musculature is well developed, and the subcutaneous tissue relatively shallow. The site is removed from major nerves and vessels and can be easily localized by palpable bony landmarks. The major hazard of this site is the inadvertent injection into the more dangerous gluteal areas. Adequate restraint and identification of pertinent landmarks is thus imperative. An assistant should be used to immobilize and divert the young child. Bone may also be penetrated in small children and infants. An additional disadvantage is that this site may be visible to the child. Postinjection discomfort may be greater than with the two lateral thigh sites.

Preparation and positioning The site is accessible from the prone, supine, standing, or lateral recumbent position. The lateral recumbent position with the knee flexed will provide maximal muscular relaxation.

Technique With the heel of the hand on the greater trochanter, the index finger is placed on the anterior superior iliac crest and the middle finger is extended along the crest of the ilium as far as possible. A triangle is formed, and the injection is given in the center of this triangle. The needle is pointed slightly toward the iliac crest at 75 to 80°.

The Dorsal Gluteal Area (Fig. A1-4)

The gluteal area is fairly expansive and extends forward to the anterior superior iliac spine. The area is not synonymous with the buttock, and injections should never be given into any quadrant. Only the inner portion of the upper outer quadrant with the anterior superior iliac crest as the outside landmark should be used. Location of the sciatic nerve and the superior gluteal artery and vein make injection into any other quadrant unsafe practice. Subcutaneous tissue in

Figure A1-3 The ventral gluteal area.

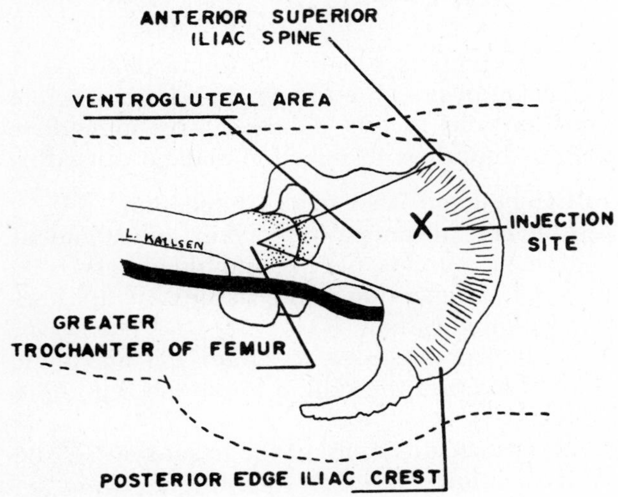

Figure A1-4 The dorsal gluteal area.

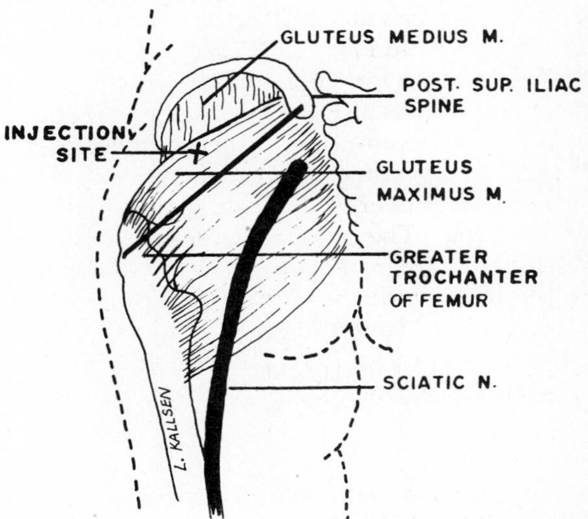

the area is thick; medication intended for intramuscular injection may be erroneously deposited into these tissues. The gluteal muscles develop with locomotion; this site should be used only, if at all, in a child who has been walking for a year or more.

Preparation and Positioning The site is accessible only from the prone position. "Toeing-in" will relax the muscles; the standing position will not permit proper relaxation of the muscle. Underwear should be removed. If pulled up from below, only the dangerous lower inner quadrant is exposed.

Technique The site is located by drawing an imaginary line connecting the posterior superior iliac spine and the greater trochanter. The injection is given lateral and superior to the line with the *syringe held perpendicular to the surface on which the person is lying.*

The Deltoid Muscle (Fig. A1-5)

Although a developed deltoid muscle appears as a large triangle on the shoulder prominence, the area available for intramuscular injection is limited by the close proximity of the brachial nerve plexus, the brachial veins and arteries, and various bony structures (the acromion process, clavicle, and humerus). This muscle is not fully developed in young children. *This site is dangerous and should be used only in the adolescent or adult with a well-developed muscle mass and then* ONLY WHEN NO OTHER SITE IS AVAILABLE. In addition, the muscle is shallow, limiting the number of injections and the volume of medication. Pain is likely to be greater at this site than at other areas.

Figure A1-5 The deltoid muscle.

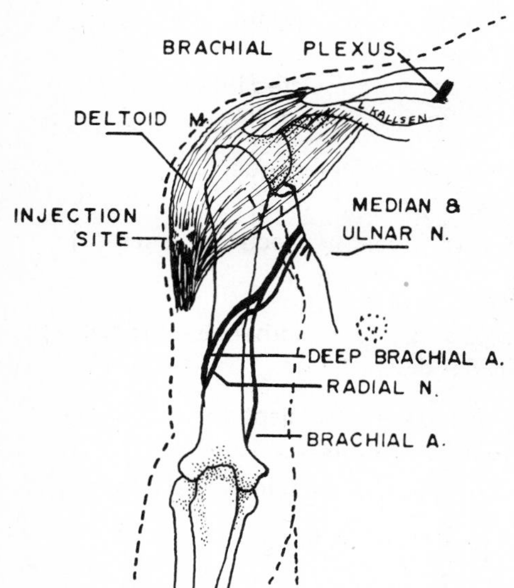

Preparation and Positioning The muscle is accessible from any position. Flexion of the arm at the elbow will aid in relaxing the muscle. Identification of pertinent landmarks necessitates exposure of the entire arm and shoulder area. "Rolling up a sleeve" is likely to expose only the inferior groove of the deltoid. Shirts or blouses should be removed for adequate visualization.

Technique The injection site is located by drawing an imaginary rectangle bounded on the top by the lower edge of the acromion process and on the bottom, by the axilla. The two side boundaries are one-third and two-thirds of the way around the lateral surface of the arm. The needle is inserted into the densest portion of the muscle, pointing slightly upward toward the shoulder. The muscle mass should be compressed and grasped between the fingers to judge muscle depth and to avoid bone in thin individuals.

REDUCTION OF PAIN

Pain receptors are randomly found in the skin, and it is not possible to select an intramuscular injection site that is painless. The immediate pain surrounding an injection may be caused by

1. Direct disturbance of a pain receptor
2. Mechanical trauma to the skin, subcutaneous tissues, muscles, nerves, and blood vessels
3. Sudden distention of the tissues by rapid entry of medication
4. Local irritation due to either the antiseptic used to clean the skin or to the medication itself
5. Abnormal sensitivity of the tissues at the site of injection

Certain methods can, however, be utilized to minimize the discomfort of an injection. These methods include

1. Using a sharp needle with the smallest gauge possible
2. Limiting the volume of drug injected into any one site. Use two injections if needed. The maximum volume to be used will depend on the size of the muscle used; 2.0 mL is an absolute maximum in children.
3. Avoiding injecting the medication rapidly
4. Keeping medications as near to room temperature as possible
5. Allowing the antiseptic to dry before the skin is penetrated

DEVELOPMENTAL CONSIDERATIONS

Few children will escape the experience of an intramuscular injection, and to the child this experience usually means one thing—pain. This pain can cause an immeasurable amount of fear, anxiety, and psychological trauma that may persist for a long time and may pervade the child's response to all health care activities. But this fear, anxiety, etc., need not be. Measures have been outlined which can help alleviate the pain. The trauma of an injection can also be dealt with effectively and can be eliminated, it is hoped, by utilizing a developmental approach. Tables A1-2 through A1-6 outline this approach. The tables take into account muscular and interactive development that may have bearing on the child's response to an intramuscular injection. The stages of Erikson have been used as a framework for interactive development. Nursing implications for administering intramuscular injections are derived.

Table A1-1 Complications of Intramuscular Injections and Implications for Prevention

Complication	Prevention
Nerve and/or tissue damage	Use an air lock. Use only drugs suitable for intramuscular injection. Carefully identify and assess injection site. Rotate sites when repeated injections necessary. Hold the needle steady when penetrating the skin and injecting. Avoid even the slightest depression of the plunger during needle insertion. Limit the volume of drug injected into one site; volume determined by muscle size.
Abscess formation	Adhere strictly to aseptic technique. Use an air lock. Rotate sites when repeated injections necessary.
Nerve damage	Carefully select injection site. Remove needle and select another site if radiating or severe pain occurs.
Inadequate absorption of drug	Rotate sites when repeated injections necessary. Avoid areas with scar tissue. Avoid injection into areas with impaired circulation.
Vascular damage; inadvertent injection into bloodstream	Always aspirate before injecting. Carefully select site.

Table A1-2 Pediatric Injection Guidelines—The Infant (0–12 Months)

Developmental Tasks and Behaviors	Nursing Implications
Muscular	
Deltoid and dorsal gluteal muscles not fully developed. Injection into either is dangerously close to major nerves and vessels.	The vastus lateralis is the preferred injection site. The ventral gluteal area may be used in well-developed infants as a second choice when repeated injections are necessary.
Interactive—Basic Trust Vs. Mistrust	
Early response to the pain of injection is diffuse and generalized, manifested by crying, startle reflex, and generalized body movement. Response may be delayed for a short period of time.	Establish an easy, nonhurried, comfortable situation. Safe restraint of the very young infant can be achieved without a second person present.
By 6–8 months of age, pain response involves active cortical participation; early memory may associate needle with pain. May recall negative experiences.	Begin to expect active rejection of an injection. An assistant may be needed for safe restraint. Early experiences with injections can have lasting effects.
Totally egocentric and dependent on mother. She is seen as an extension of child's body. She gives satisfaction and relieves tension. Recognizes trusted individuals and may exhibit stranger anxiety when separated from mother.	Allow and encourage mother to participate in the injection routine, giving the infant the source of strength needed in this threatening procedure. Mother's participation will increase the infant's confidence in having needs met and in feeling physically safe.
	Provide immediate comforting to alleviate distress. This is part of the infant's learning to form trust relationships.
	Adequate and safe restraint during the injection is important in the development of feeling physically safe.
Communication skills begin to develop. By 12 months can make simple requests by gesturing.	Be alert for the infant indicating his or her own needs.

Table A1-3 Pediatric Injection Guidelines—The Toddler (1–3 Years)

Developmental Tasks and Behaviors	Nursing Implications
Muscular	
Motor skills developing rapidly; walks (12 months), climbs (18 months) and runs without falling (24 months). Very adept at resistive behaviors.	Adequate and safe restraint mandatory. Use an assistant or parent. Figure A1-2 illustrates a position for intramuscular injection that provides safe restraint, limits immobility, and provides the security of mother's arms.
Gluteal muscles not fully developed until the toddler has been walking for at least a year. Deltoid muscles not developed.	Vastus lateralis continues as the preferred injection site.
Interactive—Autonomy Vs. Shame and Doubt	
Central to the development of autonomy is the toddler's concept of being in charge for most activities. Muscular maturation and locomotion provide the toddler with a major means of obtaining autonomy and independence. Immobility or restraining motor activity is viewed as a significant threat in itself.	Provide the toddler with opportunities for self-assertion and exhibition of graduated amounts of control. Involve toddler in part of the routine. Although some authorities recommend that the ventral gluteal muscles are sufficiently developed for safe injection, the restraint and resultant immobility necessary to keep the child in a

Table A1-3 Pediatric Injection Guidelines—The Toddler (1–3 Years) *(continued)*

Developmental Tasks and Behaviors	Nursing Implications
Interactive—Autonomy Vs. Shame and Doubt (continued)	
	supine, prone, or lateral recumbent position will add a great amount of fear to the already stressful situation. Instead, use the position illustrated in Fig. A1-2.
Temper tantrums and negativism at a peak. These behaviors are the toddler's way of controlling the environment and demonstrating assertiveness and/or aggression.	Give the toddler permission to object but be positive about your actions. Ignore resistive behaviors. Provide opportunities to play out the frustrations inherent in this painful situation.
Although does not know right from wrong, demonstrates pride in accomplished tasks. Can carry out simple directions.	Give simplified directions. Use a firm and consistent approach. Tell the toddler what is expected of him or her and follow through. The toddler must have firm, consistent expectations for protection from feelings of shame and early doubt. Give immediate comforting and praise after an injection.
Crucial to the development of autonomy is the distinction between self and nonself. Initially egocentric, the toddler refers every event to himself or herself. This develops into an awareness that things exist independently. The origins of separation anxiety are founded in this awareness of self and nonself.	
In spite of the toddler's need for self-assertion, having control, and learning self from nonself, security is still determined by the presence of the mother or another trusted person. The toddler's ability to explore the world and tolerate anxiety is impaired when mother is not present.	Presence of mother will enhance the toddler's ability to deal with the threat and pain of an injection. If this is not possible, learn what symbolic language or actions mother uses in other painful or stressful situations.
Develops a symbolic language.	
Experiments with holding on and letting go. Beginnings of the development of free choice.	Allow as much freedom as possible. Give choices. Do not give a choice if the toddler does not have one or imply a choice is possible by asking if you may proceed.
Elicits cues on how to act in specific situations from mother or other trusted individuals.	Explore mother's feelings about injections. If she is stressed, the toddler will perceive this, heightening personal anxiety.
Develops perception of objects as stable by testing and exploring from all angles (shapes, weight, etc.).	Allow the toddler to explore the equipment, aiding in the development of an accurate perception of the object. Older toddlers can be given an empty, clean syringe to take home.
Little perception of time. By 21 months can respond to "just a minute" and at 2 years, to "play after this."	Tell the toddler about the injection just before the procedure. Use perceptions of time in explaining how long it will hurt.
Does not initially realize that it is possible to be hurt or to hurt someone else. Is not intrinsically afraid of an injection for the first time but the strange environment, strange people, immobility, and limited language cause a distortion of the event. The future can become even more threatening.	Provide playful, positive, nonpainful experiences, lessening the distortion that the clinic, office, or hospital means pain and injections. NEVER TELL A CHILD THAT AN INJECTION WILL NOT HURT. To do so will forever impair his or her ability to trust the health care system.
Play is the child's work and way of learning about and coping with an environment.	Use play to elicit cooperation and allow the child to vent anxiety and aggression.

Table A1-4 Pediatric Injection Guidelines—The Preschooler (3–6 Years)

Developmental Tasks and Behaviors	Nursing Implications
Muscular	
The gluteal muscles are developed but are still relatively small, increasing the hazard of inadvertent injection into the more dangerous portions of the buttocks. Positioning for safe restraint continues as a disadvantage of the area. The deltoid muscles are not developed.	Vastus lateralis continues as the preferred injection site. The ventral gluteal area may also be used as a second choice.
Interactive—Initiative Vs. Guilt	
The stage of initiative builds upon the successes of autonomy and adds the ability to plan, undertake, and complete a task. The preschooler is eager to work cooperatively and share obligations. At no other time is the child more ready to learn, hindered only by concrete thinking and limited language.	Involve the preschooler in the routine of injection giving. Ask for child's assistance. Teaching can have long-range effects.
By 4 years, mastery of a task is most important. At 5 years the preschooler can follow rules and by age 6, engage in problem solving.	Give simple, concrete explanations of what you expect. Child can understand his or her role in the procedure.
Mastery requires that the preschooler see, feel, and handle an object before understanding it.	Provide opportunities to explore the equipment. Give the preschooler an empty syringe to take home.
Demonstrates pride in making decisions and in accomplishments.	Give a choice—"Which leg do you want the injection in?"
Beginning of the development of a sense of moral obligation.	Enlist child's assistance in holding still. Explain that it is important to hold as still as possible but that you understand this is hard. You will help. Give immediate praise and reward after an injection.
The preschooler is in control for most activities. However, limits are important to help control a frightening sense of "power." Sense of security is jeopardized when a clear understanding of the expectations of him or her are absent in a specific situation. Ability to tolerate frustration is variable.	Give the preschooler clear expectations of what is expected of him or her. Avoid prolonged bargaining. This is frustrating and frightening to the child because no one is in control.
The preschooler's time concept is sufficiently developed to allow for delayed satisfaction.	Able to understand that an injection will hurt for only a few minutes. Can count the time. Simple explanations of the reason for an injection (to help get rid of the hurting ear) may be accepted.
This time is the stage of magical thinking—"I am what I think I can be." By 3 years, fantasy precedes every action.	Explain the procedure only a few minutes before, diminishing the amount of time available for the preschooler to fantasize.
Importance of dramatic play at a peak. The preschooler copes with unfamiliar situations and stress by playing out feelings and thoughts.	Providing the tools for dramatic play will enhance the preschooler's ability to come to understand and deal with the stress of an injection.
Explores different social roles in play.	Enjoys playing hospital, nurse, doctor.
Because of newly gained control over body and its functions, maintenance of body integrity is of prime concern to the preschooler. Mutilation fears are at	Explain in simple terms what you are going to do, being sure to state that child's body will remain intact after your procedure.

Table A1-4 Pediatric Injection Guidelines—The Preschooler (3–6 Years) *(continued)*

Developmental Tasks and Behaviors	Nursing Implications
Interactive—Initiative Vs. Guilt (continued)	
a peak and any intrusive procedure is viewed as a hostile invasion.	
The preschooler has some understanding of the inside of the body—the "skin keeps it all in." Possibly believes will bleed to death when the skin is penetrated.	Applying a bandaid to the injection site will provide immeasurable relief to the preschooler. This simple plastic strip will "patch up the hole and keep the blood inside."
The young preschooler lacks the necessary cognitive skills needed to comprehend the meaning and circumstances of illness and is apt to interpret it as a result of his or her "badness" which is now being punished. Painful procedures are also interpreted as punishment of badness.	Explain to the preschooler that illness is not due to "badness" and that you are not punishing by giving an injection. This may need to be stated several times. Reassure the child that he or she is not to blame for the illness.
	Parents need to be cautioned against using a visit to the clinic, hospital, or office for an injection as a way to secure cooperation (i.e., "don't do that or you will have to get a shot").
The preschooler has many castration fears. Begins to develop modesty.	Explain carefully to the preschooler where you are giving the injection. Respect need for privacy. The vastus lateralis may be preferred over the ventral gluteal area because this site does not require removing the undergarments.

Tabel A1-5 Pediatric Injection Guidelines—The School-Age Child (6–11 Years)

Developmental Tasks and Behaviors	Nursing Implications
Muscular	
Period of refinement and further development of muscular skills. Deltoid muscles remain small.	Vastus lateralis and ventral gluteal are both acceptable sites for intramuscular injection.
Interactive—Industry Vs. Inferiority	
The major theme of middle childhood is the mastery of skills and talents. The school-age child is involved in exploring himself or herself and the world. Concern is with making and building both things and friends. Child has a good command of language; needs answers as to how and why.	The school-age child wants and needs to understand how body works. Give concise explanations of disease, the effect on him or her, and the reasons for an injection. Involve child in health care.
Strives for and is very proud of accomplishments. Thrives on praise.	Give praise for holding still and cooperating. This will give the school-age child a sense of accomplishment and will help gain cooperation in the future.
Tests limits and challenges authority.	Continue to use a consistent firm approach. Tell the child what you expect. Give choices.
Demonstrates flexibility of thought. This child is reflective and has a storage of memories to draw upon. Actions are influenced by previous experiences. The unknown is fearful.	Explore previous experiences. Resistive behavior may be due to a previous, stressful experience. The school-age child may or may not be able to understand the difference in this situation.
Applies rules of logic and demonstrates the ability to classify, group, and deal with several parts of a whole.	Draw upon the school-age child's experiences in helping child to understand this situation.
One of the main tensions of this period is the	Acknowledge that an injection hurts and that it is

Tabel A1-5 Pediatric Injection Guidelines—The School-Age Child (6–11 Years) *(continued)*

Developmental Tasks and Behaviors	Nursing Implications
Interactive—Industry Vs. Inferiority (continued)	
conflict between the desire to attain adult status and the desire to retain the privileges of earlier childhood. Regression is not uncommon when faced with stress.	not always possible to hold still—you will help. Do not shame or ridicule crying or resistive behaviors. Accept this regression and help the child understand that crying is an acceptable way of displaying emotion. But it is important to try as hard as possible to hold still. Explain the impact of untreated disease on his or her future.
The school-age child is very social, and the peer group becomes as important as family. Response to parent(s) is variable.	The school-age child may prefer to not have parent(s) present during an injection. Give child the choice.
Perception of time accurate and the child can delay gratification.	Can understand how long it will hurt. Can count the minutes.
The school-age child is very modest.	Maintain privacy. Vastus lateralis may be preferred site as it does not involve removing the undergarments. Give child the choice.
Response to illness will depend in part on the child's interpretations and in part on how his or her peer group will react. May fear being displaced from the group.	Explore the child's perceptions of illness and treatment. Explain how long the illness will last. Explore the reactions, if any, he or she expects from peer group.

Table A1-6 Pediatric Injection Guidelines—The Adolescent (11–18 Years)

Developmental Tasks and Behaviors	Nursing Implications
Muscular	
Muscle mass approaching adult levels.	The vastus lateralis, dorsal gluteal, and ventral gluteal are all suitable for intramuscular injection. The deltoid should be used only when no other site is available and then with extreme caution.
Interactive–Identity Vs. Role Confusion	
The adolescent is striving to know "who and what I am." Seeking to understand self and develop an image that is congruent with what he or she wants and with others' perception of him or her.	The adolescent needs a concise, accurate undertanding of his or her body and the impact of illness and treatment on it. Approaches to the adolescent need to be highly individualized and based on how child is feeling at that time. Listen to them.
Compares self to peers and does not want to be different.	Reassure the adolescent that his or her behavior is like others in a similar situation.
Adapts to values of peer group.	
The adolescent is responsible for own activities.	Include the adolescent in his or her health care. Give responsibilities in the injection routine.
Begins to solidify future plans.	Explore these plans. Does the current illness have any impact on these?
The adolescent can deal effectively with reality and with the abstract. Thinking can be deductive and can evaluate the logic of own thinking.	
Reality orientation will permit delayed gratification for future goals.	The adolescent can look at an injection realistically and in relation to future goals.

Table A1-6 Pediatric Injection Guidelines—The Adolescent (11–18 Years) *(continued)*

Developmental Tasks and Behaviors	Nursing Implications
Interactive–Identity Vs. Role Confusion (continued)	
Uses adult coping mechanisms. Regression may occur, and the adolescent may feel hostile and ashamed of this behavior.	Allow the adolescent to display hostility; protect him or her against feelings of shame.
The adolescent begins to loosen ties with family; still needs the security of family. May identify with other adults—the stage of "crushes."	Expect a variable response to parent(s). May be reluctant to express that he or she needs family.
The adolescent is very concerned with the dramatic physiological changes of his or her body. Uncertain at times how to deal with these changes. Illness may be very difficult because it upsets body perceptions.	Give careful explanations of body functions and the impact of illness on them. The adolescent can accept these changes better if he or she understands them.
Modesty varies and depends on child's trust of the nurse and the sex of both.	Take cues from the adolescent. Always drape him or her properly. If possible, allow child to choose the injection site.

bibliography

Brandt, P. A., et al. IM injections in children. *American Journal of Nursing,* **72**:1402–06 (1972).

Erikson, E. H. *Childhood and society* (2d ed.). New York: Norton, 1963.

Fisher, T. L. This procedure has legal as well as clinical risks. *Canadian Medical Association Journal,* **112** (3):395–396 (1975).

Hill, L. F. Intramuscular injection in infants and children. *The Journal of Pediatrics,* **70**:1012–13 (1967).

Hughes, W. T. Complications resulting from an intramuscular injection. *The Journal of Pediatrics,* **70**:1011–12 (1967).

———. *Pediatric procedures.* Philadelphia: Saunders, 1964, pp. 87–92.

Intramuscular injections. Philadelphia: Wyeth, 1970.

Johnson, E. W., and Raptou, A. D. A study of intragluteal injection. *Archives of Physical Medicine and Rehabilitation,* **46**:167–177 (1965).

Petrillo, M., and Sanger, S. *Emotional care of hospitalized children.* Philadelphia: Lippincott, 1972.

Talbert, J. L. et al Gangrene of the foot following intramuscular injection in the lateral thigh; a case report with recommendations for prevention. *The Journal of Pediatrics,* **70**:110–114 (1967).

2 Oral Medication

COLLEEN CAULFIELD/ELIZABETH ORMOND

Prescribing drugs for children only on the basis of organism culture and sensitivity, i.e., consideration of the drug only, is sure to lead to frequent therapeutic failure. A comprehensive approach to drug prescription and administration must also include the child and parent(s) (Fig. A2-1). As illustrated, the child is central; other factors must be evaluated in accord with their impact on *him* or *her*. Each of the three factors, child, parent(s), and drug is discussed in relation to information which will assist the health care provider in achieving successful drug therapy of the pediatric client.

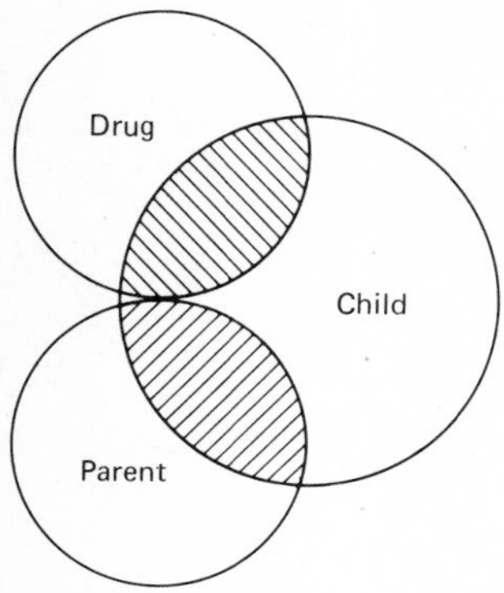

Figure A2-1 Schematic conceptualization of factors which must be considered in prescribing and administering medications.

THE CHILD

Each child is unique; no child can be considered a small adult. A developmental framework which recognizes both emotional-social and physiological development should be used. For convenience these are presented separately, though in practice they are considered simultaneously. Tables A2-1 to A2-6 cover emotional-social development relevant to the taking of medication. They extend only to age 6 years; by this age essential behaviors are achieved. Further development is highly influenced by experiences and the child's stage of industry versus inferiority (Erikson). Tables A2-7 to A2-10 cover the absorption, distribution, metabolism, and elimination of drugs during childhood. They identify altered physiology, effects of illness, and drug interactions.

THE PARENT

Children under 12 years of age are not usually independent in medication taking. The person most often responsible for this action is the parent figure. Compliance with prescribed drug treatment should never be assumed merely because an adult is involved. Overall noncompliance with oral drug therapy in outpatient settings is at least 25 to 50 percent, Figure A2-2 presents factors which influence parental readiness to follow recommended therapy, factors which may modify parent readiness, and barriers to compliance.

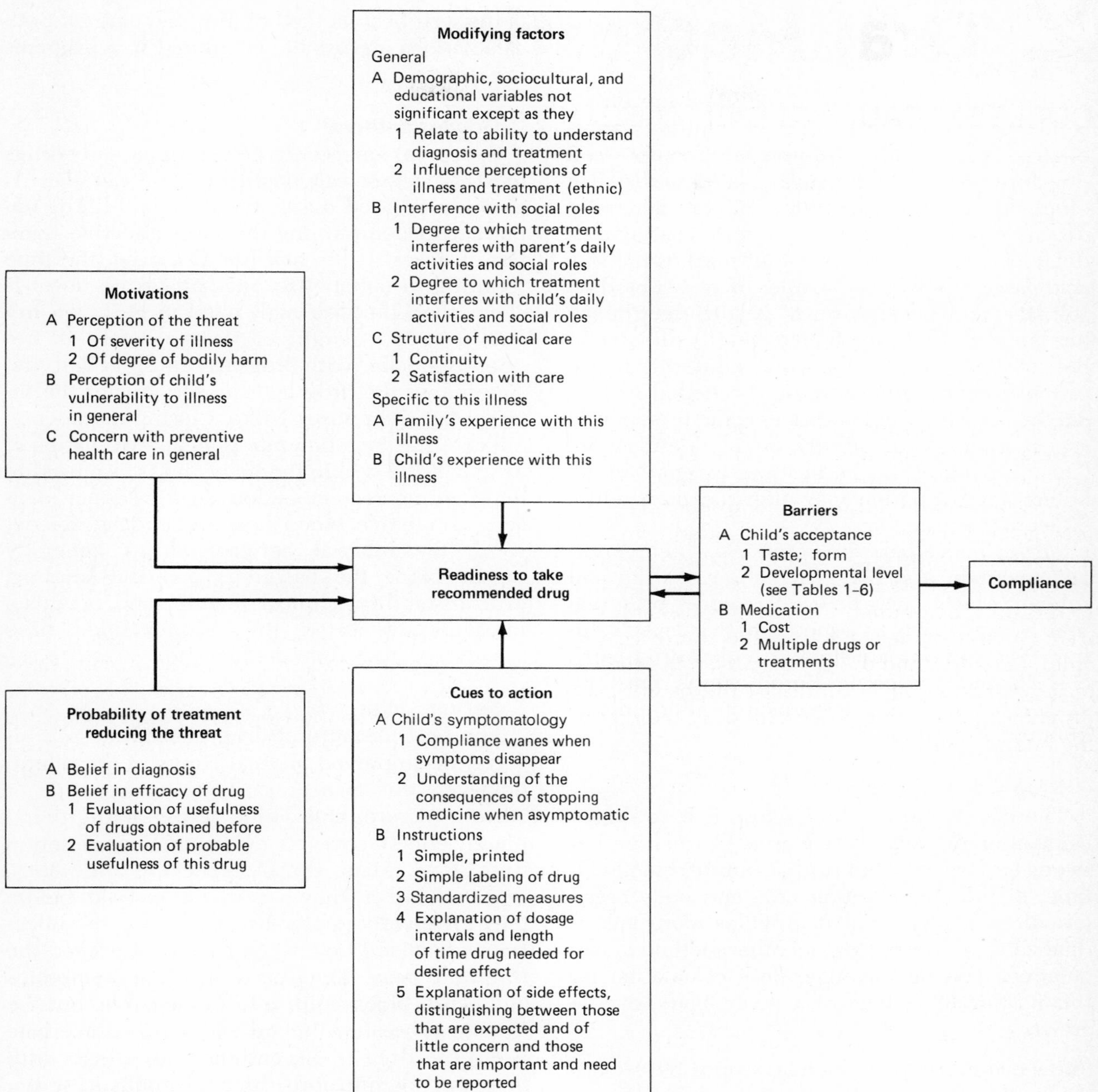

Figure A2-2 Schematic diagram of factors which influence parental compliance with drug therapy. Modified from Becker, M. H., Health Belief Model in Predicting mothers' compliance with pediatric medical regimes. *The Journal of Pediatrics*, **81**(4):843–854 (1972).

THE DRUG

Drug Form

Oral medication forms for children are either solid (tablets and capsules) or liquid (syrups, elixirs, suspensions). Tablets are compressed powders which may be sugar-coated to disguise offensive or lingering taste. Tablets generally dissolve in the stomach but enteric coating will delay dissolving until the tablet reaches the less acid large intestine. Capsules may be hard or soft; the ratio of glycerin to gelatin determines hardness of the casing; both generally dissolve in the stomach. Besides the drug, solid-form medications may contain ingredients needed in production or which enhance a specific therapeutic aspect, increase palatability, or aid identification, Changing solid-form medications by emulsifying before administration may alter the therapeutic effect of the drug.

Syrups and *elixirs* are solutions which generally maintain a stable distribution of drug and solvent. Alcohol may be used as a drug preservative. Syrup USP is an aqueous 85% sucrose solution. *Suspensions* are finely divided drug particles in an appropriate liquid which must be shaken before each use to ensure uniform distribution of drug in the liquid.

Drug Calculations

The most accurate child's dose is based upon calculation of body surface area. Correlation between surface area and cardiac output, blood volume, glomerular filtration rate, and body organ growth and development provides more individualization of dose than any other method of calculation. The best average dose calculation for infants through adults of a given body surface area is

$$\text{Surface area in square meters} \times \text{dose per square meter} = \text{dose}$$

This calculation is not reliable in the neonatal period. The West nomogram may be used to convert height and weight data to square meters (Fig. A2-3).

When does per square meter (dose/m^2) is not available or when there is a wide margin of drug safety, dose in milligrams per kilogram (mg/kg) is the next best method of drug calculation. Both calculations are usually computed in milligrams per day.

Dosage Interval

Except for emergency and one-time-only drugs most drugs are calculated on dose *per day.* If given in divided doses, the drug half-life is important in determining the most effective number of doses. If the half-life of a drug (the time required to metabolize one-half of the dose) is short, then the dose will need to be given frequently. The margin of dosage safety is frequently smaller with drugs having short half-life. The longer the drug half-life the greater the interval between doses without losing therapeutic effect. Drug excretion rate is an approximation of drug half-life within the body and is also used in determining recommended dose freqency. Unless cumulative blood levels of a drug are desired, the interval between doses generally equals twice the half-life. Chemical binding, drug instability, clinical picture, and organism idiosyncrasies cause the recommended dose schedule to vary from the half-life.

Serum Level

The best measure of drug effectiveness is always the improved clinical status of the client; however, this is necessarily a retrospective or current picture. One guide in predicting therapeutic effectiveness is determination of serum drug level. Many drugs, especially antibiotics, must exceed a known serum threshold before they effectively penetrate and destroy the infectious organism. Levels which do not exceed the threshold may temporarily alleviate symptoms and cause blood culture to be negative, but the disease process will continue or will exacerbate when the drug is discontinued. In clients with increased or impaired drug metabolism, serum levels may be especially useful in individualizing the dose to avoid drug toxicity.

Proprietary or Generic Prescriptions

Before ordering a drug it may be helpful to review the advantages of both generic and proprietary prescribing (Table A2-11).

Table A2-12 presents oral drugs of frequent

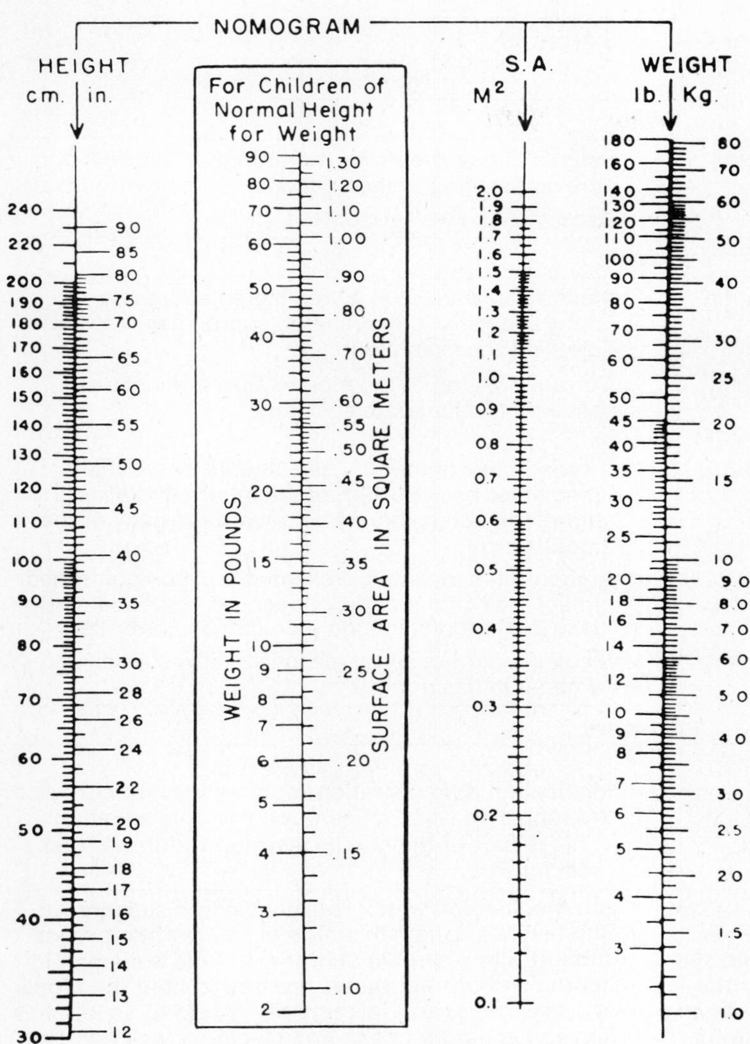

Figure A2-3 West nomogram for estimation of surface area. The surface area is indicated at the point where a straight line connecting the height and weight levels intersects the surface area (S.A.) column. For children of normal height for weight, the body surface area may be estimated from the weight alone by referring to the enclosed area at the left center of the figure. *(Modified from data of E. Boyd by C. D. West. Reproduced with permission of V. C. Vaughan and R. J. McKay (eds.), Nelson textbook of pediatrics (10th ed.), Philadelphia: Saunders, 1975, p. 1713.)*

use in children. Coverage includes drug, drug forms appropriate for pediatrics, a partial list of brand names which have suitable pediatric forms, drug uses, pediatric dosage, physiological concerns, laboratory effects, and comments relevant to administration and effectiveness.

Table A2-1 Pediatric Medication Guidelines—1 to 3 Months

Developmental Tasks and Behaviors	Nursing Implications
	Motor
Reaches randomly toward mouth; shows strong palmar grasp reflex.	Infant's hands should be monitored or controlled to prevent spilling of medications.
Head drops or exhibits bobbing control.	Head must be well supported.
	Feeding
Sucks reflexively in response to tactile stimulation.	Medication should be administered using this natural behavior: medication should be given via nipple. (See example.)
Corners of the mouth may not seal effectively and the tongue may be reflexively forced against the palate.	Correct position of the nipple, if used, must be assured for adequate sucking.
Tongue movement may project food out of mouth.	A syringe or dropper, if used, should be placed in the center back portion of the mouth. If placed along the gums, it must be toward the back of the mouth.
Sucking strength increases (3 mo).	Amount of medication presented must be controlled. Infant may choke or drool because he or she can take in more medication than can be controlled.
Stops taking fluids when full; progresses to fading of sucking reflex (3 mo).	Medication more easily given in small volumes and when infant is hungry.
	Interactive
Basic trust versus mistrust stage Infant becomes socially responsible.	Medication administration requires feeding behavior which establishes an easy, confortable situation. This is part of the child's learning to form a trust relationship.

EXAMPLE: Jonathan, 2 months, has received 125 mg of ampicillin intravenously every 4 hours for 2 weeks and by mouth every 4 hours for 2 days. Irritable and febrile on admission, his status improves after the medication starts. He becomes alert and afebrile and orders for discharge are written. He is to continue the ampicillin for 5 more days and return to the clinic in 7 days.

Jonathan's mother is very nervous about "getting him to take medicine" at home. She explains that she herself "throws up" every time she tries to drink medicine.

The nurse helps the mother prepare to give her son medication, which is available in a suspension. She teaches Jonathan's mother to draw the proper amount into a syringe and how to hold Jonathan in her lap so both her hands are free to hold the nipple and syringe. Then, touching the nipple to Jonathan's lips so his mouth opens and placing it well back in his mouth in a natural feeding position, the nurse drips the medicine into the nipple and follows it with some water to assure his getting full amount. For Jonathan this is like all feedings. Demonstrating this technique can help relieve the mother's fears and increase the likelihood of Jonathan's continued recovery as well.

Table A2-2 Pediatric Medication Guidelines—3 to 12 Months

Developmental Tasks and Behaviors	Nursing Implications
Motor	
Advances from sitting well with support (3–4 mo) to crawling (10 mo).	Safety precautions regarding where medications are placed and kept become extremely important.
Begins to develop fine motor hand control.	
Advances from lying as placed (3 mo) to standing with support (12 mo).	Child who does not want to cooperate has ability to resist with whole body.
Feeding	
Starting at 12-month-old level:	
Smacks and pouts lips in act of shifting food in mouth and in swallowing. Lower lip active in eating.	Child may spit out food and medicine not wanted.
Tongue may protrude during swallowing.	Eating is inefficient, so medications may need to be retrieved and refed. A small medicine cup may be more effective than a spoon.
Learns to drink from cup. Generally has poor approximation of corners of the mouth when drinking.	
Learns to finger-feed self.	Feeding patterns and routines at home need to be considered.
Feeding behaviors become individualized.	
Interactive	
Basic trust versus mistrust and oral sensory stages	
Communication skills develop from random social responses (3 mo) to making simple requests by gesturing (12 mo).	One must be alert for child's indicating his or her own needs (12 mo).
Is sensitive and responsive to tactile stimulation. Begins developing responsiveness to other stimuli.	Physical comforting will be most effective with child. Verbal comforting secondary.
Recognizes immediate family and, very important, may exhibit intense separation anxiety.	Exhibits early memory. May recall negative experiences, precipitating negative response in another similar situation.

EXAMPLE: Herman, age 8 months, has had recurrent otitis media, and his mother has given him medications from a syringe since he was 2 months. Currently admitted with fever, dehydration, and otitis media, he has received ampicillin intravenously. Herman's condition improves and oral fluids and medications are initiated. Knowing he drinks from a cup, the nurse pours his ampicillin suspension (200 mg) into a medicine cup. In his room she holds Herman, talks with him in a relaxed manner, then puts the cup to his mouth.

After a brief pause, Herman begins crying and reaching for his bottle. Herman's mother arrives to visit and explains that at home she uses a syringe and he does not seem to mind taking medicine. Leaving Herman with his mother, the nurse gets a syringe for the remainder of the dose, and Herman's mother then gives him a bottle of juice to drink. Familiar activities are very important to Herman. Six hours later the same approach works for the nurse. She describes Herman's familiar routine in the Kardex before going off duty.

Source: Copyright September-October 1976, The American Journal of Nursing Company. Used with permission from *MCN, The American Journal of Maternal Child Nursing,* **1**(5), (1976).

Table A2-3 Pediatric Medication Guidelines—12 to 18 Months

Developmental Tasks and Behaviors	Nursing Implications
Motor	
Advances from standing with support to independent walking.	Have the child choose a position for taking medication or hold the child to provide control and comfort. Forcing the child to take medicine when he or she is lying down takes away the child's sense of independence and will frequently result in very resistive behavior.
Feeding	
Begins independent self-feeding, but is still messy.	Home feeding habits should be considered.
Develops voluntary tongue and lip control. Spits deliberately.	Spits out disagreeable tastes effectively. Disguise crushed tablets and contents of capsules in a *small* amount of familiar solid. Be prepared to refeed.
Interactive	
Autonomy versus shame and doubt Indicates needs and wants by pointing.	
Speaks 4 to 6 words. Uses individual jargon. Responds to familiar commands.	Find out what words child uses for drinking, swallowing, and how oral medicines have been given at home.
Responds to and participates in the routines of daily living.	Let child explore an empty medication cup. He or she will likely be more cooperative if familiar items are used. When possible, involve the parents. They are familiar and trusted persons, which is an important factor during an unfamiliar experience. Tell parents and staff the approach used for medication. Report its effectiveness.
Exhibits notable independence, resistance, self-assertiveness, and ambivalence. Begins to have temper tantrums.	Allow the child as much freedom as possible. Allow the child to assert self by choosing his or her own drink to wash down the medicine. Use games to gain cooperation. Tell the child what you expect and then follow through. A consistent, firm approach is essential.

EXAMPLE: Eighteen-month-old Simon has been in the hospital 4 days with severe gastroenteritis. He has had nothing orally and has received intravenous (IV) fluids for volume replacement and ampicillin therapy. This morning his IV was discontinued and oral ampicillin started. At shift report the day nurse states he does not take his oral medication well. She reports that she gave the suspension via syringe.

Recognizing that Simon has had experience with a variety of syringes in the last few days, the evening nurse elects to try a different approach. From talking with Simon's mother she knows Simon is used to an assisted self-feeding routine—he has his own fork and spoon and his mother supplements his efforts with another spoon. Also, he enjoys apple juice and can manage a cup fairly well by himself.

Using this "at home" activity and Simon's need to feel familiar with an object to decrease his fear, the nurse allows him to play with a medication cup, drink juice from it, and watch his mother handle and use it. Later she measures the ampicillin into one now-familiar cup and apple juice into another. She allows Simon to hold the juice cup. Simon's sip of ampicillin, given by the nurse, is alternated with a self-fed sip of apple juice. He took the ampicillin without resistance. At night shift report the nurse notes this approach was effective. She encountered no resistive behavior.

Source: Copyright September-October 1976, The American Journal of Nursing Company. Used with permission from *MCN, The American Journal of Maternal Child Nursing,* **1**(5), (1976).

Table A2-4 Pediatric Medication Guidelines—18 to 30 Months

Developmental Tasks and Behaviors	Nursing Implications
Motor	
Walks, climbs into chair (18 mo). Advances to running without falling (24 mo).	Child is able to run away and kick.
Advances to obtaining and throwing small objects.	Child may throw materials placed within reach. Never leave medications sitting on the bedside stand.
Feeding	
Generally feeds self. Advances to proficiency with minimal spilling.	Allow child opportunity to drink liquids from a medicine cup by him or herself.
Second molars erupt (20–30 mo). Exhibits increased rotary chewing; manages solid food particles.	Permits greater flexibility in choosing form of medication.
Controls mouth and jaw proficiently.	Child is effective in spitting out unwanted medications and in clamping mouth tightly closed in resistance.
Interactive	
Autonomy versus shame and doubt	
Has some sense of time, but not words for time (18 mo). Then responds to "just a minute" (21 mo). Advances to understanding, "Play after you drink this." (24 mo).	Tell the child getting medicine that any bad taste will only last "a minute." Learn child's level of time awareness from nursing history.
Carries out 2 to 3 directions given one at a time.	Give simplified directions: "Open your mouth, drink, and then swallow."
Shows ability to respond to and participate in routines of daily living.	Include child in establishing medicine-taking routine.
Helps put things away; carries breakable objects.	
Exhibits independence, resistance, self-assertiveness, and ambivalence.	Use a firm, consistent approach. Resistive behaviors are at a peak.
Throws temper tantrums frequently.	
Shows pride in accomplished skills. Does not know right from wrong.	Give immediate, positive tactile and verbal response to cooperative taking of medicine. Ignore resistive behavior.
Shows conflict between holding on and letting go.	Give choices when possible: "Do you want to sit in the chair or on my lap to take your medicine?"

EXAMPLE: Barbara, 28 months, has bronchitis and was admitted to the hospital 3 days ago. She has been receiving ampicillin 250 mg by mouth every 6 hours. Usually a delightful, playful child, she has been labeled a "brat" when it comes time to take her medicine. Nurses have emptied capsules, placed the contents in chocolate syrup, and spoon-fed her with the result of most of the mixture ending up on the nurse. Suspension form has also been tried ineffectively.

Referring to the nursing history for possible help with this child, the nurse discovers that Barbara's favorite food is now candy. Since she has demonstrated proficiency in chewing solid food and candy, the nurse suspects she might take her ampicillin as a chewable tablet. The nurse also feels that involving Barbara in the ritual of medication time might be helpful. At the next medicine time the nurse allows Barbara to pick out two 125 mg tablets herself from a medication cup. Barbara then chews and swallows them. Next she throws the now empty cup into the wastebasket. The nurse gives Barbara a chaser of choice and praises her for her help. Barbara is now a "successful helper" in taking medications.

Source: Copyright September-October 1976, The American Journal of Nursing Company. Used with permission from *MCN, The American Journal of Maternal Child Nursing,* **1**(5), (1976).

Table A2-5 Pediatric Medication Guidelines—2½ to 3½ Years

Developmental Tasks and Behaviors	Nursing Implications
Motor	
Continues to develop proficiency. Basic skills have all been initiated.	Child may be quite adept in resistive behavior.
Feeding	
Becoming more proficient in skills. Eating likes and dislikes are definite but changeable.	Medication tastes can be disguised with variable effectiveness.
May be influenced by others' reactions in responding to new food experiences.	A calm, positive approach is needed to gain a cooperative response from the child; quick tense approach is likely to produce similar behavior in the child.
Interactive	
Initiative versus guilt	
Gives full name.	Begin asking for verbal identification of client before giving medications.
Is ritualistic.	Communicate administration methods.
Has little understanding of past, present, or future.	Use concrete and immediate rewards.
Shows concrete thinking, egocentricity.	Tolerates frustration poorly. Child's initial response to reason appears positive, but without consistent effect.
	Prolonged bargaining is frustrating and frightening to the child because no one is in control of the situation.
Exhibits early aggressiveness; coercive, manipulative behavior.	Give a choice when possible. Do not give a choice if the child does not have one.
Has many fantasies.	Begin giving simple, honest explanations of why the medication is given (not because the child was bad).
May be frightened by own "power."	Child's sense of security is dependent upon the nurses' consistent expectations of behavior.

EXAMPLE: Roger, 3 years old, has otitis media and ampicillin 200 mg is ordered by mouth every 6 hours. He is to get the first dose in the clinic and then treatment is to be continued at home. His mother seems reluctant to agree that he really needs the medication. Finally she says she just cannot face what she knows will be trouble because he is at "that stage" when he won't do anything he is told.

The nurse pours the ampicillin into a cup. Roger is seated on his mother's lap. The nurse says, "Roger, your ears have been hurting. This medicine will help stop the hurting. I have the medicine in a little cup for you to drink. It tastes funny, but I don't think it tastes too bad. You can hold the cup and do it yourself; your mother and I will watch." She hands Roger the cup and watches while he follows through. "Good, it's done in one big swallow. Would you like some apple juice or some water now?" the nurse asks.

When they come back in 10 days, Roger's mother reports changing from juice to gum to ice pops to lemon drops after the medication, but that the medication all went down.

Source: Copyright September-October 1976, The American Journal of Nursing Company. Used with permission from *MCN, The American Journal of Maternal Child Nursing,* **1**(5), (1976).

Table A2-6 Pediatric Medication Guidelines—3½ to 6 Years

Developmental Tasks and Behaviors	Nursing Implications
Motor	
Develops proficiency of coordination. Can identify the parts of a complete movement or task.	Child can attempt and master pill taking.
Feeding	
Exhibits olfactory, gustatory, and kinesthetic refinement.	Disguising tastes is generally less effective than it is at younger ages. Child can distinguish medical tastes and smells.
Begins to lose temporary teeth (5 yr).	Loose teeth may need to be considered with selecting form of medication.
Interactive	
Initiative versus guilt	
Makes decisions.	Child should be active in making decisions which affect him or her.
Sense of time allows enjoyment of delayed gratification. Is able to tolerate frustration. Seeks companionship. Shows pride in accomplishments.	Rewards which are not immediately received and social interaction can be used as effective motivators. Child is able to understand the purpose of medications in simple terms.
Has ability to follow directions and remember several instructions for a period of minutes to hours.	Teaching can have long-term benefits.
Exhibits developing conscience. Needs limits set to help control frightening sense of "power."	Prolonged reasoning or arguing may frighten the child; a simple command by a trusted adult may be more effective.
Exhibits genital interest, general mutilation fears.	Explain the relationship between cause, illness, and treatment. Use simple terms.
Illness often seen as punishment.	Give control when possible—child needs to make choices.
Shows changeable response to parents.	Child may be more cooperative in medicine taking for the nurse than for the parent(s).

EXAMPLE: Orlando, a 4-year-old with repeated pneumonia secondary to cystic fibrosis, has been treated repeatedly with ampicillin. The nurse remembers that previously the suspension form was used with no resistance. But with this admission Orlando has been refusing the familiar suspension.

After watching him swallow whole jelly beans during an afternoon playtime, the evening nurse tries giving him ampicillin capsules at bedtime. She explains the pills are medicine like the pink liquid but that the shells they have stop the medicine from tasting so bad. She points out that they are the same size as the jelly beans he took while playing. Other things she tells him include how he can place the capsules far back in his mouth and swallow water to help "wash" the pills down to his stomach. By bedtime the next day, medication refusal is no longer a nursing problem.

Source: Copyright September-October 1976, The American Journal of Nursing Company. Used with permission from *MCN, The American Journal of Maternal Child Nursing*, **1**(5), (1976).

Table A2-7 Absorption of Oral Drugs during Childhood

Altered Physiology	Effect of Disease	Drug Interactions
Gastric acidity is increased during the neonatal period. The gastric pH ranges from 1–2.5 during the neonatal period. A drug with a low pK_a (the pH at which 50% of the drug is ionized) will exhibit enhanced absorption (i.e., salicylate). Gastric emptying is prolonged. The effect can be either to increase the amount of drug absorbed or to decrease the rate at which absorption occurs. Drugs with a low pK_a that are better absorbed from the acid environment of the stomach will have increased absorption. Peak concentration of some drugs may be less in neonates since it takes longer to get to the highly absorptive surface of the small intestine. However, overall absorption may be similar to or greater than that of older children and adults because absorption proceeds over a longer period of time. Ampicillin and nafcillin are better absorbed in neonates and infants. Penicillin, tetracycline, cephalosporin, and chloramphenicol are rapidly and effectively absorbed in young infants due to an increased rate of absorption and a decreased rate of renal elimination and hepatic degradation. The premature infant is able to absorb both procaine penicillin and phenoxypenicillin better than full-term neonates. Digoxin is well absorbed even in the presence of congestive heart failure and diarrhea. The development of some gastric enzyme systems is incomplete.	Gastrointestinal disease may affect the absorption of oral drugs. The effects of altering gastrointestinal emptying or transit time are unpredictable and may affect the rate of absorption but not necessarily the amount absorbed. Absorption of weakly acidic drugs (i.e., acetaminophen) is delayed in conditions of prolonged gastric emptying (i.e., low gastric pH, peptic ulcers, pain and nausea, pyloric stenosis). Effective plasma concentration of chlorpromazine is decreased when transit time is prolonged because of greater time available for its enzymatic metabolism by the gut wall. A decrease in motility may lead to enhanced absorption of poorly soluble drugs. Very rapid transit time (i.e., diarrhea) may profoundly affect absorption of some drugs. Malabsorption syndromes can affect the absorption of oral drugs; the effect is unpredictable and depends on the physiochemical properties of the drug, the clinical state of the child, and the treatment regimen. Steatorrhea impairs the absorption of fat-soluble preparations of vitamins A and D. In Crohn's disease or in children with strictures of the gastrointestinal tract sustained-release tablets should be used with caution. Any disease which reduces the surface area of the gastrointestinal tract may affect the absorption of oral drugs.	Alteration in gastric pH can affect absorption. Drugs may be considered weak electrolytes; the nonionized, more lipid-soluble forms are more readily absorbed. Acidic drugs (i.e., aspirin, phenobarbital, penicillin, sulfonamide) are more readily absorbed from the stomach, where they exist in a nonionized form. Substances which increase the gastric pH (i.e., antacids) decrease the absorption of acidic drugs since a larger fraction then exists in the ionized, more lipid-soluble form. Sodium bicarbonate decreases the absorption of tetracycline by raising gastric pH. Buffered aspirin increases the rate of absorption of indomethacin. Lowering the gastric pH increases the absorption of acidic drugs. Drugs such as reserpine which stimulate gastric secretions enhance the absorption of acidic drugs. The bulk of basic drugs are absorbed from the small intestine. Weakly basic drugs form water-soluble salts with the acid environment of the stomach. After moving to the more alkaline small intestine, they are converted to nonionized, absorbable forms. Changes in the gastric pH retard the solubility of weak basic drugs. However, gastric emptying time would be faster because of the alkaline shift. Any effect of slower dissolution would be compensated for by the large absorptive surface of the small intestine. Weakly basic drugs are not as affected by changes in gastric pH as are weakly acidic drugs.

Table A2-7 Absorption of Oral Drugs during Childhood *(continued)*

Altered Physiology	Effect of Disease	Drug Interactions
Drugs that require enzymatic hydrolysis may not be adequately absorbed following oral administration.	Any interference with gastrointestinal blood (i.e., cardiac disease) may affect absorption of oral drugs. Little is known about the effect of renal disease on absorption of oral drugs.	The release characteristics of enteric-coated tablets are altered by changes in gastric pH. Enteric-coated tablets are designed so that their contents will remain intact until they reach the alkaline small intestine. This is done to prevent irritation of the gastric mucosa or inactivation in the stomach. Concurrent administration of drugs which increase gastric pH may cause premature release of the drug in the stomach. Sustained-release medications are coated with a pH-sensitive substance which causes a prolonged, gradual release of the drug. Alteration of gastric pH can cause premature wearing away of the sensitive coating, yielding release of all the drug at one time and overdosing. Drugs which affect gastrointestinal motility can influence either the rate of absorption or the amount absorbed of other drugs taken concurrently. Drugs which increase motility (i.e., the stimulant cathartics) may decrease the time other drugs are in contact with the absorptive surface of the gastrointestinal tract. This is especially detrimental in the case of drugs that require prolonged gut contact for absorption (i.e., griseofulvin) or in the case of drugs that are absorbed at specific sites in the intestine (i.e., levodopa, riboflavin). Drugs with anticholinergic effects, the opiates and aluminum hydroxide gel, diminish motility. Propantheline slows the absorption of acetaminophen but not the total amount absorbed.

Table A2-7 Absorption of Oral Drugs during Childhood *(continued)*

Altered Physiology	Effect of Disease	Drug Interactions
		By decreasing motility, propantheline increases the contact time of digoxin with the intestine wall, causing more drug to be absorbed. Bioavailability of some poorly absorbed drugs (i.e., Dicumarol) is enhanced by concurrent administration of anticholinergic drugs
		Drug complexation reactions, the chemical or physical binding or adsorption of one drug onto the surface of another, can result in sporadic or erratic absorption of one or both drugs. The ions Ca^{2+}, Mg^{2+}, and Al^{3+} present in most antacids, bind or chelate many antibiotics (especially tetracyclines) forming insoluble complexes. Doxycycline and minocycline are not chelated by Ca^{2+}. Iron and tetracycline form an insoluble complex. Aluminum hydroxide gel can adsorb other drugs (i.e., chlorpromazine, isoniazid). Magnesium trisilicate and Ca^{2+} may decrease the absorption of iron. Antidiarrheal agents which are used to adsorb toxic substances causing diarrhea may also adsorb drugs given concurrently. The claylike molecules of compounds containing kaolin-pectin may physically adsorb other drugs. The ion-exchange resins cholestyramine and colestipol bind a number of drugs including chlorothiazide, hydrochlorothiazide, phenobarbital, digitoxin, aspirin, warfarin, thyroid, and tetracycline. Complexation reactions may form soluble complexes which are more readily absorbed (i.e., caffeine and ergotamine; Dicumarol and magnesium hydroxide).

Table A2-7 Absorption of Oral Drugs during Childhood *(continued)*

Altered Physiology	Effect of Disease	Drug Interactions
		Drug-food interactions can affect the rate and amount of drug absorbed. Fatty foods and meals high in fat and low in fiber content retard gastric emptying. Drugs absorbed from the small intestine can exhibit delayed absorption under these circumstances. Food may inactivate, bind, or adsorb drugs given concurrently. Milk and dairy products interfere with the absorption of certain forms of tetracycline. Absorption of penicillin, ampicillin, lincomycin, and erythromycin (except Ilosone) is reduced by the presence of food. The antidotal effect of activated charcoal is significantly reduced when mixed with dairy products. Acid liquids (i.e., cranberry, lemon, pineapple, ginger ale) can inactivate unstable drugs.
		Long-term therapy with some drugs(*p*-aminosalicylic acid, neomycin) may cause a malabsorption syndrome, impairing absorption of other drugs.
		Suppression of gut bacterial flora by antibiotics may interfere with other drugs that are metabolized by the gut bacterial flora.

Table A2-8 Distribution of Oral Drugs During Childhood

Altered Physiology	Effect of Disease	Drug Interactions
The size of the body water compartments is relatively and absolutely different during childhood. Body composition is not constant and changes rapidly. These changes are most rapid during early life. Extracellular fluid volume decreases from 50% in prematures, to 35% in infants 4 to 6 months of age, to 20–25% in children 1 year of age and older. Total body water is also much greater and varies from 85% of body weight in small prematures, to 70% in full-term neonates, to 55% in adults. Water-soluble drugs circulate freely in the extracellular fluid. Drug dose of water-soluble drugs will decrease during childhood in relation to weight. Fat content, in contrast, is decreased in the premature compared with the normal full-term infant. Organs or tissues that accumulate high concentration of lipophilic drugs may have a decreased affinity for such compounds in prematures. Protein binding of drugs to plasma proteins is decreased in neonates and infants leading to an increase in the fraction of unbound, active drug in the plasma. There is an absolute lower concentration of plasma proteins, particularly albumin. Adult levels are reached during the first year. Plasma albumin is even lower and takes longer to achieve mature levels in the premature. There is a quantitative difference in the binding capacity of plasma proteins. Endogenous substances present during the first few days of life that have crossed the placenta	In disease states where the extracellular fluid volume falls, the usual dose of a water-soluble drug will attain a higher concentration. Conversely, the plasma concentration of a water-soluble drug is reduced in disease states where the extracellular fluid is increased. Any disease which affects plasma proteins can interfere with drug distribution. In the presence of hyperbilirubinemia protein binding is unpredictable. Bilirubin may compete for and attain binding sites, making the blood level of active, unbound drug higher than would be expected. If a drug is more strongly bound to protein than bilirubin (i.e., oxacillin, phenytoin, aspirin, sulfa, synthetic vitamin K) bilirubin may be displaced from binding sites. This would increase the amount of unbound bilirubin and could lead to kernicterus. Any disease characterized by hypoalbuminemia can decrease protein binding of drugs. Displacement of protein binding sites may occur with placental transfer of drugs. By affecting regional tissue perfusion, cardiac output, and the permeability of cell membranes, cardiovascular disease may affect distribution of drugs. Time of onset, intensity, and duration of action can be affected. In the presence of cardiac failure the volume of distribution of lidocaine, procainamide, and quinidine is decreased leading to an increased concentration of the drug in the plasma and a decreased rate of elimination if hepatic or renal blood flow is compromised.	The most important drug interactions which influence drug distribution are those in which drugs are displaced from plasma protein binding sites. Displacement can cause potentiation of one drug due to a temporary increase in the concentration of active, unbound drug. This potentiation is usually temporary since more unbound drug is available for metabolism or excretion. A steady state is gradually reached. However, serious effects may occur (as with anticoagulants) before a steady state is reached. The significance of a change in protein binding is greater with drugs that are highly protein bound. Highly bound acidic drugs that can compete with each other include salicylate, phenylbutazone, oxyphenbutazone, indomethacin, probenecid, coumarin anticoagulants, diazoxide, ethacrynic acid, furosemide, thiazide diuretics, penicillin, many sulfonamides, nalidixic acid, methotrexate, and radiographic contrast media. Basic drugs may also be highly protein bound, but significant displacement interactions have not been reported.

Table A2-8 Distribution of Oral Drugs During Childhood *(continued)*

Altered Physiology	Effect of Disease	Drug Interactions
(i.e., maternal hormones) may occupy binding sites, thus decreasing the binding capacity of drugs given during this time.	Since the extent to which ionization takes place depends on the pK_a of the drug and the pH of the solution in which it is dissolved, small changes in acid-base balance may affect distribution of drugs. Acidosis may increase the uptake of acidic drugs and decrease the uptake of basic drugs.	
The central nervous system and the blood-brain barrier is not fully developed. Access of drugs to the nervous system is more easily obtained. Lipid-soluble drugs (i.e., sedatives, analgesics, tetracycline) and other substances (unconjugated bilirubin) readily enter the central nervous system and brain. Morphine and barbiturate reach higher concentrations in infants. Infants are also more sensitive to the respiratory depressant effects of morphine.	In renal failure, the percent of protein binding of some acidic drugs is less.	
Drug receptor site sensitivity is different; some developing organs are exceptionally sensitive to certain drugs. The neonatal retina is very sensitive to high oxygen tension. Exposure to high concentrations can cause retrolental fibroplasia. Immature erythrocytes are sensitive to nitrates in water and to oxidizing drugs with the development of methemoglobinemia after limited exposure. Higher concentrations of digoxin are required in the myocardium of infants. Infants demonstrate increased responsiveness to vagal stimulation, and blockade of reflex bradycardia in neonatal anesthesia requires larger doses of atropine than would be required to suppress salivation. Neonates also tolerate relatively higher doses of adrenalin.		

Table A2-9 Metabolism of Oral Drugs During Childhood

Altered Physiology	Effect of Disease	Drug Interactions
The hepatic metabolism of drugs is generally impaired in neonates, leading to higher than expected blood levels. There is marked variation among individual infants, and liver function changes very rapidly after birth. For drugs metabolized extensively by the liver, impairment of liver metabolism is significant usually during the first few weeks of life for full-term neonates and for longer periods in prematures. Salicylate, amobarbital, phenobarbital, lidocaine, and diazepam all demonstrate deficient metabolism. Not all metabolic processes are impaired; the neonate is able to adequately metabolize many drugs (i.e., acetaminophen). Diminished hepatic metabolism is thought to be the basis for many of the adverse effects noted in infants born to mothers who received drugs during pregnancy. Continuous in utero exposure to certain drugs (i.e., phenytoin, carbamazepine, salicylate) may induce the activity of the hepatic enzyme system; the neonate may then be able to metabolize transplacentally acquired drugs or similar drugs at or close to adult rates.	The effects of liver disease on drug pharmacokinetics are complex; alteration in the rate of metabolism depends on the severity of liver disease and on whether the drug is metabolized mainly by the liver. The liver has a great reserve capacity and only in severe disease are problems likely to occur. The metabolism of phenytoin and barbiturate is abnormally slow following acute liver necrosis of acetaminophen overdose. Central nervous system depressants are most hazardous in clients with chronic liver disease. Clients in hepatic coma or hepatic precoma are extremely sensitive to morphine, paraldehyde, barbiturate, and ergot. Liver disease may also affect the rate of metabolism of lidocaine, diazepam, meperidine, chloramphenicol, and theophylline. Binding of protein-bound drugs is decreased in liver disease especially when either hypoalbuminemia or hyperbilirubinemia is present. Alcohol may have profound effects on drug metabolism. Other factors are often present in the client with liver disease that affect drug handling. These factors include chronic alcohol consumption, concurrent therapy with other drugs, altered body water compartments, hypoalbuminemia, hyperbilirubinemia, and other diseases (i.e., renal). By altering hepatic blood flow cardiovascular disease may have an effect on drug metabolism. In general the rate of metabolism is not impaired in renal disease.	One drug, called an *inducing drug,* may cause stimulation of not only its own metabolism but also stimulate the metabolism of other drugs or compounds which are substrates for liver enzymes. Known inducing drugs include barbiturates, glutethimide, meprobromate, chlorpromazine, tricyclic antidepressants, phenytoin, primidone, carbamazepine, ethchlorvynol, ethanol, antipyrine, phenylbutazone, rifampin, and griseofulvin. One of the most important induction interactions is the stimulation of the metabolism of oral anticoagulants by barbiturates and other hypnotics. More rapid metabolism and excretion of the anticoagulant occurs. Many drug metabolites produced by induction interactions have little or no pharmacologic activity. In these cases, drug effects are reduced by inducing drugs. This may explain the development of drug tolerance. The metabolites produced may be pharmacologically active and toxicity may occur. Previous exposure to inducing agents would then enhance the development of toxicity. Hepatic necrosis following acetaminophen overdose is more pronounced when inducing drugs have been used previously. Hemolysis produced by phenacetin is enhanced by prior consumption of phenobarbital. Certain drugs can inhibit the metabolism of others and result in exaggerated and prolonged response with an increaed risk of toxicity. 6-Mercaptopurine is metabolized by xanthine oxidase. Toxicity of this drug is increased if given concurrently with allopurinol, a xanthine oxidase inhibitor.

Table A2-9 Metabolism of Oral Drugs During Childhood *(continued)*

Altered Physiology	Effect of Disease	Drug Interactions
	Metabolism of some drugs (i.e., phenacetin) is normal or accelerated (i.e., phenytoin) in uremia. Reduced metabolism may occur with isoniazid, hydrocortisone, sulfisoxazole, and hydralazine.	Phenytoin toxicity may be caused by concurrent administration of isoniazid and infrequently by Dicumarol, chloramphenicol, phenylbutazone, chlorpromazine, prochlorperazine, diazepam, chlordiazepoxide, and propoxyphene. Allopurinol and chloramphenicol can inhibit the metabolism of Dicumarol.
		Changes in hepatic blood flow may affect the metabolism of drugs. By decreasing cardiac output, propranolol not only decreases hepatic blood flow and its own clearance but also decreases the clearance of other drugs which are metabolized extensively by the liver. Vasoactive drugs (i.e., glucagon, isoproterenol, phenobarbital) increase hepatic blood flow and can increase the rate of elimination of other drugs.

Table A2-10 Elimination of Oral Drugs during Childhood

Altered Physiology	Effect of Disease	Drug Interactions
The kidneys are immature at birth and demonstrate successive maturation with age. The rate of glomerular filtration and tubular secretion changes rapidly following birth. At birth, the rate of glomerular filtration and tubular secretion is 30–40% that of an adult. By day 5, the rate has increased to 50%. Adult rates are reached by 1 year of age. In adults, tubular mechanisms are important in the excretion of some drugs (i.e., penicillin), and glomerular filtration is	By changing body composition and glomerular filtration rate, any impairment of kidney function may affect the pharmacokinetic properties of a drug. In evaluating the effect of renal disease each drug must be considered separately. Many formulas and nomograms are available for calculating dose and dose intervals in clients with renal disease. However, these are based on serum creatinine, creatinine clearance, and blood urea nitrogen and assume that drug excretion is analogous to creatinine, which is not	Many acidic drugs and drug metabolites share the same active tubular secretion transport system and can compete with each for secretion, causing accumulation and toxicity. Some of the drugs transported by this mechanism that can compete with each other include phenolsulfonphthalein, sulfonamides, acetazolamide, thiazide diuretics, diazoxide, chlorpropamide, indomethacin, salicylate, phenylbutazone, oxyphenbutazone, probenecid, penicillin, Dicumarol, and methotrexate.

Table A2-10 Elimination of Oral Drugs during Childhood *(continued)*

Altered Physiology	Effect of Disease	Drug Interactions
important for other drugs. In the newborn and young infant, glomerular filtration is more important for the elimination of penicillin while tubular secretion is the prime mechanism in older infants and children. Clearance of drugs that are primarily dependent on kidney for excretion is significantly lower in neonates. Most antibiotics are eliminated by the kidney. Digoxin elimination is also governed by changing renal function. Renal clearance is low during the first month but increases with age. The plasma half-life is shorter in infants 1 month to 2 years of age than in neonates and older children. Plasma half-lives and serum concentrations are the basis for determining appropriate dose and dose intervals. These values change during childhood. For antibiotics excreted mainly by the kidney, plasma half-lives are prolonged during the first two weeks of life. The rate of elimination increases rapidly and by 4 weeks, half-lives are similar to that for adults. Serum concentrations of most antibiotics are higher and sustained for considerably longer periods of time during the first few days of life. With increasing age there is a gradual decline. Peak levels continue to be higher throughout the first months of life. Premature infants exhibit an exaggerated response. In view of these rapidly changing half-lives and serum concentrations, dose and dose intervals must be constantly reevaluated and may need to be changed from week to week.	necessarily true. Nomograms should be used only with caution in children. Any disease which alters body composition or changes renal blood flow may affect the excretion of drugs.	Many of these same drugs are capable of displacing each other for protein-binding sites and can cause dual interactions. Competition for active tubular secretion may be used therapeutically. Probenecid inhibits the renal clearance of penicillin. The serum half-life of penicillin is also prolonged by phenylbutazone, sulphinpyrazone, aspirin, indomethacin, and sulphaphenazole. Probenecid will also inhibit the renal clearance of ampicillin, cephalosporin, indomethacin, chlorothiazide, salicylic acid, and acetylate sulfonamides. Alterations in urinary pH will influence the ionization of weak acidic and basic drugs and may affect excretion. Renal clearance of weak basic drugs (pK_a7.5–10) is increased in acid urine. Acidification of urine may be used in the treatment of methadone and amphetamine intoxication. Renal clearance of weak acid drugs (pK_a3.0–7.5) is higher in alkaline urine. Alkalinization of the urine may markedly enhance urinary excretion of salicylic acid and phenobarbital; this interaction is useful in the treatment of overdoses. The solubility of some drugs may depend on urinary pH. Sulfadiazine acetate is more soluble in an alkaline urine.

Table A2-11 Advantages of Generic and Proprietary Prescriptions

Generic	Proprietary
Allows the pharmacist and client to select the least expensive preparation.	A brand which is especially palatable may be more effective than a generic drug equivalent if the child will take it.
If drug combinations require change, it may be more efficient to order each drug separately.	One multidrug medication may be easier to administer than two single-drug medications.
	Chemical, biological, and clinical equivalency may not be available in a generic preparation.

Table A2-12 Pediatric Oral Medications

Drug	Uses	Dosage
	Anticonvulsants	
Phenobarbital Tablets 8, 15, 30, 65, 100 mg Elixir 20 mg/5 mL Also available in combination with other drugs, e.g., asthmatic	Long-acting sedation, relief of anxiety, voluntary muscle relaxation, anesthesia, treatment of spinal cord irritation and convulsive states	Sedation: 180 mg/m^2 per day or 6 mg/kg per day q8h Anticonvulsant: Begin $\frac{1}{2}$ the sedative dose, increase prn
Diphenylhydantoin No suspension available		
Phenytoin Capsules 30, 100 mg Suspension 30 mg/5 mL, 125 mg/5 mL Dilantin	Control of grand mal and psychomotor seizures Tends to stabilize hyperexcitability threshold	Initial: 50 mg/kg per day q12h Maintenance: 250 mg/m^2 per day, or 3–8 mg/kg per day 1 dose Maximum: 300 mg/day
	Antidiarrheals	
Diphenoxylate hydrochloride Tablets 2.5 mg Liquid 2.5 mg/5 mL Lomotil	Diarrhea control	2–5 yr: 2 mg tid 5–8 yr: 2 mg qid 8–12 yr. 2 mg 5 times/day Adult: 5 mg 3–4 times/day

Physiological Considerations*	Laboratory Effects	Comments
	Anticonvulsants	
E: Urine S: Habituating, ataxia, respiratory depression C: Respiratory depression		Sedative effects are additive. Overdose leads to medullary depression.
M: Liver E: Urine S: Nystagmus, ataxia, slurred speech, mental confusion, nausea, vomiting, constipation, morbilliform rash, cytopenias, gingival hyperplasia, hyperglycemia. Abrupt withdrawal possible cause of status epilepticus C: History of hydantoin hypersensitivity, appearance of skin rash, or osteomalacia	Urine: Color pink to red-brown reported	Monitor serum glucose and blood cell count. Therapeutic serum drug level stabilizes in 7–10 days. Half-life is 10–42 (22) h. Gradual withdrawal is necessary. Metabolized more readily in clients weighing < 20 kg. Impairs folic acid and vitamin B_{12}. Unusually high levels are found in liver disease, congenital enzyme deficiency, drug interactions which decrease drug metabolism (coumarin anticoagulants, phenylbutazone, isoniazid, sulfaphenazole, salicylates). Unusually low levels are found in noncompliance to the drug and drug hypermetabolism by bariturates.
	Antidiarrheals	
M: Liver E: Urine S: Atropine response, sedation, nausea, vomiting, headache, pruritis, coma, dizziness, anorexia, euphoria, restlessness, respiratory depression, gum swelling, extremity numbness, paralytic ileus C: Jaundice, hypersensitivity to meperidine or atropine		Do not use in children < 2 yr old, limited margin of safety. Atropine in subtherapeutic levels is added to discourage intentional abuse. (0.025 mg/5 mL). Schedule V controlled substance. Addiction is theoretically possible. May potentiate barbiturates, alcohol, and tranquilizers. Naloxone hydrochloride (Narcan) is the injectable counteractant.

**Key:* A = absorption, M = metabolism, E = excretion, S = side effects, C = contraindications.

Table A2-12 Pediatric Oral Medications *(continued)*

Drug	Uses	Dosage
	Anti-inflammatories	
Adrenal corticosteroids *Prednisone*—tablets only Betapar 4 mg Deltasone 2.5, 5, 10, 50 mg scored Orasone 1, 5, 10, 20 mg USP 5, 10, 20 mg *Prednisolone*—similar to prednisone but slightly greater potency Ataraxoid 2.5, 5 mg Delta-Cortef 5 mg	Anti-inflammatory adjunct in treatment of rheumatic fever, rheumatoid arthritis, systemic lupus erythematosus, nephrosis, ulcerative colitis, idiopathic thrombocytopenia, hemolytic anemia, asthma, pruritis ani, atopic dermatitis	Dose for cortisone acetate: 50–80 mg/m² per day or 1.75–2 mg/kg per day q8h Prednisone dose: $\frac{1}{5}$ of cortisone dose Prednisolone dose: $\frac{1}{5}$ of cortisone dose Taper doses to discontinue to allow adrenal function to return to normal.
Aspirin—see Antipyretics		
	Antimicrobials	
Ampicillin—available as sodium trihydrate and hetacillin Capsules 250, 500 mg Chewable tablets 125 mg Suspension 125, 250, 500 mg/5 mL Drops 100 mg/mL Alpen Amcill Ampicillin Omnipen Penbritin Polycillin Principen SK/Ampicillin Supen Totacillin	A broad-based synthetic antibiotic used in the treatment of many gram-negative and gram-positive bacteria, including *Shigella;* not effective against penicillinase-producing staphylococci	50–300 mg/kg per day 4–6 doses for 10 days
Amoxicillin—analog of ampicillin trihydrate Capsules 250, 500 mg Suspension 125, 250 mg/5 mL Drops 50 mg/1 mL Amoxil Larotid Polymox	Same uses as ampicillin except is not effective against *Shigella*	450 mg/m² per day or 20–40 mg/kg per day q6h for 10 days
Cephalosporins Capsules 250, 500 mg Suspension 125, 250 mg/5 mL *Cephalexin* Keflex *Cephradine* Anspore Velosef	Respiratory streptococci; streptococci and staphylococci skin infections; and common-organism GU infections	25–50 mg/kg per day q6h

Physiological Considerations*	Laboratory Effects	Comments
	Anti-inflammatories	
E: Urine S: Cushing's syndrome with 2 weeks of therapy, adrenal suppression, hyperglycemia, glycosuria, sodium retention, hypocalcemia, peptic ulcer, osteoporosis, hidden infection C: Concomitant fungal infection. Used cautiously with psychoses and when side-effect processes are preexisting	Serum: ↑ glucose ↓ potassium ↓ cholesterol ↑ uric acid ↑ sodium False-negative LE prep. Urine: ↑ glucose	Antagonizes vitamin-D effect on calcium Half-life is 2.5–3 h. Barbiturates increase inductive phase of metabolism; phenytoin may do so. Topical vitamin A enhances wound healing in clients on steriods by reestablishing the inflammatory process. Similar effect is not seen in clients not on steroids. Take with meals to decrease GI irritation.
	Antimicrobials	
M: Liver E: Urine via active tubular secretion S: Nausea, vomiting, diarrhea, superinfection with overgrowth of gut flora, skin rash C: Penicillin allergy, superinfection not responsive to therapy	Urine: False-positive glucose with Clinitest	Periodic renal, hepatic, and serum evaluation with prolonged treatment. Rapidly and effectively absorbed. Half is excreted in 2 h. Concurrent probenecid will slow metabolism and excretion rates. Take on an empty stomach, 1 h before or 2-3 h after meals. DO NOT administer with fruit juice.
M: Liver E: Same as ampicillin S: Same as ampicillin but generally less frequent and less severe C: Same as ampicillin	Same as ampicillin	Half-life is 61.5 min. Only slightly affected by food; can be given without regard to meals.
M: Excreted unchanged E: Urine via active tubular secretion S: Nausea, vomiting, diarrhea, overgrowth of normal flora with prolonged use. Renal toxicity and blood dyscrasias rare	Serum: Possible positive direct Coombs' Urine: False-positive glucose with Clinitest	Half is excreted in $\frac{1}{2}$–1 h. Food delays but does not decrease drug absorption.

**Key:* A = absorption, M = metabolism, E = excretion, S = side effects, C = contraindications.

Table A2-12 Pediatric Oral Medications *(continued)*

Drug	Uses	Dosage
	Antimicrobials (continued)	
Clindamycin Capsules 75, 150 mg Suspension 75 mg/5 mL Cleocin	Used in treatment of staphylococci, streptococci (except enterococcus), pneumococcus, *Actinomyces,* anaerobes	8–20 mg/kg per day q6h
Erythromycin Chewable tabs 200 mg Suspension 200, 400 mg/5 mL Drops 100 mg/2.5 mL Pediamycin	Against upper and lower respiratory alpha-hemolytic streptococci, staphylococci, *Diplococcus pneumoniae, Hemophilus influenzae.* Used as an antitoxin adjunct and to prevent carriers of *Corynebacterium diphtheriae.* An alternative drug of choice in treatment of primary syphilis *(Treponema pallidum)*	Mild to moderate infections: 0.9–1.5 g/m^2 per day or 30–50 mg/kg per day q6–8h for 10 days Severe infections: double-strength Rheumatic fever prophylaxis: 200 mg/day
Griseofulvin Tablets 250, 500 mg Suspension 250 mg/5 mL Microtablets 125, 250, 500 mg Fulvicin Grifulvin	Fungal infection	Microcrystalline: 300 mg/m^2 per day or 10 mg/kg per day in 2 doses for 2–3 days Regular: doubled micro dose Course longer if hair and nails are involved
Nitrofurantoin Tablets 50, 100 mg Suspension 25 mg/5 mL Furadantin	Treatment of many urinary tract infections. Given over long periods for control of chronic UTIs.	150–200 mg/m^2 per day or 5–7 mg/kg per day q6h for 2 wk If continued, decrease to $\frac{1}{2}$ for 2 wk; if continued; decrease to $\frac{1}{4}$
Nystatin Tablets 500,000 U Suspension 100,000 U/1 mL Vaginal tablets 100,000 U Declostatin Korostatin Mycostatin Nilstat	Fungal infection, especially *Candida* and dermatophytes	Premature infants and newborns: 100,000 U q6–8h Children: 1–2 million units per day q6–8h

Physiological Considerations	Laboratory Effects	Comments
	Antimicrobials (continued)	
C: Known cephalosporin allergy; used with caution in clients with penicillin allergy		
M: Liver S: Diarrhea, occasional rash, pseudomembranous colitis	Serum: ↑SGOT, SGPT	Generally not a drug of choice but gaining in use as organisms develop resistance to other drugs.
M: Liver S: Nausea, vomiting, diarrhea, GI cramping (dose-related) C: Hypersensitivity	Serum: ↑alkaline phosphatase ↑SGOT, SGPT Urine: ↑catecholamines	Half-life is 1.4 h. *H. influenzae* and staphylococci are showing resistant strains. Best effect when taken on empty stomach. DO NOT administer with fruit juice. Alkaline urine may enhance urinary tract effect.
A: Aided by high-fat foods M: Liver E: Feces, urine S: Headache, nausea, vomiting, diarrhea, decreased taste sensitivity, unpleasant or altered taste sensations, fever, rash, serum-type sickness, leukopenia, hepatotoxicity, photosensitivity, neurologic difficulties	Serum: Positive LE prep. ↑ prothrombin time Urine: Proteinuria	Schedule regular-interval CBC, liver, and renal function tests. Binds to keratin. Topical application has little effect. Phenobarbital decreases absorption, if concomitant treatment is necessary, give griseofulvin in 3 divided doses/day.
M: Protein-bound in serum E: Urine, excreted unchanged S: Anorexia, nausea, vomiting, various allergic responses (especially skin rashes) reported	Serum: ↑SGOT, SGPT Urine: Color yellow to brown	Drug is most effective in acid urine (< 5.5 pH). Give antacids at spaced intervals.
E: Most excreted unchanged		Action limited to sites in which drug has direct contact. Vaginal tabs have been used as oral lozenges to prolong contact with oral mucosa.

Key: A = absorption, M = metabolism, E = excretion, S = side effects, C = contraindications.

Table A2-12 Pediatric Oral Medications *(continued)*

Drug	Uses	Dosage
	Antimicrobials (continued)	
Penicillin		
Isoxazolyl penicillin: *Oxacillin sodium* Capsules 250 mg Suspension 250 mg/5 mL Prostaphlin *Cloxacillin sodium* Capsules 250 mg Suspension 125 mg/5 mL Tegopen	Treatment of beta-lactamase-producing staphylococci	Oxacillin and cloxicillin: 0.6–1.5 g/m^2 per day or 50 mg/kg per day q6h
Dicloxacillin sodium monohydrate Capsules 250 mg Suspension 62.5 mg/5 mL Dynapen Pathocil *Nafcillin* Capsules 500 mg Suspension 250 mg/5 mL Unipen		Dicloxacillin and nafcillin: 0.75–1.5 g/m^2 per day or 25–50 mg/kg per day q6h
Penicillin G potassium: Tablets 250, 500 mg Suspension 125, 250 mg/5 mL Pentids QIDpen G *Phenoxymethyl penicillin:* *Potassium* (penicillin V) Tablets 250, 500 mg Suspension 125, 250 mg/5 mL Compocillin-VK Pen-Vee K Ledercillin VK Pfizerpen VK Penicillin V QIDpen VK Robicillin SK-Penicillin VK Veetids	The drug of choice against gonococci, pneumococci, streptococci, meningococci, non-beta-lactamase-producing staphylococci, many spirochetes, many gram-positive rods, *Clostridia, Listeria, Bacteroides, Streptobacillus.* Should be used only for minor infections	0.5–1 g/m^2 per day or 25,000–50,000 U/kg per day, 4 doses per day
Piperazine citrate Tablets 250, 550 mg Wafers 500 mg Syrups 110 mg/1 mL	Anthelmintic against roundworm and pinworm	Roundworm: For 2 days, once a day 75 mg/kg (maximum 4 g) Pinworm: For 2 days, once a day $<$7 kg: 250 mg 7–14 kg: 500 mg 15–27 kg: 1 g $>$27 kg: 2 m

Physiological Considerations*	Laboratory Effects	Comments
Antimicrobials (continued)		
M: Liver E: Urine via active tubular secretion, sputum, milk. Nafcillin excreted via bile S: Suppression of normal GI flora, occasionally nephritis and granulocytopenia C: Penicillin allergy	Serum: ↑SGOT, SGPT	Periodic serum and urine evaluation with long-term use. One-twentieth to one-third oral dose is absorbed. Uremia may reduce drug absorption. May displace bilirubin from protein-binding sites. Oxacillin half-life is 0.5 h. Cloxacillin half-life is 1.5 h. Administer 1 h before or 2–3 h after meals. DO NOT administer with fruit juice.
A: One-third to one-half oral dose is absorbed M: Liver E: Urine, especially via tubular secretion, sputum, milk S: Nausea, vomiting, diarrhea, overgrowth of normal flora C: Penicillin allergy	Serum: Possible ↑ prothrombin time Urine: High doses cause false-positive glucose with Clinitest, false-negative glucose with Testape	Simultaneous tetracycline or erythromycin may decrease effect of penicillins. Not for use in serious illness. Many gonococci are partially resistant to oral penicillin; use procaine penicillin. Penicillin G should be given 1 h before or 2–3 h after meals. Penicillin V is only slightly affected by foods and gastric acidity.
M: Partially in liver; part excreted unchanged E: Urine, feces S: Nausea, vomiting, diarrhea, abdominal pain, vertigo, muscular weakness, lethargy C: Renal disease, seizure disorder		May exacerbate seizure activity. Give before breakfast.

*Key: A = absorption, M = metabolism, E = excretion, S = side effects, C = contraindications.

Table A2-12 Pediatric Oral Medications *(continued)*

Drug	Uses	Dosage
	Antimicrobials (continued)	
Pyrvinium pamoate Tablets 50 mg Suspension 10 mg/1 mL Povan	Anthelmintic against pinworm	150 mg/m² or 5 mg/kg, 1 dose Repeat after 2 weeks if needed
Pyrantel pamoate Suspension 50 mg/1 mL Antiminth	Anthelmintic against roundworm and pinworm	11 mg/kg (maximum 1 g)
Sulfonamides, soluble *Sulfadiazine* Lozenges 200, 300 mg Suspension 500 mg/5 mL *Sulfisoxazole* Tablets 500 mg Suspension 500 mg/5 mL Syrup 500 mg/5 mL Gantrisin *Sulfamethoxazole (long-acting)* Tablets 500 mg Suspension 10%, 500 mg/5 mL Gantanol Bactrim *Sulfadimethoxine* Chewable tablet 250 mg Suspension 250 mg/5 mL Drops 250 mg/1 mL Madribon *Sulfamethoxypyridazine (long-acting)* Suspension 250 mg/5 mL Kynex acetyl	Effective in treatment of both gram-positive and gram-negative sensitive bacteria but especially gram-negative coliform bacteria *(Escherichia coli).* Useful in treatment of urinary tract infections, nocardiosis, toxoplasmosis, and trachoma	Do not give to neonates. 4 g/m² per day or 150 mg/kg per day q4–6h Maximum: 6 g/day Initial dose: one-half the daily dose Long-acting dose: 1.2 g/m² per day or 60 mg/kg per day q12h Initial dose: equal to daily dose
Tetracyclines *Tetracycline hydrochloride* Tablets 250 mg Syrup 125 mg/5 mL Suspension 250 mg/1 mL Drops 100 mg/1 mL Achromycin V Retet-S syrup SK/Tetracycline syrup Other formulations seem to have equal therapeutic value as the hydrochloride.	The most typical broad-spectrum antibiotic Resistant strains increasing, especially gram-negative strains This drug less often prescribed and useful than in the past	Not of use in children $<$ 12 yr 20–40 mg/kg per day q6h Dose may be increased 2–3 times for severe infection

Physiological Considerations*	Laboratory Effects	Comments
	Antimicrobials (continued)	
E: Feces, excreted unchanged S: Nausea, vomiting, diarrhea, staining of teeth if tablets chewed	Stool: Red-stained for days	Nausea and vomiting are more frequent with suspension than with tablets. Tablets have aspirin base; use suspension for aspirin-sensitive clients.
	Serum: ↑*SGOT*	
E: Urine, excreted unchanged S: Urine precipitation of drug crystals (especially in acid urine), hemolytic and aplastic anemia and jaundice. C Glomerulonephritis, pyelonephritis of pregnancy, hepatic disease, last trimester of pregnancy.	Serum: ↑ amylase ↓ PBI ↑ prothrombin time ↑ SGOT, SGPT Urine: Color rusty yellow to brown Crystalluria Proteinuria False-positive glucose with Clinitest	Periodic serum, liver, renal function evaluation with prolonged use. Abuse has increased the number of resistant strains. Generally low-cost, relatively efficient drug against common bacterial infections. PABA inhibits action. Antacids may decrease effect; space doses. Competes with bilirubin for protein-binding sites. Only soluble sulfonamides are absorbed; insoluble forms are for local GI use only. Sulfamethoxazole, sulfadimethoxine, and sulfamethoxypyridazine are long-acting sulfonamides.
M: Liver E: Urine, bile S: Nausea, vomiting, diarrhea, microflora change with superinfection, functional GI disturbances C: Hypersensitivity (unusual)	Serum: ↑ amylase Urine: False-positive glucose with Clinitest	Half-life 8.5 h. Taken on empty stomach. Divalent ions chelate the drug, as does iron; space doses Binds with calcium and is deposited in bones and teeth. May decrease vitamin K, producing bacteria in the gut.

Key: A = absorption, M = metabolism, E = excretion, S = side effects, C = contraindications.

Table A2-12 Pediatric Oral Medications *(continued)*

Drug	Uses	Dosage
	Antipyretics	
Acetaminophen Tablets 325 mg Chewable tablets 125 mg Elixir 120 mg/5 mL Drops 60 mg/0.6 mL Tylenol Tempra	Fever reduction and pain relief (especially headache and musculoskeletal pain) Drug of choice in most childhood illnesses	700 mg/m² per day or 30–60 mg/kg per day in 4–6 doses
Acetylsalicylic acid (ASA) Tablets 300 mg Chewable tablets 75 mg Commonly known as aspirin—many brands available	Analgesic, antipyretic, anti-inflammatory agent	1.5 g/m² per day or 30–65 mg/kg per day in 4–6 doses
	Behavioral Drugs	
Methylphenidate Tablets 5, 10, 20 mg Ritalin	Adjunct in treatment of minimal brain dysfunction, especially in hyperkinesis and petit mal seizure management	Begin 5 mg bid, morning and noon Increase 5 mg/dose per week prn Maximum dose 60 mg/day
	Cardiac Drugs	
Digoxin Elixir 0.5 mg/1 mL Lanoxin	Congestive heart failure (CHF), atrial fibrillation, paroxysmal atrial tachycardia	Digitalizing: 0–1 mo: 0.03–0.06 mg/kg 1–24 mo: 0.06–0.08 mg/kg 2–10 yr: 0.04–0.06 mg/kg Maintenance: 20–30% digitalizing dose in 2–4 doses per day

Physiological Considerations*	Laboratory Effects	Comments
	Antipyretics	
E: Urine S: Hypoglycemia with large doses	Serum: ↑SGOT, SGPT with overdose	Well-absorbed in neonates. Half is excreted in 2 h.
M: Liver E: Urine via active tubular secretion S: Nausea, gastric mucosa irritation, heartburn, provoke or intensify asthmatic attack C: Bleeding tendency	Serum: ↑ bleeding time ↑ amylase ↑ SGOT, SGPT ↓ potassium ↓ cholesterol ↑ or ↓ glucose Urine: Ketonuria	Salicylic acid half-life is 6–8 h. Giving with an alkaline delays absorption but decreases side effects. DO NOT give with fruit juice. Competes with bilirubin for protein binding sites. Yellow-colored soft drinks, canned vegetables, medicines may contain ASA.
	Behavioral Drugs	
M: Liver E: Urine S: Weight and height gain suppression with long-term use, anorexia, abdominal pain, insomnia, tachycardia, dry mouth C: Hypertension, seizures, hyperthyroid, anxiety, glaucoma		Monitor blood pressure. Not for use in children under 6 yr of age. Adult-type reaction begins in early teens. Acid urine (pH 5–5.6) increases excretion rate. May decrease convulsive threshold. May inhibit coumarin anticoagulants, anticonvulsants, and tricyclic antidepressants.
	Cardiac Drugs	
A: Completely and rapidly absorbed from stomach, complete liver cycle before use E: Urine, bile; most excreted unchanged S: GI, cardiac, visual disturbances. Side effects and toxic effects are difficult to separate C: Ventricular fibrillation		Monitor serum electrolytes (especially potassium) and renal function. Potassium depletion sensitizes the myocardium, potentiating effect. Advanced CHF potentiates effect. Well absorbed even in CHF and diarrhea. Narrow therapeutic margin. Early toxic symptoms (GI disturbances) are rarely identified alone in children; often more advanced symptoms are present before toxicity is identified.

**Key:* A = absorption, M = metabolism, E = excretion, S = side effects, C = contraindications.

Table A2-12 Pediatric Oral Medications *(continued)*

Drug	Uses	Dosage
	Decongestants	
Aminophylline Elixir 100, 250 mg/15 mL, 20% alcohol Lixaminol Mini-Lix	Small bronchi and smooth-muscle relaxation, to promote pulmonary artery dilatation and increase cardiac output Acts as a mild diuretic	400–500 mg/m² per day or 12–15 mg/kg per day
Theophylline Tablets 130 mg Elixirs, 10–20% alcohol with varying amounts of drug Generally available in combination, with phenobarbital, ephedrine, hydroxyine HCL, potassium iodide, guaifenesin Bronkolixir Slo-phyllin Elixophyllin Tedral Asbron Inlay Theo-Organidin Marax Mudrane Quibron Quadrinal	Same as aminophylline, effect less immediate and longer in duration	300 mg/m² per day or 10 mg/kg per day in 2–3 doses
Brompheniramine Tablets 4 mg Elixir 2 mg/5 mL Dimetane, Dimetane expectorant Dimetapp elixir 4 mg/5 mL	Antihistamine for relief of upper respiratory tract infections Not for emergency use Anticholenergic effect.	15 mg/m² per day or 0.5 mg/kg per day in 3–4 doses
Chlorpheniramine maleate Tablets 4 mg Sustained-action tablets 8, 12 mg Chlor-Trimeton	Antihistamine relief of upper respiratory tract infections Not for emergency use Anticholenergic effect	10 mg/m² per day or 0.35 mg/kg per day in 4 doses

Physiological Considerations*	Laboratory Effects	Comments
	Decongestants	
S: Stimulates gastric acid secretion, nausea, vomiting (especially with prolonged use), wakefulness, may be habit-forming C: Peptic ulcer, use of other xanthine derivatives, xanthine-free diet	Serum: False ↑ uric acid (Bittner method)	Take with meals to decrease GI irritation. Oral anticoagulation dose may need to be increased.
		Theophylline half-life is 3–9.5 h. Some preparations contain sugar; evaluate if client is diabetic.
M: Liver. S: Anticholinergic drying effect, sedation. Excitation in young children. Overdose may cause auditory and visual hallucinations, convulsions. Dimetane expectorant and Dimetapp contain phenylephrine, which can cause atrial fibrillation.		Additive effect with alcohol, hypnotics, sedatives, tranquilizers. Diminishes GI motility, which can delay absorption rate or decrease the amount absorbed.
M: Liver S: Restlessness		Less likely to cause depression than other antihistamines.

Key: A = absorption, M = metabolism, E = excretion, S = side effects, C = contraindications.

Table A2-12 Pediatric Oral Medications *(continued)*

Drug	Uses	Dosage
	Decongestants (continued)	
Diphenhydramine hydrochloride Capsules 25, 50 mg Elixir 10 mg/4 mL Benadryl	Anticholenergic antihistamine effect, sedation, local anesthesia	150 mg/m² per day or 5 mg/kg per day in 4 doses
Guaifenesin Tablets 100, 200 mg Syrup 100 mg/5 mL often containing alcohol Available in combination with many antihistamines Actol Expectran Glycotuss GG-Cen 2/G Robitussin	Used as an expectorant Causes increased formation of respiratory tract fluid	200–400 mg/m² per dose q 4–6 h
Plus antitussive action—most contain codeine or codeine derivative Expectran DM Robitussin A-C Robitussin-DM Sorbutuss Dorcol Hycotuss 2/G-DM	Should be used only when cough disrupts ability to sleep, eat	
	Phenylisopropylamines	
Ephedrine Tablets 15, 25, 30, 50, 60 mg Syrup 20 mg/5 mL Quelidrine Bronkolixir Quibron Pyribenzamine Marax Mudrane Tedral *Pseudoephedrine* Tablets 15, 25, 30, 50, 60 mg Syrup 20 mg/5 mL Actifed Deconamine Fedahist Isoclor Rondec Sudafed	Smooth-muscle relaxation, pupil dilatation, when longer effect than epinephrine is desired in treatment of nonemergency allergic response, asthma, spinal anesthetic hypotension, AV block, and nasal congestion and vasodilatation	Ephedrine: 100 mg/m² per day or 3 mg/kg per day in 4–6 doses Pseudoephedrine: 125 mg/m² per day or 4mg/kg per day in 4 doses

Physiological Considerations*	Laboratory Effects	Comments
	Decongestants (continued)	
S: Anticholinergic drying effect—dry mouth common. Blurred vision, urine retention, palpitations, and with higher doses constipation		Dimishes gastric emptying, may inhibit absorption of other drugs. Onset of action is 10-30 min. Half-life is 6 h. Sedative effect is generally perceived as unpleasant. Anesthetic effect is true for denuded skin only.
S: Codeine-type effects may occur with the expectorant-antitussives	Urine: Color interference with lab steroid tests	Also known as glyceryl guiacolate.
	Phenylisopropylamines	
E: Most excreted unchanged S: Anxiety, tremors, palpitations, insomnia, possible difficulty in initiating urination C: Angina pain may be induced in clients with angina pectoris	Serum: ↓ amylase with poisoning ↑ prothrombin time in clients on Coumadin	Side effects not uncommon with 3–4 doses/day. Side effects and toxic effects are counteracted by barbiturates. Concomitant phenobarbital may be used to limit side effects. May increase coumarin metabolism. Cardiac effect is variable and is less noted with pseudoephedrine. Additive effect with alcohol.

*Key: A = absorption, M = metabolism, E = excretion, S = side effects, C = contraindications.

Table A2-12 Pediatric Oral Medications *(continued)*

Drug	Uses	Dosage
	Phenylisopropylamines (continued)	
Also available in combinations; may be combined with phenobarbital to limit side effects		
Hydroxyamphetamine *Phenylpropanolamine* Used in combination with antihistamines	Adjunct in acute asthma attack, effect is CNS stimulation, vasoconstriction, nasal decongestion	
	Dietary Additives	
Vitamins Tablets, chewable tablets, drops A, D, C, E only: Tri-Vi-Flor Tri-Vi-Sol Novacebrin Adeflor Iberet Broad-spectrum: Vi-Penta Vi-Daylin C-B Time	Vitamin maintenance and supplement	As per RDA recommendations
Fluoride Drops In many water supplies	Protection against dental caries	Not to exceed 1 mg/day
Iron *Ferrous sulfate* Liquid 220 mg/5 mL (33.3 mg elemental iron) Feosol Available in infant formula, cereal, and with vitamin preparations *Ferrous gluconate* Tablets 320 mg Elixir 300 mg/5 mL (44 mg elemental iron) Fergon *Polysaccharide complex* Elixir 100 mg elemental iron/5 mL Nu-Iron	Preventive maintenance of iron levels and in treatment of iron-deficiency anemias	Dosage for elemental iron: Prophylaxis: 1–2 mg/kg per day for the first year of life Therapeutic: 6 mg/kg per day in 1–3 doses

Physiological Considerations*	Laboratory Effects	Comments
	Phenylisopropylamines (continued)	
C: Hypertension, hyperthyroid		Acid urine (pH 4.5–5.6) increases excretion rate.
	Dietary Additives	
E: Urine S: Hypervitaminosis, especially of fat-soluble vitamins		Administer water-soluble forms of vitamins A, D, E when fat absorption is altered.
S: Excess may cause mottling of tooth enamel. High doses over long periods may produce dental and skeletal fluorosis. Acute toxicity only with insecticide ingestion	Serum: ↓ glucose with large doses	Long-term intake of >4 mg/day causes dental fluorosis. Long-term intake of 8-20 mg/day causes skeletal fluorosis.
S: With ferrous sulfate and gluconate—nausea, abdominal cramps, constipation, diarrhea, and the elixir causes temporary staining of the teeth. With polysaccharide complex no metal aftertaste, no GI side effects, and no tooth staining, but very little iron absorption C: Hemosiderosis	Stool: False-positive benzidine test for occult blood. Use quaiac.	Ferrous sulfate is incompatible with milk and vitamin C. Ferrous gluconate absorption and possibly utilization is aided by vitamin C. Oral tetracyclines are inhibited by iron; take at spaced intervals (minimum of 2 h apart).

**Key:* A = absorption, M = metabolism, E = excretion, S = side effects, C = contraindications.

Table A2-12 Pediatric Oral Medications *(continued)*

Drug	Uses	Dosage
	Emetics	
Ipecac Syrup 32 grains/1 oz Available over-the-counter in 1-oz containers	Generally used as an emetic May also be used in very small doses as an expectorant	Emetic dose: <1 yr: 5–10 mL >1 yr: 15 mL Repeat in 20 min if no emesis Lavage if emesis does not occur Expectorant dose: 0.5 mL qid
	Fecal Softeners	
Dioctyl sodium sulfosuccinate Capsules, tablets 50, 60, 100, 150, 200, 250 mg Liquid 10 mg/1 mL Suspension 20 mg/5 mL Colace	When gross motor activity restricted for an extended period Is an anionic detergent with surface action	150 mg/m² per day or 5 mg/kg per day

bibliography

Avery, G. S. (ed.) *Drug treatment: Principles and practice of clinical pharmacology and therapeutics.* Mass.: Publishing Sciences Group, 1976.

Becker, M. H., et al. Predicting mother's compliance with pediatric medical regimens. *The Journal of Pediatrics,* **81**(4):843–854(1972).

Bergman, A. B., and Werner, R. J. Failure of children to receive penicillin by mouth. *New England Journal of Medicine,* **268**(24):1334–1338 (1963).

Black, C. D., et al. Drug interactions in the G. I. tract. *The American Journal of Nursing,* **77**:1426–1429 (1977).

Blackwell, B. Patient compliance. *New England Journal of Medicine,* **289**(5):249–252 (1973).

Chudzik, G. M., and Jaffee, S. J. Drug interaction: An important consideration for rational pediatric therapy. *Pediatric Clinics of North America,* **19**(1): 131–140 (1972).

Eisenberg, M., et. al. *Manual of antimicrobial therapy and interactions.* Seattle: University of Washington RC-02, 1979.

Erikson, E. *Childhood and society.* New York: Norton, 1950.

Francis V., et al. Gaps in doctor-patient communication; Patients' response to medical advice. *New England Journal of Medicine,* **280**(10):535–540 (1969).

Gill, S. E., and Davis, J. A. The pharmacology of the fetus, baby and growing child. In J. A. Davis and J. Dobbing (eds.). *Scientific foundations of pediatrics,* Philadelphia: Saunders, 1974.

Hansten, Philip D. *Drug Interactions* (2d ed.). Philadelphia: Lea & Febiger, 1973.

Hussar, D. A. Drug interactions: Good and bad. *Nursing 76,* **6**:61–65 (1976).

Kauffman, R. E., and Azarnoff, D. L. Drug interactions. In H. C. Shirkey (ed.), *Pediatric therapy* (5th ed.). St. Louis: Mosby, 1975, pp. 92–94.

Knoefel, Peter K. (ed.). *Absorption, distribution, transformation and excretion of drugs.* Springfield, Ill.: Charles C Thomas, 1972.

Lambert, M. L., Jr. Drug and diet interactions. *American Journal of Nursing,* **75**(3):402–406 (1975).

Martin, Eric W. *Hazards of medication.* Philadelphia: Lippincott, 1971.

Mirkin, Bernard L. Principles of drug disposition and therapy in infants and children. In A. M. Rudolph (ed.), *Pediatrics* (16th ed.). New York: Appleton Century Crofts, 1977, pp. 843–852.

———, et al. Pediatric clinical pharmacology. *Pediatric Annals,* **5**(9):12–97 (1976).

Ormond, E. A. R., and Caulfield, C. A practical guide to giving oral medications to young children. *MCN, The American Journal of Maternal Child Nursing,* **1**(5):320–325 (1976).

Physiological Considerations*	Laboratory Effects	Comments
	Emetics	
A: Can be cardiotoxic if absorbed S: Cardiotoxic if absorbed C: Ingestion of strychnine, corrosives, petroleum distillates, unconsciousness	Serum: Electrolyte imbalance if vomiting is prolonged or in young clients	Prepare for vomiting of large amounts. Follow with water and physical activity to encourage emesis. Vomiting generally occurs within 10 min.
	Fecal Softeners	
E: Stool, excreted unchanged.		

**Key:* A = absorption, M = metabolism, E = excretion, S = side effects, C = contraindications.

Ray, C. George, et al. *Manual of antimicrobial therapy.* Seattle, Wash.: 1975.

Rolewicz, T. F. A rational approach to antibiotic therapy in infants and children. *Pediatric Annals,* **5**(9):43–59 (1976).

Shirkey, H. C. *Pediatric drug handbook.* Philadelphia: Saunders, 1977.

———, *Pediatric therapy.* St. Louis: Mosby, 1975.

Smith, Stephen E., and Rawlins, Michael D. *Variability in human drug response.* London: Butterworth, 1973.

Vaughan, V. C., and McKay, R. J. *Nelson's textbook of pediatrics.* Philadelphia: Saunders, 1979.

Waring, William W., and Jeansonne, Louis O., III. *Practical manual of pediatrics.* St. Louis: Mosby, 1975,

3 Laboratory Tests

MAUREEN COLLAR

Laboratory tests such as the ones included here are to be used only as diagnostic or screening aids. The results of these tests need to be combined with the practitioner's subjective and objective findings in order to form a complete data base. Only then can one arrive at an accurate interpretation and diagnosis.

Test	Normal Value	Interpretation
	Blood	
ASO (antistreptolysin O) titer	12–166 Todd units	Increased in Rheumatic fever Rheumatoid arthritis Acute glomerulonephritis Streptococcal infection Collagen diseases
Calcium	9–11.5 mg/100 mL	Increased in Hyperparathyroidism Excess vitamin D Acute osteoporosis Idiopathic hypercalcemia of infants Decreased in Hypoparathyroidism Malabsorption of calcium and vitamin D Chronic renal disease
Carbohydrate metabolism tests		
Glucose	70–110 mg/100 mL (Newborn—40 mg/100 mL)	Increased in Diabetes mellitus Increased adrenalin Decreased in Pancreatic disorders Hepatic disorders Infant of diabetic mother Premature infant
Glucose tolerance test (oral)	125 mg/100 mL at 1 h 75 mg/100 mL at 2 h	Increased tolerance in Intestinal diseases

Test	Normal Value	Interpretation
Blood (continued)		
	90 mg/100 mL at 3 h (Peak of not more than 150 mg/100 mL; return to fasting level within 2 h)	Hypothyroidism Addison's disease Decreased tolerance in Hyperthyroidism Diabetes mellitus Steroid effect Severe liver damage
Coagulation tests		
Bleeding time	3–6 min (Ivy's method)	Prolonged in Thrombocytopenia
Thrombin time	7–15 s	Prolonged in Heparin therapy Low fibrinogen level
PTT (partial thromboplastin time)	37–50 s (with kaolin) 70–100 s (without activator)	Prolonged in Defect in factor I, II, V, VIII, IX, X, XI, or XII Normal in Thrombocytopenia Platelet dysfunction
Platelet count	150,000–350,000/mm^3	Increased in Malignancy Postsplenectomy Rheumatoid arthritis Iron-deficiency anemia Decreased in Thrombocytopenic purpura Leukemia Some viral infections
Prothrombin time	11–13 s	Prolonged in Defect in factor I, II, V, VII, or X Inadequate vitamin K Severe liver damage Anticoagulants
G-6-PD (glucose-6-phosphate dehydrogenase)	5–15 U	Increased in Pernicious anemia Idiopathic thrombocytopenic purpura Decreased in 13% of black males 3% of black females (Associated with drug-induced hemolytic anemias)
Hematocrit	Newborn 42-64% Child 34-40% Adult Male 38-52% Female 36-47%	Increased in Polycythemia Dehydration Decreased in Anemias Hemorrhage
Hemoglobin	Newborn 14–22 g/100 mL Child 12–14 g/100 mL	Increased in Intravascular hemolysis

Test	Normal Value	Interpretation
Blood (continued)		
	Adult Male 14–18 g/100 mL Female 12–16 g/100 mL	Dehydration Polycythemia Decreased in Iron-deficiency anemia Sickle-cell anemia Thalassemia Hemorrhage
Liver function tests Alkaline phosphatase	Infant 73-266 IU/L Child 57-151 IU/L Adolescent 57-258 IU/L Adult 14-38 IU/L	Increased in: Acute viral hepatitis Obstructive jaundice Cirrhosis Rickets Decreased in Hyperthyroidism
Bilirubin	Conjugated 0.1-0.4 mg/100 mL Unconjugated 0.1-0.5 mg/100 mL Total 0.2-0.9 mg/100 mL (Newborn—up to 12 mg/100 mL)	Increased in *Conjugated* Acute and chronic hepatitis Biliary duct obstruction *Unconjugated* Hemolytic disease Acute hepatitis Hereditary glucuronyl transferase deficiency
LDH (lactate dehydrogenase)	90–180 IU/L	Increased in Chronic hepatitis Hepatic cirrhosis Sickle-cell anemia Pernicious anemia
SGOT (glutamic oxalacetic transaminase)	5–40 U/mL	Increased in Acute liver disease Musculoskeletal diseases Acute pancreatitis Acute myocardial infarction
SGPT (glutamic pyruvic transaminase)	5–35 U/mL	Increased in Same as for SGOT
Mono spot (slide test)	Negative (titers up to 1:56 may be normal)	Positive = agglutination titers of 1:224 or higher in infectious mononucleosis
Phenylalanine (Guthrie test)	0-2 mg/100 mL	Increased in Greater than 15 mg/100 mL in phenylketonuria (PKU) Greater than 4 mg/100 mL = positive
Reticulocyte count	0.5–1.5% of RBC	Increased in Blood loss Increased RBC destruction Following iron therapy Decreased in Severe autoimmune type of hemolytic anemia

Test	Normal Value	Interpretation
	Blood (continued)	
Sedimentation rate	Males 0–15 mm in 1 h Females 0–20 mm in 1 h (Westergren)	Increased in Tuberculosis Bacterial infection (abscess) Acute rheumatic fever Acute pelvic inflammatory disease Rheumatoid arthritis
Sickle cell (sickledex)	Negative	Positive in Sicle cell disease Sickle cell trait False positive in Transfusion of sickling blood within 4 mo of test False negative in Transfusion of normal RBCs within 4 mo of test Newborn
Thyroid function tests T_3 (uptake in serum)	45–60%	Increased in Hyperthyroidism Thyroxine administration Steroid therapy Decreased in Hypothyroidism Estrogen therapy Pregnancy
T_4 (total thyroxine)	3.2–6.4 μg/100 mL	Increased in Hyperthyroidism Thyroxine administration Estrogen administration Pregnancy Thyrotoxicosis
T_4 (free thyroxine)	1.0–2.1 μg/100 mL	Increased in Hyperthyroidism Thyroxine administration Decreased in Hypothyroidism
Thyroid stimulating hormone	Up to 0.2 mU/mL	Decreased in Secondary (pituitary) hypothyroidism Dwarfism associated with decreased pituitary growth hormone
VDRL (Venereal Disease Research Laboratory) test	Nonreactive	Reaction in Syphilis (confirm reactive tests with FTA-ABS)
White blood cell count	Total leukocytes 5000–10,000	Increased in Intoxication Acute hemorrhage or hemolysis Bacterial infection

Test	Normal Value	Interpretation
Blood (continued)		
		Decreased in Viral infection Rickettsial infection Leukemia Aplastic anemia Pernicious anemia
Basophils	0–1% of WBCs	Increased in Polycythemia Leukemia Hodgkin's disease Chickenpox
Eosinophils	1–3% of WBCs	Increased in Allergic diseases Parasitic infections Some skin diseases
Lymphocytes	Child 31–57% of WBCs Adult 25–33% of WBCs	Increased in Pertussis Mononucleosis Infectious hepatitis Mumps Rubella Other viral infections
Monocytes	Child 6–8% of WBCs Adult 3–7% of WBCs	Increased in Leukemia Hodgkin's disease Collagen diseases
Neutrophils	Child 33–60% of WBCs Adult 57–68% of WBCs	Increased in Bacterial infection Decreased in Neutropenia associated with immune deficiencies Granulocytopenia Leukemia
Urine		
Bile (bilirubin)	0 Icto test—negative Bili-Labstix—negative	Increased in Liver disease Biliary tract obstruction
Color	Pale straw color	Dark yellow to amber Dehydration Acute febrile illness Red Hemoglobinuria Trauma Food dyes Blue or green Bilirubin Jaundice Orange Excreted drugs

Test	Normal Value	Interpretation
	Urine (continued)	
Culture	No growth Uricult—negative Culturia—negative Microstix—negative	Increased in Skin contamination Bacterial count greater than 100,000/mm³ on clean catch indicates an active urinary tract infection
Ferric chloride	Negative	Postitive in Phenylketonuria Tyrosinuria Maple syrup disease Alkaptonuria
Glucose	Up to 0.3 g/24 h Clinitest—negative Tes-tape—negative Clinistix—negative	Increased in Diabetes mellitus Liver disease Other metabolic disorders Renal tubular disease CNS disease
Ketones	0 Acetest —negative Ketostix—negative	Increased in Diabetic acidosis Starvation Fever Hyperthyroidism
Microscopic exam		
Red blood cells	Up to 1–2 RBCs/hpf (high-power field)	Increased in Acute glomerulonephritis Nephrosis Trauma Cystitis Renal stone Tuberculosis
White blood cells	Up to 1–2 WBCs/hpf	Increased in Urinary tract infection Nephrosis Pyelonephritis
Epithelial cells	Occasional/lpf (low-power field)	Increased in Renal cells—renal disease or damage Squamous cells—normal finding
Casts	0/lpf	Increased in Disorder of kidney tubules Hemorrhagic or inflammatory disease Dehydration
pH	4.6–7.0	Increased in Urinary tract infection Alkalosis Decreased in Metabolic acidosis Respiratory acidosis PKU

Test	Normal Value	Interpretation
	Urine (continued)	
Pregnancy test	Negative=no agglutination Gravindex Pregnosticon	Positive in Pregnancy Hydatidiform mole False positive Elevated protein or blood in urine Methadone therapy False negative Missed abortion Ectopic pregnancy
Protein	None to slight trace Combistix—negative Uristix—negative	Positive in Nephritis Nephrosis Renal calculi Toxemia Orthostatic proteinuria
Specific gravity	1.005–1.025	Increased in Diabetes mellitus Dehydration Glomerulonephritis Decreased in Diabetes insipidus Renal failure Nephrosis
Urobilinogen	0–4 mg/24 h	Increased in Hepatitis Cirrhosis Biliary obstruction Hemolytic diseases Severe infection
	Feces	
Blood	Negative guaiac test	Present in Ulcerative lesions of GI tract Nosebleed
Fat	Less than 6 g/24 h	Increased in Mineral oil ingestion Suppository Steatorrhea Chronic pancreatic disease Sprue
Microscopic exam White blood cells	Few/hpf	Increased in Polynuclear Shigellosis Salmonella Ulcerative colitis Monocytes Typhoid

Test	Normal Value	Interpretation
Feces (continued)		
		Decreased in Viral diarrhea Noninvasive *E. coli* Nonspecific diarrhea
Ova and parasites	None	Present in Parasitic infestations
Urobilinogen	40–280 mg/24 h	Increased in Hemolytic anemias Decreased in Biliary obstruction Liver disease Oral antibiotics
Cerebral Spinal Fluid		
Appearance	Clear, colorless	Yellow Severe jaundice Metastatic melanoma Meningitis Bloody Traumatic tap Cerebral hemorrhage Subdural hematoma with contusion
Culture and smear	No growth Negative gram stain No acid-fast bacilli	Present in Bacterial meningitis Tuberculous meningitis *(Mycobacterium tuberculosis)*
Glucose	50–75 mg/100 mL (50% of blood sugar)	Decreased in Bacterial meningitis Tuberculous meningitis
Protein	20–45 mg/100 mL	Increased in Acute encephalomyelitis Bacterial meningitis Normal or slightly increased in Aseptic meningitis Tuberculous meningitis
Total cell count	Infants 0–20/mm^3 Adults 0–10/mm^3	Increased in Lymphocytes Encephalomyelitis 25–10,000 in tuberculous meningitis Polymorphonuclear leukocytes 25–10,000 in bacterial meningitis Polymorphonuclear leukocytes then mononuclear cells Up to 500 in aseptic meningitis

Test	Normal Value	Interpretation
	Miscellaneous	
GC culture and smear	No growth on Thayer-Martin medium Gram stain negative for intracellular diplococci	Present in Gonococcal infection
KOH, west prep smear	No organisms	Present in Vaginal infection *Canadida albicans* Other yeasts Trichomonas
Pap smear	Negative No malignant cells	Positive in Carcinoma of cervix or uterus (abnormal, premalignant, or malignant cells)
Sweat chloride	4–60 meq/L	Increased in Cystic fibrosis (greater than 60 meq/L) Untreated adrenal insufficiency

bibliography

Garb, Solomon. *Laboratory tests in common use.* New York: Springer, 1976.

Headings, Dennis L. (ed.). *The Harriet Lane handbook.* Chicago: Year Book, 1975.

Kempe, C. Henry, et al. *Current pediatric diagnosis and treatment.* Los Altos, Calif.: Lange, 1978.

Wallach, Jacques. *Interpretation of diagnostic tests.* Boston:Little, Brown, 1974.

———: *Pocket book of medical tables.* Philadelphia: Smith, Kline, and French, 1976.

4 Radiologic Procedures

ERICKA K. LEIBOLD WAIDLEY

Diagnostic radiology is becoming one of the most common experiences that a child faces during hospitalization; and yet it is the most often ignored as far as preparation is concerned. A child's experience in the radiology department depends upon many factors: developmental and emotional age, the method and effectiveness of the preparation, the amount of parental support and involvement, and the professional's availability to answer questions and encourage verbalization before and after the procedure.

Many methods are available for preparing a child for procedures, and the current research supports any or all of them as being effective in certain situations. An important factor in the effectiveness of any method of preparation is that the information given must be factual. How many health professionals really know what happens to a child during an intravenous pyelogram, upper gastrointestinal series, or voiding cystourethrogram? Before a professional attempts to prepare a child for any procedure, she or he must observe the procedure, comprehend it, and document both the process and any physician idiosyncrasies for reference at a later time.

The availability of a professional person who has specific knowledge about the procedure is invaluable to both the child and the parent(s). The professional is responsible for evaluating the effectiveness of the preparation and for determining the child's readiness for the procedure. Too many times children are sent to have procedures that they either have not been prepared for or do not understand and then are chastised for becoming uncooperative and unmanageable. An assessment of the child's status prior to the procedure can often eliminate the need for cancellations and reschedulings as well as prevent the unneeded unpleasantness for the child and parent(s).

Preparation prior to any stressful event should always be augmented by a follow-up period to allow verbalization of thoughts and playing out fantasies and feelings of anger. This follow-up can be done in the safe environment of the playroom, where the child feels free to express him or her self and have his or her behavior accepted by others. Toys and dolls depicting x-ray equipment and personnel can be made available to allow the child to explore and reenact the procedure. It is important to educate the parent(s) regarding the need for this playing out behavior and encourage them to allow their child to verbalize about the procedure.

Table A4-1 presents the developmental needs of different ages of children in relation to radiologic procedures and Table A4-2, Common Pediatric X-rays, deals with specific preparation considerations and techniques that may be used. Several guidelines are included in the conclusion that can be used when planning a radiology preparation program.

CONCLUSION

Many radiologic procedures, no matter how simple, are traumatic experiences for an unprepared child, and a child has the right to know what to expect before being sent to the x-ray department. Summed up below are a few important facts that should be used as guidelines when planning a radiology preparation program.

1. Effective preparation must be timely, well-organized, complete, and factual.
2. Each child should be assessed prior to the preparation in order to determine individual needs.
3. Parental involvement during preparation and/or during the procedure, if allowed, offers the child trustworthy and reliable support before and after the x-ray.
4. Adequate time must be allotted during the preparation for questions from the child and parent(s) and answers to those questions, and after the procedure for verbalization and playing out.

references

Erikson, Erik. *Childhood and society.* New York: Norton, 1963, p. 251.

Phillips, J. *The origins of intellect piaget's theory.* San Francisco: Freeman, 1975, pp. 73, 83.

Skipper, J., and Leonard, R. Children, stress, and hospitalization: A field experiment. *Journal of Health and Social Behavior,* **9**:275–287 (1968).

Waechter, E., and Blake, F. *Nursing care of children* (9th ed.). New York: Lippincott, 1976, p. 743.

bibliography

Jacobi, C., and Paris, D. *Xray technology* (3d ed.). St. Louis: Mosby, 1964.

Petrillo, M., and Sanger, S. *Emotional care of hospitalized children.* Philadelphia: Lippincott, 1972.

Poznanski, A. *Practical approaches to pediatric radiology.* Chicago: Year Book, 1976.

Waidley, E. Preparing children for radiology procedures. *Journal of the Association for the Care of Children in Hospitals,* **6**:6–11 (1977).

Watson, J. *Patient care and special procedures in radiologic technology.* St. Louis: Mosby, 1974.

Table A4-1 Developmental Considerations in Relation to Radiologic Procedures

Developmental Considerations	Child and/or Parent Preparation
Infants (Birth to 1 Year)	
During the first year, the infant is basically egocentric and is concerned with need satisfaction and physical safety. Separation from the mother (or care giver) produces a form of primary anxiety which is behavioralized as increased tension (continued crying, frenzied movements, and rigid muscle tone). Because of this anxiety and the resulting movement, infants are usually placed on an immobilization board so that the x-ray procedure can be done successfully the first time (thus preventing further exposure to radiation due to repeated attempts to complete the procedure). One of the infant's main concerns for need satisfaction is food. For procedures that examine the digestive tract, the infant usually has to be npo for a certain length of time (Table A4-2). It is extremely important to make every attempt with the radiology department to schedule these procedures between feeding times so that the infant does not have to go for an extended period of time without adequate nutrition. If this scheduling is not possible, then the physician should be consulted as to how long the child has to be npo prior to the procedure for it to still be successful. This can range from 2 to 6 h depending on the age of the infant and the type of procedure.	It is obvious that the infant can not be emotionally prepared for the radiologic procedure, but it is important to inform and prepare the parent(s) or significant care giver. Research supports the theory that by lowering the mother's stress, the child's stress will be indirectly reduced (Skipper and Leonard, 1968). This suggests that by interacting with and preparing the mother for stressful events she will in turn interact with her child and lower his or her anxiety. If the mother is adequately prepared for what will be happening to the infant during the procedure (e.g., the immobilization board, injection of dye, etc.), and she feels able to cope with this, then she should be allowed to stay with the infant during the procedure (although many radiology departments do not allow this). Even if the mother or care giver cannot accompany the child, certain comfort measures should be considered. Most radiology departments, because of their location, are usually cold, and the infant should be well covered with blankets. Also, for the older infants a pacifier can be used to satisfy the sucking needs if feedings have had to be withheld. The infant should be clean and have dry diapers applied before being sent to the radiology department so that further delays are prevented.
Toddlers (1 to $3\frac{1}{2}$ Years)	
In this stage of development the utmost concern for the child is separation from the mother (or care giver) because she is still the main component for need satisfaction. When separation occurs, the child may appear to miss the mother and doubt that she will return. An important developmental task at this stage is muscle control of elimination and retention of urine and feces. It is difficult for the toddler to let go of this newly acquired control, which is sometimes necessary with several of the radiologic procedures and/or their preparation (barium enema, IVP, voiding cystourethrogram). With this increasing body independence, the body products become associated with sexual and aggressive behavior, and the toddler may feel a considerable loss when forced to give them up without control. Imagination also begins to play an important part in the daily life of the older toddler, and each new effort is usually preceded by fantasy play. In stressful situations this can be hazardous because the toddler may perceive the radiologic procedure as threatening to his or her well-being and may fight to maintain self-integrity. Defenses that the toddler uses to cope with this anxiety are imitation, avoidance, denial, and increasing stubbornness.	The toddler's major concerns with off-unit procedures are separation anxiety and permanent desertion by the mother. It may be important to a child in this age group to leave a note on the pillow to "tell Mommy where I am" or to encourage the parent(s) (after adequate preparation) to accompany the child to the x-ray department and wait in the waiting room (if not allowed to stay with the child) until the procedure has been completed. Another common fear is fear of strange and unfamiliar places and new people. Preparation that involves using pictures of the environment and strange equipment can help reduce some of these fears. Because the toddler has such a vivid imagination when left alone in stressful situations, he or she should be told exactly what will and will not happen. An example of this is to tell the child that the x-ray equipment can not move by itself, that it will not crush him or her, and that even though it looks and sounds scary it does not hurt. Being honest and factual with the child usually results in success. Because of the attention span of this age group, it is usually best to prepare the child 1 to 3 h prior to the procedure.

Table A4-1 Developmental Considerations in Relation to Radiologic Procedures *(continued)*

Developmental Considerations	Child and/or Parent Preparation
Preschoolers (3½ to 6½ Years)	
The preschool age is a tender time for hospitalization and diagnostic testing because of the child's limited vocabulary and ability to understand. The thinking process is still egocentric, and conclusions are based on intuitive and magical beliefs, e.g., on what the child wants to believe (preoperational thought) (Phillips, 1975, p. 73). During this stage, the child is also trying to discover what kind of a person he or she is going to be. The child is developing a conscience and a sense of autonomy (Erikson, 1963), and there is an increasing interest in competence, prowess, and dominance. Toward the end of this stage is the oedipal phase, when the child prefers the parent of the opposite sex and turns away from the parent of the same sex. This phase may also involve a fear of castration by the parent of the same sex and can be projected to include fear of harm by a technologist who is the same sex as the child. It is also during this stage of development that children begin to find pleasure in genital manipulation. They develop a sense of reward and gratification, and at the same time, a sense of guilt associated with this activity. A common radiologic procedure, the IVP, is done to determine if the kidneys, bladder, and urinary tract are functioning correctly. If the child is having an IVP and has been experimenting with masturbation the guilt and shame can be overwhelming.	The preschooler has a vivid imagination that allows fantasizing when left alone in an unfamiliar and threatening situation. Common fantasies of this age group are similar to those of the toddler: animation of the machinery with fears of mutilation and bodily harm and beliefs that the machine can "see inside the head" (thought invasion) and know what the child is thinking. The preschooler is also afraid of cutaneous invasion in procedures (e.g., IVP) that require an injection or an IV to be started. The procedures are especially stressful for children who may feel that they are being punished for bad behavior. With this age group it is often beneficial to use drawings, dolls, or actual equipment (x-ray films, syringes, "play" x-ray tables, etc.) during the preparation to help increase the child's comprehension. The preschooler is capable of understanding simple explanations of the body parts and should be shown what areas of the body the doctor needs to see. By explaining and showing the child which parts will be examined, you are helping him or her to cope with fears of mutilation and castration. This is an inquisitive age group, and all the child's questions need to be answered appropriately. Repeated reassurance and compliments on the child's ability to understand will increase his or her feelings of mastery and self-pride.
School-age (6½ to 13 Years)	
The school-age child looks to peers or a special friend for support and encouragement. This is a time when secrets are kept and only confided to each other, thought processes become more organized [concrete operational thought (Phillips, 1975, p. 83)], and a more stable self-identity begins to form. The most important task, however, is competence in school; and interruption from this can be devastating. Latency occurs between 7 and 11 years with the sexual drive being controlled and repressed. In order to do this, the child may use several unconscious mechanisms: isolation, pseudocompulsion, turning to the opposite (e.g., denying anger), and sublimation of wishes (channeling drives into acceptable outlets). In this stage the child still may fear castration, mutilation, and even death. An example of how this fear can be potentiated is when the technologist places a heavy rubber plate or "apron" over the child's genitals with an explanation that the x-ray machine may hurt these areas. It is better to offer an explanation that the doctor doesn't need to see these parts on the picture, and therefore they need to be covered.	Visual aids, equipment, and tours can be useful with this age group to increase their knowledge of health and the hospital system. It is helpful to instruct the child in the medical terminology for body parts and procedures after you have learned his or her own words for them. Many children need to know the sequence of events that will occur (including strange sounds), how it will feel (including when it will hurt), and how long it will take. By telling the child everything to expect you are providing time to rally forces and decide upon acceptable ways to cope. It is helpful to discuss with the child ways that he or she has coped with uncomfortable situations in the past. If the child is not able to think of any coping behaviors that have been successful, then the professional should offer some suggestions, e.g., counting to 10 until the injection is over, watching the minutes advance, singing a favorite song or rhyme, or practicing the multiplication tables. The child can even be encouraged to practice the chosen strategy prior to the procedure in order to be able to remember it more easily.

Table A4-1 Developmental Considerations in Relation to Radiologic Procedures *(continued)*

Developmental Considerations	Child and/or Parent Preparation
School-age ($6\frac{1}{2}$ to 13 Years) (continued)	
	The optimal time for preparing the school-age child is the night or day prior to the procedure. This gives the child enough time to think through some fears and get answers to many questions but does not allow overreaction because of excessive anticipatory fear.
Adolescents (Age Varies Depending on the Individual and the Family Environment)	
There are several psychosocial tasks that are important in this stage: emancipation from parent(s), adaptation to a rapidly changing body, development of a sexual identity, determination of values and ideals, and preparation for a future career. Hospitalization and/or illness can interrupt the normal developmental progress, causing an increase in anxiety and stress. The adolescent's move toward autonomy is also an important factor in radiologic procedures. Orders and restrictions associated with x-rays may be difficult for young adults, who are trying to be independent. Their response to these limitations is often seen as hostile and stubborn behavior, including an open refusal to cooperate. It is possible to avoid some of these problems by encouraging adolescents to be involved in the decision-making process of their care and by keeping them well-informed of the rationale for tests and procedures. Another consideration for radiologic procedures is that of the adolescent's need for adequate nutrition. This is a stage of increased physical activity and growth when the caloric intake needs to be higher than ever before. Once again higher compliance with the procedural restrictions will be reached if the adolescent is involved in choosing a diet from a list of specific alternatives.	The adolescent is very different from the other age groups in respect to need for independence and autonomy. For this reason it is usually best to do procedure preparation and teaching when the parent(s) are not present; if necessary, a separate time to talk to the parent(s) should be planned. This age group usually prefers an honest, straightforward approach, and most medical terminology is easily understood once explained. Use of anatomy and physiology textbooks, medical charts, skeleton models, and x-ray films can be beneficial. The young adult's curiosity about sex and reproduction may lead to questions about radiation exposure and damage. Factual answers to these questions are important to avoid misinterpretation and confusion. The adolescent may be embarrassed to talk about these fears but an observant practitioner and trusting atmosphere may help overcome these fears. Preparation with this age group can usually be done more in advance or during the procedure (if an emergency) without any dramatic side effects. The adolescent is able to understand cause and effect relationships and usually has established some satisfactory coping mechanisms so there may be fewer fears associated with radiologic procedures than with the other age groups.

Table A4-2 Common Pediatric X-rays

Name of Examination	Possible Purpose and/or Indications	Possible Physical Preparation Needed*
ABDOMEN		
	To detect any abnormalities (e.g., bowel obstruction) To demonstrate the presence of free air in the stomach To visualize a fluid level In newborn infants with imperforate anus, immediate preoperative films done to determine the lowest end of the colon that is patent as a guide for surgical intervention	None

Table A4-2 Common Pediatric X-rays *(continued)*

Name of Examination	Possible Purpose and/or Indications	Possible Physical Preparation Needed*
BARIUM ENEMA		
Involves the insertion of an enema tip (usually a soft rubber catheter) into the anal orifice	To visualize the large colon and detect any large-bowel obstruction; small-bowel follow-through—the visualization of the terminal ileum at the end of fluoroscopy To diagnose chronic constipation or megacolon, acute abdominal conditions, ulcerative colitis, colonic bleeding, polyps, etc.	Preparation varies with indications for exam. Check with physician for specific orders. Chronic constipation, megacolon, acute abdomen: none Ulcerative colitis Liquid diet for 12 h; npo (nothing by mouth) after midnight prior to the exam Colonic bleeding Liquid diet for 24 h prior to exam Laxative afternoon prior to exam Saline or Fleet enema at bedtime and morning of exam Other indications 0–2 yr: npo for 3 h prior to exam 2–6 yr: Clear-liquid dinner, npo for 4 h prior to exam One-half suppository at bedtime and one-half 3 h prior to exam If poor results: Fleet or normal saline enema 6–16 yr: Clear liquid dinner; npo after midnight prior to exam One suppository afternoon prior to exam One suppository morning of exam If poor results: Fleet enema
BONE AGE SERIES		
Birth to 2 yr: hands, wrists, and knees 2 yrs and older; hands and wrists	To determine if child is at desired bone growth for chronological age Evaluation of the "bone age" based on the appearance of the bones, the extent of bone formation in the epiphyses and round bones, and the extent to which the epiphyses have begun to unite with their shafts	None
CARDIAC CATHETERIZATION		
Involves the introduction of a catheter under fluoroscopic control into the blood vessels or into the chambers of the heart	To obtain samples of blood from the chambers of the heart To monitor the functioning of the heart	Sedation usually ordered npo after midnight prior to the exam

Table A4-2 Common Pediatric X-rays *(continued)*

Name of Examination	Possible Purpose and/or Indications	Possible Physical Preparation Needed*
	To obtain information for the diagnosis of congenital heart malformations, especially prior to cardiac surgery	
CHEST Usually involves immobilization of smaller children (done by placing child in or on some type of apparatus to prevent movement)	To detect any anomalies of the chest, ribs, lungs, etc. To determine the true size of the heart To visualize lung or pleural areas where extreme densities or fluid are present (including horizontal fluid levels) Contrast medium possibly used on empyema cases to show the size and position of known cavities To visualize foreign bodies in the tracheobronchial tree	None
INTRAVENOUS PYELOGRAM (IVP) Also called excretory urography	To yield information regarding renal morphology and function To visualize the collecting and transporting system of the urinary tract (e.g., the renal calyces, pelvises, and bladder); excretory capacity of the individual kidneys can be roughly determined by appearance time and concentration of the radiopaque dye as it is being excreted	In trauma cases: none Other indications 0–yr: Clear liquids in morning; npo for 3 h prior to exam 2–6 yr: Clear liquids in morning; npo for 4 h prior to exam One-half suppository at bed time One-half suppository in morning If not effective: normal saline enema in morning 6–16 yr: npo after midnight prior to exam, or clear-liquid breakfast then npo One suppository at bedtime One suppository in morning If not effective, normal saline enema in morning
KUB (KIDNEY, URETERS, BLADDER) Also called a posterior flat plate of the abdomen	To detect the presence of calculi, especially in the kidneys, ureters, or bladder To visualize any abnormalities, e.g., bowel obstruction	None

Table A4-2 Common Pediatric X-rays *(continued)*

Name of Examination	Possible Purpose and/or Indications	Possible Physical Preparation Needed*
SKULL SERIES		
Usually includes at least four different views: AP, lateral, PA, and basal (cerebellar)	To visualize and study the cranial vault, cranial bones, facial bones (including the nose, hard palate, mandible, and orbital ridges)	None
Tomography	May be used to get more information about the skull, face, and mastoid because it is easier to obtain than many of the regular views needed for these areas Often used in mastoid and temporomandibular joint problems, evaluation of facial trauma, and destructive lesions of the face and skull	Sedation that allows the child to sleep through the procedure often ordered
SPINE	To evaluate curvatures of the spine: scoliosis, kyphosis, lordosis, etc. To assess stability of the spine in spondylolysis and spondylolisthesis To evaluate meningoceles and other soft-tissue projections	None
Cervical spine	Always indicated following trauma in these circumstances: Suspected cervical spine injury Maxillofacial injury Unconsciousness Prior to general anesthesia when manipulation of the head and neck necessary for intubation	
SURVEYS		
Skeletal survey Metastatic survey Joint or arthritic survey	To detect the presence or extent of localized lesions To evaluate the degree of involvement of the skeleton in a generalized disease process Indications Metastatic surveys for neoplasms or chronic granuloma Skeletal survey for leukemia and anemia, osteochondrodystrophy, mongolism, or multiple congenital defects	None

Table A4-2 Common Pediatric X-rays *(continued)*

Name of Examination	Possible Purpose and/or Indications	Possible Physical Preparation Needed*
UPPER GASTROINTESTINAL SERIES (UGI)		
Includes pharynx, esophagus, stomach, and duodenum	In neonates and young infants: for evaluation of esophageal atresia, difficulty with feeding, regurgitation, vomiting, abdominal distention, and questionable abdominal masses In older infants or children: for evaluation of repeated pneumonias, aspiration, tracheoesophageal fistula; also for esophageal foreign bodies, vomiting, abdominal distention, failure to thrive, abdominal pain, diarrhea, and GI bleeding	0–2 yr: Clear liquids after 6 P.M. the night before exam; npo for 3 h prior to exam 2–16 yr: npo after midnight prior to exam No gum chewing on day of exam

*Preparation will vary depending on physician and/or radiologist idiosyncrasies. Always check physician's orders prior to intervention.

5 Reference Tables and Assessment and Screening Tools

NEUROLOGICAL SIGN	SCORE 0	1	2	3	4	5
POSTURE						
SQUARE WINDOW	90°	60°	45°	30°	0°	
ANKLE DORSIFLEXION	90°	75°	45°	20°	0°	
ARM RECOIL	180°	90–180°	<90°			
LEG RECOIL	180°	90–180°	<90°			
POPLITEAL ANGLE	180	160°	130°	110°	90°	<90°
HEEL TO EAR						
SCARF SIGN						
HEAD LAG						
VENTRAL SUSPENSION						

Figure A5-1 Dubowitz scoring system of neurologic signs for assessment of gestational age. *(From Dubowitz, Victor, et al. Clinical assessment of gestational age in the newborn infant. Journal of Pediatrics, 77:1–10, 1970.)*

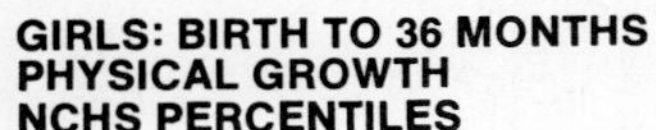

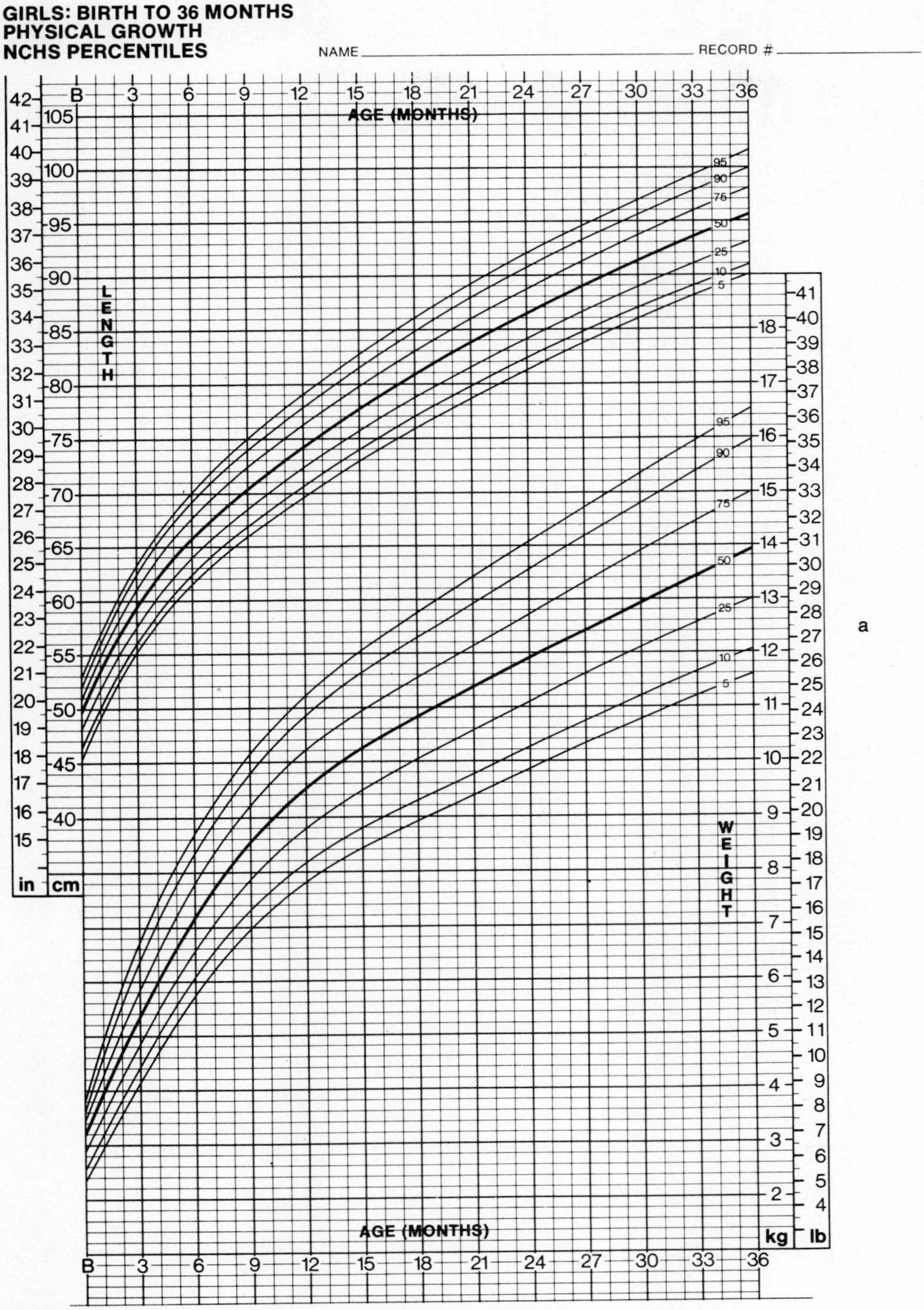

NAME ______ RECORD # ______

a

Figure A5-2 Female infant growth charts, birth to 36 months. *(a)* Lenth-age and weight-age relationships. *(b)* Head circumference-age and length-weight relationships. *(Adapted from the National Center for Health Statistics: NCHS Growth Charts, 1976. Monthly Vital Statistics Report, 25(3), Supp. (HRA) 76-1120. Data from the Fels Research Institute. Charts prepared by Ross Laboratories, Columbus, Ohio, 1976.)*

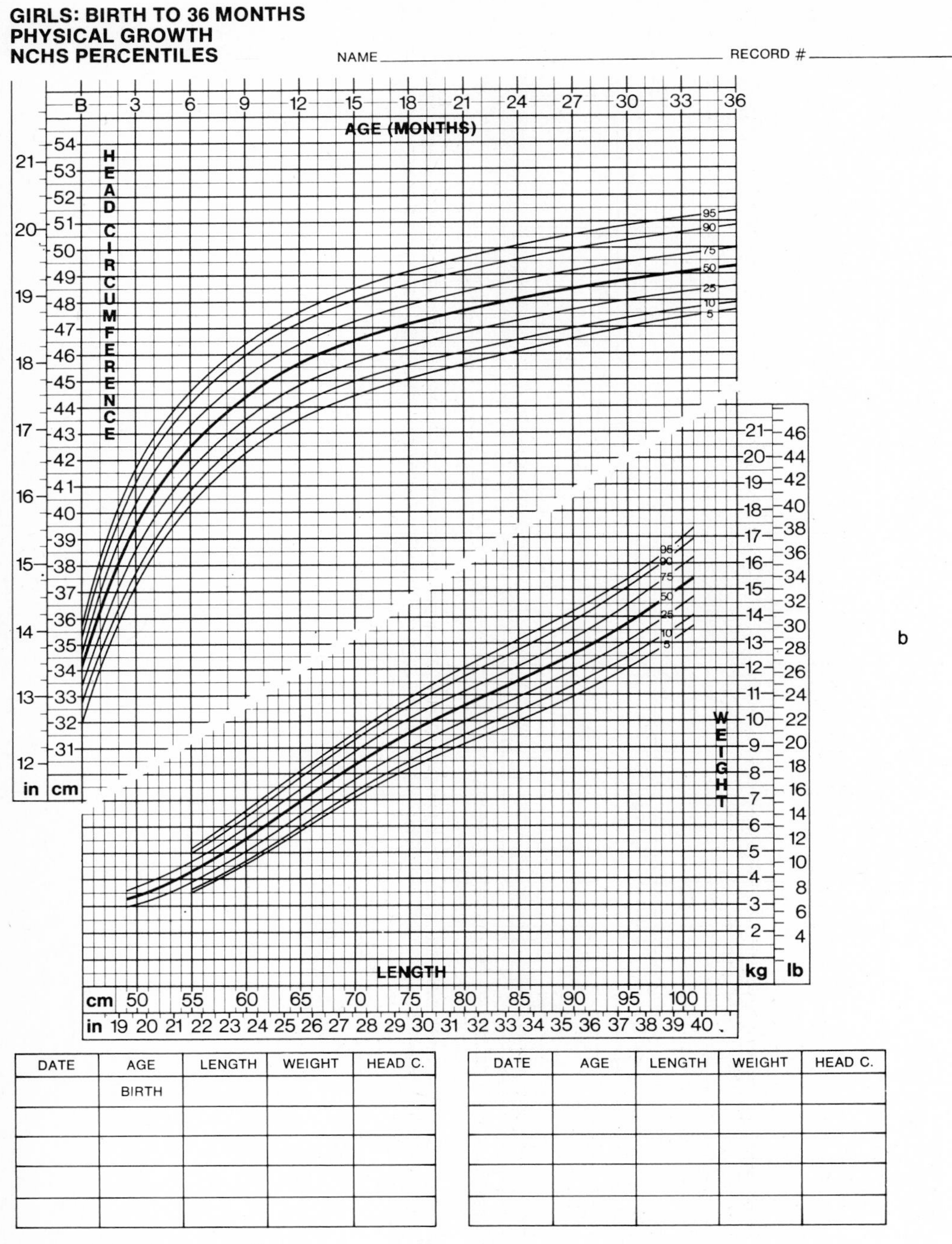

DATE	AGE	LENGTH	WEIGHT	HEAD C.
	BIRTH			

DATE	AGE	LENGTH	WEIGHT	HEAD C.

Figure A5-2 (continued)

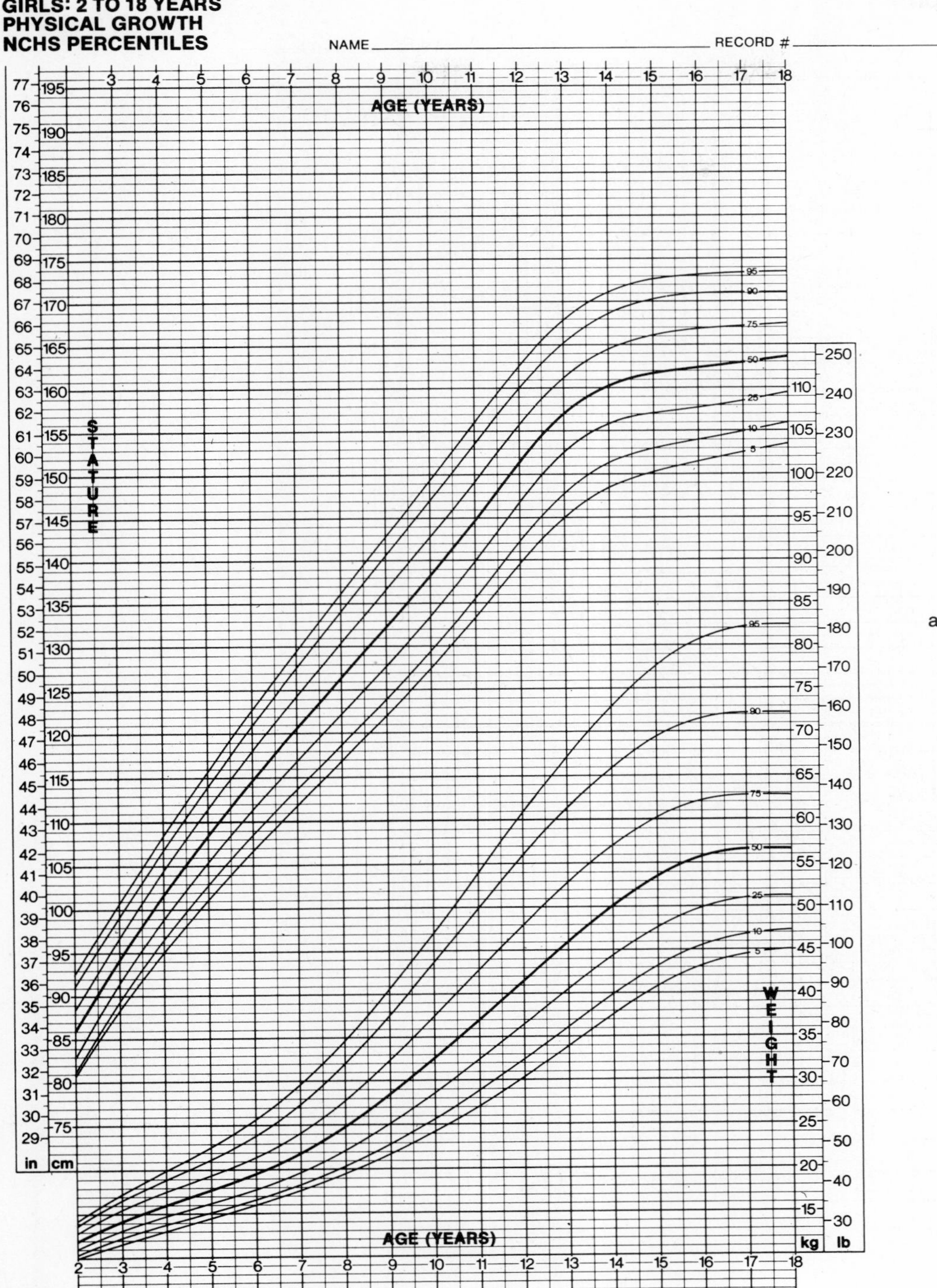

Figure A5-3 Female growth charts. *(a)* Age-weight-stature relationships, from 2 to 18 years. *(b)* Weight-stature relationships of prepubescent girls. *(Prepared by Ross Laboratories from the NCHS Growth Charts.)*

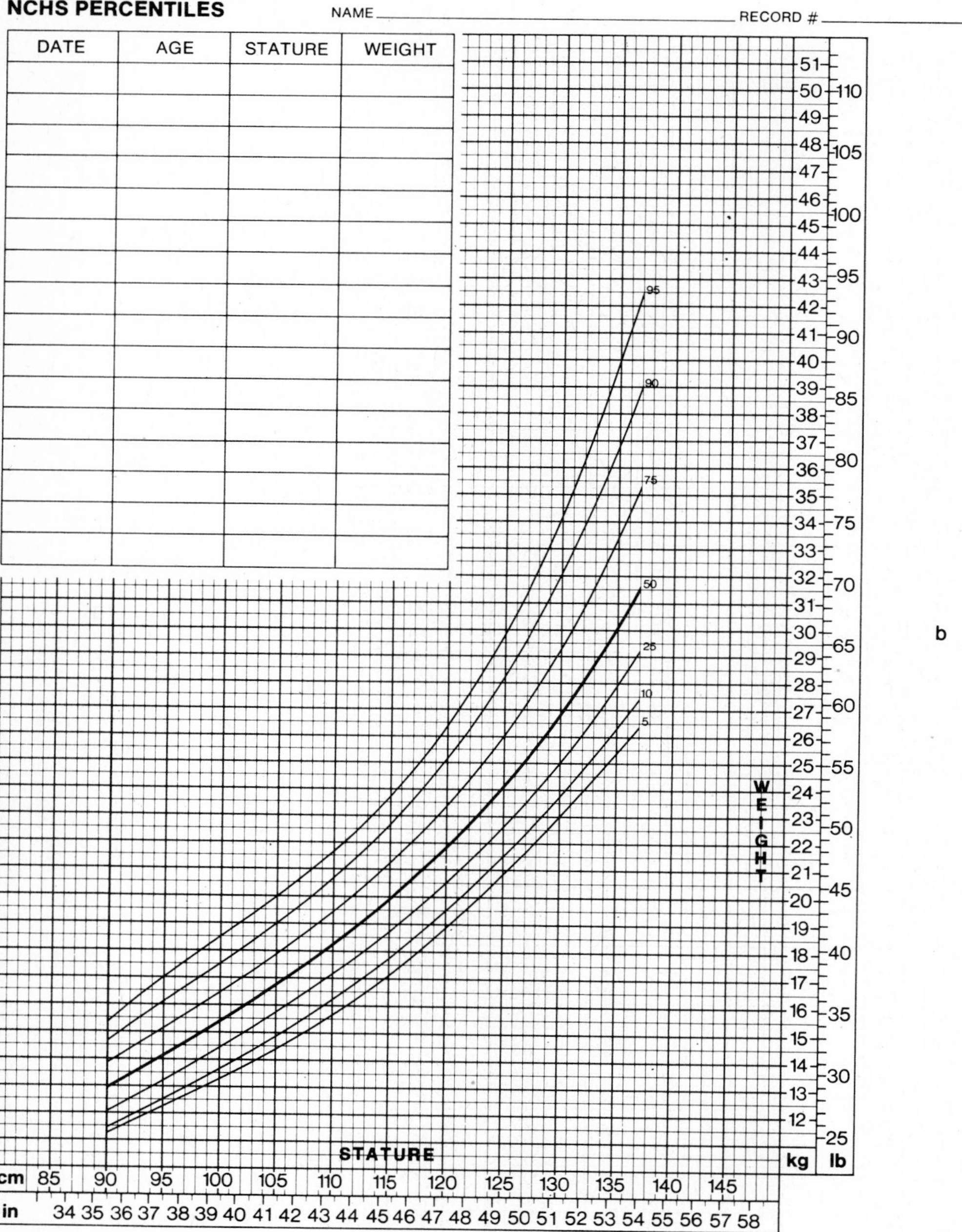

Figure A5-3 (continued)

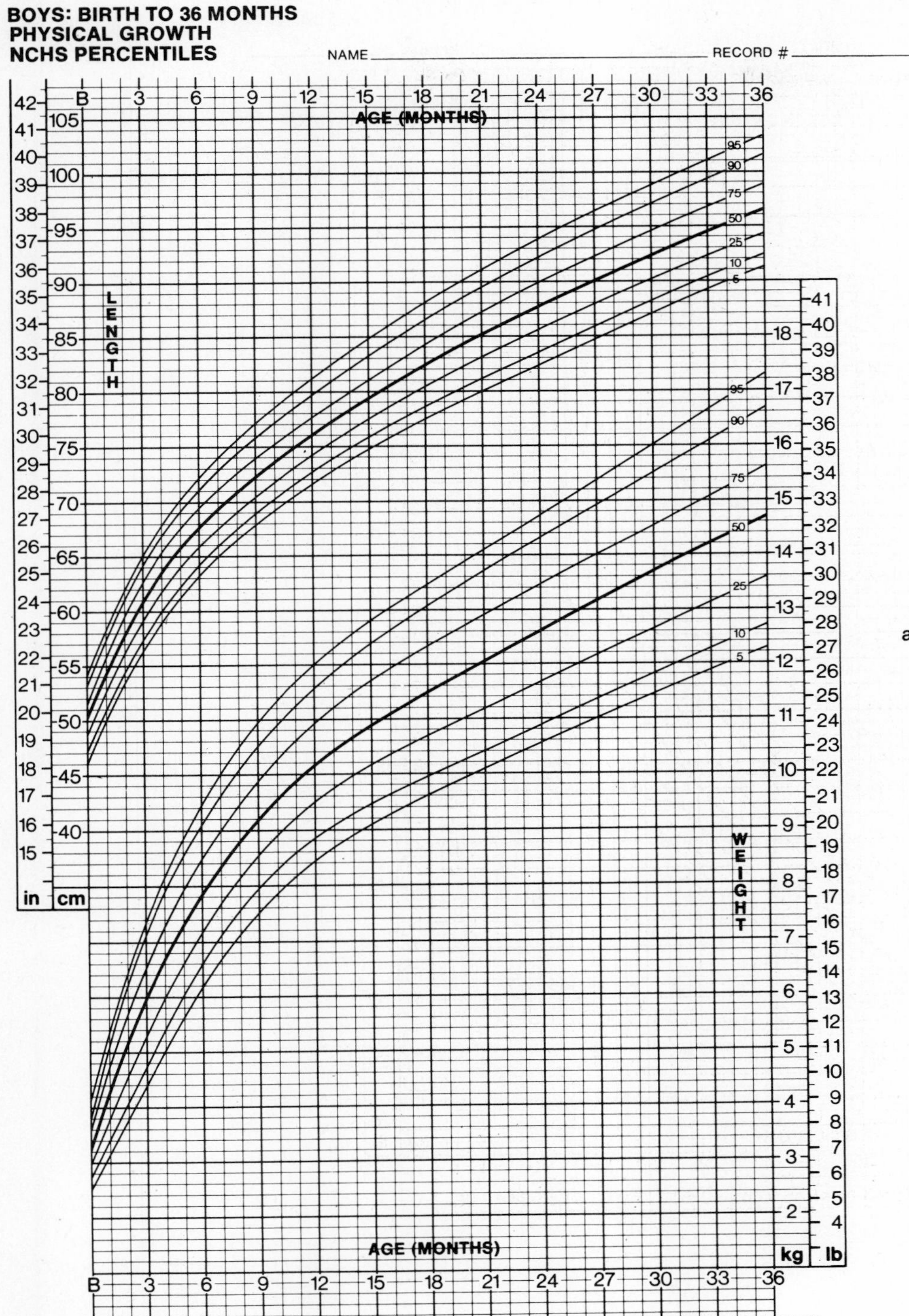

a

Figure A5-4 Male infant growth charts, birth to 36 months. *(a)* Length-age and weight-age relationships. *(b)* Head circumference-age and length-weight relationships. *(Prepared by Ross Laboratories from the NCHS Growth Charts.)*

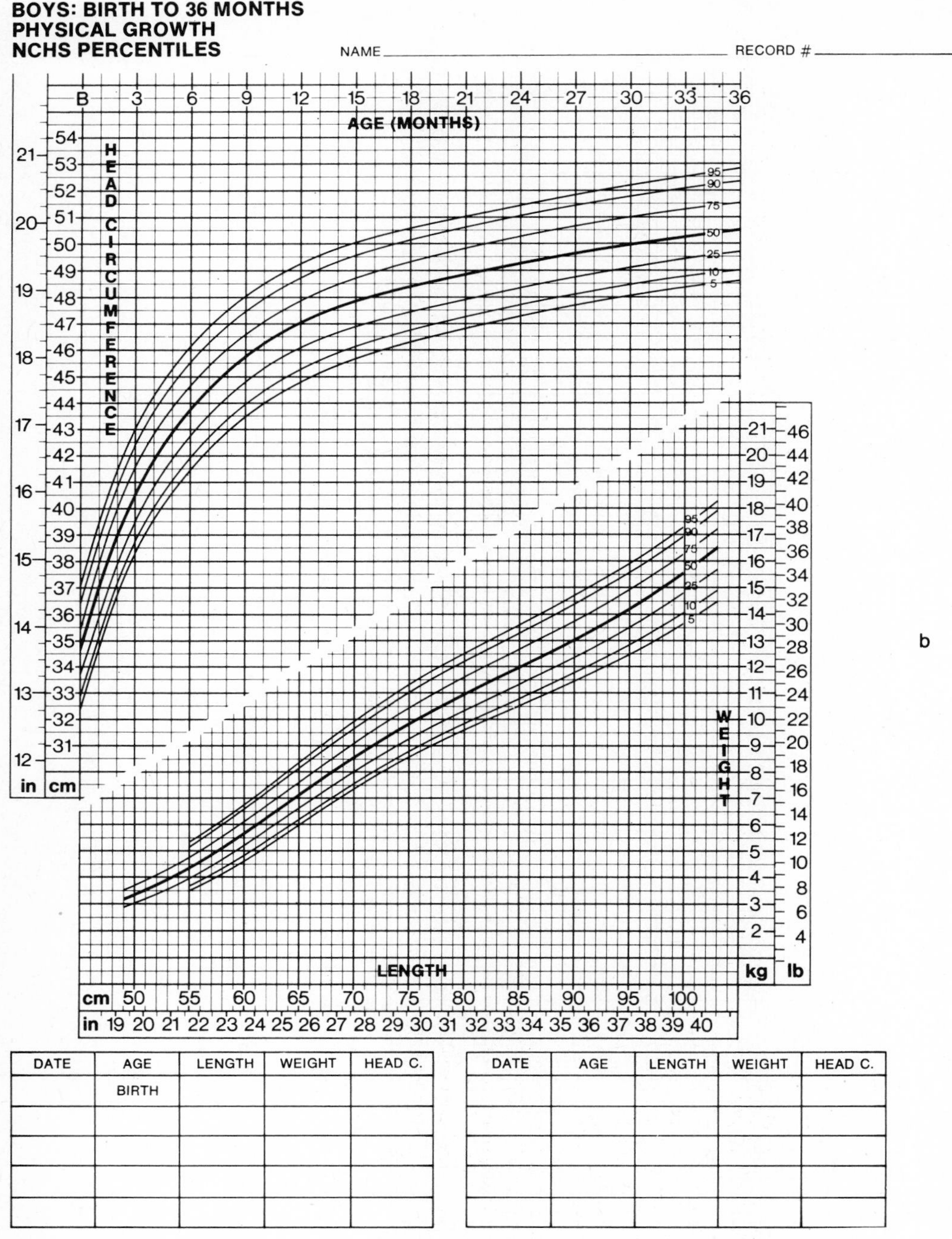

DATE	AGE	LENGTH	WEIGHT	HEAD C.
	BIRTH			

DATE	AGE	LENGTH	WEIGHT	HEAD C.

b

Figure A5-4 (continued)

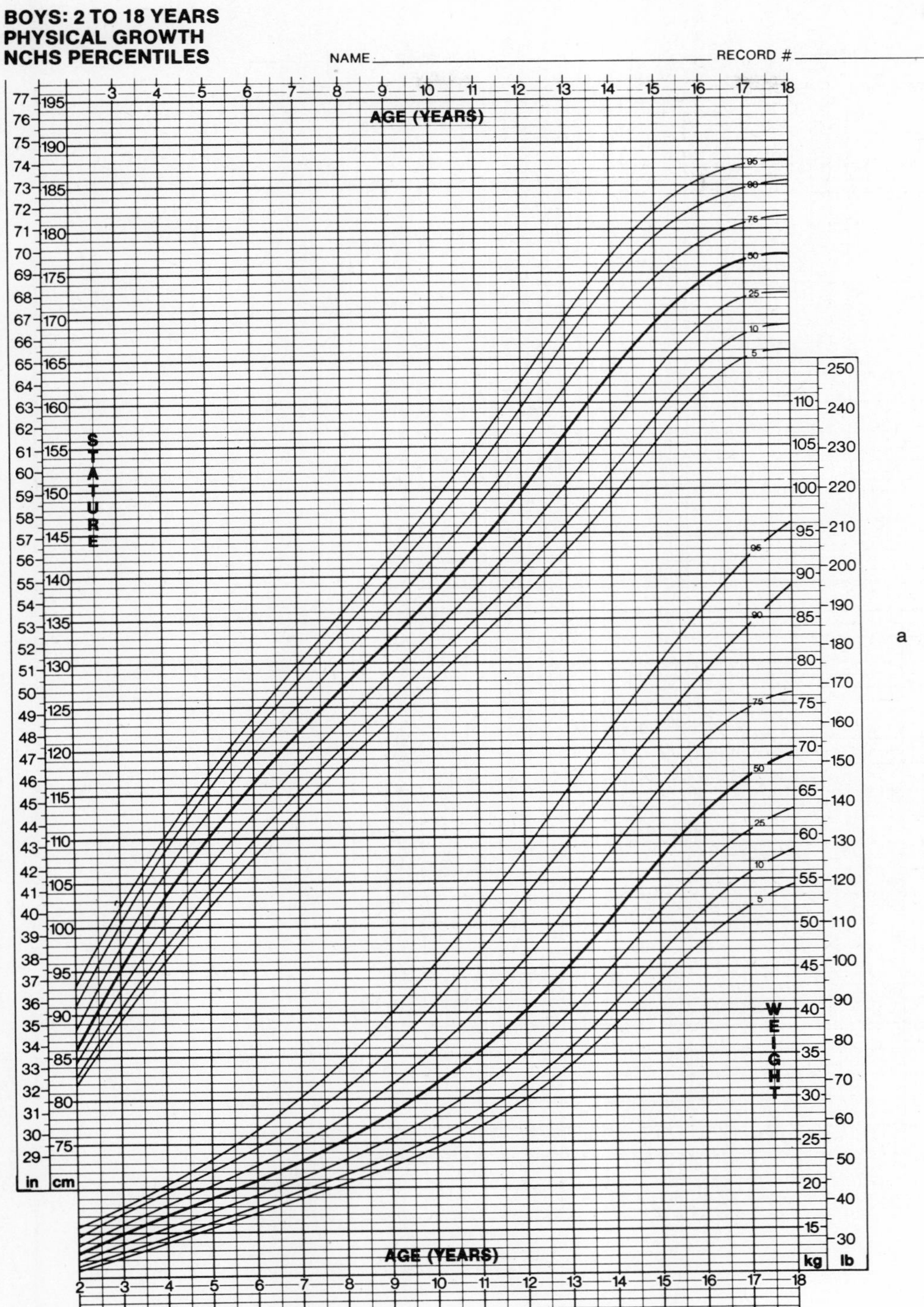

a

Figure A5-5 Male growth charts. *(a)* Age-weight-stature relationships from 2 to 18 years. *(b)* Weight-stature relationships of prepubescent boys. *(Prepared by Ross Laboratories from the NCHS Growth Charts.)*

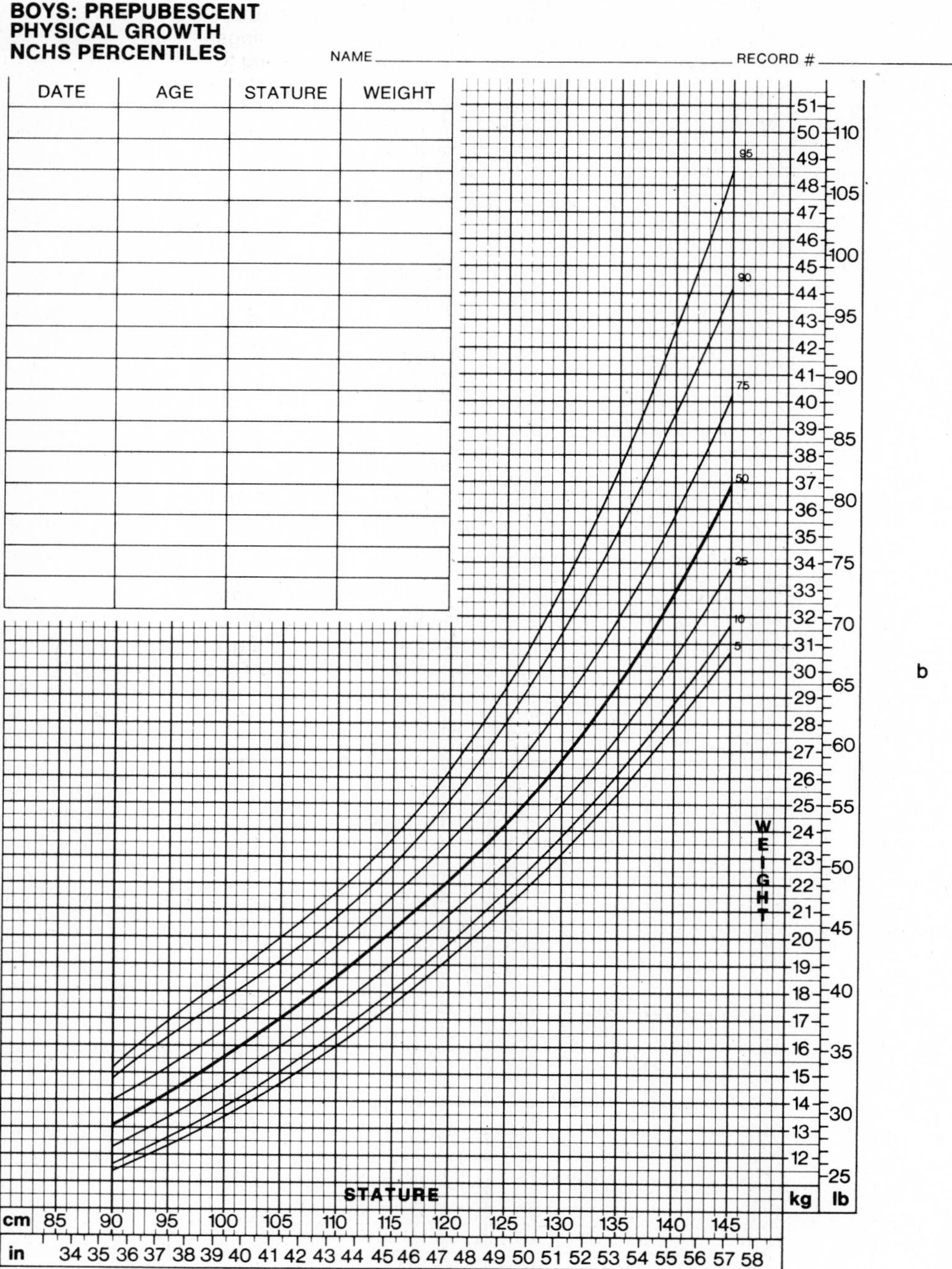

b

Figure A5-5 (continued)

Neonatal Perception Inventories (NPI) and Degree of Bother Inventory

Administration procedure (according to Broussard)

Explain to the mother that

> We are interested in learning more about the experiences of mothers and their babies during the first few weeks after delivery. The more we can learn about mothers and their babies, the better we will be able to help other mothers with their babies. We would appreciate it if you would help other mothers by answering a few questions.

As you give the mother the "Average Baby" form *(a)* say something like

> Although this is your first baby, you probably have some ideas of what most little babies are like. Will you please check the blank you *think* best describes what *most* little babies are like.

When the mother has completed the "Average Baby" form, take it and give her the "Your Baby" form *(b)* with verbal instructions such as

> While it is not possible to know for certain what your baby will be like, you probably have some ideas of what your baby will be like. Please check the blank that you *think* best describes what *your* baby will be like.

The procedure for administering the NPI is the same at 1 month as it was at 2 or 3 days postpartum, except that the examiner might now give such instructions as

> You have had a chance to live with your baby for a month now. Please check the blank you think best describes your baby.

After completion of the "Average Baby" and "Your Baby" inventories, at the 1-month test period, the mother is given the "Degree of Bother" inventory *(c)*, used to assess problems of infant behavior at 1 month of age, with the following instructions.

> Listed below are some of the things that have sometimes bothered other mothers in caring for their babies. We would like to know if you were bothered by any of these. Please place a check in the blank that best describes how much you were bothered by your baby's behavior in regard to these.

Scoring: NPI

Each of the six single-item scales is assigned a numerical weight of 1 to 5, beginning with 1 for "none" up to 5 for "a great deal." The total numerical score on each inventory is obtained, and then the total score from the "Your Baby" inventory is *subtracted* from the "Average Baby" inventory. The difference between the two scores is the NPI score. Example: If the "Average Baby" total is 20 and the "Your Baby" total is 17, the NPI score would be "+3".

A positive NPI score indicates a favorable perception and the infant is considered at low risk. When the infant is not rated as better than average (a minus score or a zero score), the infant is considered at high risk.

Scoring: Degree of Bother Inventory

The total problem score is calculated by assigning values of 1 to 4 (1 = none, 4 = a great deal) to each of the six items on the inventory. These values are totaled to give the score; the possible range is 6 to 24.

NEONATAL PERCEPTION INVENTORY II

AVERAGE BABY

How much crying do you think the average baby does?

_____ a great deal   _____ a good bit   _____ moderate amount   _____ very little   _____ none

How much trouble do you think the average baby has in feeding?

_____ a great deal   _____ a good bit   _____ moderate amount   _____ very little   _____ none

How much spitting up or vomiting do you think the average baby does?

_____ a great deal   _____ a good bit   _____ moderate amount   _____ very little   _____ none

How much difficulty do you think the average baby has in sleeping?

_____ a great deal   _____ a good bit   _____ moderate amount   _____ very little   _____ none

How much difficulty does the average baby have with bowel movements?

_____ a great deal   _____ a good bit   _____ moderate amount   _____ very little   _____ none

How much trouble do you think the average baby has in settling down to a predictable pattern of eating and sleeping?

_____ a great deal   _____ a good bit   _____ moderate amount   _____ very little   _____ none

(*a*)

Figure A5-6 (Copyright 1964–Retained, Elsie R. Broussard, M.D. University of Pittsburgh, 209 Parran Hall, Graduate School of Public Health, Pittsburgh, PA 15261.)

NEONATAL PERCEPTION INVENTORY II

YOUR BABY

How much crying has your baby done?

a great deal	a good bit	moderate amount	very little	none

How much trouble has your baby had feeding?

a great deal	a good bit	moderate amount	very little	none

How much spitting up or vomiting has your baby done?

a great deal	a good bit	moderate amount	very little	none

How much difficulty has your baby had in sleeping?

a great deal	a good bit	moderate amount	very little	none

How much difficulty has your baby had with bowel movements?

a great deal	a good bit	moderate amount	very little	none

How much trouble has your baby had in settling down to a predictable pattern of eating and sleeping?

a great deal	a good bit	moderate amount	very little	none

(*b*)

DEGREE OF BOTHER INVENTORY

Crying	a great deal	somewhat	very little	none
Spitting up or vomiting	a great deal	somewhat	very little	none
Sleeping	a great deal	somewhat	very little	none
Feeding	a great deal	somewhat	very little	none
Elimination	a great deal	somewhat	very little	none
Lack of a predictable schedule	a great deal	somewhat	very little	none
Other (specify):				
________	a great deal	somewhat	very little	none
________	a great deal	somewhat	very little	none
________	a great deal	somewhat	very little	none
________	a great deal	somewhat	very little	none

(*c*)

Figure A5-6 (continued)

Erickson's Parent-Infant Care Record

Administration procedure
Instruct the mother (care giver):

1. Note the nine circles on the clock face. Each circle represents a care activity such as feeding. Record in the appropriate circle the time care occurred, the type and length of care, and the number of times care was provided.
2. Since there is not enough space for writing, three symbols are used to record care, length of care activity, and the mood of mother and baby. An X, an arrow, and a happy or unhappy face are the symbols used.
   a. An X is placed in the appropriate circle to indicate when the infant was checked, diapered or position changed. (Explain position change to mother.)
   b. Complete arrows are drawn to show the time that the following activities begin, continue, or stop: all sleeping, feeding, parent play, holding or picking up infant, any consoling of infant for crying or fussing, and changes in the infants environment (e.g., moving infant from crib to couch or infant seat, or from chair to floor).
   c. Use a happy or sad face to report perceived mood changes of the mother (care giver) and baby throughout the 24 hr. The mother's face is drawn to the right within the outermost circle, and the infant's face is drawn to the left. The infant's face should be drawn somewhat smaller than the mother's face to aid in distinguishing between them. To indicate corresponding mood changes or lack of mood change, draw the infant's face next to the mother's.
3. Begin the daytime record at 7:30 A.M., *using a pencil,* and the nighttime record at 7:30 P.M., *using a pen.* Should day and night activities occur at the same time, record them side by side in appropriate colors.
4. Anything unusual should be mentioned as a comment.

The tool may be used by the mother to record only those activities with which she is concerned.

Interpretation
Evaluate the record for patterns of maternal-infant care, infant needs, and on-going maternal needs. Evaluate the following:

1. Time between feedings/hours of sleep.
2. Periods of happiness, day/night.
3. Recurrent periods of fussiness.
4. Amount of maternal sleep.
5. Number of diaper changes.
6. Amount of time infant is held, consoled, etc.

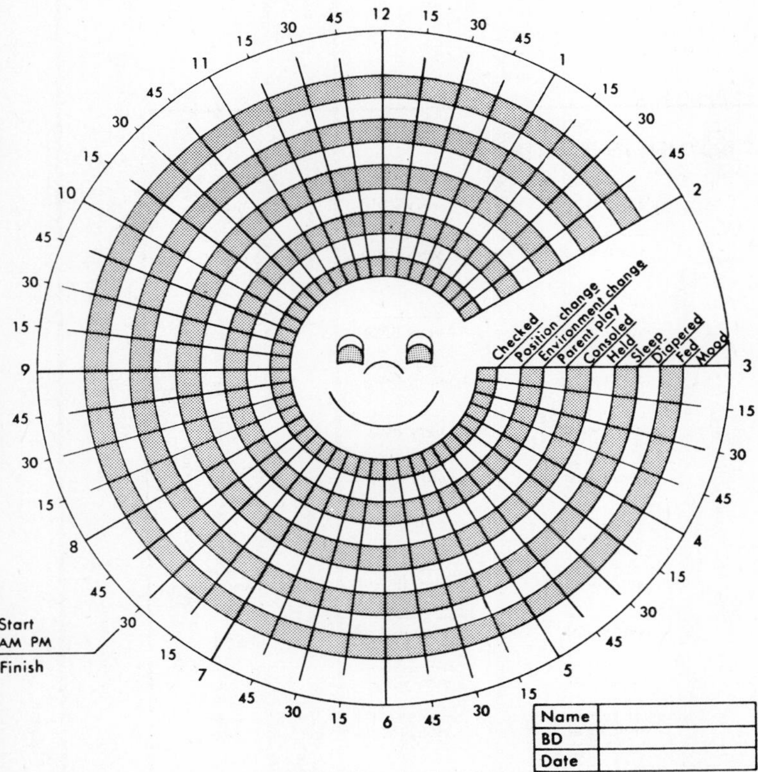

Figure A5-7 (From Erickson, Marcene L. Assessment and management of developmental changes in children. St. Louis: Mosby, 1976, pp. 110–115.)

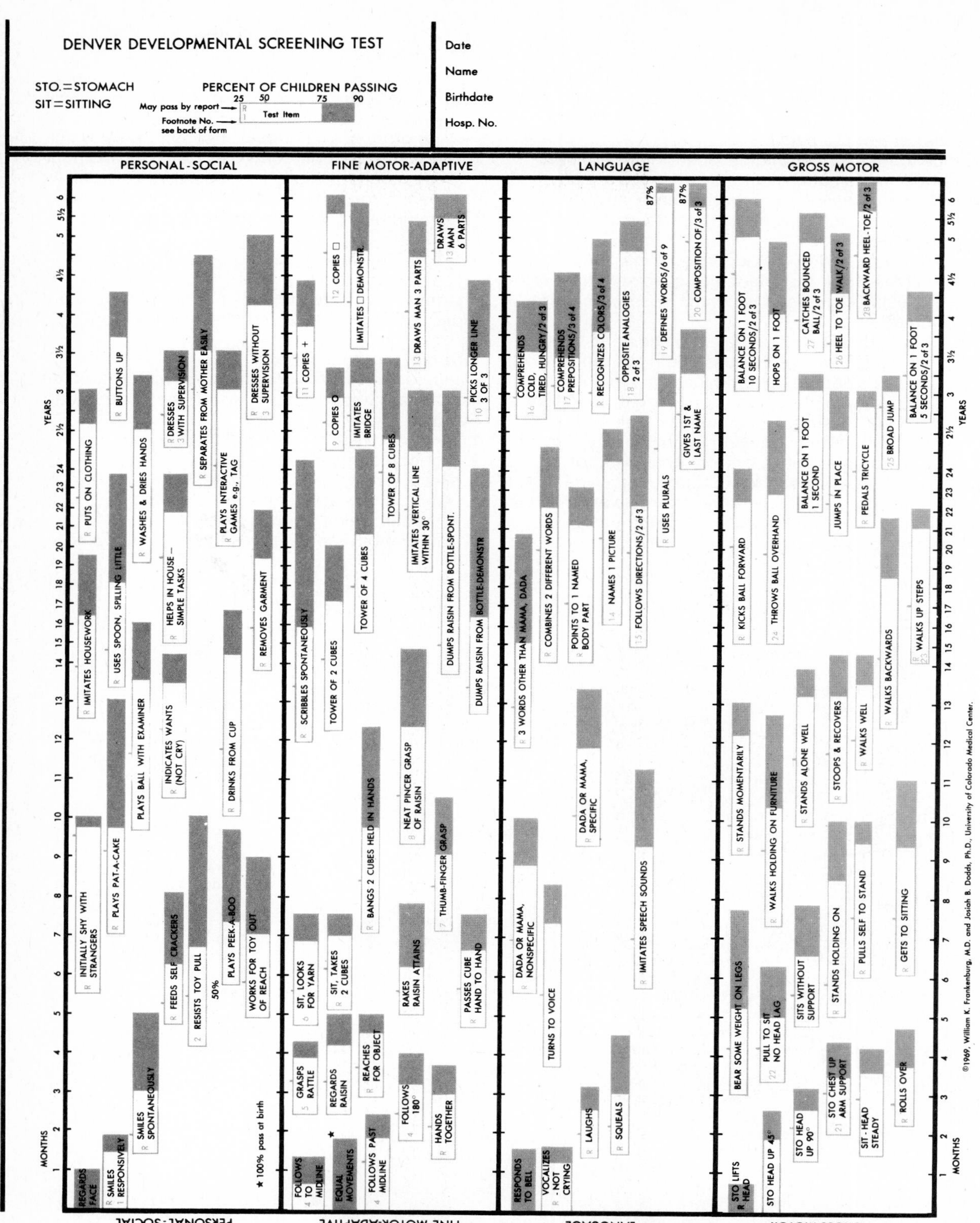

Figure A5-8 Denver Developmental Screening Test. *(Reprinted with permission. William K. Frankenburg, M.D. LADOCA Project and Publishing*

1. Try to get child to smile by smiling, talking or waving to him. Do not touch him.
2. When child is playing with toy, pull it away from him. Pass if he resists.
3. Child does not have to be able to tie shoes or button in the back.
4. Move yarn slowly in an arc from one side to the other, about 6" above child's face. Pass if eyes follow 90° to midline. (Past midline; 180°)
5. Pass if child grasps rattle when it is touched to the backs or tips of fingers.
6. Pass if child continues to look where yarn disappeared or tries to see where it went. Yarn should be dropped quickly from sight from tester's hand without arm movement.
7. Pass if child picks up raisin with any part of thumb and a finger.
8. Pass if child picks up raisin with the ends of thumb and index finger using an over hand approach.

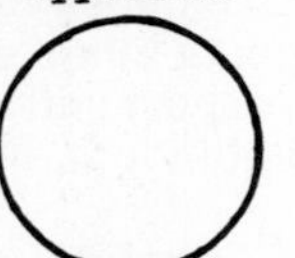

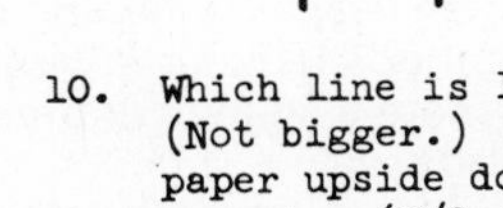

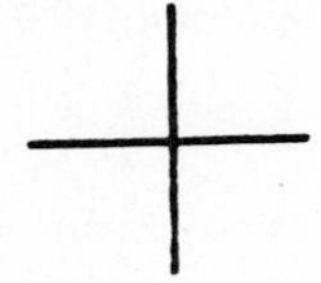

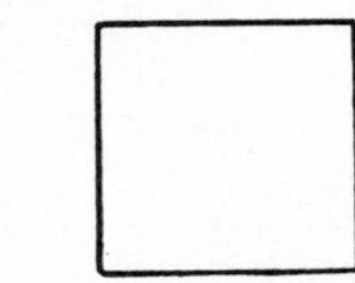

9. Pass any enclosed form. Fail continuous round motions.

10. Which line is longer? (Not bigger.) Turn paper upside down and repeat. (3/3 or 5/6)

11. Pass any crossing lines.

12. Have child copy first. If failed, demonstrate

When giving items 9, 11 and 12, do not name the forms. Do not demonstrate 9 and 11.

13. When scoring, each pair (2 arms, 2 legs, etc.) counts as one part.
14. Point to picture and have child name it. (No credit is given for sounds only.)

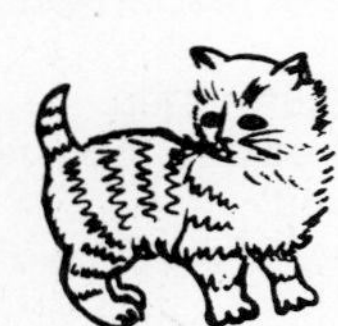

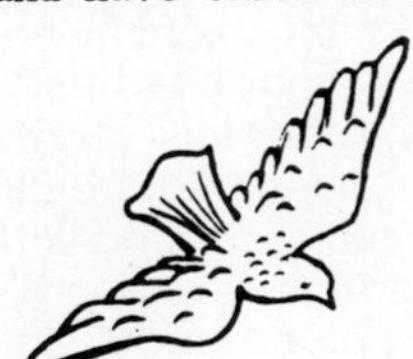

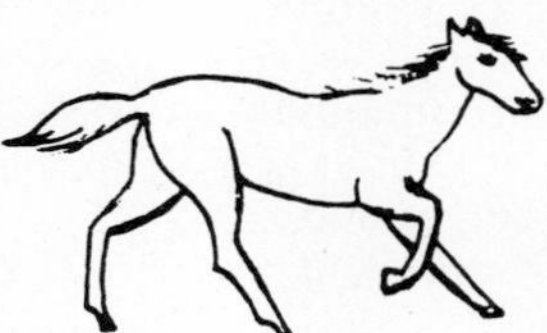

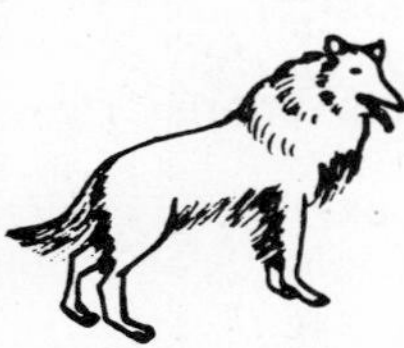

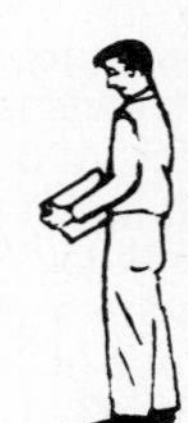

15. Tell child to: Give block to Mommie; put block on table; put block on floor. Pass 2 of 3. (Do not help child by pointing, moving head or eyes.)
16. Ask child: What do you do when you are cold? ..hungry? ..tired? Pass 2 of 3.
17. Tell child to: Put block <u>on</u> table; <u>under</u> table; <u>in</u> <u>front</u> of chair, <u>behind</u> chair. Pass 3 of 4. (Do not help child by pointing, moving head or eyes.)
18. Ask child: If fire is hot, ice is ?; Mother is a woman, Dad is a ?; a horse is big, a mouse is ?. Pass 2 of 3.
19. Ask child: What is a ball? ..lake? ..desk? ..house? ..banana? ..curtain? ..ceiling? ..hedge? ..pavement? Pass if defined in terms of use, shape, what it is made of or general category (such as banana is fruit, not just yellow). Pass 6 of 9.
20. Ask child: What is a spoon made of? ..a shoe made of? ..a door made of? (No other objects may be substituted.) Pass 3 of 3.
21. When placed on stomach, child lifts chest off table with support of forearms and/or hands.
22. When child is on back, grasp his hands and pull him to sitting. Pass if head does not hang back.
23. Child may use wall or rail only, not person. May not crawl.
24. Child must throw ball overhand 3 feet to within arm's reach of tester.
25. Child must perform standing broad jump over width of test sheet. (8-1/2 inches)
26. Tell child to walk forward, → heel within 1 inch of toe. Tester may demonstrate. Child must walk 4 consecutive steps, 2 out of 3 trials.
27. Bounce ball to child who should stand 3 feet away from tester. Child must catch ball with hands, not arms, 2 out of 3 trials.
28. Tell child to walk backward, ← toe within 1 inch of heel. Tester may demonstrate. Child must walk 4 consecutive steps, 2 out of 3 trials.

<u>DATE AND BEHAVIORAL OBSERVATIONS</u> (how child feels at time of test, relation to tester, attention span, verbal behavior, self-confidence, etc,):

Guide for Assessment of the Infant's Animate and Inanimate Environment

Observations should be carried out on the following developmental tasks, stimuli, and environments that are provided for infants, as well as on parent-infant interactions and parents' assessments of infants' stimulation.

A. Opportunities to develop head control
   1. What is infant's favorite position to be held?
   2. How often is position changed (number of times)?
   3. In what position is infant placed? Different?
   4. Is infant held in front, back, or side of parent?
   5. Is infant pulled to sitting position? How often?
   6. Is infant placed on abdomen? How often? On back? How often?
   7. How long is infant held once picked up?

B. Visual accommodation
   1. Are there varied opportunities to see? From different heights such as on floor, sofa, chair, crib?
   2. What is available to see?
   3. Is light varied?
   4. Are objects varied?
   5. How much face-to-face contact is there? Does infant follow faces and inanimate objects? What is length of time infant attends to object, face, toy, or activity?
   6. Are visual objects complex? Simple? Colorful? Bright or dull?
   7. Is infant placed in different rooms throughout the day?
   8. Does mother look directly in infant's eyes and face? Does infant focus on mother's eyes and face?

C. Motor control
   1. Is there evidence of infant play with hands, fingers, and feet?
   2. Is there evidence of encouragement and opportunity to develop head and chest control? How many times a day?
   3. Does parent place infant in a position to turn freely?
   4. Is infant ever briefly placed in standing position for weight bearing?
   5. Does mother encourage movement of infant's arms and legs while he or she is bathed, dressed, and fed?
   6. Are infant's movements restricted? Does mother interfere with or stop an activity that infant begins? Verbal restrictions (number of times)? Physical restrictions (number of times)?
   7. Does clothing or blankets impede movement?

D. Feeding
   1. How often is infant touched and mode?
   2. Is infant held in horizontal or up position?
   3. How much time is required for feeding?
   4. Does mother smile or talk? Does her affect change? Does infant's affect change?
   5. How close is infant held to mother, or if not held, what is mother's proximity while infant is being fed?
   6. Does mother hold infant, or does another person?
   7. Is infant propped?
   8. Is there evidence of face-to-face or eye-to-eye contact?
   9. Does mother observe infant's reactions?
   10. What is mother's behavior in response to infant (talking, smiling, touching, etc.)?
   11. Is technique of feeding varied (i.e., does mother offer nipple to each side of infant's mouth so that he or she gets opportunities to grasp it on right and left side of mouth, not just one side)?
   12. When is spoon-feeding begun? What is mother's technique? Infant's reaction?
   13. Is there evidence of oral-sensory stimulation?

E. Language
   1. Is there eye-to-eye contact?
   2. Is there face-to-face contact? How near is mother to infant usually when verbalizing or making sounds?
   3. Does mother repeat sounds that infant makes?
   4. Does infant's activity change in response to sounds he or she hears?
   5. Does mother talk spontaneously while washing, feeding, holding, dressing, playing, and walking around with infant?
   6. What sounds are heard? What is content of what is being said?
   7. When does infant make sounds and how often?
   8. What is total number of maternal vocalizations to infant during observation period?

F. Sleeping environment
   1. Is crib changed to different positions in room?
   2. Is surface stimulation varied? Weight of covers varied?
   3. Is room temperature varied?
   4. What is position in which baby is placed to sleep?
   5. How much time does infant spend sleeping or lying on back?
   6. How often is infant on side or abdomen?
   7. How much freedom of movement does infant have?
   8. Where does infant sleep?
   9. Are patterns of sleep similar from day to day, changing, or inconsistent?

G. General stimuli available in infant's environment
   1. How much stimulus is available for baby to see (e.g., presence of mobiles)?
   2. Are covers soft, silky, smooth, velvety, furry, rough, fuzzy, colorful, and clean?
   3. What is intensity and variability of noise levels in rooms (e.g., quiet, loud, consistent)?
   4. What is number, size, shape, and appropriateness of toys selected? Are they different textures, shapes, sizes, colors, in

Figure A5-9 (From Erickson, op. cit., pp. 107–110.)

crib, offered at appropriate times, or handed to infant? What is infant's ability to reach, grasp, and hold onto toys? Are toys alternated?

H. Tactile stimuli
   1. When held, is infant in actual contact with mother's trunk, chest, shoulders, head, and/or face?
   2. What is frequency of touching, rubbing, patting, kissing, bouncing, rocking, and holding?
   3. How long is infant usually left alone? How much time in playpen, infant seat, crib, or swing?
   4. Are specific efforts made to attend to infant while he or she is quiet and amusing him- or herself?
   5. Are infant's head, neck, trunk, and extremities supported steadily when held?
   6. How consistent is mother in her approaches to picking up and holding?
   7. Is infant moved about quickly, slowly, abruptly, or gently and held closely and firmly?
   8. How often does mother present a toy or object?
   9. Does infant experience different positions in space (e.g., lifted up, turned around, and moved in different rhythms)?

I. Movement pattern
   1. How often does infant move?
   2. What objects or persons does infant move away from?
   3. What objects or persons does infant move toward?
   4. How many different places does infant move to and from?
   5. How frequently does infant move head, chest, trunk, arms, and legs?
   6. Do activity levels change in different environmental settings or with different care providers?

J. Provision of activities for infant
   1. Does mother hold attention of infant by either nonverbal efforts, body movements, or use of toys? How often for each?
   2. Does mother hold or attempt to entertain infant by verbal attempts?
   3. If infant does not attend to mother's verbal or physical efforts, what is her response (i.e., continuation or termination of effort to get infant to respond)?
   4. Does mother offer verbal or nonverbal stimuli at a time when infant appears in an alert and attending state?
   5. Does mother respond to infant's state of alertness by providing stimulation?
   6. Does mother respond to inactive state, fatigue, or sleepy states by reducing efforts at stimulation? Is novelty of stimuli available?

K. Bathing
   1. How often is infant bathed? Length of time of bath?
   2. Who bathes infant?
   3. What is infant's reaction?
   4. What is mode and place?
   5. Are diapers changed? How often? By whom?

L. Dressing
   1. What is weight of clothes?
   2. Are they loose or tight?
   3. Are they dry and clean?
   4. How often are clothes changed?
   5. Is there variety in textures and colors of clothing?

M. Consoling
   1. What is mother's definition of "fussiness," "irritated," and "distressed," and what explanation does she give for infant's crying?
   2. What is mother's method of consoling infant when fussing and/or crying?
   3. Does mother verbalize to infant? For how long?
   4. Does mother touch infant? Where?
   5. Does mother pick infant up?
   6. Once picked up, does mother move, touch, stroke, caress, or rock infant?
   7. Does mother talk to infant while holding?
   8. Does mother distract with toys when fussing or crying occurs?
   9. At what point of fussing or crying does mother attempt to console infant? How long does it take before crying or fussiness stops?
   10. Does mother offer pacifier?
   11. Does mother offer food?
   12. Is infant placed in bed? Infant seat? Another location?
   13. Does mother attend at onset of fussing?
   14. When does infant begin to demonstrate signs of being consoled?
   15. What is mother's response?
   16. What is average number of times mother consoles infant a day?

N. Mother's assessment of infant's stimulation
   1. Has mother thought of ways to promote head control, visual development, motor control, infant feeding, language, and appropriate patterns of sleep?
   2. What has mother noted about infant's reactions to her attempts?
   3. Has mother observed changes in infant's behavior?
   4. How does mother view infant's development for his or her age? Is infant meeting mother's expectations?
   5. What behaviors of infant are most satisfying to mother? What are least satisfying?
   6. Has mother begun to consider next steps of development and ways to promote advances in infant's behavior?
   7. Does mother express positive statements about infant's growth and development and her efforts at influencing infant's behavior?

Home Observation for Measurement of the Environment (HOME) (Figures A5-10 and A5-11)

Administration

1. Make arrangements in advance with the parent(s) to go into the home when the child is awake following his or her normal daily routine. Allow 1 hour for completion.
2. Give a thorough explanation to the parent(s) prior to the home visit.
3. Strive to be objective and accepting. This is especially important when eliciting information from the parent(s) which cannot be gathered from observation.
4. Complete coding prior to leaving the house. There should be a check in either the Yes or No column for every item.

Scoring

1. The score is based on observations made and answers given by the mother or primary care giver during a semistructured interview administered within the home.
2. Each item on HOME is rated Yes or No. Interviewers should, in addition, write down additional pertinent information and general impressions following each home visit.
3. All observations refer to conditions present at the time of the home visit.
4. The score for the HOME is the total number of items marked Yes.
5. The HOME provides subscores for each subscale and a total score. Following each set of items which belong to a subscale, the total score for the particular subscale may be recorded.
6. Space is provided on the cover sheet for transcribing all raw scores for each subscale and determining the total raw score.

HOME OBSERVATION FOR MEASUREMENT OF THE ENVIRONMENT

BIRTH TO THREE

Date of interview __________

Child designee ______________________________
Name Age Sex Ethnicity

Child's birthday ____________ Birth order __________

Mother's name ____________ Father's name __________

Address ______________________________

Categories	Raw scores	Percentile scores
I. Emotional and verbal responsivity of mother		
II. Avoidance of restriction and punishment		
III. Organization of physical and temporal environment		
IV. Provision of appropriate play materials		
V. Maternal involvement with child		
VI. Opportunities for variety in daily stimulation		
Totals		

I. Emotional and verbal responsivity of mother	Yes	No
1. Mother spontaneously vocalizes to child at least twice during visit (excluding scolding).		
2. Mother responds to child's vocalizations with a verbal response.		
3. Mother tells child the name of some object during visit or says name of person or object in a "teaching" style.		
4. Mother's speech is distinct, clear, and audible.		
5. Mother initiates verbal interchanges with observer—asks questions and makes spontaneous comments.		
6. Mother expresses ideas freely and easily and uses statements of appropriate length for conversation (e.g., gives more than brief answers).		
*7. Mother permits child occasionally to engage in "messy" type of play.		
8. Mother spontaneously praises child's qualities or behavior twice during visit.		
9. When speaking of or to child, mother's voice conveys positive feeling.		
10. Mother caresses or kisses child at least once during visit.		
11. Mother shows some positive emotional responses to praise of child offered by visitor.		
Subscore		

*Items that may require direct questions.

Figure A5-10 (From Caldwell, Bettye M. Home Observation for Measurement of the Environment (birth to three). Little Rock, 1970).

HOME—cont'd

BIRTH TO THREE—cont'd

II. Avoidance of restriction and punishment

Item	Yes	No
12. Mother does not shout at child during visit.		
13. Mother does not express overt annoyance with or hostility toward child.		
14. Mother neither slaps nor spanks child during visit.		
*15. Mother reports that no more than one instance of physical punishment occurred during the past week.		
16. Mother does not scold or derogate child during visit.		
17. Mother does not interfere with child's actions or restrict child's movements more than three times during visit.		
18. At least ten books are present and visible.		
*19. Family has a pet.		
Subscore		

III. Organization of physical and temporal environment

Item	Yes	No
20. When mother is away, care is provided by one of three regular substitutes.		
21. Someone takes child into grocery store at least once a week.		
22. Child gets out of house at least four times a week.		
23. Child is taken regularly to doctor's office or clinic.		
*24. Child has a special place in which to keep his toys and "treasures."		
25. Child's play environment appears safe and free of hazards.		
Subscore		

IV. Provision of appropriate play materials

Item	Yes	No
26. Child has some muscle activity toys or equipment.		
27. Child has a push or pull toy.		
28. Child has stroller or walker, kiddie car, scooter or tricycle.		
29. Mother provides toys or interesting activities for child during interview.		
30. Provides learning equipment appropriate to age—cuddly toy or role-playing toys.		
31. Provides learning equipment appropriate to age—mobile, table and chairs, high chair, play pen.		
32. Provides eye-hand coordination toys—items to go in and out of receptacle, fit together toys, beads.		

Figure A5-10 (continued)

HOME—cont'd

BIRTH TO THREE—cont'd

IV. Provision of appropriate play materials—cont'd

	Yes	No
33. Provides eye-hand coordination toys that permit combinations—stacking or nesting toys, blocks or building toys.		
34. Provides toys for literature and music.		
Subscore		

V. Maternal involvement with child

	Yes	No
35. Mother tends to keep child within visual range and to look at him often.		
36. Mother talks to child while doing her work.		
37. Mother consciously encourages developmental advance.		
38. Mother invests "maturing" toys with value via her attention.		
39. Mother structures child's play periods.		
40. Mother provides toys that challenge child to develop new skills.		
Subscore		

VI. Opportunities for variety in daily stimulation

	Yes	No
41. Father provides some caretaking every day.		
42. Mother reads stories at least three times weekly.		
43. Child eats at least one meal per day with mother and father.		
44. Family visits or receives visits from relatives.		
45. Child has three or more books of his own.		
Subscore		

Figure A5-10 (continued)

HOME OBSERVATION FOR MEASUREMENT OF THE ENVIRONMENT

THREE TO SIX

Date of interview ____________

Child designee ____
Name   Age   Sex   Ethnicity

Child's birthday ____________________ Birth order ____________

Mother's name ____________________ Father's name ____________

Address ____

____

Categories	Raw scores	Percentile scores
I. Provision of stimulation through equipment, toys, and experiences	______	______
II. Stimulation of mature behavior	______	______
III. Provision of stimulating physical and language environment	______	______
IV. Avoidance of restriction and punishment	______	______
V. Pride, affection, and thoughtfulness	______	______
VI. Masculine stimulation	______	______
VII. Independence from parental control	______	______
Totals	______	______

I. Provision of stimulation through equipment, toys, and experiences	Yes	No
1-12 The following are present in home and either belong to child subject or he is allowed to play with them: 1. Toys to learn colors, sizes, shapes—typewriter, pressouts, play school, peg boards, etc.		
2. Toy or game facilitating learning letters (e.g., blocks with letters, toy typewriter, letter sticks, books about letters, etc.).		
3. Three or more puzzles.		
4. Two toys necessitating some finger and whole hand movements (crayons and coloring books, paper dolls, etc.).		
5. Record player and at least five children's records.		
6. Real or toy musical instrument (piano, drum, toy xylophone or guitar, etc.).		
7. Toy or game permitting free expression (finger paints, play dough, crayons or paint and paper, etc.).		
8. Toys or game necessitating refined movements (paint by number, dot book, paper dolls, crayons and coloring books).		
9. Toys to learn animals—books about animals, circus games, animal puzzles, etc.		
10. Toy or game facilitating learning numbers (e.g., blocks with numbers, books about numbers, games with numbers, etc.).		

Figure A5-11 (From Caldwell, Bettye M. Home Observation for Measurement of the Environment (three to six). Little Rock, 1976).

HOME—cont'd

THREE TO SIX—cont'd

I. Provision of stimulation through equipment, toys, and experiences—cont'd

	Yes	No
11. Building toys (blocks, tinker toys, Lincoln logs, etc.).		
12. Ten children's books.		
13. At least ten books are present and visible in the apartment.		
14. Family buys a newspaper daily and reads it.		
15. Family subscribes to at least one magazine.		
16. Family member has taken child on one outing (picnic, shopping excursion) at least every other week.		
17. Child has been taken out to eat in some kind of restaurant three-four times in the past year.		
18-20 Child has been taken by a family member to the following within the past year:		
18. Airport		
19. A trip more than 50 miles from his home (50 miles radial distance, not total distance).		
20. A scientific, historical, or art museum.		
21. Child is taken to grocery store at least once a week.		
Subscore		

II. Stimulation of mature behavior

	Yes	No
22-29 Child is encouraged to learn the following:		
22. Colors		
23. Shapes		
24. Patterned speech (nursery rhymes, prayers, songs, TV commercials, etc.)		
25. The alphabet		
26. To tell time		
27. Spatial relationships (up, down, under, big, little, etc.)		
28. Numbers		
29. To read a few words		
30. Tries to get child to pick up and put away toys after play session—without help.		
31. Child is taught rules of social behavior which involve recognition of rights of others.		
32. Parent teaches child some simple manners—to say, "Please," "Thank you," "I'm sorry."		
33. Some delay of food gratification is demanded of the child, e.g., not to whine or demand food unless within ½ hour of meal time.		
Subscore		

HOME—cont'd

THREE TO SIX—cont'd

III. Provision of a stimulating physical and language environment (observation items, except **45)	Yes	No
34. Building has no potentially dangerous structural or health defect (e.g., plaster coming down from ceiling, stairwav with boards missing, rodents, etc.).		
35. Child's outside play environment appears safe and free of hazards (no outside play area requires an automatic "No").		
36. The interior of the apartment is not dark or perceptibly monotonous.		
37. House is not overly noisy—television, shouts of children, radio, etc.		
38. Neighborhood has trees, grass, birds—is esthetically pleasing.		
39. There is at least 100 square feet of living space per person in the house.		
40. In terms of available floor space, the rooms are not overcrowded with furniture.		
41. All visible rooms of the house are reasonably clean and minimally cluttered.		
42. *Mother uses complex sentence structure and some long words in conversing.		
43. Mother uses correct grammar and pronunciation.		
44. Mother's speech is distinct, clear, and audible.		
**45. Family has TV and it is used judiciously, not left on continuously (no TV requires an automatic "No"—any scheduling scores "Yes").		
Subscore		

IV. Avoidance of restriction and punishment (observation items, except **51 and **52)	Yes	No
46. Mother does not scold or derogate child more than once during visit.		
47. Mother does not use physical restraint, shake, grab, pinch child during visit.		
48. Mother neither slaps nor spanks child during visit.		
49. Mother does not express over-annoyance with or hostility toward child—complain, say child is "bad" or won't mind.		
50. Child is not punished or ridiculed for speech.		
**51. No more than one instance of physical punishment occurred during the past week (accept parental report).		
**52. Child does not get slapped or spanked for spilling food or drink.		
Subscore		

*Throughout interview this refers to *mother* OR other *caregiver* who is present for interview.

HOME—cont'd

THREE TO SIX—cont'd

V. Pride, affection, and thoughtfulness

(observation items, except **53, **54, **55, **56, **57, **58, **59)

Item	Yes	No
**53. Parent turns on special TV program regarded as "good" for children (*Captain Kangaroo, Magic Toy Shop,* Walt Disney, *Flipper, Lassie,* educational TV, etc.).		
**54. Someone reads stories to child or shows and comments on pictures in magazines fives times weekly.		
**55. Parent encourages child to relate experiences or takes time to listen to him relate experiences.		
**56. Parent holds child close ten to fifteen minutes per day, e.g., during TV, story time, visiting.		
**57. Parent occasionally sings to child, or sings in presence of child.		
**58. Child has a special place in which to keep his toys and "treasures."		
**59. Child's art work is displayed some place in house (anything that child makes).		
60. Mother introduces interviewer to child.		
61. Mother converses with child at least twice during visit (scolding and suspicious comments not counted).		
62. Mother answers child's questions or requests verbally.		
63. Mother usually responds verbally to child's talking.		
64. Mother provides toys or interesting activities or in other ways structures situation for child during visit when her attention will be elsewhere. (To score "Yes" mother must make an active guiding gesture or suggestion to structure child's play.)		
65. Mother spontaneously praises child's qualities or behavior twice during visit.		
66. When speaking of or to child, mother's voice conveys positive feeling.		
67. Mother caresses, kisses, or cuddles child at least once during visit.		
68. Mother sets up situation that allows child to show off during visit.		
Subscore		

VI. Masculine stimulation

Item	Yes	No
69. Child sees and spends some time with father or father figure four days a week.		
70. Child eats at least one meal per day, on most days, with mother (or mother figure) and father (or father figure). (One-parent families get an automatic "No.")		

HOME—cont'd

THREE TO SIX—cont'd

VI. Masculine stimulation—cont'd

	Yes	No
71-73 The following are present in home and either belong to child subject or he is allowed to play with them: 71. Ride toy (tricycle, scooter, wagon, bike with or without training wheels).		
72. Medium wheel toys—trucks, trains, doll carriage, etc.		
73. Large muscle toy (jump rope, swing, ball, climbing object, etc.).		
Subscore		

VII. Independence from parental control

	Yes	No
74. Child is encouraged to try to dress himself.		
75. Child is permitted to choose some of his clothing to be worn except on very special occasions.		
76. Child is permitted some choice in lunch or breakfast menu.		
77. Parent lets child choose certain favorite food products or brands at grocery store.		
78. Child is permitted to go to another house to play without having the caregiver accompany him.		
79. Child can express negative feelings without harsh reprisal.		
80. Child is permitted to hit parent without harsh reprisal.		
Subscore		
Total score		

Index